AMA
AMERICAN MEDICAL
ASSOCIATION

# ICD 10-PCS 2018

## The Complete Official Codebook

D1303892

## Notice

*ICD-10-PCS: The Complete Official Codebook* is designed to be an accurate and authoritative source regarding coding and every reasonable effort has been made to ensure accuracy and completeness of the content. However, the AMA makes no guarantee, warranty, or representation that this publication is accurate, complete, or without errors. It is understood that the AMA is not rendering any legal or other professional services or advice in this publication and that the AMA bears no liability for any results or consequences that may arise from the use of this book.

## Our Commitment to Accuracy

The AMA is committed to producing accurate and reliable materials. To report corrections, please call the AMA Unified Service Center at (800) 621-8335. AMA product updates, errata, and addendum can be found at amaproductupdates.org.

To purchase additional copies, contact the American Medical Association at 800 621-8335 or visit the AMA store at amastore.com. Refer to product number OP201118.

## Copyright

© 2017 Optum360, LLC
Made in the USA
OP201118
BQ45:09/17

## Acknowledgments

Lauri Gray, RHIT, CPC, AHIMA-approved ICD-10-CM Trainer, *Product Manager*

Karen Schmidt, BSN, *Technical Director*

Anita Schmidt, BS, RHIT, AHIMA-approved ICD-10-CM/PCS Trainer, *Clinical Technical Editor*

Peggy Willard, CCS, AHIMA-approved ICD-10-CM/PCS Trainer, *Clinical Technical Editor*

Karen Krawzik, RHIT, CCS, AHIMA-approved ICD-10-CM/PCS Trainer, *Clinical Technical Editor*

Anne Kenney, BA, MBA, CCA, CCS, *Clinical Technical Editor*

Stacy Perry, *Manager, Desktop Publishing*

Tracy Betzler, *Senior Desktop Publishing Specialist*

Hope M. Dunn, *Senior Desktop Publishing Specialist*

Katie Russell, *Desktop Publishing Specialist*

Kate Holden, *Editor*

### Anita Schmidt, BS, RHIT, AHIMA-approved ICD-10-CM/PCS Trainer

Ms. Schmidt has expertise in Level I adult and pediatric trauma hospital coding, specializing in ICD-9-CM, ICD-10-CM/PCS, DRG, and CPT coding. Her experience includes analysis of medical record documentation, assignment of ICD-10-CM and PCS codes, DRG validation, as well as CPT code assignments for same-day surgery cases. She has conducted coding training and auditing, including DRG validation, conducted electronic health record training, and worked with clinical documentation specialists to identify documentation needs and potential areas for physician education. Most recently she has been developing content for resource and educational products related to ICD-10-CM and ICD-10-PCS. Ms. Schmidt is an AHIMA-approved ICD-10-CM/PCS trainer, and is an active member of the American Health Information Management Association (AHIMA) and the Minnesota Health Information Management Association (MHIMA).

### Peggy Willard, CCS, AHIMA-approved ICD-10-CM/PCS Trainer

Ms. Willard's expertise is ICD-10-CM and PCS including in-depth analysis of medical record documentation, ICD-10-CM/PCS code and DRG assignment. In recent years she has been responsible for the creation and development of several print products and e-books designed to assist with appropriate application of ICD-10-CM and PCS coding system. Ms. Willard has several years of prior experience in Level I Adult and Pediatric Trauma hospital coding, specializing in ICD-9-CM, DRG, and CPT coding with emphasis in conducting coding audits, and conducting coding training for coding staff and clinical documentation specialists. Ms. Willard is an active member of the American Health Information Management Association (AHIMA) and the Minnesota Health Information Management Association (MHIMA).

### Karen Krawzik, RHIT, CCS, AHIMA-approved ICD-10-CM/PCS Trainer

Ms. Krawzik has expertise in ICD-10-CM, ICD-9-CM, and CPT/HCPCS coding. Her coding experience includes inpatient, observation, ambulatory surgery, and ancillary and emergency room records. She has served as a DRG analyst and auditor of commercial and government payer claims, and as a contract administrator. Most recently, she was responsible for the conversion of the ICD-9-CM code set to ICD-10 and for analyzing audit results, identifying issues and trends, and developing remediation plans. Ms. Krawzik is credentialed by the American Health Information Management Association (AHIMA) as a Registered Health Information Technician (RHIT) and a Certified Coding Specialist (CCS) and is an AHIMA-approved ICD-10-CM/PCS trainer. She is an active member of AHIMA and the Missouri Health Information Management Association.

### Anne Kenney, BA, MBA, CCA, CCS

Ms. Kenney has expertise in ICD-10-CM/PCS, ICD-9-CM, DRG, and CPT coding. Most recently she has been developing content for ICD-10-CM and ICD-10-PCS applications. Her prior experience in a major teaching hospital includes assignment of ICD-9-CM codes and DRGs, CPT code assignments, and determining physician evaluation and management levels for inpatient, emergency department, and observation cases. Ms. Kenney is an active member of the American Health Information Management Association (AHIMA) and the Minnesota Health Information Management Association (MHIMA).

# Contents

# Preface

The International Classification of Diseases, 10th Revision, Procedure Coding System (ICD-10-PCS) has been developed as a replacement for volume 3 of the International Classification of Diseases, Ninth Revision (ICD-9-CM). The development of ICD-10-PCS was funded by the U.S. Centers for Medicare and Medicaid Services under contract nos. 90-1138, 91-22300 500-95-0005 and HHSM-550-2004-00011C and HHSM-500-2009-000555-C to 3M Health Information Systems. ICD-10-PCS has a multi-axial, seven-character, alphanumeric code structure that provides a unique code for all substantially different procedures and allows new procedures to be easily incorporated as new codes. The initial draft was formally tested and evaluated by an independent contractor; the final version was released in 1998, with annual updates since the final release.

# What's New for 2018

The Centers for Medicare and Medicaid Services is the agency charged with maintaining and updating ICD-10-PCS. CMS released the most current revisions, a summary of which may be found on the CMS website at: https://www.cms.gov/Medicare/Coding/ICD10/2018-ICD-10-PCS-and-GEMs.html

Due to the unique structure of ICD-10-PCS, a change in a character value may affect individual codes and several code tables.

## Change Summary Table

| 2017 Total | New Codes | Revised Titles | Deleted Codes | 2018 Total |
|---|---|---|---|---|
| 75,789 | 3,562 | 1,821 | 646 | 78,705 |

### ICD-10-PCS Code FY 2018 Totals, By Section

| | |
|---|---|
| Medical and Surgical | 68,471 |
| Obstetrics | 302 |
| Placement | 861 |
| Administration | 1,444 |
| Measurement and Monitoring | 414 |
| Extracorporeal or Systemic Assistance and Performance | 43 |
| Extracorporeal or Systemic Therapies | 46 |
| Osteopathic | 100 |
| Other Procedures | 60 |
| Chiropractic | 90 |
| Imaging | 2,941 |
| Nuclear Medicine | 463 |
| Radiation Oncology | 1,939 |
| Rehabilitation and Diagnostic Audiology | 1,380 |
| Mental Health | 30 |
| Substance Abuse Treatment | 59 |
| New Technology | 62 |
| Total | 78,705 |

### ICD-10-PCS Changes Highlights

- In the Medical and Surgical section, body part values revised or streamlined for clarity and usefulness as coded data
- Endoscopic approaches added to various tables throughout the system for completeness
- ICD-10-PCS guidelines updated with new and revised guidelines

## New Definitions Addenda

**Section Ø - Medical and Surgical**

**Root Operation**

| ICD-10-PCS Value | Definition |
|---|---|
| Dilation | Delete Includes/Examples: Percutaneous transluminal angioplasty, pyloromyotomy<br>Add Includes/Examples: Percutaneous transluminal angioplasty, internal urethrotomy |

**Section Ø - Medical and Surgical**

**Body Part Key**

| ICD-10-PCS Value | Definition |
|---|---|
| Delete Ascending Colon | Delete Hepatic flexure |
| Cervical Vertebra | Add Dens<br>Add Odontoid process<br>Add Transverse foramen<br>Add Transverse process<br>Add Vertebral body |
| Delete Epidural Space | Delete Epidural space, intracranial<br>Delete Extradural space, intracranial |
| Add Epidural Space, Intracranial | Add Extradural space, intracranial |
| Delete Frontal Bone, Left<br>Delete Frontal Bone, Right | Delete Zygomatic process of frontal bone |
| Add Frontal Bone | Add Zygomatic process of frontal bone |
| Delete Greater Omentum | Delete Gastrocolic ligament<br>Delete Gastrocolic omentum<br>Delete Gastrophrenic ligament<br>Delete Gastrosplenic ligament |
| Delete Greater Saphenous Vein, Left<br>Delete Greater Saphenous Vein, Right | Delete External pudendal vein<br>Delete Great saphenous vein<br>Delete Superficial circumflex iliac vein<br>Delete Superficial epigastric vein |
| Delete Lesser Omentum | Delete Gastrohepatic omentum<br>Delete Hepatogastric ligament |
| Delete Lesser Saphenous Vein, Left<br>Delete Lesser Saphenous Vein, Right | Delete Small saphenous vein |
| Add Lower Artery | Add Umbilical artery |

| ICD-10-PCS Value | | Definition | |
|---|---|---|---|
| Add | Lower Spine Bursa and Ligament | Add<br>Add<br>Add<br>Add<br>Add<br>Add<br>Add<br>Add<br>Add | Iliolumbar ligament<br>Interspinous ligament<br>Intertransverse ligament<br>Ligamentum flavum<br>Sacrococcygeal ligament<br>Sacroiliac ligament<br>Sacrospinous ligament<br>Sacrotuberous ligament<br>Supraspinous ligament |
| Lumbar Vertebra | | Add<br>Add | Transverse process<br>Vertebral body |
| Delete<br>Delete | Maxilla, Left<br>Maxilla, Right | Delete | Alveolar process of maxilla |
| Add | Maxilla | Add | Alveolar process of maxilla |
| Delete<br>Delete | Metacarpocarpal Joint, Left<br>Metacarpocarpal Joint, Right | Delete | Carpometacarpal (CMC) joint |
| Delete<br>Delete | Metatarsal-Tarsal Joint, Left<br>Metatarsal-Tarsal Joint, Right | Delete | Tarsometatarsal joint |
| Add | Nasal Mucosa and Soft Tissue | Add<br>Add<br>Add<br>Add<br>Add<br>Add<br>Add<br>Add | Columella<br>External naris<br>Greater alar cartilage<br>Internal naris<br>Lateral nasal cartilage<br>Lesser alar cartilage<br>Nasal cavity<br>Nostril |
| Delete | Nose | Delete<br>Delete<br>Delete<br>Delete<br>Delete<br>Delete<br>Delete<br>Delete | Columella<br>External naris<br>Greater alar cartilage<br>Internal naris<br>Lateral nasal cartilage<br>Lesser alar cartilage<br>Nasal cavity<br>Nostril |
| Delete<br>Delete | Occipital Bone, Left<br>Occipital Bone, Right | Delete | Foramen magnum |
| Add | Occipital Bone | Add | Foramen magnum |
| Add | Omentum | Add<br>Add<br>Add<br>Add<br>Add<br>Add<br>Add<br>Add | Gastrocolic ligament<br>Gastrocolic omentum<br>Gastrohepatic omentum<br>Gastrophrenic ligament<br>Gastrosplenic ligament<br>Greater Omentum<br>Hepatogastric ligament<br>Lesser Omentum |
| Pharynx | | Add | Lingual tonsil |
| Add | Rib(s) Bursa and Ligament | Add<br>Add<br>Add | Costotransverse ligament<br>Costoxiphoid ligament<br>Sternocostal ligament |

| ICD-10-PCS Value | | Definition | |
|---|---|---|---|
| Add<br>Add | Saphenous Vein, Left<br>Saphenous Vein, Right | Add<br>Add<br>Add<br>Add<br>Add<br>Add | External pudendal vein<br>Great(er) saphenous vein<br>Lesser saphenous vein<br>Small saphenous vein<br>Superficial circumflex iliac vein<br>Superficial epigastric vein |
| Delete<br>Delete | Sphenoid Bone, Left<br>Sphenoid Bone, Right | Delete<br>Delete<br>Delete<br>Delete<br>Delete | Greater wing<br>Lesser wing<br>Optic foramen<br>Pterygoid process<br>Sella turcica |
| Add | Sphenoid Bone | Add<br>Add<br>Add<br>Add<br>Add | Greater wing<br>Lesser wing<br>Optic foramen<br>Pterygoid process<br>Sella turcica |
| Add | Sternum Bursa and Ligament | Add<br>Add<br>Add | Costotransverse ligament<br>Costoxiphoid ligament<br>Sternocostal ligament |
| Delete | Subarachnoid Space | Delete | Subarachnoid space, intracranial |
| Delete | Subcutaneous Tissue and Fascia, Anterior Neck | Delete<br>Delete | Deep cervical fascia<br>Pretracheal fascia |
| Delete | Subcutaneous Tissue and Fascia, Posterior Neck | Delete | Prevertebral fascia |
| Add | Subcutaneous Tissue and Fascia, Left Neck | Add<br>Add<br>Add | Deep cervical fascia<br>Pretracheal fascia<br>Prevertebral fascia |
| Add | Subcutaneous Tissue and Fascia, Right Neck | Add<br>Add<br>Add | Deep cervical fascia<br>Pretracheal fascia<br>Prevertebral fascia |
| Delete | Subdural Space | Delete | Subdural space, intracranial |
| Thoracic Vertebra | | Add<br>Add | Transverse process<br>Vertebral body |
| Delete<br>Delete | Thorax Bursa and Ligament, Left<br>Thorax Bursa and Ligament, Right | Delete<br>Delete<br>Delete | Costotransverse ligament<br>Costoxiphoid ligament<br>Sternocostal ligament |
| Tongue | | Delete | Lingual tonsil |
| Transverse Colon | | Add | Hepatic flexure |
| Delete<br>Delete | Trunk Bursa and Ligament, Left<br>Trunk Bursa and Ligament, Right | Delete<br>Delete<br>Delete<br>Delete<br>Delete<br>Delete<br>Delete<br>Delete<br>Delete<br>Delete | Iliolumbar ligament<br>Interspinous ligament<br>Intertransverse ligament<br>Ligamentum flavum<br>Pubic ligament<br>Sacrococcygeal ligament<br>Sacroiliac ligament<br>Sacrospinous ligament<br>Sacrotuberous ligament<br>Supraspinous ligament |
| Add | Upper Spine Bursa and Ligament | Add<br>Add<br>Add<br>Add | Interspinous ligament<br>Intertransverse ligament<br>Ligamentum flavum<br>Supraspinous ligament |

## Section Ø - Medical and Surgical

### Device Key

| ICD-10-PCS Value | Definition |
|---|---|
| Delete External Heart Assist System in Heart and Great Vessels | Delete Biventricular external heart assist system<br>Delete BVS 5000 Ventricular Assist Device<br>Delete Centrimag® Blood Pump<br>Delete TandemHeart® System<br>Delete Thoratec Paracorporeal Ventricular Assist Device |
| Extraluminal Device | Delete TigerPaw® system for closure of left atrial appendage<br>Add AtriClip LAA Exclusion System |
| Implantable Heart Assist System in Heart and Great Vessels | Add HeartMate 3™ LVAS |
| Delete Neurostimulator Lead in Central Nervous System | Delete Cortical strip neurostimulator lead<br>Delete DBS lead<br>Delete Deep brain neurostimulator lead<br>Delete RNS System lead<br>Delete Spinal cord neurostimulator lead |
| Add Neurostimulator Lead in Central Nervous System and Cranial Nerves | Add Cortical strip neurostimulator lead<br>Add DBS lead<br>Add Deep brain neurostimulator lead<br>Add RNS System lead<br>Add Spinal cord neurostimulator lead |
| Add Radioactive Element, Cesium-131 Collagen Implant for Insertion in Central Nervous System and Cranial Nerves | Add Cesium-131 Collagen Implant<br>Add GammaTile(tm) |
| Add Short-term External Heart Assist System in Heart and Great Vessels | Add Biventricular external heart assist system<br>Add BVS 5000 Ventricular Assist Device<br>Add Centrimag® Blood Pump<br>Add Impella® heart pump<br>Add TandemHeart® System<br>Add Thoratec Paracorporeal Ventricular Assist Device |
| Delete Synthetic Substitute, Ceramic on Polyethylene for Replacement in Lower Joints | Delete Oxidized zirconium ceramic hip bearing surface |
| Add Synthetic Substitute, Oxidized Zirconium on Polyethylene for Replacement in Lower Joints | Add OXINIUM |
| Delete Vascular Access Device in Subcutaneous Tissue and Fascia | Delete Tunneled central venous catheter<br>Delete Vectra® Vascular Access Graft |
| Delete Vascular Access Device, Reservoir in Subcutaneous Tissue and Fascia | Delete Implanted (venous)(access) port<br>Delete Injection reservoir, port<br>Delete Subcutaneous injection reservoir, port |
| Add Vascular Access Device, Totally Implantable in Subcutaneous Tissue and Fascia | Add Implanted (venous)(access) port<br>Add Injection reservoir, port<br>Add Subcutaneous injection reservoir, port |
| Add Vascular Access Device, Tunneled in Subcutaneous Tissue and Fascia | Add Tunneled central venous catheter<br>Add Vectra® Vascular Access Graft |

## Section Ø - Medical and Surgical

### Device Aggregation Table

| Specific Device | for Operation | in Body System | General Device |
|---|---|---|---|
| Synthetic Substitute, Oxidized Zirconium on Polyethylene | Replacement | Lower Joints | J Synthetic Substitute |

## Section 1 - Obstetrics

### Root Operation

| ICD-10-PCS Value | Definition |
|---|---|
| Change | Delete Explanation: All CHANGE procedures are coded using the approach EXTERNAL |
| Drainage | Delete Explanation: The qualifier DIAGNOSTIC is used to identify drainage procedures that are biopsies |
| Extraction | Delete Explanation: The qualifier DIAGNOSTIC is used to identify extraction procedures that are biopsies |

## Section 3 - Administration

### Approach

| ICD-10-PCS Value | Definition |
|---|---|
| Add Percutaneous Endoscopic | Add Definition: Entry, by puncture or minor incision, of instrumentation through the skin or mucous membrane and any other body layers necessary to reach and visualize the site of the procedure |

### Section F - Physical Rehabilitation and Diagnostic Audiology

#### Type Qualifier

| ICD-10-PCS Value | | Definition | |
|---|---|---|---|
| Delete | Neurophysiologic Intraoperative | Delete | Definition: Monitors neural status during surgery |
| Prosthesis | | Add | Includes/Examples: Limb prosthesis, ocular prosthesis |

### Section X - New Technology

#### Root Operation

| ICD-10-PCS Value | | Definition | |
|---|---|---|---|
| Delete | Insertion | Delete | Definition: Putting in a nonbiological appliance that monitors, assists, performs, or prevents a physiological function but does not physically take the place of a body part |
| | | Delete | Includes/Examples: Insertion of radioactive implant, insertion of central venous catheter |
| Delete | Removal | Delete | Definition:Taking out or off a device from a body part |
| | | Delete | Explanation: If a device is taken out and a similar device put in without cutting or puncturing the skin or mucous membrane, the procedure is coded to the root operation CHANGE. Otherwise, the procedure for taking out a device is coded to the root operation REMOVAL |
| | | Delete | Includes/Examples: Drainage tube removal, cardiac pacemaker removal |
| Delete | Revision | Delete | Definition: Correcting, to the extent possible, a portion of a malfunctioning device or the position of a displaced device |
| | | Delete | Explanation: Revision can include correcting a malfunctioning or displaced device by taking out or putting in components of the device such as a screw or pin |
| | | Delete | Includes/Examples: Adjustment of position of pacemaker lead, recementing of hip prosthesis |

### Section X - New Technology

#### Approach

| ICD-10-PCS Value | | Definition | |
|---|---|---|---|
| Delete | Via Natural or Artificial Opening | Delete | Definition: Entry of instrumentation through a natural or artificial external opening to reach the site of the procedure |
| Delete | Via Natural or Artificial Opening Endoscopic | Delete | Definition: Entry of instrumentation through a natural or artificial external opening to reach and visualize the site of the procedure |

### Section X - New Technology

#### Device / Substance / Technology

| ICD-10-PCS Value | | Definition | |
|---|---|---|---|
| Add | Bezlotoxumab Monoclonal Antibody | Add | ZINPLAVA(tm) |
| Add | Concentrated Bone Marrow Aspirate | Add | CBMA (Concentrated Bone Marrow Aspirate) |
| Add | Cytarabine and Daunorubicin Liposome Antineoplastic | Add | VYXEOS™ |
| Add | Endothelial Damage Inhibitor | Add | DuraGraft® Endothelial Damage Inhibitor |
| Add | Engineered Autologous Chimeric Antigen Receptor Tcell Immunotherapy | Add | Axicabtagene Ciloeucel |
| Add | Interbody Fusion Device, Radiolucent Porous in New Technology | Add | COALESCE® radiolucent interbody fusion device |
| | | Add | COHERE® radiolucent interbody fusion device |
| Add | Other New Technology Therapeutic Substance | Add | STELARA® |
| | | Add | Ustekinumab |

## List of Updated Files

### 2018 Official ICD-10-PCS Coding Guidelines

- New Guideline B4.1c added in response to public comment
- Guidelines B3.3, B3.7, and B6.1a revised in response to public comment and internal review
- Downloadable PDF, file name pcs_guidelines_2018.pdf

### 2018 ICD-10-PCS Code Tables and Index (Zip file)

- Code tables for use beginning October 1, 2017
- Downloadable PDF, file name is pcs_2018.pdf
- Downloadable xml files for developers, file names are icd10pcs_tables_2018.xml, icd10pcs_index_2018.xml, icd10pcs_definitions_2018.xml
- Accompanying schema for developers, file names are icd10pcs_tables_2018.xsd, icd10pcs_index_2018.xsd, icd10pcs_definitions_2018.xsd

### 2018 ICD-10-PCS Codes File (Zip file)

- ICD-10-PCS Codes file is a simple format for non-technical uses, containing the valid FY 2018 ICD-10-PCS codes and their long titles
- File is in text file format, file name is icd10pcs_codes_2018.txt
- Accompanying documentation for codes file, file name is icd10pcsCodesFile.pdf
- Codes file addenda in text format, file name is codes_addenda_2018.txt

### 2018 ICD-10-PCS Order File (Long and Abbreviated Titles) (Zip file)

- ICD-10-PCS order file is for developers, provides a unique five-digit "order number" for each ICD-10-PCS table and code, as well as a long and abbreviated code title
- ICD-10-PCS order file name is icd10pcs_order_2018.txt
- Accompanying documentation for tabular order file, file name is icd10pcsOrderFile.pdf
- Tabular order file addenda in text format, file name is order_addenda_2018.txt

### 2018 ICD-10-PCS Final Addenda (Zip file)

- Addenda files in downloadable PDF, file names are tables_addenda_2018.pdf, index_addenda_2018.pdf, definitions_addenda_2018.pdf
- Addenda files also in machine readable text format for developers, file names are tables_addenda_2018.txt, index_addenda_2018.txt, definitions_addenda_2018.txt

### 2018 ICD-10-PCS Conversion Table (Zip file)

- ICD-10-PCS code conversion table is provided to assist users in data retrieval, in downloadable Excel spreadsheet, file name is icd10pcs_conversion_table_2018.xlsx
- Conversion table also in machine readable text format for developers, file name is icd10pcs_conversion_table_2018.txt
- Accompanying documentation for code conversion table, file name is icd10pcsConversionTable.pdf

# Introduction

## History of ICD-10-PCS

The World Health Organization has maintained the International Classification of Diseases (ICD) for recording cause of death since 1893. It has updated the ICD periodically to reflect new discoveries in epidemiology and changes in medical understanding of disease.

The International Classification of Diseases Tenth Revision (ICD-10), published in 1992, is the latest revision of the ICD. The WHO authorized the National Center for Health Statistics (NCHS) to develop a clinical modification of ICD-10 for use in the United States. This version, called ICD-10-CM, is intended to replace the previous U.S. clinical modification, ICD-9-CM, that has been in use since 1979. ICD-9-CM contains a procedure classification; ICD-10-CM does not.

CMS, the agency responsible for maintaining the inpatient procedure code set in the United States, contracted with 3M Health Information Systems in 1993 to design and then develop a procedure classification system to replace volume 3 of ICD-9-CM.

The result, ICD-10-PCS, was initially completed in 1998. The code set has been updated annually since that time to ensure that ICD-10-PCS includes classifications for new procedures, devices, and technologies.

The development of ICD-10-PCS had as its goal the incorporation of the following major attributes:

- **Completeness:** There should be a unique code for all substantially different procedures.
- **Unique definitions:** Because ICD-10-PCS codes are constructed of individual values rather than lists of fixed codes and text descriptions, the unique, stable definition of a code in the system is retained. New values may be added to the system to represent a specific new approach or device or qualifier, but whole codes by design cannot be given new meanings and reused.
- **Expandability:** As new procedures are developed, the structure of ICD-10-PCS should allow them to be easily incorporated as unique codes.
- **Multi-axial codes:** ICD-10-PCS codes should consist of independent characters, with each individual component retaining its meaning across broad ranges of codes to the extent possible.
- **Standardized terminology:** ICD-10-PCS should include definitions of the terminology used. While the meaning of specific words varies in common usage, ICD-10-PCS should not include multiple meanings for the same term, and each term must be assigned a specific meaning. There are no eponyms or common procedure terms in ICD-10-PCS.
- **Structural integrity:** ICD-10-PCS can be easily expanded without disrupting the structure of the system. ICD-10-PCS allows unique new codes to be added to the system because values for the seven characters that make up a code can be combined as needed. The system can evolve as medical technology and clinical practice evolve, without disrupting the ICD-10-PCS structure.

In the development of ICD-10-PCS, several additional general characteristics were added:

- **Diagnostic information is not included in procedure description:** When procedures are performed for specific diseases or disorders, the disease or disorder is not contained in the procedure code. The diagnosis codes, not the procedure codes, specify the disease or disorder.
- **Explicit not otherwise specified (NOS) options are restricted:** Explicit "not otherwise specified," (NOS) options are restricted in ICD-10-PCS. A minimal level of specificity is required for each component of the procedure.
- **Limited use of not elsewhere classified (NEC) option:** Because all significant components of a procedure are specified in ICD-10-PCS, there is generally no need for a "not elsewhere classified" (NEC) code option. However, limited NEC options are incorporated into ICD-10-PCS where necessary. For example, new devices are frequently developed, and therefore it is necessary to provide an "other device" option for use until the new device can be explicitly added to the coding system.
- **Level of specificity:** All procedures currently performed can be specified in ICD-10-PCS. The frequency with which a procedure is performed was not a consideration in the development of the system. A unique code is available for variations of a procedure that can be performed.

ICD-10-PCS code structure results in qualities that optimize the performance of the system in electronic applications, and maximize the usefulness of the coded healthcare data. These qualities include:

- **Optimal search capability:** ICD-10-PCS is designed for maximum versatility in the ability to aggregate coded data. Values belonging to the same character as defined in a section or sections can be easily compared, since they occupy the same position in a code. This provides a high degree of flexibility and functionality for data mining.
- **Consistent characters and values:** Stability of characters and values across vast ranges of codes provides the maximum degree of functionality and flexibility for the collection and analysis of data. Because the character definition is consistent, and only the individual values assigned to that character differ as needed, meaningful comparisons of data over time can be conducted across a virtually infinite range of procedures.
- **Code readability:** ICD-10-PCS resembles a language in the sense that it is made up of semi-independent values combined by following the rules of the system, much the way a sentence is formed by combining words and following the rules of grammar and syntax. As with words in their context, the meaning of any single value is a combination of its position in the code and any preceding values on which it may be dependent.

## ICD-10-PCS Code Structure

ICD-10-PCS has a seven-character alphanumeric code structure. Each character contains up to 34 possible values. Each value represents a specific option for the general character definition. The 10 digits Ø–9 and the 24 letters A–H, J–N, and P–Z may be used in each character. The letters O and I are not used so as to avoid confusion with the digits Ø and 1. An ICD-10-PCS code is the result of a process rather than as a single fixed set of digits or alphabetic characters. The process consists of combining semi-independent values from among a selection of values, according to the rules governing the construction of codes.

| | Section | Body System | Root Operation | Body Part | Approach | Device | Qualifier |
|---|---|---|---|---|---|---|---|
| **Characters:** | 1 | 2 | 3 | 4 | 5 | 6 | 7 |

A code is derived by choosing a specific value for each of the seven characters. Based on details about the procedure performed, values for each character specifying the section, body system, root operation, body part, approach, device, and qualifier are assigned. Because the definition of each character is also a function of its physical position in the code, the same letter or number placed in a different position in the code has a different meaning.

The seven characters that make up a complete code have specific meanings that vary for each of the 17 sections of the manual.

Procedures are then divided into sections that identify the general type of procedure (e.g., Medical and Surgical, Obstetrics, Imaging). The first character of the procedure code always specifies the section. The second through seventh characters have the same meaning within each section, but may mean different things in other sections. In all sections, the third character specifies the general type of procedure performed (e.g., Resection, Transfusion, Fluoroscopy), while the other characters give additional information such as the body part and approach.

In ICD-10-PCS, the term *procedure* refers to the complete specification of the seven characters.

## Number of Codes in ICD-10-PCS

The table structure of ICD-10-PCS permits the specification of a large number of codes on a single page. At the time of this publication, there are 78,705 codes in the 2018 ICD-10-PCS.

# ICD-10-PCS Manual

## Index

Codes may be found in the index based on the general type of procedure (e.g., resection, transfusion, fluoroscopy), or a more commonly used term (e.g., appendectomy). For example, the code for percutaneous intraluminal dilation of the coronary arteries with an intraluminal device can be found in the Index under *Dilation*, or a synonym of *Dilation* (e.g., angioplasty). The Index then specifies the first three or four values of the code or directs the user to see another term.

*Example:*

**Dilation**
  Artery
    Coronary
      One Artery Ø27Ø

Based on the first three values of the code provided in the Index, the corresponding table can be located. In the example above, the first three values indicate table Ø27 is to be referenced for code completion.

The tables and characters are arranged first by number and then by letter for each character (tables for ØØ-, Ø1-, Ø2-, etc., are followed by those for ØB-, ØC-, ØD-, etc., followed by ØB1, ØB2, etc., followed by ØBB, ØBC, ØBD, etc.).

**Note**: The Tables section must be used to construct a complete and valid code by specifying the last three or four values.

## Tables

The Tables are composed of rows that specify the valid combinations of code values. In most sections of the system, the upper portion of each table contains a description of the first three characters of the procedure code. In the Medical and Surgical section, for example, the first three characters contain the name of the section, the body system, and the root operation performed.

For instance, the values *Ø27* specify the section *Medical and Surgical* (Ø), the body system *Heart and Great Vessels* (2) and the root operation *Dilation* (7). As shown in table Ø27, the root operation (*Dilation*) is accompanied by its definition.

The lower portion of the table specifies all the valid combinations of characters 4 through 7. The four columns in the table specify the last four characters. In the Medical and Surgical section they are labeled body part, approach, device and qualifier, respectively. Each row in the table specifies the valid combination of values for characters 4 through 7.

**Table 1: Row from table Ø27**

**Ø Medical and Surgical**
**2 Heart and Great Vessels**
**7 Dilation** Definition: Expanding an orifice or the lumen of a tubular body part

Explanation: The orifice can be a natural orifice or an artificially created orifice. Accomplished by stretching a tubular body part using intraluminal pressure or by cutting part of the orifice or wall of the tubular body part.

| Body Part Character 4 | Approach Character 5 | Device Character 6 | Qualifier Character 7 |
|---|---|---|---|
| **Ø** Coronary Artery, One Artery<br>**1** Coronary Artery, Two Arteries<br>**2** Coronary Artery, Three Arteries<br>**3** Coronary Artery, Four or More Arteries | **Ø** Open<br>**3** Percutaneous<br>**4** Percutaneous Endoscopic | 4 **Intraluminal Device, Drug-eluting**<br>5 **Intraluminal Device, Drug-eluting, Two**<br>6 **Intraluminal Device, Drug-eluting, Three**<br>7 **Intraluminal Device, Drug-eluting, Four or More**<br>D **Intraluminal Device**<br>E **Intraluminal Device, Two**<br>F **Intraluminal Device, Three**<br>G **Intraluminal Device, Four or More**<br>T **Intraluminal Device, Radioactive**<br>Z **No Device** | **6** Bifurcation<br>**Z** No Qualifier |

The rows of this table can be used to construct 240 unique procedure codes. For example, code Ø27Ø3DZ specifies the procedure for dilation of one coronary artery using an intraluminal device via percutaneous approach (i.e., percutaneous transluminal coronary angioplasty with stent).

The valid codes shown in table 2 are constructed using the first body part value in table 1 (i.e., one coronary artery), combined with all the valid approaches and devices listed in the table, and the value "No Qualifier".

**Table 2: Code titles for dilation of one coronary artery (Ø27Ø)**

| | |
|---|---|
| Ø27ØØ4Z | Dilation of Coronary Artery, One Artery with Drug-eluting Intraluminal Device, Open Approach |
| Ø27ØØ5Z | Dilation of Coronary Artery, One Artery with Two Drug-eluting Intraluminal Devices, Open Approach |
| Ø27ØØ6Z | Dilation of Coronary Artery, One Artery with Three Drug-eluting Intraluminal Devices, Open Approach |
| Ø27ØØ7Z | Dilation of Coronary Artery, One Artery with Four or More Drug-eluting Intraluminal Devices, Open Approach |
| Ø27ØØDZ | Dilation of Coronary Artery, One Artery with Intraluminal Device, Open Approach |
| Ø27ØØEZ | Dilation of Coronary Artery, One Artery with Two Intraluminal Devices, Open Approach |
| Ø27ØØFZ | Dilation of Coronary Artery, One Artery with Three Intraluminal Devices, Open Approach |
| Ø27ØØGZ | Dilation of Coronary Artery, One Artery with Four or More Intraluminal Devices, Open Approach |
| Ø27ØØTZ | Dilation of Coronary Artery, One Artery with Radioactive Intraluminal Device, Open Approach |
| Ø27ØØZZ | Dilation of Coronary Artery, One Artery, Open Approach |
| Ø27Ø34Z | Dilation of Coronary Artery, One Artery with Drug-eluting Intraluminal Device, Percutaneous Approach |
| Ø27Ø35Z | Dilation of Coronary Artery, One Artery with Two Drug-eluting Intraluminal Devices, Percutaneous Approach |
| Ø27Ø36Z | Dilation of Coronary Artery, One Artery with Three Drug-eluting Intraluminal Devices, Percutaneous Approach |
| Ø27Ø37Z | Dilation of Coronary Artery, One Artery with Four or More Drug-eluting Intraluminal Devices, Percutaneous Approach |
| Ø27Ø3DZ | Dilation of Coronary Artery, One Artery with Intraluminal Device, Percutaneous Approach |
| Ø27Ø3EZ | Dilation of Coronary Artery, One Artery with Two Intraluminal Devices, Percutaneous Approach |
| Ø27Ø3FZ | Dilation of Coronary Artery, One Artery with Three Intraluminal Devices, Percutaneous Approach |
| Ø27Ø3GZ | Dilation of Coronary Artery, One Artery with Four or More Intraluminal Devices, Percutaneous Approach |
| Ø27Ø3TZ | Dilation of Coronary Artery, One Artery with Radioactive Intraluminal Device, Percutaneous Approach |
| Ø27Ø3ZZ | Dilation of Coronary Artery, One Artery, Percutaneous Approach |
| Ø27Ø44Z | Dilation of Coronary Artery, One Artery with Drug-eluting Intraluminal Device, Percutaneous Endoscopic Approach |
| Ø27Ø45Z | Dilation of Coronary Artery, One Artery with Two Drug-eluting Intraluminal Devices, Percutaneous Endoscopic Approach |
| Ø27Ø46Z | Dilation of Coronary Artery, One Artery with Three Drug-eluting Intraluminal Devices, Percutaneous Endoscopic Approach |
| Ø27Ø47Z | Dilation of Coronary Artery, One Artery with Four or More Drug-eluting Intraluminal Devices, Percutaneous Endoscopic Approach |
| Ø27Ø4DZ | Dilation of Coronary Artery, One Artery with Intraluminal Device, Percutaneous Endoscopic Approach |
| Ø27Ø4EZ | Dilation of Coronary Artery, One Artery with Two Intraluminal Devices, Percutaneous Endoscopic Approach |
| Ø27Ø4FZ | Dilation of Coronary Artery, One Artery with Three Intraluminal Devices, Percutaneous Endoscopic Approach |
| Ø27Ø4GZ | Dilation of Coronary Artery, One Artery with Four or More Intraluminal Devices, Percutaneous Endoscopic Approach |
| Ø27Ø4TZ | Dilation of Coronary Artery, One Artery with Radioactive Intraluminal Device, Percutaneous Endoscopic Approach |
| Ø27Ø4ZZ | Dilation of Coronary Artery, One Artery, Percutaneous Endoscopic Approach |

**Table 3: Rows from table Ø01**

**Ø Medical and Surgical**
**Ø Central Nervous System and Cranial Nerves**
**1 Bypass** Definition: Altering the route of passage of the contents of a tubular body part
Explanation: Rerouting contents of a body part to a downstream area of the normal route, to a similar route and body part, or to an abnormal route and dissimilar body part. Includes one or more anastomoses, with or without the use of a device.

| Body Part Character 4 | Approach Character 5 | Device Character 6 | Qualifier Character 7 |
|---|---|---|---|
| **6 Cerebral Ventricle**<br>Aqueduct of Sylvius<br>Cerebral aqueduct (Sylvius)<br>Choroid plexus<br>Ependyma<br>Foramen of Monro (intraventricular)<br>Fourth ventricle<br>Interventricular foramen (Monro)<br>Left lateral ventricle<br>Right lateral ventricle<br>Third ventricle | **Ø Open**<br>**3 Percutaneous**<br>**4 Percutaneous Endoscopic** | **7 Autologous Tissue Substitute**<br>**J Synthetic Substitute**<br>**K Nonautologous Tissue Substitute** | **Ø Nasopharynx**<br>**1 Mastoid Sinus**<br>**2 Atrium**<br>**3 Blood Vessel**<br>**4 Pleural Cavity**<br>**5 Intestine**<br>**6 Peritoneal Cavity**<br>**7 Urinary Tract**<br>**8 Bone Marrow**<br>**B Cerebral Cisterns** |
| **6 Cerebral Ventricle**<br>Aqueduct of Sylvius<br>Cerebral aqueduct (Sylvius)<br>Choroid plexus<br>Ependyma<br>Foramen of Monro (intraventricular)<br>Fourth ventricle<br>Interventricular foramen (Monro)<br>Left lateral ventricle<br>Right lateral ventricle<br>Third ventricle | **Ø Open**<br>**3 Percutaneous**<br>**4 Percutaneous Endoscopic** | **Z No Device** | **B Cerebral Cisterns** |
| **U Spinal Canal**<br>Epidural space, spinal<br>Extradural space, spinal<br>Subarachnoid space, spinal<br>Subdural space, spinal<br>Vertebral canal | **Ø Open**<br>**3 Percutaneous** | **7 Autologous Tissue Substitute**<br>**J Synthetic Substitute**<br>**K Nonautologous Tissue Substitute** | **4 Pleural Cavity**<br>**6 Peritoneal Cavity**<br>**7 Urinary Tract**<br>**9 Fallopian Tube** |

Table 3, is split into three rows; values of characters must all be selected from within the same row of the table.

Row 1 and Row 3 indicate that the body part (character 4) values *6* and *U* may both be used in combination with device values *7*, *J* or *K*. However, the approach (character 5) and qualifier (character 7) values are not the same for both rows. Body part value *U* may only be used in combination with approach values *0* and *3* and qualifier values *4, 6, 7* and *9*. In other words, code 001U473 is invalid as the approach value *4* and the qualifier value *3* are only applicable to Row 1. It would be inappropriate to build a code for body part value U from values not contained within its own row.

**Note:** In this manual, there are instances in which some tables due to length must be continued on the next page. Each section must be used separately and value selection must be made within the same row of the table.

## Character Meanings

In each section, each character has a specific meaning, and this character meaning remains constant within that section. Character meaning tables have been provided at the beginning of each section or, in the case of the Medical and Surgical section (Ø), at the beginning of each body system to help the user identify the character members available within that section. These tables have purple headers, unlike the official code tables that have green headers and **SHOULD NOT** be used to build a PCS code. Following is an excerpt of a character meaning table.

**Table 4: Rows from Central Nervous System and Cranial Nerves - Character Meanings Table**

| Operation–Character 3 | Body Part–Character 4 | Approach–Character 5 | Device–Character 6 | Qualifier–Character 7 |
|---|---|---|---|---|
| 1 Bypass | Ø Brain | Ø Open | Ø Drainage Device | Ø Nasopharynx |
| 2 Change | 1 Cerebral Meninges | 3 Percutaneous | 2 Monitoring Device | 1 Mastoid Sinus |
| 5 Destruction | 2 Dura Mater | 4 Percutaneous Endoscopic | 3 Infusion Device | 2 Atrium |
| 7 Dilation | 3 Epidural Space, Intracranial | X External | 4 Radioactive Element, Cesium-131 Collagen Implant | 3 Blood Vessel |
| 8 Division | 4 Subdural Space, Intracranial | | 7 Autologous Tissue Substitute | 4 Pleural Cavity |
| 9 Drainage | 5 Subarachnoid Space, Intracranial | | J Synthetic Substitute | 5 Intestine |
| B Excision | 6 Cerebral Ventricle | | K Nonautologous Tissue Substitute | 6 Peritoneal Cavity |
| C Extirpation | 7 Cerebral Hemisphere | | M Neurostimulator Lead | 7 Urinary Tract |
| D Extraction | 8 Basal Ganglia | | Y Other Device | 8 Bone Marrow |
| F Fragmentation | 9 Thalamus | | Z No Device | 9 Fallopian Tube |
| H Insertion | A Hypothalamus | | | B Cerebral Cisterns |
| J Inspection | B Pons | | | F Olfactory Nerve |

## Sections

Procedures are divided into sections that identify the general type of procedure (e.g., Medical and Surgical, Obstetrics, Imaging). The first character of the procedure code always specifies the section.

The sections are listed below:

**Medical and Surgical section**

Ø Medical and Surgical

**Medical and Surgical-related sections**

1 Obstetrics

2 Placement

3 Administration

4 Measurement and Monitoring

5 Extracorporeal or Systemic Assistance and Performance

6 Extracorporeal or Systemic Therapies

7 Osteopathic

8 Other Procedures

9 Chiropractic

**Ancillary Sections**

B Imaging

C Nuclear Medicine

D Radiation Therapy

F Physical Rehabilitation and Diagnostic Audiology

G Mental Health

H Substance Abuse Treatment

**New Technology Section**

X New Technology

# Medical and Surgical Section (Ø)

## Character Meaning

The seven characters for Medical and Surgical procedures have the following meaning:

| Character | Meaning |
|---|---|
| 1 | Section |
| 2 | Body System |
| 3 | Root Operation |
| 4 | Body Part |
| 5 | Approach |
| 6 | Device |
| 7 | Qualifier |

The Medical and Surgical section constitutes the vast majority of procedures reported in an inpatient setting. Medical and Surgical procedure codes all have a first character value of Ø. The second character indicates the general body system (e.g., Mouth and Throat, Gastrointestinal). The third character indicates the root operation, or specific objective, of the procedure (e.g., Excision). The fourth character indicates the specific body part on which the procedure was performed (e.g., Tonsils, Duodenum). The fifth character indicates the approach used to reach the procedure site (e.g., Open). The sixth character indicates whether a device was left in place during the procedure (e.g., Synthetic Substitute). The seventh character is qualifier, which has a specific meaning for each root operation. For example, the qualifier can be used to identify the destination site of a *Bypass*. The first through fifth characters are always assigned a specific value, but the device (sixth character) and the qualifier (seventh character) are not applicable to all procedures. The value *Z* is used for the sixth and seventh characters to indicate that a specific device or qualifier does not apply to the procedure.

## Section (Character 1)

Medical and Surgical procedure codes all have a first character value of *Ø*.

## Body Systems (Character 2)

Body systems for Medical and Surgical section codes are specified in the second character.

**Body Systems**

Ø Central Nervous System and Cranial Nerves

1 Peripheral Nervous System

2 Heart and Great Vessels

3 Upper Arteries

4 Lower Arteries

5 Upper Veins

6 Lower Veins

7 Lymphatic and Hemic Systems

8 Eye

9 Ear, Nose, Sinus

B Respiratory System

C Mouth and Throat

D Gastrointestinal System

F Hepatobiliary System and Pancreas

G Endocrine System

H Skin and Breast

J Subcutaneous Tissue and Fascia

K Muscles

L Tendons

M Bursae and Ligaments

N Head and Facial Bones

P Upper Bones

Q Lower Bones

R Upper Joints

S Lower Joints

T Urinary System

U Female Reproductive System

V Male Reproductive System

W Anatomical Regions, General

X Anatomical Regions, Upper Extremities

Y Anatomical Regions, Lower Extremities

## Root Operations (Character 3)

The root operation is specified in the third character. In the Medical and Surgical section there are 31 different root operations. The root operation identifies the objective of the procedure. Each root operation has a precise definition.

- *Alteration:* Modifying the natural anatomic structure of a body part without affecting the function of the body part
- *Bypass:* Altering the route of passage of the contents of a tubular body part
- *Change:* Taking out or off a device from a body part and putting back an identical or similar device in or on the same body part without cutting or puncturing the skin or a mucous membrane
- *Control:* Stopping, or attempting to stop, postprocedural or other acute bleeding
- *Creation:* Putting in or on biological or synthetic material to form a new body part that to the extent possible replicates the anatomic structure or function of an absent body part
- *Destruction:* Physical eradication of all or a portion of a body part by the direct use of energy, force, or a destructive agent
- *Detachment:* Cutting off all or a portion of the upper or lower extremities
- *Dilation:* Expanding an orifice or the lumen of a tubular body part
- *Division:* Cutting into a body part without draining fluids and/or gases from the body part in order to separate or transect a body part
- *Drainage:* Taking or letting out fluids and/or gases from a body part
- *Excision:* Cutting out or off, without replacement, a portion of a body part
- *Extirpation:* Taking or cutting out solid matter from a body part
- *Extraction:* Pulling or stripping out or off all or a portion of a body part by the use of force
- *Fragmentation:* Breaking solid matter in a body part into pieces
- *Fusion:* Joining together portions of an articular body part rendering the articular body part immobile
- *Insertion:* Putting in a nonbiological appliance that monitors, assists, performs, or prevents a physiological function but does not physically take the place of a body part
- *Inspection:* Visually and/or manually exploring a body part
- *Map:* Locating the route of passage of electrical impulses and/or locating functional areas in a body part
- *Occlusion:* Completely closing an orifice or lumen of a tubular body part
- *Reattachment:* Putting back in or on all or a portion of a separated body part to its normal location or other suitable location
- *Release:* Freeing a body part from an abnormal physical constraint by cutting or by use of force
- *Removal:* Taking out or off a device from a body part
- *Repair:* Restoring, to the extent possible, a body part to its normal anatomic structure and function
- *Replacement:* Putting in or on biological or synthetic material that physically takes the place and/or function of all or a portion of a body part
- *Reposition:* Moving to its normal location or other suitable location all or a portion of a body part
- *Resection:* Cutting out or off, without replacement, all of a body part
- *Restriction:* Partially closing an orifice or lumen of a tubular body part
- *Revision:* Correcting, to the extent possible, a portion of a malfunctioning device or the position of a displaced device
- *Supplement:* Putting in or on biological or synthetic material that physically reinforces and/or augments the function of a portion of a body part
- *Transfer:* Moving, without taking out, all or a portion of a body part to another location to take over the function of all or a portion of a body part
- *Transplantation:* Putting in or on all or a portion of a living body part taken from another individual or animal to physically take the place and/or function of all or a portion of a similar body part

The above definitions of root operations illustrate the precision of code values defined in the system. There is a clear distinction between each root operation.

A root operation specifies the objective of the procedure. The term *anastomosis* is not a root operation, because it is a means of joining and is always an integral part of another procedure (e.g., Bypass, Resection) with a specific objective. Similarly, *incision* is not a root operation, since it is always part of the objective of another procedure (e.g., Division, Drainage). The root operation *Repair* in the Medical and Surgical section functions as a "not elsewhere classified" option. *Repair* is used when the procedure performed is not one of the other specific root operations.

Appendix B provides additional explanation and representative examples of the Medical and Surgical root operations. Appendix C groups all root operations in the Medical and Surgical section into subcategories and provides an example of each root operation.

## Body Part (Character 4)

The body part is specified in the fourth character. The body part indicates the specific anatomical site of the body system on which the procedure was performed (e.g., Duodenum). Tubular body parts are defined in ICD-10-PCS as those hollow body parts that provide a route of passage for solids, liquids, or gases. They include the cardiovascular system and body parts such as those contained in the gastrointestinal tract, genitourinary tract, biliary tract, and respiratory tract.

## Approach (Character 5)

The technique used to reach the site of the procedure is specified in the fifth character. There are seven different approaches:

- *Open*: Cutting through the skin or mucous membrane and any other body layers necessary to expose the site of the procedure
- *Percutaneous*: Entry, by puncture or minor incision, of instrumentation through the skin or mucous membrane and any other body layers necessary to reach the site of the procedure
- *Percutaneous Endoscopic*: Entry, by puncture or minor incision, of instrumentation through the skin or mucous membrane and any other body layers necessary to reach and visualize the site of the procedure
- *Via Natural or Artificial Opening*: Entry of instrumentation through a natural or artificial external opening to reach the site of the procedure
- *Via Natural or Artificial Opening Endoscopic*: Entry of instrumentation through a natural or artificial external opening to reach and visualize the site of the procedure

- *Via Natural or Artificial Opening with Percutaneous Endoscopic Assistance:* Entry of instrumentation through a natural or artificial external opening and entry, by puncture or minor incision, of instrumentation through the skin or mucous membrane and any other body layers necessary to aid in the performance of the procedure
- *External*: Procedures performed directly on the skin or mucous membrane and procedures performed indirectly by the application of external force through the skin or mucous membrane

The approach comprises three components: the access location, method, and type of instrumentation.

**Access location:** For procedures performed on an internal body part, the access location specifies the external site through which the site of the procedure is reached. There are two general types of access locations: skin or mucous membranes, and external orifices. Every approach value except external includes one of these two access locations. The skin or mucous membrane can be cut or punctured to reach the procedure site. All open and percutaneous approach values use this access location. The site of a procedure can also be reached through an external opening. External openings can be natural (e.g., mouth) or artificial (e.g., colostomy stoma).

**Method:** For procedures performed on an internal body part, the method specifies how the external access location is entered. An open method specifies cutting through the skin or mucous membrane and any other intervening body layers necessary to expose the site of the procedure. An instrumentation method specifies the entry of instrumentation through the access location to the internal procedure site. Instrumentation can be introduced by puncture or minor incision, or through an external opening. The puncture or minor incision does not constitute an open approach because it does not expose the site of the procedure. An approach can define multiple methods. For example, *Via Natural or Artificial Opening with Percutaneous Endoscopic Assistance* includes both the initial entry of instrumentation to reach the site of the procedure, and the placement of additional percutaneous instrumentation into the body part to visualize and assist in the performance of the procedure.

**Type of instrumentation:** For procedures performed on an internal body part, instrumentation means that specialized equipment is used to perform the procedure. Instrumentation is used in all internal approaches other than the basic open approach. Instrumentation may or may not include the capacity to visualize the procedure site. For example, the instrumentation used to perform a sigmoidoscopy permits the internal site of the procedure to be visualized, while the instrumentation used to perform a needle biopsy of the liver does not. The term "endoscopic" as used in approach values refers to instrumentation that permits a site to be visualized.

Procedures performed directly on the skin or mucous membrane are identified by the external approach (e.g., skin excision). Procedures performed indirectly by the application of external force are also identified by the external approach (e.g., closed reduction of fracture).

Appendix A compares the components (access location, method, and type of instrumentation) of each approach and provides an example of each approach.

## Device (Character 6)

The device is specified in the sixth character and is used only to specify devices that remain after the procedure is completed. There are four general types of devices:

- Biological or synthetic material that takes the place of all or a portion of a body part (e.g, skin graft, joint prosthesis).
- Biological or synthetic material that assists or prevents a physiological function (e.g., IUD).
- Therapeutic material that is not absorbed by, eliminated by, or incorporated into a body part (e.g., radioactive implant).
- Mechanical or electronic appliances used to assist, monitor, take the place of or prevent a physiological function (e.g., cardiac pacemaker, orthopedic pin).

While all devices can be removed, some cannot be removed without putting in another nonbiological appliance or body-part substitute.

When a specific device value is used to identify the device for a root operation, such as *Insertion* and that same device value is not an option for a more broad range root operation such as *Removal*, select the general device value. For example, in the body system Heart and Great Vessels, the specific device character for Cardiac Lead, Pacemaker in root operation *Insertion* is J. For the root operation *Removal*, the general device character M Cardiac Lead would be selected for the pacemaker lead.

ICD-10-PCS contains a PCS Device Aggregation Table (see appendix F) that crosswalks the *specific* device character values that have been created for specific root operations and specific body part character values to the *general* device character value that would be used for root operations that represent a broad range of procedures and general body part character values, such as Removal and Revision.

Instruments used to visualize the procedure site are specified in the approach, not the device, value.

If the objective of the procedure is to put in the device, then the root operation is *Insertion*. If the device is put in to meet an objective other than *Insertion*, then the root operation defining the underlying objective of the procedure is used, with the device specified in the device character. For example, if a procedure to replace the hip joint is performed, the root operation *Replacement* is coded, and the prosthetic device is specified in the device character. Materials that are incidental to a procedure such as clips, ligatures, and sutures are not specified in the device character. Because new devices can be developed, the value *Other Device* is provided as a temporary option for use until a specific device value is added to the system.

## Qualifier (Character 7)

The qualifier is specified in the seventh character. The qualifier contains unique values for individual procedures. For example, the qualifier can be used to identify the destination site in a *Bypass*.

## Medical and Surgical Section Principles

In developing the Medical and Surgical procedure codes, several specific principles were followed.

### Composite Terms Are Not Root Operations

Composite terms such as colonoscopy, sigmoidectomy, or appendectomy do not describe root operations, but they do specify multiple components of a specific root operation. In ICD-10-PCS, the components of a procedure are defined separately by the characters making up the complete code. The only component of a procedure specified in the root operation is the objective of the procedure. With each complete code the underlying objective of the procedure is specified by the root operation (third character), the precise part is specified by the body part (fourth character), and the method used to reach and visualize the procedure site is specified by the approach (fifth character). While colonoscopy, sigmoidectomy, and appendectomy are included in the Index, they do not constitute root operations in the Tables section. The objective of colonoscopy is the visualization of the colon and the root operation (character 3) is *Inspection*. Character 4 specifies the body part, which in this case is part of the colon. These composite terms, like colonoscopy or appendectomy, are included as cross-reference only. The index provides the correct root operation reference. Examples of other types of composite terms not representative of root operations are *partial* sigmoidectomy, *total* hysterectomy, and *partial* hip replacement. Always refer to the correct root operation in the Index and Tables section.

### Root Operation Based on Objective of Procedure

The root operation is based on the objective of the procedure, such as *Resection* of transverse colon or *Dilation* of an artery. The assignment of the root operation is based on the procedure actually performed, which may or may not have been the intended procedure. If the intended procedure is modified or discontinued (e.g., excision instead of resection is performed), the root operation is determined by the procedure actually performed. If the desired result is not attained after completing the procedure (i.e., the artery does not remain expanded after the dilation procedure), the root operation is still determined by the procedure actually performed.

*Examples:*

- Dilating the urethra is coded as *Dilation* since the objective of the procedure is to dilate the urethra. If dilation of the urethra includes putting in an intraluminal stent, the root operation remains *Dilation* and not *Insertion* of the intraluminal device because the underlying objective of the procedure is dilation of the urethra. The stent is identified by the intraluminal device value in the sixth character of the dilation procedure code.
- If the objective is solely to put a radioactive element in the urethra, then the procedure is coded to the root operation *Insertion*, with the radioactive element identified in the sixth character of the code.
- If the objective of the procedure is to correct a malfunctioning or displaced device, then the procedure is coded to the root operation *Revision*. In the root operation *Revision*, the original device being revised is identified in the device character. *Revision* is typically performed on mechanical appliances (e.g., pacemaker) or materials used in replacement procedures (e.g., synthetic substitute). Typical revision procedures include adjustment of pacemaker position and correction of malfunctioning knee prosthesis.

### Combination Procedures Are Coded Separately

If multiple procedures as defined by distinct objectives are performed during an operative episode, then multiple codes are used. For example, obtaining the vein graft used for coronary bypass surgery is coded as a separate procedure from the bypass itself.

### Redo of Procedures

The complete or partial redo of the original procedure is coded to the root operation that identifies the procedure performed rather than *Revision*.

*Example:*

A complete redo of a hip replacement procedure that requires putting in a new prosthesis is coded to the root operation *Replacement* rather than *Revision*.

The correction of complications arising from the original procedure, other than device complications, is coded to the procedure performed. Correction of a malfunctioning or displaced device would be coded to the root operation *Revision*.

*Example:*

A procedure to control hemorrhage arising from the original procedure is coded to *Control* rather than *Revision*.

## Examples of Procedures Coded in the Medical Surgical Section

The following are examples of procedures from the Medical and Surgical section, coded in ICD-10-PCS.

- Suture of skin laceration, left lower arm: ØHQEXZZ

  *Medical and Surgical* section (Ø), body system *Skin and Breast* (H), root operation *Repair* (Q), body part *Skin, Left Lower Arm* (E), *External* Approach (X) *No device* (Z), and *No qualifier* (Z).
- Laparoscopic appendectomy: ØDTJ4ZZ

  *Medical and Surgical* section (Ø), body system *Gastrointestinal* (D), root operation *Resection* (T), body part *Appendix* (J), *Percutaneous Endoscopic* approach (4), No Device (Z), and No qualifier (Z).
- Sigmoidoscopy with biopsy: ØDBN8ZX

  *Medical and Surgical* section (Ø), body system *Gastrointestinal* (D), root operation *Excision* (B), body part *Sigmoid Colon* (N), *Via Natural or Artificial Opening Endoscopic* approach (8), *No Device* (Z), and with qualifier *Diagnostic* (X).
- Tracheostomy with tracheostomy tube: ØB11ØF4

  *Medical and Surgical* section (Ø), body system *Respiratory* (B), root operation *Bypass* (1), body part *Trachea* (1), *Open* approach (Ø), with *Tracheostomy Device* (F), and qualifier *Cutaneous* (4).

# Obstetrics Section (1)

## Character Meanings

The seven characters in the Obstetrics section have the same meaning as in the Medical and Surgical section.

| Character | Meaning |
|---|---|
| 1 | Section |
| 2 | Body System |
| 3 | Root Operation |
| 4 | Body Part |
| 5 | Approach |
| 6 | Device |
| 7 | Qualifier |

The Obstetrics section includes procedures performed on the products of conception only. Procedures on the pregnant female are coded in the Medical and Surgical section (e.g., episiotomy). The term "products of conception" refers to all physical components of a pregnancy, including the fetus, amnion, umbilical cord, and placenta. There is no differentiation of the products of conception based on gestational age. Thus, the specification of the products of conception as a zygote, embryo or fetus, or the trimester of the pregnancy is not part of the procedure code but can be found in the diagnosis code.

### Section (Character 1)

Obstetrics procedure codes have a first character value of *1*.

### Body System (Character 2)

The second character value for body system is *Pregnancy*.

### Root Operation (Character 3)

The root operations *Change, Drainage, Extraction, Insertion, Inspection, Removal, Repair, Reposition, Resection,* and *Transplantation* are used in the obstetrics section and have the same meaning as in the Medical and Surgical section.

The Obstetrics section also includes two additional root operations, *Abortion* and *Delivery*, defined below:

- *Abortion*: Artificially terminating a pregnancy
- *Delivery*: Assisting the passage of the products of conception from the genital canal

A cesarean section is not a separate root operation because the underlying objective is *Extraction* (i.e., pulling out all or a portion of a body part).

### Body Part (Character 4)

The body part values in the obstetrics section are:

- *Products of conception*
- *Products of conception, retained*
- *Products of conception, ectopic*

### Approach (Character 5)

The fifth character specifies approaches and is defined as are those in the Medical and Surgical section. In the case of an abortion procedure that uses a laminaria or an abortifacient, the approach is *Via Natural or Artificial Opening*.

### Device (Character 6)

The sixth character is used for devices such as fetal monitoring electrodes.

### Qualifier (Character 7)

Qualifier values are specific to the root operation and are used to specify the type of extraction (e.g., low forceps, high forceps, etc.), the type of cesarean section (e.g., classical, low cervical, etc.), or the type of fluid taken out during a drainage procedure (e.g., amniotic fluid, fetal blood, etc.).

## Placement Section (2)

### Character Meanings

The seven characters in the Placement section have the following meaning:

| Character | Meaning |
|---|---|
| 1 | Section |
| 2 | Body System |
| 3 | Root Operation |
| 4 | Body Region |
| 5 | Approach |
| 6 | Device |
| 7 | Qualifier |

Placement section codes represent procedures for putting a device in or on a body region for the purpose of protection, immobilization, stretching, compression, or packing.

### Section (Character 1)

Placement procedure codes have a first character value of *2*.

### Body System (Character 2)

The second character contains two values specifying either *Anatomical Regions* or *Anatomical Orifices.*

### Root Operation (Character 3)

The root operations in the Placement section include only those procedures that are performed without making an incision or a puncture. The root operations *Change* and *Removal* are in the Placement section and have the same meaning as in the Medical and Surgical section.

The Placement section also includes five additional root operations, defined as follows:

- *Compression*: Putting pressure on a body region
- *Dressing*: Putting material on a body region for protection
- *Immobilization*: Limiting or preventing motion of an external body region
- *Packing*: Putting material in a body region or orifice
- *Traction*: Exerting a pulling force on a body region in a distal direction

### Body Region (Character 4)

The fourth character values are either body regions (e.g., *Upper Leg*) or natural orifices (e.g., *Ear*).

### Approach (Character 5)

Since all placement procedures are performed directly on the skin or mucous membrane, or performed indirectly by applying external force through the skin or mucous membrane, the approach value is always *External.*

### Device (Character 6)

The device character is always specified (except in the case of manual traction) and indicates the device placed during the procedure (e.g., cast, splint, bandage, etc.). Except for casts for fractures and dislocations, devices in the Placement section are off the shelf and do not require any extensive design, fabrication, or fitting. Placement of devices that require extensive design, fabrication, or fitting are coded in the Rehabilitation section.

### Qualifier (Character 7)
The qualifier character is not specified in the Placement section; the qualifier value is always *No Qualifier.*

## Administration Section (3)

### Character Meanings
The seven characters in the Administration section have the following meaning:

| Character | Meaning |
|---|---|
| 1 | Section |
| 2 | Body System |
| 3 | Root Operation |
| 4 | Body System/Region |
| 5 | Approach |
| 6 | Substance |
| 7 | Qualifier |

Administration section codes represent procedures for putting in or on a therapeutic, prophylactic, protective, diagnostic, nutritional, or physiological substance. The section includes transfusions, infusions, and injections, along with other similar services such as irrigation and tattooing.

### Section (Character 1)
Administration procedure codes have a first character value of *3*.

### Body System (Character 2)
The body system character contains only three values: *Indwelling Device, Physiological Systems and Anatomical Regions,* or *Circulatory System*. The *Circulatory System* is used for transfusion procedures.

### Root Operation (Character 3)
There are three root operations in the Administration section.

- *Introduction*: Putting in or on a therapeutic, diagnostic, nutritional, physiological, or prophylactic substance except blood or blood products
- *Irrigation*: Putting in or on a cleansing substance
- *Transfusion*: Putting in blood or blood products

### Body/System Region (Character 4)
The fourth character specifies the body system/region. The fourth character identifies the site where the substance is administered, not the site where the substance administered takes effect. Sites include *Skin and Mucous Membranes, Subcutaneous Tissue,* and *Muscle.* These differentiate intradermal, subcutaneous, and intramuscular injections, respectively. Other sites include *Eye, Respiratory Tract, Peritoneal Cavity,* and *Epidural Space.*

The body systems/regions for arteries and veins are *Peripheral Artery, Central Artery, Peripheral Vein,* and *Central Vein*. The *Peripheral Artery* or *Vein* is typically used when a substance is introduced locally into an artery or vein. For example, chemotherapy is the introduction of an antineoplastic substance into a peripheral artery or vein by a percutaneous approach. In general, the substance introduced into a peripheral artery or vein has a systemic effect.

The *Central Artery* or *Vein* is typically used when the site where the substance is introduced is distant from the point of entry into the artery or vein. For example, the introduction of a substance directly at the site of a clot within an artery or vein using a catheter is coded as an introduction of a thrombolytic substance into a central artery or vein by a percutaneous approach. In general, the substance introduced into a central artery or vein has a local effect.

### Approach (Character 5)
The fifth character specifies approaches as defined in the Medical and Surgical section. The approach for intradermal, subcutaneous, and intramuscular introductions (i.e., injections) is *Percutaneous.* If a catheter is placed to introduce a substance into an internal site within the circulatory system, then the approach is also *Percutaneous.* For example, if a catheter is used to introduce contrast directly into the heart for angiography, then the procedure would be coded as a percutaneous introduction of contrast into the heart.

### Substance (Character 6)
The sixth character specifies the substance being introduced. Broad categories of substances are defined, such as anesthetic, contrast, dialysate, and blood products such as platelets.

### Qualifier (Character 7)
The seventh character is a qualifier and is used to indicate whether the substance is *Autologous* or *Nonautologous*, or to further specify the substance.

## Measurement and Monitoring Section (4)

### Character Meanings
The seven characters in the Measurement and Monitoring section have the following meaning:

| Character | Meaning |
|---|---|
| 1 | Section |
| 2 | Body System |
| 3 | Root Operation |
| 4 | Body System |
| 5 | Approach |
| 6 | Function/Device |
| 7 | Qualifier |

Measurement and Monitoring section codes represent procedures for determining the level of a physiological or physical function.

### Section (Character 1)
Measurement and Monitoring procedure codes have a first character value of *4*.

### Body System (Character 2)
The second character values for body system are A, *Physiological Systems* or *B, Physiological Devices*.

### Root Operation (Character 3)
There are two root operations in the Measurement and Monitoring section, as defined below:

- *Measurement*: Determining the level of a physiological or physical function at a point in time

- *Monitoring*: Determining the level of a physiological or physical function repetitively over a period of time

### Body System (Character 4)
The fourth character specifies the specific body system measured or monitored.

### Approach (Character 5)
The fifth character specifies approaches as defined in the Medical and Surgical section.

### Function/Device (Character 6)
The sixth character specifies the physiological or physical function being measured or monitored. Examples of physiological or physical functions are *Conductivity, Metabolism, Pulse, Temperature,* and *Volume.* If a device used to perform the measurement or monitoring is inserted and left in, then insertion of the device is coded as a separate Medical and Surgical procedure.

### Qualifier (Character 7)
The seventh character qualifier contains specific values as needed to further specify the body part (e.g., central, portal, pulmonary) or a variation of the procedure performed (e.g., ambulatory, stress). Examples of typical procedures coded in this section are EKG, EEG, and cardiac catheterization. An EKG is the measurement of cardiac electrical activity, while an EEG is the measurement of electrical activity of the central nervous system. A cardiac catheterization performed to measure the pressure in the heart is coded as the measurement of cardiac pressure by percutaneous approach.

## Extracorporeal or Systemic Assistance and Performance Section (5)

### Character Meanings
The seven characters in the Extracorporeal or Systemic Assistance and Performance section have the following meaning:

| Character | Meaning |
|---|---|
| 1 | Section |
| 2 | Body System |
| 3 | Root Operation |
| 4 | Body System |
| 5 | Duration |
| 6 | Function |
| 7 | Qualifier |

In Extracorporeal or Systemic Assistance and Performance procedures, equipment outside the body is used to assist or perform a physiological function. The section includes procedures performed in a critical care setting, such as mechanical ventilation and cardioversion; it also includes other services such as hyperbaric oxygen treatment and hemodialysis.

### Section (Character 1)
Extracorporeal or Systemic Assistance and Performance procedure codes have a first character value of *5*.

### Body System (Character 2)
The second character value for body system is A, *Physiological Systems*.

### Root Operation (Character 3)
There are three root operations in the Extracorporeal or Systemic Assistance and Performance section, as defined below.

- *Assistance*: Taking over a portion of a physiological function by extracorporeal means
- *Performance*: Completely taking over a physiological function by extracorporeal means
- *Restoration*: Returning, or attempting to return, a physiological function to its natural state by extracorporeal means

The root operation *Restoration* contains a single procedure code that identifies extracorporeal cardioversion.

### Body System (Character 4)
The fourth character specifies the body system (e.g., cardiac, respiratory) to which extracorporeal or systemic assistance or performance is applied.

### Duration (Character 5)
The fifth character specifies the duration of the procedure—*Single, Intermittent*, or *Continuous*. For respiratory ventilation assistance or performance, the duration is specified in hours— *< 24 Consecutive Hours, 24–96 Consecutive Hours*, or *> 96 Consecutive Hours*. For urinary procedures, duration is specified as *Intermittent, Less than 6 Hours Per Day; Prolonged Intermittent, 6-18 hours Per Day*; or *Continuous, Greater than 18 hours Per Day*. Value 6, *Multiple* identifies serial procedure treatment.

### Function (Character 6)
The sixth character specifies the physiological function assisted or performed (e.g., oxygenation, ventilation) during the procedure.

### Qualifier (Character 7)
The seventh character qualifier specifies the type of equipment used, if any.

## Extracorporeal or Systemic Therapies Section (6)

### Character Meanings
The seven characters in the Extracorporeal or Systemic Therapies section have the following meaning:

| Character | Meaning |
|---|---|
| 1 | Section |
| 2 | Body System |
| 3 | Root Operation |
| 4 | Body System |
| 5 | Duration |
| 6 | Qualifier |
| 7 | Qualifier |

In extracorporeal or systemic therapy, equipment outside the body is used for a therapeutic purpose that does not involve the assistance or performance of a physiological function.

### Section (Character 1)
Extracorporeal or Systemic Therapy procedure codes have a first character value of 6.

### Body System (Character 2)
The second character value for body system is *Physiological Systems*.

### Root Operation (Character 3)
There are 11 root operations in the Extracorporeal or Systemic Therapy section, as defined below.

- *Atmospheric Control*: Extracorporeal control of atmospheric pressure and composition
- *Decompression*: Extracorporeal elimination of undissolved gas from body fluids

  *Coding note:* The root operation *Decompression* involves only one type of procedure: treatment for decompression sickness (the bends) in a hyperbaric chamber.
- *Electromagnetic Therapy*: Extracorporeal treatment by electromagnetic rays
- *Hyperthermia*: Extracorporeal raising of body temperature

  *Coding note:* The term hyperthermia is used to describe both a temperature imbalance treatment and also as an adjunct radiation treatment for cancer. When treating the temperature imbalance, it is coded to this section; for the cancer treatment, it is coded in section *D Radiation Therapy.*
- *Hypothermia*: Extracorporeal lowering of body temperature
- *Perfusion*: Extracorporeal treatment by diffusion of therapeutic fluid
- *Pheresis*: Extracorporeal separation of blood products

  *Coding note: Pheresis* may be used for two main purposes: to treat diseases when too much of a blood component is produced (e.g., leukemia) and to remove a blood product such as platelets from a donor, for transfusion into another patient.
- *Phototherapy*: Extracorporeal treatment by light rays

  *Coding note:* Phototherapy involves using a machine that exposes the blood to light rays outside the body, recirculates it, and then returns it to the body.
- *Shock Wave Therapy*: Extracorporeal treatment by shock waves
- *Ultrasound Therapy*: Extracorporeal treatment by ultrasound
- *Ultraviolet Light Therapy*: Extracorporeal treatment by ultraviolet light

### Body System (Character 4)
The fourth character specifies the body system on which the extracorporeal or systemic therapy is performed (e.g., skin, circulatory).

### Duration (Character 5)
The fifth character specifies the duration of the procedure (e.g., single or intermittent).

### Qualifier (Character 6)
The sixth character for Extracorporeal or Systemic Therapies is *No Qualifier*, except for root operation Perfusion which has a sixth character qualifier of *Donor Organ*.

### Qualifier (Character 7)
The seventh character qualifier is used in the root operation *Pheresis* to specify the blood component on which pheresis is performed and in the root operation *Ultrasound Therapy* to specify site of treatment.

## Osteopathic Section (7)

### Character Meanings
The seven characters in the Osteopathic section have the following meaning:

| Character | Meaning |
|---|---|
| 1 | Section |
| 2 | Body System |
| 3 | Root Operation |
| 4 | Body Region |
| 5 | Approach |
| 6 | Method |
| 7 | Qualifier |

### Section (Character 1)
Osteopathic procedure codes have a first character value of *7*.

### Body System (Character 2)
The body system character contains the value *Anatomical Regions*.

### Root Operation (Character 3)
There is only one root operation in the Osteopathic section.

- *Treatment*: Manual treatment to eliminate or alleviate somatic dysfunction and related disorders

### Body Region (Character 4)
The fourth character specifies the body region on which the osteopathic treatment is performed.

### Approach (Character 5)
The approach for osteopathic treatment is always *External*.

### Method (Character 6)
The sixth character specifies the method by which the treatment is accomplished.

### Qualifier (Character 7)
The seventh character is not specified in the Osteopathic section and always has the value *None*.

# Other Procedures Section (8)

## Character Meanings

The seven characters in the Other Procedures section have the following meaning:

| Character | Meaning |
|---|---|
| 1 | Section |
| 2 | Body System |
| 3 | Root Operation |
| 4 | Body Region |
| 5 | Approach |
| 6 | Method |
| 7 | Qualifier |

The Other Procedures section includes acupuncture, suture removal, and in vitro fertilization.

## Section (Character 1)

Other Procedure section codes have a first character value of *8*.

## Body System (Character 2)

The second character values for body systems are *Physiological Systems and Anatomical Regions* and *Indwelling Device.*

## Root Operation (Character 3)

The Other Procedures section has only one root operation, defined as follows:

- *Other Procedures*: Methodologies that attempt to remediate or cure a disorder or disease.

## Body Region (Character 4)

The fourth character contains specified body-region values, and also the body-region value *None.*

## Approach (Character 5)

The fifth character specifies approaches as defined in the Medical and Surgical section.

## Method (Character 6)

The sixth character specifies the method (e.g., *Acupuncture, Therapeutic Massage*).

## Qualifier (Character 7)

The seventh character is a qualifier and contains specific values as needed.

# Chiropractic Section (9)

## Character Meanings

The seven characters in the Chiropractic section have the following meaning:

| Character | Meaning |
|---|---|
| 1 | Section |
| 2 | Body System |
| 3 | Root Operation |
| 4 | Body Region |
| 5 | Approach |
| 6 | Method |
| 7 | Qualifier |

## Section (Character 1)

Chiropractic section procedure codes have a first character value of *9*.

## Body System (Character 2)

The second character value for body system is *Anatomical Regions.*

## Root Operation (Character 3)

There is only one root operation in the *Chiropractic* section.

- *Manipulation:* Manual procedure that involves a directed thrust to move a joint past the physiological range of motion, without exceeding the anatomical limit.

## Body Region (Character 4)

The fourth character specifies the body region on which the chiropractic manipulation is performed.

## Approach (Character 5)

The approach for chiropractic manipulation is always *External.*

## Method (Character 6)

The sixth character is the method by which the manipulation is accomplished.

## Qualifier (Character 7)

The seventh character is not specified in the Chiropractic section and always has the value *None.*

# Imaging Section (B)

## Character Meanings

The seven characters in Imaging procedures have the following meaning:

| Character | Meaning |
|---|---|
| 1 | Section |
| 2 | Body System |
| 3 | Root Type |
| 4 | Body Part |
| 5 | Contrast |
| 6 | Qualifier |
| 7 | Qualifier |

Imaging procedures include plain radiography, fluoroscopy, CT, MRI, and ultrasound. Nuclear medicine procedures, including PET, uptakes, and scans, are in the nuclear medicine section. Therapeutic radiation procedure codes are in a separate radiation therapy section.

### Section (Character 1)

Imaging procedure codes have a first character value of *B*.

### Body System (Character 2)

In the Imaging section, the second character defines the body system, such as *Heart* or *Gastrointestinal System*.

### Root Type (Character 3)

The third character defines the type of imaging procedure (e.g., MRI, ultrasound). The following list includes all types in the *Imaging* section with a definition of each type:

- *Computerized Tomography (CT Scan)*: Computer reformatted digital display of multiplanar images developed from the capture of multiple exposures of external ionizing radiation
- *Fluoroscopy*: Single plane or bi-plane real time display of an image developed from the capture of external ionizing radiation on a fluorescent screen. The image may also be stored by either digital or analog means
- *Magnetic Resonance Imaging (MRI)*: Computer reformatted digital display of multiplanar images developed from the capture of radiofrequency signals emitted by nuclei in a body site excited within a magnetic field
- *Plain Radiography*: Planar display of an image developed from the capture of external ionizing radiation on photographic or photoconductive plate
- *Ultrasonography*: Real time display of images of anatomy or flow information developed from the capture of reflected and attenuated high frequency sound waves

### Body Part (Character 4)

The fourth character defines the body part with different values for each body system (character 2) value.

### Contrast (Character 5)

The fifth character specifies whether the contrast material used in the imaging procedure is *High Osmolar, Low Osmolar,* or *Other Contrast* when applicable.

### Qualifier (Character 6)

The sixth character qualifier provides further detail regarding the nature of the substance or technologies used, such as *Unenhanced and Enhanced (contrast), Laser, or Intravascular Optical Coherence.*

### Qualifier (Character 7)

The seventh character is a qualifier that may be used to specify certain procedural circumstances, the method by which the procedure was performed, or technologies utilized, such as *Intraoperative, Intravascular, or Transesophageal.*

## Nuclear Medicine Section (C)

### Character Meanings

The seven characters in the Nuclear Medicine section have the following meaning:

| Character | Meaning |
|---|---|
| 1 | Section |
| 2 | Body System |
| 3 | Root Type |
| 4 | Body Part |
| 5 | Radionuclide |
| 6 | Qualifier |
| 7 | Qualifier |

Nuclear Medicine is the introduction of radioactive material into the body to create an image, to diagnose and treat pathologic conditions, or to assess metabolic functions. The Nuclear Medicine section does not include the introduction of encapsulated radioactive material for the treatment of cancer. These procedures are included in the Radiation Therapy section.

### Section (Character 1)

Nuclear Medicine procedure codes have a first character value of *C*.

### Body System (Character 2)

The second character specifies the body system on which the nuclear medicine procedure is performed.

### Root Type (Character 3)

The third character indicates the type of nuclear medicine procedure (e.g., planar imaging or nonimaging uptake). The following list includes the types of nuclear medicine procedures with a definition of each type.

- *Nonimaging Nuclear Medicine Assay:* Introduction of radioactive materials into the body for the study of body fluids and blood elements, by the detection of radioactive emissions
- *Nonimaging Nuclear Medicine Probe:* Introduction of radioactive materials into the body for the study of distribution and fate of certain substances by the detection of radioactive emissions; or alternatively, measurement of absorption of radioactive emissions from an external source
- *Nonimaging Nuclear Medicine Uptake:* Introduction of radioactive materials into the body for measurements of organ function, from the detection of radioactive emissions
- *Planar Nuclear Medicine Imaging*: Introduction of radioactive materials into the body for single-plane display of images developed from the capture of radioactive emissions
- *Positron Emission Tomography (PET) Imaging:* Introduction of radioactive materials into the body for three dimensional display of images developed from the simultaneous capture, 180 degrees apart, of radioactive emissions
- *Systemic Nuclear Medicine Therapy:* Introduction of unsealed radioactive materials into the body for treatment
- *Tomographic (Tomo) Nuclear Medicine Imaging*: Introduction of radioactive materials into the body for three dimensional display of images developed from the capture of radioactive emissions

### Body Part (Character 4)

The fourth character indicates the body part or body region studied; with regional (e.g., *lower extremity veins*) and combination (e.g., *liver and spleen*) body parts commonly used.

### Radionuclide (Character 5)

The fifth character specifies the radionuclide, the radiation source. The option *Other Radionuclide* is provided in the nuclear medicine section for newly approved radionuclides until they can be added to the coding system. If more than one radiopharmaceutical is given to perform the procedure, then more than one code is used.

### Qualifier (Character 6 and 7)

The sixth and seventh characters are qualifiers but are not specified in the *Nuclear Medicine* section; the value is always *None*.

## Radiation Therapy Section (D)

### Character Meanings

The seven characters in the Radiation Therapy section have the following meaning:

| Character | Meaning |
|---|---|
| 1 | Section |
| 2 | Body System |
| 3 | Modality |
| 4 | Treatment Site |
| 5 | Modality Qualifier |
| 6 | Isotope |
| 7 | Qualifier |

### Section (Character 1)

Radiation therapy procedure codes have a first character value of *D*.

### Body System (Character 2)

The second character specifies the body system (e.g., central nervous system, musculoskeletal) irradiated.

### Root Type (Character 3)

The third character specifies the general modality used (e.g., beam radiation).

### Treatment Site (Character 4)

The fourth character specifies the body part that is the focus of the radiation therapy.

### Modality Qualifier (Character 5)

The fifth character further specifies the radiation modality used (e.g., photons, electrons).

### Isotope (Character 6)

The sixth character specifies the isotopes introduced into the body, if applicable.

### Qualifier (Character 7)

The seventh character may specify whether the procedure was performed intraoperatively.

## Physical Rehabilitation and Diagnostic Audiology Section (F)

### Character Meanings

The seven characters in the Physical Rehabilitation and Diagnostic Audiology section have the following meaning:

| Character | Meaning |
|---|---|
| 1 | Section |
| 2 | Section Qualifier |
| 3 | Root Type |
| 4 | Body System/Region |
| 5 | Type Qualifier |
| 6 | Equipment |
| 7 | Qualifier |

Physical rehabilitation procedures include physical therapy, occupational therapy, and speech-language pathology. Osteopathic procedures and chiropractic procedures are in separate sections.

### Section (Character 1)

Physical Rehabilitation and Diagnostic Audiology procedure codes have a first character value of *F*.

### Section Qualifier (Character 2)

The section qualifier *Rehabilitation* or *Diagnostic Audiology* is specified in the second character.

### Root Type (Character 3)

The third character specifies the root type. There are 14 different root type values, which can be classified into four basic types of rehabilitation and diagnostic audiology procedures, defined as follows:

*Assessment*: Includes a determination of the patient's diagnosis when appropriate, need for treatment, planning for treatment, periodic assessment, and documentation related to these activities

Assessments are further classified into more than 100 different tests or methods. The majority of these focus on the faculties of hearing and speech, but others focus on various aspects of body function, and on the patient's quality of life, such as muscle performance, neuromotor development, and reintegration skills.

- *Speech Assessment*: Measurement of speech and related functions
- *Motor and/or Nerve Function Assessment*: Measurement of motor, nerve, and related functions
- *Activities of Daily Living Assessment*: Measurement of functional level for activities of daily living
- *Hearing Assessment*: Measurement of hearing and related functions
- *Hearing Aid Assessment*: Measurement of the appropriateness and/or effectiveness of a hearing device
- *Vestibular Assessment*: Measurement of the vestibular system and related functions

*Caregiver Training*: Educating caregiver with the skills and knowledge used to interact with and assist the patient

*Caregiver Training* is divided into 18 different broad subjects taught to help a caregiver provide proper patient care.

- *Caregiver Training*: Training in activities to support patient's optimal level of function

*Fitting(s)*: Design, fabrication, modification, selection, and/or application of splint, orthosis, prosthesis, hearing aids, and/or other rehabilitation device

The fifth character used in *Device Fitting* procedures describes the device being fitted rather than the method used to fit the device. Definitions of devices, when provided, are located in the definitions portion of the ICD-10-PCS tables and index, under section F, character 5.

- *Device Fitting*: Fitting of a device designed to facilitate or support achievement of a higher level of function

*Treatment*: Use of specific activities or methods to develop, improve, and/or restore the performance of necessary functions, compensate for dysfunction and/or minimize debilitation

Treatment procedures include swallowing dysfunction exercises, bathing and showering techniques, wound management, gait training, and a host of activities typically associated with rehabilitation.

- *Speech Treatment*: Application of techniques to improve, augment, or compensate for speech and related functional impairment
- *Motor Treatment*: Exercise or activities to increase or facilitate motor function
- *Activities of Daily Living Treatment*: Exercise or activities to facilitate functional competence for activities of daily living
- *Hearing Treatment*: Application of techniques to improve, augment, or compensate for hearing and related functional impairment
- *Cochlear Implant Treatment*: Application of techniques to improve the communication abilities of individuals with cochlear implant
- *Vestibular Treatment*: Application of techniques to improve, augment, or compensate for vestibular and related functional impairment

The type of treatment includes training as well as activities that restore function.

### Body System/Region (Character 4)

The fourth character specifies the body region and/or system on which the procedure is performed.

### Type Qualifier (Character 5)

The fifth character is a type qualifier that further specifies the procedure performed. Examples include therapy to improve the range of motion and training for bathing techniques. Refer to appendix I for definitions of these types of procedures.

### Equipment (Character 6)

The sixth character specifies the equipment used. Specific equipment is not defined in the equipment value. Instead, broad categories of equipment are specified (e.g., aerobic endurance and conditioning, assistive/adaptive/supportive, etc.)

### Qualifier (Character 7)

The seventh character is not specified in the Physical Rehabilitation and Diagnostic Audiology section and always has the value *None*.

## Mental Health Section (G)

### Character Meanings

The seven characters in the Mental Health section have the following meaning:

| Character | Meaning |
|---|---|
| 1 | Section |
| 2 | Body System |
| 3 | Root Type |
| 4 | Qualifier |
| 5 | Qualifier |
| 6 | Qualifier |
| 7 | Qualifier |

### Section (Character 1)

Mental health procedure codes have a first character value of *G*.

### Body System (Character 2)

The second character is used to identify the body system elsewhere in ICD-10-PCS. In this section it always has the value *None*.

### Root Type (Character 3)

The third character specifies the procedure type, such as crisis intervention or counseling. There are 12 types of mental health procedures.

- Psychological Tests: The administration and interpretation of standardized psychological tests and measurement instruments for the assessment of psychological function
- Crisis Intervention: Treatment of a traumatized, acutely disturbed, or distressed individual for the purpose of short-term stabilization
- Medication Management: Monitoring and adjusting the use of medications for the treatment of a mental health disorder
- Individual Psychotherapy: Treatment of an individual with a mental health disorder by behavioral, cognitive, psychoanalytic, psychodynamic, or psychophysiological means to improve functioning or well-being
- Counseling: The application of psychological methods to treat an individual with normal developmental issues and psychological problems in order to increase function, improve well-being, alleviate distress, maladjustment, or resolve crises
- Family Psychotherapy: Treatment that includes one or more family members of an individual with a mental health disorder by behavioral, cognitive, psychoanalytic, psychodynamic, or psychophysiological means to improve functioning or well-being
- Electroconvulsive Therapy: The application of controlled electrical voltages to treat a mental health disorder
- Biofeedback: Provision of information from the monitoring and regulating of physiological processes in conjunction with cognitive-behavioral techniques to improve patient functioning or well-being

- Hypnosis: Induction of a state of heightened suggestibility by auditory, visual, and tactile techniques to elicit an emotional or behavioral response
- Narcosynthesis: Administration of intravenous barbiturates in order to release suppressed or repressed thoughts
- Group Psychotherapy: Treatment of two or more individuals with a mental health disorder by behavioral, cognitive, psychoanalytic, psychodynamic, or psychophysiological means to improve functioning or well-being
- Light Therapy: Application of specialized light treatments to improve functioning or well-being

### Qualifier (Character 4)

The fourth character is a qualifier to indicate that counseling was educational or vocational or to indicate type of test or method of therapy.

### Qualifier (Character 5, 6 and 7)

The fifth, sixth, and seventh characters are not specified and always have the value *None.*

## Substance Abuse Treatment Section (H)

### Character Meanings

The seven characters in the Substance Abuse Treatment section have the following meaning:

| Character | Meaning |
|---|---|
| 1 | Section |
| 2 | Body System |
| 3 | Root Type |
| 4 | Qualifier |
| 5 | Qualifier |
| 6 | Qualifier |
| 7 | Qualifier |

### Section (Character 1)

Substance Abuse Treatment codes have a first character value of *H.*

### Body System (Character 2)

The second character is used to identify the body system elsewhere in ICD-10-PCS. In this section, it always has the value *None.*

### Root Type (Character 3)

The third character specifies the procedure. There are seven root type values classified in this section, as listed below:

- Detoxification Services: Detoxification from alcohol and/or drugs
- Individual Counseling: The application of psychological methods to treat an individual with addictive behavior
- Group Counseling: The application of psychological methods to treat two or more individuals with addictive behavior
- Individual Psychotherapy: Treatment of an individual with addictive behavior by behavioral, cognitive, psychoanalytic, psychodynamic, or psychophysiological means
- Family Counseling: The application of psychological methods that includes one or more family members to treat an individual with addictive behavior
- Medication Management: Monitoring and adjusting the use of replacement medications for the treatment of addiction
- Pharmacotherapy: The use of replacement medications for the treatment of addiction

### Qualifier (Character 4)

The fourth character further specifies the procedure type. These qualifier values vary dependent upon the Root Type procedure (Character 3). Root type 2, *Detoxification Services* contains only the value Z, *None* and Root type 6, *Family Counseling* contains only the value 3, *Other Family Counseling*, whereas the remainder Root Type procedures include multiple possible values.

### Qualifier (Character 5, 6 and 7)

The fifth through seventh characters are designated as qualifiers but are never specified, so they always have the value *None*.

## New Technology Section (X)

### General Information

Section X New Technology is a section added to ICD-10-PCS beginning October 1, 2015. The new section provides a place for codes that uniquely identify procedures requested via the New Technology Application Process or that capture other new technologies not currently classified in ICD-10-PCS.

Section X does not introduce any new coding concepts or unusual guidelines for correct coding. In fact, Section X codes maintain continuity with the other sections in ICD-10-PCS by using the same root operation and body part values as their closest counterparts in other sections of ICD-10-PCS. For example, the codes for the infusion of ceftazidime-avibactam, use the same root operation (Introduction) and body part values (Central Vein and Peripheral Vein) in section X as the infusion codes in section 3 Administration, which are their closest counterparts in the other sections of ICD-10-PCS.

### Character Meanings

The seven characters in the new technology section have the following meaning:

| Character | Meaning |
|---|---|
| 1 | Section |
| 2 | Body System |
| 3 | Root Operation |
| 4 | Body Part |
| 5 | Approach |
| 6 | Device/Substance/Technology |
| 7 | Qualifier |

### Section (Character 1)

New technology procedure codes have a first character value of *X*.

### Body System (Character 2)

The second character values for body system combine the uses of body system, body region, and physiological system as specified in other sections in ICD-10-PCS.

## Root Operation (Character 3)

The third character utilizes the same root operation values as their counterparts in other sections of ICD-10-PCS.

## Body Part (Character 4)

The fourth character specifies the same body part values as their closest counterparts in other sections of ICD-10-PCS.

## Approach (Character 5)

The fifth character specifies approaches as defined in the Medical and Surgical section.

## Device/Substance/Technology (Character 6)

The sixth character specifies the key feature of the new technology procedure. It may be specified as a new device, a new substance, or other new technology. Examples of sixth character values are blinatumomab antineoplastic immunotherapy, orbital atherectomy technology, and intraoperative knee replacement sensor.

## Qualifier (Character 7)

The seventh character qualifier is used exclusively to specify the new technology group, a number or letter that changes each year that new technology codes are added to the system. For example, Section X codes added for the first year have the seventh character value 1, New Technology Group 1, and the next year that Section X codes are added have the seventh character value 2, New Technology Group 2, and so on. Changing the seventh character value to a unique letter or number every year that there are new codes in the new technology section allows the ICD-10-PCS to "recycle" the values in the third, fourth, and sixth characters as needed.

## New Technology Coding Instruction

Section X codes are standalone codes. They are not supplemental codes. Section X codes fully represent the specific procedure described in the code title, and do not require any additional codes from other sections of ICD-10-PCS. When section X contains a code title which describes a specific new technology procedure, only that X code is reported for the procedure. There is no need to report a broader, non-specific code in another section of ICD-10-PCS.

For example, code XWØ4321 Introduction of Ceftazidime-Avibactam Anti-infective into Central Vein, Percutaneous Approach, New Technology Group 1, would be reported to indicate that Ceftazidime-Avibactam Anti-infective was administered via central vein. A separate code from table 3EØ in the Administration section of ICD-10-PCS would not be reported in addition to this code. The X section code fully identifies the administration of the ceftazidime-avibactam antibiotic, and no additional code is needed.

The New Technology section codes are easily found by looking in the ICD-10-PCS Index or the Tables. In the Index, the name of the new technology device, substance or technology for a section X code is included as a main term. In addition, all codes in section X are listed under the main term New Technology. The new technology code index entry for ceftazidime-avibactam is shown below.

**Ceftazidime-Avibactam Anti-infective** XWØ

**New Technology**
Ceftazidime-Avibactam Anti-infective XWØ

# Appendixes

The resources described below have been included as appendixes for *ICD-10-PCS The Complete Official Code Set*. These resources further instruct the coder on the appropriate application of the ICD-10-PCS code set.

## Appendix A: Components of the Medical and Surgical Approach Definitions

This resource further defines the approach characters used in the Medical and Surgical (Ø) section. Complementing the detailed definition of the approach, additional information includes whether or not instrumentation is a part of the approach, the typical access location, the method used to initiate the approach, and related procedural examples, all of which will help the user determine the appropriate approach value.

## Appendix B: Root Operation Definitions

This resource is a compilation of all root operations found in the Medical and Surgical-related sections (Ø-9) of this PCS manual. It provides a definition and in some cases a more detailed explanation of the root operation, to better reflect the purpose or objective. Examples of related procedure(s) may also be provided.

## Appendix C: Comparison of Medical and Surgical Root Operations

The Medical and Surgical root operations are divided into groups that share similar attributes. These groups, and the root operations in each group, are listed in this resource along with information identifying the target of the root operation, the action used to perform the root operation, any clarification or further explanation on the objective of the root operation, and procedure examples.

## Appendix D: Body Part Key

When an anatomical term or description is provided in the documentation but does not have a specific body part character within a table, the user can reference this resource to search for the anatomical description or site noted in the documentation to determine if there is a specific PCS body part character (character 4) to which the anatomical description or site could be coded.

## Appendix E: Body Part Definitions

This resource is the reverse look-up of the Body Part Key. Each table in the Medical and Surgical section (Ø) of the PCS manual contains anatomical terms linked to a body part character or value, for example, in Table ØBB the Body Part (character 4) of 1 is Trachea. The body part Trachea may have anatomical structures or descriptions that may be used in procedure documentation instead of the term trachea. The Body Part Definitions list other anatomical structures or synonyms that are included in specific ICD-10-PCS body part values. According to the body part definitions, in the example above, cricoid cartilage is included in the Trachea (character 1) body part.

## Appendix F: Device Key and Aggregation Table

The Device Key relates specific devices used in the medical profession, such as stents or bovine pericardial valves, with the appropriate device character (character 6).

The Aggregation Table crosswalks specific device character value definitions for specific root operations in a specific body system to the more general device character value to be used when the root operation covers a wide range of body parts and the device character represents an entire family of devices.

## Appendix G: Device Definitions

This resource is a reverse look-up to the Device Key. The user may reference this resource to see all the specific devices that may be grouped to a particular device character (character 6).

## Appendix H: Substance Key/Substance Definitions

The Substance Key lists substances by trade name or synonym and relates them to a PCS character in the Administration (3) or New Technology (X) section in the sixth character Substance or seventh character Qualifier column.

The Substance Definitions table is the reverse look-up of the substance key, relating all substance categories, the sixth- or seventh character values, to all trade name or synonyms that may be classified to that particular character.

## Appendix I: Sections B-H Character Definitions

In each ancillary section (B-H) the characters in a particular column may have different meanings depending on which ancillary section the user is working from. This resource provides the values for the characters in that particular ancillary section as well as a definition of the character value.

## Appendix J: Hospital Acquired Conditions

This comprehensive table displays codes identifying conditions that are considered reasonably preventable when occurring during the hospital admission and may prevent the case from grouping to a higher-paying MS-DRG. Many of these HACs are conditional and are based on reporting of a specific ICD-10-CM diagnosis code in combination with certain ICD-10-PCS procedure codes, all of which are noted in this table.

## Appendix K: Coding Exercises with Answers

This resource provides the coding exercises with answers, and in some cases a brief explanation as to the reason that particular code was used.

## Appendix L: Procedure Combination Tables

The procedure combination tables provided in this resource illustrate certain procedure combinations that must occur in order to assign a specific MS-DRG.

## Sources

All material contained in this manual is derived from the ICD-10-PCS Coding System files, revised and distributed by the Centers for Medicare and Medicaid Services, FY 2018.

# ICD-10-PCS Index and Tabular Format

The *ICD-10-PCS: The Complete Official Code Set* is based on the official version of the International Classification of Diseases, 10th Revision, Procedure Classification System, issued by the U.S. Department of Health and Human Services, Centers for Medicare and Medicaid Services. This book is consistent with the content of the government's version of ICD-10-PCS and follows their official format.

## Index

The user can use the Alphabetic Index to locate the appropriate table containing all the information necessary to construct a procedure code. The PCS tables should always be consulted to find the most appropriate valid code. Users may choose a valid code directly from the tables—he or she need not consult the index before proceeding to the tables to complete the code.

### Main Terms

The Alphabetic Index reflects the structure of the tables. Therefore, the index is organized as an alphabetic listing. The index:

- Is based on the value of the third character
- Contains common procedure terms
- Lists anatomic sites
- Uses device terms

***The main terms in the Alphabetic Index are root operations, root procedure types, or common procedure names. In addition, anatomic sites from the Body Part Key and device terms from the Device Key have been added for ease of use.***

***Examples:***

*Resection* (root operation)

*Fluoroscopy* (root type)

*Prostatectomy* (common procedure name)

*Brachial artery* (body part)

*Bard® Dulex™ mesh* (device)

***The index provides at least the first three or four values of the code, and some entries may provide complete valid codes. However, the user should always consult the appropriate table to verify that the most appropriate valid code has been selected.***

### Root Operation and Procedure Type Main Terms

For the *Medical and Surgical* and related sections, the root operation values are used as main terms in the index. The subterms under the root operation main terms are body parts. For the Ancillary section of the tables, the main terms in the index are the general type of procedure performed.

***Examples:***

**Destruction**
Acetabulum
Left ØQ55
Right ØQ54
Adenoids ØC5Q
Ampulla of Vater ØF5C
**Biofeedback** GZC9ZZZ
**Planar Nuclear Medicine Imaging**

### *See* Reference

The second type of term in the index uses common procedure names, such as "appendectomy" or "fundoplication." These common terms are listed as main terms with a "see" reference noting the PCS root operations that are possible valid code tables based on the objective of the procedure.

***Examples:***

**Tendonectomy**
*see* Excision, Tendons ØLB
*see* Resection, Tendons ØLT

### *Use* Reference

The index also lists anatomic sites from the Body Part Key and device terms from the Device Key. These terms are listed with a "use" reference. The purpose of these references is to act as an additional reference to the terms located in the Appendix Keys. The term provided is the Body Part value or Device value to be selected when constructing a procedure code using the code tables. This type of index reference is not intended to direct the user to another term in the index, but to provide guidance regarding character value selection. Therefore, "use" references generally do not refer to specific valid code tables.

***Examples:***

**Epitrochlear lymph node**
*use* Lymphatic, Right Upper Extremity
*use* Lymphatic, Left Upper Extremity
**CoAxia NeuroFlo catheter**
*use* Intraluminal Device
**SynCardia Total Artificial Heart**
*use* Synthetic Substitute

## Code Tables

ICD-10-PCS contains 17 sections of Code Tables organized by general type of procedure. The first three characters of a procedure code define each table. The tables consist of columns providing the possible last four characters of codes and rows providing valid values for each character. Within a PCS table, valid codes include all combinations of choices in characters 4 through 7 contained in the same row of the table. All seven characters must be specified to form a valid code.

There are three main sections of tables:

- *Medical and Surgical* section:
  - *Medical and Surgical* (Ø)
- *Medical and Surgical*-related sections:
  - *Obstetrics* (1)
  - *Placement* (2)
  - *Administration* (3)
  - *Measurement and Monitoring* (4)
  - *Extracorporeal or Systemic Assistance and Performance* (5)
  - *Extracorporeal or Systemic Therapies* (6)
  - *Osteopathic* (7)
  - *Other Procedures* (8)
  - *Chiropractic* (9)

- Ancillary sections:
  - *Imaging* (B)
  - *Nuclear Medicine* (C)
  - *Radiation Therapy* (D)
  - *Physical Rehabilitation and Diagnostic Audiology* (F)
  - *Mental Health* (G)
  - *Substance Abuse Treatment* (H)
- New Technology section:
  - *New Technology* (X)

The first three character values define each table. The root operation or root type designated for each table is accompanied by its official definition.

***Example:***
Table ØØF provides codes for procedures on the central nervous system that involve breaking up of solid matter into pieces:

| | |
|---|---|
| Character 1, Section | Ø: Medical and Surgical |
| Character 2, Body System | Ø: Central Nervous System and Cranial Nerves |
| Character 3, Root Operation | F: Fragmentation: Breaking solid matter in a body part into pieces |

Tables are arranged numerically, then alphabetically.

When reviewing tables, the user should keep in mind that:

- There are multiple tables for the first three characters.
- Some tables may cover multiple pages in the code book—to ensure maximum clarity about character choices, valid entries do not split rows between pages. For instance, the entire table of valid characters completing a code beginning with 4A1 is split between two pages, but the split is between, not within, rows. This means that all the valid sixth and seventh characters for, say, body system *Arterial* (3) and approach *External* (X) are contained on one page.
- Individual entries may be listed in several horizontal "selection" lines.

When a table is continued onto another page, a note to this effect has been added in red.

**Body Part Definitions:**
An exclusive feature in the tables is the incorporation of the body part definitions provided in appendix E into the Medical and Surgical section (Ø) tables under their appropriate body part characters in the fourth column (character 4). This provides the user a direct reference to all anatomical descriptions, terms, and sites that could be coded to that particular body part value.

Paired body parts typically have values for the right and left side and in some cases a value for bilateral. These paired body parts often have the same list of inclusive body part definitions. When there are paired body parts with the same body part definitions, the first listed body part (usually the right side) contains the list of body part definitions while the second listed body part (usually the left side) contains a ***See*** instruction. This ***See*** instruction references the body part value that contains the body part definitions. In the table below, body part value P – Upper Eyelid, Left is followed by a ***See*** instruction that states ***See*** *N Upper Eyelid, Right*. All body part descriptions under value N also apply to body part value P.

***Example:***

**Ø Medical and Surgical**
**8 Eye**
**M Reattachment** Definition: Putting back in or on all or a portion of a separated body part to its normal location or other suitable location
Explanation: Vascular circulation and nervous pathways may or may not be reestablished

| Body Part Character 4 | Approach Character 5 | Device Character 6 | Qualifier Character 7 |
|---|---|---|---|
| **N Upper Eyelid, Right**<br>Lateral canthus<br>Levator palpebrae superioris muscle<br>Orbicularis oculi muscle<br>Superior tarsal plate<br>**P Upper Eyelid, Left**<br>*See N Upper Eyelid, Right*<br>**Q Lower Eyelid, Right**<br>Inferior tarsal plate<br>Medial canthus<br>**R Lower Eyelid, Left**<br>*See Q Lower Eyelid, Right* | **X External** | **Z No Device** | **Z No Qualifier** |

# ICD-10-PCS Additional Features

## Use of Official Sources

The *ICD-10-PCS: The Complete Official Code Set* contains the official U.S. Department of Health and Human Services, Tenth Revision, Procedure Classification System, effective for the current year.

Color-coding, symbol, and other annotations in this manual that identify coding and reimbursement issues are derived from various official federal government sources, including Medicare Code Editor (MCE), version 34, ICD-10 MS-DRG Definitions Manual Files, version 34, and the *Federal Register*, volume 82, number 81, April 28, 2017 ("Hospital Inpatient Prospective Payment Systems for Acute Care Hospitals and the Long Term Care Hospital Prospective Payment System and Proposed Policy Changes and Fiscal Year 2018 Rates; Proposed Rule"). For the most current files related to IPPS, please refer to the following:

https://www.cms.gov/Medicare/Medicare-Fee-for-Service-Payment/AcuteInpatientPPS/IPPS-Regulations-and-Notices.html.

## Table Notations

Many tables in ICD-10-PCS contain color or symbol annotations that may aid in code selection, provide clinical or coding information, or alert the coder to reimbursement issues affected by the PCS code assignment. These annotations are most often displayed on or next to a character 4 value. Some character 4 values may have more than one annotation.

Refer to the color/symbol legend at the bottom of each page in the tables section for an abridged description of each color and symbol.

### Annotation Box

An annotation box has been appended to all tables that contain color-coding or symbol annotations. The color bar or symbol attached to a character 4 value is provided in the box, as well as a list of the valid PCS code(s) to which that edit applies. The box may also list conditional criteria that must be met to satisfy the edit.

For example, see Table ØØF. Four character 4 body part values have a gray color bar. In the annotation box below the table, the gray color bar is defined as "Non-OR," or a nonoperating room procedure edit. Following the Non-OR annotation are the PCS codes that are considered nonoperating room procedures from that row of Table ØØF.

### Bracketed Code Notation

The use of bracketed codes is an efficient convention to provide all valid character value alternatives for a specific set of circumstances. The character values in the brackets correspond to the valid values for the character in the position the bracket appears.

***Examples:***

In the annotation box for Table ØØF the Noncovered Procedure edit (NC) applies to codes represented in the bracketed code ØØF[3,4,5,6]XZZ.

ØØF[3,4,5,6]XZZ Fragmentation in (Central Nervous System and Cranial Nerves), External Approach

The valid fourth character values (Body Part) that may be selected for this specific circumstance are as follows:

3 Epidural Space, Intracranial
4 Subdural Space, Intracranial
5 Subarachnoid Space, Intracranial
6 Cerebral Ventricle

The fragmentation of matter in the spinal canal, Body Part value U, is not included in the noncovered procedure code edits.

## Color-Coding/Symbols

### New and Revised Text

To highlight changes to the PCS tables for the current year, the new and revised text is provided in green font.

### Medicare Code Edits

Medicare administrative contractors (MACs) and many payers use Medicare code edits to check the coding accuracy on claims. The coding edits in this manual are only those directly related to ICD-10-PCS codes and are used for acute care hospital inpatient admissions.

The PCS related Medicare code edits are listed below:

- Invalid procedure code
- *Sex conflict
- *Noncovered procedure
- *Limited coverage procedure

***Starred edits above that are related to PCS issues are identified in this manual by symbols as described below.***

#### *Sex Edit Symbols*

The sex edit symbols below address MCE and are used to detect inconsistencies between the patient's sex and the procedure. The symbols below most often appear to the right of a character 4 value but may also be found to the right of a character 7 value:

Male procedure only ♂
Female procedure only ♀

#### *Noncovered Procedure* NC

Medicare does not cover all procedures. However, some noncovered procedures, due to the presence of certain diagnoses, are reimbursed.

#### *Limited Coverage* LC

For certain procedures whose medical complexity and serious nature incur extraordinary associated costs, Medicare limits coverage to a portion of the cost. The limited coverage edit indicates the type of limited coverage.

### ICD-10 MS-DRG Definitions Manual Edits

An MS-DRG is assigned based on specific patient attributes, such as principal diagnosis, secondary diagnoses, procedures, and discharge status. The attributes (edits) provided in this manual are only those directly related to ICD-10-PCS codes and are used for acute care hospital inpatient admissions.

### *Non-Operating Room Procedures Not Affecting MS-DRG Assignment* Non-OR

In the Medical and Surgical section (ØØ1-ØYW) and the Obstetric section (1Ø2-1ØY) tables **only,** ICD-10-PCS procedures codes that DO NOT affect MS-DRG assignment are identified by a **gray color bar** over the character 4 value and are considered non-operating room (non-OR) procedures.

NOTE: The majority of the ICD-10-PCS codes in the Medical and Surgical-Related, Ancillary and New Technology section tables are non-operating room procedures that do not typically affect MS-DRG assignment. Only the Valid Operating Room and DRG Non-Operating Room procedures are highlighted in these sections, *see* Non-Operating Room Procedures Affecting MS-DRG Assignment and Valid OR Procedure description below.

### *Non-Operating Room Procedures Affecting MS-DRG Assignment* DRG Non-OR

Some ICD-10-PCS procedure codes, although considered non-operating room procedures, may still affect MS-DRG assignment. In all sections of the ICD-10-PCS book, these procedures are identified by a **purple color bar** over the character 4 value.

### *Valid OR Procedure* Valid OR

In the Medical and Surgical-Related (2WØ-9WB), Ancillary (BØØ-HZ9) and New Technology (X2A-XYØ) section tables **only**, any codes that are considered a valid operating room procedure are identified with a **blue color bar** over the character 4 value and will affect MS-DRG assignment. All codes without a color bar (blue or purple) are considered non-operating room procedures.

### *Hospital-Acquired Condition Related Procedures* HAC

Procedures associated with hospital-acquired conditions (HAC) are identified with the **yellow color bar** over the body part value.

### *Combination Only* Combination Only

Some ICD-10-PCS procedure codes are considered "noncovered procedures" except when reported in combination with certain other procedure codes. Such codes are designated by a **red color bar** over the character 4 value.

### *Combination Member* ⊞

A combination member is an ICD-10-PCS procedure code that can influence MS-DRG assignment either on its own or in combination with other specific ICD-10-PCS procedure codes. Combination member codes are designated by a plus sign (⊞) to the right of the body part value.

### *See Appendix L for Procedure Combinations*

Under certain circumstances, more than one procedure code is needed in order to group to a specific MS-DRG. When codes within a table have been identified as a Combination Only (**red color bar**) or Combination Member (⊞) code, there is also a footnote instructing the coder to *see Appendix L*. Appendix L contains tables that identify the other procedure codes needed in the combination and the title and number of the MS-DRG to which the combination will group.

## Other Table Notations

### AHA Coding Clinic:

Official citations from AHA's *Coding Clinic for ICD-10-CM/PCS* have been provided at the beginning of each section, when applicable. Each specific citation is listed below a header identifying the table to which that particular *Coding Clinic* citation applies. The citations appear in purple type with the year, quarter, and page of the reference as well as the title of the question as it appears in that *Coding Clinic's* table of contents. *Coding Clinic* citations included in this edition have been updated through second quarter 2017.

## Index Notations

- Subterms under main terms may continue to the next column or page. This warning statement is a reminder to always check for additional subterms and information that may continue onto the next page or column before making a final selection.

# ICD-10-PCS Official Guidelines for Coding and Reporting 2018

Narrative changes appear in **bold** text.

The Centers for Medicare and Medicaid Services (CMS) and the National Center for Health Statistics (NCHS), two departments within the U.S. Federal Government's Department of Health and Human Services (DHHS) provide the following guidelines for coding and reporting using the International Classification of Diseases, 10th Revision, Procedure Coding System (ICD-10-PCS). These guidelines should be used as a companion document to the official version of the ICD-10-PCS as published on the CMS website. The ICD-10-PCS is a procedure classification published by the United States for classifying procedures performed in hospital inpatient health care settings.

These guidelines have been approved by the four organizations that make up the Cooperating Parties for the ICD-10-PCS: the American Hospital Association (AHA), the American Health Information Management Association (AHIMA), CMS, and NCHS.

These guidelines are a set of rules that have been developed to accompany and complement the official conventions and instructions provided within the ICD-10-PCS itself. The instructions and conventions of the classification take precedence over guidelines. These guidelines are based on the coding and sequencing instructions in the Tables, Index and Definitions of ICD-10-PCS, but provide additional instruction. Adherence to these guidelines when assigning ICD-10-PCS procedure codes is required under the Health Insurance Portability and Accountability Act (HIPAA). The procedure codes have been adopted under HIPAA for hospital inpatient healthcare settings. A joint effort between the healthcare provider and the coder is essential to achieve complete and accurate documentation, code assignment, and reporting of diagnoses and procedures. These guidelines have been developed to assist both the healthcare provider and the coder in identifying those procedures that are to be reported. The importance of consistent, complete documentation in the medical record cannot be overemphasized. Without such documentation accurate coding cannot be achieved.

## Conventions

**A1.** ICD-10-PCS codes are composed of seven characters. Each character is an axis of classification that specifies information about the procedure performed. Within a defined code range, a character specifies the same type of information in that axis of classification.

*Example:* The fifth axis of classification specifies the approach in sections 0 through 4 and 7 through 9 of the system.

**A2.** One of 34 possible values can be assigned to each axis of classification in the seven-character code: they are the numbers 0 through 9 and the alphabet (except I and O because they are easily confused with the numbers 1 and 0). The number of unique values used in an axis of classification differs as needed.

*Example:* Where the fifth axis of classification specifies the approach, seven different approach values are currently used to specify the approach.

**A3.** The valid values for an axis of classification can be added to as needed.

*Example:* If a significantly distinct type of device is used in a new procedure, a new device value can be added to the system.

**A4.** As with words in their context, the meaning of any single value is a combination of its axis of classification and any preceding values on which it may be dependent.

*Example:* The meaning of a body part value in the Medical and Surgical section is always dependent on the body system value. The body part value 0 in the Central Nervous body system specifies Brain and the body part value 0 in the Peripheral Nervous body system specifies Cervical Plexus.

**A5.** As the system is expanded to become increasingly detailed, over time more values will depend on preceding values for their meaning.

*Example:* In the Lower Joints body system, the device value 3 in the root operation Insertion specifies Infusion Device and the device value 3 in the root operation Replacement specifies Ceramic Synthetic Substitute.

**A6.** The purpose of the alphabetic index is to locate the appropriate table that contains all information necessary to construct a procedure code. The PCS Tables should always be consulted to find the most appropriate valid code.

**A7.** It is not required to consult the index first before proceeding to the tables to complete the code. A valid code may be chosen directly from the tables.

**A8.** All seven characters must be specified to be a valid code. If the documentation is incomplete for coding purposes, the physician should be queried for the necessary information.

**A9.** Within a PCS table, valid codes include all combinations of choices in characters 4 through 7 contained in the same row of the table. In the example below, ØJHT3VZ is a valid code, and ØJHW3VZ is *not* a valid code.

**Section:** **Ø** **Medical and Surgical**
**Body System:** **J** **Subcutaneous Tissue and Fascia**
**Operation:** **H** **Insertion** Putting in a nonbiological appliance that monitors, assists, performs, or prevents a physiological function but does not physically take the place of a body part

| Body Part | Approach | Device | Qualifier |
|---|---|---|---|
| **S** Subcutaneous Tissue and Fascia, Head and Neck<br>**V** Subcutaneous Tissue and Fascia, Upper Extremity<br>**W** Subcutaneous Tissue and Fascia, Lower Extremity | **Ø** Open<br>**3** Percutaneous | **1** Radioactive Element<br>**3** Infusion Device | **Z** No Qualifier |
| **T** Subcutaneous Tissue and Fascia, Trunk | **Ø** Open<br>**3** Percutaneous | **1** Radioactive Element<br>**3** Infusion Device<br>**V** Infusion Pump | **Z** No Qualifier |

**A10.** "And," when used in a code description, means "and/or."

*Example:* Lower Arm and Wrist Muscle means lower arm and/or wrist muscle.

**A11.** Many of the terms used to construct PCS codes are defined within the system. It is the coder's responsibility to determine what the documentation in the medical record equates to in the PCS definitions. The physician is not expected to use the terms used in PCS code descriptions, nor is the coder required to query the physician when the correlation between the documentation and the defined PCS terms is clear.

*Example:* When the physician documents "partial resection" the coder can independently correlate "partial resection" to the root operation Excision without querying the physician for clarification.

# Medical and Surgical Section Guidelines (section Ø)

## B2. Body System

*General guidelines*

**B2.1a.** The procedure codes in the general anatomical regions body systems can be used when the procedure is performed on an anatomical region rather than a specific body part (e.g., root operations Control and Detachment, Drainage of a body cavity) or on the rare occasion when no information is available to support assignment of a code to a specific body part.

*Examples:* Control of postoperative hemorrhage is coded to the root operation Control found in the general anatomical regions body systems.

Chest tube drainage of the pleural cavity is coded to the root operation Drainage found in the general anatomical regions body systems. Suture repair of the abdominal wall is coded to the root operation Repair in the general anatomical regions body system.

**B2.1b.** Where the general body part values "upper" and "lower" are provided as an option in the Upper Arteries, Lower Arteries, Upper Veins, Lower Veins, Muscles and Tendons body systems, "upper" or "lower "specifies body parts located above or below the diaphragm respectively.

*Example:* Vein body parts above the diaphragm are found in the Upper Veins body system; vein body parts below the diaphragm are found in the Lower Veins body system.

## B3. Root Operation

*General guidelines*

**B3.1a.** In order to determine the appropriate root operation, the full definition of the root operation as contained in the PCS Tables must be applied.

**B3.1b.** Components of a procedure specified in the root operation definition and explanation are not coded separately. Procedural steps necessary to reach the operative site and close the operative site, including anastomosis of a tubular body part, are also not coded separately.

*Examples:* Resection of a joint as part of a joint replacement procedure is included in the root operation definition of Replacement and is not coded separately.

Laparotomy performed to reach the site of an open liver biopsy is not coded separately. In a resection of sigmoid colon with anastomosis of descending colon to rectum, the anastomosis is not coded separately.

*Multiple procedures*

**B3.2.** During the same operative episode, multiple procedures are coded if:

a. The same root operation is performed on different body parts as defined by distinct values of the body part character.

   *Examples:* Diagnostic excision of liver and pancreas are coded separately.

   Excision of lesion in the ascending colon and excision of lesion in the transverse colon are coded separately.

b. The same root operation is repeated in multiple body parts, and those body parts are separate and distinct body parts classified to a single ICD-10-PCS body part value.

   *Examples:* Excision of the sartorius muscle and excision of the gracilis muscle are both included in the upper leg muscle body part value, and multiple procedures are coded.

   Extraction of multiple toenails are coded separately.

c. Multiple root operations with distinct objectives are performed on the same body part.

   *Example:* Destruction of sigmoid lesion and bypass of sigmoid colon are coded separately.

d. The intended root operation is attempted using one approach, but is converted to a different approach.

   *Example:* Laparoscopic cholecystectomy converted to an open cholecystectomy is coded as percutaneous endoscopic Inspection and open Resection.

*Discontinued **or incomplete** procedures*

**B3.3.** If the intended procedure is discontinued **or otherwise not completed**, code the procedure to the root operation performed. If a procedure is discontinued before any other root operation is performed, code the root operation Inspection of the body part or anatomical region inspected.

*Example:* A planned aortic valve replacement procedure is discontinued after the initial thoracotomy and before any incision is made in the heart muscle, when the patient becomes hemodynamically unstable. This procedure is coded as an open Inspection of the mediastinum.

*Biopsy procedures*

**B3.4a.** Biopsy procedures are coded using the root operations Excision, Extraction, or Drainage and the qualifier Diagnostic.

*Examples*: Fine needle aspiration biopsy of fluid in the lung is coded to the root operation Drainage with the qualifier Diagnostic.

Biopsy of bone marrow is coded to the root operation Extraction with the qualifier Diagnostic.

Lymph node sampling for biopsy is coded to the root operation Excision with the qualifier Diagnostic.

### *Biopsy followed by more definitive treatment*

**B3.4b.** If a diagnostic Excision, Extraction, or Drainage procedure (biopsy) is followed by a more definitive procedure, such as Destruction, Excision or Resection at the same procedure site, both the biopsy and the more definitive treatment are coded.

*Example:* Biopsy of breast followed by partial mastectomy at the same procedure site, both the biopsy and the partial mastectomy procedure are coded.

### *Overlapping body layers*

**B3.5.** If the root operations Excision, Repair or Inspection are performed on overlapping layers of the musculoskeletal system, the body part specifying the deepest layer is coded.

*Example:* Excisional debridement that includes skin and subcutaneous tissue and muscle is coded to the muscle body part.

### *Bypass procedures*

**B3.6a.** Bypass procedures are coded by identifying the body part bypassed "from" and the body part bypassed "to." The fourth character body part specifies the body part bypassed from, and the qualifier specifies the body part bypassed to.

*Example:* Bypass from stomach to jejunum, stomach is the body part and jejunum is the qualifier.

B3.6b. Coronary artery bypass procedures are coded differently than other bypass procedures as described in the previous guideline. Rather than identifying the body part bypassed from, the body part identifies the number of coronary arteries bypassed to, and the qualifier specifies the vessel bypassed from.

*Example:* Aortocoronary artery bypass of the left anterior descending coronary artery and the obtuse marginal coronary artery is classified in the body part axis of classification as two coronary arteries, and the qualifier specifies the aorta as the body part bypassed from.

**B3.6c.** If multiple coronary arteries are bypassed, a separate procedure is coded for each coronary artery that uses a different device and/or qualifier.

*Example:* Aortocoronary artery bypass and internal mammary coronary artery bypass are coded separately.

### *Control vs. more definitive root operations*

**B3.7.** The root operation Control is defined as, "Stopping, or attempting to stop, postprocedural or other acute bleeding." If an attempt to stop postprocedural or other acute bleeding is initially unsuccessful, and to stop the bleeding requires performing **a more** definitive root operation, **such as** Bypass, Detachment, Excision, Extraction, Reposition, Replacement, or Resection, then **the more definitive** root operation is coded instead of Control.

*Example:* Resection of spleen to stop bleeding is coded to Resection instead of Control.

### *Excision vs. Resection*

**B3.8.** PCS contains specific body parts for anatomical subdivisions of a body part, such as lobes of the lungs or liver and regions of the intestine. Resection of the specific body part is coded whenever all of the body part is cut out or off, rather than coding Excision of a less specific body part.

*Example:* Left upper lung lobectomy is coded to Resection of Upper Lung Lobe, Left rather than Excision of Lung, Left.

### *Excision for graft*

**B3.9.** If an autograft is obtained from a different procedure site in order to complete the objective of the procedure, a separate procedure is coded.

*Example:* Coronary bypass with excision of saphenous vein graft, excision of saphenous vein is coded separately.

### *Fusion procedures of the spine*

**B3.10a.** The body part coded for a spinal vertebral joint(s) rendered immobile by a spinal fusion procedure is classified by the level of the spine (e.g. thoracic). There are distinct body part values for a single vertebral joint and for multiple vertebral joints at each spinal level.

*Example:* Body part values specify Lumbar Vertebral Joint, Lumbar Vertebral Joints, 2 or More and Lumbosacral Vertebral Joint.

**B3.10b.** If multiple vertebral joints are fused, a separate procedure is coded for each vertebral joint that uses a different device and/or qualifier.

*Example:* Fusion of lumbar vertebral joint, posterior approach, anterior column and fusion of lumbar vertebral joint, posterior approach, posterior column are coded separately.

**B3.10c.** Combinations of devices and materials are often used on a vertebral joint to render the joint immobile. When combinations of devices are used on the same vertebral joint, the device value coded for the procedure is as follows:

- If an interbody fusion device is used to render the joint immobile (alone or containing other material like bone graft), the procedure is coded with the device value Interbody Fusion Device
- If bone graft is the *only* device used to render the joint immobile, the procedure is coded with the device value Nonautologous Tissue Substitute or Autologous Tissue Substitute
- If a mixture of autologous and nonautologous bone graft (with or without biological or synthetic extenders or binders) is used to render the joint immobile, code the procedure with the device value Autologous Tissue Substitute

*Examples:* Fusion of a vertebral joint using a cage style interbody fusion device containing morsellized bone graft is coded to the device Interbody Fusion Device.

Fusion of a vertebral joint using a bone dowel interbody fusion device made of cadaver bone and packed with a mixture of local morsellized bone and demineralized bone matrix is coded to the device Interbody Fusion Device.

Fusion of a vertebral joint using both autologous bone graft and bone bank bone graft is coded to the device Autologous Tissue Substitute.

### *Inspection procedures*

**B3.11a.** Inspection of a body part(s) performed in order to achieve the objective of a procedure is not coded separately.

*Example:* Fiberoptic bronchoscopy performed for irrigation of bronchus, only the irrigation procedure is coded.

**B3.11b.** If multiple tubular body parts are inspected, the most distal body part (the body part furthest from the starting point of the inspection) is coded. If multiple non-tubular body parts in a region are inspected, the body part that specifies the entire area inspected is coded.

*Examples:* Cystoureteroscopy with inspection of bladder and ureters is coded to the ureter body part value.

Exploratory laparotomy with general inspection of abdominal contents is coded to the peritoneal cavity body part value.

**B3.11c.** When both an Inspection procedure and another procedure are performed on the same body part during the same episode, if the Inspection procedure is performed using a different approach than the other procedure, the Inspection procedure is coded separately.

*Example:* Endoscopic Inspection of the duodenum is coded separately when open Excision of the duodenum is performed during the same procedural episode.

### *Occlusion vs. Restriction for vessel embolization procedures*

**B3.12.** If the objective of an embolization procedure is to completely close a vessel, the root operation Occlusion is coded. If the objective of an embolization procedure is to narrow the lumen of a vessel, the root operation Restriction is coded.

*Examples:* Tumor embolization is coded to the root operation Occlusion, because the objective of the procedure is to cut off the blood supply to the vessel.

Embolization of a cerebral aneurysm is coded to the root operation Restriction, because the objective of the procedure is not to close off the vessel entirely, but to narrow the lumen of the vessel at the site of the aneurysm where it is abnormally wide.

### *Release procedures*

**B3.13.** In the root operation Release, the body part value coded is the body part being freed and not the tissue being manipulated or cut to free the body part.

*Example:* Lysis of intestinal adhesions is coded to the specific intestine body part value.

### *Release vs. Division*

**B3.14.** If the sole objective of the procedure is freeing a body part without cutting the body part, the root operation is Release. If the sole objective of the procedure is separating or transecting a body part, the root operation is Division.

*Examples:* Freeing a nerve root from surrounding scar tissue to relieve pain is coded to the root operation Release.

Severing a nerve root to relieve pain is coded to the root operation Division.

### *Reposition for fracture treatment*

**B3.15.** Reduction of a displaced fracture is coded to the root operation Reposition and the application of a cast or splint in conjunction with the Reposition procedure is not coded separately. Treatment of a nondisplaced fracture is coded to the procedure performed.

*Examples:* Casting of a nondisplaced fracture is coded to the root operation Immobilization in the Placement section.

Putting a pin in a nondisplaced fracture is coded to the root operation Insertion.

### *Transplantation vs. Administration*

**B3.16.** Putting in a mature and functioning living body part taken from another individual or animal is coded to the root operation Transplantation. Putting in autologous or nonautologous cells is coded to the Administration section.

*Example:* Putting in autologous or nonautologous bone marrow, pancreatic islet cells or stem cells is coded to the Administration section.

## B4. Body Part

### *General guidelines*

**B4.1a.** If a procedure is performed on a portion of a body part that does not have a separate body part value, code the body part value corresponding to the whole body part.

*Example:* A procedure performed on the alveolar process of the mandible is coded to the mandible body part.

**B4.1b.** If the prefix "peri" is combined with a body part to identify the site of the procedure, and the site of the procedure is not further specified, then the procedure is coded to the body part named. This guideline applies only when a more specific body part value is not available.

*Examples:* A procedure site identified as perirenal is coded to the kidney body part when the site of the procedure is not further specified.

A procedure site described in the documentation as peri-urethral, and the documentation also indicates that it is the vulvar tissue and not the urethral tissue that is the site of the procedure, then the procedure is coded to the vulva body part.

**B4.1c. If a procedure is performed on a continuous section of a tubular body part, code the body part value corresponding to the furthest anatomical site from the point of entry.**

***Example:* A procedure performed on a continuous section of artery from the femoral artery to the external iliac artery with the point of entry at the femoral artery is coded to the external iliac body part.**

### *Branches of body parts*

**B4.2.** Where a specific branch of a body part does not have its own body part value in PCS, the body part is typically coded to the closest proximal branch that has a specific body part value. In the cardiovascular body systems, if a general body part is available in the correct root operation table, and coding to a proximal branch would require assigning a code in a different body system, the procedure is coded using the general body part value.

*Examples:* A procedure performed on the mandibular branch of the trigeminal nerve is coded to the trigeminal nerve body part value.

Occlusion of the bronchial artery is coded to the body part value Upper Artery in the body system Upper Arteries, and not to the body part value Thoracic Aorta, Descending in the body system Heart and Great Vessels.

### *Bilateral body part values*

**B4.3.** Bilateral body part values are available for a limited number of body parts. If the identical procedure is performed on contralateral body parts, and a bilateral body part value exists for that body part, a single procedure is coded using the bilateral body part value. If no bilateral body part value exists, each procedure is coded separately using the appropriate body part value.

*Examples:* The identical procedure performed on both fallopian tubes is coded once using the body part value Fallopian Tube, Bilateral.

The identical procedure performed on both knee joints is coded twice using the body part values Knee Joint, Right and Knee Joint, Left.

### *Coronary arteries*

**B4.4.** The coronary arteries are classified as a single body part that is further specified by number of arteries treated. One procedure code specifying multiple arteries is used when the same procedure is performed, including the same device and qualifier values.

*Examples:* Angioplasty of two distinct coronary arteries with placement of two stents is coded as Dilation of Coronary Artery, Two Arteries with Two Intraluminal Devices.

Angioplasty of two distinct coronary arteries, one with stent placed and one without, is coded separately as Dilation of Coronary Artery, One Artery with Intraluminal Device, and Dilation of Coronary Artery, One Artery with no device.

### *Tendons, ligaments, bursae and fascia near a joint*

**B4.5.** Procedures performed on tendons, ligaments, bursae and fascia supporting a joint are coded to the body part in the respective body system that is the focus of the procedure. Procedures performed on joint structures themselves are coded to the body part in the joint body systems.

*Examples:* Repair of the anterior cruciate ligament of the knee is coded to the knee bursa and ligament body part in the bursae and ligaments body system.

Knee arthroscopy with shaving of articular cartilage is coded to the knee joint body part in the Lower Joints body system.

### *Skin, subcutaneous tissue and fascia overlying a joint*

**B4.6.** If a procedure is performed on the skin, subcutaneous tissue or fascia overlying a joint, the procedure is coded to the following body part:

- Shoulder is coded to Upper Arm
- Elbow is coded to Lower Arm
- Wrist is coded to Lower Arm
- Hip is coded to Upper Leg
- Knee is coded to Lower Leg
- Ankle is coded to Foot

### *Fingers and toes*

**B4.7.** If a body system does not contain a separate body part value for fingers, procedures performed on the fingers are coded to the body part value for the hand. If a body system does not contain a separate body part value for toes, procedures performed on the toes are coded to the body part value for the foot.

*Example:* Excision of finger muscle is coded to one of the hand muscle body part values in the Muscles body system.

### *Upper and lower intestinal tract*

**B4.8.** In the Gastrointestinal body system, the general body part values Upper Intestinal Tract and Lower Intestinal Tract are provided as an option for the root operations Change, Inspection, Removal and Revision. Upper Intestinal Tract includes the portion of the gastrointestinal tract from the esophagus down to and including the duodenum, and Lower Intestinal Tract includes the portion of the gastrointestinal tract from the jejunum down to and including the rectum and anus.

*Example:* In the root operation Change table, change of a device in the jejunum is coded using the body part Lower Intestinal Tract.

## B5. Approach

### *Open approach with percutaneous endoscopic assistance*

**B5.2.** Procedures performed using the open approach with percutaneous endoscopic assistance are coded to the approach Open.

*Example:* Laparoscopic-assisted sigmoidectomy is coded to the approach Open.

### *External approach*

**B5.3a.** Procedures performed within an orifice on structures that are visible without the aid of any instrumentation are coded to the approach External.

*Example:* Resection of tonsils is coded to the approach External.

**B5.3b.** Procedures performed indirectly by the application of external force through the intervening body layers are coded to the approach External.

*Example:* Closed reduction of fracture is coded to the approach External.

### *Percutaneous procedure via device*

**B5.4.** Procedures performed percutaneously via a device placed for the procedure are coded to the approach Percutaneous.

*Example:* Fragmentation of kidney stone performed via percutaneous nephrostomy is coded to the approach Percutaneous.

## B6. Device

### *General guidelines*

**B6.1a.** A device is coded only if a device remains after the procedure is completed. If no device remains, the device value No Device is coded. **In limited root operations, the classification provides the qualifier values Temporary and Intraoperative, for specific procedures involving clinically significant devices, where the purpose of the device is to be utilized for a brief duration during the procedure or current inpatient stay.**

**B6.1b.** Materials such as sutures, ligatures, radiological markers and temporary post-operative wound drains are considered integral to the performance of a procedure and are not coded as devices.

**B6.1c.** Procedures performed on a device only and not on a body part are specified in the root operations Change, Irrigation, Removal and Revision, and are coded to the procedure performed.

*Example:* Irrigation of percutaneous nephrostomy tube is coded to the root operation Irrigation of indwelling device in the Administration section.

*Drainage device*

**B6.2.** A separate procedure to put in a drainage device is coded to the root operation Drainage with the device value Drainage Device.

# Obstetric Section Guidelines (section 1)

## Obstetrics Section

*Products of conception*

**C1.** Procedures performed on the products of conception are coded to the Obstetrics section. Procedures performed on the pregnant female other than the products of conception are coded to the appropriate root operation in the Medical and Surgical section.

*Example:* Amniocentesis is coded to the products of conception body part in the Obstetrics section. Repair of obstetric urethral laceration is coded to the urethra body part in the Medical and Surgical section.

*Procedures following delivery or abortion*

**C2.** Procedures performed following a delivery or abortion for curettage of the endometrium or evacuation of retained products of conception are all coded in the Obstetrics section, to the root operation Extraction and the body part Products of Conception, Retained.

Diagnostic or therapeutic dilation and curettage performed during times other than the postpartum or post-abortion period are all coded in the Medical and Surgical section, to the root operation Extraction and the body part Endometrium.

# New Technology Section Guidelines (section X)

## New Technology Section

*General guidelines*

**D1.** Section X codes are standalone codes. They are not supplemental codes. Section X codes fully represent the specific procedure described in the code title, and do not require any additional codes from other sections of ICD-10-PCS. When section X contains a code title which describes a specific new technology procedure, only that X code is reported for the procedure. There is no need to report a broader, non-specific code in another section of ICD-10-PCS.

*Example:* XW04321 Introduction of Ceftazidime-Avibactam Anti-infective into Central Vein, Percutaneous Approach, New Technology Group 1, can be coded to indicate that Ceftazidime-Avibactam Anti-infective was administered via a central vein. A separate code from table 3E0 in the Administration section of ICD-10-PCS is not coded in addition to this code.

# Selection of Principal Procedure

The following instructions should be applied in the selection of principal procedure and clarification on the importance of the relation to the principal diagnosis when more than one procedure is performed:

1. Procedure performed for definitive treatment of both principal diagnosis and secondary diagnosis
    a. Sequence procedure performed for definitive treatment most related to principal diagnosis as principal procedure.
2. Procedure performed for definitive treatment and diagnostic procedures performed for both principal diagnosis and secondary diagnosis.
    a. Sequence procedure performed for definitive treatment most related to principal diagnosis as principal procedure
3. A diagnostic procedure was performed for the principal diagnosis and a procedure is performed for definitive treatment of a secondary diagnosis.
    a. Sequence diagnostic procedure as principal procedure, since the procedure most related to the principal diagnosis takes precedence.
4. No procedures performed that are related to principal diagnosis; procedures performed for definitive treatment and diagnostic procedures were performed for secondary diagnosis
    a. Sequence procedure performed for definitive treatment of secondary diagnosis as principal procedure, since there are no procedures (definitive or nondefinitive treatment) related to principal diagnosis.

# #

**3f (Aortic) Bioprosthesis valve** *use* Zooplastic Tissue in Heart and Great Vessels

# A

**Abdominal aortic plexus** *use* Nerve, Abdominal Sympathetic
**Abdominal esophagus** *use* Esophagus, Lower
**Abdominohysterectomy**
*see* Resection, Cervix ØUTC
*see* Resection, Uterus ØUT9
**Abdominoplasty**
*see* Alteration, Abdominal Wall ØWØF
*see* Repair, Abdominal Wall ØWQF
*see* Supplement, Abdominal Wall ØWUF
**Abductor hallucis muscle**
*use* Foot Muscle, Left
*use* Foot Muscle, Right
**AbioCor® Total Replacement Heart** *use* Synthetic Substitute
**Ablation** *see* Destruction
**Abortion**
Abortifacient 1ØAØ7ZX
Laminaria 1ØAØ7ZW
Products of Conception 1ØAØ
Vacuum 1ØAØ7Z6
**Abrasion** *see* Extraction
**Absolute Pro Vascular (OTW) Self-Expanding Stent System** *use* Intraluminal Device
**Accessory cephalic vein**
*use* Cephalic Vein, Left
*use* Cephalic Vein, Right
**Accessory obturator nerve** *use* Lumbar Plexus
**Accessory phrenic nerve** *use* Phrenic Nerve
**Accessory spleen** *use* Spleen
**Acculink (RX) Carotid Stent System** *use* Intraluminal Device
**Acellular Hydrated Dermis** *use* Nonautologous Tissue Substitute
**Acetabular cup** *use* Liner in Lower Joints
**Acetabulectomy**
*see* Excision, Lower Bones ØQB
*see* Resection, Lower Bones ØQT
**Acetabulofemoral joint**
*use* Hip Joint, Left
*use* Hip Joint, Right
**Acetabuloplasty**
*see* Repair, Lower Bones ØQQ
*see* Replacement, Lower Bones ØQR
*see* Supplement, Lower Bones ØQU
**Achilles tendon**
*use* Lower Leg Tendon, Left
*use* Lower Leg Tendon, Right
**Achillorrhaphy** *see* Repair, Tendons ØLQ
**Achillotenotomy, achillotomy**
*see* Division, Tendons ØL8
*see* Drainage, Tendons ØL9
**Acromioclavicular ligament**
*use* Shoulder Bursa and Ligament, Left
*use* Shoulder Bursa and Ligament, Right
**Acromion (process)**
*use* Scapula, Left
*use* Scapula, Right
**Acromionectomy**
*see* Excision, Upper Joints ØRB
*see* Resection, Upper Joints ØRT
**Acromioplasty**
*see* Repair, Upper Joints ØRQ
*see* Replacement, Upper Joints ØRR
*see* Supplement, Upper Joints ØRU
**Activa PC neurostimulator** *use* Stimulator Generator, Multiple Array in ØJH
**Activa RC neurostimulator** *use* Stimulator Generator, Multiple Array Rechargeable in ØJH
**Activa SC neurostimulator** *use* Stimulator Generator, Single Array in ØJH
**Activities of Daily Living Assessment** FØ2
**Activities of Daily Living Treatment** FØ8
**ACUITY™ Steerable Lead**
*use* Cardiac Lead, Defibrillator in Ø2H
*use* Cardiac Lead, Pacemaker in Ø2H
**Acupuncture**
Breast
Anesthesia 8EØH3ØØ
No Qualifier 8EØH3ØZ
Integumentary System
Anesthesia 8EØH3ØØ
No Qualifier 8EØH3ØZ
**Adductor brevis muscle**
*use* Upper Leg Muscle, Left
*use* Upper Leg Muscle, Right
**Adductor hallucis muscle**
*use* Foot Muscle, Left
*use* Foot Muscle, Right
**Adductor longus muscle**
*use* Upper Leg Muscle, Left
*use* Upper Leg Muscle, Right
**Adductor magnus muscle**
*use* Upper Leg Muscle, Left
*use* Upper Leg Muscle, Right
**Adenohypophysis** *use* Pituitary Gland
**Adenoidectomy**
*see* Excision, Adenoids ØCBQ
*see* Resection, Adenoids ØCTQ
**Adenoidotomy** *see* Drainage, Adenoids ØC9Q
**Adhesiolysis** *see* Release
**Administration**
Blood products *see* Transfusion
Other substance *see* Introduction of substance in or on
**Adrenalectomy**
*see* Excision, Endocrine System ØGB
*see* Resection, Endocrine System ØGT
**Adrenalorrhaphy** *see* Repair, Endocrine System ØGQ
**Adrenalotomy** *see* Drainage, Endocrine System ØG9
**Advancement**
*see* Reposition
*see* Transfer
**Advisa (MRI)** *use* Pacemaker, Dual Chamber in ØJH
**AFX® Endovascular AAA System** *use* Intraluminal Device
**AIGISRx Antibacterial Envelope** *use* Anti-Infective Envelope
**Alar ligament of axis** *use* Head and Neck Bursa and Ligament
**Alfieri Stitch Valvuloplasty** *see* Restriction, Valve, Mitral Ø2VG
**Alimentation** *see* Introduction of substance in or on
**Alteration**
Abdominal Wall ØWØF
Ankle Region
Left ØYØL
Right ØYØK
Arm
Lower
Left ØXØF
Right ØXØD
Upper
Left ØXØ9
Right ØXØ8
Axilla
Left ØXØ5
Right ØXØ4
Back
Lower ØWØL
Upper ØWØK
Breast
Bilateral ØHØV
Left ØHØU
Right ØHØT
Buttock
Left ØYØ1
Right ØYØØ
Chest Wall ØWØ8
Ear
Bilateral Ø9Ø2
Left Ø9Ø1
Right Ø9ØØ
Elbow Region
Left ØXØC
Right ØXØB
Extremity
Lower
Left ØYØB
Right ØYØ9
Upper
Left ØXØ7
Right ØXØ6
**Alteration** — *continued*
Eyelid
Lower
Left Ø8ØR
Right Ø8ØQ
Upper
Left Ø8ØP
Right Ø8ØN
Face ØWØ2
Head ØWØØ
Jaw
Lower ØWØ5
Upper ØWØ4
Knee Region
Left ØYØG
Right ØYØF
Leg
Lower
Left ØYØJ
Right ØYØH
Upper
Left ØYØD
Right ØYØC
Lip
Lower ØCØ1X
Upper ØCØØX
Nasal Mucosa and Soft Tissue Ø9ØK
Neck ØWØ6
Perineum
Female ØWØN
Male ØWØM
Shoulder Region
Left ØXØ3
Right ØXØ2
Subcutaneous Tissue and Fascia
Abdomen ØJØ8
Back ØJØ7
Buttock ØJØ9
Chest ØJØ6
Face ØJØ1
Lower Arm
Left ØJØH
Right ØJØG
Lower Leg
Left ØJØP
Right ØJØN
Neck
Left ØJØ5
Right ØJØ4
Upper Arm
Left ØJØF
Right ØJØD
Upper Leg
Left ØJØM
Right ØJØL
Wrist Region
Left ØXØH
Right ØXØG
**Alveolar process of mandible**
*use* Mandible, Left
*use* Mandible, Right
**Alveolar process of maxilla** *use* Maxilla
**Alveolectomy**
*see* Excision, Head and Facial Bones ØNB
*see* Resection, Head and Facial Bones ØNT
**Alveoloplasty**
*see* Repair, Head and Facial Bones ØNQ
*see* Replacement, Head and Facial Bones ØNR
*see* Supplement, Head and Facial Bones ØNU
**Alveolotomy**
*see* Division, Head and Facial Bones ØN8
*see* Drainage, Head and Facial Bones ØN9
**Ambulatory cardiac monitoring** 4A12X45
**Amniocentesis** *see* Drainage, Products of Conception 1Ø9Ø
**Amnioinfusion** *see* Introduction of substance in or on, Products of Conception 3EØE
**Amnioscopy** 1ØJØ8ZZ
**Amniotomy** *see* Drainage, Products of Conception 1Ø9Ø
**AMPLATZER® Muscular VSD Occluder** *use* Synthetic Substitute
**Amputation** *see* Detachment
**AMS 8ØØ® Urinary Control System** *use* Artificial Sphincter in Urinary System
**Anal orifice** *use* Anus
**Analog radiography** *see* Plain Radiography
**Analog radiology** *see* Plain Radiography
**Anastomosis** *see* Bypass

**Anatomical snuffbox**
*use* Lower Arm and Wrist Muscle, Left
*use* Lower Arm and Wrist Muscle, Right
**Andexanet Alfa, Factor Xa Inhibitor Reversal Agent** XWØ
**AneuRx® AAA Advantage®** *use* Intraluminal Device
**Angiectomy**
*see* Excision, Heart and Great Vessels Ø2B
*see* Excision, Lower Arteries Ø4B
*see* Excision, Lower Veins Ø6B
*see* Excision, Upper Arteries Ø3B
*see* Excision, Upper Veins Ø5B
**Angiocardiography**
Combined right and left heart *see* Fluoroscopy, Heart, Right and Left B216
Left Heart *see* Fluoroscopy, Heart, Left B215
Right Heart *see* Fluoroscopy, Heart, Right B214
SPY system intravascular fluorescence *see* Monitoring, Physiological Systems 4A1
**Angiography**
*see* Fluoroscopy, Heart B21
*see* Plain Radiography, Heart B2Ø
**Angioplasty**
*see* Dilation, Heart and Great Vessels Ø27
*see* Dilation, Lower Arteries Ø47
*see* Dilation, Upper Arteries Ø37
*see* Repair, Heart and Great Vessels Ø2Q
*see* Repair, Lower Arteries Ø4Q
*see* Repair, Upper Arteries Ø3Q
*see* Replacement, Heart and Great Vessels Ø2R
*see* Replacement, Lower Arteries Ø4R
*see* Replacement, Upper Arteries Ø3R
*see* Supplement, Heart and Great Vessels Ø2U
*see* Supplement, Lower Arteries Ø4U
*see* Supplement, Upper Arteries Ø3U
**Angiorrhaphy**
*see* Repair, Heart and Great Vessels Ø2Q
*see* Repair, Lower Arteries Ø4Q
*see* Repair, Upper Arteries Ø3Q
**Angioscopy** Ø4JY4ZZ
**Angiotripsy**
*see* Occlusion, Lower Arteries Ø4L
*see* Occlusion, Upper Arteries Ø3L
**Angular artery** *use* Artery, Face
**Angular vein**
*use* Face Vein, Left
*use* Face Vein, Right
**Annular ligament**
*use* Elbow Bursa and Ligament, Left
*use* Elbow Bursa and Ligament, Right
**Annuloplasty**
*see* Repair, Heart and Great Vessels Ø2Q
*see* Supplement, Heart and Great Vessels Ø2U
**Annuloplasty ring** *use* Synthetic Substitute
**Anoplasty**
*see* Repair, Anus ØDQQ
*see* Supplement, Anus ØDUQ
**Anorectal junction** *use* Rectum
**Anoscopy** ØDJD8ZZ
**Ansa cervicalis** *use* Cervical Plexus
**Antabuse therapy** HZ93ZZZ
**Antebrachial fascia**
*use* Subcutaneous Tissue and Fascia, Left Lower Arm
*use* Subcutaneous Tissue and Fascia, Right Lower Arm
**Anterior cerebral artery** *use* Intracranial Artery
**Anterior cerebral vein** *use* Intracranial Vein
**Anterior choroidal artery** *use* Intracranial Artery
**Anterior circumflex humeral artery**
*use* Axillary Artery, Left
*use* Axillary Artery, Right
**Anterior communicating artery** *use* Intracranial Artery
**Anterior cruciate ligament (ACL)**
*use* Knee Bursa and Ligament, Left
*use* Knee Bursa and Ligament, Right
**Anterior crural nerve** *use* Femoral Nerve
**Anterior facial vein**
*use* Face Vein, Left
*use* Face Vein, Right
**Anterior intercostal artery**
*use* Internal Mammary Artery, Left
*use* Internal Mammary Artery, Right
**Anterior interosseous nerve** *use* Median Nerve
**Anterior lateral malleolar artery**
*use* Anterior Tibial Artery, Left
*use* Anterior Tibial Artery, Right
**Anterior lingual gland** *use* Minor Salivary Gland
**Anterior (pectoral) lymph node**
*use* Lymphatic, Left Axillary
*use* Lymphatic, Right Axillary
**Anterior medial malleolar artery**
*use* Anterior Tibial Artery, Left
*use* Anterior Tibial Artery, Right
**Anterior spinal artery**
*use* Vertebral Artery, Left
*use* Vertebral Artery, Right
**Anterior tibial recurrent artery**
*use* Anterior Tibial Artery, Left
*use* Anterior Tibial Artery, Right
**Anterior ulnar recurrent artery**
*use* Ulnar Artery, Left
*use* Ulnar Artery, Right
**Anterior vagal trunk** *use* Vagus Nerve
**Anterior vertebral muscle**
*use* Neck Muscle, Left
*use*Neck Muscle, Right
**Antigen-free air conditioning** *see* Atmospheric Control, Physiological Systems 6AØ
**Antihelix**
*use* External Ear, Bilateral
*use* External Ear, Left
*use* External Ear, Right
**Antimicrobial envelope** *use* Anti-Infective Envelope
**Antitragus**
*use* External Ear, Bilateral
*use* External Ear, Left
*use* External Ear, Right
**Antrostomy** *see* Drainage, Ear, Nose, Sinus Ø99
**Antrotomy** *see* Drainage, Ear, Nose, Sinus Ø99
**Antrum of Highmore**
*use* Maxillary Sinus, Left
*use* Maxillary Sinus, Right
**Aortic annulus** *use* Aortic Valve
**Aortic arch** *use* Thoracic Aorta, Ascending/Arch
**Aortic intercostal artery** *use* Upper Artery
**Aortography**
*see* Fluoroscopy, Lower Arteries B41
*see* Fluoroscopy, Upper Arteries B31
*see* Plain Radiography, Lower Arteries B4Ø
*see* Plain Radiography, Upper Arteries B3Ø
**Aortoplasty**
*see* Repair, Aorta, Abdominal Ø4QØ
*see* Repair, Aorta, Thoracic, Ascending/Arch Ø2QX
*see* Repair, Aorta, Thoracic, Descending Ø2QW
*see* Replacement, Aorta, Abdominal Ø4RØ
*see* Replacement, Aorta, Thoracic, Ascending/Arch Ø2RX
*see* Replacement, Aorta, Thoracic, Descending Ø2RW
*see* Supplement, Aorta, Abdominal Ø4UØ
*see* Supplement, Aorta, Thoracic, Ascending/Arch Ø2UX
*see* Supplement, Aorta, Thoracic, Descending Ø2UW
**Apical (subclavicular) lymph node**
*use* Lymphatic, Left Axillary
*use* Lymphatic, Right Axillary
**Apneustic center** *use* Pons
**Appendectomy**
*see* Excision, Appendix ØDBJ
*see* Resection, Appendix ØDTJ
**Appendicolysis** *see* Release, Appendix ØDNJ
**Appendicotomy** *see* Drainage, Appendix ØD9J
**Application** *see* Introduction of substance in or on
**Aquapheresis** 6A55ØZ3
**Aqueduct of Sylvius** *use* Cerebral Ventricle
**Aqueous humour**
*use* Anterior Chamber, Left
*use* Anterior Chamber, Right
**Arachnoid mater, intracranial** *use* Cerebral Meninges
**Arachnoid mater, spinal** *use* Spinal Meninges
**Arcuate artery**
*use* Foot Artery, Left
*use* Foot Artery, Right
**Areola**
*use* Nipple, Left
*use* Nipple, Right
**AROM (artificial rupture of membranes)** 1Ø9Ø7ZC
**Arterial canal (duct)** *use* Pulmonary Artery, Left
**Arterial pulse tracing** *see* Measurement, Arterial 4AØ3
**Arteriectomy**
*see* Excision, Heart and Great Vessels Ø2B
*see* Excision, Lower Arteries Ø4B
*see* Excision, Upper Arteries Ø3B
**Arteriography**
*see* Fluoroscopy, Heart B21
**Arteriography** — *continued*
*see* Fluoroscopy, Lower Arteries B41
*see* Fluoroscopy, Upper Arteries B31
*see* Plain Radiography, Heart B2Ø
*see* Plain Radiography, Lower Arteries B4Ø
*see* Plain Radiography, Upper Arteries B3Ø
**Arterioplasty**
*see* Repair, Heart and Great Vessels Ø2Q
*see* Repair, Lower Arteries Ø4Q
*see* Repair, Upper Arteries Ø3Q
*see* Replacement, Heart and Great Vessels Ø2R
*see* Replacement, Lower Arteries Ø4R
*see* Replacement, Upper Arteries Ø3R
*see* Supplement, Heart and Great Vessels Ø2U
*see* Supplement, Lower Arteries Ø4U
*see* Supplement, Upper Arteries Ø3U
**Arteriorrhaphy**
*see* Repair, Heart and Great Vessels Ø2Q
*see* Repair, Lower Arteries Ø4Q
*see* Repair, Upper Arteries Ø3Q
**Arterioscopy**
*see* Inspection, Artery, Lower Ø4JY
*see* Inspection, Artery, Upper Ø3JY
*see* Inspection, Great Vessel Ø2JY
**Arthrectomy**
*see* Excision, Lower Joints ØSB
*see* Excision, Upper Joints ØRB
*see* Resection, Lower Joints ØST
*see* Resection, Upper Joints ØRT
**Arthrocentesis**
*see* Drainage, Lower Joints ØS9
*see* Drainage, Upper Joints ØR9
**Arthrodesis**
*see* Fusion, Lower Joints ØSG
*see* Fusion, Upper Joints ØRG
**Arthrography**
*see* Plain Radiography, Non-Axial Lower Bones BQØ
*see* Plain Radiography, Non-Axial Upper Bones BPØ
*see* Plain Radiography, Skull and Facial Bones BNØ
**Arthrolysis**
*see* Release, Lower Joints ØSN
*see* Release, Upper Joints ØRN
**Arthropexy**
*see* Repair, Lower Joints ØSQ
*see* Repair, Upper Joints ØRQ
*see* Reposition, Lower Joints ØSS
*see* Reposition, Upper Joints ØRS
**Arthroplasty**
*see* Repair, Lower Joints ØSQ
*see* Repair, Upper Joints ØRQ
*see* Replacement, Lower Joints ØSR
*see* Replacement, Upper Joints ØRR
*see* Supplement, Lower Joints ØSU
*see* Supplement, Upper Joints ØRU
**Arthroscopy**
*see* Inspection, Lower Joints ØSJ
*see* Inspection, Upper Joints ØRJ
**Arthrotomy**
*see* Drainage, Lower Joints ØS9
*see* Drainage, Upper Joints ØR9
**Artificial anal sphincter (AAS)** *use* Artificial Sphincter in Gastrointestinal System
**Artificial bowel sphincter (neosphincter)** *use* Artificial Sphincter in Gastrointestinal System
**Artificial Sphincter**
Insertion of device in
Anus ØDHQ
Bladder ØTHB
Bladder Neck ØTHC
Urethra ØTHD
Removal of device from
Anus ØDPQ
Bladder ØTPB
Urethra ØTPD
Revision of device in
Anus ØDWQ
Bladder ØTWB
Urethra ØTWD
**Artificial urinary sphincter (AUS)** *use* Artificial Sphincter in Urinary System
**Aryepiglottic fold** *use* Larynx
**Arytenoid cartilage** *use* Larynx
**Arytenoid muscle**
*use* Neck Muscle, Left
*use* Neck Muscle, Right
**Arytenoidectomy** *see* Excision, Larynx ØCBS
**Arytenoidopexy** *see* Repair, Larynx ØCQS

**Ascenda Intrathecal Catheter** *use* Infusion Device
**Ascending aorta** *use* Thoracic Aorta, Ascending/Arch
**Ascending palatine artery** *use* Face Artery
**Ascending pharyngeal artery**
- *use* External Carotid Artery, Left
- *use* External Carotid Artery, Right

**Aspiration, fine needle**
- fluid or gas *see* Drainage
- tissue *see* Excision

**Assessment**
- Activities of daily living *see* Activities of Daily Living Assessment, Rehabilitation FØ2
- Hearing *see* Hearing Assessment, Diagnostic Audiology F13
- Hearing aid *see* Hearing Aid Assessment, Diagnostic Audiology F14
- Intravascular perfusion, using indocyanine green (ICG) dye *see* Monitoring, Physiological Systems 4A1
- Motor function *see* Motor Function Assessment, Rehabilitation FØ1
- Nerve function *see* Motor Function Assessment, Rehabilitation FØ1
- Speech *see* Speech Assessment, Rehabilitation FØØ
- Vestibular *see* Vestibular Assessment, Diagnostic Audiology F15
- Vocational *see* Activities of Daily Living Treatment, Rehabilitation FØ8

**Assistance**
- Cardiac
  - Continuous
    - Balloon Pump 5AØ221Ø
    - Impeller Pump 5AØ221D
    - Other Pump 5AØ2216
    - Pulsatile Compression 5AØ2215
  - Intermittent
    - Balloon Pump 5AØ211Ø
    - Impeller Pump 5AØ211D
    - Other Pump 5AØ2116
    - Pulsatile Compression 5AØ2115
- Circulatory
  - Continuous
    - Hyperbaric 5AØ5221
    - Supersaturated 5AØ522C
  - Intermittent
    - Hyperbaric 5AØ5121
    - Supersaturated 5AØ512C
- Respiratory
  - 24-96 Consecutive Hours
    - Continuous Negative Airway Pressure 5AØ9459
    - Continuous Positive Airway Pressure 5AØ9457
    - Intermittent Negative Airway Pressure 5AØ945B
    - Intermittent Positive Airway Pressure 5AØ9458
    - No Qualifier 5AØ945Z
  - Continuous, Filtration 5AØ92ØZ
  - Greater than 96 Consecutive Hours
    - Continuous Negative Airway Pressure 5AØ9559
    - Continuous Positive Airway Pressure 5AØ9557
    - Intermittent Negative Airway Pressure 5AØ955B
    - Intermittent Positive Airway Pressure 5AØ9558
    - No Qualifier 5AØ955Z
  - Less than 24 Consecutive Hours
    - Continuous Negative Airway Pressure 5AØ9359
    - Continuous Positive Airway Pressure 5AØ9357
    - Intermittent Negative Airway Pressure 5AØ935B
    - Intermittent Positive Airway Pressure 5AØ9358
    - No Qualifier 5AØ935Z

**Assurant (Cobalt) stent** *use* Intraluminal Device
**Atherectomy**
- *see* Extirpation, Heart and Great Vessels Ø2C
- *see* Extirpation, Lower Arteries Ø4C
- *see* Extirpation, Upper Arteries Ø3C

**Atlantoaxial joint** *use* Cervical Vertebral Joint
**Atmospheric Control** 6AØZ
**AtriClip LAA Exclusion System** *use* Extraluminal Device
**Atrioseptoplasty**
- *see* Repair, Heart and Great Vessels Ø2Q
- *see* Replacement, Heart and Great Vessels Ø2R
- *see* Supplement, Heart and Great Vessels Ø2U

**Atrioventricular node** *use* Conduction Mechanism
**Atrium dextrum cordis** *use* Atrium, Right
**Atrium pulmonale** *use* Atrium, Left
**Attain Ability® lead** Ø2H
- *use* Cardiac Lead, Defibrillator in Ø2H
- *use* Cardiac Lead, Pacemaker in Ø2H

**Attain Starfix® (OTW) lead**
- *use* Cardiac Lead, Defibrillator in Ø2H
- *use* Cardiac Lead, Pacemaker in Ø2H

**Audiology, diagnostic**
- *see* Hearing Aid Assessment, Diagnostic Audiology F14
- *see* Hearing Assessment, Diagnostic Audiology F13
- *see* Vestibular Assessment, Diagnostic Audiology F15

**Audiometry** *see* Hearing Assessment, Diagnostic Audiology F13
**Auditory tube**
- *use* Eustachian Tube, Left
- *use* Eustachian Tube, Right

**Auerbach's (myenteric) plexus** *use* Abdominal Sympathetic Nerve
**Auricle**
- *use* External Ear, Bilateral
- *use* External Ear, Left
- *use* External Ear, Right

**Auricularis muscle** *use* Head Muscle
**Autograft** *use* Autologous Tissue Substitute
**Autologous artery graft**
- *use* Autologous Arterial Tissue in Heart and Great Vessels
- *use* Autologous Arterial Tissue in Lower Arteries
- *use* Autologous Arterial Tissue in Lower Veins
- *use* Autologous Arterial Tissue in Upper Arteries
- *use* Autologous Arterial Tissue in Upper Veins

**Autologous vein graft**
- *use* Autologous Venous Tissue in Heart and Great Vessels
- *use* Autologous Venous Tissue in Lower Arteries
- *use* Autologous Venous Tissue in Lower Veins
- *use* Autologous Venous Tissue in Upper Arteries
- *use* Autologous Venous Tissue in Upper Veins

**Autotransfusion** *see* Transfusion
**Autotransplant**
- Adrenal tissue *see* Reposition, Endocrine System ØGS
- Kidney *see* Reposition, Urinary System ØTS
- Pancreatic tissue *see* Reposition, Pancreas ØFSG
- Parathyroid tissue *see* Reposition, Endocrine System ØGS
- Thyroid tissue *see* Reposition, Endocrine System ØGS
- Tooth *see* Reattachment, Mouth and Throat ØCM

**Avulsion** *see* Extraction
**Axial Lumbar Interbody Fusion System** *use* Interbody Fusion Device in Lower Joints
**AxiaLIF® System** *use* Interbody Fusion Device in Lower Joints
**Axicabtagene Ciloeucel** *use* Engineered Autologous Chimeric Antigen Receptor T-cell Immunotherapy
**Axillary fascia**
- *use* Subcutaneous Tissue and Fascia, Left Upper Arm
- *use* Subcutaneous Tissue and Fascia, Right Upper Arm

**Axillary nerve** *use* Brachial Plexus

## B

**BAK/C® Interbody Cervical Fusion System** *use* Interbody Fusion Device in Upper Joints
**BAL (bronchial alveolar lavage), diagnostic** *see* Drainage, Respiratory System ØB9
**Balanoplasty**
- *see* Repair, Penis ØVQS
- *see* Supplement, Penis ØVUS

**Balloon atrial septostomy (BAS)** Ø2163Z7
**Balloon Pump**
- Continuous, Output 5AØ221Ø
- Intermittent, Output 5AØ211Ø

**Bandage, Elastic** *see* Compression
**Banding**
- *see* Occlusion
- *see* Restriction

**Banding, esophageal varices** *see* Occlusion, Vein, Esophageal Ø6L3
**Banding, laparoscopic (adjustable) gastric**
- Adjustment/revision ØDW64CZ
- Initial procedure ØDV64CZ

**Bard® Composix® Kugel® patch** *use* Synthetic Substitute
**Bard® Composix® (E/X) (LP) mesh** *use* Synthetic Substitute
**Bard® Dulex™ mesh** *use* Synthetic Substitute
**Bard® Ventralex™ Hernia Patch** *use* Synthetic Substitute
**Barium swallow** *see* Fluoroscopy, Gastrointestinal System BD1
**Baroreflex Activation Therapy® (BAT®)**
- *use* Stimulator Generator in Subcutaneous Tissue and Fascia

**Baroreflex Activation Therapy® (BAT®)** — *continued*
- *use* Stimulator Lead in Upper Arteries

**Bartholin's (greater vestibular) gland** *use* Vestibular Gland
**Basal (internal) cerebral vein** *use* Intracranial Vein
**Basal metabolic rate (BMR)** *see* Measurement, Physiological Systems 4AØZ
**Basal nuclei** *use* Basal Ganglia
**Base of Tongue** *use* Pharynx
**Basilar artery** *use* Intracranial Artery
**Basis pontis** *use* Pons
**Beam Radiation**
- Abdomen DWØ3
  - Intraoperative DWØ33ZØ
- Adrenal Gland DGØ2
  - Intraoperative DGØ23ZØ
- Bile Ducts DFØ2
  - Intraoperative DFØ23ZØ
- Bladder DTØ2
  - Intraoperative DTØ23ZØ
- Bone
  - Intraoperative DPØC3ZØ
  - Other DPØC
- Bone Marrow D7ØØ
  - Intraoperative D7ØØ3ZØ
- Brain DØØØ
  - Intraoperative DØØØ3ZØ
- Brain Stem DØØ1
  - Intraoperative DØØ13ZØ
- Breast
  - Left DMØØ
    - Intraoperative DMØØ3ZØ
  - Right DMØ1
    - Intraoperative DMØ13ZØ
- Bronchus DBØ1
  - Intraoperative DBØ13ZØ
- Cervix DUØ1
  - Intraoperative DUØ13ZØ
- Chest DWØ2
  - Intraoperative DWØ23ZØ
- Chest Wall DBØ7
  - Intraoperative DBØ73ZØ
- Colon DDØ5
  - Intraoperative DDØ53ZØ
- Diaphragm DBØ8
  - Intraoperative DBØ83ZØ
- Duodenum DDØ2
  - Intraoperative DDØ23ZØ
- Ear D9ØØ
  - Intraoperative D9ØØ3ZØ
- Esophagus DDØØ
  - Intraoperative DDØØ3ZØ
- Eye D8ØØ
  - Intraoperative D8ØØ3ZØ
- Femur DPØ9
  - Intraoperative DPØ93ZØ
- Fibula DPØB
  - Intraoperative DPØB3ZØ
- Gallbladder DFØ1
  - Intraoperative DFØ13ZØ
- Gland
  - Adrenal DGØ2
    - Intraoperative DGØ23ZØ
  - Parathyroid DGØ4
    - Intraoperative DGØ43ZØ
  - Pituitary DGØØ
    - Intraoperative DGØØ3ZØ
  - Thyroid DGØ5
    - Intraoperative DGØ53ZØ
- Glands
  - Intraoperative D9Ø63ZØ
  - Salivary D9Ø6
- Head and Neck DWØ1
  - Intraoperative DWØ13ZØ
- Hemibody DWØ4
  - Intraoperative DWØ43ZØ
- Humerus DPØ6
  - Intraoperative DPØ63ZØ
- Hypopharynx D9Ø3
  - Intraoperative D9Ø33ZØ
- Ileum DDØ4
  - Intraoperative DDØ43ZØ
- Jejunum DDØ3
  - Intraoperative DDØ33ZØ
- Kidney DTØØ
  - Intraoperative DTØØ3ZØ
- Larynx D9ØB

**Beam Radiation** — *continued*
Larynx — *continued*
Intraoperative D9ØB3ZØ
Liver DFØØ
Intraoperative DFØØ3ZØ
Lung DBØ2
Intraoperative DBØ23ZØ
Lymphatics
Abdomen D7Ø6
Intraoperative D7Ø63ZØ
Axillary D7Ø4
Intraoperative D7Ø43ZØ
Inguinal D7Ø8
Intraoperative D7Ø83ZØ
Neck D7Ø3
Intraoperative D7Ø33ZØ
Pelvis D7Ø7
Intraoperative D7Ø73ZØ
Thorax D7Ø5
Intraoperative D7Ø53ZØ
Mandible DPØ3
Intraoperative DPØ33ZØ
Maxilla DPØ2
Intraoperative DPØ23ZØ
Mediastinum DBØ6
Intraoperative DBØ63ZØ
Mouth D9Ø4
Intraoperative D9Ø43ZØ
Nasopharynx D9ØD
Intraoperative D9ØD3ZØ
Neck and Head DWØ1
Intraoperative DWØ13ZØ
Nerve
Intraoperative DØØ73ZØ
Peripheral DØØ7
Nose D9Ø1
Intraoperative D9Ø13ZØ
Oropharynx D9ØF
Intraoperative D9ØF3ZØ
Ovary DUØØ
Intraoperative DUØØ3ZØ
Palate
Hard D9Ø8
Intraoperative D9Ø83ZØ
Soft D9Ø9
Intraoperative D9Ø93ZØ
Pancreas DFØ3
Intraoperative DFØ33ZØ
Parathyroid Gland DGØ4
Intraoperative DGØ43ZØ
Pelvic Bones DPØ8
Intraoperative DPØ83ZØ
Pelvic Region DWØ6
Intraoperative DWØ63ZØ
Pineal Body DGØ1
Intraoperative DGØ13ZØ
Pituitary Gland DGØØ
Intraoperative DGØØ3ZØ
Pleura DBØ5
Intraoperative DBØ53ZØ
Prostate DVØØ
Intraoperative DVØØ3ZØ
Radius DPØ7
Intraoperative DPØ73ZØ
Rectum DDØ7
Intraoperative DDØ73ZØ
Rib DPØ5
Intraoperative DPØ53ZØ
Sinuses D9Ø7
Intraoperative D9Ø73ZØ
Skin
Abdomen DHØ8
Intraoperative DHØ83ZØ
Arm DHØ4
Intraoperative DHØ43ZØ
Back DHØ7
Intraoperative DHØ73ZØ
Buttock DHØ9
Intraoperative DHØ93ZØ
Chest DHØ6
Intraoperative DHØ63ZØ
Face DHØ2
Intraoperative DHØ23ZØ
Leg DHØB
Intraoperative DHØB3ZØ
Neck DHØ3
Intraoperative DHØ33ZØ
Skull DPØØ
Intraoperative DPØØ3ZØ

**Beam Radiation** — *continued*
Spinal Cord DØØ6
Intraoperative DØØ63ZØ
Spleen D7Ø2
Intraoperative D7Ø23ZØ
Sternum DPØ4
Intraoperative DPØ43ZØ
Stomach DDØ1
Intraoperative DDØ13ZØ
Testis DVØ1
Intraoperative DVØ13ZØ
Thymus D7Ø1
Intraoperative D7Ø13ZØ
Thyroid Gland DGØ5
Intraoperative DGØ53ZØ
Tibia DPØB
Intraoperative DPØB3ZØ
Tongue D9Ø5
Intraoperative D9Ø53ZØ
Trachea DBØØ
Intraoperative DBØØ3ZØ
Ulna DPØ7
Intraoperative DPØ73ZØ
Ureter DTØ1
Intraoperative DTØ13ZØ
Urethra DTØ3
Intraoperative DTØ33ZØ
Uterus DUØ2
Intraoperative DUØ23ZØ
Whole Body DWØ5
Intraoperative DWØ53ZØ
**Bedside swallow** FØØZJWZ
**Berlin Heart Ventricular Assist Device** *use* Implantable Heart Assist System in Heart and Great Vessels
**Bezlotoxumab Monoclonal Antibody** XWØ
**Biceps brachii muscle**
*use* Upper Arm Muscle, Left
*use* Upper Arm Muscle, Right
**Biceps femoris muscle**
*use* Upper Leg Muscle, Left
*use* Upper Leg Muscle, Right
**Bicipital aponeurosis**
*use* Subcutaneous Tissue and Fascia, Left Lower Arm
*use* Subcutaneous Tissue and Fascia, Right Lower Arm
**Bicuspid valve** *use* Mitral Valve
**Bililite therapy** *see* Ultraviolet Light Therapy, Skin 6A8Ø
**Bioactive embolization coil(s)** *use* Intraluminal Device, Bioactive in Upper Arteries
**Biofeedback** GZC9ZZZ
**Biopsy**
*see* Drainage with qualifier Diagnostic
*see* Excision with qualifier Diagnostic
Bone Marrow *see* Extraction with qualifier Diagnostic
**BiPAP** *see* Assistance, Respiratory 5AØ9
**Bisection** *see* Division
**Biventricular external heart assist system** *use* Short-term External Heart Assist System in Heart and Great Vessels
**Blepharectomy**
*see* Excision, Eye Ø8B
*see* Resection, Eye Ø8T
**Blepharoplasty**
*see* Repair, Eye Ø8Q
*see* Replacement, Eye Ø8R
*see* Reposition, Eye Ø8S
*see* Supplement, Eye Ø8U
**Blepharorrhaphy** *see* Repair, Eye Ø8Q
**Blepharotomy** *see* Drainage, Eye Ø89
**Blinatumomab Antineoplastic Immunotherapy** XWØ
**Block, Nerve, anesthetic injection**
**Blood glucose monitoring system** *use* Monitoring Device
**Blood pressure** *see* Measurement, Arterial 4AØ3
**BMR (basal metabolic rate)** *see* Measurement, Physiological Systems 4AØZ
**Body of femur**
*use* Femoral Shaft, Left
*use* Femoral Shaft, Right
**Body of fibula**
*use* Fibula, Left
*use* Fibula, Right
**Bone anchored hearing device**
*use* Hearing Device, Bone Conduction in Ø9H
*use* Hearing Device in Head and Facial Bones
**Bone bank bone graft** *use* Nonautologous Tissue Substitute

**Bone Growth Stimulator**
Insertion of device in
Bone
Facial ØNHW
Lower ØQHY
Nasal ØNHB
Upper ØPHY
Skull ØNHØ
Removal of device from
Bone
Facial ØNPW
Lower ØQPY
Nasal ØNPB
Upper ØPPY
Skull ØNPØ
Revision of device in
Bone
Facial ØNWW
Lower ØQWY
Nasal ØNWB
Upper ØPWY
Skull ØNWØ
**Bone marrow transplant** *see* Transfusion, Circulatory 3Ø2
**Bone morphogenetic protein 2 (BMP 2)** *use* Recombinant Bone Morphogenetic Protein
**Bone screw (interlocking) (lag) (pedicle) (recessed)**
*use* Internal Fixation Device in Head and Facial Bones
*use* Internal Fixation Device in Lower Bones
*use* Internal Fixation Device in Upper Bones
**Bony labyrinth**
*use* Inner Ear, Left
*use* Inner Ear, Right
**Bony orbit**
*use* Orbit, Left
*use* Orbit, Right
**Bony vestibule**
*use* Inner Ear, Left
*use* Inner Ear, Right
**Botallo's duct** *use* Artery, Pulmonary, Left
**Bovine pericardial valve** *use* Zooplastic Tissue in Heart and Great Vessels
**Bovine pericardium graft** *use* Zooplastic Tissue in Heart and Great Vessels
**BP (blood pressure)** *see* Measurement, Arterial 4AØ3
**Brachial (lateral) lymph node**
*use* Lymphatic, Left Axillary
*use* Lymphatic, Right Axillary
**Brachialis muscle**
*use* Upper Arm Muscle, Left
*use* Upper Arm Muscle, Right
**Brachiocephalic artery** *use* Innominate Artery
**Brachiocephalic trunk** *use* Innominate Artery
**Brachiocephalic vein**
*use* Innominate Vein, Left
*use* Innominate Vein, Right
**Brachioradialis muscle**
*use* Lower Arm and Wrist Muscle, Left
*use* Lower Arm and Wrist Muscle, Right
**Brachytherapy**
Abdomen DW13
Adrenal Gland DG12
Bile Ducts DF12
Bladder DT12
Bone Marrow D71Ø
Brain DØ1Ø
Brain Stem DØ11
Breast
Left DM1Ø
Right DM11
Bronchus DB11
Cervix DU11
Chest DW12
Chest Wall DB17
Colon DD15
Diaphragm DB18
Duodenum DD12
Ear D91Ø
Esophagus DD1Ø
Eye D81Ø
Gallbladder DF11
Gland
Adrenal DG12
Parathyroid DG14
Pituitary DG1Ø
Thyroid DG15
Glands, Salivary D916
Head and Neck DW11

**Brachytherapy** — *continued*
Hypopharynx D913
Ileum DD14
Jejunum DD13
Kidney DT1Ø
Larynx D91B
Liver DF1Ø
Lung DB12
Lymphatics
Abdomen D716
Axillary D714
Inguinal D718
Neck D713
Pelvis D717
Thorax D715
Mediastinum DB16
Mouth D914
Nasopharynx D91D
Neck and Head DW11
Nerve, Peripheral DØ17
Nose D911
Oropharynx D91F
Ovary DU1Ø
Palate
Hard D918
Soft D919
Pancreas DF13
Parathyroid Gland DG14
Pelvic Region DW16
Pineal Body DG11
Pituitary Gland DG1Ø
Pleura DB15
Prostate DV1Ø
Rectum DD17
Sinuses D917
Spinal Cord DØ16
Spleen D712
Stomach DD11
Testis DV11
Thymus D711
Thyroid Gland DG15
Tongue D915
Trachea DB1Ø
Ureter DT11
Urethra DT13
Uterus DU12
**Brachytherapy seeds** *use* Radioactive Element
**Broad ligament** *use* Uterine Supporting Structure
**Bronchial artery** *use* Upper Artery
**Bronchography**
*see* Fluoroscopy, Respiratory System BB1
*see* Plain Radiography, Respiratory System BBØ
**Bronchoplasty**
*see* Repair, Respiratory System ØBQ
*see* Supplement, Respiratory System ØBU
**Bronchorrhaphy** *see* Repair, Respiratory System ØBQ
**Bronchoscopy** ØBJØ8ZZ
**Bronchotomy** *see* Drainage, Respiratory System ØB9
**Bronchus Intermedius** *use* Main Bronchus, Right
**BRYAN® Cervical Disc System** *use* Synthetic Substitute
**Buccal gland** *use* Buccal Mucosa
**Buccinator lymph node** *use* Lymphatic, Head
**Buccinator muscle** *use* Facial Muscle
**Buckling, scleral with implant** *see* Supplement, Eye Ø8U
**Bulbospongiosus muscle** *use* Perineum Muscle
**Bulbourethral (Cowper's) gland** *use* Urethra
**Bundle of His** *use* Conduction Mechanism
**Bundle of Kent** *use* Conduction Mechanism
**Bunionectomy** *see* Excision, Lower Bones ØQB
**Bursectomy**
*see* Excision, Bursae and Ligaments ØMB
*see* Resection, Bursae and Ligaments ØMT
**Bursocentesis** *see* Drainage, Bursae and Ligaments ØM9
**Bursography**
*see* Plain Radiography, Non-Axial Lower Bones BQØ
*see* Plain Radiography, Non-Axial Upper Bones BPØ
**Bursotomy**
*see* Division, Bursae and Ligaments ØM8
*see* Drainage, Bursae and Ligaments ØM9
**BVS 5ØØØ Ventricular Assist Device** *use* Short-term External Heart Assist System in Heart and Great Vessels
**Bypass**
Anterior Chamber
Left Ø8133
Right Ø8123

**Bypass** — *continued*
Aorta
Abdominal Ø41Ø
Thoracic
Ascending/Arch Ø21X
Descending Ø21W
Artery
Axillary
Left Ø316Ø
Right Ø315Ø
Brachial
Left Ø318Ø
Right Ø317Ø
Common Carotid
Left Ø31JØ
Right Ø31HØ
Common Iliac
Left Ø41D
Right Ø41C
Coronary
Four or More Arteries Ø213
One Artery Ø21Ø
Three Arteries Ø212
Two Arteries Ø211
External Carotid
Left Ø31NØ
Right Ø31MØ
External Iliac
Left Ø41J
Right Ø41H
Femoral
Left Ø41L
Right Ø41K
Foot
Left Ø41W
Right Ø41V
Hepatic Ø413
Innominate Ø312Ø
Internal Carotid
Left Ø31LØ
Right Ø31KØ
Internal Iliac
Left Ø41F
Right Ø41E
Intracranial Ø31GØ
Peroneal
Left Ø41U
Right Ø41T
Popliteal
Left Ø41N
Right Ø41M
Pulmonary
Left Ø21R
Right Ø21Q
Pulmonary Trunk Ø21P
Radial
Left Ø31CØ
Right Ø31BØ
Splenic Ø414
Subclavian
Left Ø314Ø
Right Ø313Ø
Temporal
Left Ø31TØ
Right Ø31SØ
Ulnar
Left Ø31AØ
Right Ø319Ø
Atrium
Left Ø217
Right Ø216
Bladder ØT1B
Cavity, Cranial ØW11ØJ
Cecum ØD1H
Cerebral Ventricle ØØ16
Colon
Ascending ØD1K
Descending ØD1M
Sigmoid ØD1N
Transverse ØD1L
Duct
Common Bile ØF19
Cystic ØF18
Hepatic
Common ØF17
Left ØF16
Right ØF15
Lacrimal
Left Ø81Y

**Bypass** — *continued*
Duct — *continued*
Lacrimal — *continued*
Right Ø81X
Pancreatic ØF1D
Accessory ØF1F
Duodenum ØD19
Ear
Left Ø91EØ
Right Ø91DØ
Esophagus ØD15
Lower ØD13
Middle ØD12
Upper ØD11
Fallopian Tube
Left ØU16
Right ØU15
Gallbladder ØF14
Ileum ØD1B
Jejunum ØD1A
Kidney Pelvis
Left ØT14
Right ØT13
Pancreas ØF1G
Pelvic Cavity ØW1J
Peritoneal Cavity ØW1G
Pleural Cavity
Left ØW1B
Right ØW19
Spinal Canal ØØ1U
Stomach ØD16
Trachea ØB11
Ureter
Left ØT17
Right ØT16
Ureters, Bilateral ØT18
Vas Deferens
Bilateral ØV1Q
Left ØV1P
Right ØV1N
Vein
Axillary
Left Ø518
Right Ø517
Azygos Ø51Ø
Basilic
Left Ø51C
Right Ø51B
Brachial
Left Ø51A
Right Ø519
Cephalic
Left Ø51F
Right Ø51D
Colic Ø617
Common Iliac
Left Ø61D
Right Ø61C
Esophageal Ø613
External Iliac
Left Ø61G
Right Ø61F
External Jugular
Left Ø51Q
Right Ø51P
Face
Left Ø51V
Right Ø51T
Femoral
Left Ø61N
Right Ø61M
Foot
Left Ø61V
Right Ø61T
Gastric Ø612
Hand
Left Ø51H
Right Ø51G
Hemiazygos Ø511
Hepatic Ø614
Hypogastric
Left Ø61J
Right Ø61H
Inferior Mesenteric Ø616
Innominate
Left Ø514
Right Ø513
Internal Jugular
Left Ø51N

**Bypass** — *continued*
Vein — *continued*
Internal Jugular — *continued*
Right Ø51M
Intracranial Ø51L
Portal Ø618
Renal
Left Ø61B
Right Ø619
Saphenous
Left Ø61Q
Right Ø61P
Splenic Ø611
Subclavian
Left Ø516
Right Ø515
Superior Mesenteric Ø615
Vertebral
Left Ø51S
Right Ø51R
Vena Cava
Inferior Ø61Ø
Superior Ø21V
Ventricle
Left Ø21L
Right Ø21K
**Bypass, cardiopulmonary** 5A1221Z

# C

**Caesarean section** *see* Extraction, Products of Conception 1ØDØ
**Calcaneocuboid joint**
*use* Tarsal Joint, Left
*use* Tarsal Joint, Right
**Calcaneocuboid ligament**
*use* Foot Bursa and Ligament, Left
*use* Foot Bursa and Ligament, Right
**Calcaneofibular ligament**
*use* Ankle Bursa and Ligament, Left
*use* Ankle Bursa and Ligament, Right
**Calcaneus**
*use* Tarsal, Left
*use* Tarsal, Right
**Cannulation**
*see* Bypass
*see* Dilation
*see* Drainage
*see* Irrigation
**Canthorrhaphy** *see* Repair, Eye Ø8Q
**Canthotomy** *see* Release, Eye Ø8N
**Capitate bone**
*use* Carpal, Left
*use* Carpal, Right
**Capsulectomy, lens** *see* Excision, Eye Ø8B
**Capsulorrhaphy, joint**
*see* Repair, Lower Joints ØSQ
*see* Repair, Upper Joints ØRQ
**Cardia** *use* Esophagogastric Junction
**Cardiac contractility modulation lead** *use* Cardiac Lead in Heart and Great Vessels
**Cardiac event recorder** *use* Monitoring Device
**Cardiac Lead**
Defibrillator
Atrium
Left Ø2H7
Right Ø2H6
Pericardium Ø2HN
Vein, Coronary Ø2H4
Ventricle
Left Ø2HL
Right Ø2HK
Insertion of device in
Atrium
Left Ø2H7
Right Ø2H6
Pericardium Ø2HN
Vein, Coronary Ø2H4
Ventricle
Left Ø2HL
Right Ø2HK
Pacemaker
Atrium
Left Ø2H7
Right Ø2H6
Pericardium Ø2HN
Vein, Coronary Ø2H4
**Cardiac Lead** — *continued*
Pacemaker — *continued*
Ventricle
Left Ø2HL
Right Ø2HK
Removal of device from, Heart Ø2PA
Revision of device in, Heart Ø2WA
**Cardiac plexus** *use* Thoracic Sympathetic Nerve
**Cardiac Resynchronization Defibrillator Pulse Generator**
Abdomen ØJH8
Chest ØJH6
**Cardiac Resynchronization Pacemaker Pulse Generator**
Abdomen ØJH8
Chest ØJH6
**Cardiac resynchronization therapy (CRT) lead**
*use* Cardiac Lead, Defibrillator in Ø2H
*use* Cardiac Lead, Pacemaker in Ø2H
**Cardiac Rhythm Related Device**
Insertion of device in
Abdomen ØJH8
Chest ØJH6
Removal of device from, Subcutaneous Tissue and Fascia, Trunk ØJPT
Revision of device in, Subcutaneous Tissue and Fascia, Trunk ØJWT
**Cardiocentesis** *see* Drainage, Pericardial Cavity ØW9D
**Cardioesophageal junction** *use* Esophagogastric Junction
**Cardiolysis** *see* Release, Heart and Great Vessels Ø2N
**CardioMEMS® pressure sensor** *use* Monitoring Device, Pressure Sensor in Ø2H
**Cardiomyotomy** *see* Division, Esophagogastric Junction ØD84
**Cardioplegia** *see* Introduction of substance in or on, Heart 3EØ8
**Cardiorrhaphy** *see* Repair, Heart and Great Vessels Ø2Q
**Cardioversion** 5A22Ø4Z
**Caregiver Training** FØFZ
**Caroticotympanic artery**
*use* Internal Carotid Artery, Left
*use* Internal Carotid Artery, Right
**Carotid glomus**
*use* Carotid Bodies, Bilateral
*use* Carotid Body, Left
*use* Carotid Body, Right
**Carotid sinus**
*use* Internal Carotid Artery, Left
*use* Internal Carotid Artery, Right
**Carotid (artery) sinus (baroreceptor) lead** *use* Stimulator Lead in Upper Arteries
**Carotid sinus nerve** *use* Glossopharyngeal Nerve
**Carotid WALLSTENT® Monorail® Endoprosthesis** *use* Intraluminal Device
**Carpectomy**
*see* Excision, Upper Bones ØPB
*see* Resection, Upper Bones ØPT
**Carpometacarpal ligament**
*use* Hand Bursa and Ligament, Left
*use* Hand Bursa and Ligament, Right
**Casting** *see* Immobilization
**CAT scan** *see* Computerized Tomography (CT Scan)
**Catheterization**
*see* Dilation
*see* Drainage
*see* Insertion of device in
*see* Irrigation
Heart *see* Measurement, Cardiac 4AØ2
Umbilical vein, for infusion Ø6HØ33T
**Cauda equina** *use* Spinal Cord, Lumbar
**Cauterization**
*see* Destruction
*see* Repair
**Cavernous plexus** *use* Head and Neck Sympathetic Nerve
**CBMA (Concentrated Bone Marrow Aspirate)** *use* Concentrated Bone Marrow Aspirate
**CBMA (Concentrated Bone Marrow Aspirate) injection, intramuscular** XKØ23Ø3
**Cecectomy**
*see* Excision, Cecum ØDBH
*see* Resection, Cecum ØDTH
**Cecocolostomy**
*see* Bypass, Gastrointestinal System ØD1
*see* Drainage, Gastrointestinal System ØD9
**Cecopexy**
*see* Repair, Cecum ØDQH
**Cecopexy** — *continued*
*see* Reposition, Cecum ØDSH
**Cecoplication** *see* Restriction, Cecum ØDVH
**Cecorrhaphy** *see* Repair, Cecum ØDQH
**Cecostomy**
*see* Bypass, Cecum ØD1H
*see* Drainage, Cecum ØD9H
**Cecotomy** *see* Drainage, Cecum ØD9H
**Ceftazidime-Avibactam Anti-infective** XWØ
**Celiac ganglion** *use* Abdominal Sympathetic Nerve
**Celiac lymph node** *use* Lymphatic, Aortic
**Celiac (solar) plexus** *use* Abdominal Sympathetic Nerve
**Celiac trunk** *use* Celiac Artery
**Central axillary lymph node**
*use* Lymphatic, Left Axillary
*use* Lymphatic, Right Axillary
**Central venous pressure** *see* Measurement, Venous 4AØ4
**Centrimag® Blood Pump** *use* Short-term External Heart Assist System in Heart and Great Vessels
**Cephalogram** BNØØZZZ
**Ceramic on ceramic bearing surface** *use* Synthetic Substitute, Ceramic in ØSR
**Cerclage** *see* Restriction
**Cerebral aqueduct (Sylvius)** *use* Cerebral Ventricle
**Cerebral Embolic Filtration, Dual Filter** X2A5312
**Cerebrum** *use* Brain
**Cervical esophagus** *use* Esophagus, Upper
**Cervical facet joint**
*use* Cervical Vertebral Joint
*use* Cervical Vertebral Joint, 2 or more
**Cervical ganglion** *use* Head and Neck Sympathetic Nerve
**Cervical interspinous ligament** *use* Bursa and Ligament, Head and Neck
**Cervical intertransverse ligament** *use* Bursa and Ligament, Head and Neck
**Cervical ligamentum flavum** *use* Bursa and Ligament, Head and Neck
**Cervical lymph node**
*use* Lymphatic, Left Neck
*use* Lymphatic, Right Neck
**Cervicectomy**
*see* Excision, Cervix ØUBC
*see* Resection, Cervix ØUTC
**Cervicothoracic facet joint** *use* Cervicothoracic Vertebral Joint
**Cesarean section** *see* Extraction, Products of Conception 1ØDØ
**Cesium-131 Collagen Implant** *use* Radioactive Element, Cesium-131 Collagen Implant in ØØH
**Change device in**
Abdominal Wall ØW2FX
Back
Lower ØW2LX
Upper ØW2KX
Bladder ØT2BX
Bone
Facial ØN2WX
Lower ØQ2YX
Nasal ØN2BX
Upper ØP2YX
Bone Marrow Ø72TX
Brain ØØ2ØX
Breast
Left ØH2UX
Right ØH2TX
Bursa and Ligament
Lower ØM2YX
Upper ØM2XX
Cavity, Cranial ØW21X
Chest Wall ØW28X
Cisterna Chyli Ø72LX
Diaphragm ØB2TX
Duct
Hepatobiliary ØF2BX
Pancreatic ØF2DX
Ear
Left Ø92JX
Right Ø92HX
Epididymis and Spermatic Cord ØV2MX
Extremity
Lower
Left ØY2BX
Right ØY29X
Upper
Left ØX27X
Right ØX26X

**Change device in** — *continued*
  Eye
    Left Ø821X
    Right Ø82ØX
  Face ØW22X
  Fallopian Tube ØU28X
  Gallbladder ØF24X
  Gland
    Adrenal ØG25X
    Endocrine ØG2SX
    Pituitary ØG2ØX
    Salivary ØC2AX
  Head ØW2ØX
  Intestinal Tract
    Lower ØD2DXUZ
    Upper ØD2ØXUZ
  Jaw
    Lower ØW25X
    Upper ØW24X
  Joint
    Lower ØS2YX
    Upper ØR2YX
  Kidney ØT25X
  Larynx ØC2SX
  Liver ØF2ØX
  Lung
    Left ØB2LX
    Right ØB2KX
  Lymphatic Ø72NX
    Thoracic Duct Ø72KX
  Mediastinum ØW2CX
  Mesentery ØD2VX
  Mouth and Throat ØC2YX
  Muscle
    Lower ØK2YX
    Upper ØK2XX
  Nasal Mucosa and Soft Tissue Ø92KX
  Neck ØW26X
  Nerve
    Cranial ØØ2EX
    Peripheral Ø12YX
  Omentum ØD2UX
  Ovary ØU23X
  Pancreas ØF2GX
  Parathyroid Gland ØG2RX
  Pelvic Cavity ØW2JX
  Penis ØV2SX
  Pericardial Cavity ØW2DX
  Perineum
    Female ØW2NX
    Male ØW2MX
  Peritoneal Cavity ØW2GX
  Peritoneum ØD2WX
  Pineal Body ØG21X
  Pleura ØB2QX
  Pleural Cavity
    Left ØW2BX
    Right ØW29X
  Products of Conception 1Ø2Ø7
  Prostate and Seminal Vesicles ØV24X
  Retroperitoneum ØW2HX
  Scrotum and Tunica Vaginalis ØV28X
  Sinus Ø92YX
  Skin ØH2PX
  Skull ØN2ØX
  Spinal Canal ØØ2UX
  Spleen Ø72PX
  Subcutaneous Tissue and Fascia
    Head and Neck ØJ2SX
    Lower Extremity ØJ2WX
    Trunk ØJ2TX
    Upper Extremity ØJ2VX
  Tendon
    Lower ØL2YX
    Upper ØL2XX
  Testis ØV2DX
  Thymus Ø72MX
  Thyroid Gland ØG2KX
  Trachea ØB21
  Tracheobronchial Tree ØB2ØX
  Ureter ØT29X
  Urethra ØT2DX
  Uterus and Cervix ØU2DXHZ
  Vagina and Cul-de-sac ØU2HXGZ
  Vas Deferens ØV2RX
  Vulva ØU2MX
**Change device in or on**
  Abdominal Wall 2WØ3X
  Anorectal 2YØ3X5Z

**Change device in or on** — *continued*
  Arm
    Lower
      Left 2WØDX
      Right 2WØCX
    Upper
      Left 2WØBX
      Right 2WØAX
  Back 2WØ5X
  Chest Wall 2WØ4X
  Ear 2YØ2X5Z
  Extremity
    Lower
      Left 2WØMX
      Right 2WØLX
    Upper
      Left 2WØ9X
      Right 2WØ8X
  Face 2WØ1X
  Finger
    Left 2WØKX
    Right 2WØJX
  Foot
    Left 2WØTX
    Right 2WØSX
  Genital Tract, Female 2YØ4X5Z
  Hand
    Left 2WØFX
    Right 2WØEX
  Head 2WØØX
  Inguinal Region
    Left 2WØ7X
    Right 2WØ6X
  Leg
    Lower
      Left 2WØRX
      Right 2WØQX
    Upper
      Left 2WØPX
      Right 2WØNX
  Mouth and Pharynx 2YØØX5Z
  Nasal 2YØ1X5Z
  Neck 2WØ2X
  Thumb
    Left 2WØHX
    Right 2WØGX
  Toe
    Left 2WØVX
    Right 2WØUX
  Urethra 2YØ5X5Z
**Chemoembolization** *see* Introduction of substance in or on
**Chemosurgery, Skin** 3EØØXTZ
**Chemothalamectomy** *see* Destruction, Thalamus ØØ59
**Chemotherapy, Infusion for cancer** *see* Introduction of substance in or on
**Chest x-ray** *see* Plain Radiography, Chest BWØ3
**Chiropractic Manipulation**
  Abdomen 9WB9X
  Cervical 9WB1X
  Extremities
    Lower 9WB6X
    Upper 9WB7X
  Head 9WBØX
  Lumbar 9WB3X
  Pelvis 9WB5X
  Rib Cage 9WB8X
  Sacrum 9WB4X
  Thoracic 9WB2X
**Choana** *use* Nasopharynx
**Cholangiogram**
  *see* Fluoroscopy, Hepatobiliary System and Pancreas BF1
  *see* Plain Radiography, Hepatobiliary System and Pancreas BFØ
**Cholecystectomy**
  *see* Excision, Gallbladder ØFB4
  *see* Resection, Gallbladder ØFT4
**Cholecystojejunostomy**
  *see* Bypass, Hepatobiliary System and Pancreas ØF1
  *see* Drainage, Hepatobiliary System and Pancreas ØF9
**Cholecystopexy**
  *see* Repair, Gallbladder ØFQ4
  *see* Reposition, Gallbladder ØFS4
**Cholecystoscopy** ØFJ44ZZ
**Cholecystostomy**
  *see* Bypass, Gallbladder ØF14
  *see* Drainage, Gallbladder ØF94

**Cholecystotomy** *see* Drainage, Gallbladder ØF94
**Choledochectomy**
  *see* Excision, Hepatobiliary System and Pancreas ØFB
  *see* Resection, Hepatobiliary System and Pancreas ØFT
**Choledocholithotomy** *see* Extirpation, Duct, Common Bile ØFC9
**Choledochoplasty**
  *see* Repair, Hepatobiliary System and Pancreas ØFQ
  *see* Replacement, Hepatobiliary System and Pancreas ØFR
  *see* Supplement, Hepatobiliary System and Pancreas ØFU
**Choledochoscopy** ØFJB8ZZ
**Choledochotomy** *see* Drainage, Hepatobiliary System and Pancreas ØF9
**Cholelithotomy** *see* Extirpation, Hepatobiliary System and Pancreas ØFC
**Chondrectomy**
  *see* Excision, Lower Joints ØSB
  *see* Excision, Upper Joints ØRB
  Knee *see* Excision, Lower Joints ØSB
  Semilunar cartilage *see* Excision, Lower Joints ØSB
**Chondroglossus muscle** *use* Tongue, Palate, Pharynx Muscle
**Chorda tympani** *use* Nerve, Facial
**Chordotomy** *see* Division, Central Nervous System and Cranial Nerves ØØ8
**Choroid plexus** *use* Cerebral Ventricle
**Choroidectomy**
  *see* Excision, Eye Ø8B
  *see* Resection, Eye Ø8T
**Ciliary body**
  *use* Eye, Left
  *use* Eye, Right
**Ciliary ganglion** *use* Head and Neck Sympathetic Nerve
**Circle of Willis** *use* Intracranial Artery
**Circumcision** ØVTTXZZ
**Circumflex iliac artery**
  *use* Femoral Artery, Left
  *use* Femoral Artery, Right
**Clamp and rod internal fixation system (CRIF)**
  *use* Internal Fixation Device in Lower Bones
  *use* Internal Fixation Device in Upper Bones
**Clamping** *see* Occlusion
**Claustrum** *use* Basal Ganglia
**Claviculectomy**
  *see* Excision, Upper Bones ØPB
  *see* Resection, Upper Bones ØPT
**Claviculotomy**
  *see* Division, Upper Bones ØP8
  *see* Drainage, Upper Bones ØP9
**Clipping, aneurysm**
  *see* Occlusion using Extraluminal Device
  *see* Restriction using Extraluminal Device
**Clitorectomy, clitoridectomy**
  *see* Excision, Clitoris ØUBJ
  *see* Resection, Clitoris ØUTJ
**Clolar** *use* Clofarabine
**Closure**
  *see* Occlusion
  *see* Repair
**Clysis** *see* Introduction of substance in or on
**Coagulation** *see* Destruction
**COALESCE® radiolucent interbody fusion device** *use* Interbody Fusion Device, Radiolucent Porous in New Technology
**CoAxia NeuroFlo catheter** *use* Intraluminal Device
**Cobalt/chromium head and polyethylene socket** *use* Synthetic Substitute, Metal on Polyethylene in ØSR
**Cobalt/chromium head and socket** *use* Synthetic Substitute, Metal in ØSR
**Coccygeal body** *use* Coccygeal Glomus
**Coccygeus muscle**
  *use* Trunk Muscle, Left
  *use* Trunk Muscle, Right
**Cochlea**
  *use* Inner Ear, Left
  *use* Inner Ear, Right
**Cochlear implant (CI), multiple channel (electrode)**
  *use* Hearing Device, Multiple Channel Cochlear Prosthesis in Ø9H
**Cochlear implant (CI), single channel (electrode)** *use* Hearing Device, Single Channel Cochlear Prosthesis in Ø9H
**Cochlear Implant Treatment** FØBZØ
**Cochlear nerve** *use* Acoustic Nerve

**COGNIS® CRT-D** *use* Cardiac Resynchronization Defibrillator Pulse Generator in ØJH
**COHERE® radiolucent interbody fusion device** *use* Interbody Fusion Device, Radiolucent Porous in New Technology
**Colectomy**
*see* Excision, Gastrointestinal System ØDB
*see* Resection, Gastrointestinal System ØDT
**Collapse** *see* Occlusion
**Collection from**
Breast, Breast Milk 8EØHX62
Indwelling Device
Circulatory System
Blood 8CØ2X6K
Other Fluid 8CØ2X6L
Nervous System
Cerebrospinal Fluid 8CØ1X6J
Other Fluid 8CØ1X6L
Integumentary System, Breast Milk 8EØHX62
Reproductive System, Male, Sperm 8EØVX63
**Colocentesis** *see* Drainage, Gastrointestinal System ØD9
**Colofixation**
*see* Repair, Gastrointestinal System ØDQ
*see* Reposition, Gastrointestinal System ØDS
**Cololysis** *see* Release, Gastrointestinal System ØDN
**Colonic Z-Stent®** *use* Intraluminal Device
**Colonoscopy** ØDJD8ZZ
**Colopexy**
*see* Repair, Gastrointestinal System ØDQ
*see* Reposition, Gastrointestinal System ØDS
**Coloplication** *see* Restriction, Gastrointestinal System ØDV
**Coloproctectomy**
*see* Excision, Gastrointestinal System ØDB
*see* Resection, Gastrointestinal System ØDT
**Coloproctostomy**
*see* Bypass, Gastrointestinal System ØD1
*see* Drainage, Gastrointestinal System ØD9
**Colopuncture** *see* Drainage, Gastrointestinal System ØD9
**Colorrhaphy** *see* Repair, Gastrointestinal System ØDQ
**Colostomy**
*see* Bypass, Gastrointestinal System ØD1
*see* Drainage, Gastrointestinal System ØD9
**Colpectomy**
*see* Excision, Vagina ØUBG
*see* Resection, Vagina ØUTG
**Colpocentesis** *see* Drainage, Vagina ØU9G
**Colpopexy**
*see* Repair, Vagina ØUQG
*see* Reposition, Vagina ØUSG
**Colpoplasty**
*see* Repair, Vagina ØUQG
*see* Supplement, Vagina ØUUG
**Colporrhaphy** *see* Repair, Vagina ØUQG
**Colposcopy** ØUJH8ZZ
**Columella** *use* Nasal Mucosa and Soft Tissue
**Common digital vein**
*use* Foot Vein, Left
*use* Foot Vein, Right
**Common facial vein**
*use* Face Vein, Left
*use* Face Vein, Right
**Common fibular nerve** *use* Peroneal Nerve
**Common hepatic artery** *use* Hepatic Artery
**Common iliac (subaortic) lymph node** *use* Lymphatic, Pelvis
**Common interosseous artery**
*use* Ulnar Artery, Left
*use* Ulnar Artery, Right
**Common peroneal nerve** *use* Peroneal Nerve
**Complete (SE) stent** *use* Intraluminal Device
**Compression**
*see* Restriction
Abdominal Wall 2W13X
Arm
Lower
Left 2W1DX
Right 2W1CX
Upper
Left 2W1BX
Right 2W1AX
Back 2W15X
Chest Wall 2W14X
Extremity
Lower
Left 2W1MX
Right 2W1LX

**Compression** — *continued*
Extremity — *continued*
Upper
Left 2W19X
Right 2W18X
Face 2W11X
Finger
Left 2W1KX
Right 2W1JX
Foot
Left 2W1TX
Right 2W1SX
Hand
Left 2W1FX
Right 2W1EX
Head 2W1ØX
Inguinal Region
Left 2W17X
Right 2W16X
Leg
Lower
Left 2W1RX
Right 2W1QX
Upper
Left 2W1PX
Right 2W1NX
Neck 2W12X
Thumb
Left 2W1HX
Right 2W1GX
Toe
Left 2W1VX
Right 2W1UX
**Computer Assisted Procedure**
Extremity
Lower
With Computerized Tomography 8EØYXBG
With Fluoroscopy 8EØYXBF
With Magnetic Resonance Imaging 8EØYXBH
No Qualifier 8EØYXBZ
Upper
With Computerized Tomography 8EØXXBG
With Fluoroscopy 8EØXXBF
With Magnetic Resonance Imaging 8EØXXBH
No Qualifier 8EØXXBZ
Head and Neck Region
With Computerized Tomography 8EØ9XBG
With Fluoroscopy 8EØ9XBF
With Magnetic Resonance Imaging 8EØ9XBH
No Qualifier 8EØ9XBZ
Trunk Region
With Computerized Tomography 8EØWXBG
With Fluoroscopy 8EØWXBF
With Magnetic Resonance Imaging 8EØWXBH
No Qualifier 8EØWXBZ
**Computerized Tomography (CT Scan)**
Abdomen BW2Ø
Chest and Pelvis BW25
Abdomen and Chest BW24
Abdomen and Pelvis BW21
Airway, Trachea BB2F
Ankle
Left BQ2H
Right BQ2G
Aorta
Abdominal B42Ø
Intravascular Optical Coherence B42ØZ2Z
Thoracic B32Ø
Intravascular Optical Coherence B32ØZ2Z
Arm
Left BP2F
Right BP2E
Artery
Celiac B421
Intravascular Optical Coherence B421Z2Z
Common Carotid
Bilateral B325
Intravascular Optical Coherence B325Z2Z
Coronary
Bypass Graft
Intravascular Optical Coherence B223Z2Z
Multiple B223
Multiple B221
Intravascular Optical Coherence B221Z2Z
Internal Carotid
Bilateral B328
Intravascular Optical Coherence B328Z2Z
Intracranial B32R
Intravascular Optical Coherence B32RZ2Z

**Computerized Tomography (CT Scan)** — *continued*
Artery — *continued*
Lower Extremity
Bilateral B42H
Intravascular Optical Coherence B42HZ2Z
Left B42G
Intravascular Optical Coherence B42GZ2Z
Right B42F
Intravascular Optical Coherence B42FZ2Z
Pelvic B42C
Intravascular Optical Coherence B42CZ2Z
Pulmonary
Left B32T
Intravascular Optical Coherence B32TZ2Z
Right B32S
Intravascular Optical Coherence B32SZ2Z
Renal
Bilateral B428
Intravascular Optical Coherence B428Z2Z
Transplant B42M
Intravascular Optical Coherence B42MZ2Z
Superior Mesenteric B424
Intravascular Optical Coherence B424Z2Z
Vertebral
Bilateral B32G
Intravascular Optical Coherence B32GZ2Z
Bladder BT2Ø
Bone
Facial BN25
Temporal BN2F
Brain BØ2Ø
Calcaneus
Left BQ2K
Right BQ2J
Cerebral Ventricle BØ28
Chest, Abdomen and Pelvis BW25
Chest and Abdomen BW24
Cisterna BØ27
Clavicle
Left BP25
Right BP24
Coccyx BR2F
Colon BD24
Ear B92Ø
Elbow
Left BP2H
Right BP2G
Extremity
Lower
Left BQ2S
Right BQ2R
Upper
Bilateral BP2V
Left BP2U
Right BP2T
Eye
Bilateral B827
Left B826
Right B825
Femur
Left BQ24
Right BQ23
Fibula
Left BQ2C
Right BQ2B
Finger
Left BP2S
Right BP2R
Foot
Left BQ2M
Right BQ2L
Forearm
Left BP2K
Right BP2J
Gland
Adrenal, Bilateral BG22
Parathyroid BG23
Parotid, Bilateral B926
Salivary, Bilateral B92D
Submandibular, Bilateral B929
Thyroid BG24
Hand
Left BP2P
Right BP2N
Hands and Wrists, Bilateral BP2Q
Head BW28
Head and Neck BW29
Heart
Intravascular Optical Coherence B226Z2Z





Subterms under main terms may continue to next column or page

**Continuous Negative Airway Pressure**
24-96 Consecutive Hours, Ventilation 5AØ9459
Greater than 96 Consecutive Hours, Ventilation 5AØ9559
Less than 24 Consecutive Hours, Ventilation 5AØ9359
**Continuous Positive Airway Pressure**
24-96 Consecutive Hours, Ventilation 5AØ9457
Greater than 96 Consecutive Hours, Ventilation 5AØ9557
Less than 24 Consecutive Hours, Ventilation 5AØ9357
**Continuous renal replacement therapy (CRRT)** 5A1D90Z
**Contraceptive Device**
Change device in, Uterus and Cervix ØU2DXHZ
Insertion of device in
Cervix ØUHC
Subcutaneous Tissue and Fascia
Abdomen ØJH8
Chest ØJH6
Lower Arm
Left ØJHH
Right ØJHG
Lower Leg
Left ØJHP
Right ØJHN
Upper Arm
Left ØJHF
Right ØJHD
Upper Leg
Left ØJHM
Right ØJHL
Uterus ØUH9
Removal of device from
Subcutaneous Tissue and Fascia
Lower Extremity ØJPW
Trunk ØJPT
Upper Extremity ØJPV
Uterus and Cervix ØUPD
Revision of device in
Subcutaneous Tissue and Fascia
Lower Extremity ØJWW
Trunk ØJWT
Upper Extremity ØJWV
Uterus and Cervix ØUWD
**Contractility Modulation Device**
Abdomen ØJH8
Chest ØJH6
**Control bleeding in**
Abdominal Wall ØW3F
Ankle Region
Left ØY3L
Right ØY3K
Arm
Lower
Left ØX3F
Right ØX3D
Upper
Left ØX39
Right ØX38
Axilla
Left ØX35
Right ØX34
Back
Lower ØW3L
Upper ØW3K
Buttock
Left ØY31
Right ØY3Ø
Cavity, Cranial ØW31
Chest Wall ØW38
Elbow Region
Left ØX3C
Right ØX3B
Extremity
Lower
Left ØY3B
Right ØY39
Upper
Left ØX37
Right ØX36
Face ØW32
Femoral Region
Left ØY38
Right ØY37
Foot
Left ØY3N
Right ØY3M
Gastrointestinal Tract ØW3P
Genitourinary Tract ØW3R
**Control bleeding in** — *continued*
Hand
Left ØX3K
Right ØX3J
Head ØW3Ø
Inguinal Region
Left ØY36
Right ØY35
Jaw
Lower ØW35
Upper ØW34
Knee Region
Left ØY3G
Right ØY3F
Leg
Lower
Left ØY3J
Right ØY3H
Upper
Left ØY3D
Right ØY3C
Mediastinum ØW3C
Neck ØW36
Oral Cavity and Throat ØW33
Pelvic Cavity ØW3J
Pericardial Cavity ØW3D
Perineum
Female ØW3N
Male ØW3M
Peritoneal Cavity ØW3G
Pleural Cavity
Left ØW3B
Right ØW39
Respiratory Tract ØW3Q
Retroperitoneum ØW3H
Shoulder Region
Left ØX33
Right ØX32
Wrist Region
Left ØX3H
Right ØX3G
**Conus arteriosus** *use* Ventricle, Right
**Conus medullaris** *use* Lumbar Spinal Cord
**Conversion**
Cardiac rhythm 5A22Ø4Z
Gastrostomy to jejunostomy feeding device *see* Insertion of device in, Jejunum ØDHA
**Cook Biodesign® Fistula Plug(s)** *use* Nonautologous Tissue Substitute
**Cook Biodesign® Hernia Graft(s)** *use* Nonautologous Tissue Substitute
**Cook Biodesign® Layered Graft(s)** *use* Nonautologous Tissue Substitute
**Cook Zenaprom™ Layered Graft(s)** *use* Nonautologous Tissue Substitute
**Cook Zenith AAA Endovascular Graft**
*use* Intraluminal Device
*use* Intraluminal Device, Branched or Fenestrated, One or Two Arteries in Ø4V
*use* Intraluminal Device, Branched or Fenestrated, Three or More Arteries in Ø4V
**Coracoacromial ligament**
*use* Shoulder Bursa and Ligament, Left
*use* Shoulder Bursa and Ligament, Right
**Coracobrachialis muscle**
*use* Upper Arm Muscle, Left
*use* Upper Arm Muscle, Right
**Coracoclavicular ligament**
*use* Shoulder Bursa and Ligament, Left
*use* Shoulder Bursa and Ligament, Right
**Coracohumeral ligament**
*use* Shoulder Bursa and Ligament, Left
*use* Shoulder Bursa and Ligament, Right
**Coracoid process**
*use* Scapula, Left
*use* Scapula, Right
**Cordotomy** *see* Division, Central Nervous System and Cranial Nerves ØØ8
**Core needle biopsy** *see* Excision with qualifier Diagnostic
**CoreValve transcatheter aortic valve** *use* Zooplastic Tissue in Heart and Great Vessels
**Cormet Hip Resurfacing System** *use* Resurfacing Device in Lower Joints
**Corniculate cartilage** *use* Larynx
**CoRoent® XL** *use* Interbody Fusion Device in Lower Joints
**Coronary arteriography**
*see* Fluoroscopy, Heart B21
*see* Plain Radiography, Heart B2Ø
**Corox (OTW) Bipolar Lead**
*use* Cardiac Lead, Defibrillator in Ø2H
*use* Cardiac Lead, Pacemaker in Ø2H
**Corpus callosum** *use* Brain
**Corpus cavernosum** *use* Penis
**Corpus spongiosum** *use* Penis
**Corpus striatum** *use* Basal Ganglia
**Corrugator supercilii muscle** *use* Facial Muscle
**Cortical strip neurostimulator lead** *use* Neurostimulator Lead in Central Nervous System and Cranial Nerves
**Costatectomy**
*see* Excision, Upper Bones ØPB
*see* Resection, Upper Bones ØPT
**Costectomy**
*see* Excision, Upper Bones ØPB
*see* Resection, Upper Bones ØPT
**Costocervical trunk**
*use* Subclavian Artery, Left
*use* Subclavian Artery, Right
**Costochondrectomy**
*see* Excision, Upper Bones ØPB
*see* Resection, Upper Bones ØPT
**Costoclavicular ligament**
*use* Shoulder Bursa and Ligament, Left
*use* Shoulder Bursa and Ligament, Right
**Costosternoplasty**
*see* Repair, Upper Bones ØPQ
*see* Replacement, Upper Bones ØPR
*see* Supplement, Upper Bones ØPU
**Costotomy**
*see* Division, Upper Bones ØP8
*see* Drainage, Upper Bones ØP9
**Costotransverse joint** *use* Joint, Thoracic Vertebral
**Costotransverse ligament**
*use* Rib(s) Bursa and Ligament
*use* Sternum Bursa and Ligament
**Costovertebral joint** *use* Thoracic Vertebral Joint
**Costoxiphoid ligament**
*use* Rib(s) Bursa and Ligament
*use* Sternum Bursa and Ligament
**Counseling**
Family, for substance abuse, Other Family Counseling HZ63ZZZ
Group
12-Step HZ43ZZZ
Behavioral HZ41ZZZ
Cognitive HZ4ØZZZ
Cognitive-Behavioral HZ42ZZZ
Confrontational HZ48ZZZ
Continuing Care HZ49ZZZ
Infectious Disease
Post-Test HZ4CZZZ
Pre-Test HZ4CZZZ
Interpersonal HZ44ZZZ
Motivational Enhancement HZ47ZZZ
Psychoeducation HZ46ZZZ
Spiritual HZ4BZZZ
Vocational HZ45ZZZ
Individual
12-Step HZ33ZZZ
Behavioral HZ31ZZZ
Cognitive HZ3ØZZZ
Cognitive-Behavioral HZ32ZZZ
Confrontational HZ38ZZZ
Continuing Care HZ39ZZZ
Infectious Disease
Post-Test HZ3CZZZ
Pre-Test HZ3CZZZ
Interpersonal HZ34ZZZ
Motivational Enhancement HZ37ZZZ
Psychoeducation HZ36ZZZ
Spiritual HZ3BZZZ
Vocational HZ35ZZZ
Mental Health Services
Educational GZ6ØZZZ
Other Counseling GZ63ZZZ
Vocational GZ61ZZZ
**Countershock, cardiac** 5A22Ø4Z
**Cowper's (bulbourethral) gland** *use* Urethra
**CPAP (continuous positive airway pressure)** *see* Assistance, Respiratory 5AØ9
**Craniectomy**
*see* Excision, Head and Facial Bones ØNB
*see* Resection, Head and Facial Bones ØNT
**Cranioplasty**
*see* Repair, Head and Facial Bones ØNQ

**Cranioplasty** — *continued*
*see* Replacement, Head and Facial Bones ØNR
*see* Supplement, Head and Facial Bones ØNU
**Craniotomy**
*see* Division, Head and Facial Bones ØN8
*see* Drainage, Central Nervous System and Cranial Nerves ØØ9
*see* Drainage, Head and Facial Bones ØN9
**Creation**
Perineum
Female ØW4NØ
Male ØW4MØ
Valve
Aortic Ø24FØ
Mitral Ø24GØ
Tricuspid Ø24JØ
**Cremaster muscle** *use* Muscle, Perineum
**Cribriform plate**
*use* Bone, Ethmoid, Left
*use* Bone, Ethmoid, Right
**Cricoid cartilage** *use* Trachea
**Cricoidectomy** *see* Excision, Larynx ØCBS
**Cricothyroid artery**
*use* Artery, Thyroid, Left
*use* Artery, Thyroid, Right
**Cricothyroid muscle**
*use* Muscle, Neck, Left
*use* Muscle, Neck, Right
**Crisis Intervention** GZ2ZZZZ
**CRRT (Continuous renal replacement therapy)** 5A1D90Z
**Crural fascia**
*use* Subcutaneous Tissue and Fascia, Upper Leg, Left
*use* Subcutaneous Tissue and Fascia, Upper Leg, Right
**Crushing, nerve**
Cranial *see* Destruction, Central Nervous System and Cranial Nerves ØØ5
Peripheral *see* Destruction, Peripheral Nervous System Ø15
**Cryoablation** *see* Destruction
**Cryotherapy** *see* Destruction
**Cryptorchidectomy**
*see* Excision, Male Reproductive System ØVB
*see* Resection, Male Reproductive System ØVT
**Cryptorchiectomy**
*see* Excision, Male Reproductive System ØVB
*see* Resection, Male Reproductive System ØVT
**Cryptotomy**
*see* Division, Gastrointestinal System ØD8
*see* Drainage, Gastrointestinal System ØD9
**CT scan** *see* Computerized Tomography (CT Scan)
**CT sialogram** *see* Computerized Tomography (CT Scan), Ear, Nose, Mouth and Throat B92
**Cubital lymph node**
*use* Lymphatic, Upper Extremity, Left
*use* Lymphatic, Upper Extremity, Right
**Cubital nerve** *use* Nerve, Ulnar
**Cuboid bone**
*use* Tarsal, Left
*use* Tarsal, Right
**Cuboideonavicular joint**
*use* Joint, Tarsal, Left
*use* Joint, Tarsal, Right
**Culdocentesis** *see* Drainage, Cul-de-sac ØU9F
**Culdoplasty**
*see* Repair, Cul-de-sac ØUQF
*see* Supplement, Cul-de-sac ØUUF
**Culdoscopy** ØUJH8ZZ
**Culdotomy** *see* Drainage, Cul-de-sac ØU9F
**Culmen** *use* Cerebellum
**Cultured epidermal cell autograft** *use* Autologous Tissue Substitute
**Cuneiform cartilage** *use* Larynx
**Cuneonavicular joint**
*use* Joint, Tarsal, Left
*use* Joint, Tarsal, Right
**Cuneonavicular ligament**
*use* Bursa and Ligament, Foot, Left
*use* Bursa and Ligament, Foot, Right
**Curettage**
*see* Excision
*see* Extraction
**Cutaneous (transverse) cervical nerve** *use* Nerve, Cervical Plexus
**CVP (central venous pressure)** *see* Measurement, Venous 4AØ4
**Cyclodiathermy** *see* Destruction, Eye Ø85
**Cyclophotocoagulation** *see* Destruction, Eye Ø85
**CYPHER® Stent** *use* Intraluminal Device, Drug-eluting in Heart and Great Vessels
**Cystectomy**
*see* Excision, Bladder ØTBB
*see* Resection, Bladder ØTTB
**Cystocele repair** *see* Repair, Subcutaneous Tissue and Fascia, Pelvic Region ØJQC
**Cystography**
*see* Fluoroscopy, Urinary System BT1
*see* Plain Radiography, Urinary System BTØ
**Cystolithotomy** *see* Extirpation, Bladder ØTCB
**Cystopexy**
*see* Repair, Bladder ØTQB
*see* Reposition, Bladder ØTSB
**Cystoplasty**
*see* Repair, Bladder ØTQB
*see* Replacement, Bladder ØTRB
*see* Supplement, Bladder ØTUB
**Cystorrhaphy** *see* Repair, Bladder ØTQB
**Cystoscopy** ØTJB8ZZ
**Cystostomy** *see* Bypass, Bladder ØT1B
**Cystostomy tube** *use* Drainage Device
**Cystotomy** *see* Drainage, Bladder ØT9B
**Cystourethrography**
*see* Fluoroscopy, Urinary System BT1
*see* Plain Radiography, Urinary System BTØ
**Cystourethroplasty**
*see* Repair, Urinary System ØTQ
*see* Replacement, Urinary System ØTR
*see* Supplement, Urinary System ØTU
**Cytarabine and Daunorubicin Liposome Antineoplastic** XWØ

# D

**DBS lead** *use* Neurostimulator Lead in Central Nervous System and Cranial Nerves
**DeBakey Left Ventricular Assist Device** *use* Implantable Heart Assist System in Heart and Great Vessels
**Debridement**
Excisional *see* Excision
Non-excisional *see* Extraction
**Decompression, Circulatory** 6A15
**Decortication, lung**
*see* Extirpation, Respiratory System ØBC
*see* Release, Respiratory System ØBN
**Deep brain neurostimulator lead** *use* Neurostimulator Lead in Central Nervous System and Cranial Nerves
**Deep cervical fascia**
*use* Subcutaneous Tissue and Fascia, Left Neck
*use* Subcutaneous Tissue and Fascia, Right Neck
**Deep cervical vein**
*use* Vein, Vertebral, Left
*use* Vein, Vertebral, Right
**Deep circumflex iliac artery**
*use* Artery, External Iliac, Left
*use* Artery, External Iliac, Right
**Deep facial vein**
*use* Vein, Face, Left
*use* Vein, Face, Right
**Deep femoral artery**
*use* Artery, Femoral, Left
*use* Artery, Femoral, Right
**Deep femoral (profunda femoris) vein**
*use* Vein, Femoral, Left
*use* Vein, Femoral, Right
**Deep Inferior Epigastric Artery Perforator Flap**
Replacement
Bilateral ØHRVØ77
Left ØHRUØ77
Right ØHRTØ77
Transfer
Left ØKXG
Right ØKXF
**Deep palmar arch**
*use* Artery, Hand, Left
*use* Artery, Hand, Right
**Deep transverse perineal muscle** *use* Muscle, Perineum
**Deferential artery**
*use* Artery, Internal Iliac, Left
*use* Artery, Internal Iliac, Right
**Defibrillator Generator**
Abdomen ØJH8
**Defibrillator Generator** — *continued*
Chest ØJH6
**Defibrotide Sodium Anticoagulant** XWØ
**Defitelio** *use* Defibrotide Sodium Anticoagulant
**Delivery**
Cesarean *see* Extraction, Products of Conception 1ØDØ
Forceps *see* Extraction, Products of Conception 1ØDØ
Manually assisted 1ØEØXZZ
Products of Conception 1ØEØXZZ
Vacuum assisted *see* Extraction, Products of Conception 1ØDØ
**Delta frame external fixator**
*use* External Fixation Device, Hybrid in ØPH
*use* External Fixation Device, Hybrid in ØPS
*use* External Fixation Device, Hybrid in ØQH
*use* External Fixation Device, Hybrid in ØQS
**Delta III Reverse shoulder prosthesis** *use* Synthetic Substitute, Reverse Ball and Socket in ØRR
**Deltoid fascia**
*use* Subcutaneous Tissue and Fascia, Upper Arm, Left
*use* Subcutaneous Tissue and Fascia, Upper Arm, Right
**Deltoid ligament**
*use* Bursa and Ligament, Ankle, Left
*use* Bursa and Ligament, Ankle, Right
**Deltoid muscle**
*use* Muscle, Shoulder, Left
*use* Muscle, Shoulder, Right
**Deltopectoral (infraclavicular) lymph node**
*use* Lymphatic, Upper Extremity, Left
*use* Lymphatic, Upper Extremity, Right
**Denervation**
Cranial nerve *see* Destruction, Central Nervous System and Cranial Nerves ØØ5
Peripheral nerve *see* Destruction, Peripheral Nervous System Ø15
**Dens** *use* Cervical Vertebra
**Densitometry**
Plain Radiography
Femur
Left BQ04ZZ1
Right BQ03ZZ1
Hip
Left BQ01ZZ1
Right BQ00ZZ1
Spine
Cervical BRØØZZ1
Lumbar BRØ9ZZ1
Thoracic BRØ7ZZ1
Whole BRØGZZ1
Ultrasonography
Elbow
Left BP4HZZ1
Right BP4GZZ1
Hand
Left BP4PZZ1
Right BP4NZZ1
Shoulder
Left BP49ZZ1
Right BP48ZZ1
Wrist
Left BP4MZZ1
Right BP4LZZ1
**Denticulate (dentate) ligament** *use* Spinal Meninges
**Depressor anguli oris muscle** *use* Muscle, Facial
**Depressor labii inferioris muscle** *use* Muscle, Facial
**Depressor septi nasi muscle** *use* Muscle, Facial
**Depressor supercilii muscle** *use* Muscle, Facial
**Dermabrasion** *see* Extraction, Skin and Breast ØHD
**Dermis** *use* Skin
**Descending genicular artery**
*use* Artery, Femoral, Left
*use* Artery, Femoral, Right
**Destruction**
Acetabulum
Left ØQ55
Right ØQ54
Adenoids ØC5Q
Ampulla of Vater ØF5C
Anal Sphincter ØD5R
Anterior Chamber
Left Ø8533ZZ
Right Ø8523ZZ
Anus ØD5Q
Aorta
Abdominal
Thoracic
Ascending/Arch Ø25X

**Destruction** — *continued*
Aorta — *continued*
Thoracic — *continued*
Descending Ø25W
Aortic Body ØG5D
Appendix ØD5J
Artery
Anterior Tibial
Left Ø45Q
Right Ø45P
Axillary
Left Ø356
Right Ø355
Brachial
Left Ø358
Right Ø357
Celiac Ø451
Colic
Left Ø457
Middle Ø458
Right Ø456
Common Carotid
Left Ø35J
Right Ø35H
Common Iliac
Left Ø45D
Right Ø45C
External Carotid
Left Ø35N
Right Ø35M
External Iliac
Left Ø45J
Right Ø45H
Face Ø35R
Femoral
Left Ø45L
Right Ø45K
Foot
Left Ø45W
Right Ø45V
Gastric Ø452
Hand
Left Ø35F
Right Ø35D
Hepatic Ø453
Inferior Mesenteric Ø45B
Innominate Ø352
Internal Carotid
Left Ø35L
Right Ø35K
Internal Iliac
Left Ø45F
Right Ø45E
Internal Mammary
Left Ø351
Right Ø35Ø
Intracranial Ø35G
Lower Ø45Y
Peroneal
Left Ø45U
Right Ø45T
Popliteal
Left Ø45N
Right Ø45M
Posterior Tibial
Left Ø45S
Right Ø45R
Pulmonary
Left Ø25R
Right Ø25Q
Pulmonary Trunk Ø25P
Radial
Left Ø35C
Right Ø35B
Renal
Left Ø45A
Right Ø459
Splenic Ø454
Subclavian
Left Ø354
Right Ø353
Superior Mesenteric Ø455
Temporal
Left Ø35T
Right Ø35S
Thyroid
Left Ø35V
Right Ø35U

**Destruction** — *continued*
Artery — *continued*
Ulnar
Left Ø35A
Right Ø359
Upper Ø35Y
Vertebral
Left Ø35Q
Right Ø35P
Atrium
Left Ø257
Right Ø256
Auditory Ossicle
Left Ø95A
Right Ø959
Basal Ganglia ØØ58
Bladder ØT5B
Bladder Neck ØT5C
Bone
Ethmoid
Left ØN5G
Right ØN5F
Frontal ØN51
Hyoid ØN5X
Lacrimal
Left ØN5J
Right ØN5H
Nasal ØN5B
Occipital ØN57
Palatine
Left ØN5L
Right ØN5K
Parietal
Left ØN54
Right ØN53
Pelvic
Left ØQ53
Right ØQ52
Sphenoid ØN5C
Temporal
Left ØN56
Right ØN55
Zygomatic
Left ØN5N
Right ØN5M
Brain ØØ5Ø
Breast
Bilateral ØH5V
Left ØH5U
Right ØH5T
Bronchus
Lingula ØB59
Lower Lobe
Left ØB5B
Right ØB56
Main
Left ØB57
Right ØB53
Middle Lobe, Right ØB55
Upper Lobe
Left ØB58
Right ØB54
Buccal Mucosa ØC54
Bursa and Ligament
Abdomen
Left ØM5J
Right ØM5H
Ankle
Left ØM5R
Right ØM5Q
Elbow
Left ØM54
Right ØM53
Foot
Left ØM5T
Right ØM5S
Hand
Left ØM58
Right ØM57
Head and Neck ØM5Ø
Hip
Left ØM5M
Right ØM5L
Knee
Left ØM5P
Right ØM5N
Lower Extremity
Left ØM5W
Right ØM5V

**Destruction** — *continued*
Bursa and Ligament — *continued*
Perineum ØM5K
Rib(s) ØM5G
Shoulder
Left ØM52
Right ØM51
Spine
Lower ØM5D
Upper ØM5C
Sternum ØM5F
Upper Extremity
Left ØM5B
Right ØM59
Wrist
Left ØM56
Right ØM55
Carina ØB52
Carotid Bodies, Bilateral ØG58
Carotid Body
Left ØG56
Right ØG57
Carpal
Left ØP5N
Right ØP5M
Cecum ØD5H
Cerebellum ØØ5C
Cerebral Hemisphere ØØ57
Cerebral Meninges ØØ51
Cerebral Ventricle ØØ56
Cervix ØU5C
Chordae Tendineae Ø259
Choroid
Left Ø85B
Right Ø85A
Cisterna Chyli Ø75L
Clavicle
Left ØP5B
Right ØP59
Clitoris ØU5J
Coccygeal Glomus ØG5B
Coccyx ØQ5S
Colon
Ascending ØD5K
Descending ØD5M
Sigmoid ØD5N
Transverse ØD5L
Conduction Mechanism Ø258
Conjunctiva
Left Ø85TXZZ
Right Ø85SXZZ
Cord
Bilateral ØV5H
Left ØV5G
Right ØV5F
Cornea
Left Ø859XZZ
Right Ø858XZZ
Cul-de-sac ØU5F
Diaphragm ØB5T
Disc
Cervical Vertebral ØR53
Cervicothoracic Vertebral ØR55
Lumbar Vertebral ØS52
Lumbosacral ØS54
Thoracic Vertebral ØR59
Thoracolumbar Vertebral ØR5B
Duct
Common Bile ØF59
Cystic ØF58
Hepatic
Common ØF57
Left ØF56
Right ØF55
Lacrimal
Left Ø85Y
Right Ø85X
Pancreatic ØF5D
Accessory ØF5F
Parotid
Left ØC5C
Right ØC5B
Duodenum ØD59
Dura Mater ØØ52
Ear
External
Left Ø951
Right Ø95Ø

**Destruction** — *continued*
Ear — *continued*
External Auditory Canal
Left Ø954
Right Ø953
Inner
Left Ø95E
Right Ø95D
Middle
Left Ø956
Right Ø955
Endometrium ØU5B
Epididymis
Bilateral ØV5L
Left ØV5K
Right ØV5J
Epiglottis ØC5R
Esophagogastric Junction ØD54
Esophagus ØD55
Lower ØD53
Middle ØD52
Upper ØD51
Eustachian Tube
Left Ø95G
Right Ø95F
Eye
Left Ø851XZZ
Right Ø85ØXZZ
Eyelid
Lower
Left Ø85R
Right Ø85Q
Upper
Left Ø85P
Right Ø85N
Fallopian Tube
Left ØU56
Right ØU55
Fallopian Tubes, Bilateral ØU57
Femoral Shaft
Left ØQ59
Right ØQ58
Femur
Lower
Left ØQ5C
Right ØQ5B
Upper
Left ØQ57
Right ØQ56
Fibula
Left ØQ5K
Right ØQ5J
Finger Nail ØH5QXZZ
Gallbladder ØF54
Gingiva
Lower ØC56
Upper ØC55
Gland
Adrenal
Bilateral ØG54
Left ØG52
Right ØG53
Lacrimal
Left Ø85W
Right Ø85V
Minor Salivary ØC5J
Parotid
Left ØC59
Right ØC58
Pituitary ØG5Ø
Sublingual
Left ØC5F
Right ØC5D
Submaxillary
Left ØC5H
Right ØC5G
Vestibular ØU5L
Glenoid Cavity
Left ØP58
Right ØP57
Glomus Jugulare ØG5C
Humeral Head
Left ØP5D
Right ØP5C
Humeral Shaft
Left ØP5G
Right ØP5F
Hymen ØU5K
Hypothalamus ØØ5A

**Destruction** — *continued*
Ileocecal Valve ØD5C
Ileum ØD5B
Intestine
Large ØD5E
Left ØD5G
Right ØD5F
Small ØD58
Iris
Left Ø85D3ZZ
Right Ø85C3ZZ
Jejunum ØD5A
Joint
Acromioclavicular
Left ØR5H
Right ØR5G
Ankle
Left ØS5G
Right ØS5F
Carpal
Left ØR5R
Right ØR5Q
Carpometacarpal
Left ØR5T
Right ØR5S
Cervical Vertebral ØR51
Cervicothoracic Vertebral ØR54
Coccygeal ØS56
Elbow
Left ØR5M
Right ØR5L
Finger Phalangeal
Left ØR5X
Right ØR5W
Hip
Left ØS5B
Right ØS59
Knee
Left ØS5D
Right ØS5C
Lumbar Vertebral ØS5Ø
Lumbosacral ØS53
Metacarpophalangeal
Left ØR5V
Right ØR5U
Metatarsal-Phalangeal
Left ØS5N
Right ØS5M
Occipital-cervical ØR5Ø
Sacrococcygeal ØS55
Sacroiliac
Left ØS58
Right ØS57
Shoulder
Left ØR5K
Right ØR5J
Sternoclavicular
Left ØR5F
Right ØR5E
Tarsal
Left ØS5J
Right ØS5H
Tarsometatarsal
Left ØS5L
Right ØS5K
Temporomandibular
Left ØR5D
Right ØR5C
Thoracic Vertebral ØR56
Thoracolumbar Vertebral ØR5A
Toe Phalangeal
Left ØS5Q
Right ØS5P
Wrist
Left ØR5P
Right ØR5N
Kidney
Left ØT51
Right ØT5Ø
Kidney Pelvis
Left ØT54
Right ØT53
Larynx ØC5S
Lens
Left Ø85K3ZZ
Right Ø85J3ZZ
Lip
Lower ØC51
Upper ØC5Ø

**Destruction** — *continued*
Liver ØF5Ø
Left Lobe ØF52
Right Lobe ØF51
Lung
Bilateral ØB5M
Left ØB5L
Lower Lobe
Left ØB5J
Right ØB5F
Middle Lobe, Right ØB5D
Right ØB5K
Upper Lobe
Left ØB5G
Right ØB5C
Lung Lingula ØB5H
Lymphatic
Aortic Ø75D
Axillary
Left Ø756
Right Ø755
Head Ø75Ø
Inguinal
Left Ø75J
Right Ø75H
Internal Mammary
Left Ø759
Right Ø758
Lower Extremity
Left Ø75G
Right Ø75F
Mesenteric Ø75B
Neck
Left Ø752
Right Ø751
Pelvis Ø75C
Thoracic Duct Ø75K
Thorax Ø757
Upper Extremity
Left Ø754
Right Ø753
Mandible
Left ØN5V
Right ØN5T
Maxilla ØN5R
Medulla Oblongata ØØ5D
Mesentery ØD5V
Metacarpal
Left ØP5Q
Right ØP5P
Metatarsal
Left ØQ5P
Right ØQ5N
Muscle
Abdomen
Left ØK5L
Right ØK5K
Extraocular
Left Ø85M
Right Ø85L
Facial ØK51
Foot
Left ØK5W
Right ØK5V
Hand
Left ØK5D
Right ØK5C
Head ØK5Ø
Hip
Left ØK5P
Right ØK5N
Lower Arm and Wrist
Left ØK5B
Right ØK59
Lower Leg
Left ØK5T
Right ØK5S
Neck
Left ØK53
Right ØK52
Papillary Ø25D
Perineum ØK5M
Shoulder
Left ØK56
Right ØK55
Thorax
Left ØK5J
Right ØK5H
Tongue, Palate, Pharynx ØK54

**Destruction** — *continued*
Muscle — *continued*
Trunk
Left ØK5G
Right ØK5F
Upper Arm
Left ØK58
Right ØK57
Upper Leg
Left ØK5R
Right ØK5Q
Nasal Mucosa and Soft Tissue Ø95K
Nasopharynx Ø95N
Nerve
Abdominal Sympathetic Ø15M
Abducens ØØ5L
Accessory ØØ5R
Acoustic ØØ5N
Brachial Plexus Ø153
Cervical Ø151
Cervical Plexus Ø15Ø
Facial ØØ5M
Femoral Ø15D
Glossopharyngeal ØØ5P
Head and Neck Sympathetic Ø15K
Hypoglossal ØØ5S
Lumbar Ø15B
Lumbar Plexus Ø159
Lumbar Sympathetic Ø15N
Lumbosacral Plexus Ø15A
Median Ø155
Oculomotor ØØ5H
Olfactory ØØ5F
Optic ØØ5G
Peroneal Ø15H
Phrenic Ø152
Pudendal Ø15C
Radial Ø156
Sacral Ø15R
Sacral Plexus Ø15Q
Sacral Sympathetic Ø15P
Sciatic Ø15F
Thoracic Ø158
Thoracic Sympathetic Ø15L
Tibial Ø15G
Trigeminal ØØ5K
Trochlear ØØ5J
Ulnar Ø154
Vagus ØØ5Q
Nipple
Left ØH5X
Right ØH5W
Omentum ØD5U
Orbit
Left ØN5Q
Right ØN5P
Ovary
Bilateral ØU52
Left ØU51
Right ØU5Ø
Palate
Hard ØC52
Soft ØC53
Pancreas ØF5G
Para-aortic Body ØG59
Paraganglion Extremity ØG5F
Parathyroid Gland ØG5R
Inferior
Left ØG5P
Right ØG5N
Multiple ØG5Q
Superior
Left ØG5M
Right ØG5L
Patella
Left ØQ5F
Right ØQ5D
Penis ØV5S
Pericardium Ø25N
Peritoneum ØD5W
Phalanx
Finger
Left ØP5V
Right ØP5T
Thumb
Left ØP5S
Right ØP5R
Toe
Left ØQ5R

**Destruction** — *continued*
Phalanx — *continued*
Toe — *continued*
Right ØQ5Q
Pharynx ØC5M
Pineal Body ØG51
Pleura
Left ØB5P
Right ØB5N
Pons ØØ5B
Prepuce ØV5T
Prostate ØV5Ø
Radius
Left ØP5J
Right ØP5H
Rectum ØD5P
Retina
Left Ø85F3ZZ
Right Ø85E3ZZ
Retinal Vessel
Left Ø85H3ZZ
Right Ø85G3ZZ
Ribs
1 to 2 ØP51
3 or More ØP52
Sacrum ØQ51
Scapula
Left ØP56
Right ØP55
Sclera
Left Ø857XZZ
Right Ø856XZZ
Scrotum ØV55
Septum
Atrial Ø255
Nasal Ø95M
Ventricular Ø25M
Sinus
Accessory Ø95P
Ethmoid
Left Ø95V
Right Ø95U
Frontal
Left Ø95T
Right Ø95S
Mastoid
Left Ø95C
Right Ø95B
Maxillary
Left Ø95R
Right Ø95Q
Sphenoid
Left Ø95X
Right Ø95W
Skin
Abdomen ØH57XZ
Back ØH56XZ
Buttock ØH58XZ
Chest ØH55XZ
Ear
Left ØH53XZ
Right ØH52XZ
Face ØH51XZ
Foot
Left ØH5NXZ
Right ØH5MXZ
Hand
Left ØH5GXZ
Right ØH5FXZ
Inguinal ØH5AXZ
Lower Arm
Left ØH5EXZ
Right ØH5DXZ
Lower Leg
Left ØH5LXZ
Right ØH5KXZ
Neck ØH54XZ
Perineum ØH59XZ
Scalp ØH5ØXZ
Upper Arm
Left ØH5CXZ
Right ØH5BXZ
Upper Leg
Left ØH5JXZ
Right ØH5HXZ
Skull ØN5Ø
Spinal Cord
Cervical ØØ5W
Lumbar ØØ5Y

**Destruction** — *continued*
Spinal Cord — *continued*
Thoracic ØØ5X
Spinal Meninges ØØ5T
Spleen Ø75P
Sternum ØP5Ø
Stomach ØD56
Pylorus ØD57
Subcutaneous Tissue and Fascia
Abdomen ØJ58
Back ØJ57
Buttock ØJ59
Chest ØJ56
Face ØJ51
Foot
Left ØJ5R
Right ØJ5Q
Hand
Left ØJ5K
Right ØJ5J
Lower Arm
Left ØJ5H
Right ØJ5G
Lower Leg
Left ØJ5P
Right ØJ5N
Neck
Left ØJ55
Right ØJ54
Pelvic Region ØJ5C
Perineum ØJ5B
Scalp ØJ5Ø
Upper Arm
Left ØJ5F
Right ØJ5D
Upper Leg
Left ØJ5M
Right ØJ5L
Tarsal
Left ØQ5M
Right ØQ5L
Tendon
Abdomen
Left ØL5G
Right ØL5F
Ankle
Left ØL5T
Right ØL5S
Foot
Left ØL5W
Right ØL5V
Hand
Left ØL58
Right ØL57
Head and Neck ØL5Ø
Hip
Left ØL5K
Right ØL5J
Knee
Left ØL5R
Right ØL5Q
Lower Arm and Wrist
Left ØL56
Right ØL55
Lower Leg
Left ØL5P
Right ØL5N
Perineum ØL5H
Shoulder
Left ØL52
Right ØL51
Thorax
Left ØL5D
Right ØL5C
Trunk
Left ØL5B
Right ØL59
Upper Arm
Left ØL54
Right ØL53
Upper Leg
Left ØL5M
Right ØL5L
Testis
Bilateral ØV5C
Left ØV5B
Right ØV59
Thalamus ØØ59
Thymus Ø75M

**Destruction** — *continued*
Thyroid Gland ØG5K
Left Lobe ØG5G
Right Lobe ØG5H
Tibia
Left ØQ5H
Right ØQ5G
Toe Nail ØH5RXZZ
Tongue ØC57
Tonsils ØC5P
Tooth
Lower ØC5X
Upper ØC5W
Trachea ØB51
Tunica Vaginalis
Left ØV57
Right ØV56
Turbinate, Nasal Ø95L
Tympanic Membrane
Left Ø958
Right Ø957
Ulna
Left ØP5L
Right ØP5K
Ureter
Left ØT57
Right ØT56
Urethra ØT5D
Uterine Supporting Structure ØU54
Uterus ØU59
Uvula ØC5N
Vagina ØU5G
Valve
Aortic Ø25F
Mitral Ø25G
Pulmonary Ø25H
Tricuspid Ø25J
Vas Deferens
Bilateral ØV5Q
Left ØV5P
Right ØV5N
Vein
Axillary
Left Ø558
Right Ø557
Azygos Ø55Ø
Basilic
Left Ø55C
Right Ø55B
Brachial
Left Ø55A
Right Ø559
Cephalic
Left Ø55F
Right Ø55D
Colic Ø657
Common Iliac
Left Ø65D
Right Ø65C
Coronary Ø254
Esophageal Ø653
External Iliac
Left Ø65G
Right Ø65F
External Jugular
Left Ø55Q
Right Ø55P
Face
Left Ø55V
Right Ø55T
Femoral
Left Ø65N
Right Ø65M
Foot
Left Ø65V
Right Ø65T
Gastric Ø652
Hand
Left Ø55H
Right Ø55G
Hemiazygos Ø551
Hepatic Ø654
Hypogastric
Left Ø65J
Right Ø65H
Inferior Mesenteric Ø656
Innominate
Left Ø554
Right Ø553

**Destruction** — *continued*
Vein — *continued*
Internal Jugular
Left Ø55N
Right Ø55M
Intracranial Ø55L
Lower Ø65Y
Portal Ø658
Pulmonary
Left Ø25T
Right Ø25S
Renal
Left Ø65B
Right Ø659
Saphenous
Left Ø65Q
Right Ø65P
Splenic Ø651
Subclavian
Left Ø556
Right Ø555
Superior Mesenteric Ø655
Upper Ø55Y
Vertebral
Left Ø55S
Right Ø55R
Vena Cava
Inferior Ø65Ø
Superior Ø25V
Ventricle
Left Ø25L
Right Ø25K
Vertebra
Cervical ØP53
Lumbar ØQ5Ø
Thoracic ØP54
Vesicle
Bilateral ØV53
Left ØV52
Right ØV51
Vitreous
Left Ø8553ZZ
Right Ø8543ZZ
Vocal Cord
Left ØC5V
Right ØC5T
Vulva ØU5M
**Detachment**
Arm
Lower
Left ØX6FØZ
Right ØX6DØZ
Upper
Left ØX69ØZ
Right ØX68ØZ
Elbow Region
Left ØX6CØZZ
Right ØX6BØZZ
Femoral Region
Left ØY68ØZZ
Right ØY67ØZZ
Finger
Index
Left ØX6PØZ
Right ØX6NØZ
Little
Left ØX6WØZ
Right ØX6VØZ
Middle
Left ØX6RØZ
Right ØX6QØZ
Ring
Left ØX6TØZ
Right ØX6SØZ
Foot
Left ØY6NØZ
Right ØY6MØZ
Forequarter
Left ØX61ØZZ
Right ØX6ØØZZ
Hand
Left ØX6KØZ
Right ØX6JØZ
Hindquarter
Bilateral ØY64ØZZ
Left ØY63ØZZ
Right ØY62ØZZ
Knee Region
Left ØY6GØZZ

**Detachment** — *continued*
Knee Region — *continued*
Right ØY6FØZZ
Leg
Lower
Left ØY6JØZ
Right ØY6HØZ
Upper
Left ØY6DØZ
Right ØY6CØZ
Shoulder Region
Left ØX63ØZZ
Right ØX62ØZZ
Thumb
Left ØX6MØZ
Right ØX6LØZ
Toe
1st
Left ØY6QØZ
Right ØY6PØZ
2nd
Left ØY6SØZ
Right ØY6RØZ
3rd
Left ØY6UØZ
Right ØY6TØZ
4th
Left ØY6WØZ
Right ØY6VØZ
5th
Left ØY6YØZ
Right ØY6XØZ
**Determination, Mental status** GZ14ZZZ
**Detorsion**
*see* Release
*see* Reposition
**Detoxification Services, for substance abuse** HZ2ZZZZ
**Device Fitting** FØDZ
**Diagnostic Audiology** *see* Audiology, Diagnostic
**Diagnostic imaging** *see* Imaging, Diagnostic
**Diagnostic radiology** *see* Imaging, Diagnostic
**Dialysis**
Hemodialysis *see* Performance, Urinary 5A1D
Peritoneal 3E1M39Z
**Diaphragma sellae** *use* Dura Mater
**Diaphragmatic pacemaker generator** *use* Stimulator Generator in Subcutaneous Tissue and Fascia
**Diaphragmatic Pacemaker Lead**
Insertion of device in, Diaphragm ØBHT
Removal of device from, Diaphragm ØBPT
Revision of device in, Diaphragm ØBWT
**Digital radiography, plain** *see* Plain Radiography
**Dilation**
Ampulla of Vater ØF7C
Anus ØD7Q
Aorta
Abdominal
Thoracic
Ascending/Arch Ø27X
Descending Ø27W
Artery
Anterior Tibial
Left Ø47Q
Right Ø47P
Axillary
Left Ø376
Right Ø375
Brachial
Left Ø378
Right Ø377
Celiac Ø471
Colic
Left Ø477
Middle Ø478
Right Ø476
Common Carotid
Left Ø37J
Right Ø37H
Common Iliac
Left Ø47D
Right Ø47C
Coronary
Four or More Arteries Ø273
One Artery Ø27Ø
Three Arteries Ø272
Two Arteries Ø271

**Dilation** — *continued*
Artery — *continued*
External Carotid
Left Ø37N
Right Ø37M
External Iliac
Left Ø47J
Right Ø47H
Face Ø37R
Femoral
Left Ø47L
Right Ø47K
Foot
Left Ø47W
Right Ø47V
Gastric Ø472
Hand
Left Ø37F
Right Ø37D
Hepatic Ø473
Inferior Mesenteric Ø47B
Innominate Ø372
Internal Carotid
Left Ø37L
Right Ø37K
Internal Iliac
Left Ø47F
Right Ø47E
Internal Mammary
Left Ø371
Right Ø370
Intracranial Ø37G
Lower Ø47Y
Peroneal
Left Ø47U
Right Ø47T
Popliteal
Left Ø47N
Right Ø47M
Posterior Tibial
Left Ø47S
Right Ø47R
Pulmonary
Left Ø27R
Right Ø27Q
Pulmonary Trunk Ø27P
Radial
Left Ø37C
Right Ø37B
Renal
Left Ø47A
Right Ø479
Splenic Ø474
Subclavian
Left Ø374
Right Ø373
Superior Mesenteric Ø475
Temporal
Left Ø37T
Right Ø37S
Thyroid
Left Ø37V
Right Ø37U
Ulnar
Left Ø37A
Right Ø379
Upper Ø37Y
Vertebral
Left Ø37Q
Right Ø37P
Bladder ØT7B
Bladder Neck ØT7C
Bronchus
Lingula ØB79
Lower Lobe
Left ØB7B
Right ØB76
Main
Left ØB77
Right ØB73
Middle Lobe, Right ØB75
Upper Lobe
Left ØB78
Right ØB74
Carina ØB72
Cecum ØD7H
Cerebral Ventricle ØØ76
Cervix ØU7C

**Dilation** — *continued*
Colon
Ascending ØD7K
Descending ØD7M
Sigmoid ØD7N
Transverse ØD7L
Duct
Common Bile ØF79
Cystic ØF78
Hepatic
Common ØF77
Left ØF76
Right ØF75
Lacrimal
Left Ø87Y
Right Ø87X
Pancreatic ØF7D
Accessory ØF7F
Parotid
Left ØC7C
Right ØC7B
Duodenum ØD79
Esophagogastric Junction ØD74
Esophagus ØD75
Lower ØD73
Middle ØD72
Upper ØD71
Eustachian Tube
Left Ø97G
Right Ø97F
Fallopian Tube
Left ØU76
Right ØU75
Fallopian Tubes, Bilateral ØU77
Hymen ØU7K
Ileocecal Valve ØD7C
Ileum ØD7B
Intestine
Large ØD7E
Left ØD7G
Right ØD7F
Small ØD78
Jejunum ØD7A
Kidney Pelvis
Left ØT74
Right ØT73
Larynx ØC7S
Pharynx ØC7M
Rectum ØD7P
Stomach ØD76
Pylorus ØD77
Trachea ØB71
Ureter
Left ØT77
Right ØT76
Ureters, Bilateral ØT78
Urethra ØT7D
Uterus ØU79
Vagina ØU7G
Valve
Aortic Ø27F
Mitral Ø27G
Pulmonary Ø27H
Tricuspid Ø27J
Vas Deferens
Bilateral ØV7Q
Left ØV7P
Right ØV7N
Vein
Axillary
Left Ø578
Right Ø577
Azygos Ø570
Basilic
Left Ø57C
Right Ø57B
Brachial
Left Ø57A
Right Ø579
Cephalic
Left Ø57F
Right Ø57D
Colic Ø677
Common Iliac
Left Ø67D
Right Ø67C
Esophageal Ø673
External Iliac
Left Ø67G

**Dilation** — *continued*
Vein — *continued*
External Iliac — *continued*
Right Ø67F
External Jugular
Left Ø57Q
Right Ø57P
Face
Left Ø57V
Right Ø57T
Femoral
Left Ø67N
Right Ø67M
Foot
Left Ø67V
Right Ø67T
Gastric Ø672
Hand
Left Ø57H
Right Ø57G
Hemiazygos Ø571
Hepatic Ø674
Hypogastric
Left Ø67J
Right Ø67H
Inferior Mesenteric Ø676
Innominate
Left Ø574
Right Ø573
Internal Jugular
Left Ø57N
Right Ø57M
Intracranial Ø57L
Lower Ø67Y
Portal Ø678
Pulmonary
Left Ø27T
Right Ø27S
Renal
Left Ø67B
Right Ø679
Saphenous
Left Ø67Q
Right Ø67P
Splenic Ø671
Subclavian
Left Ø576
Right Ø575
Superior Mesenteric Ø675
Upper Ø57Y
Vertebral
Left Ø57S
Right Ø57R
Vena Cava
Inferior Ø670
Superior Ø27V
Ventricle
Left Ø27L
Right Ø27K
**Direct Lateral Interbody Fusion (DLIF) device** *use* Interbody Fusion Device in Lower Joints
**Disarticulation** *see* Detachment
**Discectomy, diskectomy**
*see* Excision, Lower Joints ØSB
*see* Excision, Upper Joints ØRB
*see* Resection, Lower Joints ØST
*see* Resection, Upper Joints ØRT
**Discography**
*see* Fluoroscopy, Axial Skeleton, Except Skull and Facial Bones BR1
*see* Plain Radiography, Axial Skeleton, Except Skull and Facial Bones BRØ
**Distal humerus**
*use* Humeral Shaft, Left
*use* Humeral Shaft, Right
**Distal humerus, involving joint**
*use* Joint, Elbow, Left
*use* Joint, Elbow, Right
**Distal radioulnar joint**
*use* Joint, Wrist, Left
*use* Joint, Wrist, Right
**Diversion** *see* Bypass
**Diverticulectomy** *see* Excision, Gastrointestinal System ØDB
**Division**
Acetabulum
Left ØQ85
Right ØQ84

**Division** — *continued*
- Anal Sphincter ØD8R
- Basal Ganglia ØØ88
- Bladder Neck ØT8C
- Bone
  - Ethmoid
    - Left ØN8G
    - Right ØN8F
  - Frontal ØN81
  - Hyoid ØN8X
  - Lacrimal
    - Left ØN8J
    - Right ØN8H
  - Nasal ØN8B
  - Occipital ØN87
  - Palatine
    - Left ØN8L
    - Right ØN8K
  - Parietal
    - Left ØN84
    - Right ØN83
  - Pelvic
    - Left ØQ83
    - Right ØQ82
  - Sphenoid ØN8C
  - Temporal
    - Left ØN86
    - Right ØN85
  - Zygomatic
    - Left ØN8N
    - Right ØN8M
- Brain ØØ8Ø
- Bursa and Ligament
  - Abdomen
    - Left ØM8J
    - Right ØM8H
  - Ankle
    - Left ØM8R
    - Right ØM8Q
  - Elbow
    - Left ØM84
    - Right ØM83
  - Foot
    - Left ØM8T
    - Right ØM8S
  - Hand
    - Left ØM88
    - Right ØM87
  - Head and Neck ØM8Ø
  - Hip
    - Left ØM8M
    - Right ØM8L
  - Knee
    - Left ØM8P
    - Right ØM8N
  - Lower Extremity
    - Left ØM8W
    - Right ØM8V
  - Perineum ØM8K
  - Rib(s) ØM8G
  - Shoulder
    - Left ØM82
    - Right ØM81
  - Spine
    - Lower ØM8D
    - Upper ØM8C
  - Sternum ØM8F
  - Upper Extremity
    - Left ØM8B
    - Right ØM89
  - Wrist
    - Left ØM86
    - Right ØM85
- Carpal
  - Left ØP8N
  - Right ØP8M
- Cerebral Hemisphere ØØ87
- Chordae Tendineae Ø289
- Clavicle
  - Left ØP8B
  - Right ØP89
- Coccyx ØQ8S
- Conduction Mechanism Ø288
- Esophagogastric Junction ØD84
- Femoral Shaft
  - Left ØQ89
  - Right ØQ88

**Division** — *continued*
- Femur
  - Lower
    - Left ØQ8C
    - Right ØQ8B
  - Upper
    - Left ØQ87
    - Right ØQ86
- Fibula
  - Left ØQ8K
  - Right ØQ8J
- Gland, Pituitary ØG8Ø
- Glenoid Cavity
  - Left ØP88
  - Right ØP87
- Humeral Head
  - Left ØP8D
  - Right ØP8C
- Humeral Shaft
  - Left ØP8G
  - Right ØP8F
- Hymen ØU8K
- Kidneys, Bilateral ØT82
- Mandible
  - Left ØN8V
  - Right ØN8T
- Maxilla ØN8R
- Metacarpal
  - Left ØP8Q
  - Right ØP8P
- Metatarsal
  - Left ØQ8P
  - Right ØQ8N
- Muscle
  - Abdomen
    - Left ØK8L
    - Right ØK8K
  - Facial ØK81
  - Foot
    - Left ØK8W
    - Right ØK8V
  - Hand
    - Left ØK8D
    - Right ØK8C
  - Head ØK8Ø
  - Hip
    - Left ØK8P
    - Right ØK8N
  - Lower Arm and Wrist
    - Left ØK8B
    - Right ØK89
  - Lower Leg
    - Left ØK8T
    - Right ØK8S
  - Neck
    - Left ØK83
    - Right ØK82
  - Papillary Ø28D
  - Perineum ØK8M
  - Shoulder
    - Left ØK86
    - Right ØK85
  - Thorax
    - Left ØK8J
    - Right ØK8H
  - Tongue, Palate, Pharynx ØK84
  - Trunk
    - Left ØK8G
    - Right ØK8F
  - Upper Arm
    - Left ØK88
    - Right ØK87
  - Upper Leg
    - Left ØK8R
    - Right ØK8Q
- Nerve
  - Abdominal Sympathetic Ø18M
  - Abducens ØØ8L
  - Accessory ØØ8R
  - Acoustic ØØ8N
  - Brachial Plexus Ø183
  - Cervical Ø181
  - Cervical Plexus Ø18Ø
  - Facial ØØ8M
  - Femoral Ø18D
  - Glossopharyngeal ØØ8P
  - Head and Neck Sympathetic Ø18K
  - Hypoglossal ØØ8S
  - Lumbar Ø18B

**Division** — *continued*
- Nerve — *continued*
  - Lumbar Plexus Ø189
  - Lumbar Sympathetic Ø18N
  - Lumbosacral Plexus Ø18A
  - Median Ø185
  - Oculomotor ØØ8H
  - Olfactory ØØ8F
  - Optic ØØ8G
  - Peroneal Ø18H
  - Phrenic Ø182
  - Pudendal Ø18C
  - Radial Ø186
  - Sacral Ø18R
  - Sacral Plexus Ø18Q
  - Sacral Sympathetic Ø18P
  - Sciatic Ø18F
  - Thoracic Ø188
  - Thoracic Sympathetic Ø18L
  - Tibial Ø18G
  - Trigeminal ØØ8K
  - Trochlear ØØ8J
  - Ulnar Ø184
  - Vagus ØØ8Q
- Orbit
  - Left ØN8Q
  - Right ØN8P
- Ovary
  - Bilateral ØU82
  - Left ØU81
  - Right ØU8Ø
- Pancreas ØF8G
- Patella
  - Left ØQ8F
  - Right ØQ8D
- Perineum, Female ØW8NXZZ
- Phalanx
  - Finger
    - Left ØP8V
    - Right ØP8T
  - Thumb
    - Left ØP8S
    - Right ØP8R
  - Toe
    - Left ØQ8R
    - Right ØQ8Q
- Radius
  - Left ØP8J
  - Right ØP8H
- Ribs
  - 1 to 2 ØP81
  - 3 or More ØP82
- Sacrum ØQ81
- Scapula
  - Left ØP86
  - Right ØP85
- Skin
  - Abdomen ØH87XZZ
  - Back ØH86XZZ
  - Buttock ØH88XZZ
  - Chest ØH85XZZ
  - Ear
    - Left ØH83XZZ
    - Right ØH82XZZ
  - Face ØH81XZZ
  - Foot
    - Left ØH8NXZZ
    - Right ØH8MXZZ
  - Hand
    - Left ØH8GXZZ
    - Right ØH8FXZZ
  - Inguinal ØH8AXZZ
  - Lower Arm
    - Left ØH8EXZZ
    - Right ØH8DXZZ
  - Lower Leg
    - Left ØH8LXZZ
    - Right ØH8KXZZ
  - Neck ØH84XZZ
  - Perineum ØH89XZZ
  - Scalp ØH8ØXZZ
  - Upper Arm
    - Left ØH8CXZZ
    - Right ØH8BXZZ
  - Upper Leg
    - Left ØH8JXZZ
    - Right ØH8HXZZ
- Skull ØN8Ø

**Division** — *continued*
Spinal Cord
Cervical ØØ8W
Lumbar ØØ8Y
Thoracic ØØ8X
Sternum ØP8Ø
Stomach, Pylorus ØD87
Subcutaneous Tissue and Fascia
Abdomen ØJ88
Back ØJ87
Buttock ØJ89
Chest ØJ86
Face ØJ81
Foot
Left ØJ8R
Right ØJ8Q
Hand
Left ØJ8K
Right ØJ8J
Head and Neck ØJ8S
Lower Arm
Left ØJ8H
Right ØJ8G
Lower Extremity ØJ8W
Lower Leg
Left ØJ8P
Right ØJ8N
Neck
Left ØJ85
Right ØJ84
Pelvic Region ØJ8C
Perineum ØJ8B
Scalp ØJ8Ø
Trunk ØJ8T
Upper Arm
Left ØJ8F
Right ØJ8D
Upper Extremity ØJ8V
Upper Leg
Left ØJ8M
Right ØJ8L
Tarsal
Left ØQ8M
Right ØQ8L
Tendon
Abdomen
Left ØL8G
Right ØL8F
Ankle
Left ØL8T
Right ØL8S
Foot
Left ØL8W
Right ØL8V
Hand
Left ØL88
Right ØL87
Head and Neck ØL8Ø
Hip
Left ØL8K
Right ØL8J
Knee
Left ØL8R
Right ØL8Q
Lower Arm and Wrist
Left ØL86
Right ØL85
Lower Leg
Left ØL8P
Right ØL8N
Perineum ØL8H
Shoulder
Left ØL82
Right ØL81
Thorax
Left ØL8D
Right ØL8C
Trunk
Left ØL8B
Right ØL89
Upper Arm
Left ØL84
Right ØL83
Upper Leg
Left ØL8M
Right ØL8L
Thyroid Gland Isthmus ØG8J
Tibia
Left ØQ8H

**Division** — *continued*
Tibia — *continued*
Right ØQ8G
Turbinate, Nasal Ø98L
Ulna
Left ØP8L
Right ØP8K
Uterine Supporting Structure ØU84
Vertebra
Cervical ØP83
Lumbar ØQ8Ø
Thoracic ØP84
**Doppler study** *see* Ultrasonography
**Dorsal digital nerve** *use* Nerve, Radial
**Dorsal metacarpal vein**
*use* Vein, Hand, Left
*use* Vein, Hand, Right
**Dorsal metatarsal artery**
*use* Artery, Foot, Left
*use* Artery, Foot, Right
**Dorsal metatarsal vein**
*use* Vein, Foot, Left
*use* Vein, Foot, Right
**Dorsal scapular artery**
*use* Artery, Subclavian, Left
*use* Artery, Subclavian, Right
**Dorsal scapular nerve** *use* Nerve, Brachial Plexus
**Dorsal venous arch**
*use* Vein, Foot, Left
*use* Vein, Foot, Right
**Dorsalis pedis artery**
*use* Artery, Anterior Tibial, Left
*use* Artery, Anterior Tibial, Right
**Drainage**
Abdominal Wall ØW9F
Acetabulum
Left ØQ95
Right ØQ94
Adenoids ØC9Q
Ampulla of Vater ØF9C
Anal Sphincter ØD9R
Ankle Region
Left ØY9L
Right ØY9K
Anterior Chamber
Left Ø893
Right Ø892
Anus ØD9Q
Aorta, Abdominal Ø49Ø
Aortic Body ØG9D
Appendix ØD9J
Arm
Lower
Left ØX9F
Right ØX9D
Upper
Left ØX99
Right ØX98
Artery
Anterior Tibial
Left Ø49Q
Right Ø49P
Axillary
Left Ø396
Right Ø395
Brachial
Left Ø398
Right Ø397
Celiac Ø491
Colic
Left Ø497
Middle Ø498
Right Ø496
Common Carotid
Left Ø39J
Right Ø39H
Common Iliac
Left Ø49D
Right Ø49C
External Carotid
Left Ø39N
Right Ø39M
External Iliac
Left Ø49J
Right Ø49H
Face Ø39R
Femoral
Left Ø49L

**Drainage** — *continued*
Artery — *continued*
Femoral — *continued*
Right Ø49K
Foot
Left Ø49W
Right Ø49V
Gastric Ø492
Hand
Left Ø39F
Right Ø39D
Hepatic Ø493
Inferior Mesenteric Ø49B
Innominate Ø392
Internal Carotid
Left Ø39L
Right Ø39K
Internal Iliac
Left Ø49F
Right Ø49E
Internal Mammary
Left Ø391
Right Ø39Ø
Intracranial Ø39G
Lower Ø49Y
Peroneal
Left Ø49U
Right Ø49T
Popliteal
Left Ø49N
Right Ø49M
Posterior Tibial
Left Ø49S
Right Ø49R
Radial
Left Ø39C
Right Ø39B
Renal
Left Ø49A
Right Ø499
Splenic Ø494
Subclavian
Left Ø394
Right Ø393
Superior Mesenteric Ø495
Temporal
Left Ø39T
Right Ø39S
Thyroid
Left Ø39V
Right Ø39U
Ulnar
Left Ø39A
Right Ø399
Upper Ø39Y
Vertebral
Left Ø39Q
Right Ø39P
Auditory Ossicle
Left Ø99A
Right Ø999
Axilla
Left ØX95
Right ØX94
Back
Lower ØW9L
Upper ØW9K
Basal Ganglia ØØ98
Bladder ØT9B
Bladder Neck ØT9C
Bone
Ethmoid
Left ØN9G
Right ØN9F
Frontal ØN91
Hyoid ØN9X
Lacrimal
Left ØN9J
Right ØN9H
Nasal ØN9B
Occipital ØN97
Palatine
Left ØN9L
Right ØN9K
Parietal
Left ØN94
Right ØN93
Pelvic
Left ØQ93

**Drainage** — *continued*
Bone — *continued*
Pelvic — *continued*
Right ØQ92
Sphenoid ØN9C
Temporal
Left ØN96
Right ØN95
Zygomatic
Left ØN9N
Right ØN9M
Bone Marrow Ø79T
Brain ØØ9Ø
Breast
Bilateral ØH9V
Left ØH9U
Right ØH9T
Bronchus
Lingula ØB99
Lower Lobe
Left ØB9B
Right ØB96
Main
Left ØB97
Right ØB93
Middle Lobe, Right ØB95
Upper Lobe
Left ØB98
Right ØB94
Buccal Mucosa ØC94
Bursa and Ligament
Abdomen
Left ØM9J
Right ØM9H
Ankle
Left ØM9R
Right ØM9Q
Elbow
Left ØM94
Right ØM93
Foot
Left ØM9T
Right ØM9S
Hand
Left ØM98
Right ØM97
Head and Neck ØM9Ø
Hip
Left ØM9M
Right ØM9L
Knee
Left ØM9P
Right ØM9N
Lower Extremity
Left ØM9W
Right ØM9V
Perineum ØM9K
Rib(s) ØM9G
Shoulder
Left ØM92
Right ØM91
Spine
Lower ØM9D
Upper ØM9C
Sternum ØM9F
Upper Extremity
Left ØM9B
Right ØM99
Wrist
Left ØM96
Right ØM95
Buttock
Left ØY91
Right ØY9Ø
Carina ØB92
Carotid Bodies, Bilateral ØG98
Carotid Body
Left ØG96
Right ØG97
Carpal
Left ØP9N
Right ØP9M
Cavity, Cranial ØW91
Cecum ØD9H
Cerebellum ØØ9C
Cerebral Hemisphere ØØ97
Cerebral Meninges ØØ91
Cerebral Ventricle ØØ96
Cervix ØU9C

**Drainage** — *continued*
Chest Wall ØW98
Choroid
Left Ø89B
Right Ø89A
Cisterna Chyli Ø79L
Clavicle
Left ØP9B
Right ØP99
Clitoris ØU9J
Coccygeal Glomus ØG9B
Coccyx ØQ9S
Colon
Ascending ØD9K
Descending ØD9M
Sigmoid ØD9N
Transverse ØD9L
Conjunctiva
Left Ø89T
Right Ø89S
Cord
Bilateral ØV9H
Left ØV9G
Right ØV9F
Cornea
Left Ø899
Right Ø898
Cul-de-sac ØU9F
Diaphragm ØB9T
Disc
Cervical Vertebral ØR93
Cervicothoracic Vertebral ØR95
Lumbar Vertebral ØS92
Lumbosacral ØS94
Thoracic Vertebral ØR99
Thoracolumbar Vertebral ØR9B
Duct
Common Bile ØF99
Cystic ØF98
Hepatic
Common ØF97
Left ØF96
Right ØF95
Lacrimal
Left Ø89Y
Right Ø89X
Pancreatic ØF9D
Accessory ØF9F
Parotid
Left ØC9C
Right ØC9B
Duodenum ØD99
Dura Mater ØØ92
Ear
External
Left Ø991
Right Ø99Ø
External Auditory Canal
Left Ø994
Right Ø993
Inner
Left Ø99E
Right Ø99D
Middle
Left Ø996
Right Ø995
Elbow Region
Left ØX9C
Right ØX9B
Epididymis
Bilateral ØV9L
Left ØV9K
Right ØV9J
Epidural Space, Intracranial ØØ93
Epiglottis ØC9R
Esophagogastric Junction ØD94
Esophagus ØD95
Lower ØD93
Middle ØD92
Upper ØD91
Eustachian Tube
Left Ø99G
Right Ø99F
Extremity
Lower
Left ØY9B
Right ØY99
Upper
Left ØX97

**Drainage** — *continued*
Extremity — *continued*
Upper — *continued*
Right ØX96
Eye
Left Ø891
Right Ø89Ø
Eyelid
Lower
Left Ø89R
Right Ø89Q
Upper
Left Ø89P
Right Ø89N
Face ØW92
Fallopian Tube
Left ØU96
Right ØU95
Fallopian Tubes, Bilateral ØU97
Femoral Region
Left ØY98
Right ØY97
Femoral Shaft
Left ØQ99
Right ØQ98
Femur
Lower
Left ØQ9C
Right ØQ9B
Upper
Left ØQ97
Right ØQ96
Fibula
Left ØQ9K
Right ØQ9J
Finger Nail ØH9Q
Foot
Left ØY9N
Right ØY9M
Gallbladder ØF94
Gingiva
Lower ØC96
Upper ØC95
Gland
Adrenal
Bilateral ØG94
Left ØG92
Right ØG93
Lacrimal
Left Ø89W
Right Ø89V
Minor Salivary ØC9J
Parotid
Left ØC99
Right ØC98
Pituitary ØG9Ø
Sublingual
Left ØC9F
Right ØC9D
Submaxillary
Left ØC9H
Right ØC9G
Vestibular ØU9L
Glenoid Cavity
Left ØP98
Right ØP97
Glomus Jugulare ØG9C
Hand
Left ØX9K
Right ØX9J
Head ØW9Ø
Humeral Head
Left ØP9D
Right ØP9C
Humeral Shaft
Left ØP9G
Right ØP9F
Hymen ØU9K
Hypothalamus ØØ9A
Ileocecal Valve ØD9C
Ileum ØD9B
Inguinal Region
Left ØY96
Right ØY95
Intestine
Large ØD9E
Left ØD9G
Right ØD9F
Small ØD98

- **Drainage** — *continued*
  - Iris
    - Left Ø89D
    - Right Ø89C
  - Jaw
    - Lower ØW95
    - Upper ØW94
  - Jejunum ØD9A
  - Joint
    - Acromioclavicular
      - Left ØR9H
      - Right ØR9G
    - Ankle
      - Left ØS9G
      - Right ØS9F
    - Carpal
      - Left ØR9R
      - Right ØR9Q
    - Carpometacarpal
      - Left ØR9T
      - Right ØR9S
    - Cervical Vertebral ØR91
    - Cervicothoracic Vertebral ØR94
    - Coccygeal ØS96
    - Elbow
      - Left ØR9M
      - Right ØR9L
    - Finger Phalangeal
      - Left ØR9X
      - Right ØR9W
    - Hip
      - Left ØS9B
      - Right ØS99
    - Knee
      - Left ØS9D
      - Right ØS9C
    - Lumbar Vertebral ØS9Ø
    - Lumbosacral ØS93
    - Metacarpophalangeal
      - Left ØR9V
      - Right ØR9U
    - Metatarsal-Phalangeal
      - Left ØS9N
      - Right ØS9M
    - Occipital-cervical ØR9Ø
    - Sacrococcygeal ØS95
    - Sacroiliac
      - Left ØS98
      - Right ØS97
    - Shoulder
      - Left ØR9K
      - Right ØR9J
    - Sternoclavicular
      - Left ØR9F
      - Right ØR9E
    - Tarsal
      - Left ØS9J
      - Right ØS9H
    - Tarsometatarsal
      - Left ØS9L
      - Right ØS9K
    - Temporomandibular
      - Left ØR9D
      - Right ØR9C
    - Thoracic Vertebral ØR96
    - Thoracolumbar Vertebral ØR9A
    - Toe Phalangeal
      - Left ØS9Q
      - Right ØS9P
    - Wrist
      - Left ØR9P
      - Right ØR9N
  - Kidney
    - Left ØT91
    - Right ØT9Ø
  - Kidney Pelvis
    - Left ØT94
    - Right ØT93
  - Knee Region
    - Left ØY9G
    - Right ØY9F
  - Larynx ØC9S
  - Leg
    - Lower
      - Left ØY9J
      - Right ØY9H
    - Upper
      - Left ØY9D
      - Right ØY9C

- **Drainage** — *continued*
  - Lens
    - Left Ø89K
    - Right Ø89J
  - Lip
    - Lower ØC91
    - Upper ØC9Ø
  - Liver ØF9Ø
    - Left Lobe ØF92
    - Right Lobe ØF91
  - Lung
    - Bilateral ØB9M
    - Left ØB9L
    - Lower Lobe
      - Left ØB9J
      - Right ØB9F
    - Middle Lobe, Right ØB9D
    - Right ØB9K
    - Upper Lobe
      - Left ØB9G
      - Right ØB9C
  - Lung Lingula ØB9H
  - Lymphatic
    - Aortic Ø79D
    - Axillary
      - Left Ø796
      - Right Ø795
    - Head Ø79Ø
    - Inguinal
      - Left Ø79J
      - Right Ø79H
    - Internal Mammary
      - Left Ø799
      - Right Ø798
    - Lower Extremity
      - Left Ø79G
      - Right Ø79F
    - Mesenteric Ø79B
    - Neck
      - Left Ø792
      - Right Ø791
    - Pelvis Ø79C
    - Thoracic Duct Ø79K
    - Thorax Ø797
    - Upper Extremity
      - Left Ø794
      - Right Ø793
  - Mandible
    - Left ØN9V
    - Right ØN9T
  - Maxilla ØN9R
  - Mediastinum ØW9C
  - Medulla Oblongata ØØ9D
  - Mesentery ØD9V
  - Metacarpal
    - Left ØP9Q
    - Right ØP9P
  - Metatarsal
    - Left ØQ9P
    - Right ØQ9N
  - Muscle
    - Abdomen
      - Left ØK9L
      - Right ØK9K
    - Extraocular
      - Left Ø89M
      - Right Ø89L
    - Facial ØK91
    - Foot
      - Left ØK9W
      - Right ØK9V
    - Hand
      - Left ØK9D
      - Right ØK9C
    - Head ØK9Ø
    - Hip
      - Left ØK9P
      - Right ØK9N
    - Lower Arm and Wrist
      - Left ØK9B
      - Right ØK99
    - Lower Leg
      - Left ØK9T
      - Right ØK9S
    - Neck
      - Left ØK93
      - Right ØK92
    - Perineum ØK9M

- **Drainage** — *continued*
  - Muscle — *continued*
    - Shoulder
      - Left ØK96
      - Right ØK95
    - Thorax
      - Left ØK9J
      - Right ØK9H
    - Tongue, Palate, Pharynx ØK94
    - Trunk
      - Left ØK9G
      - Right ØK9F
    - Upper Arm
      - Left ØK98
      - Right ØK97
    - Upper Leg
      - Left ØK9R
      - Right ØK9Q
  - Nasal Mucosa and Soft Tissue Ø99K
  - Nasopharynx Ø99N
  - Neck ØW96
  - Nerve
    - Abdominal Sympathetic Ø19M
    - Abducens ØØ9L
    - Accessory ØØ9R
    - Acoustic ØØ9N
    - Brachial Plexus Ø193
    - Cervical Ø191
    - Cervical Plexus Ø19Ø
    - Facial ØØ9M
    - Femoral Ø19D
    - Glossopharyngeal ØØ9P
    - Head and Neck Sympathetic Ø19K
    - Hypoglossal ØØ9S
    - Lumbar Ø19B
    - Lumbar Plexus Ø199
    - Lumbar Sympathetic Ø19N
    - Lumbosacral Plexus Ø19A
    - Median Ø195
    - Oculomotor ØØ9H
    - Olfactory ØØ9F
    - Optic ØØ9G
    - Peroneal Ø19H
    - Phrenic Ø192
    - Pudendal Ø19C
    - Radial Ø196
    - Sacral Ø19R
    - Sacral Plexus Ø19Q
    - Sacral Sympathetic Ø19P
    - Sciatic Ø19F
    - Thoracic Ø198
    - Thoracic Sympathetic Ø19L
    - Tibial Ø19G
    - Trigeminal ØØ9K
    - Trochlear ØØ9J
    - Ulnar Ø194
    - Vagus ØØ9Q
  - Nipple
    - Left ØH9X
    - Right ØH9W
  - Omentum ØD9U
  - Oral Cavity and Throat ØW93
  - Orbit
    - Left ØN9Q
    - Right ØN9P
  - Ovary
    - Bilateral ØU92
    - Left ØU91
    - Right ØU9Ø
  - Palate
    - Hard ØC92
    - Soft ØC93
  - Pancreas ØF9G
  - Para-aortic Body ØG99
  - Paraganglion Extremity ØG9F
  - Parathyroid Gland ØG9R
    - Inferior
      - Left ØG9P
      - Right ØG9N
    - Multiple ØG9Q
    - Superior
      - Left ØG9M
      - Right ØG9L
  - Patella
    - Left ØQ9F
    - Right ØQ9D
  - Pelvic Cavity ØW9J
  - Penis ØV9S
  - Pericardial Cavity ØW9D

- **Drainage** — *continued*
  - Perineum
    - Female ØW9N
    - Male ØW9M
  - Peritoneal Cavity ØW9G
  - Peritoneum ØD9W
  - Phalanx
    - Finger
      - Left ØP9V
      - Right ØP9T
    - Thumb
      - Left ØP9S
      - Right ØP9R
    - Toe
      - Left ØQ9R
      - Right ØQ9Q
  - Pharynx ØC9M
  - Pineal Body ØG91
  - Pleura
    - Left ØB9P
    - Right ØB9N
  - Pleural Cavity
    - Left ØW9B
    - Right ØW99
  - Pons ØØ9B
  - Prepuce ØV9T
  - Products of Conception
    - Amniotic Fluid
      - Diagnostic 1Ø9Ø
      - Therapeutic 1Ø9Ø
    - Fetal Blood 1Ø9Ø
    - Fetal Cerebrospinal Fluid 1Ø9Ø
    - Fetal Fluid, Other 1Ø9Ø
    - Fluid, Other 1Ø9Ø
  - Prostate ØV9Ø
  - Radius
    - Left ØP9J
    - Right ØP9H
  - Rectum ØD9P
  - Retina
    - Left Ø89F
    - Right Ø89E
  - Retinal Vessel
    - Left Ø89H
    - Right Ø89G
  - Retroperitoneum ØW9H
  - Ribs
    - 1 to 2 ØP91
    - 3 or More ØP92
  - Sacrum ØQ91
  - Scapula
    - Left ØP96
    - Right ØP95
  - Sclera
    - Left Ø897
    - Right Ø896
  - Scrotum ØV95
  - Septum, Nasal Ø99M
  - Shoulder Region
    - Left ØX93
    - Right ØX92
  - Sinus
    - Accessory Ø99P
    - Ethmoid
      - Left Ø99V
      - Right Ø99U
    - Frontal
      - Left Ø99T
      - Right Ø99S
    - Mastoid
      - Left Ø99C
      - Right Ø99B
    - Maxillary
      - Left Ø99R
      - Right Ø99Q
    - Sphenoid
      - Left Ø99X
      - Right Ø99W
  - Skin
    - Abdomen ØH97
    - Back ØH96
    - Buttock ØH98
    - Chest ØH95
    - Ear
      - Left ØH93
      - Right ØH92
    - Face ØH91
    - Foot
      - Left ØH9N

- **Drainage** — *continued*
  - Skin — *continued*
    - Foot — *continued*
      - Right ØH9M
    - Hand
      - Left ØH9G
      - Right ØH9F
    - Inguinal ØH9A
    - Lower Arm
      - Left ØH9E
      - Right ØH9D
    - Lower Leg
      - Left ØH9L
      - Right ØH9K
    - Neck ØH94
    - Perineum ØH99
    - Scalp ØH9Ø
    - Upper Arm
      - Left ØH9C
      - Right ØH9B
    - Upper Leg
      - Left ØH9J
      - Right ØH9H
  - Skull ØN9Ø
  - Spinal Canal ØØ9U
  - Spinal Cord
    - Cervical ØØ9W
    - Lumbar ØØ9Y
    - Thoracic ØØ9X
  - Spinal Meninges ØØ9T
  - Spleen Ø79P
  - Sternum ØP9Ø
  - Stomach ØD96
    - Pylorus ØD97
  - Subarachnoid Space, Intracranial ØØ95
  - Subcutaneous Tissue and Fascia
    - Abdomen ØJ98
    - Back ØJ97
    - Buttock ØJ99
    - Chest ØJ96
    - Face ØJ91
    - Foot
      - Left ØJ9R
      - Right ØJ9Q
    - Hand
      - Left ØJ9K
      - Right ØJ9J
    - Lower Arm
      - Left ØJ9H
      - Right ØJ9G
    - Lower Leg
      - Left ØJ9P
      - Right ØJ9N
    - Neck
      - Left ØJ95
      - Right ØJ94
    - Pelvic Region ØJ9C
    - Perineum ØJ9B
    - Scalp ØJ9Ø
    - Upper Arm
      - Left ØJ9F
      - Right ØJ9D
    - Upper Leg
      - Left ØJ9M
      - Right ØJ9L
  - Subdural Space, Intracranial ØØ94
  - Tarsal
    - Left ØQ9M
    - Right ØQ9L
  - Tendon
    - Abdomen
      - Left ØL9G
      - Right ØL9F
    - Ankle
      - Left ØL9T
      - Right ØL9S
    - Foot
      - Left ØL9W
      - Right ØL9V
    - Hand
      - Left ØL98
      - Right ØL97
    - Head and Neck ØL9Ø
    - Hip
      - Left ØL9K
      - Right ØL9J
    - Knee
      - Left ØL9R
      - Right ØL9Q

- **Drainage** — *continued*
  - Tendon — *continued*
    - Lower Arm and Wrist
      - Left ØL96
      - Right ØL95
    - Lower Leg
      - Left ØL9P
      - Right ØL9N
    - Perineum ØL9H
    - Shoulder
      - Left ØL92
      - Right ØL91
    - Thorax
      - Left ØL9D
      - Right ØL9C
    - Trunk
      - Left ØL9B
      - Right ØL99
    - Upper Arm
      - Left ØL94
      - Right ØL93
    - Upper Leg
      - Left ØL9M
      - Right ØL9L
  - Testis
    - Bilateral ØV9C
    - Left ØV9B
    - Right ØV99
  - Thalamus ØØ99
  - Thymus Ø79M
  - Thyroid Gland ØG9K
    - Left Lobe ØG9G
    - Right Lobe ØG9H
  - Tibia
    - Left ØQ9H
    - Right ØQ9G
  - Toe Nail ØH9R
  - Tongue ØC97
  - Tonsils ØC9P
  - Tooth
    - Lower ØC9X
    - Upper ØC9W
  - Trachea ØB91
  - Tunica Vaginalis
    - Left ØV97
    - Right ØV96
  - Turbinate, Nasal Ø99L
  - Tympanic Membrane
    - Left Ø998
    - Right Ø997
  - Ulna
    - Left ØP9L
    - Right ØP9K
  - Ureter
    - Left ØT97
    - Right ØT96
  - Ureters, Bilateral ØT98
  - Urethra ØT9D
  - Uterine Supporting Structure ØU94
  - Uterus ØU99
  - Uvula ØC9N
  - Vagina ØU9G
  - Vas Deferens
    - Bilateral ØV9Q
    - Left ØV9P
    - Right ØV9N
  - Vein
    - Axillary
      - Left Ø598
      - Right Ø597
    - Azygos Ø59Ø
    - Basilic
      - Left Ø59C
      - Right Ø59B
    - Brachial
      - Left Ø59A
      - Right Ø599
    - Cephalic
      - Left Ø59F
      - Right Ø59D
    - Colic Ø697
    - Common Iliac
      - Left Ø69D
      - Right Ø69C
    - Esophageal Ø693
    - External Iliac
      - Left Ø69G
      - Right Ø69F

**Drainage** — *continued*
Vein — *continued*
External Jugular
Left Ø59Q
Right Ø59P
Face
Left Ø59V
Right Ø59T
Femoral
Left Ø69N
Right Ø69M
Foot
Left Ø69V
Right Ø69T
Gastric Ø692
Hand
Left Ø59H
Right Ø59G
Hemiazygos Ø591
Hepatic Ø694
Hypogastric
Left Ø69J
Right Ø69H
Inferior Mesenteric Ø696
Innominate
Left Ø594
Right Ø593
Internal Jugular
Left Ø59N
Right Ø59M
Intracranial Ø59L
Lower Ø69Y
Portal Ø698
Renal
Left Ø69B
Right Ø699
Saphenous
Left Ø69Q
Right Ø69P
Splenic Ø691
Subclavian
Left Ø596
Right Ø595
Superior Mesenteric Ø695
Upper Ø59Y
Vertebral
Left Ø59S
Right Ø59R
Vena Cava, Inferior Ø69Ø
Vertebra
Cervical ØP93
Lumbar ØQ9Ø
Thoracic ØP94
Vesicle
Bilateral ØV93
Left ØV92
Right ØV91
Vitreous
Left Ø895
Right Ø894
Vocal Cord
Left ØC9V
Right ØC9T
Vulva ØU9M
Wrist Region
Left ØX9H
Right ØX9G
**Dressing**
Abdominal Wall 2W23X4Z
Arm
Lower
Left 2W2DX4Z
Right 2W2CX4Z
Upper
Left 2W2BX4Z
Right 2W2AX4Z
Back 2W25X4Z
Chest Wall 2W24X4Z
Extremity
Lower
Left 2W2MX4Z
Right 2W2LX4Z
Upper
Left 2W29X4Z
Right 2W28X4Z
Face 2W21X4Z
Finger
Left 2W2KX4Z
Right 2W2JX4Z

**Dressing** — *continued*
Foot
Left 2W2TX4Z
Right 2W2SX4Z
Hand
Left 2W2FX4Z
Right 2W2EX4Z
Head 2W2ØX4Z
Inguinal Region
Left 2W27X4Z
Right 2W26X4Z
Leg
Lower
Left 2W2RX4Z
Right 2W2QX4Z
Upper
Left 2W2PX4Z
Right 2W2NX4Z
Neck 2W22X4Z
Thumb
Left 2W2HX4Z
Right 2W2GX4Z
Toe
Left 2W2VX4Z
Right 2W2UX4Z
**Driver stent (RX) (OTW)** *use* Intraluminal Device
**Drotrecogin alfa** *see* Introduction of Recombinant Human-activated Protein C
**Duct of Santorini** *use* Duct, Pancreatic, Accessory
**Duct of Wirsung** *use* Duct, Pancreatic
**Ductogram, mammary** *see* Plain Radiography, Skin, Subcutaneous Tissue and Breast BHØ
**Ductography, mammary** *see* Plain Radiography, Skin, Subcutaneous Tissue and Breast BHØ
**Ductus deferens**
*use* Vas Deferens
*use* Vas Deferens, Bilateral
*use* Vas Deferens, Left
*use* Vas Deferens, Right
**Duodenal ampulla** *use* Ampulla of Vater
**Duodenectomy**
*see* Excision, Duodenum ØDB9
*see* Resection, Duodenum ØDT9
**Duodenocholedochotomy** *see* Drainage, Gallbladder ØF94
**Duodenocystostomy**
*see* Bypass, Gallbladder ØF14
*see* Drainage, Gallbladder ØF94
**Duodenoenterostomy**
*see* Bypass, Gastrointestinal System ØD1
*see* Drainage, Gastrointestinal System ØD9
**Duodenojejunal flexure** *use* Jejunum
**Duodenolysis** *see* Release, Duodenum ØDN9
**Duodenorrhaphy** *see* Repair, Duodenum ØDQ9
**Duodenostomy**
*see* Bypass, Duodenum ØD19
*see* Drainage, Duodenum ØD99
**Duodenotomy** *see* Drainage, Duodenum ØD99
**Dura mater, intracranial** *use* Dura Mater
**Dura mater, spinal** *use* Spinal Meninges
**DuraGraft® Endothelial Damage Inhibitor** *use* Endothelial Damage Inhibitor
**DuraHeart Left Ventricular Assist System** *use* Implantable Heart Assist System in Heart and Great Vessels
**Dural venous sinus** *use* Vein, Intracranial
**Durata® Defibrillation Lead** *use* Cardiac Lead, Defibrillator in Ø2H
**Dynesys® Dynamic Stabilization System**
*use* Spinal Stabilization Device, Pedicle-Based in ØRH
*use* Spinal Stabilization Device, Pedicle-Based in ØSH

# E

**Earlobe**
*use* Ear, External, Bilateral
*use* Ear, External, Left
*use* Ear, External, Right
**ECCO2R (Extracorporeal Carbon Dioxide Removal)** 5A092ØZ
**Echocardiogram** *see* Ultrasonography, Heart B24
**Echography** *see* Ultrasonography
**ECMO** *see* Performance, Circulatory 5A15
**EDWARDS INTUITY Elite valve system** *use* Zooplastic Tissue, Rapid Deployment Technique in New Technology
**EEG (electroencephalogram)** *see* Measurement, Central Nervous 4AØØ
**EGD (esophagogastroduodenoscopy)** ØDJØ8ZZ
**Eighth cranial nerve** *use* Nerve, Acoustic
**Ejaculatory duct**
*use* Vas Deferens
*use* Vas Deferens, Bilateral
*use* Vas Deferens, Left
*use* Vas Deferens, Right
**EKG (electrocardiogram)** *see* Measurement, Cardiac 4AØ2
**Electrical bone growth stimulator (EBGS)**
*use* Bone Growth Stimulator in Head and Facial Bones
*use* Bone Growth Stimulator in Lower Bones
*use* Bone Growth Stimulator in Upper Bones
**Electrical muscle stimulation (EMS) lead** *use* Stimulator Lead in Muscles
**Electrocautery**
Destruction *see* Destruction
Repair *see* Repair
**Electroconvulsive Therapy**
Bilateral-Multiple Seizure GZB3ZZZ
Bilateral-Single Seizure GZB2ZZZ
Electroconvulsive Therapy, Other GZB4ZZZ
Unilateral-Multiple Seizure GZB1ZZZ
Unilateral-Single Seizure GZBØZZZ
**Electroencephalogram (EEG)** *see* Measurement, Central Nervous 4AØØ
**Electromagnetic Therapy**
Central Nervous 6A22
Urinary 6A21
**Electronic muscle stimulator lead** *use* Stimulator Lead in Muscles
**Electrophysiologic stimulation (EPS)** *see* Measurement, Cardiac 4AØ2
**Electroshock therapy** *see* Electroconvulsive Therapy
**Elevation, bone fragments, skull** *see* Reposition, Head and Facial Bones ØNS
**Eleventh cranial nerve** *use* Nerve, Accessory
**E-Luminexx™ (Biliary) (Vascular) Stent** *use* Intraluminal Device
**Embolectomy** *see* Extirpation
**Embolization**
*see* Occlusion
*see* Restriction
**Embolization coil(s)** *use* Intraluminal Device
**EMG (electromyogram)** *see* Measurement, Musculoskeletal 4AØF
**Encephalon** *use* Brain
**Endarterectomy**
*see* Extirpation, Lower Arteries Ø4C
*see* Extirpation, Upper Arteries Ø3C
**Endeavor® (III) (IV) (Sprint) Zotarolimus-eluting Coronary Stent System** *use* Intraluminal Device, Drug-eluting in Heart and Great Vessels
**Endologix® AFX Endovascular AAA System** *use* Intraluminal Device
**EndoSure® sensor** *use* Monitoring Device, Pressure Sensor in Ø2H
**ENDOTAK RELIANCE® (G) Defibrillation Lead** *use* Cardiac Lead, Defibrillator in Ø2H
**Endothelial damage inhibitor, applied to vein graft** XYØVX83
**Endotracheal tube (cuffed) (double-lumen)** *use* Intraluminal Device, Endotracheal Airway in Respiratory System
**Endurant® Endovascular Stent Graft** *use* Intraluminal Device
**Endurant® II AAA stent graft system** *use* Intraluminal Device
**Engineered Autologous Chimeric Antigen Receptor T-cell Immunotherapy** XWØ
**Enlargement**
*see* Dilation
*see* Repair
**EnRhythm** *use* Pacemaker, Dual Chamber in ØJH
**Enterorrhaphy** *see* Repair, Gastrointestinal System ØDQ
**Enterra gastric neurostimulator** *use* Stimulator Generator, Multiple Array in ØJH
**Enucleation**
Eyeball *see* Resection, Eye Ø8T
Eyeball with prosthetic implant *see* Replacement, Eye Ø8R
**Ependyma** *use* Cerebral Ventricle
**Epicel® cultured epidermal autograft** *use* Autologous Tissue Substitute




Subterms under main terms may continue to next column or page

**Epic™ Stented Tissue Valve (aortic)** *use* Zooplastic Tissue in Heart and Great Vessels
**Epidermis** *use* Skin
**Epididymectomy**
*see* Excision, Male Reproductive System ØVB
*see* Resection, Male Reproductive System ØVT
**Epididymoplasty**
*see* Repair, Male Reproductive System ØVQ
*see* Supplement, Male Reproductive System ØVU
**Epididymorrhaphy** *see* Repair, Male Reproductive System ØVQ
**Epididymotomy** *see* Drainage, Male Reproductive System ØV9
**Epidural space, spinal** *use* Spinal Canal
**Epiphysiodesis**
*see* Insertion of device in, Lower Bones ØQH
*see* Insertion of device in, Upper Bones ØPH
*see* Repair, Lower Bones ØQQ
*see* Repair, Upper Bones ØPQ
**Epiploic foramen** *use* Peritoneum
**Epiretinal Visual Prosthesis**
Left Ø8H1Ø5Z
Right Ø8HØØ5Z
**Episiorrhaphy** *see* Repair, Perineum, Female ØWQN
**Episiotomy** *see* Division, Perineum, Female ØW8N
**Epithalamus** *use* Thalamus
**Epitrochlear lymph node**
*use* Lymphatic, Upper Extremity, Left
*use* Lymphatic, Upper Extremity, Right
**EPS (electrophysiologic stimulation)** *see* Measurement, Cardiac 4AØ2
**Eptifibatide, infusion** *see* Introduction of Platelet Inhibitor
**ERCP (endoscopic retrograde cholangiopancreatography)** *see* Fluoroscopy, Hepatobiliary System and Pancreas BF1
**Erector spinae muscle**
*use* Muscle, Trunk, Left
*use* Muscle, Trunk, Right
**Esophageal artery** *use* Upper Artery
**Esophageal obturator airway (EOA)** *use* Intraluminal Device, Airway in Gastrointestinal System
**Esophageal plexus** *use* Nerve, Thoracic Sympathetic
**Esophagectomy**
*see* Excision, Gastrointestinal System ØDB
*see* Resection, Gastrointestinal System ØDT
**Esophagocoloplasty**
*see* Repair, Gastrointestinal System ØDQ
*see* Supplement, Gastrointestinal System ØDU
**Esophagoenterostomy**
*see* Bypass, Gastrointestinal System ØD1
*see* Drainage, Gastrointestinal System ØD9
**Esophagoesophagostomy**
*see* Bypass, Gastrointestinal System ØD1
*see* Drainage, Gastrointestinal System ØD9
**Esophagogastrectomy**
*see* Excision, Gastrointestinal System ØDB
*see* Resection, Gastrointestinal System ØDT
**Esophagogastroduodenoscopy (EGD)** ØDJØ8ZZ
**Esophagogastroplasty**
*see* Repair, Gastrointestinal System ØDQ
*see* Supplement, Gastrointestinal System ØDU
**Esophagogastroscopy** ØDJ68ZZ
**Esophagogastrostomy**
*see* Bypass, Gastrointestinal System ØD1
*see* Drainage, Gastrointestinal System ØD9
**Esophagojejunoplasty** *see* Supplement, Gastrointestinal System ØDU
**Esophagojejunostomy**
*see* Bypass, Gastrointestinal System ØD1
*see* Drainage, Gastrointestinal System ØD9
**Esophagomyotomy** *see* Division, Esophagogastric Junction ØD84
**Esophagoplasty**
*see* Repair, Gastrointestinal System ØDQ
*see* Replacement, Esophagus ØDR5
*see* Supplement, Gastrointestinal System ØDU
**Esophagoplication** *see* Restriction, Gastrointestinal System ØDV
**Esophagorrhaphy** *see* Repair, Gastrointestinal System ØDQ
**Esophagoscopy** ØDJØ8ZZ
**Esophagotomy** *see* Drainage, Gastrointestinal System ØD9
**Esteem® implantable hearing system** *use* Hearing Device in Ear, Nose, Sinus
**ESWL (extracorporeal shock wave lithotripsy)** *see* Fragmentation
**Ethmoidal air cell**
*use* Sinus, Ethmoid, Left
*use* Sinus, Ethmoid, Right
**Ethmoidectomy**
*see* Excision, Ear, Nose, Sinus Ø9B
*see* Excision, Head and Facial Bones ØNB
*see* Resection, Ear, Nose, Sinus Ø9T
*see* Resection, Head and Facial Bones ØNT
**Ethmoidotomy** *see* Drainage, Ear, Nose, Sinus Ø99
**Evacuation**
Hematoma *see* Extirpation
Other Fluid *see* Drainage
**Evera (XT) (S) (DR/VR)** *use* Defibrillator Generator in ØJH
**Everolimus-eluting coronary stent** *use* Intraluminal Device, Drug-eluting in Heart and Great Vessels
**Evisceration**
Eyeball *see* Resection, Eye Ø8T
Eyeball with prosthetic implant *see* Replacement, Eye Ø8R
**Examination** *see* Inspection
**Exchange** *see* Change device in
**Excision**
Abdominal Wall ØWBF
Acetabulum
Left ØQB5
Right ØQB4
Adenoids ØCBQ
Ampulla of Vater ØFBC
Anal Sphincter ØDBR
Ankle Region
Left ØYBL
Right ØYBK
Anus ØDBQ
Aorta
Abdominal
Thoracic
Ascending/Arch Ø2BX
Descending Ø2BW
Aortic Body ØGBD
Appendix ØDBJ
Arm
Lower
Left ØXBF
Right ØXBD
Upper
Left ØXB9
Right ØXB8
Artery
Anterior Tibial
Left Ø4BQ
Right Ø4BP
Axillary
Left Ø3B6
Right Ø3B5
Brachial
Left Ø3B8
Right Ø3B7
Celiac Ø4B1
Colic
Left Ø4B7
Middle Ø4B8
Right Ø4B6
Common Carotid
Left Ø3BJ
Right Ø3BH
Common Iliac
Left Ø4BD
Right Ø4BC
External Carotid
Left Ø3BN
Right Ø3BM
External Iliac
Left Ø4BJ
Right Ø4BH
Face Ø3BR
Femoral
Left Ø4BL
Right Ø4BK
Foot
Left Ø4BW
Right Ø4BV
Gastric Ø4B2
Hand
Left Ø3BF
Right Ø3BD
Hepatic Ø4B3
**Excision** — *continued*
Artery — *continued*
Inferior Mesenteric Ø4BB
Innominate Ø3B2
Internal Carotid
Left Ø3BL
Right Ø3BK
Internal Iliac
Left Ø4BF
Right Ø4BE
Internal Mammary
Left Ø3B1
Right Ø3BØ
Intracranial Ø3BG
Lower Ø4BY
Peroneal
Left Ø4BU
Right Ø4BT
Popliteal
Left Ø4BN
Right Ø4BM
Posterior Tibial
Left Ø4BS
Right Ø4BR
Pulmonary
Left Ø2BR
Right Ø2BQ
Pulmonary Trunk Ø2BP
Radial
Left Ø3BC
Right Ø3BB
Renal
Left Ø4BA
Right Ø4B9
Splenic Ø4B4
Subclavian
Left Ø3B4
Right Ø3B3
Superior Mesenteric Ø4B5
Temporal
Left Ø3BT
Right Ø3BS
Thyroid
Left Ø3BV
Right Ø3BU
Ulnar
Left Ø3BA
Right Ø3B9
Upper Ø3BY
Vertebral
Left Ø3BQ
Right Ø3BP
Atrium
Left Ø2B7
Right Ø2B6
Auditory Ossicle
Left Ø9BA
Right Ø9B9
Axilla
Left ØXB5
Right ØXB4
Back
Lower ØWBL
Upper ØWBK
Basal Ganglia ØØB8
Bladder ØTBB
Bladder Neck ØTBC
Bone
Ethmoid
Left ØNBG
Right ØNBF
Frontal ØNB1
Hyoid ØNBX
Lacrimal
Left ØNBJ
Right ØNBH
Nasal ØNBB
Occipital ØNB7
Palatine
Left ØNBL
Right ØNBK
Parietal
Left ØNB4
Right ØNB3
Pelvic
Left ØQB3
Right ØQB2
Sphenoid ØNBC

Subterms under main terms may continue to next column or page

**Excision** — *continued*
Bone — *continued*
Temporal
Left ØNB6
Right ØNB5
Zygomatic
Left ØNBN
Right ØNBM
Brain ØØBØ
Breast
Bilateral ØHBV
Left ØHBU
Right ØHBT
Supernumerary ØHBY
Bronchus
Lingula ØBB9
Lower Lobe
Left ØBBB
Right ØBB6
Main
Left ØBB7
Right ØBB3
Middle Lobe, Right ØBB5
Upper Lobe
Left ØBB8
Right ØBB4
Buccal Mucosa ØCB4
Bursa and Ligament
Abdomen
Left ØMBJ
Right ØMBH
Ankle
Left ØMBR
Right ØMBQ
Elbow
Left ØMB4
Right ØMB3
Foot
Left ØMBT
Right ØMBS
Hand
Left ØMB8
Right ØMB7
Head and Neck ØMBØ
Hip
Left ØMBM
Right ØMBL
Knee
Left ØMBP
Right ØMBN
Lower Extremity
Left ØMBW
Right ØMBV
Perineum ØMBK
Rib(s) ØMBG
Shoulder
Left ØMB2
Right ØMB1
Spine
Lower ØMBD
Upper ØMBC
Sternum ØMBF
Upper Extremity
Left ØMBB
Right ØMB9
Wrist
Left ØMB6
Right ØMB5
Buttock
Left ØYB1
Right ØYBØ
Carina ØBB2
Carotid Bodies, Bilateral ØGB8
Carotid Body
Left ØGB6
Right ØGB7
Carpal
Left ØPBN
Right ØPBM
Cecum ØDBH
Cerebellum ØØBC
Cerebral Hemisphere ØØB7
Cerebral Meninges ØØB1
Cerebral Ventricle ØØB6
Cervix ØUBC
Chest Wall ØWB8
Chordae Tendineae Ø2B9
Choroid
Left Ø8BB

**Excision** — *continued*
Choroid — *continued*
Right Ø8BA
Cisterna Chyli Ø7BL
Clavicle
Left ØPBB
Right ØPB9
Clitoris ØUBJ
Coccygeal Glomus ØGBB
Coccyx ØQBS
Colon
Ascending ØDBK
Descending ØDBM
Sigmoid ØDBN
Transverse ØDBL
Conduction Mechanism Ø2B8
Conjunctiva
Left Ø8BTXZ
Right Ø8BSXZ
Cord
Bilateral ØVBH
Left ØVBG
Right ØVBF
Cornea
Left Ø8B9XZ
Right Ø8B8XZ
Cul-de-sac ØUBF
Diaphragm ØBBT
Disc
Cervical Vertebral ØRB3
Cervicothoracic Vertebral ØRB5
Lumbar Vertebral ØSB2
Lumbosacral ØSB4
Thoracic Vertebral ØRB9
Thoracolumbar Vertebral ØRBB
Duct
Common Bile ØFB9
Cystic ØFB8
Hepatic
Common ØFB7
Left ØFB6
Right ØFB5
Lacrimal
Left Ø8BY
Right Ø8BX
Pancreatic ØFBD
Accessory ØFBF
Parotid
Left ØCBC
Right ØCBB
Duodenum ØDB9
Dura Mater ØØB2
Ear
External
Left Ø9B1
Right Ø9BØ
External Auditory Canal
Left Ø9B4
Right Ø9B3
Inner
Left Ø9BE
Right Ø9BD
Middle
Left Ø9B6
Right Ø9B5
Elbow Region
Left ØXBC
Right ØXBB
Epididymis
Bilateral ØVBL
Left ØVBK
Right ØVBJ
Epiglottis ØCBR
Esophagogastric Junction ØDB4
Esophagus ØDB5
Lower ØDB3
Middle ØDB2
Upper ØDB1
Eustachian Tube
Left Ø9BG
Right Ø9BF
Extremity
Lower
Left ØYBB
Right ØYB9
Upper
Left ØXB7
Right ØXB6

**Excision** — *continued*
Eye
Left Ø8B1
Right Ø8BØ
Eyelid
Lower
Left Ø8BR
Right Ø8BQ
Upper
Left Ø8BP
Right Ø8BN
Face ØWB2
Fallopian Tube
Left ØUB6
Right ØUB5
Fallopian Tubes, Bilateral ØUB7
Femoral Region
Left ØYB8
Right ØYB7
Femoral Shaft
Left ØQB9
Right ØQB8
Femur
Lower
Left ØQBC
Right ØQBB
Upper
Left ØQB7
Right ØQB6
Fibula
Left ØQBK
Right ØQBJ
Finger Nail ØHBQXZ
Floor of mouth *see* Excision, Oral Cavity and Throat ØWB3
Foot
Left ØYBN
Right ØYBM
Gallbladder ØFB4
Gingiva
Lower ØCB6
Upper ØCB5
Gland
Adrenal
Bilateral ØGB4
Left ØGB2
Right ØGB3
Lacrimal
Left Ø8BW
Right Ø8BV
Minor Salivary ØCBJ
Parotid
Left ØCB9
Right ØCB8
Pituitary ØGBØ
Sublingual
Left ØCBF
Right ØCBD
Submaxillary
Left ØCBH
Right ØCBG
Vestibular ØUBL
Glenoid Cavity
Left ØPB8
Right ØPB7
Glomus Jugulare ØGBC
Hand
Left ØXBK
Right ØXBJ
Head ØWBØ
Humeral Head
Left ØPBD
Right ØPBC
Humeral Shaft
Left ØPBG
Right ØPBF
Hymen ØUBK
Hypothalamus ØØBA
Ileocecal Valve ØDBC
Ileum ØDBB
Inguinal Region
Left ØYB6
Right ØYB5
Intestine
Large ØDBE
Left ØDBG
Right ØDBF
Small ØDB8

**Excision** — *continued*
Iris
Left Ø8BD3Z
Right Ø8BC3Z
Jaw
Lower ØWB5
Upper ØWB4
Jejunum ØDBA
Joint
Acromioclavicular
Left ØRBH
Right ØRBG
Ankle
Left ØSBG
Right ØSBF
Carpal
Left ØRBR
Right ØRBQ
Carpometacarpal
Left ØRBT
Right ØRBS
Cervical Vertebral ØRB1
Cervicothoracic Vertebral ØRB4
Coccygeal ØSB6
Elbow
Left ØRBM
Right ØRBL
Finger Phalangeal
Left ØRBX
Right ØRBW
Hip
Left ØSBB
Right ØSB9
Knee
Left ØSBD
Right ØSBC
Lumbar Vertebral ØSBØ
Lumbosacral ØSB3
Metacarpophalangeal
Left ØRBV
Right ØRBU
Metatarsal-Phalangeal
Left ØSBN
Right ØSBM
Occipital-cervical ØRBØ
Sacrococcygeal ØSB5
Sacroiliac
Left ØSB8
Right ØSB7
Shoulder
Left ØRBK
Right ØRBJ
Sternoclavicular
Left ØRBF
Right ØRBE
Tarsal
Left ØSBJ
Right ØSBH
Tarsometatarsal
Left ØSBL
Right ØSBK
Temporomandibular
Left ØRBD
Right ØRBC
Thoracic Vertebral ØRB6
Thoracolumbar Vertebral ØRBA
Toe Phalangeal
Left ØSBQ
Right ØSBP
Wrist
Left ØRBP
Right ØRBN
Kidney
Left ØTB1
Right ØTBØ
Kidney Pelvis
Left ØTB4
Right ØTB3
Knee Region
Left ØYBG
Right ØYBF
Larynx ØCBS
Leg
Lower
Left ØYBJ
Right ØYBH
Upper
Left ØYBD
Right ØYBC

**Excision** — *continued*
Lens
Left Ø8BK3Z
Right Ø8BJ3Z
Lip
Lower ØCB1
Upper ØCBØ
Liver ØFBØ
Left Lobe ØFB2
Right Lobe ØFB1
Lung
Bilateral ØBBM
Left ØBBL
Lower Lobe
Left ØBBJ
Right ØBBF
Middle Lobe, Right ØBBD
Right ØBBK
Upper Lobe
Left ØBBG
Right ØBBC
Lung Lingula ØBBH
Lymphatic
Aortic Ø7BD
Axillary
Left Ø7B6
Right Ø7B5
Head Ø7BØ
Inguinal
Left Ø7BJ
Right Ø7BH
Internal Mammary
Left Ø7B9
Right Ø7B8
Lower Extremity
Left Ø7BG
Right Ø7BF
Mesenteric Ø7BB
Neck
Left Ø7B2
Right Ø7B1
Pelvis Ø7BC
Thoracic Duct Ø7BK
Thorax Ø7B7
Upper Extremity
Left Ø7B4
Right Ø7B3
Mandible
Left ØNBV
Right ØNBT
Maxilla ØNBR
Mediastinum ØWBC
Medulla Oblongata ØØBD
Mesentery ØDBV
Metacarpal
Left ØPBQ
Right ØPBP
Metatarsal
Left ØQBP
Right ØQBN
Muscle
Abdomen
Left ØKBL
Right ØKBK
Extraocular
Left Ø8BM
Right Ø8BL
Facial ØKB1
Foot
Left ØKBW
Right ØKBV
Hand
Left ØKBD
Right ØKBC
Head ØKBØ
Hip
Left ØKBP
Right ØKBN
Lower Arm and Wrist
Left ØKBB
Right ØKB9
Lower Leg
Left ØKBT
Right ØKBS
Neck
Left ØKB3
Right ØKB2
Papillary Ø2BD
Perineum ØKBM

**Excision** — *continued*
Muscle — *continued*
Shoulder
Left ØKB6
Right ØKB5
Thorax
Left ØKBJ
Right ØKBH
Tongue, Palate, Pharynx ØKB4
Trunk
Left ØKBG
Right ØKBF
Upper Arm
Left ØKB8
Right ØKB7
Upper Leg
Left ØKBR
Right ØKBQ
Nasal Mucosa and Soft Tissue Ø9BK
Nasopharynx Ø9BN
Neck ØWB6
Nerve
Abdominal Sympathetic Ø1BM
Abducens ØØBL
Accessory ØØBR
Acoustic ØØBN
Brachial Plexus Ø1B3
Cervical Ø1B1
Cervical Plexus Ø1BØ
Facial ØØBM
Femoral Ø1BD
Glossopharyngeal ØØBP
Head and Neck Sympathetic Ø1BK
Hypoglossal ØØBS
Lumbar Ø1BB
Lumbar Plexus Ø1B9
Lumbar Sympathetic Ø1BN
Lumbosacral Plexus Ø1BA
Median Ø1B5
Oculomotor ØØBH
Olfactory ØØBF
Optic ØØBG
Peroneal Ø1BH
Phrenic Ø1B2
Pudendal Ø1BC
Radial Ø1B6
Sacral Ø1BR
Sacral Plexus Ø1BQ
Sacral Sympathetic Ø1BP
Sciatic Ø1BF
Thoracic Ø1B8
Thoracic Sympathetic Ø1BL
Tibial Ø1BG
Trigeminal ØØBK
Trochlear ØØBJ
Ulnar Ø1B4
Vagus ØØBQ
Nipple
Left ØHBX
Right ØHBW
Omentum ØDBU
Oral Cavity and Throat ØWB3
Orbit
Left ØNBQ
Right ØNBP
Ovary
Bilateral ØUB2
Left ØUB1
Right ØUBØ
Palate
Hard ØCB2
Soft ØCB3
Pancreas ØFBG
Para-aortic Body ØGB9
Paraganglion Extremity ØGBF
Parathyroid Gland ØGBR
Inferior
Left ØGBP
Right ØGBN
Multiple ØGBQ
Superior
Left ØGBM
Right ØGBL
Patella
Left ØQBF
Right ØQBD
Penis ØVBS
Pericardium Ø2BN

**Excision** — *continued*
- Perineum
  - Female ØWBN
  - Male ØWBM
- Peritoneum ØDBW
- Phalanx
  - Finger
    - Left ØPBV
    - Right ØPBT
  - Thumb
    - Left ØPBS
    - Right ØPBR
  - Toe
    - Left ØQBR
    - Right ØQBQ
- Pharynx ØCBM
- Pineal Body ØGB1
- Pleura
  - Left ØBBP
  - Right ØBBN
- Pons ØØBB
- Prepuce ØVBT
- Prostate ØVBØ
- Radius
  - Left ØPBJ
  - Right ØPBH
- Rectum ØDBP
- Retina
  - Left Ø8BF3Z
  - Right Ø8BE3Z
- Retroperitoneum ØWBH
- Ribs
  - 1 to 2 ØPB1
  - 3 or More ØPB2
- Sacrum ØQB1
- Scapula
  - Left ØPB6
  - Right ØPB5
- Sclera
  - Left Ø8B7XZ
  - Right Ø8B6XZ
- Scrotum ØVB5
- Septum
  - Atrial Ø2B5
  - Nasal Ø9BM
  - Ventricular Ø2BM
- Shoulder Region
  - Left ØXB3
  - Right ØXB2
- Sinus
  - Accessory Ø9BP
  - Ethmoid
    - Left Ø9BV
    - Right Ø9BU
  - Frontal
    - Left Ø9BT
    - Right Ø9BS
  - Mastoid
    - Left Ø9BC
    - Right Ø9BB
  - Maxillary
    - Left Ø9BR
    - Right Ø9BQ
  - Sphenoid
    - Left Ø9BX
    - Right Ø9BW
- Skin
  - Abdomen ØHB7XZ
  - Back ØHB6XZ
  - Buttock ØHB8XZ
  - Chest ØHB5XZ
  - Ear
    - Left ØHB3XZ
    - Right ØHB2XZ
  - Face ØHB1XZ
  - Foot
    - Left ØHBNXZ
    - Right ØHBMXZ
  - Hand
    - Left ØHBGXZ
    - Right ØHBFXZ
  - Inguinal ØHBAXZ
  - Lower Arm
    - Left ØHBEXZ
    - Right ØHBDXZ
  - Lower Leg
    - Left ØHBLXZ
    - Right ØHBKXZ
  - Neck ØHB4XZ

**Excision** — *continued*
- Skin — *continued*
  - Perineum ØHB9XZ
  - Scalp ØHBØXZ
  - Upper Arm
    - Left ØHBCXZ
    - Right ØHBBXZ
  - Upper Leg
    - Left ØHBJXZ
    - Right ØHBHXZ
- Skull ØNBØ
- Spinal Cord
  - Cervical ØØBW
  - Lumbar ØØBY
  - Thoracic ØØBX
- Spinal Meninges ØØBT
- Spleen Ø7BP
- Sternum ØPBØ
- Stomach ØDB6
  - Pylorus ØDB7
- Subcutaneous Tissue and Fascia
  - Abdomen ØJB8
  - Back ØJB7
  - Buttock ØJB9
  - Chest ØJB6
  - Face ØJB1
  - Foot
    - Left ØJBR
    - Right ØJBQ
  - Hand
    - Left ØJBK
    - Right ØJBJ
  - Lower Arm
    - Left ØJBH
    - Right ØJBG
  - Lower Leg
    - Left ØJBP
    - Right ØJBN
  - Neck
    - Left ØJB5
    - Right ØJB4
  - Pelvic Region ØJBC
  - Perineum ØJBB
  - Scalp ØJBØ
  - Upper Arm
    - Left ØJBF
    - Right ØJBD
  - Upper Leg
    - Left ØJBM
    - Right ØJBL
- Tarsal
  - Left ØQBM
  - Right ØQBL
- Tendon
  - Abdomen
    - Left ØLBG
    - Right ØLBF
  - Ankle
    - Left ØLBT
    - Right ØLBS
  - Foot
    - Left ØLBW
    - Right ØLBV
  - Hand
    - Left ØLB8
    - Right ØLB7
  - Head and Neck ØLBØ
  - Hip
    - Left ØLBK
    - Right ØLBJ
  - Knee
    - Left ØLBR
    - Right ØLBQ
  - Lower Arm and Wrist
    - Left ØLB6
    - Right ØLB5
  - Lower Leg
    - Left ØLBP
    - Right ØLBN
  - Perineum ØLBH
  - Shoulder
    - Left ØLB2
    - Right ØLB1
  - Thorax
    - Left ØLBD
    - Right ØLBC
  - Trunk
    - Left ØLBB
    - Right ØLB9

**Excision** — *continued*
- Tendon — *continued*
  - Upper Arm
    - Left ØLB4
    - Right ØLB3
  - Upper Leg
    - Left ØLBM
    - Right ØLBL
- Testis
  - Bilateral ØVBC
  - Left ØVBB
  - Right ØVB9
- Thalamus ØØB9
- Thymus Ø7BM
- Thyroid Gland
  - Left Lobe ØGBG
  - Right Lobe ØGBH
- Thyroid Gland Isthmus ØGBJ
- Tibia
  - Left ØQBH
  - Right ØQBG
- Toe Nail ØHBRXZ
- Tongue ØCB7
- Tonsils ØCBP
- Tooth
  - Lower ØCBX
  - Upper ØCBW
- Trachea ØBB1
- Tunica Vaginalis
  - Left ØVB7
  - Right ØVB6
- Turbinate, Nasal Ø9BL
- Tympanic Membrane
  - Left Ø9B8
  - Right Ø9B7
- Ulna
  - Left ØPBL
  - Right ØPBK
- Ureter
  - Left ØTB7
  - Right ØTB6
- Urethra ØTBD
- Uterine Supporting Structure ØUB4
- Uterus ØUB9
- Uvula ØCBN
- Vagina ØUBG
- Valve
  - Aortic Ø2BF
  - Mitral Ø2BG
  - Pulmonary Ø2BH
  - Tricuspid Ø2BJ
- Vas Deferens
  - Bilateral ØVBQ
  - Left ØVBP
  - Right ØVBN
- Vein
  - Axillary
    - Left Ø5B8
    - Right Ø5B7
  - Azygos Ø5BØ
  - Basilic
    - Left Ø5BC
    - Right Ø5BB
  - Brachial
    - Left Ø5BA
    - Right Ø5B9
  - Cephalic
    - Left Ø5BF
    - Right Ø5BD
  - Colic Ø6B7
  - Common Iliac
    - Left Ø6BD
    - Right Ø6BC
  - Coronary Ø2B4
  - Esophageal Ø6B3
  - External Iliac
    - Left Ø6BG
    - Right Ø6BF
  - External Jugular
    - Left Ø5BQ
    - Right Ø5BP
  - Face
    - Left Ø5BV
    - Right Ø5BT
  - Femoral
    - Left Ø6BN
    - Right Ø6BM
  - Foot
    - Left Ø6BV

**Excision** — *continued*
Vein — *continued*
Foot — *continued*
Right Ø6BT
Gastric Ø6B2
Hand
Left Ø5BH
Right Ø5BG
Hemiazygos Ø5B1
Hepatic Ø6B4
Hypogastric
Left Ø6BJ
Right Ø6BH
Inferior Mesenteric Ø6B6
Innominate
Left Ø5B4
Right Ø5B3
Internal Jugular
Left Ø5BN
Right Ø5BM
Intracranial Ø5BL
Lower Ø6BY
Portal Ø6B8
Pulmonary
Left Ø2BT
Right Ø2BS
Renal
Left Ø6BB
Right Ø6B9
Saphenous
Left Ø6BQ
Right Ø6BP
Splenic Ø6B1
Subclavian
Left Ø5B6
Right Ø5B5
Superior Mesenteric Ø6B5
Upper Ø5BY
Vertebral
Left Ø5BS
Right Ø5BR
Vena Cava
Inferior Ø6BØ
Superior Ø2BV
Ventricle
Left Ø2BL
Right Ø2BK
Vertebra
Cervical ØPB3
Lumbar ØQBØ
Thoracic ØPB4
Vesicle
Bilateral ØVB3
Left ØVB2
Right ØVB1
Vitreous
Left Ø8B53Z
Right Ø8B43Z
Vocal Cord
Left ØCBV
Right ØCBT
Vulva ØUBM
Wrist Region
Left ØXBH
Right ØXBG
**EXCLUDER® AAA Endoprosthesis**
*use* Intraluminal Device
*use* Intraluminal Device, Branched or Fenestrated, One or Two Arteries in Ø4V
*use* Intraluminal Device, Branched or Fenestrated, Three or More Arteries in Ø4V
**EXCLUDER® IBE Endoprosthesis** *use* Intraluminal Device, Branched or Fenestrated, One or Two Arteries in Ø4V
**Exclusion, Left atrial appendage (LAA)** *see* Occlusion, Atrium, Left Ø2L7
**Exercise, rehabilitation** *see* Motor Treatment, Rehabilitation FØ7
**Exploration** *see* Inspection
**Express® Biliary SD Monorail® Premounted Stent System** *use* Intraluminal Device
**Express® (LD) Premounted Stent System** *use* Intraluminal Device
**Express® SD Renal Monorail® Premounted Stent System** *use* Intraluminal Device
**Ex-PRESS™ mini glaucoma shunt** *use* Synthetic Substitute
**Extensor carpi radialis muscle**
*use* Muscle, Lower Arm and Wrist, Left
*use* Muscle, Lower Arm and Wrist, Right
**Extensor carpi ulnaris muscle**
*use* Muscle, Lower Arm and Wrist, Left
*use* Muscle, Lower Arm and Wrist, Right
**Extensor digitorum brevis muscle**
*use* Muscle, Foot, Left
*use* Muscle, Foot, Right
**Extensor digitorum longus muscle**
*use* Muscle, Lower Leg, Left
*use* Muscle, Lower Leg, Right
**Extensor hallucis brevis muscle**
*use* Muscle, Foot, Left
*use* Muscle, Foot, Right
**Extensor hallucis longus muscle**
*use* Muscle, Lower Leg, Left
*use* Muscle, Lower Leg, Right
**External anal sphincter** *use* Anal Sphincter
**External auditory meatus**
*use* Ear, External Auditory Canal, Left
*use* Ear, External Auditory Canal, Right
**External fixator**
*use* External Fixation Device in Head and Facial Bones
*use* External Fixation Device in Lower Bones
*use* External Fixation Device in Lower Joints
*use* External Fixation Device in Upper Bones
*use* External Fixation Device in Upper Joints
**External maxillary artery** *use* Artery, Face
**External naris** *use* Nasal Mucosa and Soft Tissue
**External oblique aponeurosis** *use* Subcutaneous Tissue and Fascia, Trunk
**External oblique muscle**
*use* Muscle, Abdomen, Left
*use* Muscle, Abdomen, Right
**External popliteal nerve** *use* Nerve, Peroneal
**External pudendal artery**
*use* Artery, Femoral, Left
*use* Artery, Femoral, Right
**External pudendal vein**
*use* Saphenous Vein, Left
*use* Saphenous Vein, Right
**External urethral sphincter** *use* Urethra
**Extirpation**
Acetabulum
Left ØQC5
Right ØQC4
Adenoids ØCCQ
Ampulla of Vater ØFCC
Anal Sphincter ØDCR
Anterior Chamber
Left Ø8C3
Right Ø8C2
Anus ØDCQ
Aorta
Abdominal Ø4CØ
Thoracic
Ascending/Arch Ø2CX
Descending Ø2CW
Aortic Body ØGCD
Appendix ØDCJ
Artery
Anterior Tibial
Left Ø4CQ
Right Ø4CP
Axillary
Left Ø3C6
Right Ø3C5
Brachial
Left Ø3C8
Right Ø3C7
Celiac Ø4C1
Colic
Left Ø4C7
Middle Ø4C8
Right Ø4C6
Common Carotid
Left Ø3CJ
Right Ø3CH
Common Iliac
Left Ø4CD
Right Ø4CC
Coronary
Four or More Arteries Ø2C3
One Artery Ø2CØ
Three Arteries Ø2C2
Two Arteries Ø2C1
**Extirpation** — *continued*
Artery — *continued*
External Carotid
Left Ø3CN
Right Ø3CM
External Iliac
Left Ø4CJ
Right Ø4CH
Face Ø3CR
Femoral
Left Ø4CL
Right Ø4CK
Foot
Left Ø4CW
Right Ø4CV
Gastric Ø4C2
Hand
Left Ø3CF
Right Ø3CD
Hepatic Ø4C3
Inferior Mesenteric Ø4CB
Innominate Ø3C2
Internal Carotid
Left Ø3CL
Right Ø3CK
Internal Iliac
Left Ø4CF
Right Ø4CE
Internal Mammary
Left Ø3C1
Right Ø3CØ
Intracranial Ø3CG
Lower Ø4CY
Peroneal
Left Ø4CU
Right Ø4CT
Popliteal
Left Ø4CN
Right Ø4CM
Posterior Tibial
Left Ø4CS
Right Ø4CR
Pulmonary
Left Ø2CR
Right Ø2CQ
Pulmonary Trunk Ø2CP
Radial
Left Ø3CC
Right Ø3CB
Renal
Left Ø4CA
Right Ø4C9
Splenic Ø4C4
Subclavian
Left Ø3C4
Right Ø3C3
Superior Mesenteric Ø4C5
Temporal
Left Ø3CT
Right Ø3CS
Thyroid
Left Ø3CV
Right Ø3CU
Ulnar
Left Ø3CA
Right Ø3C9
Upper Ø3CY
Vertebral
Left Ø3CQ
Right Ø3CP
Atrium
Left Ø2C7
Right Ø2C6
Auditory Ossicle
Left Ø9CA
Right Ø9C9
Basal Ganglia ØØC8
Bladder ØTCB
Bladder Neck ØTCC
Bone
Ethmoid
Left ØNCG
Right ØNCF
Frontal ØNC1
Hyoid ØNCX
Lacrimal
Left ØNCJ
Right ØNCH
Nasal ØNCB

**Extirpation** — *continued*
Bone — *continued*
Occipital ØNC7
Palatine
Left ØNCL
Right ØNCK
Parietal
Left ØNC4
Right ØNC3
Pelvic
Left ØQC3
Right ØQC2
Sphenoid ØNCC
Temporal
Left ØNC6
Right ØNC5
Zygomatic
Left ØNCN
Right ØNCM
Brain ØØCØ
Breast
Bilateral ØHCV
Left ØHCU
Right ØHCT
Bronchus
Lingula ØBC9
Lower Lobe
Left ØBCB
Right ØBC6
Main
Left ØBC7
Right ØBC3
Middle Lobe, Right ØBC5
Upper Lobe
Left ØBC8
Right ØBC4
Buccal Mucosa ØCC4
Bursa and Ligament
Abdomen
Left ØMCJ
Right ØMCH
Ankle
Left ØMCR
Right ØMCQ
Elbow
Left ØMC4
Right ØMC3
Foot
Left ØMCT
Right ØMCS
Hand
Left ØMC8
Right ØMC7
Head and Neck ØMCØ
Hip
Left ØMCM
Right ØMCL
Knee
Left ØMCP
Right ØMCN
Lower Extremity
Left ØMCW
Right ØMCV
Perineum ØMCK
Rib(s) ØMCG
Shoulder
Left ØMC2
Right ØMC1
Spine
Lower ØMCD
Upper ØMCC
Sternum ØMCF
Upper Extremity
Left ØMCB
Right ØMC9
Wrist
Left ØMC6
Right ØMC5
Carina ØBC2
Carotid Bodies, Bilateral ØGC8
Carotid Body
Left ØGC6
Right ØGC7
Carpal
Left ØPCN
Right ØPCM
Cavity, Cranial ØWC1
Cecum ØDCH
Cerebellum ØØCC

**Extirpation** — *continued*
Cerebral Hemisphere ØØC7
Cerebral Meninges ØØC1
Cerebral Ventricle ØØC6
Cervix ØUCC
Chordae Tendineae Ø2C9
Choroid
Left Ø8CB
Right Ø8CA
Cisterna Chyli Ø7CL
Clavicle
Left ØPCB
Right ØPC9
Clitoris ØUCJ
Coccygeal Glomus ØGCB
Coccyx ØQCS
Colon
Ascending ØDCK
Descending ØDCM
Sigmoid ØDCN
Transverse ØDCL
Conduction Mechanism Ø2C8
Conjunctiva
Left Ø8CTXZZ
Right Ø8CSXZZ
Cord
Bilateral ØVCH
Left ØVCG
Right ØVCF
Cornea
Left Ø8C9XZZ
Right Ø8C8XZZ
Cul-de-sac ØUCF
Diaphragm ØBCT
Disc
Cervical Vertebral ØRC3
Cervicothoracic Vertebral ØRC5
Lumbar Vertebral ØSC2
Lumbosacral ØSC4
Thoracic Vertebral ØRC9
Thoracolumbar Vertebral ØRCB
Duct
Common Bile ØFC9
Cystic ØFC8
Hepatic
Common ØFC7
Left ØFC6
Right ØFC5
Lacrimal
Left Ø8CY
Right Ø8CX
Pancreatic ØFCD
Accessory ØFCF
Parotid
Left ØCCC
Right ØCCB
Duodenum ØDC9
Dura Mater ØØC2
Ear
External
Left Ø9C1
Right Ø9CØ
External Auditory Canal
Left Ø9C4
Right Ø9C3
Inner
Left Ø9CE
Right Ø9CD
Middle
Left Ø9C6
Right Ø9C5
Endometrium ØUCB
Epididymis
Bilateral ØVCL
Left ØVCK
Right ØVCJ
Epidural Space, Intracranial ØØC3
Epiglottis ØCCR
Esophagogastric Junction ØDC4
Esophagus ØDC5
Lower ØDC3
Middle ØDC2
Upper ØDC1
Eustachian Tube
Left Ø9CG
Right Ø9CF
Eye
Left Ø8C1XZZ
Right Ø8CØXZZ

**Extirpation** — *continued*
Eyelid
Lower
Left Ø8CR
Right Ø8CQ
Upper
Left Ø8CP
Right Ø8CN
Fallopian Tube
Left ØUC6
Right ØUC5
Fallopian Tubes, Bilateral ØUC7
Femoral Shaft
Left ØQC9
Right ØQC8
Femur
Lower
Left ØQCC
Right ØQCB
Upper
Left ØQC7
Right ØQC6
Fibula
Left ØQCK
Right ØQCJ
Finger Nail ØHCQXZZ
Gallbladder ØFC4
Gastrointestinal Tract ØWCP
Genitourinary Tract ØWCR
Gingiva
Lower ØCC6
Upper ØCC5
Gland
Adrenal
Bilateral ØGC4
Left ØGC2
Right ØGC3
Lacrimal
Left Ø8CW
Right Ø8CV
Minor Salivary ØCCJ
Parotid
Left ØCC9
Right ØCC8
Pituitary ØGCØ
Sublingual
Left ØCCF
Right ØCCD
Submaxillary
Left ØCCH
Right ØCCG
Vestibular ØUCL
Glenoid Cavity
Left ØPC8
Right ØPC7
Glomus Jugulare ØGCC
Humeral Head
Left ØPCD
Right ØPCC
Humeral Shaft
Left ØPCG
Right ØPCF
Hymen ØUCK
Hypothalamus ØØCA
Ileocecal Valve ØDCC
Ileum ØDCB
Intestine
Large ØDCE
Left ØDCG
Right ØDCF
Small ØDC8
Iris
Left Ø8CD
Right Ø8CC
Jejunum ØDCA
Joint
Acromioclavicular
Left ØRCH
Right ØRCG
Ankle
Left ØSCG
Right ØSCF
Carpal
Left ØRCR
Right ØRCQ
Carpometacarpal
Left ØRCT
Right ØRCS
Cervical Vertebral ØRC1

- **Extirpation** — *continued*
  - Joint — *continued*
    - Cervicothoracic Vertebral ØRC4
    - Coccygeal ØSC6
    - Elbow
      - Left ØRCM
      - Right ØRCL
    - Finger Phalangeal
      - Left ØRCX
      - Right ØRCW
    - Hip
      - Left ØSCB
      - Right ØSC9
    - Knee
      - Left ØSCD
      - Right ØSCC
    - Lumbar Vertebral ØSCØ
    - Lumbosacral ØSC3
    - Metacarpophalangeal
      - Left ØRCV
      - Right ØRCU
    - Metatarsal-Phalangeal
      - Left ØSCN
      - Right ØSCM
    - Occipital-cervical ØRCØ
    - Sacrococcygeal ØSC5
    - Sacroiliac
      - Left ØSC8
      - Right ØSC7
    - Shoulder
      - Left ØRCK
      - Right ØRCJ
    - Sternoclavicular
      - Left ØRCF
      - Right ØRCE
    - Tarsal
      - Left ØSCJ
      - Right ØSCH
    - Tarsometatarsal
      - Left ØSCL
      - Right ØSCK
    - Temporomandibular
      - Left ØRCD
      - Right ØRCC
    - Thoracic Vertebral ØRC6
    - Thoracolumbar Vertebral ØRCA
    - Toe Phalangeal
      - Left ØSCQ
      - Right ØSCP
    - Wrist
      - Left ØRCP
      - Right ØRCN
  - Kidney
    - Left ØTC1
    - Right ØTCØ
  - Kidney Pelvis
    - Left ØTC4
    - Right ØTC3
  - Larynx ØCCS
  - Lens
    - Left Ø8CK
    - Right Ø8CJ
  - Lip
    - Lower ØCC1
    - Upper ØCCØ
  - Liver ØFCØ
    - Left Lobe ØFC2
    - Right Lobe ØFC1
  - Lung
    - Bilateral ØBCM
    - Left ØBCL
    - Lower Lobe
      - Left ØBCJ
      - Right ØBCF
    - Middle Lobe, Right ØBCD
    - Right ØBCK
    - Upper Lobe
      - Left ØBCG
      - Right ØBCC
  - Lung Lingula ØBCH
  - Lymphatic
    - Aortic Ø7CD
    - Axillary
      - Left Ø7C6
      - Right Ø7C5
    - Head Ø7CØ
    - Inguinal
      - Left Ø7CJ
      - Right Ø7CH

- **Extirpation** — *continued*
  - Lymphatic — *continued*
    - Internal Mammary
      - Left Ø7C9
      - Right Ø7C8
    - Lower Extremity
      - Left Ø7CG
      - Right Ø7CF
    - Mesenteric Ø7CB
    - Neck
      - Left Ø7C2
      - Right Ø7C1
    - Pelvis Ø7CC
    - Thoracic Duct Ø7CK
    - Thorax Ø7C7
    - Upper Extremity
      - Left Ø7C4
      - Right Ø7C3
  - Mandible
    - Left ØNCV
    - Right ØNCT
  - Maxilla ØNCR
  - Mediastinum ØWCC
  - Medulla Oblongata ØØCD
  - Mesentery ØDCV
  - Metacarpal
    - Left ØPCQ
    - Right ØPCP
  - Metatarsal
    - Left ØQCP
    - Right ØQCN
  - Muscle
    - Abdomen
      - Left ØKCL
      - Right ØKCK
    - Extraocular
      - Left Ø8CM
      - Right Ø8CL
    - Facial ØKC1
    - Foot
      - Left ØKCW
      - Right ØKCV
    - Hand
      - Left ØKCD
      - Right ØKCC
    - Head ØKCØ
    - Hip
      - Left ØKCP
      - Right ØKCN
    - Lower Arm and Wrist
      - Left ØKCB
      - Right ØKC9
    - Lower Leg
      - Left ØKCT
      - Right ØKCS
    - Neck
      - Left ØKC3
      - Right ØKC2
    - Papillary Ø2CD
    - Perineum ØKCM
    - Shoulder
      - Left ØKC6
      - Right ØKC5
    - Thorax
      - Left ØKCJ
      - Right ØKCH
    - Tongue, Palate, Pharynx ØKC4
    - Trunk
      - Left ØKCG
      - Right ØKCF
    - Upper Arm
      - Left ØKC8
      - Right ØKC7
    - Upper Leg
      - Left ØKCR
      - Right ØKCQ
  - Nasal Mucosa and Soft Tissue Ø9CK
  - Nasopharynx Ø9CN
  - Nerve
    - Abdominal Sympathetic Ø1CM
    - Abducens ØØCL
    - Accessory ØØCR
    - Acoustic ØØCN
    - Brachial Plexus Ø1C3
    - Cervical Ø1C1
    - Cervical Plexus Ø1CØ
    - Facial ØØCM
    - Femoral Ø1CD
    - Glossopharyngeal ØØCP

- **Extirpation** — *continued*
  - Nerve — *continued*
    - Head and Neck Sympathetic Ø1CK
    - Hypoglossal ØØCS
    - Lumbar Ø1CB
    - Lumbar Plexus Ø1C9
    - Lumbar Sympathetic Ø1CN
    - Lumbosacral Plexus Ø1CA
    - Median Ø1C5
    - Oculomotor ØØCH
    - Olfactory ØØCF
    - Optic ØØCG
    - Peroneal Ø1CH
    - Phrenic Ø1C2
    - Pudendal Ø1CC
    - Radial Ø1C6
    - Sacral Ø1CR
    - Sacral Plexus Ø1CQ
    - Sacral Sympathetic Ø1CP
    - Sciatic Ø1CF
    - Thoracic Ø1C8
    - Thoracic Sympathetic Ø1CL
    - Tibial Ø1CG
    - Trigeminal ØØCK
    - Trochlear ØØCJ
    - Ulnar Ø1C4
    - Vagus ØØCQ
  - Nipple
    - Left ØHCX
    - Right ØHCW
  - Omentum ØDCU
  - Oral Cavity and Throat ØWC3
  - Orbit
    - Left ØNCQ
    - Right ØNCP
  - Orbital Atherectomy Technology X2C
  - Ovary
    - Bilateral ØUC2
    - Left ØUC1
    - Right ØUCØ
  - Palate
    - Hard ØCC2
    - Soft ØCC3
  - Pancreas ØFCG
  - Para-aortic Body ØGC9
  - Paraganglion Extremity ØGCF
  - Parathyroid Gland ØGCR
    - Inferior
      - Left ØGCP
      - Right ØGCN
    - Multiple ØGCQ
    - Superior
      - Left ØGCM
      - Right ØGCL
  - Patella
    - Left ØQCF
    - Right ØQCD
  - Pelvic Cavity ØWCJ
  - Penis ØVCS
  - Pericardial Cavity ØWCD
  - Pericardium Ø2CN
  - Peritoneal Cavity ØWCG
  - Peritoneum ØDCW
  - Phalanx
    - Finger
      - Left ØPCV
      - Right ØPCT
    - Thumb
      - Left ØPCS
      - Right ØPCR
    - Toe
      - Left ØQCR
      - Right ØQCQ
  - Pharynx ØCCM
  - Pineal Body ØGC1
  - Pleura
    - Left ØBCP
    - Right ØBCN
  - Pleural Cavity
    - Left ØWCB
    - Right ØWC9
  - Pons ØØCB
  - Prepuce ØVCT
  - Prostate ØVCØ
  - Radius
    - Left ØPCJ
    - Right ØPCH
  - Rectum ØDCP
  - Respiratory Tract ØWCQ

**Extirpation** — *continued*
Retina
Left Ø8CF
Right Ø8CE
Retinal Vessel
Left Ø8CH
Right Ø8CG
Retroperitoneum ØWCH
Ribs
1 to 2 ØPC1
3 or More ØPC2
Sacrum ØQC1
Scapula
Left ØPC6
Right ØPC5
Sclera
Left Ø8C7XZZ
Right Ø8C6XZZ
Scrotum ØVC5
Septum
Atrial Ø2C5
Nasal Ø9CM
Ventricular Ø2CM
Sinus
Accessory Ø9CP
Ethmoid
Left Ø9CV
Right Ø9CU
Frontal
Left Ø9CT
Right Ø9CS
Mastoid
Left Ø9CC
Right Ø9CB
Maxillary
Left Ø9CR
Right Ø9CQ
Sphenoid
Left Ø9CX
Right Ø9CW
Skin
Abdomen ØHC7XZZ
Back ØHC6XZZ
Buttock ØHC8XZZ
Chest ØHC5XZZ
Ear
Left ØHC3XZZ
Right ØHC2XZZ
Face ØHC1XZZ
Foot
Left ØHCNXZZ
Right ØHCMXZZ
Hand
Left ØHCGXZZ
Right ØHCFXZZ
Inguinal ØHCAXZZ
Lower Arm
Left ØHCEXZZ
Right ØHCDXZZ
Lower Leg
Left ØHCLXZZ
Right ØHCKXZZ
Neck ØHC4XZZ
Perineum ØHC9XZZ
Scalp ØHCØXZZ
Upper Arm
Left ØHCCXZZ
Right ØHCBXZZ
Upper Leg
Left ØHCJXZZ
Right ØHCHXZZ
Spinal Canal ØØCU
Spinal Cord
Cervical ØØCW
Lumbar ØØCY
Thoracic ØØCX
Spinal Meninges ØØCT
Spleen Ø7CP
Sternum ØPCØ
Stomach ØDC6
Pylorus ØDC7
Subarachnoid Space, Intracranial ØØC5
Subcutaneous Tissue and Fascia
Abdomen ØJC8
Back ØJC7
Buttock ØJC9
Chest ØJC6
Face ØJC1

**Extirpation** — *continued*
Subcutaneous Tissue and Fascia — *continued*
Foot
Left ØJCR
Right ØJCQ
Hand
Left ØJCK
Right ØJCJ
Lower Arm
Left ØJCH
Right ØJCG
Lower Leg
Left ØJCP
Right ØJCN
Neck
Left ØJC5
Right ØJC4
Pelvic Region ØJCC
Perineum ØJCB
Scalp ØJCØ
Upper Arm
Left ØJCF
Right ØJCD
Upper Leg
Left ØJCM
Right ØJCL
Subdural Space, Intracranial ØØC4
Tarsal
Left ØQCM
Right ØQCL
Tendon
Abdomen
Left ØLCG
Right ØLCF
Ankle
Left ØLCT
Right ØLCS
Foot
Left ØLCW
Right ØLCV
Hand
Left ØLC8
Right ØLC7
Head and Neck ØLCØ
Hip
Left ØLCK
Right ØLCJ
Knee
Left ØLCR
Right ØLCQ
Lower Arm and Wrist
Left ØLC6
Right ØLC5
Lower Leg
Left ØLCP
Right ØLCN
Perineum ØLCH
Shoulder
Left ØLC2
Right ØLC1
Thorax
Left ØLCD
Right ØLCC
Trunk
Left ØLCB
Right ØLC9
Upper Arm
Left ØLC4
Right ØLC3
Upper Leg
Left ØLCM
Right ØLCL
Testis
Bilateral ØVCC
Left ØVCB
Right ØVC9
Thalamus ØØC9
Thymus Ø7CM
Thyroid Gland ØGCK
Left Lobe ØGCG
Right Lobe ØGCH
Tibia
Left ØQCH
Right ØQCG
Toe Nail ØHCRXZZ
Tongue ØCC7
Tonsils ØCCP
Tooth
Lower ØCCX

**Extirpation** — *continued*
Tooth — *continued*
Upper ØCCW
Trachea ØBC1
Tunica Vaginalis
Left ØVC7
Right ØVC6
Turbinate, Nasal Ø9CL
Tympanic Membrane
Left Ø9C8
Right Ø9C7
Ulna
Left ØPCL
Right ØPCK
Ureter
Left ØTC7
Right ØTC6
Urethra ØTCD
Uterine Supporting Structure ØUC4
Uterus ØUC9
Uvula ØCCN
Vagina ØUCG
Valve
Aortic Ø2CF
Mitral Ø2CG
Pulmonary Ø2CH
Tricuspid Ø2CJ
Vas Deferens
Bilateral ØVCQ
Left ØVCP
Right ØVCN
Vein
Axillary
Left Ø5C8
Right Ø5C7
Azygos Ø5CØ
Basilic
Left Ø5CC
Right Ø5CB
Brachial
Left Ø5CA
Right Ø5C9
Cephalic
Left Ø5CF
Right Ø5CD
Colic Ø6C7
Common Iliac
Left Ø6CD
Right Ø6CC
Coronary Ø2C4
Esophageal Ø6C3
External Iliac
Left Ø6CG
Right Ø6CF
External Jugular
Left Ø5CQ
Right Ø5CP
Face
Left Ø5CV
Right Ø5CT
Femoral
Left Ø6CN
Right Ø6CM
Foot
Left Ø6CV
Right Ø6CT
Gastric Ø6C2
Hand
Left Ø5CH
Right Ø5CG
Hemiazygos Ø5C1
Hepatic Ø6C4
Hypogastric
Left Ø6CJ
Right Ø6CH
Inferior Mesenteric Ø6C6
Innominate
Left Ø5C4
Right Ø5C3
Internal Jugular
Left Ø5CN
Right Ø5CM
Intracranial Ø5CL
Lower Ø6CY
Portal Ø6C8
Pulmonary
Left Ø2CT
Right Ø2CS

**Extirpation** — *continued*
Vein — *continued*
Renal
Left Ø6CB
Right Ø6C9
Saphenous
Left Ø6CQ
Right Ø6CP
Splenic Ø6C1
Subclavian
Left Ø5C6
Right Ø5C5
Superior Mesenteric Ø6C5
Upper Ø5CY
Vertebral
Left Ø5CS
Right Ø5CR
Vena Cava
Inferior Ø6CØ
Superior Ø2CV
Ventricle
Left Ø2CL
Right Ø2CK
Vertebra
Cervical ØPC3
Lumbar ØQCØ
Thoracic ØPC4
Vesicle
Bilateral ØVC3
Left ØVC2
Right ØVC1
Vitreous
Left Ø8C5
Right Ø8C4
Vocal Cord
Left ØCCV
Right ØCCT
Vulva ØUCM
**Extracorporeal Carbon Dioxide Removal (ECCO2R)** 5AØ92ØZ
**Extracorporeal shock wave lithotripsy** *see* Fragmentation
**Extracranial-intracranial bypass (EC-IC)** *see* Bypass, Upper Arteries Ø31
**Extraction**
Acetabulum
Left ØQD5ØZZ
Right ØQD4ØZZ
Anus ØDDQ
Appendix ØDDJ
Auditory Ossicle
Left Ø9DAØZZ
Right Ø9D9ØZZ
Bone
Ethmoid
Left ØNDGØZZ
Right ØNDFØZZ
Frontal ØND1ØZZ
Hyoid ØNDXØZZ
Lacrimal
Left ØNDJØZZ
Right ØNDHØZZ
Nasal ØNDBØZZ
Occipital ØND7ØZZ
Palatine
Left ØNDLØZZ
Right ØNDKØZZ
Parietal
Left ØND4ØZZ
Right ØND3ØZZ
Pelvic
Left ØQD3ØZZ
Right ØQD2ØZZ
Sphenoid ØNDCØZZ
Temporal
Left ØND6ØZZ
Right ØND5ØZZ
Zygomatic
Left ØNDNØZZ
Right ØNDMØZZ
Bone Marrow
Iliac Ø7DR
Sternum Ø7DQ
Vertebral Ø7DS
Bronchus
Lingula ØBD9
Lower Lobe
Left ØBDB
Right ØBD6

**Extraction** — *continued*
Bronchus — *continued*
Main
Left ØBD7
Right ØBD3
Middle Lobe, Right ØBD5
Upper Lobe
Left ØBD8
Right ØBD4
Bursa and Ligament
Abdomen
Left ØMDJ
Right ØMDH
Ankle
Left ØMDR
Right ØMDQ
Elbow
Left ØMD4
Right ØMD3
Foot
Left ØMDT
Right ØMDS
Hand
Left ØMD8
Right ØMD7
Head and Neck ØMDØ
Hip
Left ØMDM
Right ØMDL
Knee
Left ØMDP
Right ØMDN
Lower Extremity
Left ØMDW
Right ØMDV
Perineum ØMDK
Rib(s) ØMDG
Shoulder
Left ØMD2
Right ØMD1
Spine
Lower ØMDD
Upper ØMDC
Sternum ØMDF
Upper Extremity
Left ØMDB
Right ØMD9
Wrist
Left ØMD6
Right ØMD5
Carina ØBD2
Carpal
Left ØPDNØZZ
Right ØPDMØZZ
Cecum ØDDH
Cerebral Meninges ØØD1
Cisterna Chyli Ø7DL
Clavicle
Left ØPDBØZZ
Right ØPD9ØZZ
Coccyx ØQDSØZZ
Colon
Ascending ØDDK
Descending ØDDM
Sigmoid ØDDN
Transverse ØDDL
Cornea
Left Ø8D9XZ
Right Ø8D8XZ
Duodenum ØDD9
Dura Mater ØØD2
Endometrium ØUDB
Esophagogastric Junction ØDD4
Esophagus ØDD5
Lower ØDD3
Middle ØDD2
Upper ØDD1
Femoral Shaft
Left ØQD9ØZZ
Right ØQD8ØZZ
Femur
Lower
Left ØQDCØZZ
Right ØQDBØZZ
Upper
Left ØQD7ØZZ
Right ØQD6ØZZ
Fibula
Left ØQDKØZZ

**Extraction** — *continued*
Fibula — *continued*
Right ØQDJØZZ
Finger Nail ØHDQXZZ
Glenoid Cavity
Left ØPD8ØZZ
Right ØPD7ØZZ
Hair ØHDSXZZ
Humeral Head
Left ØPDDØZZ
Right ØPDCØZZ
Humeral Shaft
Left ØPDGØZZ
Right ØPDFØZZ
Ileocecal Valve ØDDC
Ileum ØDDB
Intestine
Large ØDDE
Left ØDDG
Right ØDDF
Small ØDD8
Jejunum ØDDA
Kidney
Left ØTD1
Right ØTDØ
Lens
Left Ø8DK3ZZ
Right Ø8DJ3ZZ
Lung
Bilateral ØBDM
Left ØBDL
Lower Lobe
Left ØBDJ
Right ØBDF
Middle Lobe, Right ØBDD
Right ØBDK
Upper Lobe
Left ØBDG
Right ØBDC
Lung Lingula ØBDH
Lymphatic
Aortic Ø7DD
Axillary
Left Ø7D6
Right Ø7D5
Head Ø7DØ
Inguinal
Left Ø7DJ
Right Ø7DH
Internal Mammary
Left Ø7D9
Right Ø7D8
Lower Extremity
Left Ø7DG
Right Ø7DF
Mesenteric Ø7DB
Neck
Left Ø7D2
Right Ø7D1
Pelvis Ø7DC
Thoracic Duct Ø7DK
Thorax Ø7D7
Upper Extremity
Left Ø7D4
Right Ø7D3
Mandible
Left ØNDVØZZ
Right ØNDTØZZ
Maxilla ØNDRØZZ
Metacarpal
Left ØPDQØZZ
Right ØPDPØZZ
Metatarsal
Left ØQDPØZZ
Right ØQDNØZZ
Muscle
Abdomen
Left ØKDLØZZ
Right ØKDKØZZ
Facial ØKD1ØZZ
Foot
Left ØKDWØZZ
Right ØKDVØZZ
Hand
Left ØKDDØZZ
Right ØKDCØZZ
Head ØKDØØZZ
Hip
Left ØKDPØZZ

- **Extraction** — *continued*
  - Muscle — *continued*
    - Hip — *continued*
      - Right ØKDNØZZ
    - Lower Arm and Wrist
      - Left ØKDBØZZ
      - Right ØKD9ØZZ
    - Lower Leg
      - Left ØKDTØZZ
      - Right ØKDSØZZ
    - Neck
      - Left ØKD3ØZZ
      - Right ØKD2ØZZ
    - Perineum ØKDMØZZ
    - Shoulder
      - Left ØKD6ØZZ
      - Right ØKD5ØZZ
    - Thorax
      - Left ØKDJØZZ
      - Right ØKDHØZZ
    - Tongue, Palate, Pharynx ØKD4ØZZ
    - Trunk
      - Left ØKDGØZZ
      - Right ØKDFØZZ
    - Upper Arm
      - Left ØKD8ØZZ
      - Right ØKD7ØZZ
    - Upper Leg
      - Left ØKDRØZZ
      - Right ØKDQØZZ
  - Nerve
    - Abdominal Sympathetic Ø1DM
    - Abducens ØØDL
    - Accessory ØØDR
    - Acoustic ØØDN
    - Brachial Plexus Ø1D3
    - Cervical Ø1D1
    - Cervical Plexus Ø1DØ
    - Facial ØØDM
    - Femoral Ø1DD
    - Glossopharyngeal ØØDP
    - Head and Neck Sympathetic Ø1DK
    - Hypoglossal ØØDS
    - Lumbar Ø1DB
    - Lumbar Plexus Ø1D9
    - Lumbar Sympathetic Ø1DN
    - Lumbosacral Plexus Ø1DA
    - Median Ø1D5
    - Oculomotor ØØDH
    - Olfactory ØØDF
    - Optic ØØDG
    - Peroneal Ø1DH
    - Phrenic Ø1D2
    - Pudendal Ø1DC
    - Radial Ø1D6
    - Sacral Ø1DR
    - Sacral Plexus Ø1DQ
    - Sacral Sympathetic Ø1DP
    - Sciatic Ø1DF
    - Thoracic Ø1D8
    - Thoracic Sympathetic Ø1DL
    - Tibial Ø1DG
    - Trigeminal ØØDK
    - Trochlear ØØDJ
    - Ulnar Ø1D4
    - Vagus ØØDQ
  - Orbit
    - Left ØNDQØZZ
    - Right ØNDPØZZ
  - Ova ØUDN
  - Patella
    - Left ØQDFØZZ
    - Right ØQDDØZZ
  - Phalanx
    - Finger
      - Left ØPDVØZZ
      - Right ØPDTØZZ
    - Thumb
      - Left ØPDSØZZ
      - Right ØPDRØZZ
    - Toe
      - Left ØQDRØZZ
      - Right ØQDQØZZ
  - Pleura
    - Left ØBDP
    - Right ØBDN
  - Products of Conception
    - Classical 1ØDØØZØ
    - Ectopic 1ØD2

- **Extraction** — *continued*
  - Products of Conception — *continued*
    - Extraperitoneal 1ØDØØZ2
    - High Forceps 1ØDØ7Z5
    - Internal Version 1ØDØ7Z7
    - Low Cervical 1ØDØØZ1
    - Low Forceps 1ØDØ7Z3
    - Mid Forceps 1ØDØ7Z4
    - Other 1ØDØ7Z8
    - Retained 1ØD1
    - Vacuum 1ØDØ7Z6
  - Radius
    - Left ØPDJØZZ
    - Right ØPDHØZZ
  - Rectum ØDDP
  - Ribs
    - 1 to 2 ØPD1ØZZ
    - 3 or More ØPD2ØZZ
  - Sacrum ØQD1ØZZ
  - Scapula
    - Left ØPD6ØZZ
    - Right ØPD5ØZZ
  - Septum, Nasal Ø9DM
  - Sinus
    - Accessory Ø9DP
    - Ethmoid
      - Left Ø9DV
      - Right Ø9DU
    - Frontal
      - Left Ø9DT
      - Right Ø9DS
    - Mastoid
      - Left Ø9DC
      - Right Ø9DB
    - Maxillary
      - Left Ø9DR
      - Right Ø9DQ
    - Sphenoid
      - Left Ø9DX
      - Right Ø9DW
  - Skin
    - Abdomen ØHD7XZZ
    - Back ØHD6XZZ
    - Buttock ØHD8XZZ
    - Chest ØHD5XZZ
    - Ear
      - Left ØHD3XZZ
      - Right ØHD2XZZ
    - Face ØHD1XZZ
    - Foot
      - Left ØHDNXZZ
      - Right ØHDMXZZ
    - Hand
      - Left ØHDGXZZ
      - Right ØHDFXZZ
    - Inguinal ØHDAXZZ
    - Lower Arm
      - Left ØHDEXZZ
      - Right ØHDDXZZ
    - Lower Leg
      - Left ØHDLXZZ
      - Right ØHDKXZZ
    - Neck ØHD4XZZ
    - Perineum ØHD9XZZ
    - Scalp ØHDØXZZ
    - Upper Arm
      - Left ØHDCXZZ
      - Right ØHDBXZZ
    - Upper Leg
      - Left ØHDJXZZ
      - Right ØHDHXZZ
  - Skull ØNDØØZZ
  - Spinal Meninges ØØDT
  - Spleen Ø7DP
  - Sternum ØPDØØZZ
  - Stomach ØDD6
    - Pylorus ØDD7
  - Subcutaneous Tissue and Fascia
    - Abdomen ØJD8
    - Back ØJD7
    - Buttock ØJD9
    - Chest ØJD6
    - Face ØJD1
    - Foot
      - Left ØJDR
      - Right ØJDQ
    - Hand
      - Left ØJDK
      - Right ØJDJ

- **Extraction** — *continued*
  - Subcutaneous Tissue and Fascia — *continued*
    - Lower Arm
      - Left ØJDH
      - Right ØJDG
    - Lower Leg
      - Left ØJDP
      - Right ØJDN
    - Neck
      - Left ØJD5
      - Right ØJD4
    - Pelvic Region ØJDC
    - Perineum ØJDB
    - Scalp ØJDØ
    - Upper Arm
      - Left ØJDF
      - Right ØJDD
    - Upper Leg
      - Left ØJDM
      - Right ØJDL
  - Tarsal
    - Left ØQDMØZZ
    - Right ØQDLØZZ
  - Tendon
    - Abdomen
      - Left ØLDGØZZ
      - Right ØLDFØZZ
    - Ankle
      - Left ØLDTØZZ
      - Right ØLDSØZZ
    - Foot
      - Left ØLDWØZZ
      - Right ØLDVØZZ
    - Hand
      - Left ØLD8ØZZ
      - Right ØLD7ØZZ
    - Head and Neck ØLDØØZZ
    - Hip
      - Left ØLDKØZZ
      - Right ØLDJØZZ
    - Knee
      - Left ØLDRØZZ
      - Right ØLDQØZZ
    - Lower Arm and Wrist
      - Left ØLD6ØZZ
      - Right ØLD5ØZZ
    - Lower Leg
      - Left ØLDPØZZ
      - Right ØLDNØZZ
    - Perineum ØLDHØZZ
    - Shoulder
      - Left ØLD2ØZZ
      - Right ØLD1ØZZ
    - Thorax
      - Left ØLDDØZZ
      - Right ØLDCØZZ
    - Trunk
      - Left ØLDBØZZ
      - Right ØLD9ØZZ
    - Upper Arm
      - Left ØLD4ØZZ
      - Right ØLD3ØZZ
    - Upper Leg
      - Left ØLDMØZZ
      - Right ØDLLØZZ
  - Thymus Ø7DM
  - Tibia
    - Left ØQDHØZZ
    - Right ØQDGØZZ
  - Toe Nail ØHDRXZZ
  - Tooth
    - Lower ØCDXXZ
    - Upper ØCDWXZ
  - Trachea ØBD1
  - Turbinate, Nasal Ø9DL
  - Tympanic Membrane
    - Left Ø9D8
    - Right Ø9D7
  - Ulna
    - Left ØPDLØZZ
    - Right ØPDKØZZ
  - Vein
    - Basilic
      - Left Ø5DC
      - Right Ø5DB
    - Brachial
      - Left Ø5DA
      - Right Ø5D9

**Extraction** — *continued*
Vein — *continued*
Cephalic
Left Ø5DF
Right Ø5DD
Femoral
Left Ø6DN
Right Ø6DM
Foot
Left Ø6DV
Right Ø6DT
Hand
Left Ø5DH
Right Ø5DG
Lower Ø6DY
Saphenous
Left Ø6DQ
Right Ø6DP
Upper Ø5DY
Vertebra
Cervical ØPD3ØZZ
Lumbar ØQDØØZZ
Thoracic ØPD4ØZZ
Vocal Cord
Left ØCDV
Right ØCDT
**Extradural space, intracranial** *use* Epidural Space, Intracranial
**Extradural space, spinal** *use* Spinal Canal
**EXtreme Lateral Interbody Fusion (XLIF) device** *use* Interbody Fusion Device in Lower Joints

# F

**Face lift** *see* Alteration, Face ØWØ2
**Facet replacement spinal stabilization device**
*use* Spinal Stabilization Device, Facet Replacement in ØRH
*use* Spinal Stabilization Device, Facet Replacement in ØSH
**Facial artery** *use* Artery, Face
**Factor Xa Inhibitor Reversal Agent, Andexanet Alfa**
*use* Andexanet Alfa, Factor Xa Inhibitor Reversal Agent
**False vocal cord** *use* Larynx
**Falx cerebri** *use* Dura Mater
**Fascia lata**
*use* Subcutaneous Tissue and Fascia, Upper Leg, Left
*use* Subcutaneous Tissue and Fascia, Upper Leg, Right
**Fasciaplasty, fascioplasty**
*see* Repair, Subcutaneous Tissue and Fascia ØJQ
*see* Replacement, Subcutaneous Tissue and Fascia ØJR
**Fasciectomy** *see* Excision, Subcutaneous Tissue and Fascia ØJB
**Fasciorrhaphy** *see* Repair, Subcutaneous Tissue and Fascia ØJQ
**Fasciotomy**
*see* Division, Subcutaneous Tissue and Fascia ØJ8
*see* Drainage, Subcutaneous Tissue and Fascia ØJ9
*see* Release
**Feeding Device**
Change device in
Lower ØD2DXUZ
Upper ØD2ØXUZ
Insertion of device in
Duodenum ØDH9
Esophagus ØDH5
Ileum ØDHB
Intestine, Small ØDH8
Jejunum ØDHA
Stomach ØDH6
Removal of device from
Esophagus ØDP5
Intestinal Tract
Lower ØDPD
Upper ØDPØ
Stomach ØDP6
Revision of device in
Intestinal Tract
Lower ØDWD
Upper ØDWØ
Stomach ØDW6
**Femoral head**
*use* Femur, Upper, Left
*use* Femur, Upper, Right
**Femoral lymph node**
*use* Lymphatic, Lower Extremity, Left
**Femoral lymph node** — *continued*
*use* Lymphatic, Lower Extremity, Right
**Femoropatellar joint**
*use* Joint, Knee, Left
*use* Joint, Knee, Left, Tibial Surface
*use* Joint, Knee, Right
*use* Joint, Knee, Right, Femoral Surface
**Femorotibial joint**
*use* Joint, Knee, Left
*use* Joint, Knee, Left, Tibial Surface
*use* Joint, Knee, Right
*use* Joint, Knee, Right, Tibial Surface
**Fibular artery**
*use* Artery, Peroneal, Left
*use* Artery, Peroneal, Right
**Fibularis brevis muscle**
*use* Muscle, Lower Leg, Left
*use* Muscle, Lower Leg, Right
**Fibularis longus muscle**
*use* Muscle, Lower Leg, Left
*use* Muscle, Lower Leg, Right
**Fifth cranial nerve** *use* Nerve, Trigeminal
**Filum terminale** *use* Spinal Meninges
**Fimbriectomy**
*see* Excision, Female Reproductive System ØUB
*see* Resection, Female Reproductive System ØUT
**Fine needle aspiration**
fluid or gas *see* Drainage
tissue *see* Excision
**First cranial nerve** *use* Nerve, Olfactory
**First intercostal nerve** *use* Nerve, Brachial Plexus
**Fistulization**
*see* Bypass
*see* Drainage
*see* Repair
**Fitting**
Arch bars, for fracture reduction *see* Reposition, Mouth and Throat ØCS
Arch bars, for immobilization *see* Immobilization, Face 2W31
Artificial limb *see* Device Fitting, Rehabilitation FØD
Hearing aid *see* Device Fitting, Rehabilitation FØD
Ocular prosthesis FØDZ8UZ
Prosthesis, limb *see* Device Fitting, Rehabilitation FØD
Prosthesis, ocular FØDZ8UZ
**Fixation, bone**
External, with fracture reduction *see* Reposition
External, without fracture reduction *see* Insertion
Internal, with fracture reduction *see* Reposition
Internal, without fracture reduction *see* Insertion
**FLAIR® Endovascular Stent Graft** *use* Intraluminal Device
**Flexible Composite Mesh** *use* Synthetic Substitute
**Flexor carpi radialis muscle**
*use* Muscle, Lower Arm and Wrist, Left
*use* Muscle, Lower Arm and Wrist, Right
**Flexor carpi ulnaris muscle**
*use* Muscle, Lower Arm and Wrist, Left
*use* Muscle, Lower Arm and Wrist, Right
**Flexor digitorum brevis muscle**
*use* Muscle, Foot, Left
*use* Muscle, Foot, Right
**Flexor digitorum longus muscle**
*use* Muscle, Lower Leg, Left
*use* Muscle, Lower Leg, Right
**Flexor hallucis brevis muscle**
*use* Muscle, Foot, Left
*use* Muscle, Foot, Right
**Flexor hallucis longus muscle**
*use* Muscle, Lower Leg, Left
*use* Muscle, Lower Leg, Right
**Flexor pollicis longus muscle**
*use* Muscle, Lower Arm and Wrist, Left
*use* Muscle, Lower Arm and Wrist, Right
**Fluoroscopy**
Abdomen and Pelvis BW11
Airway, Upper BB1DZZZ
Ankle
Left BQ1H
Right BQ1G
Aorta
Abdominal B41Ø
Laser, Intraoperative B41Ø
Thoracic B31Ø
Laser, Intraoperative B31Ø
Thoraco-Abdominal B31P
Laser, Intraoperative B31P
**Fluoroscopy** — *continued*
Aorta and Bilateral Lower Extremity Arteries B41D
Laser, Intraoperative B41D
Arm
Left BP1FZZZ
Right BP1EZZZ
Artery
Brachiocephalic-Subclavian
Laser, Intraoperative B311
Right B311
Bronchial B31L
Laser, Intraoperative B31L
Bypass Graft, Other B21F
Cervico-Cerebral Arch B31Q
Laser, Intraoperative B31Q
Common Carotid
Bilateral B315
Laser, Intraoperative B315
Left B314
Laser, Intraoperative B314
Right B313
Laser, Intraoperative B313
Coronary
Bypass Graft
Multiple B213
Laser, Intraoperative B213
Single B212
Laser, Intraoperative B212
Multiple B211
Laser, Intraoperative B211
Single B21Ø
Laser, Intraoperative B21Ø
External Carotid
Bilateral B31C
Laser, Intraoperative B31C
Left B31B
Laser, Intraoperative B31B
Right B319
Laser, Intraoperative B319
Hepatic B412
Laser, Intraoperative B412
Inferior Mesenteric B415
Laser, Intraoperative B415
Intercostal B31L
Laser, Intraoperative B31L
Internal Carotid
Bilateral B318
Laser, Intraoperative B318
Left B317
Laser, Intraoperative B317
Right B316
Laser, Intraoperative B316
Internal Mammary Bypass Graft
Left B218
Right B217
Intra-Abdominal
Laser, Intraoperative B41B
Other B41B
Intracranial B31R
Laser, Intraoperative B31R
Lower
Laser, Intraoperative B41J
Other B41J
Lower Extremity
Bilateral and Aorta B41D
Laser, Intraoperative B41D
Left B41G
Laser, Intraoperative B41G
Right B41F
Laser, Intraoperative B41F
Lumbar B419
Laser, Intraoperative B419
Pelvic B41C
Laser, Intraoperative B41C
Pulmonary
Left B31T
Laser, Intraoperative B31T
Right B31S
Laser, Intraoperative B31S
Pulmonary Trunk B31U
Laser, Intraoperative B31U
Renal
Bilateral B418
Laser, Intraoperative B418
Left B417
Laser, Intraoperative B417
Right B416
Laser, Intraoperative B416
Spinal B31M

**Fluoroscopy** — *continued*
Artery — *continued*
Spinal — *continued*
Laser, Intraoperative B31M
Splenic B413
Laser, Intraoperative B413
Subclavian
Laser, Intraoperative B312
Left B312
Superior Mesenteric B414
Laser, Intraoperative B414
Upper
Laser, Intraoperative B31N
Other B31N
Upper Extremity
Bilateral B31K
Laser, Intraoperative B31K
Left B31J
Laser, Intraoperative B31J
Right B31H
Laser, Intraoperative B31H
Vertebral
Bilateral B31G
Laser, Intraoperative B31G
Left B31F
Laser, Intraoperative B31F
Right B31D
Laser, Intraoperative B31D
Bile Duct BF1Ø
Pancreatic Duct and Gallbladder BF14
Bile Duct and Gallbladder BF13
Biliary Duct BF11
Bladder BT1Ø
Kidney and Ureter BT14
Left BT1F
Right BT1D
Bladder and Urethra BT1B
Bowel, Small BD1
Calcaneus
Left BQ1KZZZ
Right BQ1JZZZ
Clavicle
Left BP15ZZZ
Right BP14ZZZ
Coccyx BR1F
Colon BD14
Corpora Cavernosa BV1Ø
Dialysis Fistula B51W
Dialysis Shunt B51W
Diaphragm BB16ZZZ
Disc
Cervical BR11
Lumbar BR13
Thoracic BR12
Duodenum BD19
Elbow
Left BP1H
Right BP1G
Epiglottis B91G
Esophagus BD11
Extremity
Lower BW1C
Upper BW1J
Facet Joint
Cervical BR14
Lumbar BR16
Thoracic BR15
Fallopian Tube
Bilateral BU12
Left BU11
Right BU1Ø
Fallopian Tube and Uterus BU18
Femur
Left BQ14ZZZ
Right BQ13ZZZ
Finger
Left BP1SZZZ
Right BP1RZZZ
Foot
Left BQ1MZZZ
Right BQ1LZZZ
Forearm
Left BP1KZZZ
Right BP1JZZZ
Gallbladder BF12
Bile Duct and Pancreatic Duct BF14
Gallbladder and Bile Duct BF13
Gastrointestinal, Upper BD1

**Fluoroscopy** — *continued*
Hand
Left BP1PZZZ
Right BP1NZZZ
Head and Neck BW19
Heart
Left B215
Right B214
Right and Left B216
Hip
Left BQ11
Right BQ1Ø
Humerus
Left BP1BZZZ
Right BP1AZZZ
Ileal Diversion Loop BT1C
Ileal Loop, Ureters and Kidney BT1G
Intracranial Sinus B512
Joint
Acromioclavicular, Bilateral BP13ZZZ
Finger
Left BP1D
Right BP1C
Foot
Left BQ1Y
Right BQ1X
Hand
Left BP1D
Right BP1C
Lumbosacral BR1B
Sacroiliac BR1D
Sternoclavicular
Bilateral BP12ZZZ
Left BP11ZZZ
Right BP1ØZZZ
Temporomandibular
Bilateral BN19
Left BN18
Right BN17
Thoracolumbar BR18
Toe
Left BQ1Y
Right BQ1X
Kidney
Bilateral BT13
Ileal Loop and Ureter BT1G
Left BT12
Right BT11
Ureter and Bladder BT14
Left BT1F
Right BT1D
Knee
Left BQ18
Right BQ17
Larynx B91J
Leg
Left BQ1FZZZ
Right BQ1DZZZ
Lung
Bilateral BB14ZZZ
Left BB13ZZZ
Right BB12ZZZ
Mediastinum BB1CZZZ
Mouth BD1B
Neck and Head BW19
Oropharynx BD1B
Pancreatic Duct BF1
Gallbladder and Bile Buct BF14
Patella
Left BQ1WZZZ
Right BQ1VZZZ
Pelvis BR1C
Pelvis and Abdomen BW11
Pharynx B91G
Ribs
Left BP1YZZZ
Right BP1XZZZ
Sacrum BR1F
Scapula
Left BP17ZZZ
Right BP16ZZZ
Shoulder
Left BP19
Right BP18
Sinus, Intracranial B512
Spinal Cord BØ1B
Spine
Cervical BR1Ø
Lumbar BR19

**Fluoroscopy** — *continued*
Spine — *continued*
Thoracic BR17
Whole BR1G
Sternum BR1H
Stomach BD12
Toe
Left BQ1QZZZ
Right BQ1PZZZ
Tracheobronchial Tree
Bilateral BB19YZZ
Left BB18YZZ
Right BB17YZZ
Ureter
Ileal Loop and Kidney BT1G
Kidney and Bladder BT14
Left BT1F
Right BT1D
Left BT17
Right BT16
Urethra BT15
Urethra and Bladder BT1B
Uterus BU16
Uterus and Fallopian Tube BU18
Vagina BU19
Vasa Vasorum BV18
Vein
Cerebellar B511
Cerebral B511
Epidural B51Ø
Jugular
Bilateral B515
Left B514
Right B513
Lower Extremity
Bilateral B51D
Left B51C
Right B51B
Other B51V
Pelvic (Iliac)
Left B51G
Right B51F
Pelvic (Iliac) Bilateral B51H
Portal B51T
Pulmonary
Bilateral B51S
Left B51R
Right B51Q
Renal
Bilateral B51L
Left B51K
Right B51J
Spanchnic B51T
Subclavian
Left B517
Right B516
Upper Extremity
Bilateral B51P
Left B51N
Right B51M
Vena Cava
Inferior B519
Superior B518
Wrist
Left BP1M
Right BP1L
**Fluoroscopy, laser intraoperative**
*see* Fluoroscopy, Heart B21
*see* Fluoroscopy, Lower Arteries B41
*see* Fluoroscopy, Upper Arteries B31
**Flushing** *see* Irrigation
**Foley catheter** *use* Drainage Device
**Fontan completion procedure Stage II** *see* Bypass, Vena Cava, Inferior Ø61Ø
**Foramen magnum** *use* Occipital Bone
**Foramen of Monro (intraventricular)** *use* Cerebral Ventricle
**Foreskin** *use* Prepuce
**Formula™ Balloon-Expandable Renal Stent System** *use* Intraluminal Device
**Fossa of Rosenmuller** *use* Nasopharynx
**Fourth cranial nerve** *use* Nerve, Trochlear
**Fourth ventricle** *use* Cerebral Ventricle
**Fovea**
*use* Retina, Left
*use* Retina, Right
**Fragmentation**
Ampulla of Vater ØFFC

**Fragmentation** — *continued*
Anus ØDFQ
Appendix ØDFJ
Bladder ØTFB
Bladder Neck ØTFC
Bronchus
Lingula ØBF9
Lower Lobe
Left ØBFB
Right ØBF6
Main
Left ØBF7
Right ØBF3
Middle Lobe, Right ØBF5
Upper Lobe
Left ØBF8
Right ØBF4
Carina ØBF2
Cavity, Cranial ØWF1
Cecum ØDFH
Cerebral Ventricle ØØF6
Colon
Ascending ØDFK
Descending ØDFM
Sigmoid ØDFN
Transverse ØDFL
Duct
Common Bile ØFF9
Cystic ØFF8
Hepatic
Common ØFF7
Left ØFF6
Right ØFF5
Pancreatic ØFFD
Accessory ØFFF
Parotid
Left ØCFC
Right ØCFB
Duodenum ØDF9
Epidural Space, Intracranial ØØF3
Esophagus ØDF5
Fallopian Tube
Left ØUF6
Right ØUF5
Fallopian Tubes, Bilateral ØUF7
Gallbladder ØFF4
Gastrointestinal Tract ØWFP
Genitourinary Tract ØWFR
Ileum ØDFB
Intestine
Large ØDFE
Left ØDFG
Right ØDFF
Small ØDF8
Jejunum ØDFA
Kidney Pelvis
Left ØTF4
Right ØTF3
Mediastinum ØWFC
Oral Cavity and Throat ØWF3
Pelvic Cavity ØWFJ
Pericardial Cavity ØWFD
Pericardium Ø2FN
Peritoneal Cavity ØWFG
Pleural Cavity
Left ØWFB
Right ØWF9
Rectum ØDFP
Respiratory Tract ØWFQ
Spinal Canal ØØFU
Stomach ØDF6
Subarachnoid Space, Intracranial ØØF5
Subdural Space, Intracranial ØØF4
Trachea ØBF1
Ureter
Left ØTF7
Right ØTF6
Urethra ØTFD
Uterus ØUF9
Vitreous
Left Ø8F5
Right Ø8F4
**Freestyle (Stentless) Aortic Root Bioprosthesis** *use* Zooplastic Tissue in Heart and Great Vessels
**Frenectomy**
*see* Excision, Mouth and Throat ØCB
*see* Resection, Mouth and Throat ØCT
**Frenoplasty, frenuloplasty**
*see* Repair, Mouth and Throat ØCQ
*see* Replacement, Mouth and Throat ØCR
*see* Supplement, Mouth and Throat ØCU
**Frenotomy**
*see* Drainage, Mouth and Throat ØC9
*see* Release, Mouth and Throat ØCN
**Frenulotomy**
*see* Drainage, Mouth and Throat ØC9
*see* Release, Mouth and Throat ØCN
**Frenulum labii inferioris** *use* Lip, Lower
**Frenulum labii superioris** *use* Lip, Upper
**Frenulum linguae** *use* Tongue
**Frenulumectomy**
*see* Excision, Mouth and Throat ØCB
*see* Resection, Mouth and Throat ØCT
**Frontal lobe** *use* Cerebral Hemisphere
**Frontal vein**
*use* Vein, Face, Left
*use* Vein, Face, Right
**Fulguration** *see* Destruction
**Fundoplication, gastroesophageal** *see* Restriction, Esophagogastric Junction ØDV4
**Fundus uteri** *use* Uterus
**Fusion**
Acromioclavicular
Left ØRGH
Right ØRGG
Ankle
Left ØSGG
Right ØSGF
Carpal
Left ØRGR
Right ØRGQ
Carpometacarpal
Left ØRGT
Right ØRGS
Cervical Vertebral ØRG1
2 or more ØRG2
Interbody Fusion Device
Nanotextured Surface XRG2Ø92
Radiolucent Porous XRG2ØF3
Interbody Fusion Device
Nanotextured Surface XRG1Ø92
Radiolucent Porous XRG1ØF3
Cervicothoracic Vertebral ØRG4
Interbody Fusion Device
Nanotextured Surface XRG4Ø92
Radiolucent Porous XRG4ØF3
Coccygeal ØSG6
Elbow
Left ØRGM
Right ØRGL
Finger Phalangeal
Left ØRGX
Right ØRGW
Hip
Left ØSGB
Right ØSG9
Knee
Left ØSGD
Right ØSGC
Lumbar Vertebral ØSGØ
2 or more ØSG1
Interbody Fusion Device
Nanotextured Surface XRGCØ92
Radiolucent Porous XRGCØF3
Interbody Fusion Device
Nanotextured Surface XRGBØ92
Radiolucent Porous XRGBØF3
Lumbosacral ØSG3
Interbody Fusion Device
Nanotextured Surface XRGDØ92
Radiolucent Porous XRGDØF3
Metacarpophalangeal
Left ØRGV
Right ØRGU
Metatarsal-Phalangeal
Left ØSGN
Right ØSGM
Occipital-cervical ØRGØ
Interbody Fusion Device
Nanotextured Surface XRGØØ92
Radiolucent Porous XRGØØF3
Sacrococcygeal ØSG5
Sacroiliac
Left ØSG8
Right ØSG7
**Fusion** — *continued*
Shoulder
Left ØRGK
Right ØRGJ
Sternoclavicular
Left ØRGF
Right ØRGE
Tarsal
Left ØSGJ
Right ØSGH
Tarsometatarsal
Left ØSGL
Right ØSGK
Temporomandibular
Left ØRGD
Right ØRGC
Thoracic Vertebral ØRG6
2 to 7 ØRG7
Interbody Fusion Device
Nanotextured Surface XRG7Ø92
Radiolucent Porous XRG7ØF3
8 or more ØRG8
Interbody Fusion Device
Nanotextured Surface XRG8Ø92
Radiolucent Porous XRG8ØF3
Interbody Fusion Device
Nanotextured Surface XRG6Ø92
Radiolucent Porous XRG6ØF3
Thoracolumbar Vertebral ØRGA
Interbody Fusion Device
Nanotextured Surface XRGAØ92
Radiolucent Porous XRGAØF3
Toe Phalangeal
Left ØSGQ
Right ØSGP
Wrist
Left ØRGP
Right ØRGN
**Fusion screw (compression) (lag) (locking)**
*use* Internal Fixation Device in Lower Joints
*use* Internal Fixation Device in Upper Joints

## G

**Gait training** *see* Motor Treatment, Rehabilitation FØ7
**Galea aponeurotica** *use* Subcutaneous Tissue and Fascia, Scalp
**GammaTile™** *use* Radioactive Element, Cesium-131 Collagen Implant in ØØH
**Ganglion impar (ganglion of Walther)** *use* Nerve, Sacral Sympathetic
**Ganglionectomy**
Destruction of lesion *see* Destruction
Excision of lesion *see* Excision
**Gasserian ganglion** *use* Nerve, Trigeminal
**Gastrectomy**
Partial *see* Excision, Stomach ØDB6
Total *see* Resection, Stomach ØDT6
Vertical (sleeve) *see* Excision, Stomach ØDB6
**Gastric electrical stimulation (GES) lead** *use* Stimulator Lead in Gastrointestinal System
**Gastric lymph node** *use* Lymphatic, Aortic
**Gastric pacemaker lead** *use* Stimulator Lead in Gastrointestinal System
**Gastric plexus** *use* Nerve, Abdominal Sympathetic
**Gastrocnemius muscle**
*use* Muscle, Lower Leg, Left
*use* Muscle, Lower Leg, Right
**Gastrocolic ligament** *use* Omentum
**Gastrocolic omentum** *use* Omentum
**Gastrocolostomy**
*see* Bypass, Gastrointestinal System ØD1
*see* Drainage, Gastrointestinal System ØD9
**Gastroduodenal artery** *use* Artery, Hepatic
**Gastroduodenectomy**
*see* Excision, Gastrointestinal System ØDB
*see* Resection, Gastrointestinal System ØDT
**Gastroduodenoscopy** ØDJØ8ZZ
**Gastroenteroplasty**
*see* Repair, Gastrointestinal System ØDQ
*see* Supplement, Gastrointestinal System ØDU
**Gastroenterostomy**
*see* Bypass, Gastrointestinal System ØD1
*see* Drainage, Gastrointestinal System ØD9
**Gastroesophageal (GE) junction** *use* Esophagogastric Junction

**Gastrogastrostomy**
*see* Bypass, Stomach ØD16
*see* Drainage, Stomach ØD96
**Gastrohepatic omentum** *use* Omentum
**Gastrojejunostomy**
*see* Bypass, Stomach ØD16
*see* Drainage, Stomach ØD96
**Gastrolysis** *see* Release, Stomach ØDN6
**Gastropexy**
*see* Repair, Stomach ØDQ6
*see* Reposition, Stomach ØDS6
**Gastrophrenic ligament** *use* Omentum
**Gastroplasty**
*see* Repair, Stomach ØDQ6
*see* Supplement, Stomach ØDU6
**Gastroplication** *see* Restriction, Stomach ØDV6
**Gastropylorectomy** *see* Excision, Gastrointestinal System ØDB
**Gastrorrhaphy** *see* Repair, Stomach ØDQ6
**Gastroscopy** ØDJ68ZZ
**Gastrosplenic ligament** *use* Omentum
**Gastrostomy**
*see* Bypass, Stomach ØD16
*see* Drainage, Stomach ØD96
**Gastrotomy** *see* Drainage, Stomach ØD96
**Gemellus muscle**
*use* Muscle, Hip, Left
*use* Muscle, Hip, Right
**Geniculate ganglion** *use* Nerve, Facial
**Geniculate nucleus** *use* Thalamus
**Genioglossus muscle** *use* Muscle, Tongue, Palate, Pharynx
**Genioplasty** *see* Alteration, Jaw, Lower ØWØ5
**Genitofemoral nerve** *use* Nerve, Lumbar Plexus
**Gingivectomy** *see* Excision, Mouth and Throat ØCB
**Gingivoplasty**
*see* Repair, Mouth and Throat ØCQ
*see* Replacement, Mouth and Throat ØCR
*see* Supplement, Mouth and Throat ØCU
**Glans penis** *use* Prepuce
**Glenohumeral joint**
*use* Joint, Shoulder, Left
*use* Joint, Shoulder, Right
**Glenohumeral ligament**
*use* Bursa and Ligament, Shoulder, Left
*use* Bursa and Ligament, Shoulder, Right
**Glenoid fossa (of scapula)**
*use* Glenoid Cavity, Left
*use* Glenoid Cavity, Right
**Glenoid ligament (labrum)**
*use* Shoulder Joint, Left
*use* Shoulder Joint, Right
**Globus pallidus** *use* Basal Ganglia
**Glomectomy**
*see* Excision, Endocrine System ØGB
*see* Resection, Endocrine System ØGT
**Glossectomy**
*see* Excision, Tongue ØCB7
*see* Resection, Tongue ØCT7
**Glossoepiglottic fold** *use* Epiglottis
**Glossopexy**
*see* Repair, Tongue ØCQ7
*see* Reposition, Tongue ØCS7
**Glossoplasty**
*see* Repair, Tongue ØCQ7
*see* Replacement, Tongue ØCR7
*see* Supplement, Tongue ØCU7
**Glossorrhaphy** *see* Repair, Tongue ØCQ7
**Glossotomy** *see* Drainage, Tongue ØC97
**Glottis** *use* Larynx
**Gluteal Artery Perforator Flap**
Replacement
Bilateral ØHRVØ79
Left ØHRUØ79
Right ØHRTØ79
Transfer
Left ØKXG
Right ØKXF
**Gluteal lymph node** *use* Lymphatic, Pelvis
**Gluteal vein**
*use* Vein, Hypogastric, Left
*use* Vein, Hypogastric, Right
**Gluteus maximus muscle**
*use* Muscle, Hip, Left
*use* Muscle, Hip, Right
**Gluteus medius muscle**
*use* Muscle, Hip, Left
*use* Muscle, Hip, Right
**Gluteus minimus muscle**
*use* Muscle, Hip, Left
*use* Muscle, Hip, Right
**GORE EXCLUDER® AAA Endoprosthesis**
*use* Intraluminal Device
*use* Intraluminal Device, Branched or Fenestrated, One or Two Arteries in Ø4V
*use* Intraluminal Device, Branched or Fenestrated, Three or More Arteries in Ø4V
**GORE EXCLUDER® IBE Endoprosthesis** *use* Intraluminal Device, Branched or Fenestrated, One or Two Arteries in Ø4V
**GORE TAG® Thoracic Endoprosthesis** *use* Intraluminal Device
**GORE® DUALMESH®** *use* Synthetic Substitute
**Gracilis muscle**
*use* Muscle, Upper Leg, Left
*use* Muscle, Upper Leg, Right
**Graft**
*see* Replacement
*see* Supplement
**Great auricular nerve** *use* Nerve, Cervical Plexus
**Great cerebral vein** *use* Vein, Intracranial
**Great(er) saphenous vein**
*use* Saphenous Vein, Left
*use* Saphenous Vein, Right
**Greater alar cartilage** *use* Nasal Mucosa and Soft Tissue
**Greater occipital nerve** *use* Nerve, Cervical
**Greater Omentum** *use* Omentum
**Greater splanchnic nerve** *use* Nerve, Thoracic Sympathetic
**Greater superficial petrosal nerve** *use* Nerve, Facial
**Greater trochanter**
*use* Femur, Upper, Left
*use* Femur, Upper, Right
**Greater tuberosity**
*use* Humeral Head, Left
*use* Humeral Head, Right
**Greater vestibular (Bartholin's) gland** *use* Gland, Vestibular
**Greater wing** *use* Sphenoid Bone
**Guedel airway** *use* Intraluminal Device, Airway in Mouth and Throat
**Guidance, catheter placement**
EKG *see* Measurement, Physiological Systems 4AØ
Fluoroscopy *see* Fluoroscopy, Veins B51
Ultrasound *see* Ultrasonography, Veins B54

# H

**Hallux**
*use* Toe, 1st, Left
*use* Toe, 1st, Right
**Hamate bone**
*use* Carpal, Left
*use* Carpal, Right
**Hancock Bioprosthesis (aortic) (mitral) valve** *use* Zooplastic Tissue in Heart and Great Vessels
**Hancock Bioprosthetic Valved Conduit** *use* Zooplastic Tissue in Heart and Great Vessels
**Harvesting, stem cells** *see* Pheresis, Circulatory 6A55
**Head of fibula**
*use* Fibula, Left
*use* Fibula, Right
**Hearing Aid Assessment** F14Z
**Hearing Assessment** F13Z
**Hearing Device**
Bone Conduction
Left Ø9HE
Right Ø9HD
Insertion of device in
Left ØNH6
Right ØNH5
Multiple Channel Cochlear Prosthesis
Left Ø9HE
Right Ø9HD
Removal of device from, Skull ØNPØ
Revision of device in, Skull ØNWØ
Single Channel Cochlear Prosthesis
Left Ø9HE
Right Ø9HD
**Hearing Treatment** FØ9Z
**Heart Assist System**
Implantable
Insertion of device in, Heart Ø2HA
Removal of device from, Heart Ø2PA
Revision of device in, Heart Ø2WA
Short-term External
Insertion of device in, Heart Ø2HA
Removal of device from, Heart Ø2PA
Revision of device in, Heart Ø2WA
**HeartMate 3™ LVAS** *use* Implantable Heart Assist System in Heart and Great Vessels
**HeartMate II® Left Ventricular Assist Device (LVAD)** *use* Implantable Heart Assist System in Heart and Great Vessels
**HeartMate XVE® Left Ventricular Assist Device (LVAD)** *use* Implantable Heart Assist System in Heart and Great Vessels
**HeartMate® implantable heart assist system** *see* Insertion of device in, Heart Ø2HA
**Helix**
*use* Ear, External, Bilateral
*use* Ear, External, Left
*use* Ear, External, Right
**Hematopoietic cell transplant (HCT)** *see* Transfusion, Circulatory 3Ø2
**Hemicolectomy** *see* Resection, Gastrointestinal System ØDT
**Hemicystectomy** *see* Excision, Urinary System ØTB
**Hemigastrectomy** *see* Excision, Gastrointestinal System ØDB
**Hemiglossectomy** *see* Excision, Mouth and Throat ØCB
**Hemilaminectomy**
*see* Excision, Lower Bones ØQB
*see* Excision, Upper Bones ØPB
**Hemilaminotomy**
*see* Drainage, Lower Bones ØQ9
*see* Drainage, Upper Bones ØP9
*see* Excision, Lower Bones ØQB
*see* Excision, Upper Bones ØPB
*see* Release, Central Nervous System and Cranial Nerves ØØN
*see* Release, Lower Bones ØQN
*see* Release, Peripheral Nervous System Ø1N
*see* Release, Upper Bones ØPN
**Hemilaryngectomy** *see* Excision, Larynx ØCBS
**Hemimandibulectomy** *see* Excision, Head and Facial Bones ØNB
**Hemimaxillectomy** *see* Excision, Head and Facial Bones ØNB
**Hemipylorectomy** *see* Excision, Gastrointestinal System ØDB
**Hemispherectomy**
*see* Excision, Central Nervous System and Cranial Nerves ØØB
*see* Resection, Central Nervous System and Cranial Nerves ØØT
**Hemithyroidectomy**
*see* Excision, Endocrine System ØGB
*see* Resection, Endocrine System ØGT
**Hemodialysis** *see* Performance, Urinary 5A1D
**Hemolung® Respiratory Assist System (RAS)** 5AØ92ØZ
**Hepatectomy**
*see* Excision, Hepatobiliary System and Pancreas ØFB
*see* Resection, Hepatobiliary System and Pancreas ØFT
**Hepatic artery proper** *use* Artery, Hepatic
**Hepatic flexure** *use* Transverse Colon
**Hepatic lymph node** *use* Lymphatic, Aortic
**Hepatic plexus** *use* Nerve, Abdominal Sympathetic
**Hepatic portal vein** *use* Vein, Portal
**Hepaticoduodenostomy**
*see* Bypass, Hepatobiliary System and Pancreas ØF1
*see* Drainage, Hepatobiliary System and Pancreas ØF9
**Hepaticotomy** *see* Drainage, Hepatobiliary System and Pancreas ØF9
**Hepatocholedochostomy** *see* Drainage, Duct, Common Bile ØF99
**Hepatogastric ligament** *use* Omentum
**Hepatopancreatic ampulla** *use* Ampulla of Vater
**Hepatopexy**
*see* Repair, Hepatobiliary System and Pancreas ØFQ
*see* Reposition, Hepatobiliary System and Pancreas ØFS
**Hepatorrhaphy** *see* Repair, Hepatobiliary System and Pancreas ØFQ
**Hepatotomy** *see* Drainage, Hepatobiliary System and Pancreas ØF9
**Herculink (RX) Elite Renal Stent System** *use* Intraluminal Device

**Herniorrhaphy**
with synthetic substitute
*see* Supplement, Anatomical Regions, General ØWU
*see* Supplement, Anatomical Regions, Lower Extremities ØYU
*see* Repair, Anatomical Regions, General ØWQ
*see* Repair, Anatomical Regions, Lower Extremities ØYQ
**Hip (joint) liner** *use* Liner in Lower Joints
**Holter monitoring** 4A12X45
**Holter valve ventricular shunt** *use* Synthetic Substitute
**Humeroradial joint**
*use* Joint, Elbow, Left
*use* Joint, Elbow, Right
**Humeroulnar joint**
*use* Joint, Elbow, Left
*use* Joint, Elbow, Right
**Humerus, distal**
*use* Humeral Shaft, Left
*use* Humeral Shaft, Right
**Hydrocelectomy** *see* Excision, Male Reproductive System ØVB
**Hydrotherapy**
Assisted exercise in pool *see* Motor Treatment, Rehabilitation FØ7
Whirlpool *see* Activities of Daily Living Treatment, Rehabilitation FØ8
**Hymenectomy**
*see* Excision, Hymen ØUBK
*see* Resection, Hymen ØUTK
**Hymenoplasty**
*see* Repair, Hymen ØUQK
*see* Supplement, Hymen ØUUK
**Hymenorrhaphy** *see* Repair, Hymen ØUQK
**Hymenotomy**
*see* Division, Hymen ØU8K
*see* Drainage, Hymen ØU9K
**Hyoglossus muscle** *use* Muscle, Tongue, Palate, Pharynx
**Hyoid artery**
*use* Artery, Thyroid, Left
*use* Artery, Thyroid, Right
**Hyperalimentation** *see* Introduction of substance in or on
**Hyperbaric oxygenation**
Decompression sickness treatment *see* Decompression, Circulatory 6A15
Wound treatment *see* Assistance, Circulatory 5AØ5
**Hyperthermia**
Radiation Therapy
Abdomen DWY38ZZ
Adrenal Gland DGY28ZZ
Bile Ducts DFY28ZZ
Bladder DTY28ZZ
Bone Marrow D7YØ8ZZ
Bone, Other DPYC8ZZ
Brain DØYØ8ZZ
Brain Stem DØY18ZZ
Breast
Left DMYØ8ZZ
Right DMY18ZZ
Bronchus DBY18ZZ
Cervix DUY18ZZ
Chest DWY28ZZ
Chest Wall DBY78ZZ
Colon DDY58ZZ
Diaphragm DBY88ZZ
Duodenum DDY28ZZ
Ear D9YØ8ZZ
Esophagus DDYØ8ZZ
Eye D8YØ8ZZ
Femur DPY98ZZ
Fibula DPYB8ZZ
Gallbladder DFY18ZZ
Gland
Adrenal DGY28ZZ
Parathyroid DGY48ZZ
Pituitary DGYØ8ZZ
Thyroid DGY58ZZ
Glands, Salivary D9Y68ZZ
Head and Neck DWY18ZZ
Hemibody DWY48ZZ
Humerus DPY68ZZ
Hypopharynx D9Y38ZZ
Ileum DDY48ZZ
Jejunum DDY38ZZ
Kidney DTYØ8ZZ
Larynx D9YB8ZZ
Liver DFYØ8ZZ

**Hyperthermia** — *continued*
Radiation Therapy — *continued*
Lung DBY28ZZ
Lymphatics
Abdomen D7Y68ZZ
Axillary D7Y48ZZ
Inguinal D7Y88ZZ
Neck D7Y38ZZ
Pelvis D7Y78ZZ
Thorax D7Y58ZZ
Mandible DPY38ZZ
Maxilla DPY28ZZ
Mediastinum DBY68ZZ
Mouth D9Y48ZZ
Nasopharynx D9YD8ZZ
Neck and Head DWY18ZZ
Nerve, Peripheral DØY78ZZ
Nose D9Y18ZZ
Oropharynx D9YF8ZZ
Ovary DUYØ8ZZ
Palate
Hard D9Y88ZZ
Soft D9Y98ZZ
Pancreas DFY38ZZ
Parathyroid Gland DGY48ZZ
Pelvic Bones DPY88ZZ
Pelvic Region DWY68ZZ
Pineal Body DGY18ZZ
Pituitary Gland DGYØ8ZZ
Pleura DBY58ZZ
Prostate DVYØ8ZZ
Radius DPY78ZZ
Rectum DDY78ZZ
Rib DPY58ZZ
Sinuses D9Y78ZZ
Skin
Abdomen DHY88ZZ
Arm DHY48ZZ
Back DHY78ZZ
Buttock DHY98ZZ
Chest DHY68ZZ
Face DHY28ZZ
Leg DHYB8ZZ
Neck DHY38ZZ
Skull DPYØ8ZZ
Spinal Cord DØY68ZZ
Spleen D7Y28ZZ
Sternum DPY48ZZ
Stomach DDY18ZZ
Testis DVY18ZZ
Thymus D7Y18ZZ
Thyroid Gland DGY58ZZ
Tibia DPYB8ZZ
Tongue D9Y58ZZ
Trachea DBYØ8ZZ
Ulna DPY78ZZ
Ureter DTY18ZZ
Urethra DTY38ZZ
Uterus DUY28ZZ
Whole Body DWY58ZZ
Whole Body 6A3Z
**Hypnosis** GZFZZZZ
**Hypogastric artery**
*use* Artery, Internal Iliac, Left
*use* Artery, Internal Iliac, Right
**Hypopharynx** *use* Pharynx
**Hypophysectomy**
*see* Excision, Gland, Pituitary ØGBØ
*see* Resection, Gland, Pituitary ØGTØ
**Hypophysis** *use* Gland, Pituitary
**Hypothalamotomy** *see* Destruction, Thalamus ØØ59
**Hypothenar muscle**
*use* Muscle, Hand, Left
*use* Muscle, Hand, Right
**Hypothermia, Whole Body** 6A4Z
**Hysterectomy**
supracervical *see* Resection, Uterus ØUT9
total *see* Resection, Uterus ØUT9
**Hysterolysis** *see* Release, Uterus ØUN9
**Hysteropexy**
*see* Repair, Uterus ØUQ9
*see* Reposition, Uterus ØUS9
**Hysteroplasty** *see* Repair, Uterus ØUQ9
**Hysterorrhaphy** *see* Repair, Uterus ØUQ9
**Hysteroscopy** ØUJD8ZZ
**Hysterotomy** *see* Drainage, Uterus ØU99
**Hysterotrachelectomy**
*see* Resection, Cervix ØUTC

**Hysterotrachelectomy** — *continued*
*see* Resection, Uterus ØUT9
**Hysterotracheloplasty** *see* Repair, Uterus ØUQ9
**Hysterotrachelorrhaphy** *see* Repair, Uterus ØUQ9

## I

**IABP (Intra-aortic balloon pump)** *see* Assistance, Cardiac 5AØ2
**IAEMT (Intraoperative anesthetic effect monitoring and titration)** *see* Monitoring, Central Nervous 4A1Ø
**Idarucizumab, Dabigatran Reversal Agent** XWØ
**IHD (Intermittent hemodialysis)** 5A1D7ØZ
**Ileal artery** *use* Artery, Superior Mesenteric
**Ileectomy**
*see* Excision, Ileum ØDBB
*see* Resection, Ileum ØDTB
**Ileocolic artery** *use* Artery, Superior Mesenteric
**Ileocolic vein** *use* Vein, Colic
**Ileopexy**
*see* Repair, Ileum ØDQB
*see* Reposition, Ileum ØDSB
**Ileorrhaphy** *see* Repair, Ileum ØDQB
**Ileoscopy** ØDJD8ZZ
**Ileostomy**
*see* Bypass, Ileum ØD1B
*see* Drainage, Ileum ØD9B
**Ileotomy** *see* Drainage, Ileum ØD9B
**Ileoureterostomy** *see* Bypass, Urinary System ØT1
**Iliac crest**
*use* Bone, Pelvic, Left
*use* Bone, Pelvic, Right
**Iliac fascia**
*use* Subcutaneous Tissue and Fascia, Upper Leg, Left
*use* Subcutaneous Tissue and Fascia, Upper Leg, Right
**Iliac lymph node** *use* Lymphatic, Pelvis
**Iliacus muscle**
*use* Muscle, Hip, Left
*use* Muscle, Hip, Right
**Iliofemoral ligament**
*use* Bursa and Ligament, Hip, Left
*use* Bursa and Ligament, Hip, Right
**Iliohypogastric nerve** *use* Nerve, Lumbar Plexus
**Ilioinguinal nerve** *use* Nerve, Lumbar Plexus
**Iliolumbar artery**
*use* Artery, Internal Iliac, Left
*use* Artery, Internal Iliac, Right
**Iliolumbar ligament** *use* Lower Spine Bursa and Ligament
**Iliotibial tract (band)**
*use* Subcutaneous Tissue and Fascia, Upper Leg, Left
*use* Subcutaneous Tissue and Fascia, Upper Leg, Right
**Ilium**
*use* Bone, Pelvic, Left
*use* Bone, Pelvic, Right
**Ilizarov external fixator**
*use* External Fixation Device, Ring in ØPH
*use* External Fixation Device, Ring in ØPS
*use* External Fixation Device, Ring in ØQH
*use* External Fixation Device, Ring in ØQS
**Ilizarov-Vecklich device**
*use* External Fixation Device, Limb Lengthening in ØPH
*use* External Fixation Device, Limb Lengthening in ØQH
**Imaging, diagnostic**
*see* Computerized Tomography (CT Scan)
*see* Fluoroscopy
*see* Magnetic Resonance Imaging (MRI)
*see* Plain Radiography
*see* Ultrasonography
**Immobilization**
Abdominal Wall 2W33X
Arm
Lower
Left 2W3DX
Right 2W3CX
Upper
Left 2W3BX
Right 2W3AX
Back 2W35X
Chest Wall 2W34X
Extremity
Lower
Left 2W3MX
Right 2W3LX

Index
Herniorrhaphy — Immobilization

**Immobilization** — *continued*
Extremity — *continued*
Upper
Left 2W39X
Right 2W38X
Face 2W31X
Finger
Left 2W3KX
Right 2W3JX
Foot
Left 2W3TX
Right 2W3SX
Hand
Left 2W3FX
Right 2W3EX
Head 2W30X
Inguinal Region
Left 2W37X
Right 2W36X
Leg
Lower
Left 2W3RX
Right 2W3QX
Upper
Left 2W3PX
Right 2W3NX
Neck 2W32X
Thumb
Left 2W3HX
Right 2W3GX
Toe
Left 2W3VX
Right 2W3UX
**Immunization** *see* Introduction of Serum, Toxoid, and Vaccine
**Immunotherapy** *see* Introduction of Immunotherapeutic Substance
**Immunotherapy, antineoplastic**
Interferon *see* Introduction of Low-dose Interleukin-2
Interleukin-2, high-dose *see* Introduction of High-dose Interleukin-2
Interleukin-2, low-dose *see* Introduction of Low-dose Interleukin-2
Monoclonal antibody *see* Introduction of Monoclonal Antibody
Proleukin, high-dose *see* Introduction of High-dose Interleukin-2
Proleukin, low-dose *see* Introduction of Low-dose Interleukin-2
**Impella® heart pump** *use* Short-term External Heart Assist System in Heart and Great Vessels
**Impeller Pump**
Continuous, Output 5A0221D
Intermittent, Output 5A0211D
**Implantable cardioverter-defibrillator (ICD)** *use* Defibrillator Generator in 0JH
**Implantable drug infusion pump (anti-spasmodic) (chemotherapy) (pain)** *use* Infusion Device, Pump in Subcutaneous Tissue and Fascia
**Implantable glucose monitoring device** *use* Monitoring Device
**Implantable hemodynamic monitor (IHM)** *use* Monitoring Device, Hemodynamic in 0JH
**Implantable hemodynamic monitoring system (IHMS)** *use* Monitoring Device, Hemodynamic in 0JH
**Implantable Miniature Telescope™ (IMT)** *use* Synthetic Substitute, Intraocular Telescope in 08R
**Implantation**
*see* Insertion
*see* Replacement
**Implanted (venous)(access) port** *use* Vascular Access Device, Totally Implantable in Subcutaneous Tissue and Fascia
**IMV (intermittent mandatory ventilation)** *see* Assistance, Respiratory 5A09
**In Vitro Fertilization** 8E0ZXY1
**Incision, abscess** *see* Drainage
**Incudectomy**
*see* Excision, Ear, Nose, Sinus 09B
*see* Resection, Ear, Nose, Sinus 09T
**Incudopexy**
*see* Repair, Ear, Nose, Sinus 09Q
*see* Reposition, Ear, Nose, Sinus 09S
**Incus**
*use* Auditory Ossicle, Left
*use* Auditory Ossicle, Right
**Induction of labor**
Artificial rupture of membranes *see* Drainage, Pregnancy 109
Oxytocin *see* Introduction of Hormone
**InDura, intrathecal catheter (1P) (spinal)** *use* Infusion Device
**Inferior cardiac nerve** *use* Nerve, Thoracic Sympathetic
**Inferior cerebellar vein** *use* Vein, Intracranial
**Inferior cerebral vein** *use* Vein, Intracranial
**Inferior epigastric artery**
*use* Artery, External Iliac, Left
*use* Artery, External Iliac, Right
**Inferior epigastric lymph node** *use* Lymphatic, Pelvis
**Inferior genicular artery**
*use* Artery, Popliteal, Left
*use* Artery, Popliteal, Right
**Inferior gluteal artery**
*use* Artery, Internal Iliac, Left
*use* Artery, Internal Iliac, Right
**Inferior gluteal nerve** *use* Nerve, Sacral Plexus
**Inferior hypogastric plexus** *use* Nerve, Abdominal Sympathetic
**Inferior labial artery** *use* Artery, Face
**Inferior longitudinal muscle** *use* Muscle, Tongue, Palate, Pharynx
**Inferior mesenteric ganglion** *use* Nerve, Abdominal Sympathetic
**Inferior mesenteric lymph node** *use* Lymphatic, Mesenteric
**Inferior mesenteric plexus** *use* Nerve, Abdominal Sympathetic
**Inferior oblique muscle**
*use* Muscle, Extraocular, Left
*use* Muscle, Extraocular, Right
**Inferior pancreaticoduodenal artery** *use* Artery, Superior Mesenteric
**Inferior phrenic artery** *use* Aorta, Abdominal
**Inferior rectus muscle**
*use* Muscle, Extraocular, Left
*use* Muscle, Extraocular, Right
**Inferior suprarenal artery**
*use* Artery, Renal, Left
*use* Artery, Renal, Right
**Inferior tarsal plate**
*use* Eyelid, Lower, Left
*use* Eyelid, Lower, Right
**Inferior thyroid vein**
*use* Vein, Innominate, Left
*use* Vein, Innominate, Right
**Inferior tibiofibular joint**
*use* Joint, Ankle, Left
*use* Joint, Ankle, Right
**Inferior turbinate** *use* Turbinate, Nasal
**Inferior ulnar collateral artery**
*use* Artery, Brachial, Left
*use* Artery, Brachial, Right
**Inferior vesical artery**
*use* Artery, Internal Iliac, Left
*use* Artery, Internal Iliac, Right
**Infraauricular lymph node** *use* Lymphatic, Head
**Infraclavicular (deltopectoral) lymph node**
*use* Lymphatic, Upper Extremity, Left
*use* Lymphatic, Upper Extremity, Right
**Infrahyoid muscle**
*use* Muscle, Neck, Left
*use* Muscle, Neck, Right
**Infraparotid lymph node** *use* Lymphatic, Head
**Infraspinatus fascia**
*use* Subcutaneous Tissue and Fascia, Upper Arm, Left
*use* Subcutaneous Tissue and Fascia, Upper Arm, Right
**Infraspinatus muscle**
*use* Muscle, Shoulder, Left
*use* Muscle, Shoulder, Right
**Infundibulopelvic ligament** *use* Uterine Supporting Structure
**Infusion** *see* Introduction of substance in or on
**Infusion Device, Pump**
Insertion of device in
Abdomen 0JH8
Back 0JH7
Chest 0JH6
Lower Arm
Left 0JHH
Right 0JHG
Lower Leg
Left 0JHP
Right 0JHN
**Infusion Device, Pump** — *continued*
Insertion of device in — *continued*
Trunk 0JHT
Upper Arm
Left 0JHF
Right 0JHD
Upper Leg
Left 0JHM
Right 0JHL
Removal of device from
Lower Extremity 0JPW
Trunk 0JPT
Upper Extremity 0JPV
Revision of device in
Lower Extremity 0JWW
Trunk 0JWT
Upper Extremity 0JWV
**Infusion, glucarpidase**
Central Vein 3E043GQ
Peripheral Vein 3E033GQ
**Inguinal canal**
*use* Inguinal Region, Bilateral
*use* Inguinal Region, Left
*use* Inguinal Region, Right
**Inguinal triangle**
*use* Inguinal Region, Bilateral
*use* Inguinal Region, Left
*use* Inguinal Region, Right
**Injection** *see* Introduction of substance in or on
**Injection, Concentrated Bone Marrow Aspirate (CBMA), intramuscular** XK02303
**Injection reservoir, port** *use* Vascular Access Device, Totally Implantable in Subcutaneous Tissue and Fascia
**Insemination, artificial** 3E0P7LZ
**Insertion**
Antimicrobial envelope *see* Introduction of Anti-infective
Aqueous drainage shunt
*see* Bypass, Eye 081
*see* Drainage, Eye 089
Products of Conception 10H0
Spinal Stabilization Device
*see* Insertion of device in, Lower Joints 0SH
*see* Insertion of device in, Upper Joints 0RH
**Insertion of device in**
Abdominal Wall 0WHF
Acetabulum
Left 0QH5
Right 0QH4
Anal Sphincter 0DHR
Ankle Region
Left 0YHL
Right 0YHK
Anus 0DHQ
Aorta
Abdominal 04H0
Thoracic
Ascending/Arch 02HX
Descending 02HW
Arm
Lower
Left 0XHF
Right 0XHD
Upper
Left 0XH9
Right 0XH8
Artery
Anterior Tibial
Left 04HQ
Right 04HP
Axillary
Left 03H6
Right 03H5
Brachial
Left 03H8
Right 03H7
Celiac 04H1
Colic
Left 04H7
Middle 04H8
Right 04H6
Common Carotid
Left 03HJ
Right 03HH
Common Iliac
Left 04HD
Right 04HC





Subterms under main terms may continue to next column or page

**Insertion of device in** — *continued*
Artery — *continued*
External Carotid
Left Ø3HN
Right Ø3HM
External Iliac
Left Ø4HJ
Right Ø4HH
Face Ø3HR
Femoral
Left Ø4HL
Right Ø4HK
Foot
Left Ø4HW
Right Ø4HV
Gastric Ø4H2
Hand
Left Ø3HF
Right Ø3HD
Hepatic Ø4H3
Inferior Mesenteric Ø4HB
Innominate Ø3H2
Internal Carotid
Left Ø3HL
Right Ø3HK
Internal Iliac
Left Ø4HF
Right Ø4HE
Internal Mammary
Left Ø3H1
Right Ø3HØ
Intracranial Ø3HG
Lower Ø4HY
Peroneal
Left Ø4HU
Right Ø4HT
Popliteal
Left Ø4HN
Right Ø4HM
Posterior Tibial
Left Ø4HS
Right Ø4HR
Pulmonary
Left Ø2HR
Right Ø2HQ
Pulmonary Trunk Ø2HP
Radial
Left Ø3HC
Right Ø3HB
Renal
Left Ø4HA
Right Ø4H9
Splenic Ø4H4
Subclavian
Left Ø3H4
Right Ø3H3
Superior Mesenteric Ø4H5
Temporal
Left Ø3HT
Right Ø3HS
Thyroid
Left Ø3HV
Right Ø3HU
Ulnar
Left Ø3HA
Right Ø3H9
Upper Ø3HY
Vertebral
Left Ø3HQ
Right Ø3HP
Atrium
Left Ø2H7
Right Ø2H6
Axilla
Left ØXH5
Right ØXH4
Back
Lower ØWHL
Upper ØWHK
Bladder ØTHB
Bladder Neck ØTHC
Bone
Ethmoid
Left ØNHG
Right ØNHF
Facial ØNHW
Frontal ØNH1
Hyoid ØNHX

**Insertion of device in** — *continued*
Bone — *continued*
Lacrimal
Left ØNHJ
Right ØNHH
Lower ØQHY
Nasal ØNHB
Occipital ØNH7
Palatine
Left ØNHL
Right ØNHK
Parietal
Left ØNH4
Right ØNH3
Pelvic
Left ØQH3
Right ØQH2
Sphenoid ØNHC
Temporal
Left ØNH6
Right ØNH5
Upper ØPHY
Zygomatic
Left ØNHN
Right ØNHM
Brain ØØHØ
Breast
Bilateral ØHHV
Left ØHHU
Right ØHHT
Bronchus
Lingula ØBH9
Lower Lobe
Left ØBHB
Right ØBH6
Main
Left ØBH7
Right ØBH3
Middle Lobe, Right ØBH5
Upper Lobe
Left ØBH8
Right ØBH4
Bursa and Ligament
Lower ØMHY
Upper ØMHX
Buttock
Left ØYH1
Right ØYHØ
Carpal
Left ØPHN
Right ØPHM
Cavity, Cranial ØWH1
Cerebral Ventricle ØØH6
Cervix ØUHC
Chest Wall ØWH8
Cisterna Chyli Ø7HL
Clavicle
Left ØPHB
Right ØPH9
Coccyx ØQHS
Cul-de-sac ØUHF
Diaphragm ØBHT
Disc
Cervical Vertebral ØRH3
Cervicothoracic Vertebral ØRH5
Lumbar Vertebral ØSH2
Lumbosacral ØSH4
Thoracic Vertebral ØRH9
Thoracolumbar Vertebral ØRHB
Duct
Hepatobiliary ØFHB
Pancreatic ØFHD
Duodenum ØDH9
Ear
Inner
Left Ø9HE
Right Ø9HD
Left Ø9HJ
Right Ø9HH
Elbow Region
Left ØXHC
Right ØXHB
Epididymis and Spermatic Cord ØVHM
Esophagus ØDH5
Extremity
Lower
Left ØYHB
Right ØYH9

**Insertion of device in** — *continued*
Extremity — *continued*
Upper
Left ØXH7
Right ØXH6
Eye
Left Ø8H1
Right Ø8HØ
Face ØWH2
Fallopian Tube ØUH8
Femoral Region
Left ØYH8
Right ØYH7
Femoral Shaft
Left ØQH9
Right ØQH8
Femur
Lower
Left ØQHC
Right ØQHB
Upper
Left ØQH7
Right ØQH6
Fibula
Left ØQHK
Right ØQHJ
Foot
Left ØYHN
Right ØYHM
Gallbladder ØFH4
Gastrointestinal Tract ØWHP
Genitourinary Tract ØWHR
Gland
Endocrine ØGHS
Salivary ØCHA
Glenoid Cavity
Left ØPH8
Right ØPH7
Hand
Left ØXHK
Right ØXHJ
Head ØWHØ
Heart Ø2HA
Humeral Head
Left ØPHD
Right ØPHC
Humeral Shaft
Left ØPHG
Right ØPHF
Ileum ØDHB
Inguinal Region
Left ØYH6
Right ØYH5
Intestinal Tract
Lower ØDHD
Upper ØDHØ
Intestine
Large ØDHE
Small ØDH8
Jaw
Lower ØWH5
Upper ØWH4
Jejunum ØDHA
Joint
Acromioclavicular
Left ØRHH
Right ØRHG
Ankle
Left ØSHG
Right ØSHF
Carpal
Left ØRHR
Right ØRHQ
Carpometacarpal
Left ØRHT
Right ØRHS
Cervical Vertebral ØRH1
Cervicothoracic Vertebral ØRH4
Coccygeal ØSH6
Elbow
Left ØRHM
Right ØRHL
Finger Phalangeal
Left ØRHX
Right ØRHW
Hip
Left ØSHB
Right ØSH9

Insertion of device in — continued
Joint — continued
Knee
Left ØSHD
Right ØSHC
Lumbar Vertebral ØSHØ
Lumbosacral ØSH3
Metacarpophalangeal
Left ØRHV
Right ØRHU
Metatarsal-Phalangeal
Left ØSHN
Right ØSHM
Occipital-cervical ØRHØ
Sacrococcygeal ØSH5
Sacroiliac
Left ØSH8
Right ØSH7
Shoulder
Left ØRHK
Right ØRHJ
Sternoclavicular
Left ØRHF
Right ØRHE
Tarsal
Left ØSHJ
Right ØSHH
Tarsometatarsal
Left ØSHL
Right ØSHK
Temporomandibular
Left ØRHD
Right ØRHC
Thoracic Vertebral ØRH6
Thoracolumbar Vertebral ØRHA
Toe Phalangeal
Left ØSHQ
Right ØSHP
Wrist
Left ØRHP
Right ØRHN
Kidney ØTH5
Knee Region
Left ØYHG
Right ØYHF
Larynx ØCHS
Leg
Lower
Left ØYHJ
Right ØYHH
Upper
Left ØYHD
Right ØYHC
Liver ØFHØ
Left Lobe ØFH2
Right Lobe ØFH1
Lung
Left ØBHL
Right ØBHK
Lymphatic Ø7HN
Thoracic Duct Ø7HK
Mandible
Left ØNHV
Right ØNHT
Maxilla ØNHR
Mediastinum ØWHC
Metacarpal
Left ØPHQ
Right ØPHP
Metatarsal
Left ØQHP
Right ØQHN
Mouth and Throat ØCHY
Muscle
Lower ØKHY
Upper ØKHX
Nasal Mucosa and Soft Tissue Ø9HK
Nasopharynx Ø9HN
Neck ØWH6
Nerve
Cranial ØØHE
Peripheral Ø1HY
Nipple
Left ØHHX
Right ØHHW
Oral Cavity and Throat ØWH3
Orbit
Left ØNHQ
Right ØNHP

Insertion of device in — continued
Ovary ØUH3
Pancreas ØFHG
Patella
Left ØQHF
Right ØQHD
Pelvic Cavity ØWHJ
Penis ØVHS
Pericardial Cavity ØWHD
Pericardium Ø2HN
Perineum
Female ØWHN
Male ØWHM
Peritoneal Cavity ØWHG
Phalanx
Finger
Left ØPHV
Right ØPHT
Thumb
Left ØPHS
Right ØPHR
Toe
Left ØQHR
Right ØQHQ
Pleura ØBHQ
Pleural Cavity
Left ØWHB
Right ØWH9
Prostate ØVHØ
Prostate and Seminal Vesicles ØVH4
Radius
Left ØPHJ
Right ØPHH
Rectum ØDHP
Respiratory Tract ØWHQ
Retroperitoneum ØWHH
Ribs
1 to 2 ØPH1
3 or More ØPH2
Sacrum ØQH1
Scapula
Left ØPH6
Right ØPH5
Scrotum and Tunica Vaginalis ØVH8
Shoulder Region
Left ØXH3
Right ØXH2
Sinus Ø9HY
Skin ØHHPXYZ
Skull ØNHØ
Spinal Canal ØØHU
Spinal Cord ØØHV
Spleen Ø7HP
Sternum ØPHØ
Stomach ØDH6
Subcutaneous Tissue and Fascia
Abdomen ØJH8
Back ØJH7
Buttock ØJH9
Chest ØJH6
Face ØJH1
Foot
Left ØJHR
Right ØJHQ
Hand
Left ØJHK
Right ØJHJ
Head and Neck ØJHS
Lower Arm
Left ØJHH
Right ØJHG
Lower Extremity ØJHW
Lower Leg
Left ØJHP
Right ØJHN
Neck
Left ØJH5
Right ØJH4
Pelvic Region ØJHC
Perineum ØJHB
Scalp ØJHØ
Tendon
Lower ØLHY
Upper ØLHX
Trunk ØJHT
Upper Arm
Left ØJHF
Right ØJHD
Upper Extremity ØJHV

Insertion of device in — continued
Subcutaneous Tissue and Fascia — continued
Upper Leg
Left ØJHM
Right ØJHL
Tarsal
Left ØQHM
Right ØQHL
Tendon
Lower ØLHY
Upper ØLHX
Testis ØVHD
Thymus Ø7HM
Tibia
Left ØQHH
Right ØQHG
Tongue ØCH7
Trachea ØBH1
Tracheobronchial Tree ØBHØ
Ulna
Left ØPHL
Right ØPHK
Ureter ØTH9
Urethra ØTHD
Uterus ØUH9
Uterus and Cervix ØUHD
Vagina ØUHG
Vagina and Cul-de-sac ØUHH
Vas Deferens ØVHR
Vein
Axillary
Left Ø5H8
Right Ø5H7
Azygos Ø5HØ
Basilic
Left Ø5HC
Right Ø5HB
Brachial
Left Ø5HA
Right Ø5H9
Cephalic
Left Ø5HF
Right Ø5HD
Colic Ø6H7
Common Iliac
Left Ø6HD
Right Ø6HC
Coronary Ø2H4
Esophageal Ø6H3
External Iliac
Left Ø6HG
Right Ø6HF
External Jugular
Left Ø5HQ
Right Ø5HP
Face
Left Ø5HV
Right Ø5HT
Femoral
Left Ø6HN
Right Ø6HM
Foot
Left Ø6HV
Right Ø6HT
Gastric Ø6H2
Hand
Left Ø5HH
Right Ø5HG
Hemiazygos Ø5H1
Hepatic Ø6H4
Hypogastric
Left Ø6HJ
Right Ø6HH
Inferior Mesenteric Ø6H6
Innominate
Left Ø5H4
Right Ø5H3
Internal Jugular
Left Ø5HN
Right Ø5HM
Intracranial Ø5HL
Lower Ø6HY
Portal Ø6H8
Pulmonary
Left Ø2HT
Right Ø2HS
Renal
Left Ø6HB
Right Ø6H9

**Insertion of device in** — *continued*
Vein — *continued*
Saphenous
Left Ø6HQ
Right Ø6HP
Splenic Ø6H1
Subclavian
Left Ø5H6
Right Ø5H5
Superior Mesenteric Ø6H5
Upper Ø5HY
Vertebral
Left Ø5HS
Right Ø5HR
Vena Cava
Inferior Ø6HØ
Superior Ø2HV
Ventricle
Left Ø2HL
Right Ø2HK
Vertebra
Cervical ØPH3
Lumbar ØQHØ
Thoracic ØPH4
Wrist Region
Left ØXHH
Right ØXHG
**Inspection**
Abdominal Wall ØWJF
Ankle Region
Left ØYJL
Right ØYJK
Arm
Lower
Left ØXJF
Right ØXJD
Upper
Left ØXJ9
Right ØXJ8
Artery
Lower Ø4JY
Upper Ø3JY
Axilla
Left ØXJ5
Right ØXJ4
Back
Lower ØWJL
Upper ØWJK
Bladder ØTJB
Bone
Facial ØNJW
Lower ØQJY
Nasal ØNJB
Upper ØPJY
Bone Marrow Ø7JT
Brain ØØJØ
Breast
Left ØHJU
Right ØHJT
Bursa and Ligament
Lower ØMJY
Upper ØMJX
Buttock
Left ØYJ1
Right ØYJØ
Cavity, Cranial ØWJ1
Chest Wall ØWJ8
Cisterna Chyli Ø7JL
Diaphragm ØBJT
Disc
Cervical Vertebral ØRJ3
Cervicothoracic Vertebral ØRJ5
Lumbar Vertebral ØSJ2
Lumbosacral ØSJ4
Thoracic Vertebral ØRJ9
Thoracolumbar Vertebral ØRJB
Duct
Hepatobiliary ØFJB
Pancreatic ØFJD
Ear
Inner
Left Ø9JE
Right Ø9JD
Left Ø9JJ
Right Ø9JH
Elbow Region
Left ØXJC
Right ØXJB
Epididymis and Spermatic Cord ØVJM

**Inspection** — *continued*
Extremity
Lower
Left ØYJB
Right ØYJ9
Upper
Left ØXJ7
Right ØXJ6
Eye
Left Ø8J1XZZ
Right Ø8JØXZZ
Face ØWJ2
Fallopian Tube ØUJ8
Femoral Region
Bilateral ØYJE
Left ØYJ8
Right ØYJ7
Finger Nail ØHJQXZZ
Foot
Left ØYJN
Right ØYJM
Gallbladder ØFJ4
Gastrointestinal Tract ØWJP
Genitourinary Tract ØWJR
Gland
Adrenal ØGJ5
Endocrine ØGJS
Pituitary ØGJØ
Salivary ØCJA
Great Vessel Ø2JY
Hand
Left ØXJK
Right ØXJJ
Head ØWJØ
Heart Ø2JA
Inguinal Region
Bilateral ØYJA
Left ØYJ6
Right ØYJ5
Intestinal Tract
Lower ØDJD
Upper ØDJØ
Jaw
Lower ØWJ5
Upper ØWJ4
Joint
Acromioclavicular
Left ØRJH
Right ØRJG
Ankle
Left ØSJG
Right ØSJF
Carpal
Left ØRJR
Right ØRJQ
Carpometacarpal
Left ØRJT
Right ØRJS
Cervical Vertebral ØRJ1
Cervicothoracic Vertebral ØRJ4
Coccygeal ØSJ6
Elbow
Left ØRJM
Right ØRJL
Finger Phalangeal
Left ØRJX
Right ØRJW
Hip
Left ØSJB
Right ØSJ9
Knee
Left ØSJD
Right ØSJC
Lumbar Vertebral ØSJØ
Lumbosacral ØSJ3
Metacarpophalangeal
Left ØRJV
Right ØRJU
Metatarsal-Phalangeal
Left ØSJN
Right ØSJM
Occipital-cervical ØRJØ
Sacrococcygeal ØSJ5
Sacroiliac
Left ØSJ8
Right ØSJ7
Shoulder
Left ØRJK
Right ØRJJ

**Inspection** — *continued*
Joint — *continued*
Sternoclavicular
Left ØRJF
Right ØRJE
Tarsal
Left ØSJJ
Right ØSJH
Tarsometatarsal
Left ØSJL
Right ØSJK
Temporomandibular
Left ØRJD
Right ØRJC
Thoracic Vertebral ØRJ6
Thoracolumbar Vertebral ØRJA
Toe Phalangeal
Left ØSJQ
Right ØSJP
Wrist
Left ØRJP
Right ØRJN
Kidney ØTJ5
Knee Region
Left ØYJG
Right ØYJF
Larynx ØCJS
Leg
Lower
Left ØYJJ
Right ØYJH
Upper
Left ØYJD
Right ØYJC
Lens
Left Ø8JKXZZ
Right Ø8JJXZZ
Liver ØFJØ
Lung
Left ØBJL
Right ØBJK
Lymphatic Ø7JN
Thoracic Duct Ø7JK
Mediastinum ØWJC
Mesentery ØDJV
Mouth and Throat ØCJY
Muscle
Extraocular
Left Ø8JM
Right Ø8JL
Lower ØKJY
Upper ØKJX
Nasal Mucosa and Soft Tissue Ø9JK
Neck ØWJ6
Nerve
Cranial ØØJE
Peripheral Ø1JY
Omentum ØDJU
Oral Cavity and Throat ØWJ3
Ovary ØUJ3
Pancreas ØFJG
Parathyroid Gland ØGJR
Pelvic Cavity ØWJJ
Penis ØVJS
Pericardial Cavity ØWJD
Perineum
Female ØWJN
Male ØWJM
Peritoneal Cavity ØWJG
Peritoneum ØDJW
Pineal Body ØGJ1
Pleura ØBJQ
Pleural Cavity
Left ØWJB
Right ØWJ9
Products of Conception 1ØJØ
Ectopic 1ØJ2
Retained 1ØJ1
Prostate and Seminal Vesicles ØVJ4
Respiratory Tract ØWJQ
Retroperitoneum ØWJH
Scrotum and Tunica Vaginalis ØVJ8
Shoulder Region
Left ØXJ3
Right ØXJ2
Sinus Ø9JY
Skin ØHJPXZZ
Skull ØNJØ
Spinal Canal ØØJU

**Inspection** — *continued*
Spinal Cord ØØJV
Spleen Ø7JP
Stomach ØDJ6
Subcutaneous Tissue and Fascia
Head and Neck ØJJS
Lower Extremity ØJJW
Trunk ØJJT
Upper Extremity ØJJV
Tendon
Lower ØLJY
Upper ØLJX
Testis ØVJD
Thymus Ø7JM
Thyroid Gland ØGJK
Toe Nail ØHJRXZZ
Trachea ØBJ1
Tracheobronchial Tree ØBJØ
Tympanic Membrane
Left Ø9J8
Right Ø9J7
Ureter ØTJ9
Urethra ØTJD
Uterus and Cervix ØUJD
Vagina and Cul-de-sac ØUJH
Vas Deferens ØVJR
Vein
Lower Ø6JY
Upper Ø5JY
Vulva ØUJM
Wrist Region
Left ØXJH
Right ØXJG
**Instillation** *see* Introduction of substance in or on
**Insufflation** *see* Introduction of substance in or on
**Interatrial septum** *use* Septum, Atrial
**Interbody fusion (spine) cage**
*use* Interbody Fusion Device in Lower Joints
*use* Interbody Fusion Device in Upper Joints
**Interbody Fusion Device**
Nanotextured Surface
Cervical Vertebral XRG1Ø92
2 or more XRG2Ø92
Cervicothoracic Vertebral XRG4Ø92
Lumbar Vertebral XRGBØ92
2 or more XRGCØ92
Lumbosacral XRGDØ92
Occipital-cervical XRGØØ92
Thoracic Vertebral XRG6Ø92
2 to 7 XRG7Ø92
8 or more XRG8Ø92
Thoracolumbar Vertebral XRGAØ92
Radiolucent Porous
Cervical Vertebral XRG1ØF3
2 or more XRG2ØF3
Cervicothoracic Vertebral XRG4ØF3
Lumbar Vertebral XRGBØF3
2 or more XRGCØF3
Lumbosacral XRGDØF3
Occipital-cervical XRGØØF3
Thoracic Vertebral XRG6ØF3
2 to 7 XRG7ØF3
8 or more XRG8ØF3
Thoracolumbar Vertebral XRGAØF3
**Intercarpal joint**
*use* Joint, Carpal, Left
*use* Joint, Carpal, Right
**Intercarpal ligament**
*use* Bursa and Ligament, Hand, Left
*use* Bursa and Ligament, Hand, Right
**Interclavicular ligament**
*use* Bursa and Ligament, Shoulder, Left
*use* Bursa and Ligament, Shoulder, Right
**Intercostal lymph node** *use* Lymphatic, Thorax
**Intercostal muscle**
*use* Muscle, Thorax, Left
*use* Muscle, Thorax, Right
**Intercostal nerve** *use* Nerve, Thoracic
**Intercostobrachial nerve** *use* Nerve, Thoracic
**Intercuneiform joint**
*use* Joint, Tarsal, Left
*use* Joint, Tarsal, Right
**Intercuneiform ligament**
*use* Bursa and Ligament, Foot, Left
*use* Bursa and Ligament, Foot, Right
**Intermediate bronchus** *use* Main Bronchus, Right
**Intermediate cuneiform bone**
*use* Tarsal, Left
**Intermediate cuneiform bone** — *continued*
*use* Tarsal, Right
**Intermittent hemodialysis (IHD)** 5A1D7ØZ
**Intermittent mandatory ventilation** *see* Assistance, Respiratory 5AØ9
**Intermittent Negative Airway Pressure**
24-96 Consecutive Hours, Ventilation 5AØ945B
Greater than 96 Consecutive Hours, Ventilation 5AØ955B
Less than 24 Consecutive Hours, Ventilation 5AØ935B
**Intermittent Positive Airway Pressure**
24-96 Consecutive Hours, Ventilation 5AØ9458
Greater than 96 Consecutive Hours, Ventilation 5AØ9558
Less than 24 Consecutive Hours, Ventilation 5AØ9358
**Intermittent positive pressure breathing** *see* Assistance, Respiratory 5AØ9
**Internal anal sphincter** *use* Anal Sphincter
**Internal carotid artery, intracranial portion** *use* Intracranial Artery
**Internal carotid plexus** *use* Nerve, Head and Neck Sympathetic
**Internal (basal) cerebral vein** *use* Vein, Intracranial
**Internal iliac vein**
*use* Vein, Hypogastric, Left
*use* Vein, Hypogastric, Right
**Internal maxillary artery**
*use* Artery, External Carotid, Left
*use* Artery, External Carotid, Right
**Internal naris** *use* Nasal Mucosa and Soft Tissue
**Internal oblique muscle**
*use* Muscle, Abdomen, Left
*use* Muscle, Abdomen, Right
**Internal pudendal artery**
*use* Artery, Internal Iliac, Left
*use* Artery, Internal Iliac, Right
**Internal pudendal vein**
*use* Vein, Hypogastric, Left
*use* Vein, Hypogastric, Right
**Internal thoracic artery**
*use* Artery, Internal Mammary, Left
*use* Artery, Internal Mammary, Right
*use* Artery, Subclavian, Left
*use* Artery, Subclavian, Right
**Internal urethral sphincter** *use* Urethra
**Interphalangeal (IP) joint**
*use* Joint, Finger Phalangeal, Left
*use* Joint, Finger Phalangeal, Right
*use* Joint, Toe Phalangeal, Left
*use* Joint, Toe Phalangeal, Right
**Interphalangeal ligament**
*use* Bursa and Ligament, Foot, Left
*use* Bursa and Ligament, Foot, Right
*use* Bursa and Ligament, Hand, Left
*use* Bursa and Ligament, Hand, Right
**Interrogation, cardiac rhythm related device**
With cardiac function testing *see* Measurement, Cardiac 4AØ2
Interrogation only *see* Measurement, Cardiac 4BØ2
**Interruption** *see* Occlusion
**Interspinalis muscle**
*use* Muscle, Trunk, Left
*use* Muscle, Trunk, Right
**Interspinous ligament**
*use* Head and Neck Bursa and Ligament
*use* Lower Spine Bursa and Ligament
*use* Upper Spine Bursa and Ligament
**Interspinous process spinal stabilization device**
*use* Spinal Stabilization Device, Interspinous Process in ØRH
*use* Spinal Stabilization Device, Interspinous Process in ØSH
**InterStim® Therapy lead** *use* Neurostimulator Lead in Peripheral Nervous System
**InterStim® Therapy neurostimulator** *use* Stimulator Generator, Single Array in ØJH
**Intertransversarius muscle**
*use* Muscle, Trunk, Left
*use* Muscle, Trunk, Right
**Intertransverse ligament**
*use* Lower Spine Bursa and Ligament
*use* Upper Spine Bursa and Ligament
**Interventricular foramen (Monro)** *use* Cerebral Ventricle
**Interventricular septum** *use* Septum, Ventricular
**Intestinal lymphatic trunk** *use* Cisterna Chyli
**Intraluminal Device**
Airway
Esophagus ØDH5
Mouth and Throat ØCHY
Nasopharynx Ø9HN
Bioactive
Occlusion
Common Carotid
Left Ø3LJ
Right Ø3LH
External Carotid
Left Ø3LN
Right Ø3LM
Internal Carotid
Left Ø3LL
Right Ø3LK
Intracranial Ø3LG
Vertebral
Left Ø3LQ
Right Ø3LP
Restriction
Common Carotid
Left Ø3VJ
Right Ø3VH
External Carotid
Left Ø3VN
Right Ø3VM
Internal Carotid
Left Ø3VL
Right Ø3VK
Intracranial Ø3VG
Vertebral
Left Ø3VQ
Right Ø3VP
Endobronchial Valve
Lingula ØBH9
Lower Lobe
Left ØBHB
Right ØBH6
Main
Left ØBH7
Right ØBH3
Middle Lobe, Right ØBH5
Upper Lobe
Left ØBH8
Right ØBH4
Endotracheal Airway
Change device in, Trachea ØB21XEZ
Insertion of device in, Trachea ØBH1
Pessary
Change device in, Vagina and Cul-de-sac ØU2HXGZ
Insertion of device in
Cul-de-sac ØUHF
Vagina ØUHG
**Intramedullary (IM) rod (nail)**
*use* Internal Fixation Device, Intramedullary in Lower Bones
*use* Internal Fixation Device, Intramedullary in Upper Bones
**Intramedullary skeletal kinetic distractor (ISKD)**
*use* Internal Fixation Device, Intramedullary in Lower Bones
*use* Internal Fixation Device, Intramedullary in Upper Bones
**Intraocular Telescope**
Left Ø8RK3ØZ
Right Ø8RJ3ØZ
**Intraoperative Knee Replacement Sensor** XR2
**Intraoperative Radiation Therapy (IORT)**
Anus DDY8CZZ
Bile Ducts DFY2CZZ
Bladder DTY2CZZ
Cervix DUY1CZZ
Colon DDY5CZZ
Duodenum DDY2CZZ
Gallbladder DFY1CZZ
Ileum DDY4CZZ
Jejunum DDY3CZZ
Kidney DTYØCZZ
Larynx D9YBCZZ
Liver DFYØCZZ
Mouth D9Y4CZZ
Nasopharynx D9YDCZZ
Ovary DUYØCZZ
Pancreas DFY3CZZ
Pharynx D9YCCZZ
Prostate DVYØCZZ
Rectum DDY7CZZ

**Intraoperative Radiation Therapy (IORT)** — *continued*
Stomach DDY1CZZ
Ureter DTY1CZZ
Urethra DTY3CZZ
Uterus DUY2CZZ
**Intrauterine Device (IUD)** *use* Contraceptive Device in Female Reproductive System
**Intravascular fluorescence angiography (IFA)** *see* Monitoring, Physiological Systems 4A1
**Introduction of substance in or on**
Artery
Central 3E06
Analgesics 3E06
Anesthetic, Intracirculatory 3E06
Antiarrhythmic 3E06
Anti-infective 3E06
Anti-inflammatory 3E06
Antineoplastic 3E06
Destructive Agent 3E06
Diagnostic Substance, Other 3E06
Electrolytic Substance 3E06
Hormone 3E06
Hypnotics 3E06
Immunotherapeutic 3E06
Nutritional Substance 3E06
Platelet Inhibitor 3E06
Radioactive Substance 3E06
Sedatives 3E06
Serum 3E06
Thrombolytic 3E06
Toxoid 3E06
Vaccine 3E06
Vasopressor 3E06
Water Balance Substance 3E06
Coronary 3E07
Diagnostic Substance, Other 3E07
Platelet Inhibitor 3E07
Thrombolytic 3E07
Peripheral 3E05
Analgesics 3E05
Anesthetic, Intracirculatory 3E05
Antiarrhythmic 3E05
Anti-infective 3E05
Anti-inflammatory 3E05
Antineoplastic 3E05
Destructive Agent 3E05
Diagnostic Substance, Other 3E05
Electrolytic Substance 3E05
Hormone 3E05
Hypnotics 3E05
Immunotherapeutic 3E05
Nutritional Substance 3E05
Platelet Inhibitor 3E05
Radioactive Substance 3E05
Sedatives 3E05
Serum 3E05
Thrombolytic 3E05
Toxoid 3E05
Vaccine 3E05
Vasopressor 3E05
Water Balance Substance 3E05
Biliary Tract 3E0J
Analgesics 3E0J
Anesthetic Agent 3E0J
Anti-infective 3E0J
Anti-inflammatory 3E0J
Antineoplastic 3E0J
Destructive Agent 3E0J
Diagnostic Substance, Other 3E0J
Electrolytic Substance 3E0J
Gas 3E0J
Hypnotics 3E0J
Islet Cells, Pancreatic 3E0J
Nutritional Substance 3E0J
Radioactive Substance 3E0J
Sedatives 3E0J
Water Balance Substance 3E0J
Bone 3E0V
Analgesics 3E0V3NZ
Anesthetic Agent 3E0V3BZ
Anti-infective 3E0V32
Anti-inflammatory 3E0V33Z
Antineoplastic 3E0V30
Destructive Agent 3E0V3TZ
Diagnostic Substance, Other 3E0V3KZ
Electrolytic Substance 3E0V37Z
Hypnotics 3E0V3NZ
Nutritional Substance 3E0V36Z

**Introduction of substance in or on** — *continued*
Bone — *continued*
Radioactive Substance 3E0V3HZ
Sedatives 3E0V3NZ
Water Balance Substance 3E0V37Z
Bone Marrow 3E0A3GC
Antineoplastic 3E0A30
Brain 3E0Q
Analgesics 3E0Q
Anesthetic Agent 3E0Q
Anti-infective 3E0Q
Anti-inflammatory 3E0Q
Antineoplastic 3E0Q
Destructive Agent 3E0Q
Diagnostic Substance, Other 3E0Q
Electrolytic Substance 3E0Q
Gas 3E0Q
Hypnotics 3E0Q
Nutritional Substance 3E0Q
Radioactive Substance 3E0Q
Sedatives 3E0Q
Stem Cells
Embryonic 3E0Q
Somatic 3E0Q
Water Balance Substance 3E0Q
Cranial Cavity 3E0Q
Analgesics 3E0Q
Anesthetic Agent 3E0Q
Anti-infective 3E0Q
Anti-inflammatory 3E0Q
Antineoplastic 3E0Q
Destructive Agent 3E0Q
Diagnostic Substance, Other 3E0Q
Electrolytic Substance 3E0Q
Gas 3E0Q
Hypnotics 3E0Q
Nutritional Substance 3E0Q
Radioactive Substance 3E0Q
Sedatives 3E0Q
Stem Cells
Embryonic 3E0Q
Somatic 3E0Q
Water Balance Substance 3E0Q
Ear 3E0B
Analgesics 3E0B
Anesthetic Agent 3E0B
Anti-infective 3E0B
Anti-inflammatory 3E0B
Antineoplastic 3E0B
Destructive Agent 3E0B
Diagnostic Substance, Other 3E0B
Hypnotics 3E0B
Radioactive Substance 3E0B
Sedatives 3E0B
Epidural Space 3E0S3GC
Analgesics 3E0S3NZ
Anesthetic Agent 3E0S3BZ
Anti-infective 3E0S32
Anti-inflammatory 3E0S33Z
Antineoplastic 3E0S30
Destructive Agent 3E0S3TZ
Diagnostic Substance, Other 3E0S3KZ
Electrolytic Substance 3E0S37Z
Gas 3E0S
Hypnotics 3E0S3NZ
Nutritional Substance 3E0S36Z
Radioactive Substance 3E0S3HZ
Sedatives 3E0S3NZ
Water Balance Substance 3E0S37Z
Eye 3E0C
Analgesics 3E0C
Anesthetic Agent 3E0C
Anti-infective 3E0C
Anti-inflammatory 3E0C
Antineoplastic 3E0C
Destructive Agent 3E0C
Diagnostic Substance, Other 3E0C
Gas 3E0C
Hypnotics 3E0C
Pigment 3E0C
Radioactive Substance 3E0C
Sedatives 3E0C
Gastrointestinal Tract
Lower 3E0H
Analgesics 3E0H
Anesthetic Agent 3E0H
Anti-infective 3E0H
Anti-inflammatory 3E0H
Antineoplastic 3E0H

**Introduction of substance in or on** — *continued*
Gastrointestinal Tract — *continued*
Lower — *continued*
Destructive Agent 3E0H
Diagnostic Substance, Other 3E0H
Electrolytic Substance 3E0H
Gas 3E0H
Hypnotics 3E0H
Nutritional Substance 3E0H
Radioactive Substance 3E0H
Sedatives 3E0H
Water Balance Substance 3E0H
Upper 3E0G
Analgesics 3E0G
Anesthetic Agent 3E0G
Anti-infective 3E0G
Anti-inflammatory 3E0G
Antineoplastic 3E0G
Destructive Agent 3E0G
Diagnostic Substance, Other 3E0G
Electrolytic Substance 3E0G
Gas 3E0G
Hypnotics 3E0G
Nutritional Substance 3E0G
Radioactive Substance 3E0G
Sedatives 3E0G
Water Balance Substance 3E0G
Genitourinary Tract 3E0K
Analgesics 3E0K
Anesthetic Agent 3E0K
Anti-infective 3E0K
Anti-inflammatory 3E0K
Antineoplastic 3E0K
Destructive Agent 3E0K
Diagnostic Substance, Other 3E0K
Electrolytic Substance 3E0K
Gas 3E0K
Hypnotics 3E0K
Nutritional Substance 3E0K
Radioactive Substance 3E0K
Sedatives 3E0K
Water Balance Substance 3E0K
Heart 3E08
Diagnostic Substance, Other 3E08
Platelet Inhibitor 3E08
Thrombolytic 3E08
Joint 3E0U
Analgesics 3E0U3NZ
Anesthetic Agent 3E0U3BZ
Anti-infective 3E0U
Anti-inflammatory 3E0U33Z
Antineoplastic 3E0U30
Destructive Agent 3E0U3TZ
Diagnostic Substance, Other 3E0U3KZ
Electrolytic Substance 3E0U37Z
Gas 3E0U3SF
Hypnotics 3E0U3NZ
Nutritional Substance 3E0U36Z
Radioactive Substance 3E0U3HZ
Sedatives 3E0U3NZ
Water Balance Substance 3E0U37Z
Lymphatic 3E0W3GC
Analgesics 3E0W3NZ
Anesthetic Agent 3E0W3BZ
Anti-infective 3E0W32
Anti-inflammatory 3E0W33Z
Antineoplastic 3E0W30
Destructive Agent 3E0W3TZ
Diagnostic Substance, Other 3E0W3KZ
Electrolytic Substance 3E0W37Z
Hypnotics 3E0W3NZ
Nutritional Substance 3E0W36Z
Radioactive Substance 3E0W3HZ
Sedatives 3E0W3NZ
Water Balance Substance 3E0W37Z
Mouth 3E0D
Analgesics 3E0D
Anesthetic Agent 3E0D
Antiarrhythmic 3E0D
Anti-infective 3E0D
Anti-inflammatory 3E0D
Antineoplastic 3E0D
Destructive Agent 3E0D
Diagnostic Substance, Other 3E0D
Electrolytic Substance 3E0D
Hypnotics 3E0D
Nutritional Substance 3E0D
Radioactive Substance 3E0D
Sedatives 3E0D

**Introduction of substance in or on** — *continued*
Mouth — *continued*
Serum 3EØD
Toxoid 3EØD
Vaccine 3EØD
Water Balance Substance 3EØD
Mucous Membrane 3EØØXGC
Analgesics 3EØØXNZ
Anesthetic Agent 3EØØXBZ
Anti-infective 3EØØX2
Anti-inflammatory 3EØØX3Z
Antineoplastic 3EØØXØ
Destructive Agent 3EØØXTZ
Diagnostic Substance, Other 3EØØXKZ
Hypnotics 3EØØXNZ
Pigment 3EØØXMZ
Sedatives 3EØØXNZ
Serum 3EØØX4Z
Toxoid 3EØØX4Z
Vaccine 3EØØX4Z
Muscle 3EØ23GC
Analgesics 3EØ23NZ
Anesthetic Agent 3EØ23BZ
Anti-infective 3EØ232
Anti-inflammatory 3EØ233Z
Antineoplastic 3EØ23Ø
Destructive Agent 3EØ23TZ
Diagnostic Substance, Other 3EØ23KZ
Electrolytic Substance 3EØ237Z
Hypnotics 3EØ23NZ
Nutritional Substance 3EØ236Z
Radioactive Substance 3EØ23HZ
Sedatives 3EØ23NZ
Serum 3EØ234Z
Toxoid 3EØ234Z
Vaccine 3EØ234Z
Water Balance Substance 3EØ237Z
Nerve
Cranial 3EØX3GC
Anesthetic Agent 3EØX3BZ
Anti-inflammatory 3EØX33Z
Destructive Agent 3EØX3TZ
Peripheral 3EØT3GC
Anesthetic Agent 3EØT3BZ
Anti-inflammatory 3EØT33Z
Destructive Agent 3EØT3TZ
Plexus 3EØT3GC
Anesthetic Agent 3EØT3BZ
Anti-inflammatory 3EØT33Z
Destructive Agent 3EØT3TZ
Nose 3EØ9
Analgesics 3EØ9
Anesthetic Agent 3EØ9
Anti-infective 3EØ9
Anti-inflammatory 3EØ9
Antineoplastic 3EØ9
Destructive Agent 3EØ9
Diagnostic Substance, Other 3EØ9
Hypnotics 3EØ9
Radioactive Substance 3EØ9
Sedatives 3EØ9
Serum 3EØ9
Toxoid 3EØ9
Vaccine 3EØ9
Pancreatic Tract 3EØJ
Analgesics 3EØJ
Anesthetic Agent 3EØJ
Anti-infective 3EØJ
Anti-inflammatory 3EØJ
Antineoplastic 3EØJ
Destructive Agent 3EØJ
Diagnostic Substance, Other 3EØJ
Electrolytic Substance 3EØJ
Gas 3EØJ
Hypnotics 3EØJ
Islet Cells, Pancreatic 3EØJ
Nutritional Substance 3EØJ
Radioactive Substance 3EØJ
Sedatives 3EØJ
Water Balance Substance 3EØJ
Pericardial Cavity 3EØY
Analgesics 3EØY3NZ
Anesthetic Agent 3EØY3BZ
Anti-infective 3EØY32
Anti-inflammatory 3EØY33Z
Antineoplastic 3EØY
Destructive Agent 3EØY3TZ
Diagnostic Substance, Other 3EØY3KZ
Electrolytic Substance 3EØY37Z

**Introduction of substance in or on** — *continued*
Pericardial Cavity — *continued*
Gas 3EØY
Hypnotics 3EØY3NZ
Nutritional Substance 3EØY36Z
Radioactive Substance 3EØY3HZ
Sedatives 3EØY3NZ
Water Balance Substance 3EØY37Z
Peritoneal Cavity 3EØM
Adhesion Barrier 3EØM
Analgesics 3EØM3NZ
Anesthetic Agent 3EØM3BZ
Anti-infective 3EØM32
Anti-inflammatory 3EØM33Z
Antineoplastic 3EØM
Destructive Agent 3EØM3TZ
Diagnostic Substance, Other 3EØM3KZ
Electrolytic Substance 3EØM37Z
Gas 3EØM
Hypnotics 3EØM3NZ
Nutritional Substance 3EØM36Z
Radioactive Substance 3EØM3HZ
Sedatives 3EØM3NZ
Water Balance Substance 3EØM37Z
Pharynx 3EØD
Analgesics 3EØD
Anesthetic Agent 3EØD
Antiarrhythmic 3EØD
Anti-infective 3EØD
Anti-inflammatory 3EØD
Antineoplastic 3EØD
Destructive Agent 3EØD
Diagnostic Substance, Other 3EØD
Electrolytic Substance 3EØD
Hypnotics 3EØD
Nutritional Substance 3EØD
Radioactive Substance 3EØD
Sedatives 3EØD
Serum 3EØD
Toxoid 3EØD
Vaccine 3EØD
Water Balance Substance 3EØD
Pleural Cavity 3EØL
Adhesion Barrier 3EØL
Analgesics 3EØL3NZ
Anesthetic Agent 3EØL3BZ
Anti-infective 3EØL32
Anti-inflammatory 3EØL33Z
Antineoplastic 3EØL
Destructive Agent 3EØL3TZ
Diagnostic Substance, Other 3EØL3KZ
Electrolytic Substance 3EØL37Z
Gas 3EØL
Hypnotics 3EØL3NZ
Nutritional Substance 3EØL36Z
Radioactive Substance 3EØL3HZ
Sedatives 3EØL3NZ
Water Balance Substance 3EØL37Z
Products of Conception 3EØE
Analgesics 3EØE
Anesthetic Agent 3EØE
Anti-infective 3EØE
Anti-inflammatory 3EØE
Antineoplastic 3EØE
Destructive Agent 3EØE
Diagnostic Substance, Other 3EØE
Electrolytic Substance 3EØE
Gas 3EØE
Hypnotics 3EØE
Nutritional Substance 3EØE
Radioactive Substance 3EØE
Sedatives 3EØE
Water Balance Substance 3EØE
Reproductive
Female 3EØP
Adhesion Barrier 3EØP
Analgesics 3EØP
Anesthetic Agent 3EØP
Anti-infective 3EØP
Anti-inflammatory 3EØP
Antineoplastic 3EØP
Destructive Agent 3EØP
Diagnostic Substance, Other 3EØP
Electrolytic Substance 3EØP
Gas 3EØP
Hormone 3EØP
Hypnotics 3EØP
Nutritional Substance 3EØP
Ovum, Fertilized 3EØP

**Introduction of substance in or on** — *continued*
Reproductive — *continued*
Female — *continued*
Radioactive Substance 3EØP
Sedatives 3EØP
Sperm 3EØP
Water Balance Substance 3EØP
Male 3EØN
Analgesics 3EØN
Anesthetic Agent 3EØN
Anti-infective 3EØN
Anti-inflammatory 3EØN
Antineoplastic 3EØN
Destructive Agent 3EØN
Diagnostic Substance, Other 3EØN
Electrolytic Substance 3EØN
Gas 3EØN
Hypnotics 3EØN
Nutritional Substance 3EØN
Radioactive Substance 3EØN
Sedatives 3EØN
Water Balance Substance 3EØN
Respiratory Tract 3EØF
Analgesics 3EØF
Anesthetic Agent 3EØF
Anti-infective 3EØF
Anti-inflammatory 3EØF
Antineoplastic 3EØF
Destructive Agent 3EØF
Diagnostic Substance, Other 3EØF
Electrolytic Substance 3EØF
Gas 3EØF
Hypnotics 3EØF
Nutritional Substance 3EØF
Radioactive Substance 3EØF
Sedatives 3EØF
Water Balance Substance 3EØF
Skin 3EØØXGC
Analgesics 3EØØXNZ
Anesthetic Agent 3EØØXBZ
Anti-infective 3EØØX2
Anti-inflammatory 3EØØX3Z
Antineoplastic 3EØØXØ
Destructive Agent 3EØØXTZ
Diagnostic Substance, Other 3EØØXKZ
Hypnotics 3EØØXNZ
Pigment 3EØØXMZ
Sedatives 3EØØXNZ
Serum 3EØØX4Z
Toxoid 3EØØX4Z
Vaccine 3EØØX4Z
Spinal Canal 3EØR3GC
Analgesics 3EØR3NZ
Anesthetic Agent 3EØR3BZ
Anti-infective 3EØR32
Anti-inflammatory 3EØR33Z
Antineoplastic 3EØR3Ø
Destructive Agent 3EØR3TZ
Diagnostic Substance, Other 3EØR3KZ
Electrolytic Substance 3EØR37Z
Gas 3EØR
Hypnotics 3EØR3NZ
Nutritional Substance 3EØR36Z
Radioactive Substance 3EØR3HZ
Sedatives 3EØR3NZ
Stem Cells
Embryonic 3EØR
Somatic 3EØR
Water Balance Substance 3EØR37Z
Subcutaneous Tissue 3EØ13GC
Analgesics 3EØ13NZ
Anesthetic Agent 3EØ13BZ
Anti-infective 3EØ1
Anti-inflammatory 3EØ133Z
Antineoplastic 3EØ13Ø
Destructive Agent 3EØ13TZ
Diagnostic Substance, Other 3EØ13KZ
Electrolytic Substance 3EØ137Z
Hormone 3EØ13V
Hypnotics 3EØ13NZ
Nutritional Substance 3EØ136Z
Radioactive Substance 3EØ13HZ
Sedatives 3EØ13NZ
Serum 3EØ134Z
Toxoid 3EØ134Z
Vaccine 3EØ134Z
Water Balance Substance 3EØ137Z
Vein
Central 3EØ4

**Introduction of substance in or on** — *continued*
Vein — *continued*
Central — *continued*
Analgesics 3E04
Anesthetic, Intracirculatory 3E04
Antiarrhythmic 3E04
Anti-infective 3E04
Anti-inflammatory 3E04
Antineoplastic 3E04
Destructive Agent 3E04
Diagnostic Substance, Other 3E04
Electrolytic Substance 3E04
Hormone 3E04
Hypnotics 3E04
Immunotherapeutic 3E04
Nutritional Substance 3E04
Platelet Inhibitor 3E04
Radioactive Substance 3E04
Sedatives 3E04
Serum 3E04
Thrombolytic 3E04
Toxoid 3E04
Vaccine 3E04
Vasopressor 3E04
Water Balance Substance 3E04
Peripheral 3E03
Analgesics 3E03
Anesthetic, Intracirculatory 3E03
Antiarrhythmic 3E03
Anti-infective 3E03
Anti-inflammatory 3E03
Antineoplastic 3E03
Destructive Agent 3E03
Diagnostic Substance, Other 3E03
Electrolytic Substance 3E03
Hormone 3E03
Hypnotics 3E03
Immunotherapeutic 3E03
Islet Cells, Pancreatic 3E03
Nutritional Substance 3E03
Platelet Inhibitor 3E03
Radioactive Substance 3E03
Sedatives 3E03
Serum 3E03
Thrombolytic 3E03
Toxoid 3E03
Vaccine 3E03
Vasopressor 3E03
Water Balance Substance 3E03
**Intubation**
Airway
*see* Insertion of device in, Esophagus 0DH5
*see* Insertion of device in, Mouth and Throat 0CHY
*see* Insertion of device in, Trachea 0BH1
Drainage device *see* Drainage
Feeding Device *see* Insertion of device in, Gastrointestinal System 0DH
**INTUITY Elite valve system, EDWARDS** *use* Zooplastic Tissue, Rapid Deployment Technique in New Technology
**IPPB (intermittent positive pressure breathing)** *see* Assistance, Respiratory 5A09
**Iridectomy**
*see* Excision, Eye 08B
*see* Resection, Eye 08T
**Iridoplasty**
*see* Repair, Eye 08Q
*see* Replacement, Eye 08R
*see* Supplement, Eye 08U
**Iridotomy** *see* Drainage, Eye 089
**Irrigation**
Biliary Tract, Irrigating Substance 3E1J
Brain, Irrigating Substance 3E1Q38Z
Cranial Cavity, Irrigating Substance 3E1Q38Z
Ear, Irrigating Substance 3E1B
Epidural Space, Irrigating Substance 3E1S38Z
Eye, Irrigating Substance 3E1C
Gastrointestinal Tract
Lower, Irrigating Substance 3E1H
Upper, Irrigating Substance 3E1G
Genitourinary Tract, Irrigating Substance 3E1K
Irrigating Substance 3C1ZX8Z
Joint, Irrigating Substance 3E1U38Z
Mucous Membrane, Irrigating Substance 3E10
Nose, Irrigating Substance 3E19
Pancreatic Tract, Irrigating Substance 3E1J
Pericardial Cavity, Irrigating Substance 3E1Y38Z
**Irrigation** — *continued*
Peritoneal Cavity
Dialysate 3E1M39Z
Irrigating Substance 3E1M38Z
Pleural Cavity, Irrigating Substance 3E1L38Z
Reproductive
Female, Irrigating Substance 3E1P
Male, Irrigating Substance 3E1N
Respiratory Tract, Irrigating Substance 3E1F
Skin, Irrigating Substance 3E10
Spinal Canal, Irrigating Substance 3E1R38Z
**Isavuconazole Anti-infective** XW0
**Ischiatic nerve** *use* Nerve, Sciatic
**Ischiocavernosus muscle** *use* Muscle, Perineum
**Ischiofemoral ligament**
*use* Bursa and Ligament, Hip, Left
*use* Bursa and Ligament, Hip, Right
**Ischium**
*use* Bone, Pelvic, Left
*use* Bone, Pelvic, Right
**Isolation** 8E0ZXY6
**Isotope Administration, Whole Body** DWY5G
**Itrel (3) (4) neurostimulator** *use* Stimulator Generator, Single Array 0JH

## J

**Jejunal artery** *use* Artery, Superior Mesenteric
**Jejunectomy**
*see* Excision, Jejunum 0DBA
*see* Resection, Jejunum 0DTA
**Jejunocolostomy**
*see* Bypass, Gastrointestinal System 0D1
*see* Drainage, Gastrointestinal System 0D9
**Jejunopexy**
*see* Repair, Jejunum 0DQA
*see* Reposition, Jejunum 0DSA
**Jejunostomy**
*see* Bypass, Jejunum 0D1A
*see* Drainage, Jejunum 0D9A
**Jejunotomy** *see* Drainage, Jejunum 0D9A
**Joint fixation plate**
*use* Internal Fixation Device in Lower Joints
*use* Internal Fixation Device in Upper Joints
**Joint liner (insert)** *use* Liner in Lower Joints
**Joint spacer (antibiotic)**
*use* Spacer in Lower Joints
*use* Spacer in Upper Joints
**Jugular body** *use* Glomus Jugulare
**Jugular lymph node**
*use* Lymphatic, Neck, Left
*use* Lymphatic, Neck, Right

## K

**Kappa** *use* Pacemaker, Dual Chamber in 0JH
**Kcentra** *use* 4-Factor Prothrombin Complex Concentrate
**Keratectomy, kerectomy**
*see* Excision, Eye 08B
*see* Resection, Eye 08T
**Keratocentesis** *see* Drainage, Eye 089
**Keratoplasty**
*see* Repair, Eye 08Q
*see* Replacement, Eye 08R
*see* Supplement, Eye 08U
**Keratotomy**
*see* Drainage, Eye 089
*see* Repair, Eye 08Q
**Kirschner wire (K-wire)**
*use* Internal Fixation Device in Head and Facial Bones
*use* Internal Fixation Device in Lower Bones
*use* Internal Fixation Device in Lower Joints
*use* Internal Fixation Device in Upper Bones
*use* Internal Fixation Device in Upper Joints
**Knee (implant) insert** *use* Liner in Lower Joints
**KUB x-ray** *see* Plain Radiography, Kidney, Ureter and Bladder BT04
**Kuntscher nail**
*use* Internal Fixation Device, Intramedullary in Lower Bones
*use* Internal Fixation Device, Intramedullary in Upper Bones

## L

**Labia majora** *use* Vulva
**Labia minora** *use* Vulva
**Labial gland**
*use* Lip, Lower
*use* Lip, Upper
**Labiectomy**
*see* Excision, Female Reproductive System 0UB
*see* Resection, Female Reproductive System 0UT
**Lacrimal canaliculus**
*use* Duct, Lacrimal, Left
*use* Duct, Lacrimal, Right
**Lacrimal punctum**
*use* Duct, Lacrimal, Left
*use* Duct, Lacrimal, Right
**Lacrimal sac**
*use* Duct, Lacrimal, Left
*use* Duct, Lacrimal, Right
**LAGB (laparoscopic adjustable gastric banding)**
Adjustment/revision 0DW64CZ
Initial procedure 0DV64CZ
**Laminectomy**
*see* Excision, Lower Bones 0QB
*see* Excision, Upper Bones 0PB
*see* Release, Central Nervous System and Cranial Nerves 00N
*see* Release, Peripheral Nervous System 01N
**Laminotomy**
*see* Drainage, Lower Bones 0Q9
*see* Drainage, Upper Bones 0P9
*see* Excision, Lower Bones 0QB
*see* Excision, Upper Bones 0PB
*see* Release, Central Nervous System and Cranial Nerves 00N
*see* Release, Lower Bones 0QN
*see* Release, Peripheral Nervous System 01N
*see* Release, Upper Bones 0PN
**Laparoscopic-assisted transanal pull-through**
*see* Excision, Gastrointestinal System 0DB
*see* Resection, Gastrointestinal System 0DT
**Laparoscopy** *see* Inspection
**Laparotomy**
Drainage *see* Drainage, Peritoneal Cavity 0W9G
Exploratory *see* Inspection, Peritoneal Cavity 0WJG
**LAP-BAND® Adjustable Gastric Banding System** *use* Extraluminal Device
**Laryngectomy**
*see* Excision, Larynx 0CBS
*see* Resection, Larynx 0CTS
**Laryngocentesis** *see* Drainage, Larynx 0C9S
**Laryngogram** *see* Fluoroscopy, Larynx B91J
**Laryngopexy** *see* Repair, Larynx 0CQS
**Laryngopharynx** *use* Pharynx
**Laryngoplasty**
*see* Repair, Larynx 0CQS
*see* Replacement, Larynx 0CRS
*see* Supplement, Larynx 0CUS
**Laryngorrhaphy** *see* Repair, Larynx 0CQS
**Laryngoscopy** 0CJS8ZZ
**Laryngotomy** *see* Drainage, Larynx 0C9S
**Laser Interstitial Thermal Therapy**
Adrenal Gland DGY2KZZ
Anus DDY8KZZ
Bile Ducts DFY2KZZ
Brain D0Y0KZZ
Brain Stem D0Y1KZZ
Breast
Left DMY0KZZ
Right DMY1KZZ
Bronchus DBY1KZZ
Chest Wall DBY7KZZ
Colon DDY5KZZ
Diaphragm DBY8KZZ
Duodenum DDY2KZZ
Esophagus DDY0KZZ
Gallbladder DFY1KZZ
Gland
Adrenal DGY2KZZ
Parathyroid DGY4KZZ
Pituitary DGY0KZZ
Thyroid DGY5KZZ
Ileum DDY4KZZ
Jejunum DDY3KZZ
Liver DFY0KZZ
Lung DBY2KZZ

**Laser Interstitial Thermal Therapy** — *continued*
Mediastinum DBY6KZZ
Nerve, Peripheral DØY7KZZ
Pancreas DFY3KZZ
Parathyroid Gland DGY4KZZ
Pineal Body DGY1KZZ
Pituitary Gland DGYØKZZ
Pleura DBY5KZZ
Prostate DVYØKZZ
Rectum DDY7KZZ
Spinal Cord DØY6KZZ
Stomach DDY1KZZ
Thyroid Gland DGY5KZZ
Trachea DBYØKZZ
**Lateral canthus**
*use* Eyelid, Upper, Left
*use* Eyelid, Upper, Right
**Lateral collateral ligament (LCL)**
*use* Bursa and Ligament, Knee, Left
*use* Bursa and Ligament, Knee, Right
**Lateral condyle of femur**
*use* Femur, Lower, Left
*use* Femur, Lower, Right
**Lateral condyle of tibia**
*use* Tibia, Left
*use* Tibia, Right
**Lateral cuneiform bone**
*use* Tarsal, Left
*use* Tarsal, Right
**Lateral epicondyle of femur**
*use* Femur, Lower, Left
*use* Femur, Lower, Right
**Lateral epicondyle of humerus**
*use* Humeral Shaft, Left
*use* Humeral Shaft, Right
**Lateral femoral cutaneous nerve** *use* Nerve, Lumbar Plexus
**Lateral (brachial) lymph node**
*use* Lymphatic, Axillary, Left
*use* Lymphatic, Axillary, Right
**Lateral malleolus**
*use* Fibula, Left
*use* Fibula, Right
**Lateral meniscus**
*use* Joint, Knee, Left
*use* Joint, Knee, Right
**Lateral nasal cartilage** *use* Nasal Mucosa and Soft Tissue
**Lateral plantar artery**
*use* Artery, Foot, Left
*use* Artery, Foot, Right
**Lateral plantar nerve** *use* Nerve, Tibial
**Lateral rectus muscle**
*use* Muscle, Extraocular, Left
*use* Muscle, Extraocular, Right
**Lateral sacral artery**
*use* Artery, Internal Iliac, Left
*use* Artery, Internal Iliac, Right
**Lateral sacral vein**
*use* Vein, Hypogastric, Left
*use* Vein, Hypogastric, Right
**Lateral sural cutaneous nerve** *use* Nerve, Peroneal
**Lateral tarsal artery**
*use* Artery, Foot, Left
*use* Artery, Foot, Right
**Lateral temporomandibular ligament** *use* Bursa and Ligament, Head and Neck
**Lateral thoracic artery**
*use* Artery, Axillary, Left
*use* Artery, Axillary, Right
**Latissimus dorsi muscle**
*use* Muscle, Trunk, Left
*use* Muscle, Trunk, Right
**Latissimus Dorsi Myocutaneous Flap**
Replacement
Bilateral ØHRVØ75
Left ØHRUØ75
Right ØHRTØ75
Transfer
Left ØKXG
Right ØKXF
**Lavage**
*see* Irrigation
Bronchial alveolar, diagnostic *see* Drainage, Respiratory System ØB9
**Least splanchnic nerve** *use* Nerve, Thoracic Sympathetic
**Left ascending lumbar vein** *use* Vein, Hemiazygos
**Left atrioventricular valve** *use* Valve, Mitral
**Left auricular appendix** *use* Atrium, Left
**Left colic vein** *use* Vein, Colic
**Left coronary sulcus** *use* Heart, Left
**Left gastric artery** *use* Artery, Gastric
**Left gastroepiploic artery** *use* Artery, Splenic
**Left gastroepiploic vein** *use* Vein, Splenic
**Left inferior phrenic vein** *use* Vein, Renal, Left
**Left inferior pulmonary vein** *use* Vein, Pulmonary, Left
**Left jugular trunk** *use* Lymphatic, Thoracic Duct
**Left lateral ventricle** *use* Cerebral Ventricle
**Left ovarian vein** *use* Vein, Renal, Left
**Left second lumbar vein** *use* Vein, Renal, Left
**Left subclavian trunk** *use* Lymphatic, Thoracic Duct
**Left subcostal vein** *use* Vein, Hemiazygos
**Left superior pulmonary vein** *use* Vein, Pulmonary, Left
**Left suprarenal vein** *use* Vein, Renal, Left
**Left testicular vein** *use* Vein, Renal, Left
**Lengthening**
Bone, with device *see* Insertion of Limb Lengthening Device
Muscle, by incision *see* Division, Muscles ØK8
Tendon, by incision *see* Division, Tendons ØL8
**Leptomeninges, intracranial** *use* Cerebral Meninges
**Leptomeninges, spinal** *use* Spinal Meninges
**Lesser alar cartilage** *use* Nasal Mucosa and Soft Tissue
**Lesser occipital nerve** *use* Nerve, Cervical Plexus
**Lesser Omentum** *use* Omentum
**Lesser saphenous vein**
*use* Saphenous Vein, Left
*use* Saphenous Vein, Right
**Lesser splanchnic nerve** *use* Nerve, Thoracic Sympathetic
**Lesser trochanter**
*use* Femur, Upper, Left
*use* Femur, Upper, Right
**Lesser tuberosity**
*use* Humeral Head, Left
*use* Humeral Head, Right
**Lesser wing** *use* Sphenoid Bone
**Leukopheresis, therapeutic** *see* Pheresis, Circulatory 6A55
**Levator anguli oris muscle** *use* Muscle, Facial
**Levator ani muscle** *use* Perineum Muscle
**Levator labii superioris alaeque nasi muscle** *use* Muscle, Facial
**Levator labii superioris muscle** *use* Muscle, Facial
**Levator palpebrae superioris muscle**
*use* Eyelid, Upper, Left
*use* Eyelid, Upper, Right
**Levator scapulae muscle**
*use* Muscle, Neck, Left
*use* Muscle, Neck, Right
**Levator veli palatini muscle** *use* Muscle, Tongue, Palate, Pharynx
**Levatores costarum muscle**
*use* Muscle, Thorax, Left
*use* Muscle, Thorax, Right
**LifeStent® (Flexstar) (XL) Vascular Stent System** *use* Intraluminal Device
**Ligament of head of fibula**
*use* Bursa and Ligament, Knee, Left
*use* Bursa and Ligament, Knee, Right
**Ligament of the lateral malleolus**
*use* Bursa and Ligament, Ankle, Left
*use* Bursa and Ligament, Ankle, Right
**Ligamentum flavum**
*use* Lower Spine Bursa and Ligament
*use* Upper Spine Bursa and Ligament
**Ligation** *see* Occlusion
**Ligation, hemorrhoid** *see* Occlusion, Lower Veins, Hemorrhoidal Plexus
**Light Therapy** GZJZZZZ
**Liner**
Removal of device from
Hip
Left ØSPBØ9Z
Right ØSP9Ø9Z
Knee
Left ØSPDØ9Z
Right ØSPCØ9Z
Revision of device in
Hip
Left ØSWBØ9Z
Right ØSW9Ø9Z
Knee
Left ØSWDØ9Z
**Liner** — *continued*
Revision of device in — *continued*
Knee — *continued*
Right ØSWCØ9Z
Supplement
Hip
Left ØSUBØ9Z
Acetabular Surface ØSUEØ9Z
Femoral Surface ØSUSØ9Z
Right ØSU9Ø9Z
Acetabular Surface ØSUAØ9Z
Femoral Surface ØSURØ9Z
Knee
Left ØSUDØ9
Femoral Surface ØSUUØ9Z
Tibial Surface ØSUWØ9Z
Right ØSUCØ9
Femoral Surface ØSUTØ9Z
Tibial Surface ØSUVØ9Z
**Lingual artery**
*use* Artery, External Carotid, Left
*use* Artery, External Carotid, Right
**Lingual tonsil** *use* Pharynx
**Lingulectomy, lung**
*see* Excision, Lung Lingula ØBBH
*see* Resection, Lung Lingula ØBTH
**Lithotripsy**
With removal of fragments *see* Extirpation
*see* Fragmentation
**LITT (laser interstitial thermal therapy)** *see* Laser Interstitial Thermal Therapy
**LIVIAN™ CRT-D** *use* Cardiac Resynchronization Defibrillator Pulse Generator in ØJH
**Lobectomy**
*see* Excision, Central Nervous System and Cranial Nerves ØØB
*see* Excision, Endocrine System ØGB
*see* Excision, Hepatobiliary System and Pancreas ØFB
*see* Excision, Respiratory System ØBB
*see* Resection, Endocrine System ØGT
*see* Resection, Hepatobiliary System and Pancreas ØFT
*see* Resection, Respiratory System ØBT
**Lobotomy** *see* Division, Brain ØØ8Ø
**Localization**
*see* Imaging
*see* Map
**Locus ceruleus** *use* Pons
**Long thoracic nerve** *use* Nerve, Brachial Plexus
**Loop ileostomy** *see* Bypass, Ileum ØD1B
**Loop recorder, implantable** *use* Monitoring Device
**Lower GI series** *see* Fluoroscopy, Colon BD14
**Lumbar artery** *use* Aorta, Abdominal
**Lumbar facet joint** *use* Joint, Lumbar Vertebral
**Lumbar ganglion** *use* Nerve, Lumbar Sympathetic
**Lumbar lymph node** *use* Lymphatic, Aortic
**Lumbar lymphatic trunk** *use* Cisterna Chyli
**Lumbar splanchnic nerve** *use* Nerve, Lumbar Sympathetic
**Lumbosacral facet joint** *use* Joint, Lumbosacral
**Lumbosacral trunk** *use* Nerve, Lumbar
**Lumpectomy** *see* Excision
**Lunate bone**
*use* Carpal, Left
*use* Carpal, Right
**Lunotriquetral ligament**
*use* Bursa and Ligament, Hand, Left
*use* Bursa and Ligament, Hand, Right
**Lymphadenectomy**
*see* Excision, Lymphatic and Hemic Systems Ø7B
*see* Resection, Lymphatic and Hemic Systems Ø7T
**Lymphadenotomy** *see* Drainage, Lymphatic and Hemic Systems Ø79
**Lymphangiectomy**
*see* Excision, Lymphatic and Hemic Systems Ø7B
*see* Resection, Lymphatic and Hemic Systems Ø7T
**Lymphangiogram** *see* Plain Radiography, Lymphatic System B7Ø
**Lymphangioplasty**
*see* Repair, Lymphatic and Hemic Systems Ø7Q
*see* Supplement, Lymphatic and Hemic Systems Ø7U
**Lymphangiorrhaphy** *see* Repair, Lymphatic and Hemic Systems Ø7Q
**Lymphangiotomy** *see* Drainage, Lymphatic and Hemic Systems Ø79
**Lysis** *see* Release

# M

**Macula**
*use* Retina, Left
*use* Retina, Right
**MAGEC® Spinal Bracing and Distraction System** *use* Magnetically Controlled Growth Rod(s) in New Technology
**Magnet extraction, ocular foreign body** *see* Extirpation, Eye Ø8C
**Magnetic Resonance Imaging (MRI)**
Abdomen BW3Ø
Ankle
Left BQ3H
Right BQ3G
Aorta
Abdominal B43Ø
Thoracic B33Ø
Arm
Left BP3F
Right BP3E
Artery
Celiac B431
Cervico-Cerebral Arch B33Q
Common Carotid, Bilateral B335
Coronary
Bypass Graft, Multiple B233
Multiple B231
Internal Carotid, Bilateral B338
Intracranial B33R
Lower Extremity
Bilateral B43H
Left B43G
Right B43F
Pelvic B43C
Renal, Bilateral B438
Spinal B33M
Superior Mesenteric B434
Upper Extremity
Bilateral B33K
Left B33J
Right B33H
Vertebral, Bilateral B33G
Bladder BT3Ø
Brachial Plexus BW3P
Brain BØ3Ø
Breast
Bilateral BH32
Left BH31
Right BH3Ø
Calcaneus
Left BQ3K
Right BQ3J
Chest BW33Y
Coccyx BR3F
Connective Tissue
Lower Extremity BL31
Upper Extremity BL3Ø
Corpora Cavernosa BV3Ø
Disc
Cervical BR31
Lumbar BR33
Thoracic BR32
Ear B93Ø
Elbow
Left BP3H
Right BP3G
Eye
Bilateral B837
Left B836
Right B835
Femur
Left BQ34
Right BQ33
Fetal Abdomen BY33
Fetal Extremity BY35
Fetal Head BY3Ø
Fetal Heart BY31
Fetal Spine BY34
Fetal Thorax BY32
Fetus, Whole BY36
Foot
Left BQ3M
Right BQ3L
Forearm
Left BP3K
Right BP3J

**Magnetic Resonance Imaging (MRI)** — *continued*
Gland
Adrenal, Bilateral BG32
Parathyroid BG33
Parotid, Bilateral B936
Salivary, Bilateral B93D
Submandibular, Bilateral B939
Thyroid BG34
Head BW38
Heart, Right and Left B236
Hip
Left BQ31
Right BQ3Ø
Intracranial Sinus B532
Joint
Finger
Left BP3D
Right BP3C
Hand
Left BP3D
Right BP3C
Temporomandibular, Bilateral BN39
Kidney
Bilateral BT33
Left BT32
Right BT31
Transplant BT39
Knee
Left BQ38
Right BQ37
Larynx B93J
Leg
Left BQ3F
Right BQ3D
Liver BF35
Liver and Spleen BF36
Lung Apices BB3G
Nasopharynx B93F
Neck BW3F
Nerve
Acoustic BØ3C
Brachial Plexus BW3P
Oropharynx B93F
Ovary
Bilateral BU35
Left BU34
Right BU33
Ovary and Uterus BU3C
Pancreas BF37
Patella
Left BQ3W
Right BQ3V
Pelvic Region BW3G
Pelvis BR3C
Pituitary Gland BØ39
Plexus, Brachial BW3P
Prostate BV33
Retroperitoneum BW3H
Sacrum BR3F
Scrotum BV34
Sella Turcica BØ39
Shoulder
Left BP39
Right BP38
Sinus
Intracranial B532
Paranasal B932
Spinal Cord BØ3B
Spine
Cervical BR3Ø
Lumbar BR39
Thoracic BR37
Spleen and Liver BF36
Subcutaneous Tissue
Abdomen BH3H
Extremity
Lower BH3J
Upper BH3F
Head BH3D
Neck BH3D
Pelvis BH3H
Thorax BH3G
Tendon
Lower Extremity BL33
Upper Extremity BL32
Testicle
Bilateral BV37
Left BV36
Right BV35

**Magnetic Resonance Imaging (MRI)** — *continued*
Toe
Left BQ3Q
Right BQ3P
Uterus BU36
Pregnant BU3B
Uterus and Ovary BU3C
Vagina BU39
Vein
Cerebellar B531
Cerebral B531
Jugular, Bilateral B535
Lower Extremity
Bilateral B53D
Left B53C
Right B53B
Other B53V
Pelvic (Iliac) Bilateral B53H
Portal B53T
Pulmonary, Bilateral B53S
Renal, Bilateral B53L
Spanchnic B53T
Upper Extremity
Bilateral B53P
Left B53N
Right B53M
Vena Cava
Inferior B539
Superior B538
Wrist
Left BP3M
Right BP3L
**Magnetically Controlled Growth Rod(s)**
Cervical XNS3
Lumbar XNSØ
Thoracic XNS4
**Malleotomy** *see* Drainage, Ear, Nose, Sinus Ø99
**Malleus**
*use* Auditory Ossicle, Left
*use* Auditory Ossicle, Right
**Mammaplasty, mammoplasty**
*see* Alteration, Skin and Breast ØHØ
*see* Repair, Skin and Breast ØHQ
*see* Replacement, Skin and Breast ØHR
*see* Supplement, Skin and Breast ØHU
**Mammary duct**
*use* Breast, Bilateral
*use* Breast, Left
*use* Breast, Right
**Mammary gland**
*use* Breast, Bilateral
*use* Breast, Left
*use* Breast, Right
**Mammectomy**
*see* Excision, Skin and Breast ØHB
*see* Resection, Skin and Breast ØHT
**Mammillary body** *use* Hypothalamus
**Mammography** *see* Plain Radiography, Skin, Subcutaneous Tissue and Breast BHØ
**Mammotomy** *see* Drainage, Skin and Breast ØH9
**Mandibular nerve** *use* Nerve, Trigeminal
**Mandibular notch**
*use* Mandible, Left
*use* Mandible, Right
**Mandibulectomy**
*see* Excision, Head and Facial Bones ØNB
*see* Resection, Head and Facial Bones ØNT
**Manipulation**
Adhesions *see* Release
Chiropractic *see* Chiropractic Manipulation
**Manual removal, retained placenta** *see* Extraction, Products of Conception, Retained 1ØD1
**Manubrium** *use* Sternum
**Map**
Basal Ganglia ØØK8
Brain ØØKØ
Cerebellum ØØKC
Cerebral Hemisphere ØØK7
Conduction Mechanism Ø2K8
Hypothalamus ØØKA
Medulla Oblongata ØØKD
Pons ØØKB
Thalamus ØØK9
**Mapping**
Doppler ultrasound *see* Ultrasonography
Electrocardiogram only *see* Measurement, Cardiac 4AØ2

**Mark IV Breathing Pacemaker System** *use* Stimulator Generator in Subcutaneous Tissue and Fascia
**Marsupialization**
*see* Drainage
*see* Excision
**Massage, cardiac**
External 5A12012
Open Ø2QAØZZ
**Masseter muscle** *use* Muscle, Head
**Masseteric fascia** *use* Subcutaneous Tissue and Fascia, Face
**Mastectomy**
*see* Excision, Skin and Breast ØHB
*see* Resection, Skin and Breast ØHT
**Mastoid air cells**
*use* Sinus, Mastoid, Left
*use* Sinus, Mastoid, Right
**Mastoid (postauricular) lymph node**
*use* Lymphatic, Neck, Left
*use* Lymphatic, Neck, Right
**Mastoid process**
*use* Bone, Temporal, Left
*use* Bone, Temporal, Right
**Mastoidectomy**
*see* Excision, Ear, Nose, Sinus Ø9B
*see* Resection, Ear, Nose, Sinus Ø9T
**Mastoidotomy** *see* Drainage, Ear, Nose, Sinus Ø99
**Mastopexy**
*see* Repair, Skin and Breast ØHQ
*see* Reposition, Skin and Breast ØHS
**Mastorrhaphy** *see* Repair, Skin and Breast ØHQ
**Mastotomy** *see* Drainage, Skin and Breast ØH9
**Maxillary artery**
*use* Artery, External Carotid, Left
*use* Artery, External Carotid, Right
**Maxillary nerve** *use* Nerve, Trigeminal
**Maximo II DR (VR)** *use* Defibrillator Generator in ØJH
**Maximo II DR CRT-D** *use* Cardiac Resynchronization Defibrillator Pulse Generator in ØJH
**Measurement**
Arterial
Flow
Coronary 4AØ3
Peripheral 4AØ3
Pulmonary 4AØ3
Pressure
Coronary 4AØ3
Peripheral 4AØ3
Pulmonary 4AØ3
Thoracic, Other 4AØ3
Pulse
Coronary 4AØ3
Peripheral 4AØ3
Pulmonary 4AØ3
Saturation, Peripheral 4AØ3
Sound, Peripheral 4AØ3
Biliary
Flow 4AØC
Pressure 4AØC
Cardiac
Action Currents 4AØ2
Defibrillator 4BØ2XTZ
Electrical Activity 4AØ2
Guidance 4AØ2X4A
No Qualifier 4AØ2X4Z
Output 4AØ2
Pacemaker 4BØ2XSZ
Rate 4AØ2
Rhythm 4AØ2
Sampling and Pressure
Bilateral 4AØ2
Left Heart 4AØ2
Right Heart 4AØ2
Sound 4AØ2
Total Activity, Stress 4AØ2XM4
Central Nervous
Conductivity 4AØØ
Electrical Activity 4AØØ
Pressure 4AØØØBZ
Intracranial 4AØØ
Saturation, Intracranial 4AØØ
Stimulator 4BØØXVZ
Temperature, Intracranial 4AØØ
Circulatory, Volume 4AØ5XLZ
Gastrointestinal
Motility 4AØB
Pressure 4AØB
Secretion 4AØB
**Measurement** — *continued*
Lymphatic
Flow 4AØ6
Pressure 4AØ6
Metabolism 4AØZ
Musculoskeletal
Contractility 4AØF
Stimulator 4BØFXVZ
Olfactory, Acuity 4AØ8XØZ
Peripheral Nervous
Conductivity
Motor 4AØ1
Sensory 4AØ1
Electrical Activity 4AØ1
Stimulator 4BØ1XVZ
Products of Conception
Cardiac
Electrical Activity 4AØH
Rate 4AØH
Rhythm 4AØH
Sound 4AØH
Nervous
Conductivity 4AØJ
Electrical Activity 4AØJ
Pressure 4AØJ
Respiratory
Capacity 4AØ9
Flow 4AØ9
Pacemaker 4BØ9XSZ
Rate 4AØ9
Resistance 4AØ9
Total Activity 4AØ9
Volume 4AØ9
Sleep 4AØZXQZ
Temperature 4AØZ
Urinary
Contractility 4AØD
Flow 4AØD
Pressure 4AØD
Resistance 4AØD
Volume 4AØD
Venous
Flow
Central 4AØ4
Peripheral 4AØ4
Portal 4AØ4
Pulmonary 4AØ4
Pressure
Central 4AØ4
Peripheral 4AØ4
Portal 4AØ4
Pulmonary 4AØ4
Pulse
Central 4AØ4
Peripheral 4AØ4
Portal 4AØ4
Pulmonary 4AØ4
Saturation, Peripheral 4AØ4
Visual
Acuity 4AØ7XØZ
Mobility 4AØ7X7Z
Pressure 4AØ7XBZ
**Meatoplasty, urethra** *see* Repair, Urethra ØTQD
**Meatotomy** *see* Drainage, Urinary System ØT9
**Mechanical ventilation** *see* Performance, Respiratory 5A19
**Medial canthus**
*use* Eyelid, Lower, Left
*use* Eyelid, Lower, Right
**Medial collateral ligament (MCL)**
*use* Bursa and Ligament, Knee, Left
*use* Bursa and Ligament, Knee, Right
**Medial condyle of femur**
*use* Femur, Lower, Left
*use* Femur, Lower, Right
**Medial condyle of tibia**
*use* Tibia, Left
*use* Tibia, Right
**Medial cuneiform bone**
*use* Tarsal, Left
*use* Tarsal, Right
**Medial epicondyle of femur**
*use* Femur, Lower, Left
*use* Femur, Lower, Right
**Medial epicondyle of humerus**
*use* Humeral Shaft, Left
*use* Humeral Shaft, Right
**Medial malleolus**
*use* Tibia, Left
*use* Tibia, Right
**Medial meniscus**
*use* Joint, Knee, Left
*use* Joint, Knee, Right
**Medial plantar artery**
*use* Artery, Foot, Left
*use* Artery, Foot, Right
**Medial plantar nerve** *use* Nerve, Tibial
**Medial popliteal nerve** *use* Nerve, Tibial
**Medial rectus muscle**
*use* Muscle, Extraocular, Left
*use* Muscle, Extraocular, Right
**Medial sural cutaneous nerve** *use* Nerve, Tibial
**Median antebrachial vein**
*use* Vein, Basilic, Left
*use* Vein, Basilic, Right
**Median cubital vein**
*use* Vein, Basilic, Left
*use* Vein, Basilic, Right
**Median sacral artery** *use* Aorta, Abdominal
**Mediastinal lymph node** *use* Lymphatic, Thorax
**Mediastinoscopy** ØWJC4ZZ
**Medication Management** GZ3ZZZZ
for substance abuse
Antabuse HZ83ZZZ
Bupropion HZ87ZZZ
Clonidine HZ86ZZZ
Levo-alpha-acetyl-methadol (LAAM) HZ82ZZZ
Methadone Maintenance HZ81ZZZ
Naloxone HZ85ZZZ
Naltrexone HZ84ZZZ
Nicotine Replacement HZ8ØZZZ
Other Replacement Medication HZ89ZZZ
Psychiatric Medication HZ88ZZZ
**Meditation** 8EØZXY5
**Medtronic Endurant® II AAA stent graft system** *use* Intraluminal Device
**Meissner's (submucous) plexus** *use* Nerve, Abdominal Sympathetic
**Melody® transcatheter pulmonary valve** *use* Zooplastic Tissue in Heart and Great Vessels
**Membranous urethra** *use* Urethra
**Meningeorrhaphy**
*see* Repair, Cerebral Meninges ØØQ1
*see* Repair, Spinal Meninges ØØQT
**Meniscectomy, knee**
*see* Excision, Joint, Knee, Left ØSBD
*see* Excision, Joint, Knee, Right ØSBC
**Mental foramen**
*use* Mandible, Left
*use* Mandible, Right
**Mentalis muscle** *use* Muscle, Facial
**Mentoplasty** *see* Alteration, Jaw, Lower ØWØ5
**Mesenterectomy** *see* Excision, Mesentery ØDBV
**Mesenteriorrhaphy, mesenterorrhaphy** *see* Repair, Mesentery ØDQV
**Mesenteriplication** *see* Repair, Mesentery ØDQV
**Mesoappendix** *use* Mesentery
**Mesocolon** *use* Mesentery
**Metacarpal ligament**
*use* Bursa and Ligament, Hand, Left
*use* Bursa and Ligament, Hand, Right
**Metacarpophalangeal ligament**
*use* Bursa and Ligament, Hand, Left
*use* Bursa and Ligament, Hand, Right
**Metal on metal bearing surface** *use* Synthetic Substitute, Metal in ØSR
**Metatarsal ligament**
*use* Bursa and Ligament, Foot, Left
*use* Bursa and Ligament, Foot, Right
**Metatarsectomy**
*see* Excision, Lower Bones ØQB
*see* Resection, Lower Bones ØQT
**Metatarsophalangeal (MTP) joint**
*use* Joint, Metatarsal-Phalangeal, Left
*use* Joint, Metatarsal-Phalangeal, Right
**Metatarsophalangeal ligament**
*use* Bursa and Ligament, Foot, Left
*use* Bursa and Ligament, Foot, Right
**Metathalamus** *use* Thalamus
**Micro-Driver stent (RX) (OTW)** *use* Intraluminal Device
**MicroMed HeartAssist** *use* Implantable Heart Assist System in Heart and Great Vessels
**Micrus CERECYTE Microcoil** *use* Intraluminal Device, Bioactive in Upper Arteries





Subterms under main terms may continue to next column or page

**Midcarpal joint**
*use* Joint, Carpal, Left
*use* Joint, Carpal, Right
**Middle cardiac nerve** *use* Nerve, Thoracic Sympathetic
**Middle cerebral artery** *use* Artery, Intracranial
**Middle cerebral vein** *use* Vein, Intracranial
**Middle colic vein** *use* Vein, Colic
**Middle genicular artery**
*use* Artery, Popliteal, Left
*use* Artery, Popliteal, Right
**Middle hemorrhoidal vein**
*use* Vein, Hypogastric, Left
*use* Vein, Hypogastric, Right
**Middle rectal artery**
*use* Artery, Internal Iliac, Left
*use* Artery, Internal Iliac, Right
**Middle suprarenal artery** *use* Aorta, Abdominal
**Middle temporal artery**
*use* Artery, Temporal, Left
*use* Artery, Temporal, Right
**Middle turbinate** *use* Turbinate, Nasal
**MIRODERM™ Biologic Wound Matrix** *use* Skin Substitute, Porcine Liver Derived in New Technology
**MitraClip valve repair system** *use* Synthetic Substitute
**Mitral annulus** *use* Valve, Mitral
**Mitroflow® Aortic Pericardial Heart Valve** *use* Zooplastic Tissue in Heart and Great Vessels
**Mobilization, adhesions** *see* Release
**Molar gland** *use* Buccal Mucosa
**Monitoring**
Arterial
Flow
Coronary 4A13
Peripheral 4A13
Pulmonary 4A13
Pressure
Coronary 4A13
Peripheral 4A13
Pulmonary 4A13
Pulse
Coronary 4A13
Peripheral 4A13
Pulmonary 4A13
Saturation, Peripheral 4A13
Sound, Peripheral 4A13
Cardiac
Electrical Activity 4A12
Ambulatory 4A12X45
No Qualifier 4A12X4Z
Output 4A12
Rate 4A12
Rhythm 4A12
Sound 4A12
Total Activity, Stress 4A12XM4
Vascular Perfusion, Indocyanine Green Dye 4A12XSH
Central Nervous
Conductivity 4A10
Electrical Activity
Intraoperative 4A10
No Qualifier 4A10
Pressure 4A100BZ
Intracranial 4A10
Saturation, Intracranial 4A10
Temperature, Intracranial 4A10
Gastrointestinal
Motility 4A1B
Pressure 4A1B
Secretion 4A1B
Vascular Perfusion, Indocyanine Green Dye 4A1BXSH
Intraoperative Knee Replacement Sensor XR2
Lymphatic
Flow 4A16
Pressure 4A16
Peripheral Nervous
Conductivity
Motor 4A11
Sensory 4A11
Electrical Activity
Intraoperative 4A11
No Qualifier 4A11
Products of Conception
Cardiac
Electrical Activity 4A1H
Rate 4A1H
Rhythm 4A1H
Sound 4A1H

**Monitoring** — *continued*
Products of Conception — *continued*
Nervous
Conductivity 4A1J
Electrical Activity 4A1J
Pressure 4A1J
Respiratory
Capacity 4A19
Flow 4A19
Rate 4A19
Resistance 4A19
Volume 4A19
Skin and Breast, Vascular Perfusion, Indocyanine Green Dye 4A1GXSH
Sleep 4A1ZXQZ
Temperature 4A1Z
Urinary
Contractility 4A1D
Flow 4A1D
Pressure 4A1D
Resistance 4A1D
Volume 4A1D
Venous
Flow
Central 4A14
Peripheral 4A14
Portal 4A14
Pulmonary 4A14
Pressure
Central 4A14
Peripheral 4A14
Portal 4A14
Pulmonary 4A14
Pulse
Central 4A14
Peripheral 4A14
Portal 4A14
Pulmonary 4A14
Saturation
Central 4A14
Portal 4A14
Pulmonary 4A14
**Monitoring Device, Hemodynamic**
Abdomen 0JH8
Chest 0JH6
**Mosaic Bioprosthesis (aortic) (mitral) valve** *use* Zooplastic Tissue in Heart and Great Vessels
**Motor Function Assessment** F01
**Motor Treatment** F07
**MR Angiography**
*see* Magnetic Resonance Imaging (MRI), Heart B23
*see* Magnetic Resonance Imaging (MRI), Lower Arteries B43
*see* Magnetic Resonance Imaging (MRI), Upper Arteries B33
**MULTI-LINK (VISION) (MINI-VISION) (ULTRA) Coronary Stent System** *use* Intraluminal Device
**Multiple sleep latency test** 4A0ZXQZ
**Musculocutaneous nerve** *use* Nerve, Brachial Plexus
**Musculopexy**
*see* Repair, Muscles 0KQ
*see* Reposition, Muscles 0KS
**Musculophrenic artery**
*use* Artery, Internal Mammary, Left
*use* Artery, Internal Mammary, Right
**Musculoplasty**
*see* Repair, Muscles 0KQ
*see* Supplement, Muscles 0KU
**Musculorrhaphy** *see* Repair, Muscles 0KQ
**Musculospiral nerve** *use* Nerve, Radial
**Myectomy**
*see* Excision, Muscles 0KB
*see* Resection, Muscles 0KT
**Myelencephalon** *use* Medulla Oblongata
**Myelogram**
CT *see* Computerized Tomography (CT Scan), Central Nervous System B02
MRI *see* Magnetic Resonance Imaging (MRI), Central Nervous System B03
**Myenteric (Auerbach's) plexus** *use* Nerve, Abdominal Sympathetic
**Myocardial Bridge Release** *see* Release, Artery, Coronary
**Myomectomy** *see* Excision, Female Reproductive System 0UB
**Myometrium** *use* Uterus
**Myopexy**
*see* Repair, Muscles 0KQ
*see* Reposition, Muscles 0KS

**Myoplasty**
*see* Repair, Muscles 0KQ
*see* Supplement, Muscles 0KU
**Myorrhaphy** *see* Repair, Muscles 0KQ
**Myoscopy** *see* Inspection, Muscles 0KJ
**Myotomy**
*see* Division, Muscles 0K8
*see* Drainage, Muscles 0K9
**Myringectomy**
*see* Excision, Ear, Nose, Sinus 09B
*see* Resection, Ear, Nose, Sinus 09T
**Myringoplasty**
*see* Repair, Ear, Nose, Sinus 09Q
*see* Replacement, Ear, Nose, Sinus 09R
*see* Supplement, Ear, Nose, Sinus 09U
**Myringostomy** *see* Drainage, Ear, Nose, Sinus 099
**Myringotomy** *see* Drainage, Ear, Nose, Sinus 099

# N

**Nail bed**
*use* Finger Nail
*use* Toe Nail
**Nail plate**
*use* Finger Nail
*use* Toe Nail
**nanoLOCK™ interbody fusion device** *use* Interbody Fusion Device, Nanotextured Surface in New Technology
**Narcosynthesis** GZGZZZZ
**Nasal cavity** *use* Nasal Mucosa and Soft Tissue
**Nasal concha** *use* Turbinate, Nasal
**Nasalis muscle** *use* Muscle, Facial
**Nasolacrimal duct**
*use* Duct, Lacrimal, Left
*use* Duct, Lacrimal, Right
**Nasopharyngeal airway (NPA)** *use* Intraluminal Device, Airway in Ear, Nose, Sinus
**Navicular bone**
*use* Tarsal, Left
*use* Tarsal, Right
**Near Infrared Spectroscopy, Circulatory System** 8E023DZ
**Neck of femur**
*use* Femur, Upper, Left
*use* Femur, Upper, Right
**Neck of humerus (anatomical) (surgical)**
*use* Humeral Head, Left
*use* Humeral Head, Right
**Nephrectomy**
*see* Excision, Urinary System 0TB
*see* Resection, Urinary System 0TT
**Nephrolithotomy** *see* Extirpation, Urinary System 0TC
**Nephrolysis** *see* Release, Urinary System 0TN
**Nephropexy**
*see* Repair, Urinary System 0TQ
*see* Reposition, Urinary System 0TS
**Nephroplasty**
*see* Repair, Urinary System 0TQ
*see* Supplement, Urinary System 0TU
**Nephropyeloureterostomy**
*see* Bypass, Urinary System 0T1
*see* Drainage, Urinary System 0T9
**Nephrorrhaphy** *see* Repair, Urinary System 0TQ
**Nephroscopy, transurethral** 0TJ58ZZ
**Nephrostomy**
*see* Bypass, Urinary System 0T1
*see* Drainage, Urinary System 0T9
**Nephrotomography**
*see* Fluoroscopy, Urinary System BT1
*see* Plain Radiography, Urinary System BT0
**Nephrotomy**
*see* Division, Urinary System 0T8
*see* Drainage, Urinary System 0T9
**Nerve conduction study**
*see* Measurement, Central Nervous 4A00
*see* Measurement, Peripheral Nervous 4A01
**Nerve Function Assessment** F01
**Nerve to the stapedius** *use* Nerve, Facial
**Nesiritide** *use* Human B-Type Natriuretic Peptide
**Neurectomy**
*see* Excision, Central Nervous System and Cranial Nerves 00B
*see* Excision, Peripheral Nervous System 01B

**Neurexeresis**
*see* Extraction, Central Nervous System and Cranial Nerves ØØD
*see* Extraction, Peripheral Nervous System Ø1D
**Neurohypophysis** *use* Gland, Pituitary
**Neurolysis**
*see* Release, Central Nervous System and Cranial Nerves ØØN
*see* Release, Peripheral Nervous System Ø1N
**Neuromuscular electrical stimulation (NEMS) lead** *use* Stimulator Lead in Muscles
**Neurophysiologic monitoring** *see* Monitoring, Central Nervous 4A1Ø
**Neuroplasty**
*see* Repair, Central Nervous System and Cranial Nerves ØØQ
*see* Repair, Peripheral Nervous System Ø1Q
*see* Supplement, Central Nervous System and Cranial Nerves ØØU
*see* Supplement, Peripheral Nervous System Ø1U
**Neurorrhaphy**
*see* Repair, Central Nervous System and Cranial Nerves ØØQ
*see* Repair, Peripheral Nervous System Ø1Q
**Neurostimulator Generator**
Insertion of device in, Skull ØNHØØNZ
Removal of device from, Skull ØNPØØNZ
Revision of device in, Skull ØNWØØNZ
**Neurostimulator generator, multiple channel** *use* Stimulator Generator, Multiple Array in ØJH
**Neurostimulator generator, multiple channel rechargeable** *use* Stimulator Generator, Multiple Array Rechargeable in ØJH
**Neurostimulator generator, single channel** *use* Stimulator Generator, Single Array in ØJH
**Neurostimulator generator, single channel rechargeable** *use* Stimulator Generator, Single Array Rechargeable in ØJH
**Neurostimulator Lead**
Insertion of device in
Brain ØØHØ
Cerebral Ventricle ØØH6
Nerve
Cranial ØØHE
Peripheral Ø1HY
Spinal Canal ØØHU
Spinal Cord ØØHV
Vein
Azygos Ø5HØ
Innominate
Left Ø5H4
Right Ø5H3
Removal of device from
Brain ØØPØ
Cerebral Ventricle ØØP6
Nerve
Cranial ØØPE
Peripheral Ø1PY
Spinal Canal ØØPU
Spinal Cord ØØPV
Vein
Azygos Ø5PØ
Innominate
Left Ø5P4
Right Ø5P3
Revision of device in
Brain ØØWØ
Cerebral Ventricle ØØW6
Nerve
Cranial ØØWE
Peripheral Ø1WY
Spinal Canal ØØWU
Spinal Cord ØØWV
Vein
Azygos Ø5WØ
Innominate
Left Ø5W4
Right Ø5W3
**Neurotomy**
*see* Division, Central Nervous System and Cranial Nerves ØØ8
*see* Division, Peripheral Nervous System Ø18
**Neurotripsy**
*see* Destruction, Central Nervous System and Cranial Nerves ØØ5
*see* Destruction, Peripheral Nervous System Ø15
**Neutralization plate**
*use* Internal Fixation Device in Head and Facial Bones
**Neutralization plate** — *continued*
*use* Internal Fixation Device in Lower Bones
*use* Internal Fixation Device in Upper Bones
**New Technology**
Andexanet Alfa, Factor Xa Inhibitor Reversal Agent XWØ
Bezlotoxumab Monoclonal Antibody XWØ
Blinatumomab Antineoplastic Immunotherapy XWØ
Ceftazidime-Avibactam Anti-infective XWØ
Cerebral Embolic Filtration, Dual Filter X2A5312
Concentrated Bone Marrow Aspirate XKØ23Ø3
Cytarabine and Daunorubicin Liposome Antineoplastic XWØ
Defibrotide Sodium Anticoagulant XWØ
Endothelial Damage Inhibitor XYØVX83
Engineered Autologous Chimeric Antigen Receptor T-cell Immunotherapy XWØ
Fusion
Cervical Vertebral
2 or more
Nanotextured Surface XRG2Ø92
Radiolucent Porous XRG2ØF3
Interbody Fusion Device
Nanotextured Surface XRG1Ø92
Radiolucent Porous XRG1ØF3
Cervicothoracic Vertebral
Nanotextured Surface XRG4Ø92
Radiolucent Porous XRG4ØF3
Lumbar Vertebral
2 or more
Nanotextured Surface XRGCØ92
Radiolucent Porous XRGCØF3
Interbody Fusion Device
Nanotextured Surface XRGBØ92
Radiolucent Porous XRGBØF3
Lumbosacral
Nanotextured Surface XRGDØ92
Radiolucent Porous XRGDØF3
Occipital-cervical
Nanotextured Surface XRGØØ92
Radiolucent Porous XRGØØF3
Thoracic Vertebral
2 to 7
Nanotextured Surface XRG7Ø92
Radiolucent Porous XRG7ØF3
8 or more
Nanotextured Surface XRG8Ø92
Radiolucent Porous XRG8ØF3
Interbody Fusion Device
Nanotextured Surface XRG6Ø92
Radiolucent Porous XRG6ØF3
Thoracolumbar Vertebral
Nanotextured Surface XRGAØ92
Radiolucent Porous XRGAØF3
Idarucizumab, Dabigatran Reversal Agent XWØ
Intraoperative Knee Replacement Sensor XR2
Isavuconazole Anti-infective XWØ
Orbital Atherectomy Technology X2C
Other New Technology Therapeutic Substance XWØ
Replacement
Skin Substitute, Porcine Liver Derived XHRPXL2
Zooplastic Tissue, Rapid Deployment Technique X2RF
Reposition
Cervical, Magnetically Controlled Growth Rod(s) XNS3
Lumbar, Magnetically Controlled Growth Rod(s) XNSØ
Thoracic, Magnetically Controlled Growth Rod(s) XNS4
Uridine Triacetate XWØDX82
**Ninth cranial nerve** *use* Nerve, Glossopharyngeal
**Nitinol framed polymer mesh** *use* Synthetic Substitute
**Nonimaging Nuclear Medicine Assay**
Bladder, Kidneys and Ureters CT63
Blood C763
Kidneys, Ureters and Bladder CT63
Lymphatics and Hematologic System C76YYZZ
Ureters, Kidneys and Bladder CT63
Urinary System CT6YYZZ
**Nonimaging Nuclear Medicine Probe**
Abdomen CW5Ø
Abdomen and Chest CW54
Abdomen and Pelvis CW51
Brain CØ5Ø
Central Nervous System CØ5YYZZ
Chest CW53
Chest and Abdomen CW54
**Nonimaging Nuclear Medicine Probe** — *continued*
Chest and Neck CW56
Extremity
Lower CP5PZZZ
Upper CP5NZZZ
Head and Neck CW5B
Heart C25YYZZ
Right and Left C256
Lymphatics
Head C75J
Head and Neck C755
Lower Extremity C75P
Neck C75K
Pelvic C75D
Trunk C75M
Upper Chest C75L
Upper Extremity C75N
Lymphatics and Hematologic System C75YYZZ
Musculoskeletal System, Other CP5YYZZ
Neck and Chest CW56
Neck and Head CW5B
Pelvic Region CW5J
Pelvis and Abdomen CW51
Spine CP55ZZZ
**Nonimaging Nuclear Medicine Uptake**
Endocrine System CG4YYZZ
Gland, Thyroid CG42
**Non-tunneled central venous catheter** *use* Infusion Device
**Nostril** *use* Nasal Mucosa and Soft Tissue
**Novacor Left Ventricular Assist Device** *use* Implantable Heart Assist System in Heart and Great Vessels
**Novation® Ceramic AHS® (Articulation Hip System)** *use* Synthetic Substitute, Ceramic in ØSR
**Nuclear medicine**
*see* Nonimaging Nuclear Medicine Assay
*see* Nonimaging Nuclear Medicine Probe
*see* Nonimaging Nuclear Medicine Uptake
*see* Planar Nuclear Medicine Imaging
*see* Positron Emission Tomographic (PET) Imaging
*see* Systemic Nuclear Medicine Therapy
*see* Tomographic (Tomo) Nuclear Medicine Imaging
**Nuclear scintigraphy** *see* Nuclear Medicine
**Nutrition, concentrated substances**
Enteral infusion 3EØG36Z
Parenteral (peripheral) infusion *see* Introduction of Nutritional Substance

# O

**Obliteration** *see* Destruction
**Obturator artery**
*use* Artery, Internal Iliac, Left
*use* Artery, Internal Iliac, Right
**Obturator lymph node** *use* Lymphatic, Pelvis
**Obturator muscle**
*use* Muscle, Hip, Left
*use* Muscle, Hip, Right
**Obturator nerve** *use* Nerve, Lumbar Plexus
**Obturator vein**
*use* Vein, Hypogastric, Left
*use* Vein, Hypogastric, Right
**Obtuse margin** *use* Heart, Left
**Occipital artery**
*use* Artery, External Carotid, Left
*use* Artery, External Carotid, Right
**Occipital lobe** *use* Cerebral Hemisphere
**Occipital lymph node**
*use* Lymphatic, Neck, Left
*use* Lymphatic, Neck, Right
**Occipitofrontalis muscle** *use* Muscle, Facial
**Occlusion**
Ampulla of Vater ØFLC
Anus ØDLQ
Aorta
Abdominal Ø4LØ
Thoracic, Descending Ø2LW3DJ
Artery
Anterior Tibial
Left Ø4LQ
Right Ø4LP
Axillary
Left Ø3L6
Right Ø3L5
Brachial
Left Ø3L8

**Occlusion** — *continued*
Artery — *continued*
Brachial — *continued*
Right Ø3L7
Celiac Ø4L1
Colic
Left Ø4L7
Middle Ø4L8
Right Ø4L6
Common Carotid
Left Ø3LJ
Right Ø3LH
Common Iliac
Left Ø4LD
Right Ø4LC
External Carotid
Left Ø3LN
Right Ø3LM
External Iliac
Left Ø4LJ
Right Ø4LH
Face Ø3LR
Femoral
Left Ø4LL
Right Ø4LK
Foot
Left Ø4LW
Right Ø4LV
Gastric Ø4L2
Hand
Left Ø3LF
Right Ø3LD
Hepatic Ø4L3
Inferior Mesenteric Ø4LB
Innominate Ø3L2
Internal Carotid
Left Ø3LL
Right Ø3LK
Internal Iliac
Left Ø4LF
Right Ø4LE
Internal Mammary
Left Ø3L1
Right Ø3LØ
Intracranial Ø3LG
Lower Ø4LY
Peroneal
Left Ø4LU
Right Ø4LT
Popliteal
Left Ø4LN
Right Ø4LM
Posterior Tibial
Left Ø4LS
Right Ø4LR
Pulmonary
Left Ø2LR
Right Ø2LQ
Pulmonary Trunk Ø2LP
Radial
Left Ø3LC
Right Ø3LB
Renal
Left Ø4LA
Right Ø4L9
Splenic Ø4L4
Subclavian
Left Ø3L4
Right Ø3L3
Superior Mesenteric Ø4L5
Temporal
Left Ø3LT
Right Ø3LS
Thyroid
Left Ø3LV
Right Ø3LU
Ulnar
Left Ø3LA
Right Ø3L9
Upper Ø3LY
Vertebral
Left Ø3LQ
Right Ø3LP
Atrium, Left Ø2L7
Bladder ØTLB
Bladder Neck ØTLC
Bronchus
Lingula ØBL9

**Occlusion** — *continued*
Bronchus — *continued*
Lower Lobe
Left ØBLB
Right ØBL6
Main
Left ØBL7
Right ØBL3
Middle Lobe, Right ØBL5
Upper Lobe
Left ØBL8
Right ØBL4
Carina ØBL2
Cecum ØDLH
Cisterna Chyli Ø7LL
Colon
Ascending ØDLK
Descending ØDLM
Sigmoid ØDLN
Transverse ØDLL
Cord
Bilateral ØVLH
Left ØVLG
Right ØVLF
Cul-de-sac ØULF
Duct
Common Bile ØFL9
Cystic ØFL8
Hepatic
Common ØFL7
Left ØFL6
Right ØFL5
Lacrimal
Left Ø8LY
Right Ø8LX
Pancreatic ØFLD
Accessory ØFLF
Parotid
Left ØCLC
Right ØCLB
Duodenum ØDL9
Esophagogastric Junction ØDL4
Esophagus ØDL5
Lower ØDL3
Middle ØDL2
Upper ØDL1
Fallopian Tube
Left ØUL6
Right ØUL5
Fallopian Tubes, Bilateral ØUL7
Ileocecal Valve ØDLC
Ileum ØDLB
Intestine
Large ØDLE
Left ØDLG
Right ØDLF
Small ØDL8
Jejunum ØDLA
Kidney Pelvis
Left ØTL4
Right ØTL3
Left atrial appendage (LAA) *see* Occlusion, Atrium, Left Ø2L7
Lymphatic
Aortic Ø7LD
Axillary
Left Ø7L6
Right Ø7L5
Head Ø7LØ
Inguinal
Left Ø7LJ
Right Ø7LH
Internal Mammary
Left Ø7L9
Right Ø7L8
Lower Extremity
Left Ø7LG
Right Ø7LF
Mesenteric Ø7LB
Neck
Left Ø7L2
Right Ø7L1
Pelvis Ø7LC
Thoracic Duct Ø7LK
Thorax Ø7L7
Upper Extremity
Left Ø7L4
Right Ø7L3
Rectum ØDLP

**Occlusion** — *continued*
Stomach ØDL6
Pylorus ØDL7
Trachea ØBL1
Ureter
Left ØTL7
Right ØTL6
Urethra ØTLD
Vagina ØULG
Valve, Pulmonary Ø2LH
Vas Deferens
Bilateral ØVLQ
Left ØVLP
Right ØVLN
Vein
Axillary
Left Ø5L8
Right Ø5L7
Azygos Ø5LØ
Basilic
Left Ø5LC
Right Ø5LB
Brachial
Left Ø5LA
Right Ø5L9
Cephalic
Left Ø5LF
Right Ø5LD
Colic Ø6L7
Common Iliac
Left Ø6LD
Right Ø6LC
Esophageal Ø6L3
External Iliac
Left Ø6LG
Right Ø6LF
External Jugular
Left Ø5LQ
Right Ø5LP
Face
Left Ø5LV
Right Ø5LT
Femoral
Left Ø6LN
Right Ø6LM
Foot
Left Ø6LV
Right Ø6LT
Gastric Ø6L2
Hand
Left Ø5LH
Right Ø5LG
Hemiazygos Ø5L1
Hepatic Ø6L4
Hypogastric
Left Ø6LJ
Right Ø6LH
Inferior Mesenteric Ø6L6
Innominate
Left Ø5L4
Right Ø5L3
Internal Jugular
Left Ø5LN
Right Ø5LM
Intracranial Ø5LL
Lower Ø6LY
Portal Ø6L8
Pulmonary
Left Ø2LT
Right Ø2LS
Renal
Left Ø6LB
Right Ø6L9
Saphenous
Left Ø6LQ
Right Ø6LP
Splenic Ø6L1
Subclavian
Left Ø5L6
Right Ø5L5
Superior Mesenteric Ø6L5
Upper Ø5LY
Vertebral
Left Ø5LS
Right Ø5LR
Vena Cava
Inferior Ø6LØ
Superior Ø2LV

**Occlusion, REBOA (resuscitative endovascular balloon occlusion of the aorta)**
02LW3DJ
04L03DJ
**Occupational therapy** *see* Activities of Daily Living Treatment, Rehabilitation F08
**Odentectomy**
*see* Excision, Mouth and Throat 0CB
*see* Resection, Mouth and Throat 0CT
**Odontoid process** *use* Cervical Vertebra
**Olecranon bursa**
*use* Bursa and Ligament, Elbow, Left
*use* Bursa and Ligament, Elbow, Right
**Olecranon process**
*use* Ulna, Left
*use* Ulna, Right
**Olfactory bulb** *use* Nerve, Olfactory
**Omentectomy, omentumectomy**
*see* Excision, Gastrointestinal System 0DB
*see* Resection, Gastrointestinal System 0DT
**Omentofixation** *see* Repair, Gastrointestinal System 0DQ
**Omentoplasty**
*see* Repair, Gastrointestinal System 0DQ
*see* Replacement, Gastrointestinal System 0DR
*see* Supplement, Gastrointestinal System 0DU
**Omentorrhaphy** *see* Repair, Gastrointestinal System 0DQ
**Omentotomy** *see* Drainage, Gastrointestinal System 0D9
**Omnilink Elite Vascular Balloon Expandable Stent System** *use* Intraluminal Device
**Onychectomy**
*see* Excision, Skin and Breast 0HB
*see* Resection, Skin and Breast 0HT
**Onychoplasty**
*see* Repair, Skin and Breast 0HQ
*see* Replacement, Skin and Breast 0HR
**Onychotomy** *see* Drainage, Skin and Breast 0H9
**Oophorectomy**
*see* Excision, Female Reproductive System 0UB
*see* Resection, Female Reproductive System 0UT
**Oophoropexy**
*see* Repair, Female Reproductive System 0UQ
*see* Reposition, Female Reproductive System 0US
**Oophoroplasty**
*see* Repair, Female Reproductive System 0UQ
*see* Supplement, Female Reproductive System 0UU
**Oophororrhaphy** *see* Repair, Female Reproductive System 0UQ
**Oophorostomy** *see* Drainage, Female Reproductive System 0U9
**Oophorotomy**
*see* Division, Female Reproductive System 0U8
*see* Drainage, Female Reproductive System 0U9
**Oophorrhaphy** *see* Repair, Female Reproductive System 0UQ
**Open Pivot Aortic Valve Graft (AVG)** *use* Synthetic Substitute
**Open Pivot (mechanical) Valve** *use* Synthetic Substitute
**Ophthalmic artery** *use* Intracranial Artery
**Ophthalmic nerve** *use* Nerve, Trigeminal
**Ophthalmic vein** *use* Vein, Intracranial
**Opponensplasty**
Tendon replacement *see* Replacement, Tendons 0LR
Tendon transfer *see* Transfer, Tendons 0LX
**Optic chiasma** *use* Nerve, Optic
**Optic disc**
*use* Retina, Left
*use* Retina, Right
**Optic foramen** *use* Sphenoid Bone
**Optical coherence tomography, intravascular** *see* Computerized Tomography (CT Scan)
**Optimizer™ III implantable pulse generator** *use* Contractility Modulation Device in 0JH
**Orbicularis oculi muscle**
*use* Eyelid, Upper, Left
*use* Eyelid, Upper, Right
**Orbicularis oris muscle** *use* Muscle, Facial
**Orbital Atherectomy Technology** X2C
**Orbital fascia** *use* Subcutaneous Tissue and Fascia, Face
**Orbital portion of ethmoid bone**
*use* Orbit, Left
*use* Orbit, Right
**Orbital portion of frontal bone**
*use* Orbit, Left
*use* Orbit, Right
**Orbital portion of lacrimal bone**
*use* Orbit, Left
**Orbital portion of lacrimal bone** — *continued*
*use* Orbit, Right
**Orbital portion of maxilla**
*use* Orbit, Left
*use* Orbit, Right
**Orbital portion of palatine bone**
*use* Orbit, Left
*use* Orbit, Right
**Orbital portion of sphenoid bone**
*use* Orbit, Left
*use* Orbit, Right
**Orbital portion of zygomatic bone**
*use* Orbit, Left
*use* Orbit, Right
**Orchectomy, orchidectomy, orchiectomy**
*see* Excision, Male Reproductive System 0VB
*see* Resection, Male Reproductive System 0VT
**Orchidoplasty, orchioplasty**
*see* Repair, Male Reproductive System 0VQ
*see* Replacement, Male Reproductive System 0VR
*see* Supplement, Male Reproductive System 0VU
**Orchidorrhaphy, orchiorrhaphy** *see* Repair, Male Reproductive System 0VQ
**Orchidotomy, orchiotomy, orchotomy** *see* Drainage, Male Reproductive System 0V9
**Orchiopexy**
*see* Repair, Male Reproductive System 0VQ
*see* Reposition, Male Reproductive System 0VS
**Oropharyngeal airway (OPA)** *use* Intraluminal Device, Airway in Mouth and Throat
**Oropharynx** *use* Pharynx
**Ossiculectomy**
*see* Excision, Ear, Nose, Sinus 09B
*see* Resection, Ear, Nose, Sinus 09T
**Ossiculotomy** *see* Drainage, Ear, Nose, Sinus 099
**Ostectomy**
*see* Excision, Head and Facial Bones 0NB
*see* Excision, Lower Bones 0QB
*see* Excision, Upper Bones 0PB
*see* Resection, Head and Facial Bones 0NT
*see* Resection, Lower Bones 0QT
*see* Resection, Upper Bones 0PT
**Osteoclasis**
*see* Division, Head and Facial Bones 0N8
*see* Division, Lower Bones 0Q8
*see* Division, Upper Bones 0P8
**Osteolysis**
*see* Release, Head and Facial Bones 0NN
*see* Release, Lower Bones 0QN
*see* Release, Upper Bones 0PN
**Osteopathic Treatment**
Abdomen 7W09X
Cervical 7W01X
Extremity
Lower 7W06X
Upper 7W07X
Head 7W00X
Lumbar 7W03X
Pelvis 7W05X
Rib Cage 7W08X
Sacrum 7W04X
Thoracic 7W02X
**Osteopexy**
*see* Repair, Head and Facial Bones 0NQ
*see* Repair, Lower Bones 0QQ
*see* Repair, Upper Bones 0PQ
*see* Reposition, Head and Facial Bones 0NS
*see* Reposition, Lower Bones 0QS
*see* Reposition, Upper Bones 0PS
**Osteoplasty**
*see* Repair, Head and Facial Bones 0NQ
*see* Repair, Lower Bones 0QQ
*see* Repair, Upper Bones 0PQ
*see* Replacement, Head and Facial Bones 0NR
*see* Replacement, Lower Bones 0QR
*see* Replacement, Upper Bones 0PR
*see* Supplement, Head and Facial Bones 0NU
*see* Supplement, Lower Bones 0QU
*see* Supplement, Upper Bones 0PU
**Osteorrhaphy**
*see* Repair, Head and Facial Bones 0NQ
*see* Repair, Lower Bones 0QQ
*see* Repair, Upper Bones 0PQ
**Osteotomy, ostotomy**
*see* Division, Head and Facial Bones 0N8
*see* Division, Lower Bones 0Q8
**Osteotomy, ostotomy** — *continued*
*see* Division, Upper Bones 0P8
*see* Drainage, Head and Facial Bones 0N9
*see* Drainage, Lower Bones 0Q9
*see* Drainage, Upper Bones 0P9
**Otic ganglion** *use* Nerve, Head and Neck Sympathetic
**Otoplasty**
*see* Repair, Ear, Nose, Sinus 09Q
*see* Replacement, Ear, Nose, Sinus 09R
*see* Supplement, Ear, Nose, Sinus 09U
**Otoscopy** *see* Inspection, Ear, Nose, Sinus 09J
**Oval window**
*use* Ear, Middle, Left
*use* Ear, Middle, Right
**Ovarian artery** *use* Aorta, Abdominal
**Ovarian ligament** *use* Uterine Supporting Structure
**Ovariectomy**
*see* Excision, Female Reproductive System 0UB
*see* Resection, Female Reproductive System 0UT
**Ovariocentesis** *see* Drainage, Female Reproductive System 0U9
**Ovariopexy**
*see* Repair, Female Reproductive System 0UQ
*see* Reposition, Female Reproductive System 0US
**Ovariotomy**
*see* Division, Female Reproductive System 0U8
*see* Drainage, Female Reproductive System 0U9
**Ovatio™ CRT-D** *use* Cardiac Resynchronization Defibrillator Pulse Generator in 0JH
**Oversewing**
Gastrointestinal ulcer *see* Repair, Gastrointestinal System 0DQ
Pleural bleb *see* Repair, Respiratory System 0BQ
**Oviduct**
*use* Fallopian Tube, Left
*use* Fallopian Tube, Right
**Oximetry, Fetal pulse** 10H073Z
**OXINIUM** *use* Synthetic Substitute, Oxidized Zirconium on Polyethylene in 0SR
**Oxygenation**
Extracorporeal membrane (ECMO) *see* Performance, Circulatory 5A15
Hyperbaric *see* Assistance, Circulatory 5A05
Supersaturated *see* Assistance, Circulatory 5A05

# P

**Pacemaker**
Dual Chamber
Abdomen 0JH8
Chest 0JH6
Intracardiac
Insertion of device in
Atrium
Left 02H7
Right 02H6
Vein, Coronary 02H4
Ventricle
Left 02HL
Right 02HK
Removal of device from, Heart 02PA
Revision of device in, Heart 02WA
Single Chamber
Abdomen 0JH8
Chest 0JH6
Single Chamber Rate Responsive
Abdomen 0JH8
Chest 0JH6
**Packing**
Abdominal Wall 2W43X5Z
Anorectal 2Y43X5Z
Arm
Lower
Left 2W4DX5Z
Right 2W4CX5Z
Upper
Left 2W4BX5Z
Right 2W4AX5Z
Back 2W45X5Z
Chest Wall 2W44X5Z
Ear 2Y42X5Z
Extremity
Lower
Left 2W4MX5Z
Right 2W4LX5Z
Upper
Left 2W49X5Z

**Packing** — *continued*
Extremity — *continued*
Upper — *continued*
Right 2W48X5Z
Face 2W41X5Z
Finger
Left 2W4KX5Z
Right 2W4JX5Z
Foot
Left 2W4TX5Z
Right 2W4SX5Z
Genital Tract, Female 2Y44X5Z
Hand
Left 2W4FX5Z
Right 2W4EX5Z
Head 2W40X5Z
Inguinal Region
Left 2W47X5Z
Right 2W46X5Z
Leg
Lower
Left 2W4RX5Z
Right 2W4QX5Z
Upper
Left 2W4PX5Z
Right 2W4NX5Z
Mouth and Pharynx 2Y40X5Z
Nasal 2Y41X5Z
Neck 2W42X5Z
Thumb
Left 2W4HX5Z
Right 2W4GX5Z
Toe
Left 2W4VX5Z
Right 2W4UX5Z
Urethra 2Y45X5Z
**Paclitaxel-eluting coronary stent** *use* Intraluminal Device, Drug-eluting in Heart and Great Vessels
**Paclitaxel-eluting peripheral stent**
*use* Intraluminal Device, Drug-eluting in Lower Arteries
*use* Intraluminal Device, Drug-eluting in Upper Arteries
**Palatine gland** *use* Buccal Mucosa
**Palatine tonsil** *use* Tonsils
**Palatine uvula** *use* Uvula
**Palatoglossal muscle** *use* Muscle, Tongue, Palate, Pharynx
**Palatopharyngeal muscle** *use* Muscle, Tongue, Palate, Pharynx
**Palatoplasty**
*see* Repair, Mouth and Throat 0CQ
*see* Replacement, Mouth and Throat 0CR
*see* Supplement, Mouth and Throat 0CU
**Palatorrhaphy** *see* Repair, Mouth and Throat 0CQ
**Palmar cutaneous nerve**
*use* Nerve, Median
*use* Nerve, Radial
**Palmar (volar) digital vein**
*use* Vein, Hand, Left
*use* Vein, Hand, Right
**Palmar fascia (aponeurosis)**
*use* Subcutaneous Tissue and Fascia, Hand, Left
*use* Subcutaneous Tissue and Fascia, Hand, Right
**Palmar interosseous muscle**
*use* Muscle, Hand, Left
*use* Muscle, Hand, Right
**Palmar (volar) metacarpal vein**
*use* Vein, Hand, Left
*use* Vein, Hand, Right
**Palmar ulnocarpal ligament**
*use* Bursa and Ligament, Wrist, Left
*use* Bursa and Ligament, Wrist, Right
**Palmaris longus muscle**
*use* Muscle, Lower Arm and Wrist, Left
*use* Muscle, Lower Arm and Wrist, Right
**Pancreatectomy**
*see* Excision, Pancreas 0FBG
*see* Resection, Pancreas 0FTG
**Pancreatic artery** *use* Artery, Splenic
**Pancreatic plexus** *use* Nerve, Abdominal Sympathetic
**Pancreatic vein** *use* Vein, Splenic
**Pancreaticoduodenostomy** *see* Bypass, Hepatobiliary System and Pancreas 0F1
**Pancreaticosplenic lymph node** *use* Lymphatic, Aortic
**Pancreatogram, endoscopic retrograde** *see* Fluoroscopy, Pancreatic Duct BF18
**Pancreatolithotomy** *see* Extirpation, Pancreas 0FCG
**Pancreatotomy**
*see* Division, Pancreas 0F8G
*see* Drainage, Pancreas 0F9G
**Panniculectomy**
*see* Excision, Abdominal Wall 0WBF
*see* Excision, Skin, Abdomen 0HB7
**Paraaortic lymph node** *use* Lymphatic, Aortic
**Paracentesis**
Eye *see* Drainage, Eye 089
Peritoneal Cavity *see* Drainage, Peritoneal Cavity 0W9G
Tympanum *see* Drainage, Ear, Nose, Sinus 099
**Pararectal lymph node** *use* Lymphatic, Mesenteric
**Parasternal lymph node** *use* Lymphatic, Thorax
**Parathyroidectomy**
*see* Excision, Endocrine System 0GB
*see* Resection, Endocrine System 0GT
**Paratracheal lymph node** *use* Lymphatic, Thorax
**Paraurethral (Skene's) gland** *use* Gland, Vestibular
**Parenteral nutrition, total** *see* Introduction of Nutritional Substance
**Parietal lobe** *use* Cerebral Hemisphere
**Parotid lymph node** *use* Lymphatic, Head
**Parotid plexus** *use* Nerve, Facial
**Parotidectomy**
*see* Excision, Mouth and Throat 0CB
*see* Resection, Mouth and Throat 0CT
**Pars flaccida**
*use* Tympanic Membrane, Left
*use* Tympanic Membrane, Right
**Partial joint replacement**
Hip *see* Replacement, Lower Joints 0SR
Knee *see* Replacement, Lower Joints 0SR
Shoulder *see* Replacement, Upper Joints 0RR
**Partially absorbable mesh** *use* Synthetic Substitute
**Patch, blood, spinal** 3E0S3GC
**Patellapexy**
*see* Repair, Lower Bones 0QQ
*see* Reposition, Lower Bones 0QS
**Patellaplasty**
*see* Repair, Lower Bones 0QQ
*see* Replacement, Lower Bones 0QR
*see* Supplement, Lower Bones 0QU
**Patellar ligament**
*use* Bursa and Ligament, Knee, Left
*use* Bursa and Ligament, Knee, Right
**Patellar tendon**
*use* Tendon, Knee, Left
*use* Tendon, Knee, Right
**Patellectomy**
*see* Excision, Lower Bones 0QB
*see* Resection, Lower Bones 0QT
**Patellofemoral joint**
*use* Joint, Knee, Left
*use* Joint, Knee, Left, Femoral Surface
*use* Joint, Knee, Right
*use* Joint, Knee, Right, Femoral Surface
**Pectineus muscle**
*use* Muscle, Upper Leg, Left
*use* Muscle, Upper Leg, Right
**Pectoral fascia** *use* Subcutaneous Tissue and Fascia, Chest
**Pectoral (anterior) lymph node**
*use* Lymphatic, Axillary, Left
*use* Lymphatic, Axillary, Right
**Pectoralis major muscle**
*use* Muscle, Thorax, Left
*use* Muscle, Thorax, Right
**Pectoralis minor muscle**
*use* Muscle, Thorax, Left
*use* Muscle, Thorax, Right
**Pedicle-based dynamic stabilization device**
*use* Spinal Stabilization Device, Pedicle-Based in 0SH
*use* Spinal Stabilization Device, Pedicle-Based in 0RH
**PEEP (positive end expiratory pressure)** *see* Assistance, Respiratory 5A09
**PEG (percutaneous endoscopic gastrostomy)** 0DH63UZ
**PEJ (percutaneous endoscopic jejunostomy)** 0DHA3UZ
**Pelvic splanchnic nerve**
*use* Nerve, Abdominal Sympathetic
*use* Nerve, Sacral Sympathetic
**Penectomy**
*see* Excision, Male Reproductive System 0VB
*see* Resection, Male Reproductive System 0VT
**Penile urethra** *use* Urethra
**Perceval sutureless valve** *use* Zooplastic Tissue, Rapid Deployment Technique in New Technology
**Percutaneous endoscopic gastrojejunostomy (PEG/J) tube** *use* Feeding Device in Gastrointestinal System
**Percutaneous endoscopic gastrostomy (PEG) tube** *use* Feeding Device in Gastrointestinal System
**Percutaneous nephrostomy catheter** *use* Drainage Device
**Percutaneous transluminal coronary angioplasty (PTCA)** *see* Dilation, Heart and Great Vessels 027
**Performance**
Biliary
Multiple, Filtration 5A1C60Z
Single, Filtration 5A1C00Z
Cardiac
Continuous
Output 5A1221Z
Pacing 5A1223Z
Intermittent, Pacing 5A1213Z
Single, Output, Manual 5A12012
Circulatory, Continuous, Oxygenation, Membrane 5A15223
Respiratory
24-96 Consecutive Hours, Ventilation 5A1945Z
Greater than 96 Consecutive Hours, Ventilation 5A1955Z
Less than 24 Consecutive Hours, Ventilation 5A1935Z
Single, Ventilation, Nonmechanical 5A19054
Urinary
Continuous, Greater than 18 hours per day, Filtration 5A1D90Z
Intermittent, Less than 6 Hours Per Day, Filtration 5A1D70Z
Prolonged Intermittent, 6-18 hours per day, Filtration 5A1D80Z
**Perfusion** *see* Introduction of substance in or on
**Perfusion, donor organ**
Heart 6AB50BZ
Kidney(s) 6ABT0BZ
Liver 6ABF0BZ
Lung(s) 6ABB0BZ
**Pericardiectomy**
*see* Excision, Pericardium 02BN
*see* Resection, Pericardium 02TN
**Pericardiocentesis** *see* Drainage, Pericardial Cavity 0W9D
**Pericardiolysis** *see* Release, Pericardium 02NN
**Pericardiophrenic artery**
*use* Artery, Internal Mammary, Left
*use* Artery, Internal Mammary, Right
**Pericardioplasty**
*see* Repair, Pericardium 02QN
*see* Replacement, Pericardium 02RN
*see* Supplement, Pericardium 02UN
**Pericardiorrhaphy** *see* Repair, Pericardium 02QN
**Pericardiostomy** *see* Drainage, Pericardial Cavity 0W9D
**Pericardiotomy** *see* Drainage, Pericardial Cavity 0W9D
**Perimetrium** *use* Uterus
**Peripheral parenteral nutrition** *see* Introduction of Nutritional Substance
**Peripherally inserted central catheter (PICC)** *use* Infusion Device
**Peritoneal dialysis** 3E1M39Z
**Peritoneocentesis**
*see* Drainage, Peritoneal Cavity 0W9G
*see* Drainage, Peritoneum 0D9W
**Peritoneoplasty**
*see* Repair, Peritoneum 0DQW
*see* Replacement, Peritoneum 0DRW
*see* Supplement, Peritoneum 0DUW
**Peritoneoscopy** 0DJW4ZZ
**Peritoneotomy** *see* Drainage, Peritoneum 0D9W
**Peritoneumectomy** *see* Excision, Peritoneum 0DBW
**Peroneus brevis muscle**
*use* Muscle, Lower Leg, Left
*use* Muscle, Lower Leg, Right
**Peroneus longus muscle**
*use* Muscle, Lower Leg, Left
*use* Muscle, Lower Leg, Right
**Pessary ring** *use* Intraluminal Device, Pessary in Female Reproductive System
**PET scan** *see* Positron Emission Tomographic (PET) Imaging
**Petrous part of temporal bone**
*use* Bone, Temporal, Left
*use* Bone, Temporal, Right

**Phacoemulsification, lens**
With IOL implant *see* Replacement, Eye Ø8R
Without IOL implant *see* Extraction, Eye Ø8D
**Phalangectomy**
*see* Excision, Lower Bones ØQB
*see* Excision, Upper Bones ØPB
*see* Resection, Lower Bones ØQT
*see* Resection, Upper Bones ØPT
**Phallectomy**
*see* Excision, Penis ØVBS
*see* Resection, Penis ØVTS
**Phalloplasty**
*see* Repair, Penis ØVQS
*see* Supplement, Penis ØVUS
**Phallotomy** *see* Drainage, Penis ØV9S
**Pharmacotherapy, for substance abuse**
Antabuse HZ93ZZZ
Bupropion HZ97ZZZ
Clonidine HZ96ZZZ
Levo-alpha-acetyl-methadol (LAAM) HZ92ZZZ
Methadone Maintenance HZ91ZZZ
Naloxone HZ95ZZZ
Naltrexone HZ94ZZZ
Nicotine Replacement HZ90ZZZ
Psychiatric Medication HZ98ZZZ
Replacement Medication, Other HZ99ZZZ
**Pharyngeal constrictor muscle** *use* Muscle, Tongue, Palate, Pharynx
**Pharyngeal plexus** *use* Nerve, Vagus
**Pharyngeal recess** *use* Nasopharynx
**Pharyngeal tonsil** *use* Adenoids
**Pharyngogram** *see* Fluoroscopy, Pharynix B91G
**Pharyngoplasty**
*see* Repair, Mouth and Throat ØCQ
*see* Replacement, Mouth and Throat ØCR
*see* Supplement, Mouth and Throat ØCU
**Pharyngorrhaphy** *see* Repair, Mouth and Throat ØCQ
**Pharyngotomy** *see* Drainage, Mouth and Throat ØC9
**Pharyngotympanic tube**
*use* Eustachian Tube, Left
*use* Eustachian Tube, Right
**Pheresis**
Erythrocytes 6A55
Leukocytes 6A55
Plasma 6A55
Platelets 6A55
Stem Cells
Cord Blood 6A55
Hematopoietic 6A55
**Phlebectomy**
*see* Excision, Lower Veins Ø6B
*see* Excision, Upper Veins Ø5B
*see* Extraction, Lower Veins Ø6D
*see* Extraction, Upper Veins Ø5D
**Phlebography**
*see* Plain Radiography, Veins B5Ø
Impedance 4AØ4X51
**Phleborrhaphy**
*see* Repair, Lower Veins Ø6Q
*see* Repair, Upper Veins Ø5Q
**Phlebotomy**
*see* Drainage, Lower Veins Ø69
*see* Drainage, Upper Veins Ø59
**Photocoagulation**
for Destruction *see* Destruction
for Repair *see* Repair
**Photopheresis, therapeutic** *see* Phototherapy, Circulatory 6A65
**Phototherapy**
Circulatory 6A65
Skin 6A6Ø
Ultraviolet light *see* Ultraviolet Light Therapy, Physiological Systems 6A8
**Phrenectomy, phrenoneurectomy** *see* Excision, Nerve, Phrenic Ø1B2
**Phrenemphraxis** *see* Destruction, Nerve, Phrenic Ø152
**Phrenic nerve stimulator generator** *use* Stimulator Generator in Subcutaneous Tissue and Fascia
**Phrenic nerve stimulator lead** *use* Diaphragmatic Pacemaker Lead in Respiratory System
**Phreniclasis** *see* Destruction, Nerve, Phrenic Ø152
**Phrenicoexeresis** *see* Extraction, Nerve, Phrenic Ø1D2
**Phrenicotomy** *see* Division, Nerve, Phrenic Ø182
**Phrenicotripsy** *see* Destruction, Nerve, Phrenic Ø152
**Phrenoplasty**
*see* Repair, Respiratory System ØBQ
*see* Supplement, Respiratory System ØBU
**Phrenotomy** *see* Drainage, Respiratory System ØB9
**Physiatry** *see* Motor Treatment, Rehabilitation FØ7
**Physical medicine** *see* Motor Treatment, Rehabilitation FØ7
**Physical therapy** *see* Motor Treatment, Rehabilitation FØ7
**PHYSIOMESH™ Flexible Composite Mesh** *use* Synthetic Substitute
**Pia mater, intracranial** *use* Cerebral Meninges
**Pia mater, spinal** *use* Spinal Meninges
**Pinealectomy**
*see* Excision, Pineal Body ØGB1
*see* Resection, Pineal Body ØGT1
**Pinealoscopy** ØGJ14ZZ
**Pinealotomy** *see* Drainage, Pineal Body ØG91
**Pinna**
*use* Ear, External, Bilateral
*use* Ear, External, Left
*use* Ear, External, Right
**Pipeline™ Embolization device (PED)** *use* Intraluminal Device
**Piriform recess (sinus)** *use* Pharynx
**Piriformis muscle**
*use* Muscle, Hip, Left
*use* Muscle, Hip, Right
**PIRRT (Prolonged intermittent renal replacement therapy)** 5A1D8ØZ
**Pisiform bone**
*use* Carpal, Left
*use* Carpal, Right
**Pisohamate ligament**
*use* Bursa and Ligament, Hand, Left
*use* Bursa and Ligament, Hand, Right
**Pisometacarpal ligament**
*use* Bursa and Ligament, Hand, Left
*use* Bursa and Ligament, Hand, Right
**Pituitectomy**
*see* Excision, Gland, Pituitary ØGBØ
*see* Resection, Gland, Pituitary ØGTØ
**Plain film radiology** *see* Plain Radiography
**Plain Radiography**
Abdomen BWØØZZZ
Abdomen and Pelvis BWØ1ZZZ
Abdominal Lymphatic
Bilateral B7Ø1
Unilateral B7ØØ
Airway, Upper BBØDZZZ
Ankle
Left BQØH
Right BQØG
Aorta
Abdominal B4ØØ
Thoracic B3ØØ
Thoraco-Abdominal B3ØP
Aorta and Bilateral Lower Extremity Arteries B4ØD
Arch
Bilateral BNØDZZZ
Left BNØCZZZ
Right BNØBZZZ
Arm
Left BPØFZZZ
Right BPØEZZZ
Artery
Brachiocephalic-Subclavian, Right B3Ø1
Bronchial B3ØL
Bypass Graft, Other B2ØF
Cervico-Cerebral Arch B3ØQ
Common Carotid
Bilateral B3Ø5
Left B3Ø4
Right B3Ø3
Coronary
Bypass Graft
Multiple B2Ø3
Single B2Ø2
Multiple B2Ø1
Single B2ØØ
External Carotid
Bilateral B3ØC
Left B3ØB
Right B3Ø9
Hepatic B4Ø2
Inferior Mesenteric B4Ø5
Intercostal B3ØL
Internal Carotid
Bilateral B3Ø8
Left B3Ø7
Right B3Ø6

**Plain Radiography** — *continued*
Artery — *continued*
Internal Mammary Bypass Graft
Left B2Ø8
Right B2Ø7
Intra-Abdominal, Other B4ØB
Intracranial B3ØR
Lower Extremity
Bilateral and Aorta B4ØD
Left B4ØG
Right B4ØF
Lower, Other B4ØJ
Lumbar B4Ø9
Pelvic B4ØC
Pulmonary
Left B3ØT
Right B3ØS
Renal
Bilateral B4Ø8
Left B4Ø7
Right B4Ø6
Transplant B4ØM
Spinal B3ØM
Splenic B4Ø3
Subclavian, Left B3Ø2
Superior Mesenteric B4Ø4
Upper Extremity
Bilateral B3ØK
Left B3ØJ
Right B3ØH
Upper, Other B3ØN
Vertebral
Bilateral B3ØG
Left B3ØF
Right B3ØD
Bile Duct BFØØ
Bile Duct and Gallbladder BFØ3
Bladder BTØØ
Kidney and Ureter BTØ4
Bladder and Urethra BTØB
Bone
Facial BNØ5ZZZ
Nasal BNØ4ZZZ
Bones, Long, All BWØBZZZ
Breast
Bilateral BHØ2ZZZ
Left BHØ1ZZZ
Right BHØØZZZ
Calcaneus
Left BQØKZZZ
Right BQØJZZZ
Chest BWØ3ZZZ
Clavicle
Left BPØ5ZZZ
Right BPØ4ZZZ
Coccyx BRØFZZZ
Corpora Cavernosa BVØØ
Dialysis Fistula B5ØW
Dialysis Shunt B5ØW
Disc
Cervical BRØ1
Lumbar BRØ3
Thoracic BRØ2
Duct
Lacrimal
Bilateral B8Ø2
Left B8Ø1
Right B8ØØ
Mammary
Multiple
Left BHØ6
Right BHØ5
Single
Left BHØ4
Right BHØ3
Elbow
Left BPØH
Right BPØG
Epididymis
Left BVØ2
Right BVØ1
Extremity
Lower BWØCZZZ
Upper BWØJZZZ
Eye
Bilateral B8Ø7ZZZ
Left B8Ø6ZZZ
Right B8Ø5ZZZ

**Plain Radiography** — *continued*
Facet Joint
Cervical BRØ4
Lumbar BRØ6
Thoracic BRØ5
Fallopian Tube
Bilateral BUØ2
Left BUØ1
Right BUØØ
Fallopian Tube and Uterus BUØ8
Femur
Left, Densitometry BQØ4ZZ1
Right, Densitometry BQØ3ZZ1
Finger
Left BPØSZZZ
Right BPØRZZZ
Foot
Left BQØMZZZ
Right BQØLZZZ
Forearm
Left BPØKZZZ
Right BPØJZZZ
Gallbladder and Bile Duct BFØ3
Gland
Parotid
Bilateral B9Ø6
Left B9Ø5
Right B9Ø4
Salivary
Bilateral B9ØD
Left B9ØC
Right B9ØB
Submandibular
Bilateral B9Ø9
Left B9Ø8
Right B9Ø7
Hand
Left BPØPZZZ
Right BPØNZZZ
Heart
Left B2Ø5
Right B2Ø4
Right and Left B2Ø6
Hepatobiliary System, All BFØC
Hip
Left BQØ1
Densitometry BQØ1ZZ1
Right BQØØ
Densitometry BQØØZZ1
Humerus
Left BPØBZZZ
Right BPØAZZZ
Ileal Diversion Loop BTØC
Intracranial Sinus B5Ø2
Joint
Acromioclavicular, Bilateral BPØ3ZZZ
Finger
Left BPØD
Right BPØC
Foot
Left BQØY
Right BQØX
Hand
Left BPØD
Right BPØC
Lumbosacral BRØBZZZ
Sacroiliac BRØD
Sternoclavicular
Bilateral BPØ2ZZZ
Left BPØ1ZZZ
Right BPØØZZZ
Temporomandibular
Bilateral BNØ9
Left BNØ8
Right BNØ7
Thoracolumbar BRØ8ZZZ
Toe
Left BQØY
Right BQØX
Kidney
Bilateral BTØ3
Left BTØ2
Right BTØ1
Ureter and Bladder BTØ4
Knee
Left BQØ8
Right BQØ7
Leg
Left BQØFZZZ

**Plain Radiography** — *continued*
Leg — *continued*
Right BQØDZZZ
Lymphatic
Head B7Ø4
Lower Extremity
Bilateral B7ØB
Left B7Ø9
Right B7Ø8
Neck B7Ø4
Pelvic B7ØC
Upper Extremity
Bilateral B7Ø7
Left B7Ø6
Right B7Ø5
Mandible BNØ6ZZZ
Mastoid B9ØHZZZ
Nasopharynx B9ØFZZZ
Optic Foramina
Left B8Ø4ZZZ
Right B8Ø3ZZZ
Orbit
Bilateral BNØ3ZZZ
Left BNØ2ZZZ
Right BNØ1ZZZ
Oropharynx B9ØFZZZ
Patella
Left BQØWZZZ
Right BQØVZZZ
Pelvis BRØCZZZ
Pelvis and Abdomen BWØ1ZZZ
Prostate BVØ3
Retroperitoneal Lymphatic
Bilateral B7Ø1
Unilateral B7ØØ
Ribs
Left BPØYZZZ
Right BPØXZZZ
Sacrum BRØFZZZ
Scapula
Left BPØ7ZZZ
Right BPØ6ZZZ
Shoulder
Left BPØ9
Right BPØ8
Sinus
Intracranial B5Ø2
Paranasal B9Ø2ZZZ
Skull BNØØZZZ
Spinal Cord BØØB
Spine
Cervical, Densitometry BRØØZZ1
Lumbar, Densitometry BRØ9ZZ1
Thoracic, Densitometry BRØ7ZZ1
Whole, Densitometry BRØGZZ1
Sternum BRØHZZZ
Teeth
All BNØJZZZ
Multiple BNØHZZZ
Testicle
Left BVØ6
Right BVØ5
Toe
Left BQØQZZZ
Right BQØPZZZ
Tooth, Single BNØGZZZ
Tracheobronchial Tree
Bilateral BBØ9YZZ
Left BBØ8YZZ
Right BBØ7YZZ
Ureter
Bilateral BTØ8
Kidney and Bladder BTØ4
Left BTØ7
Right BTØ6
Urethra BTØ5
Urethra and Bladder BTØB
Uterus BUØ6
Uterus and Fallopian Tube BUØ8
Vagina BUØ9
Vasa Vasorum BVØ8
Vein
Cerebellar B5Ø1
Cerebral B5Ø1
Epidural B5ØØ
Jugular
Bilateral B5Ø5
Left B5Ø4
Right B5Ø3

**Plain Radiography** — *continued*
Vein — *continued*
Lower Extremity
Bilateral B5ØD
Left B5ØC
Right B5ØB
Other B5ØV
Pelvic (Iliac)
Left B5ØG
Right B5ØF
Pelvic (Iliac) Bilateral B5ØH
Portal B5ØT
Pulmonary
Bilateral B5ØS
Left B5ØR
Right B5ØQ
Renal
Bilateral B5ØL
Left B5ØK
Right B5ØJ
Spanchnic B5ØT
Subclavian
Left B5Ø7
Right B5Ø6
Upper Extremity
Bilateral B5ØP
Left B5ØN
Right B5ØM
Vena Cava
Inferior B5Ø9
Superior B5Ø8
Whole Body BWØKZZZ
Infant BWØMZZZ
Whole Skeleton BWØLZZZ
Wrist
Left BPØM
Right BPØL

**Planar Nuclear Medicine Imaging**
Abdomen CW1Ø
Abdomen and Chest CW14
Abdomen and Pelvis CW11
Anatomical Region, Other CW1ZZZZ
Anatomical Regions, Multiple CW1YYZZ
Bladder and Ureters CT1H
Bladder, Kidneys and Ureters CT13
Blood C713
Bone Marrow C71Ø
Brain CØ1Ø
Breast CH1YYZZ
Bilateral CH12
Left CH11
Right CH1Ø
Bronchi and Lungs CB12
Central Nervous System CØ1YYZZ
Cerebrospinal Fluid CØ15
Chest CW13
Chest and Abdomen CW14
Chest and Neck CW16
Digestive System CD1YYZZ
Ducts, Lacrimal, Bilateral C819
Ear, Nose, Mouth and Throat C91YYZZ
Endocrine System CG1YYZZ
Extremity
Lower CW1D
Bilateral CP1F
Left CP1D
Right CP1C
Upper CW1M
Bilateral CP1B
Left CP19
Right CP18
Eye C81YYZZ
Gallbladder CF14
Gastrointestinal Tract CD17
Upper CD15
Gland
Adrenal, Bilateral CG14
Parathyroid CG11
Thyroid CG12
Glands, Salivary, Bilateral C91B
Head and Neck CW1B
Heart C21YYZZ
Right and Left C216
Hepatobiliary System, All CF1C
Hepatobiliary System and Pancreas CF1YYZZ
Kidneys, Ureters and Bladder CT13
Liver CF15
Liver and Spleen CF16
Lungs and Bronchi CB12

**Planar Nuclear Medicine Imaging** — *continued*
Lymphatics
Head C71J
Head and Neck C715
Lower Extremity C71P
Neck C71K
Pelvic C71D
Trunk C71M
Upper Chest C71L
Upper Extremity C71N
Lymphatics and Hematologic System C71YYZZ
Musculoskeletal System
All CP1Z
Other CP1YYZZ
Myocardium C21G
Neck and Chest CW16
Neck and Head CW1B
Pancreas and Hepatobiliary System CF1YYZZ
Pelvic Region CW1J
Pelvis CP16
Pelvis and Abdomen CW11
Pelvis and Spine CP17
Reproductive System, Male CV1YYZZ
Respiratory System CB1YYZZ
Skin CH1YYZZ
Skull CP11
Spine CP15
Spine and Pelvis CP17
Spleen C712
Spleen and Liver CF16
Subcutaneous Tissue CH1YYZZ
Testicles, Bilateral CV19
Thorax CP14
Ureters and Bladder CT1H
Ureters, Kidneys and Bladder CT13
Urinary System CT1YYZZ
Veins C51YYZZ
Central C51R
Lower Extremity
Bilateral C51D
Left C51C
Right C51B
Upper Extremity
Bilateral C51Q
Left C51P
Right C51N
Whole Body CW1N
**Plantar digital vein**
*use* Vein, Foot, Left
*use* Vein, Foot, Right
**Plantar fascia (aponeurosis)**
*use* Subcutaneous Tissue and Fascia, Foot, Left
*use* Subcutaneous Tissue and Fascia, Foot, Right
**Plantar metatarsal vein**
*use* Vein, Foot, Left
*use* Vein, Foot, Right
**Plantar venous arch**
*use* Vein, Foot, Left
*use* Vein, Foot, Right
**Plaque Radiation**
Abdomen DWY3FZZ
Adrenal Gland DGY2FZZ
Anus DDY8FZZ
Bile Ducts DFY2FZZ
Bladder DTY2FZZ
Bone Marrow D7YØFZZ
Bone, Other DPYCFZZ
Brain DØYØFZZ
Brain Stem DØY1FZZ
Breast
Left DMYØFZZ
Right DMY1FZZ
Bronchus DBY1FZZ
Cervix DUY1FZZ
Chest DWY2FZZ
Chest Wall DBY7FZZ
Colon DDY5FZZ
Diaphragm DBY8FZZ
Duodenum DDY2FZZ
Ear D9YØFZZ
Esophagus DDYØFZZ
Eye D8YØFZZ
Femur DPY9FZZ
Fibula DPYBFZZ
Gallbladder DFY1FZZ
Gland
Adrenal DGY2FZZ
Parathyroid DGY4FZZ

**Plaque Radiation** — *continued*
Gland — *continued*
Pituitary DGYØFZZ
Thyroid DGY5FZZ
Glands, Salivary D9Y6FZZ
Head and Neck DWY1FZZ
Hemibody DWY4FZZ
Humerus DPY6FZZ
Ileum DDY4FZZ
Jejunum DDY3FZZ
Kidney DTYØFZZ
Larynx D9YBFZZ
Liver DFYØFZZ
Lung DBY2FZZ
Lymphatics
Abdomen D7Y6FZZ
Axillary D7Y4FZZ
Inguinal D7Y8FZZ
Neck D7Y3FZZ
Pelvis D7Y7FZZ
Thorax D7Y5FZZ
Mandible DPY3FZZ
Maxilla DPY2FZZ
Mediastinum DBY6FZZ
Mouth D9Y4FZZ
Nasopharynx D9YDFZZ
Neck and Head DWY1FZZ
Nerve, Peripheral DØY7FZZ
Nose D9Y1FZZ
Ovary DUYØFZZ
Palate
Hard D9Y8FZZ
Soft D9Y9FZZ
Pancreas DFY3FZZ
Parathyroid Gland DGY4FZZ
Pelvic Bones DPY8FZZ
Pelvic Region DWY6FZZ
Pharynx D9YCFZZ
Pineal Body DGY1FZZ
Pituitary Gland DGYØFZZ
Pleura DBY5FZZ
Prostate DVYØFZZ
Radius DPY7FZZ
Rectum DDY7FZZ
Rib DPY5FZZ
Sinuses D9Y7FZZ
Skin
Abdomen DHY8FZZ
Arm DHY4FZZ
Back DHY7FZZ
Buttock DHY9FZZ
Chest DHY6FZZ
Face DHY2FZZ
Foot DHYCFZZ
Hand DHY5FZZ
Leg DHYBFZZ
Neck DHY3FZZ
Skull DPYØFZZ
Spinal Cord DØY6FZZ
Spleen D7Y2FZZ
Sternum DPY4FZZ
Stomach DDY1FZZ
Testis DVY1FZZ
Thymus D7Y1FZZ
Thyroid Gland DGY5FZZ
Tibia DPYBFZZ
Tongue D9Y5FZZ
Trachea DBYØFZZ
Ulna DPY7FZZ
Ureter DTY1FZZ
Urethra DTY3FZZ
Uterus DUY2FZZ
Whole Body DWY5FZZ
**Plasmapheresis, therapeutic** *see* Pheresis, Physiological Systems 6A5
**Plateletpheresis, therapeutic** *see* Pheresis, Physiological Systems 6A5
**Platysma muscle**
*use* Muscle, Neck, Left
*use* Muscle, Neck, Right
**Pleurectomy**
*see* Excision, Respiratory System ØBB
*see* Resection, Respiratory System ØBT
**Pleurocentesis** *see* Drainage, Anatomical Regions, General ØW9
**Pleurodesis, pleurosclerosis**
Chemical injection *see* Introduction of Substance in or on, Pleural Cavity 3EØL

**Pleurodesis, pleurosclerosis** — *continued*
Surgical *see* Destruction, Respiratory System ØB5
**Pleurolysis** *see* Release, Respiratory System ØBN
**Pleuroscopy** ØBJQ4ZZ
**Pleurotomy** *see* Drainage, Respiratory System ØB9
**Plica semilunaris**
*use* Conjunctiva, Left
*use* Conjunctiva, Right
**Plication** *see* Restriction
**Pneumectomy**
*see* Excision, Respiratory System ØBB
*see* Resection, Respiratory System ØBT
**Pneumocentesis** *see* Drainage, Respiratory System ØB9
**Pneumogastric nerve** *use* Nerve, Vagus
**Pneumolysis** *see* Release, Respiratory System ØBN
**Pneumonectomy** *see* Resection, Respiratory System ØBT
**Pneumonolysis** *see* Release, Respiratory System ØBN
**Pneumonopexy**
*see* Repair, Respiratory System ØBQ
*see* Reposition, Respiratory System ØBS
**Pneumonorrhaphy** *see* Repair, Respiratory System ØBQ
**Pneumonotomy** *see* Drainage, Respiratory System ØB9
**Pneumotaxic center** *use* Pons
**Pneumotomy** *see* Drainage, Respiratory System ØB9
**Pollicization** *see* Transfer, Anatomical Regions, Upper Extremities ØXX
**Polyethylene socket** *use* Synthetic Substitute, Polyethylene in ØSR
**Polymethylmethacrylate (PMMA)** *use* Synthetic Substitute
**Polypectomy, gastrointestinal** *see* Excision, Gastrointestinal System ØDB
**Polypropylene mesh** *use* Synthetic Substitute
**Polysomnogram** 4A1ZXQZ
**Pontine tegmentum** *use* Pons
**Popliteal ligament**
*use* Bursa and Ligament, Knee, Left
*use* Bursa and Ligament, Knee, Right
**Popliteal lymph node**
*use* Lymphatic, Lower Extremity, Left
*use* Lymphatic, Lower Extremity, Right
**Popliteal vein**
*use* Vein, Femoral, Left
*use* Vein, Femoral, Right
**Popliteus muscle**
*use* Muscle, Lower Leg, Left
*use* Muscle, Lower Leg, Right
**Porcine (bioprosthetic) valve** *use* Zooplastic Tissue in Heart and Great Vessels
**Positive end expiratory pressure** *see* Performance, Respiratory 5A19
**Positron Emission Tomographic (PET) Imaging**
Brain CØ3Ø
Bronchi and Lungs CB32
Central Nervous System CØ3YYZZ
Heart C23YYZZ
Lungs and Bronchi CB32
Myocardium C23G
Respiratory System CB3YYZZ
Whole Body CW3NYZZ
**Positron emission tomography** *see* Positron Emission Tomographic (PET) Imaging
**Postauricular (mastoid) lymph node**
*use* Lymphatic, Neck, Left
*use* Lymphatic, Neck, Right
**Postcava** *use* Vena Cava, Inferior
**Posterior auricular artery**
*use* Artery, External Carotid, Left
*use* Artery, External Carotid, Right
**Posterior auricular nerve** *use* Nerve, Facial
**Posterior auricular vein**
*use* Vein, External Jugular, Left
*use* Vein, External Jugular, Right
**Posterior cerebral artery** *use* Artery, Intracranial
**Posterior chamber**
*use* Eye, Left
*use* Eye, Right
**Posterior circumflex humeral artery**
*use* Artery, Axillary, Left
*use* Artery, Axillary, Right
**Posterior communicating artery** *use* Artery, Intracranial
**Posterior cruciate ligament (PCL)**
*use* Bursa and Ligament, Knee, Left
*use* Bursa and Ligament, Knee, Right
**Posterior facial (retromandibular) vein**
*use* Vein, Face, Left

**Posterior facial (retromandibular) vein** — *continued*
*use* Vein, Face, Right
**Posterior femoral cutaneous nerve** *use* Nerve, Sacral Plexus
**Posterior inferior cerebellar artery (PICA)** *use* Artery, Intracranial
**Posterior interosseous nerve** *use* Nerve, Radial
**Posterior labial nerve** *use* Nerve, Pudendal
**Posterior (subscapular) lymph node**
*use* Lymphatic, Axillary, Left
*use* Lymphatic, Axillary, Right
**Posterior scrotal nerve** *use* Nerve, Pudendal
**Posterior spinal artery**
*use* Artery, Vertebral, Left
*use* Artery, Vertebral, Right
**Posterior tibial recurrent artery**
*use* Artery, Anterior Tibial, Left
*use* Artery, Anterior Tibial, Right
**Posterior ulnar recurrent artery**
*use* Artery, Ulnar, Left
*use* Artery, Ulnar, Right
**Posterior vagal trunk** *use* Nerve, Vagus
**PPN (peripheral parenteral nutrition)** *see* Introduction of Nutritional Substance
**Preauricular lymph node** *use* Lymphatic, Head
**Precava** *use* Vena Cava, Superior
**Prepatellar bursa**
*use* Bursa and Ligament, Knee, Left
*use* Bursa and Ligament, Knee, Right
**Preputiotomy** *see* Drainage, Male Reproductive System ØV9
**Pressure support ventilation** *see* Performance, Respiratory 5A19
**PRESTIGE® Cervical Disc** *use* Synthetic Substitute
**Pretracheal fascia**
*use* Subcutaneous Tissue and Fascia, Left Neck
*use* Subcutaneous Tissue and Fascia, Right Neck
**Prevertebral fascia**
*use* Subcutaneous Tissue and Fascia, Left Neck
*use* Subcutaneous Tissue and Fascia, Right Neck
**PrimeAdvanced neurostimulator (SureScan) (MRI Safe)** *use* Stimulator Generator, Multiple Array in ØJH
**Princeps pollicis artery**
*use* Artery, Hand, Left
*use* Artery, Hand, Right
**Probing, duct**
Diagnostic *see* Inspection
Dilation *see* Dilation
**PROCEED™ Ventral Patch** *use* Synthetic Substitute
**Procerus muscle** *use* Muscle, Facial
**Proctectomy**
*see* Excision, Rectum ØDBP
*see* Resection, Rectum ØDTP
**Proctoclysis** *see* Introduction of substance in or on, Gastrointestinal Tract, Lower 3EØH
**Proctocolectomy**
*see* Excision, Gastrointestinal System ØDB
*see* Resection, Gastrointestinal System ØDT
**Proctocolpoplasty**
*see* Repair, Gastrointestinal System ØDQ
*see* Supplement, Gastrointestinal System ØDU
**Proctoperineoplasty**
*see* Repair, Gastrointestinal System ØDQ
*see* Supplement, Gastrointestinal System ØDU
**Proctoperineorrhaphy** *see* Repair, Gastrointestinal System ØDQ
**Proctopexy**
*see* Repair, Rectum ØDQP
*see* Reposition, Rectum ØDSP
**Proctoplasty**
*see* Repair, Rectum ØDQP
*see* Supplement, Rectum ØDUP
**Proctorrhaphy** *see* Repair, Rectum ØDQP
**Proctoscopy** ØDJD8ZZ
**Proctosigmoidectomy**
*see* Excision, Gastrointestinal System ØDB
*see* Resection, Gastrointestinal System ØDT
**Proctosigmoidoscopy** ØDJD8ZZ
**Proctostomy** *see* Drainage, Rectum ØD9P
**Proctotomy** *see* Drainage, Rectum ØD9P
**Prodisc-C** *use* Synthetic Substitute
**Prodisc-L** *use* Synthetic Substitute
**Production, atrial septal defect** *see* Excision, Septum, Atrial Ø2B5
**Profunda brachii**
*use* Artery, Brachial, Left
*use* Artery, Brachial, Right
**Profunda femoris (deep femoral) vein**
*use* Vein, Femoral, Left
*use* Vein, Femoral, Right
**PROLENE Polypropylene Hernia System (PHS)** *use* Synthetic Substitute
**Prolonged intermittent renal replacement therapy (PIRRT)** 5A1D8ØZ
**Pronator quadratus muscle**
*use* Muscle, Lower Arm and Wrist, Left
*use* Muscle, Lower Arm and Wrist, Right
**Pronator teres muscle**
*use* Muscle, Lower Arm and Wrist, Left
*use* Muscle, Lower Arm and Wrist, Right
**Prostatectomy**
*see* Excision, Prostate ØVBØ
*see* Resection, Prostate ØVTØ
**Prostatic urethra** *use* Urethra
**Prostatomy, prostatotomy** *see* Drainage, Prostate ØV9Ø
**Protecta XT CRT-D** *use* Cardiac Resynchronization Defibrillator Pulse Generator in ØJH
**Protecta XT DR (XT VR)** *use* Defibrillator Generator in ØJH
**Protégé® RX Carotid Stent System** *use* Intraluminal Device
**Proximal radioulnar joint**
*use* Joint, Elbow, Left
*use* Joint, Elbow, Right
**Psoas muscle**
*use* Muscle, Hip, Left
*use* Muscle, Hip, Right
**PSV (pressure support ventilation)** *see* Performance, Respiratory 5A19
**Psychoanalysis** GZ54ZZZ
**Psychological Tests**
Cognitive Status GZ14ZZZ
Developmental GZ1ØZZZ
Intellectual and Psychoeducational GZ12ZZZ
Neurobehavioral Status GZ14ZZZ
Neuropsychological GZ13ZZZ
Personality and Behavioral GZ11ZZZ
**Psychotherapy**
Family, Mental Health Services GZ72ZZZ
Group GZHZZZZ
Mental Health Services GZHZZZZ
Individual
*see* Psychotherapy, Individual, Mental Health Services
for substance abuse
12-Step HZ53ZZZ
Behavioral HZ51ZZZ
Cognitive HZ5ØZZZ
Cognitive-Behavioral HZ52ZZZ
Confrontational HZ58ZZZ
Interactive HZ55ZZZ
Interpersonal HZ54ZZZ
Motivational Enhancement HZ57ZZZ
Psychoanalysis HZ5BZZZ
Psychodynamic HZ5CZZZ
Psychoeducation HZ56ZZZ
Psychophysiological HZ5DZZZ
Supportive HZ59ZZZ
Mental Health Services
Behavioral GZ51ZZZ
Cognitive GZ52ZZZ
Cognitive-Behavioral GZ58ZZZ
Interactive GZ5ØZZZ
Interpersonal GZ53ZZZ
Psychoanalysis GZ54ZZZ
Psychodynamic GZ55ZZZ
Psychophysiological GZ59ZZZ
Supportive GZ56ZZZ
**PTCA (percutaneous transluminal coronary angioplasty)** *see* Dilation, Heart and Great Vessels Ø27
**Pterygoid muscle** *use* Muscle, Head
**Pterygoid process** *use* Sphenoid Bone
**Pterygopalatine (sphenopalatine) ganglion** *use* Nerve, Head and Neck Sympathetic
**Pubis**
*use* Bone, Pelvic, Left
*use* Bone, Pelvic, Right
**Pubofemoral ligament**
*use* Bursa and Ligament, Hip, Left
*use* Bursa and Ligament, Hip, Right
**Pudendal nerve** *use* Nerve, Sacral Plexus
**Pull-through, laparoscopic-assisted transanal**
*see* Excision, Gastrointestinal System ØDB
*see* Resection, Gastrointestinal System ØDT
**Pull-through, rectal** *see* Resection, Rectum ØDTP
**Pulmoaortic canal** *use* Artery, Pulmonary, Left
**Pulmonary annulus** *use* Valve, Pulmonary
**Pulmonary artery wedge monitoring** *see* Monitoring, Arterial 4A13
**Pulmonary plexus**
*use* Nerve, Thoracic Sympathetic
*use* Nerve, Vagus
**Pulmonic valve** *use* Valve, Pulmonary
**Pulpectomy** *see* Excision, Mouth and Throat ØCB
**Pulverization** *see* Fragmentation
**Pulvinar** *use* Thalamus
**Pump reservoir** *use* Infusion Device, Pump in Subcutaneous Tissue and Fascia
**Punch biopsy** *see* Excision with qualifier Diagnostic
**Puncture** *see* Drainage
**Puncture, lumbar** *see* Drainage, Spinal Canal ØØ9U
**Pyelography**
*see* Fluoroscopy, Urinary System BT1
*see* Plain Radiography, Urinary System BTØ
**Pyeloileostomy, urinary diversion** *see* Bypass, Urinary System ØT1
**Pyeloplasty**
*see* Repair, Urinary System ØTQ
*see* Replacement, Urinary System ØTR
*see* Supplement, Urinary System ØTU
**Pyelorrhaphy** *see* Repair, Urinary System ØTQ
**Pyeloscopy** ØTJ58ZZ
**Pyelostomy**
*see* Bypass, Urinary System ØT1
*see* Drainage, Urinary System ØT9
**Pyelotomy** *see* Drainage, Urinary System ØT9
**Pylorectomy**
*see* Excision, Stomach, Pylorus ØDB7
*see* Resection, Stomach, Pylorus ØDT7
**Pyloric antrum** *use* Stomach, Pylorus
**Pyloric canal** *use* Stomach, Pylorus
**Pyloric sphincter** *use* Stomach, Pylorus
**Pylorodiosis** *see* Dilation, Stomach, Pylorus ØD77
**Pylorogastrectomy**
*see* Excision, Gastrointestinal System ØDB
*see* Resection, Gastrointestinal System ØDT
**Pyloroplasty**
*see* Repair, Stomach, Pylorus ØDQ7
*see* Supplement, Stomach, Pylorus ØDU7
**Pyloroscopy** ØDJ68ZZ
**Pylorotomy** *see* Drainage, Stomach, Pylorus ØD97
**Pyramidalis muscle**
*use* Muscle, Abdomen, Left
*use* Muscle, Abdomen, Right

# Q

**Quadrangular cartilage** *use* Septum, Nasal
**Quadrant resection of breast** *see* Excision, Skin and Breast ØHB
**Quadrate lobe** *use* Liver
**Quadratus femoris muscle**
*use* Muscle, Hip, Left
*use* Muscle, Hip, Right
**Quadratus lumborum muscle**
*use* Muscle, Trunk, Left
*use* Muscle, Trunk, Right
**Quadratus plantae muscle**
*use* Muscle, Foot, Left
*use* Muscle, Foot, Right
**Quadriceps (femoris)**
*use* Muscle, Upper Leg, Left
*use* Muscle, Upper Leg, Right
**Quarantine** 8EØZXY6

# R

**Radial collateral carpal ligament**
*use* Bursa and Ligament, Wrist, Left
*use* Bursa and Ligament, Wrist, Right
**Radial collateral ligament**
*use* Bursa and Ligament, Elbow, Left
*use* Bursa and Ligament, Elbow, Right
**Radial notch**
*use* Ulna, Left
*use* Ulna, Right

**Radial recurrent artery**
*use* Artery, Radial, Left
*use* Artery, Radial, Right
**Radial vein**
*use* Vein, Brachial, Left
*use* Vein, Brachial, Right
**Radialis indicis**
*use* Artery, Hand, Left
*use* Artery, Hand, Right
**Radiation Therapy**
*see* Beam Radiation
*see* Brachytherapy
*see* Stereotactic Radiosurgery
**Radiation treatment** *see* Radiation Therapy
**Radiocarpal joint**
*use* Joint, Wrist, Left
*use* Joint, Wrist, Right
**Radiocarpal ligament**
*use* Bursa and Ligament, Wrist, Left
*use* Bursa and Ligament, Wrist, Right
**Radiography** *see* Plain Radiography
**Radiology, analog** *see* Plain Radiography
**Radiology, diagnostic** *see* Imaging, Diagnostic
**Radioulnar ligament**
*use* Bursa and Ligament, Wrist, Left
*use* Bursa and Ligament, Wrist, Right
**Range of motion testing** *see* Motor Function Assessment, Rehabilitation FØ1
**REALIZE® Adjustable Gastric Band** *use* Extraluminal Device
**Reattachment**
Abdominal Wall ØWMFØZZ
Ampulla of Vater ØFMC
Ankle Region
Left ØYMLØZZ
Right ØYMKØZZ
Arm
Lower
Left ØXMFØZZ
Right ØXMDØZZ
Upper
Left ØXM9ØZZ
Right ØXM8ØZZ
Axilla
Left ØXM5ØZZ
Right ØXM4ØZZ
Back
Lower ØWMLØZZ
Upper ØWMKØZZ
Bladder ØTMB
Bladder Neck ØTMC
Breast
Bilateral ØHMVXZZ
Left ØHMUXZZ
Right ØHMTXZZ
Bronchus
Lingula ØBM9ØZZ
Lower Lobe
Left ØBMBØZZ
Right ØBM6ØZZ
Main
Left ØBM7ØZZ
Right ØBM3ØZZ
Middle Lobe, Right ØBM5ØZZ
Upper Lobe
Left ØBM8ØZZ
Right ØBM4ØZZ
Bursa and Ligament
Abdomen
Left ØMMJ
Right ØMMH
Ankle
Left ØMMR
Right ØMMQ
Elbow
Left ØMM4
Right ØMM3
Foot
Left ØMMT
Right ØMMS
Hand
Left ØMM8
Right ØMM7
Head and Neck ØMMØ
Hip
Left ØMMM
Right ØMML

**Reattachment** — *continued*
Bursa and Ligament — *continued*
Knee
Left ØMMP
Right ØMMN
Lower Extremity
Left ØMMW
Right ØMMV
Perineum ØMMK
Rib(s) ØMMG
Shoulder
Left ØMM2
Right ØMM1
Spine
Lower ØMMD
Upper ØMMC
Sternum ØMMF
Upper Extremity
Left ØMMB
Right ØMM9
Wrist
Left ØMM6
Right ØMM5
Buttock
Left ØYM1ØZZ
Right ØYMØØZZ
Carina ØBM2ØZZ
Cecum ØDMH
Cervix ØUMC
Chest Wall ØWM8ØZZ
Clitoris ØUMJXZZ
Colon
Ascending ØDMK
Descending ØDMM
Sigmoid ØDMN
Transverse ØDML
Cord
Bilateral ØVMH
Left ØVMG
Right ØVMF
Cul-de-sac ØUMF
Diaphragm ØBMTØZZ
Duct
Common Bile ØFM9
Cystic ØFM8
Hepatic
Common ØFM7
Left ØFM6
Right ØFM5
Pancreatic ØFMD
Accessory ØFMF
Duodenum ØDM9
Ear
Left Ø9M1XZZ
Right Ø9MØXZZ
Elbow Region
Left ØXMCØZZ
Right ØXMBØZZ
Esophagus ØDM5
Extremity
Lower
Left ØYMBØZZ
Right ØYM9ØZZ
Upper
Left ØXM7ØZZ
Right ØXM6ØZZ
Eyelid
Lower
Left Ø8MRXZZ
Right Ø8MQXZZ
Upper
Left Ø8MPXZZ
Right Ø8MNXZZ
Face ØWM2ØZZ
Fallopian Tube
Left ØUM6
Right ØUM5
Fallopian Tubes, Bilateral ØUM7
Femoral Region
Left ØYM8ØZZ
Right ØYM7ØZZ
Finger
Index
Left ØXMPØZZ
Right ØXMNØZZ
Little
Left ØXMWØZZ
Right ØXMVØZZ

**Reattachment** — *continued*
Finger — *continued*
Middle
Left ØXMRØZZ
Right ØXMQØZZ
Ring
Left ØXMTØZZ
Right ØXMSØZZ
Foot
Left ØYMNØZZ
Right ØYMMØZZ
Forequarter
Left ØXM1ØZZ
Right ØXMØØZZ
Gallbladder ØFM4
Gland
Left ØGM2
Right ØGM3
Hand
Left ØXMKØZZ
Right ØXMJØZZ
Hindquarter
Bilateral ØYM4ØZZ
Left ØYM3ØZZ
Right ØYM2ØZZ
Hymen ØUMK
Ileum ØDMB
Inguinal Region
Left ØYM6ØZZ
Right ØYM5ØZZ
Intestine
Large ØDME
Left ØDMG
Right ØDMF
Small ØDM8
Jaw
Lower ØWM5ØZZ
Upper ØWM4ØZZ
Jejunum ØDMA
Kidney
Left ØTM1
Right ØTMØ
Kidney Pelvis
Left ØTM4
Right ØTM3
Kidneys, Bilateral ØTM2
Knee Region
Left ØYMGØZZ
Right ØYMFØZZ
Leg
Lower
Left ØYMJØZZ
Right ØYMHØZZ
Upper
Left ØYMDØZZ
Right ØYMCØZZ
Lip
Lower ØCM1ØZZ
Upper ØCMØØZZ
Liver ØFMØ
Left Lobe ØFM2
Right Lobe ØFM1
Lung
Left ØBMLØZZ
Lower Lobe
Left ØBMJØZZ
Right ØBMFØZZ
Middle Lobe, Right ØBMDØZZ
Right ØBMKØZZ
Upper Lobe
Left ØBMGØZZ
Right ØBMCØZZ
Lung Lingula ØBMHØZZ
Muscle
Abdomen
Left ØKML
Right ØKMK
Facial ØKM1
Foot
Left ØKMW
Right ØKMV
Hand
Left ØKMD
Right ØKMC
Head ØKMØ
Hip
Left ØKMP
Right ØKMN

- **Reattachment** — *continued*
  - Muscle — *continued*
    - Lower Arm and Wrist
      - Left ØKMB
      - Right ØKM9
    - Lower Leg
      - Left ØKMT
      - Right ØKMS
    - Neck
      - Left ØKM3
      - Right ØKM2
    - Perineum ØKMM
    - Shoulder
      - Left ØKM6
      - Right ØKM5
    - Thorax
      - Left ØKMJ
      - Right ØKMH
    - Tongue, Palate, Pharynx ØKM4
    - Trunk
      - Left ØKMG
      - Right ØKMF
    - Upper Arm
      - Left ØKM8
      - Right ØKM7
    - Upper Leg
      - Left ØKMR
      - Right ØKMQ
  - Nasal Mucosa and Soft Tissue Ø9MKXZZ
  - Neck ØWM6ØZZ
  - Nipple
    - Left ØHMXXZZ
    - Right ØHMWXZZ
  - Ovary
    - Bilateral ØUM2
    - Left ØUM1
    - Right ØUMØ
  - Palate, Soft ØCM3ØZZ
  - Pancreas ØFMG
  - Parathyroid Gland ØGMR
    - Inferior
      - Left ØGMP
      - Right ØGMN
    - Multiple ØGMQ
    - Superior
      - Left ØGMM
      - Right ØGML
  - Penis ØVMSXZZ
  - Perineum
    - Female ØWMNØZZ
    - Male ØWMMØZZ
  - Rectum ØDMP
  - Scrotum ØVM5XZZ
  - Shoulder Region
    - Left ØXM3ØZZ
    - Right ØXM2ØZZ
  - Skin
    - Abdomen ØHM7XZZ
    - Back ØHM6XZZ
    - Buttock ØHM8XZZ
    - Chest ØHM5XZZ
    - Ear
      - Left ØHM3XZZ
      - Right ØHM2XZZ
    - Face ØHM1XZZ
    - Foot
      - Left ØHMNXZZ
      - Right ØHMMXZZ
    - Hand
      - Left ØHMGXZZ
      - Right ØHMFXZZ
    - Inguinal ØHMAXZZ
    - Lower Arm
      - Left ØHMEXZZ
      - Right ØHMDXZZ
    - Lower Leg
      - Left ØHMLXZZ
      - Right ØHMKXZZ
    - Neck ØHM4XZZ
    - Perineum ØHM9XZZ
    - Scalp ØHMØXZZ
    - Upper Arm
      - Left ØHMCXZZ
      - Right ØHMBXZZ
    - Upper Leg
      - Left ØHMJXZZ
      - Right ØHMHXZZ
  - Stomach ØDM6

- **Reattachment** — *continued*
  - Tendon
    - Abdomen
      - Left ØLMG
      - Right ØLMF
    - Ankle
      - Left ØLMT
      - Right ØLMS
    - Foot
      - Left ØLMW
      - Right ØLMV
    - Hand
      - Left ØLM8
      - Right ØLM7
    - Head and Neck ØLMØ
    - Hip
      - Left ØLMK
      - Right ØLMJ
    - Knee
      - Left ØLMR
      - Right ØLMQ
    - Lower Arm and Wrist
      - Left ØLM6
      - Right ØLM5
    - Lower Leg
      - Left ØLMP
      - Right ØLMN
    - Perineum ØLMH
    - Shoulder
      - Left ØLM2
      - Right ØLM1
    - Thorax
      - Left ØLMD
      - Right ØLMC
    - Trunk
      - Left ØLMB
      - Right ØLM9
    - Upper Arm
      - Left ØLM4
      - Right ØLM3
    - Upper Leg
      - Left ØLMM
      - Right ØLML
  - Testis
    - Bilateral ØVMC
    - Left ØVMB
    - Right ØVM9
  - Thumb
    - Left ØXMMØZZ
    - Right ØXMLØZZ
  - Thyroid Gland
    - Left Lobe ØGMG
    - Right Lobe ØGMH
  - Toe
    - 1st
      - Left ØYMQØZZ
      - Right ØYMPØZZ
    - 2nd
      - Left ØYMSØZZ
      - Right ØYMRØZZ
    - 3rd
      - Left ØYMUØZZ
      - Right ØYMTØZZ
    - 4th
      - Left ØYMWØZZ
      - Right ØYMVØZZ
    - 5th
      - Left ØYMYØZZ
      - Right ØYMXØZZ
  - Tongue ØCM7ØZZ
  - Tooth
    - Lower ØCMX
    - Upper ØCMW
  - Trachea ØBM1ØZZ
  - Tunica Vaginalis
    - Left ØVM7
    - Right ØVM6
  - Ureter
    - Left ØTM7
    - Right ØTM6
  - Ureters, Bilateral ØTM8
  - Urethra ØTMD
  - Uterine Supporting Structure ØUM4
  - Uterus ØUM9
  - Uvula ØCMNØZZ
  - Vagina ØUMG
  - Vulva ØUMMXZZ
  - Wrist Region
    - Left ØXMHØZZ

- **Reattachment** — *continued*
  - Wrist Region — *continued*
    - Right ØXMGØZZ
- **REBOA (resuscitative endovascular balloon occlusion of the aorta)**
  - Ø2LW3DJ
  - Ø4LØ3DJ
- **Rebound HRD® (Hernia Repair Device)** *use* Synthetic Substitute
- **Recession**
  - *see* Repair
  - *see* Reposition
- **Reclosure, disrupted abdominal wall** ØWQFXZZ
- **Reconstruction**
  - *see* Repair
  - *see* Replacement
  - *see* Supplement
- **Rectectomy**
  - *see* Excision, Rectum ØDBP
  - *see* Resection, Rectum ØDTP
- **Rectocele repair** *see* Repair, Subcutaneous Tissue and Fascia, Pelvic Region ØJQC
- **Rectopexy**
  - *see* Repair, Gastrointestinal System ØDQ
  - *see* Reposition, Gastrointestinal System ØDS
- **Rectoplasty**
  - *see* Repair, Gastrointestinal System ØDQ
  - *see* Supplement, Gastrointestinal System ØDU
- **Rectorrhaphy** *see* Repair, Gastrointestinal System ØDQ
- **Rectoscopy** ØDJD8ZZ
- **Rectosigmoid junction** *use* Colon, Sigmoid
- **Rectosigmoidectomy**
  - *see* Excision, Gastrointestinal System ØDB
  - *see* Resection, Gastrointestinal System ØDT
- **Rectostomy** *see* Drainage, Rectum ØD9P
- **Rectotomy** *see* Drainage, Rectum ØD9P
- **Rectus abdominis muscle**
  - *use* Muscle, Abdomen, Left
  - *use* Muscle, Abdomen, Right
- **Rectus femoris muscle**
  - *use* Muscle, Upper Leg, Left
  - *use* Muscle, Upper Leg, Right
- **Recurrent laryngeal nerve** *use* Nerve, Vagus
- **Reduction**
  - Dislocation *see* Reposition
  - Fracture *see* Reposition
  - Intussusception, intestinal *see* Reposition, Gastrointestinal System ØDS
  - Mammoplasty *see* Excision, Skin and Breast ØHB
  - Prolapse *see* Reposition
  - Torsion *see* Reposition
  - Volvulus, gastrointestinal *see* Reposition, Gastrointestinal System ØDS
- **Refusion** *see* Fusion
- **Rehabilitation**
  - *see* Activities of Daily Living Assessment, Rehabilitation FØ2
  - *see* Activities of Daily Living Treatment, Rehabilitation FØ8
  - *see* Caregiver Training, Rehabilitation FØF
  - *see* Cochlear Implant Treatment, Rehabilitation FØB
  - *see* Device Fitting, Rehabilitation FØD
  - *see* Hearing Treatment, Rehabilitation FØ9
  - *see* Motor Function Assessment, Rehabilitation FØ1
  - *see* Motor Treatment, Rehabilitation FØ7
  - *see* Speech Assessment, Rehabilitation FØØ
  - *see* Speech Treatment, Rehabilitation FØ6
  - *see* Vestibular Treatment, Rehabilitation FØC
- **Reimplantation**
  - *see* Reattachment
  - *see* Reposition
  - *see* Transfer
- **Reinforcement**
  - *see* Repair
  - *see* Supplement
- **Relaxation, scar tissue** *see* Release
- **Release**
  - Acetabulum
    - Left ØQN5
    - Right ØQN4
  - Adenoids ØCNQ
  - Ampulla of Vater ØFNC
  - Anal Sphincter ØDNR
  - Anterior Chamber
    - Left Ø8N33ZZ
    - Right Ø8N23ZZ
  - Anus ØDNQ

**Release** — *continued*
Aorta
Abdominal Ø4NØ
Thoracic
Ascending/Arch Ø2NX
Descending Ø2NW
Aortic Body ØGND
Appendix ØDNJ
Artery
Anterior Tibial
Left Ø4NQ
Right Ø4NP
Axillary
Left Ø3N6
Right Ø3N5
Brachial
Left Ø3N8
Right Ø3N7
Celiac Ø4N1
Colic
Left Ø4N7
Middle Ø4N8
Right Ø4N6
Common Carotid
Left Ø3NJ
Right Ø3NH
Common Iliac
Left Ø4ND
Right Ø4NC
Coronary
Four or More Arteries Ø2N3
One Artery Ø2NØ
Three Arteries Ø2N2
Two Arteries Ø2N1
External Carotid
Left Ø3NN
Right Ø3NM
External Iliac
Left Ø4NJ
Right Ø4NH
Face Ø3NR
Femoral
Left Ø4NL
Right Ø4NK
Foot
Left Ø4NW
Right Ø4NV
Gastric Ø4N2
Hand
Left Ø3NF
Right Ø3ND
Hepatic Ø4N3
Inferior Mesenteric Ø4NB
Innominate Ø3N2
Internal Carotid
Left Ø3NL
Right Ø3NK
Internal Iliac
Left Ø4NF
Right Ø4NE
Internal Mammary
Left Ø3N1
Right Ø3NØ
Intracranial Ø3NG
Lower Ø4NY
Peroneal
Left Ø4NU
Right Ø4NT
Popliteal
Left Ø4NN
Right Ø4NM
Posterior Tibial
Left Ø4NS
Right Ø4NR
Pulmonary
Left Ø2NR
Right Ø2NQ
Pulmonary Trunk Ø2NP
Radial
Left Ø3NC
Right Ø3NB
Renal
Left Ø4NA
Right Ø4N9
Splenic Ø4N4
Subclavian
Left Ø3N4
Right Ø3N3
Superior Mesenteric Ø4N5

**Release** — *continued*
Artery — *continued*
Temporal
Left Ø3NT
Right Ø3NS
Thyroid
Left Ø3NV
Right Ø3NU
Ulnar
Left Ø3NA
Right Ø3N9
Upper Ø3NY
Vertebral
Left Ø3NQ
Right Ø3NP
Atrium
Left Ø2N7
Right Ø2N6
Auditory Ossicle
Left Ø9NA
Right Ø9N9
Basal Ganglia ØØN8
Bladder ØTNB
Bladder Neck ØTNC
Bone
Ethmoid
Left ØNNG
Right ØNNF
Frontal ØNN1
Hyoid ØNNX
Lacrimal
Left ØNNJ
Right ØNNH
Nasal ØNNB
Occipital ØNN7
Palatine
Left ØNNL
Right ØNNK
Parietal
Left ØNN4
Right ØNN3
Pelvic
Left ØQN3
Right ØQN2
Sphenoid ØNNC
Temporal
Left ØNN6
Right ØNN5
Zygomatic
Left ØNNN
Right ØNNM
Brain ØØNØ
Breast
Bilateral ØHNV
Left ØHNU
Right ØHNT
Bronchus
Lingula ØBN9
Lower Lobe
Left ØBNB
Right ØBN6
Main
Left ØBN7
Right ØBN3
Middle Lobe, Right ØBN5
Upper Lobe
Left ØBN8
Right ØBN4
Buccal Mucosa ØCN4
Bursa and Ligament
Abdomen
Left ØMNJ
Right ØMNH
Ankle
Left ØMNR
Right ØMNQ
Elbow
Left ØMN4
Right ØMN3
Foot
Left ØMNT
Right ØMNS
Hand
Left ØMN8
Right ØMN7
Head and Neck ØMNØ
Hip
Left ØMNM
Right ØMNL

**Release** — *continued*
Bursa and Ligament — *continued*
Knee
Left ØMNP
Right ØMNN
Lower Extremity
Left ØMNW
Right ØMNV
Perineum ØMNK
Rib(s) ØMNG
Shoulder
Left ØMN2
Right ØMN1
Spine
Lower ØMND
Upper ØMNC
Sternum ØMNF
Upper Extremity
Left ØMNB
Right ØMN9
Wrist
Left ØMN6
Right ØMN5
Carina ØBN2
Carotid Bodies, Bilateral ØGN8
Carotid Body
Left ØGN6
Right ØGN7
Carpal
Left ØPNN
Right ØPNM
Cecum ØDNH
Cerebellum ØØNC
Cerebral Hemisphere ØØN7
Cerebral Meninges ØØN1
Cerebral Ventricle ØØN6
Cervix ØUNC
Chordae Tendineae Ø2N9
Choroid
Left Ø8NB
Right Ø8NA
Cisterna Chyli Ø7NL
Clavicle
Left ØPNB
Right ØPN9
Clitoris ØUNJ
Coccygeal Glomus ØGNB
Coccyx ØQNS
Colon
Ascending ØDNK
Descending ØDNM
Sigmoid ØDNN
Transverse ØDNL
Conduction Mechanism Ø2N8
Conjunctiva
Left Ø8NTXZZ
Right Ø8NSXZZ
Cord
Bilateral ØVNH
Left ØVNG
Right ØVNF
Cornea
Left Ø8N9XZZ
Right Ø8N8XZZ
Cul-de-sac ØUNF
Diaphragm ØBNT
Disc
Cervical Vertebral ØRN3
Cervicothoracic Vertebral ØRN5
Lumbar Vertebral ØSN2
Lumbosacral ØSN4
Thoracic Vertebral ØRN9
Thoracolumbar Vertebral ØRNB
Duct
Common Bile ØFN9
Cystic ØFN8
Hepatic
Common ØFN7
Left ØFN6
Right ØFN5
Lacrimal
Left Ø8NY
Right Ø8NX
Pancreatic ØFND
Accessory ØFNF
Parotid
Left ØCNC
Right ØCNB
Duodenum ØDN9

**Release** — *continued*
Dura Mater ØØN2
Ear
External
Left Ø9N1
Right Ø9NØ
External Auditory Canal
Left Ø9N4
Right Ø9N3
Inner
Left Ø9NE
Right Ø9ND
Middle
Left Ø9N6
Right Ø9N5
Epididymis
Bilateral ØVNL
Left ØVNK
Right ØVNJ
Epiglottis ØCNR
Esophagogastric Junction ØDN4
Esophagus ØDN5
Lower ØDN3
Middle ØDN2
Upper ØDN1
Eustachian Tube
Left Ø9NG
Right Ø9NF
Eye
Left Ø8N1XZZ
Right Ø8NØXZZ
Eyelid
Lower
Left Ø8NR
Right Ø8NQ
Upper
Left Ø8NP
Right Ø8NN
Fallopian Tube
Left ØUN6
Right ØUN5
Fallopian Tubes, Bilateral ØUN7
Femoral Shaft
Left ØQN9
Right ØQN8
Femur
Lower
Left ØQNC
Right ØQNB
Upper
Left ØQN7
Right ØQN6
Fibula
Left ØQNK
Right ØQNJ
Finger Nail ØHNQXZZ
Gallbladder ØFN4
Gingiva
Lower ØCN6
Upper ØCN5
Gland
Adrenal
Bilateral ØGN4
Left ØGN2
Right ØGN3
Lacrimal
Left Ø8NW
Right Ø8NV
Minor Salivary ØCNJ
Parotid
Left ØCN9
Right ØCN8
Pituitary ØGNØ
Sublingual
Left ØCNF
Right ØCND
Submaxillary
Left ØCNH
Right ØCNG
Vestibular ØUNL
Glenoid Cavity
Left ØPN8
Right ØPN7
Glomus Jugulare ØGNC
Humeral Head
Left ØPND
Right ØPNC
Humeral Shaft
Left ØPNG

**Release** — *continued*
Humeral Shaft — *continued*
Right ØPNF
Hymen ØUNK
Hypothalamus ØØNA
Ileocecal Valve ØDNC
Ileum ØDNB
Intestine
Large ØDNE
Left ØDNG
Right ØDNF
Small ØDN8
Iris
Left Ø8ND3ZZ
Right Ø8NC3ZZ
Jejunum ØDNA
Joint
Acromioclavicular
Left ØRNH
Right ØRNG
Ankle
Left ØSNG
Right ØSNF
Carpal
Left ØRNR
Right ØRNQ
Carpometacarpal
Left ØRNT
Right ØRNS
Cervical Vertebral ØRN1
Cervicothoracic Vertebral ØRN4
Coccygeal ØSN6
Elbow
Left ØRNM
Right ØRNL
Finger Phalangeal
Left ØRNX
Right ØRNW
Hip
Left ØSNB
Right ØSN9
Knee
Left ØSND
Right ØSNC
Lumbar Vertebral ØSNØ
Lumbosacral ØSN3
Metacarpophalangeal
Left ØRNV
Right ØRNU
Metatarsal-Phalangeal
Left ØSNN
Right ØSNM
Occipital-cervical ØRNØ
Sacrococcygeal ØSN5
Sacroiliac
Left ØSN8
Right ØSN7
Shoulder
Left ØRNK
Right ØRNJ
Sternoclavicular
Left ØRNF
Right ØRNE
Tarsal
Left ØSNJ
Right ØSNH
Tarsometatarsal
Left ØSNL
Right ØSNK
Temporomandibular
Left ØRND
Right ØRNC
Thoracic Vertebral ØRN6
Thoracolumbar Vertebral ØRNA
Toe Phalangeal
Left ØSNQ
Right ØSNP
Wrist
Left ØRNP
Right ØRNN
Kidney
Left ØTN1
Right ØTNØ
Kidney Pelvis
Left ØTN4
Right ØTN3
Larynx ØCNS
Lens
Left Ø8NK3ZZ

**Release** — *continued*
Lens — *continued*
Right Ø8NJ3ZZ
Lip
Lower ØCN1
Upper ØCNØ
Liver ØFNØ
Left Lobe ØFN2
Right Lobe ØFN1
Lung
Bilateral ØBNM
Left ØBNL
Lower Lobe
Left ØBNJ
Right ØBNF
Middle Lobe, Right ØBND
Right ØBNK
Upper Lobe
Left ØBNG
Right ØBNC
Lung Lingula ØBNH
Lymphatic
Aortic Ø7ND
Axillary
Left Ø7N6
Right Ø7N5
Head Ø7NØ
Inguinal
Left Ø7NJ
Right Ø7NH
Internal Mammary
Left Ø7N9
Right Ø7N8
Lower Extremity
Left Ø7NG
Right Ø7NF
Mesenteric Ø7NB
Neck
Left Ø7N2
Right Ø7N1
Pelvis Ø7NC
Thoracic Duct Ø7NK
Thorax Ø7N7
Upper Extremity
Left Ø7N4
Right Ø7N3
Mandible
Left ØNNV
Right ØNNT
Maxilla ØNNR
Medulla Oblongata ØØND
Mesentery ØDNV
Metacarpal
Left ØPNQ
Right ØPNP
Metatarsal
Left ØQNP
Right ØQNN
Muscle
Abdomen
Left ØKNL
Right ØKNK
Extraocular
Left Ø8NM
Right Ø8NL
Facial ØKN1
Foot
Left ØKNW
Right ØKNV
Hand
Left ØKND
Right ØKNC
Head ØKNØ
Hip
Left ØKNP
Right ØKNN
Lower Arm and Wrist
Left ØKNB
Right ØKN9
Lower Leg
Left ØKNT
Right ØKNS
Neck
Left ØKN3
Right ØKN2
Papillary Ø2ND
Perineum ØKNM
Shoulder
Left ØKN6

Index

Release — Release

Subterms under main terms may continue to next column or page

**Release** — *continued*
Muscle — *continued*
Shoulder — *continued*
Right ØKN5
Thorax
Left ØKNJ
Right ØKNH
Tongue, Palate, Pharynx ØKN4
Trunk
Left ØKNG
Right ØKNF
Upper Arm
Left ØKN8
Right ØKN7
Upper Leg
Left ØKNR
Right ØKNQ
Myocardial Bridge *see* Release, Artery, Coronary
Nasal Mucosa and Soft Tissue Ø9NK
Nasopharynx Ø9NN
Nerve
Abdominal Sympathetic Ø1NM
Abducens ØØNL
Accessory ØØNR
Acoustic ØØNN
Brachial Plexus Ø1N3
Cervical Ø1N1
Cervical Plexus Ø1NØ
Facial ØØNM
Femoral Ø1ND
Glossopharyngeal ØØNP
Head and Neck Sympathetic Ø1NK
Hypoglossal ØØNS
Lumbar Ø1NB
Lumbar Plexus Ø1N9
Lumbar Sympathetic Ø1NN
Lumbosacral Plexus Ø1NA
Median Ø1N5
Oculomotor ØØNH
Olfactory ØØNF
Optic ØØNG
Peroneal Ø1NH
Phrenic Ø1N2
Pudendal Ø1NC
Radial Ø1N6
Sacral Ø1NR
Sacral Plexus Ø1NQ
Sacral Sympathetic Ø1NP
Sciatic Ø1NF
Thoracic Ø1N8
Thoracic Sympathetic Ø1NL
Tibial Ø1NG
Trigeminal ØØNK
Trochlear ØØNJ
Ulnar Ø1N4
Vagus ØØNQ
Nipple
Left ØHNX
Right ØHNW
Omentum ØDNU
Orbit
Left ØNNQ
Right ØNNP
Ovary
Bilateral ØUN2
Left ØUN1
Right ØUNØ
Palate
Hard ØCN2
Soft ØCN3
Pancreas ØFNG
Para-aortic Body ØGN9
Paraganglion Extremity ØGNF
Parathyroid Gland ØGNR
Inferior
Left ØGNP
Right ØGNN
Multiple ØGNQ
Superior
Left ØGNM
Right ØGNL
Patella
Left ØQNF
Right ØQND
Penis ØVNS
Pericardium Ø2NN
Peritoneum ØDNW

**Release** — *continued*
Phalanx
Finger
Left ØPNV
Right ØPNT
Thumb
Left ØPNS
Right ØPNR
Toe
Left ØQNR
Right ØQNQ
Pharynx ØCNM
Pineal Body ØGN1
Pleura
Left ØBNP
Right ØBNN
Pons ØØNB
Prepuce ØVNT
Prostate ØVNØ
Radius
Left ØPNJ
Right ØPNH
Rectum ØDNP
Retina
Left Ø8NF3ZZ
Right Ø8NE3ZZ
Retinal Vessel
Left Ø8NH3ZZ
Right Ø8NG3ZZ
Ribs
1 to 2 ØPN1
3 or More ØPN2
Sacrum ØQN1
Scapula
Left ØPN6
Right ØPN5
Sclera
Left Ø8N7XZZ
Right Ø8N6XZZ
Scrotum ØVN5
Septum
Atrial Ø2N5
Nasal Ø9NM
Ventricular Ø2NM
Sinus
Accessory Ø9NP
Ethmoid
Left Ø9NV
Right Ø9NU
Frontal
Left Ø9NT
Right Ø9NS
Mastoid
Left Ø9NC
Right Ø9NB
Maxillary
Left Ø9NR
Right Ø9NQ
Sphenoid
Left Ø9NX
Right Ø9NW
Skin
Abdomen ØHN7XZZ
Back ØHN6XZZ
Buttock ØHN8XZZ
Chest ØHN5XZZ
Ear
Left ØHN3XZZ
Right ØHN2XZZ
Face ØHN1XZZ
Foot
Left ØHNNXZZ
Right ØHNMXZZ
Hand
Left ØHNGXZZ
Right ØHNFXZZ
Inguinal ØHNAXZZ
Lower Arm
Left ØHNEXZZ
Right ØHNDXZZ
Lower Leg
Left ØHNLXZZ
Right ØHNKXZZ
Neck ØHN4XZZ
Perineum ØHN9XZZ
Scalp ØHNØXZZ
Upper Arm
Left ØHNCXZZ
Right ØHNBXZZ

**Release** — *continued*
Skin — *continued*
Upper Leg
Left ØHNJXZZ
Right ØHNHXZZ
Spinal Cord
Cervical ØØNW
Lumbar ØØNY
Thoracic ØØNX
Spinal Meninges ØØNT
Spleen Ø7NP
Sternum ØPNØ
Stomach ØDN6
Pylorus ØDN7
Subcutaneous Tissue and Fascia
Abdomen ØJN8
Back ØJN7
Buttock ØJN9
Chest ØJN6
Face ØJN1
Foot
Left ØJNR
Right ØJNQ
Hand
Left ØJNK
Right ØJNJ
Lower Arm
Left ØJNH
Right ØJNG
Lower Leg
Left ØJNP
Right ØJNN
Neck
Left ØJN5
Right ØJN4
Pelvic Region ØJNC
Perineum ØJNB
Scalp ØJNØ
Upper Arm
Left ØJNF
Right ØJND
Upper Leg
Left ØJNM
Right ØJNL
Tarsal
Left ØQNM
Right ØQNL
Tendon
Abdomen
Left ØLNG
Right ØLNF
Ankle
Left ØLNT
Right ØLNS
Foot
Left ØLNW
Right ØLNV
Hand
Left ØLN8
Right ØLN7
Head and Neck ØLNØ
Hip
Left ØLNK
Right ØLNJ
Knee
Left ØLNR
Right ØLNQ
Lower Arm and Wrist
Left ØLN6
Right ØLN5
Lower Leg
Left ØLNP
Right ØLNN
Perineum ØLNH
Shoulder
Left ØLN2
Right ØLN1
Thorax
Left ØLND
Right ØLNC
Trunk
Left ØLNB
Right ØLN9
Upper Arm
Left ØLN4
Right ØLN3
Upper Leg
Left ØLNM
Right ØLNL

**Release** — *continued*
Testis
Bilateral ØVNC
Left ØVNB
Right ØVN9
Thalamus ØØN9
Thymus Ø7NM
Thyroid Gland ØGNK
Left Lobe ØGNG
Right Lobe ØGNH
Tibia
Left ØQNH
Right ØQNG
Toe Nail ØHNRXZZ
Tongue ØCN7
Tonsils ØCNP
Tooth
Lower ØCNX
Upper ØCNW
Trachea ØBN1
Tunica Vaginalis
Left ØVN7
Right ØVN6
Turbinate, Nasal Ø9NL
Tympanic Membrane
Left Ø9N8
Right Ø9N7
Ulna
Left ØPNL
Right ØPNK
Ureter
Left ØTN7
Right ØTN6
Urethra ØTND
Uterine Supporting Structure ØUN4
Uterus ØUN9
Uvula ØCNN
Vagina ØUNG
Valve
Aortic Ø2NF
Mitral Ø2NG
Pulmonary Ø2NH
Tricuspid Ø2NJ
Vas Deferens
Bilateral ØVNQ
Left ØVNP
Right ØVNN
Vein
Axillary
Left Ø5N8
Right Ø5N7
Azygos Ø5NØ
Basilic
Left Ø5NC
Right Ø5NB
Brachial
Left Ø5NA
Right Ø5N9
Cephalic
Left Ø5NF
Right Ø5ND
Colic Ø6N7
Common Iliac
Left Ø6ND
Right Ø6NC
Coronary Ø2N4
Esophageal Ø6N3
External Iliac
Left Ø6NG
Right Ø6NF
External Jugular
Left Ø5NQ
Right Ø5NP
Face
Left Ø5NV
Right Ø5NT
Femoral
Left Ø6NN
Right Ø6NM
Foot
Left Ø6NV
Right Ø6NT
Gastric Ø6N2
Hand
Left Ø5NH
Right Ø5NG
Hemiazygos Ø5N1
Hepatic Ø6N4

**Release** — *continued*
Vein — *continued*
Hypogastric
Left Ø6NJ
Right Ø6NH
Inferior Mesenteric Ø6N6
Innominate
Left Ø5N4
Right Ø5N3
Internal Jugular
Left Ø5NN
Right Ø5NM
Intracranial Ø5NL
Lower Ø6NY
Portal Ø6N8
Pulmonary
Left Ø2NT
Right Ø2NS
Renal
Left Ø6NB
Right Ø6N9
Saphenous
Left Ø6NQ
Right Ø6NP
Splenic Ø6N1
Subclavian
Left Ø5N6
Right Ø5N5
Superior Mesenteric Ø6N5
Upper Ø5NY
Vertebral
Left Ø5NS
Right Ø5NR
Vena Cava
Inferior Ø6NØ
Superior Ø2NV
Ventricle
Left Ø2NL
Right Ø2NK
Vertebra
Cervical ØPN3
Lumbar ØQNØ
Thoracic ØPN4
Vesicle
Bilateral ØVN3
Left ØVN2
Right ØVN1
Vitreous
Left Ø8N53ZZ
Right Ø8N43ZZ
Vocal Cord
Left ØCNV
Right ØCNT
Vulva ØUNM
**Relocation** *see* Reposition
**Removal**
Abdominal Wall 2W53X
Anorectal 2Y53X5Z
Arm
Lower
Left 2W5DX
Right 2W5CX
Upper
Left 2W5BX
Right 2W5AX
Back 2W55X
Chest Wall 2W54X
Ear 2Y52X5Z
Extremity
Lower
Left 2W5MX
Right 2W5LX
Upper
Left 2W59X
Right 2W58X
Face 2W51X
Finger
Left 2W5KX
Right 2W5JX
Foot
Left 2W5TX
Right 2W5SX
Genital Tract, Female 2Y54X5Z
Hand
Left 2W5FX
Right 2W5EX
Head 2W5ØX
Inguinal Region
Left 2W57X

**Removal** — *continued*
Inguinal Region — *continued*
Right 2W56X
Leg
Lower
Left 2W5RX
Right 2W5QX
Upper
Left 2W5PX
Right 2W5NX
Mouth and Pharynx 2Y5ØX5Z
Nasal 2Y51X5Z
Neck 2W52X
Thumb
Left 2W5HX
Right 2W5GX
Toe
Left 2W5VX
Right 2W5UX
Urethra 2Y55X5Z
**Removal of device from**
Abdominal Wall ØWPF
Acetabulum
Left ØQP5
Right ØQP4
Anal Sphincter ØDPR
Anus ØDPQ
Artery
Lower Ø4PY
Upper Ø3PY
Back
Lower ØWPL
Upper ØWPK
Bladder ØTPB
Bone
Facial ØNPW
Lower ØQPY
Nasal ØNPB
Pelvic
Left ØQP3
Right ØQP2
Upper ØPPY
Bone Marrow Ø7PT
Brain ØØPØ
Breast
Left ØHPU
Right ØHPT
Bursa and Ligament
Lower ØMPY
Upper ØMPX
Carpal
Left ØPPN
Right ØPPM
Cavity, Cranial ØWP1
Cerebral Ventricle ØØP6
Chest Wall ØWP8
Cisterna Chyli Ø7PL
Clavicle
Left ØPPB
Right ØPP9
Coccyx ØQPS
Diaphragm ØBPT
Disc
Cervical Vertebral ØRP3
Cervicothoracic Vertebral ØRP5
Lumbar Vertebral ØSP2
Lumbosacral ØSP4
Thoracic Vertebral ØRP9
Thoracolumbar Vertebral ØRPB
Duct
Hepatobiliary ØFPB
Pancreatic ØFPD
Ear
Left Ø9PJ
Right Ø9PH
Epididymis and Spermatic Cord ØVPM
Esophagus ØDP5
Extremity
Lower
Left ØYPB
Right ØYP9
Upper
Left ØXP7
Right ØXP6
Eye
Left Ø8P1
Right Ø8PØ
Face ØWP2
Fallopian Tube ØUP8

**Removal of device from** — *continued*
Femoral Shaft
Left ØQP9
Right ØQP8
Femur
Lower
Left ØQPC
Right ØQPB
Upper
Left ØQP7
Right ØQP6
Fibula
Left ØQPK
Right ØQPJ
Finger Nail ØHPQX
Gallbladder ØFP4
Gastrointestinal Tract ØWPP
Genitourinary Tract ØWPR
Gland
Adrenal ØGP5
Endocrine ØGPS
Pituitary ØGPØ
Salivary ØCPA
Glenoid Cavity
Left ØPP8
Right ØPP7
Great Vessel Ø2PY
Hair ØHPSX
Head ØWPØ
Heart Ø2PA
Humeral Head
Left ØPPD
Right ØPPC
Humeral Shaft
Left ØPPG
Right ØPPF
Intestinal Tract
Lower ØDPD
Upper ØDPØ
Jaw
Lower ØWP5
Upper ØWP4
Joint
Acromioclavicular
Left ØRPH
Right ØRPG
Ankle
Left ØSPG
Right ØSPF
Carpal
Left ØRPR
Right ØRPQ
Carpometacarpal
Left ØRPT
Right ØRPS
Cervical Vertebral ØRP1
Cervicothoracic Vertebral ØRP4
Coccygeal ØSP6
Elbow
Left ØRPM
Right ØRPL
Finger Phalangeal
Left ØRPX
Right ØRPW
Hip
Left ØSPB
Acetabular Surface ØSPE
Femoral Surface ØSPS
Right ØSP9
Acetabular Surface ØSPA
Femoral Surface ØSPR
Knee
Left ØSPD
Femoral Surface ØSPU
Tibial Surface ØSPW
Right ØSPC
Femoral Surface ØSPT
Tibial Surface ØSPV
Lumbar Vertebral ØSPØ
Lumbosacral ØSP3
Metacarpophalangeal
Left ØRPV
Right ØRPU
Metatarsal-Phalangeal
Left ØSPN
Right ØSPM
Occipital-cervical ØRPØ
Sacrococcygeal ØSP5

**Removal of device from** — *continued*
Joint — *continued*
Sacroiliac
Left ØSP8
Right ØSP7
Shoulder
Left ØRPK
Right ØRPJ
Sternoclavicular
Left ØRPF
Right ØRPE
Tarsal
Left ØSPJ
Right ØSPH
Tarsometatarsal
Left ØSPL
Right ØSPK
Temporomandibular
Left ØRPD
Right ØRPC
Thoracic Vertebral ØRP6
Thoracolumbar Vertebral ØRPA
Toe Phalangeal
Left ØSPQ
Right ØSPP
Wrist
Left ØRPP
Right ØRPN
Kidney ØTP5
Larynx ØCPS
Lens
Left Ø8PK3
Right Ø8PJ3
Liver ØFPØ
Lung
Left ØBPL
Right ØBPK
Lymphatic Ø7PN
Thoracic Duct Ø7PK
Mediastinum ØWPC
Mesentery ØDPV
Metacarpal
Left ØPPQ
Right ØPPP
Metatarsal
Left ØQPP
Right ØQPN
Mouth and Throat ØCPY
Muscle
Extraocular
Left Ø8PM
Right Ø8PL
Lower ØKPY
Upper ØKPX
Nasal Mucosa and Soft Tissue Ø9PK
Neck ØWP6
Nerve
Cranial ØØPE
Peripheral Ø1PY
Omentum ØDPU
Ovary ØUP3
Pancreas ØFPG
Parathyroid Gland ØGPR
Patella
Left ØQPF
Right ØQPD
Pelvic Cavity ØWPJ
Penis ØVPS
Pericardial Cavity ØWPD
Perineum
Female ØWPN
Male ØWPM
Peritoneal Cavity ØWPG
Peritoneum ØDPW
Phalanx
Finger
Left ØPPV
Right ØPPT
Thumb
Left ØPPS
Right ØPPR
Toe
Left ØQPR
Right ØQPQ
Pineal Body ØGP1
Pleura ØBPQ
Pleural Cavity
Left ØWPB
Right ØWP9

**Removal of device from** — *continued*
Products of Conception 1ØPØ
Prostate and Seminal Vesicles ØVP4
Radius
Left ØPPJ
Right ØPPH
Rectum ØDPP
Respiratory Tract ØWPQ
Retroperitoneum ØWPH
Ribs
1 to 2 ØPP1
3 or More ØPP2
Sacrum ØQP1
Scapula
Left ØPP6
Right ØPP5
Scrotum and Tunica Vaginalis ØVP8
Sinus Ø9PY
Skin ØHPPX
Skull ØNPØ
Spinal Canal ØØPU
Spinal Cord ØØPV
Spleen Ø7PP
Sternum ØPPØ
Stomach ØDP6
Subcutaneous Tissue and Fascia
Head and Neck ØJPS
Lower Extremity ØJPW
Trunk ØJPT
Upper Extremity ØJPV
Tarsal
Left ØQPM
Right ØQPL
Tendon
Lower ØLPY
Upper ØLPX
Testis ØVPD
Thymus Ø7PM
Thyroid Gland ØGPK
Tibia
Left ØQPH
Right ØQPG
Toe Nail ØHPRX
Trachea ØBP1
Tracheobronchial Tree ØBPØ
Tympanic Membrane
Left Ø9P8
Right Ø9P7
Ulna
Left ØPPL
Right ØPPK
Ureter ØTP9
Urethra ØTPD
Uterus and Cervix ØUPD
Vagina and Cul-de-sac ØUPH
Vas Deferens ØVPR
Vein
Azygos Ø5PØ
Innominate
Left Ø5P4
Right Ø5P3
Lower Ø6PY
Upper Ø5PY
Vertebra
Cervical ØPP3
Lumbar ØQPØ
Thoracic ØPP4
Vulva ØUPM
**Renal calyx**
*use* Kidney
*use* Kidney, Left
*use* Kidney, Right
*use* Kidneys, Bilateral
**Renal capsule**
*use* Kidney
*use* Kidney, Left
*use* Kidney, Right
*use* Kidneys, Bilateral
**Renal cortex**
*use* Kidney
*use* Kidney, Left
*use* Kidney, Right
*use* Kidneys, Bilateral
**Renal dialysis** *see* Performance, Urinary 5A1D
**Renal plexus** *use* Nerve, Abdominal Sympathetic
**Renal segment**
*use* Kidney
*use* Kidney, Left

**Renal segment** — *continued*
*use* Kidney, Right
*use* Kidneys, Bilateral
**Renal segmental artery**
*use* Artery, Renal, Left
*use* Artery, Renal, Right
**Reopening, operative site**
Control of bleeding *see* Control bleeding in
Inspection only *see* Inspection
**Repair**
Abdominal Wall ØWQF
Acetabulum
Left ØQQ5
Right ØQQ4
Adenoids ØCQQ
Ampulla of Vater ØFQC
Anal Sphincter ØDQR
Ankle Region
Left ØYQL
Right ØYQK
Anterior Chamber
Left Ø8Q33ZZ
Right Ø8Q23ZZ
Anus ØDQQ
Aorta
Abdominal Ø4QØ
Thoracic
Ascending/Arch Ø2QX
Descending Ø2QW
Aortic Body ØGQD
Appendix ØDQJ
Arm
Lower
Left ØXQF
Right ØXQD
Upper
Left ØXQ9
Right ØXQ8
Artery
Anterior Tibial
Left Ø4QQ
Right Ø4QP
Axillary
Left Ø3Q6
Right Ø3Q5
Brachial
Left Ø3Q8
Right Ø3Q7
Celiac Ø4Q1
Colic
Left Ø4Q7
Middle Ø4Q8
Right Ø4Q6
Common Carotid
Left Ø3QJ
Right Ø3QH
Common Iliac
Left Ø4QD
Right Ø4QC
Coronary
Four or More Arteries Ø2Q3
One Artery Ø2QØ
Three Arteries Ø2Q2
Two Arteries Ø2Q1
External Carotid
Left Ø3QN
Right Ø3QM
External Iliac
Left Ø4QJ
Right Ø4QH
Face Ø3QR
Femoral
Left Ø4QL
Right Ø4QK
Foot
Left Ø4QW
Right Ø4QV
Gastric Ø4Q2
Hand
Left Ø3QF
Right Ø3QD
Hepatic Ø4Q3
Inferior Mesenteric Ø4QB
Innominate Ø3Q2
Internal Carotid
Left Ø3QL
Right Ø3QK

**Repair** — *continued*
Artery — *continued*
Internal Iliac
Left Ø4QF
Right Ø4QE
Internal Mammary
Left Ø3Q1
Right Ø3QØ
Intracranial Ø3QG
Lower Ø4QY
Peroneal
Left Ø4QU
Right Ø4QT
Popliteal
Left Ø4QN
Right Ø4QM
Posterior Tibial
Left Ø4QS
Right Ø4QR
Pulmonary
Left Ø2QR
Right Ø2QQ
Pulmonary Trunk Ø2QP
Radial
Left Ø3QC
Right Ø3QB
Renal
Left Ø4QA
Right Ø4Q9
Splenic Ø4Q4
Subclavian
Left Ø3Q4
Right Ø3Q3
Superior Mesenteric Ø4Q5
Temporal
Left Ø3QT
Right Ø3QS
Thyroid
Left Ø3QV
Right Ø3QU
Ulnar
Left Ø3QA
Right Ø3Q9
Upper Ø3QY
Vertebral
Left Ø3QQ
Right Ø3QP
Atrium
Left Ø2Q7
Right Ø2Q6
Auditory Ossicle
Left Ø9QA
Right Ø9Q9
Axilla
Left ØXQ5
Right ØXQ4
Back
Lower ØWQL
Upper ØWQK
Basal Ganglia ØØQ8
Bladder ØTQB
Bladder Neck ØTQC
Bone
Ethmoid
Left ØNQG
Right ØNQF
Frontal ØNQ1
Hyoid ØNQX
Lacrimal
Left ØNQJ
Right ØNQH
Nasal ØNQB
Occipital ØNQ7
Palatine
Left ØNQL
Right ØNQK
Parietal
Left ØNQ4
Right ØNQ3
Pelvic
Left ØQQ3
Right ØQQ2
Sphenoid ØNQC
Temporal
Left ØNQ6
Right ØNQ5
Zygomatic
Left ØNQN
Right ØNQM

**Repair** — *continued*
Brain ØØQØ
Breast
Bilateral ØHQV
Left ØHQU
Right ØHQT
Supernumerary ØHQY
Bronchus
Lingula ØBQ9
Lower Lobe
Left ØBQB
Right ØBQ6
Main
Left ØBQ7
Right ØBQ3
Middle Lobe, Right ØBQ5
Upper Lobe
Left ØBQ8
Right ØBQ4
Buccal Mucosa ØCQ4
Bursa and Ligament
Abdomen
Left ØMQJ
Right ØMQH
Ankle
Left ØMQR
Right ØMQQ
Elbow
Left ØMQ4
Right ØMQ3
Foot
Left ØMQT
Right ØMQS
Hand
Left ØMQ8
Right ØMQ7
Head and Neck ØMQØ
Hip
Left ØMQM
Right ØMQL
Knee
Left ØMQP
Right ØMQN
Lower Extremity
Left ØMQW
Right ØMQV
Perineum ØMQK
Rib(s) ØMQG
Shoulder
Left ØMQ2
Right ØMQ1
Spine
Lower ØMQD
Upper ØMQC
Sternum ØMQF
Upper Extremity
Left ØMQB
Right ØMQ9
Wrist
Left ØMQ6
Right ØMQ5
Buttock
Left ØYQ1
Right ØYQØ
Carina ØBQ2
Carotid Bodies, Bilateral ØGQ8
Carotid Body
Left ØGQ6
Right ØGQ7
Carpal
Left ØPQN
Right ØPQM
Cecum ØDQH
Cerebellum ØØQC
Cerebral Hemisphere ØØQ7
Cerebral Meninges ØØQ1
Cerebral Ventricle ØØQ6
Cervix ØUQC
Chest Wall ØWQ8
Chordae Tendineae Ø2Q9
Choroid
Left Ø8QB
Right Ø8QA
Cisterna Chyli Ø7QL
Clavicle
Left ØPQB
Right ØPQ9
Clitoris ØUQJ
Coccygeal Glomus ØGQB

**Repair** — *continued*
Coccyx ØQQS
Colon
Ascending ØDQK
Descending ØDQM
Sigmoid ØDQN
Transverse ØDQL
Conduction Mechanism Ø2Q8
Conjunctiva
Left Ø8QTXZZ
Right Ø8QSXZZ
Cord
Bilateral ØVQH
Left ØVQG
Right ØVQF
Cornea
Left Ø8Q9XZZ
Right Ø8Q8XZZ
Cul-de-sac ØUQF
Diaphragm ØBQT
Disc
Cervical Vertebral ØRQ3
Cervicothoracic Vertebral ØRQ5
Lumbar Vertebral ØSQ2
Lumbosacral ØSQ4
Thoracic Vertebral ØRQ9
Thoracolumbar Vertebral ØRQB
Duct
Common Bile ØFQ9
Cystic ØFQ8
Hepatic
Common ØFQ7
Left ØFQ6
Right ØFQ5
Lacrimal
Left Ø8QY
Right Ø8QX
Pancreatic ØFQD
Accessory ØFQF
Parotid
Left ØCQC
Right ØCQB
Duodenum ØDQ9
Dura Mater ØØQ2
Ear
External
Bilateral Ø9Q2
Left Ø9Q1
Right Ø9QØ
External Auditory Canal
Left Ø9Q4
Right Ø9Q3
Inner
Left Ø9QE
Right Ø9QD
Middle
Left Ø9Q6
Right Ø9Q5
Elbow Region
Left ØXQC
Right ØXQB
Epididymis
Bilateral ØVQL
Left ØVQK
Right ØVQJ
Epiglottis ØCQR
Esophagogastric Junction ØDQ4
Esophagus ØDQ5
Lower ØDQ3
Middle ØDQ2
Upper ØDQ1
Eustachian Tube
Left Ø9QG
Right Ø9QF
Extremity
Lower
Left ØYQB
Right ØYQ9
Upper
Left ØXQ7
Right ØXQ6
Eye
Left Ø8Q1XZZ
Right Ø8QØXZZ
Eyelid
Lower
Left Ø8QR
Right Ø8QQ

**Repair** — *continued*
Eyelid — *continued*
Upper
Left Ø8QP
Right Ø8QN
Face ØWQ2
Fallopian Tube
Left ØUQ6
Right ØUQ5
Fallopian Tubes, Bilateral ØUQ7
Femoral Region
Bilateral ØYQE
Left ØYQ8
Right ØYQ7
Femoral Shaft
Left ØQQ9
Right ØQQ8
Femur
Lower
Left ØQQC
Right ØQQB
Upper
Left ØQQ7
Right ØQQ6
Fibula
Left ØQQK
Right ØQQJ
Finger
Index
Left ØXQP
Right ØXQN
Little
Left ØXQW
Right ØXQV
Middle
Left ØXQR
Right ØXQQ
Ring
Left ØXQT
Right ØXQS
Finger Nail ØHQQXZZ
Floor of mouth *see* Repair, Oral Cavity and Throat ØWQ3
Foot
Left ØYQN
Right ØYQM
Gallbladder ØFQ4
Gingiva
Lower ØCQ6
Upper ØCQ5
Gland
Adrenal
Bilateral ØGQ4
Left ØGQ2
Right ØGQ3
Lacrimal
Left Ø8QW
Right Ø8QV
Minor Salivary ØCQJ
Parotid
Left ØCQ9
Right ØCQ8
Pituitary ØGQØ
Sublingual
Left ØCQF
Right ØCQD
Submaxillary
Left ØCQH
Right ØCQG
Vestibular ØUQL
Glenoid Cavity
Left ØPQ8
Right ØPQ7
Glomus Jugulare ØGQC
Hand
Left ØXQK
Right ØXQJ
Head ØWQØ
Heart Ø2QA
Left Ø2QC
Right Ø2QB
Humeral Head
Left ØPQD
Right ØPQC
Humeral Shaft
Left ØPQG
Right ØPQF
Hymen ØUQK
Hypothalamus ØØQA

**Repair** — *continued*
Ileocecal Valve ØDQC
Ileum ØDQB
Inguinal Region
Bilateral ØYQA
Left ØYQ6
Right ØYQ5
Intestine
Large ØDQE
Left ØDQG
Right ØDQF
Small ØDQ8
Iris
Left Ø8QD3ZZ
Right Ø8QC3ZZ
Jaw
Lower ØWQ5
Upper ØWQ4
Jejunum ØDQA
Joint
Acromioclavicular
Left ØRQH
Right ØRQG
Ankle
Left ØSQG
Right ØSQF
Carpal
Left ØRQR
Right ØRQQ
Carpometacarpal
Left ØRQT
Right ØRQS
Cervical Vertebral ØRQ1
Cervicothoracic Vertebral ØRQ4
Coccygeal ØSQ6
Elbow
Left ØRQM
Right ØRQL
Finger Phalangeal
Left ØRQX
Right ØRQW
Hip
Left ØSQB
Right ØSQ9
Knee
Left ØSQD
Right ØSQC
Lumbar Vertebral ØSQØ
Lumbosacral ØSQ3
Metacarpophalangeal
Left ØRQV
Right ØRQU
Metatarsal-Phalangeal
Left ØSQN
Right ØSQM
Occipital-cervical ØRQØ
Sacrococcygeal ØSQ5
Sacroiliac
Left ØSQ8
Right ØSQ7
Shoulder
Left ØRQK
Right ØRQJ
Sternoclavicular
Left ØRQF
Right ØRQE
Tarsal
Left ØSQJ
Right ØSQH
Tarsometatarsal
Left ØSQL
Right ØSQK
Temporomandibular
Left ØRQD
Right ØRQC
Thoracic Vertebral ØRQ6
Thoracolumbar Vertebral ØRQA
Toe Phalangeal
Left ØSQQ
Right ØSQP
Wrist
Left ØRQP
Right ØRQN
Kidney
Left ØTQ1
Right ØTQØ
Kidney Pelvis
Left ØTQ4
Right ØTQ3

**Repair** — *continued*
- Knee Region
  - Left ØYQG
  - Right ØYQF
- Larynx ØCQS
- Leg
  - Lower
    - Left ØYQJ
    - Right ØYQH
  - Upper
    - Left ØYQD
    - Right ØYQC
- Lens
  - Left Ø8QK3ZZ
  - Right Ø8QJ3ZZ
- Lip
  - Lower ØCQ1
  - Upper ØCQØ
- Liver ØFQØ
  - Left Lobe ØFQ2
  - Right Lobe ØFQ1
- Lung
  - Bilateral ØBQM
  - Left ØBQL
  - Lower Lobe
    - Left ØBQJ
    - Right ØBQF
  - Middle Lobe, Right ØBQD
  - Right ØBQK
  - Upper Lobe
    - Left ØBQG
    - Right ØBQC
- Lung Lingula ØBQH
- Lymphatic
  - Aortic Ø7QD
  - Axillary
    - Left Ø7Q6
    - Right Ø7Q5
  - Head Ø7QØ
  - Inguinal
    - Left Ø7QJ
    - Right Ø7QH
  - Internal Mammary
    - Left Ø7Q9
    - Right Ø7Q8
  - Lower Extremity
    - Left Ø7QG
    - Right Ø7QF
  - Mesenteric Ø7QB
  - Neck
    - Left Ø7Q2
    - Right Ø7Q1
  - Pelvis Ø7QC
  - Thoracic Duct Ø7QK
  - Thorax Ø7Q7
  - Upper Extremity
    - Left Ø7Q4
    - Right Ø7Q3
- Mandible
  - Left ØNQV
  - Right ØNQT
- Maxilla ØNQR
- Mediastinum ØWQC
- Medulla Oblongata ØØQD
- Mesentery ØDQV
- Metacarpal
  - Left ØPQQ
  - Right ØPQP
- Metatarsal
  - Left ØQQP
  - Right ØQQN
- Muscle
  - Abdomen
    - Left ØKQL
    - Right ØKQK
  - Extraocular
    - Left Ø8QM
    - Right Ø8QL
  - Facial ØKQ1
  - Foot
    - Left ØKQW
    - Right ØKQV
  - Hand
    - Left ØKQD
    - Right ØKQC
  - Head ØKQØ
  - Hip
    - Left ØKQP
    - Right ØKQN

**Repair** — *continued*
- Muscle — *continued*
  - Lower Arm and Wrist
    - Left ØKQB
    - Right ØKQ9
  - Lower Leg
    - Left ØKQT
    - Right ØKQS
  - Neck
    - Left ØKQ3
    - Right ØKQ2
  - Papillary Ø2QD
  - Perineum ØKQM
  - Shoulder
    - Left ØKQ6
    - Right ØKQ5
  - Thorax
    - Left ØKQJ
    - Right ØKQH
  - Tongue, Palate, Pharynx ØKQ4
  - Trunk
    - Left ØKQG
    - Right ØKQF
  - Upper Arm
    - Left ØKQ8
    - Right ØKQ7
  - Upper Leg
    - Left ØKQR
    - Right ØKQQ
- Nasal Mucosa and Soft Tissue Ø9QK
- Nasopharynx Ø9QN
- Neck ØWQ6
- Nerve
  - Abdominal Sympathetic Ø1QM
  - Abducens ØØQL
  - Accessory ØØQR
  - Acoustic ØØQN
  - Brachial Plexus Ø1Q3
  - Cervical Ø1Q1
  - Cervical Plexus Ø1QØ
  - Facial ØØQM
  - Femoral Ø1QD
  - Glossopharyngeal ØØQP
  - Head and Neck Sympathetic Ø1QK
  - Hypoglossal ØØQS
  - Lumbar Ø1QB
  - Lumbar Plexus Ø1Q9
  - Lumbar Sympathetic Ø1QN
  - Lumbosacral Plexus Ø1QA
  - Median Ø1Q5
  - Oculomotor ØØQH
  - Olfactory ØØQF
  - Optic ØØQG
  - Peroneal Ø1QH
  - Phrenic Ø1Q2
  - Pudendal Ø1QC
  - Radial Ø1Q6
  - Sacral Ø1QR
  - Sacral Plexus Ø1QQ
  - Sacral Sympathetic Ø1QP
  - Sciatic Ø1QF
  - Thoracic Ø1Q8
  - Thoracic Sympathetic Ø1QL
  - Tibial Ø1QG
  - Trigeminal ØØQK
  - Trochlear ØØQJ
  - Ulnar Ø1Q4
  - Vagus ØØQQ
- Nipple
  - Left ØHQX
  - Right ØHQW
- Omentum ØDQU
- Oral Cavity and Throat ØWQ3
- Orbit
  - Left ØNQQ
  - Right ØNQP
- Ovary
  - Bilateral ØUQ2
  - Left ØUQ1
  - Right ØUQØ
- Palate
  - Hard ØCQ2
  - Soft ØCQ3
- Pancreas ØFQG
- Para-aortic Body ØGQ9
- Paraganglion Extremity ØGQF
- Parathyroid Gland ØGQR
  - Inferior
    - Left ØGQP

**Repair** — *continued*
- Parathyroid Gland — *continued*
  - Inferior — *continued*
    - Right ØGQN
  - Multiple ØGQQ
  - Superior
    - Left ØGQM
    - Right ØGQL
- Patella
  - Left ØQQF
  - Right ØQQD
- Penis ØVQS
- Pericardium Ø2QN
- Perineum
  - Female ØWQN
  - Male ØWQM
- Peritoneum ØDQW
- Phalanx
  - Finger
    - Left ØPQV
    - Right ØPQT
  - Thumb
    - Left ØPQS
    - Right ØPQR
  - Toe
    - Left ØQQR
    - Right ØQQQ
- Pharynx ØCQM
- Pineal Body ØGQ1
- Pleura
  - Left ØBQP
  - Right ØBQN
- Pons ØØQB
- Prepuce ØVQT
- Products of Conception 1ØQØ
- Prostate ØVQØ
- Radius
  - Left ØPQJ
  - Right ØPQH
- Rectum ØDQP
- Retina
  - Left Ø8QF3ZZ
  - Right Ø8QE3ZZ
- Retinal Vessel
  - Left Ø8QH3ZZ
  - Right Ø8QG3ZZ
- Ribs
  - 1 to 2 ØPQ1
  - 3 or More ØPQ2
- Sacrum ØQQ1
- Scapula
  - Left ØPQ6
  - Right ØPQ5
- Sclera
  - Left Ø8Q7XZZ
  - Right Ø8Q6XZZ
- Scrotum ØVQ5
- Septum
  - Atrial Ø2Q5
  - Nasal Ø9QM
  - Ventricular Ø2QM
- Shoulder Region
  - Left ØXQ3
  - Right ØXQ2
- Sinus
  - Accessory Ø9QP
  - Ethmoid
    - Left Ø9QV
    - Right Ø9QU
  - Frontal
    - Left Ø9QT
    - Right Ø9QS
  - Mastoid
    - Left Ø9QC
    - Right Ø9QB
  - Maxillary
    - Left Ø9QR
    - Right Ø9QQ
  - Sphenoid
    - Left Ø9QX
    - Right Ø9QW
- Skin
  - Abdomen ØHQ7XZZ
  - Back ØHQ6XZZ
  - Buttock ØHQ8XZZ
  - Chest ØHQ5XZZ
  - Ear
    - Left ØHQ3XZZ
    - Right ØHQ2XZZ

**Repair** — *continued*
Skin — *continued*
Face ØHQ1XZZ
Foot
Left ØHQNXZZ
Right ØHQMXZZ
Hand
Left ØHQGXZZ
Right ØHQFXZZ
Inguinal ØHQAXZZ
Lower Arm
Left ØHQEXZZ
Right ØHQDXZZ
Lower Leg
Left ØHQLXZZ
Right ØHQKXZZ
Neck ØHQ4XZZ
Perineum ØHQ9XZZ
Scalp ØHQØXZZ
Upper Arm
Left ØHQCXZZ
Right ØHQBXZZ
Upper Leg
Left ØHQJXZZ
Right ØHQHXZZ
Skull ØNQØ
Spinal Cord
Cervical ØØQW
Lumbar ØØQY
Thoracic ØØQX
Spinal Meninges ØØQT
Spleen Ø7QP
Sternum ØPQØ
Stomach ØDQ6
Pylorus ØDQ7
Subcutaneous Tissue and Fascia
Abdomen ØJQ8
Back ØJQ7
Buttock ØJQ9
Chest ØJQ6
Face ØJQ1
Foot
Left ØJQR
Right ØJQQ
Hand
Left ØJQK
Right ØJQJ
Lower Arm
Left ØJQH
Right ØJQG
Lower Leg
Left ØJQP
Right ØJQN
Neck
Left ØJQ5
Right ØJQ4
Pelvic Region ØJQC
Perineum ØJQB
Scalp ØJQØ
Upper Arm
Left ØJQF
Right ØJQD
Upper Leg
Left ØJQM
Right ØJQL
Tarsal
Left ØQQM
Right ØQQL
Tendon
Abdomen
Left ØLQG
Right ØLQF
Ankle
Left ØLQT
Right ØLQS
Foot
Left ØLQW
Right ØLQV
Hand
Left ØLQ8
Right ØLQ7
Head and Neck ØLQØ
Hip
Left ØLQK
Right ØLQJ
Knee
Left ØLQR
Right ØLQQ

**Repair** — *continued*
Tendon — *continued*
Lower Arm and Wrist
Left ØLQ6
Right ØLQ5
Lower Leg
Left ØLQP
Right ØLQN
Perineum ØLQH
Shoulder
Left ØLQ2
Right ØLQ1
Thorax
Left ØLQD
Right ØLQC
Trunk
Left ØLQB
Right ØLQ9
Upper Arm
Left ØLQ4
Right ØLQ3
Upper Leg
Left ØLQM
Right ØLQL
Testis
Bilateral ØVQC
Left ØVQB
Right ØVQ9
Thalamus ØØQ9
Thumb
Left ØXQM
Right ØXQL
Thymus Ø7QM
Thyroid Gland ØGQK
Left Lobe ØGQG
Right Lobe ØGQH
Thyroid Gland Isthmus ØGQJ
Tibia
Left ØQQH
Right ØQQG
Toe
1st
Left ØYQQ
Right ØYQP
2nd
Left ØYQS
Right ØYQR
3rd
Left ØYQU
Right ØYQT
4th
Left ØYQW
Right ØYQV
5th
Left ØYQY
Right ØYQX
Toe Nail ØHQRXZZ
Tongue ØCQ7
Tonsils ØCQP
Tooth
Lower ØCQX
Upper ØCQW
Trachea ØBQ1
Tunica Vaginalis
Left ØVQ7
Right ØVQ6
Turbinate, Nasal Ø9QL
Tympanic Membrane
Left Ø9Q8
Right Ø9Q7
Ulna
Left ØPQL
Right ØPQK
Ureter
Left ØTQ7
Right ØTQ6
Urethra ØTQD
Uterine Supporting Structure ØUQ4
Uterus ØUQ9
Uvula ØCQN
Vagina ØUQG
Valve
Aortic Ø2QF
Mitral Ø2QG
Pulmonary Ø2QH
Tricuspid Ø2QJ
Vas Deferens
Bilateral ØVQQ
Left ØVQP

**Repair** — *continued*
Vas Deferens — *continued*
Right ØVQN
Vein
Axillary
Left Ø5Q8
Right Ø5Q7
Azygos Ø5QØ
Basilic
Left Ø5QC
Right Ø5QB
Brachial
Left Ø5QA
Right Ø5Q9
Cephalic
Left Ø5QF
Right Ø5QD
Colic Ø6Q7
Common Iliac
Left Ø6QD
Right Ø6QC
Coronary Ø2Q4
Esophageal Ø6Q3
External Iliac
Left Ø6QG
Right Ø6QF
External Jugular
Left Ø5QQ
Right Ø5QP
Face
Left Ø5QV
Right Ø5QT
Femoral
Left Ø6QN
Right Ø6QM
Foot
Left Ø6QV
Right Ø6QT
Gastric Ø6Q2
Hand
Left Ø5QH
Right Ø5QG
Hemiazygos Ø5Q1
Hepatic Ø6Q4
Hypogastric
Left Ø6QJ
Right Ø6QH
Inferior Mesenteric Ø6Q6
Innominate
Left Ø5Q4
Right Ø5Q3
Internal Jugular
Left Ø5QN
Right Ø5QM
Intracranial Ø5QL
Lower Ø6QY
Portal Ø6Q8
Pulmonary
Left Ø2QT
Right Ø2QS
Renal
Left Ø6QB
Right Ø6Q9
Saphenous
Left Ø6QQ
Right Ø6QP
Splenic Ø6Q1
Subclavian
Left Ø5Q6
Right Ø5Q5
Superior Mesenteric Ø6Q5
Upper Ø5QY
Vertebral
Left Ø5QS
Right Ø5QR
Vena Cava
Inferior Ø6QØ
Superior Ø2QV
Ventricle
Left Ø2QL
Right Ø2QK
Vertebra
Cervical ØPQ3
Lumbar ØQQØ
Thoracic ØPQ4
Vesicle
Bilateral ØVQ3
Left ØVQ2
Right ØVQ1

**Repair** — *continued*
Vitreous
Left Ø8Q53ZZ
Right Ø8Q43ZZ
Vocal Cord
Left ØCQV
Right ØCQT
Vulva ØUQM
Wrist Region
Left ØXQH
Right ØXQG
**Repair, obstetric laceration, periurethral** ØUQMXZZ
**Replacement**
Acetabulum
Left ØQR5
Right ØQR4
Ampulla of Vater ØFRC
Anal Sphincter ØDRR
Aorta
Abdominal Ø4RØ
Thoracic
Ascending/Arch Ø2RX
Descending Ø2RW
Artery
Anterior Tibial
Left Ø4RQ
Right Ø4RP
Axillary
Left Ø3R6
Right Ø3R5
Brachial
Left Ø3R8
Right Ø3R7
Celiac Ø4R1
Colic
Left Ø4R7
Middle Ø4R8
Right Ø4R6
Common Carotid
Left Ø3RJ
Right Ø3RH
Common Iliac
Left Ø4RD
Right Ø4RC
External Carotid
Left Ø3RN
Right Ø3RM
External Iliac
Left Ø4RJ
Right Ø4RH
Face Ø3RR
Femoral
Left Ø4RL
Right Ø4RK
Foot
Left Ø4RW
Right Ø4RV
Gastric Ø4R2
Hand
Left Ø3RF
Right Ø3RD
Hepatic Ø4R3
Inferior Mesenteric Ø4RB
Innominate Ø3R2
Internal Carotid
Left Ø3RL
Right Ø3RK
Internal Iliac
Left Ø4RF
Right Ø4RE
Internal Mammary
Left Ø3R1
Right Ø3RØ
Intracranial Ø3RG
Lower Ø4RY
Peroneal
Left Ø4RU
Right Ø4RT
Popliteal
Left Ø4RN
Right Ø4RM
Posterior Tibial
Left Ø4RS
Right Ø4RR
Pulmonary
Left Ø2RR
Right Ø2RQ
Pulmonary Trunk Ø2RP

**Replacement** — *continued*
Artery — *continued*
Radial
Left Ø3RC
Right Ø3RB
Renal
Left Ø4RA
Right Ø4R9
Splenic Ø4R4
Subclavian
Left Ø3R4
Right Ø3R3
Superior Mesenteric Ø4R5
Temporal
Left Ø3RT
Right Ø3RS
Thyroid
Left Ø3RV
Right Ø3RU
Ulnar
Left Ø3RA
Right Ø3R9
Upper Ø3RY
Vertebral
Left Ø3RQ
Right Ø3RP
Atrium
Left Ø2R7
Right Ø2R6
Auditory Ossicle
Left Ø9RAØ
Right Ø9R9Ø
Bladder ØTRB
Bladder Neck ØTRC
Bone
Ethmoid
Left ØNRG
Right ØNRF
Frontal ØNR1
Hyoid ØNRX
Lacrimal
Left ØNRJ
Right ØNRH
Nasal ØNRB
Occipital ØNR7
Palatine
Left ØNRL
Right ØNRK
Parietal
Left ØNR4
Right ØNR3
Pelvic
Left ØQR3
Right ØQR2
Sphenoid ØNRC
Temporal
Left ØNR6
Right ØNR5
Zygomatic
Left ØNRN
Right ØNRM
Breast
Bilateral ØHRV
Left ØHRU
Right ØHRT
Bronchus
Lingula ØBR9
Lower Lobe
Left ØBRB
Right ØBR6
Main
Left ØBR7
Right ØBR3
Middle Lobe, Right ØBR5
Upper Lobe
Left ØBR8
Right ØBR4
Buccal Mucosa ØCR4
Bursa and Ligament
Abdomen
Left ØMRJ
Right ØMRH
Ankle
Left ØMRR
Right ØMRQ
Elbow
Left ØMR4
Right ØMR3

**Replacement** — *continued*
Bursa and Ligament — *continued*
Foot
Left ØMRT
Right ØMRS
Hand
Left ØMR8
Right ØMR7
Head and Neck ØMRØ
Hip
Left ØMRM
Right ØMRL
Knee
Left ØMRP
Right ØMRN
Lower Extremity
Left ØMRW
Right ØMRV
Perineum ØMRK
Rib(s) ØMRG
Shoulder
Left ØMR2
Right ØMR1
Spine
Lower ØMRD
Upper ØMRC
Sternum ØMRF
Upper Extremity
Left ØMRB
Right ØMR9
Wrist
Left ØMR6
Right ØMR5
Carina ØBR2
Carpal
Left ØPRN
Right ØPRM
Cerebral Meninges ØØR1
Cerebral Ventricle ØØR6
Chordae Tendineae Ø2R9
Choroid
Left Ø8RB
Right Ø8RA
Clavicle
Left ØPRB
Right ØPR9
Coccyx ØQRS
Conjunctiva
Left Ø8RTX
Right Ø8RSX
Cornea
Left Ø8R9
Right Ø8R8
Diaphragm ØBRT
Disc
Cervical Vertebral ØRR3Ø
Cervicothoracic Vertebral ØRR5Ø
Lumbar Vertebral ØSR2Ø
Lumbosacral ØSR4Ø
Thoracic Vertebral ØRR9Ø
Thoracolumbar Vertebral ØRRBØ
Duct
Common Bile ØFR9
Cystic ØFR8
Hepatic
Common ØFR7
Left ØFR6
Right ØFR5
Lacrimal
Left Ø8RY
Right Ø8RX
Pancreatic ØFRD
Accessory ØFRF
Parotid
Left ØCRC
Right ØCRB
Dura Mater ØØR2
Ear
External
Bilateral Ø9R2
Left Ø9R1
Right Ø9RØ
Inner
Left Ø9REØ
Right Ø9RDØ
Middle
Left Ø9R6Ø
Right Ø9R5Ø
Epiglottis ØCRR

**Replacement** — *continued*
Esophagus ØDR5
Eye
Left Ø8R1
Right Ø8RØ
Eyelid
Lower
Left Ø8RR
Right Ø8RQ
Upper
Left Ø8RP
Right Ø8RN
Femoral Shaft
Left ØQR9
Right ØQR8
Femur
Lower
Left ØQRC
Right ØQRB
Upper
Left ØQR7
Right ØQR6
Fibula
Left ØQRK
Right ØQRJ
Finger Nail ØHRQX
Gingiva
Lower ØCR6
Upper ØCR5
Glenoid Cavity
Left ØPR8
Right ØPR7
Hair ØHRSX
Humeral Head
Left ØPRD
Right ØPRC
Humeral Shaft
Left ØPRG
Right ØPRF
Iris
Left Ø8RD3
Right Ø8RC3
Joint
Acromioclavicular
Left ØRRHØ
Right ØRRGØ
Ankle
Left ØSRG
Right ØSRF
Carpal
Left ØRRRØ
Right ØRRQØ
Carpometacarpal
Left ØRRTØ
Right ØRRSØ
Cervical Vertebral ØRR1Ø
Cervicothoracic Vertebral ØRR4Ø
Coccygeal ØSR6Ø
Elbow
Left ØRRMØ
Right ØRRLØ
Finger Phalangeal
Left ØRRXØ
Right ØRRWØ
Hip
Left ØSRB
Acetabular Surface ØSRE
Femoral Surface ØSRS
Right ØSR9
Acetabular Surface ØSRA
Femoral Surface ØSRR
Knee
Left ØSRD
Femoral Surface ØSRU
Tibial Surface ØSRW
Right ØSRC
Femoral Surface ØSRT
Tibial Surface ØSRV
Lumbar Vertebral ØSRØØ
Lumbosacral ØSR3Ø
Metacarpophalangeal
Left ØRRVØ
Right ØRRUØ
Metatarsal-Phalangeal
Left ØSRNØ
Right ØSRMØ
Occipital-cervical ØRRØØ
Sacrococcygeal ØSR5Ø

**Replacement** — *continued*
Joint — *continued*
Sacroiliac
Left ØSR8Ø
Right ØSR7Ø
Shoulder
Left ØRRK
Right ØRRJ
Sternoclavicular
Left ØRRFØ
Right ØRREØ
Tarsal
Left ØSRJØ
Right ØSRHØ
Tarsometatarsal
Left ØSRLØ
Right ØSRKØ
Temporomandibular
Left ØRRDØ
Right ØRRCØ
Thoracic Vertebral ØRR6Ø
Thoracolumbar Vertebral ØRRAØ
Toe Phalangeal
Left ØSRQØ
Right ØSRPØ
Wrist
Left ØRRPØ
Right ØRRNØ
Kidney Pelvis
Left ØTR4
Right ØTR3
Larynx ØCRS
Lens
Left Ø8RK3ØZ
Right Ø8RJ3ØZ
Lip
Lower ØCR1
Upper ØCRØ
Mandible
Left ØNRV
Right ØNRT
Maxilla ØNRR
Mesentery ØDRV
Metacarpal
Left ØPRQ
Right ØPRP
Metatarsal
Left ØQRP
Right ØQRN
Muscle
Abdomen
Left ØKRL
Right ØKRK
Facial ØKR1
Foot
Left ØKRW
Right ØKRV
Hand
Left ØKRD
Right ØKRC
Head ØKRØ
Hip
Left ØKRP
Right ØKRN
Lower Arm and Wrist
Left ØKRB
Right ØKR9
Lower Leg
Left ØKRT
Right ØKRS
Neck
Left ØKR3
Right ØKR2
Papillary Ø2RD
Perineum ØKRM
Shoulder
Left ØKR6
Right ØKR5
Thorax
Left ØKRJ
Right ØKRH
Tongue, Palate, Pharynx ØKR4
Trunk
Left ØKRG
Right ØKRF
Upper Arm
Left ØKR8
Right ØKR7

**Replacement** — *continued*
Muscle — *continued*
Upper Leg
Left ØKRR
Right ØKRQ
Nasal Mucosa and Soft Tissue Ø9RK
Nasopharynx Ø9RN
Nerve
Abducens ØØRL
Accessory ØØRR
Acoustic ØØRN
Cervical Ø1R1
Facial ØØRM
Femoral Ø1RD
Glossopharyngeal ØØRP
Hypoglossal ØØRS
Lumbar Ø1RB
Median Ø1R5
Oculomotor ØØRH
Olfactory ØØRF
Optic ØØRG
Peroneal Ø1RH
Phrenic Ø1R2
Pudendal Ø1RC
Radial Ø1R6
Sacral Ø1RR
Sciatic Ø1RF
Thoracic Ø1R8
Tibial Ø1RG
Trigeminal ØØRK
Trochlear ØØRJ
Ulnar Ø1R4
Vagus ØØRQ
Nipple
Left ØHRX
Right ØHRW
Omentum ØDRU
Orbit
Left ØNRQ
Right ØNRP
Palate
Hard ØCR2
Soft ØCR3
Patella
Left ØQRF
Right ØQRD
Pericardium Ø2RN
Peritoneum ØDRW
Phalanx
Finger
Left ØPRV
Right ØPRT
Thumb
Left ØPRS
Right ØPRR
Toe
Left ØQRR
Right ØQRQ
Pharynx ØCRM
Radius
Left ØPRJ
Right ØPRH
Retinal Vessel
Left Ø8RH3
Right Ø8RG3
Ribs
1 to 2 ØPR1
3 or More ØPR2
Sacrum ØQR1
Scapula
Left ØPR6
Right ØPR5
Sclera
Left Ø8R7X
Right Ø8R6X
Septum
Atrial Ø2R5
Nasal Ø9RM
Ventricular Ø2RM
Skin
Abdomen ØHR7
Back ØHR6
Buttock ØHR8
Chest ØHR5
Ear
Left ØHR3
Right ØHR2
Face ØHR1

**Replacement** — *continued*
Skin — *continued*
Foot
Left ØHRN
Right ØHRM
Hand
Left ØHRG
Right ØHRF
Inguinal ØHRA
Lower Arm
Left ØHRE
Right ØHRD
Lower Leg
Left ØHRL
Right ØHRK
Neck ØHR4
Perineum ØHR9
Scalp ØHRØ
Upper Arm
Left ØHRC
Right ØHRB
Upper Leg
Left ØHRJ
Right ØHRH
Skin Substitute, Porcine Liver Derived XHRPXL2
Skull ØNRØ
Spinal Meninges ØØRT
Sternum ØPRØ
Subcutaneous Tissue and Fascia
Abdomen ØJR8
Back ØJR7
Buttock ØJR9
Chest ØJR6
Face ØJR1
Foot
Left ØJRR
Right ØJRQ
Hand
Left ØJRK
Right ØJRJ
Lower Arm
Left ØJRH
Right ØJRG
Lower Leg
Left ØJRP
Right ØJRN
Neck
Left ØJR5
Right ØJR4
Pelvic Region ØJRC
Perineum ØJRB
Scalp ØJRØ
Upper Arm
Left ØJRF
Right ØJRD
Upper Leg
Left ØJRM
Right ØJRL
Tarsal
Left ØQRM
Right ØQRL
Tendon
Abdomen
Left ØLRG
Right ØLRF
Ankle
Left ØLRT
Right ØLRS
Foot
Left ØLRW
Right ØLRV
Hand
Left ØLR8
Right ØLR7
Head and Neck ØLRØ
Hip
Left ØLRK
Right ØLRJ
Knee
Left ØLRR
Right ØLRQ
Lower Arm and Wrist
Left ØLR6
Right ØLR5
Lower Leg
Left ØLRP
Right ØLRN
Perineum ØLRH

**Replacement** — *continued*
Tendon — *continued*
Shoulder
Left ØLR2
Right ØLR1
Thorax
Left ØLRD
Right ØLRC
Trunk
Left ØLRB
Right ØLR9
Upper Arm
Left ØLR4
Right ØLR3
Upper Leg
Left ØLRM
Right ØLRL
Testis
Bilateral ØVRCØJZ
Left ØVRBØJZ
Right ØVR9ØJZ
Thumb
Left ØXRM
Right ØXRL
Tibia
Left ØQRH
Right ØQRG
Toe Nail ØHRRX
Tongue ØCR7
Tooth
Lower ØCRX
Upper ØCRW
Trachea ØBR1
Turbinate, Nasal Ø9RL
Tympanic Membrane
Left Ø9R8
Right Ø9R7
Ulna
Left ØPRL
Right ØPRK
Ureter
Left ØTR7
Right ØTR6
Urethra ØTRD
Uvula ØCRN
Valve
Aortic Ø2RF
Mitral Ø2RG
Pulmonary Ø2RH
Tricuspid Ø2RJ
Vein
Axillary
Left Ø5R8
Right Ø5R7
Azygos Ø5RØ
Basilic
Left Ø5RC
Right Ø5RB
Brachial
Left Ø5RA
Right Ø5R9
Cephalic
Left Ø5RF
Right Ø5RD
Colic Ø6R7
Common Iliac
Left Ø6RD
Right Ø6RC
Esophageal Ø6R3
External Iliac
Left Ø6RG
Right Ø6RF
External Jugular
Left Ø5RQ
Right Ø5RP
Face
Left Ø5RV
Right Ø5RT
Femoral
Left Ø6RN
Right Ø6RM
Foot
Left Ø6RV
Right Ø6RT
Gastric Ø6R2
Hand
Left Ø5RH
Right Ø5RG
Hemiazygos Ø5R1

**Replacement** — *continued*
Vein — *continued*
Hepatic Ø6R4
Hypogastric
Left Ø6RJ
Right Ø6RH
Inferior Mesenteric Ø6R6
Innominate
Left Ø5R4
Right Ø5R3
Internal Jugular
Left Ø5RN
Right Ø5RM
Intracranial Ø5RL
Lower Ø6RY
Portal Ø6R8
Pulmonary
Left Ø2RT
Right Ø2RS
Renal
Left Ø6RB
Right Ø6R9
Saphenous
Left Ø6RQ
Right Ø6RP
Splenic Ø6R1
Subclavian
Left Ø5R6
Right Ø5R5
Superior Mesenteric Ø6R5
Upper Ø5RY
Vertebral
Left Ø5RS
Right Ø5RR
Vena Cava
Inferior Ø6RØ
Superior Ø2RV
Ventricle
Left Ø2RL
Right Ø2RK
Vertebra
Cervical ØPR3
Lumbar ØQRØ
Thoracic ØPR4
Vitreous
Left Ø8R53
Right Ø8R43
Vocal Cord
Left ØCRV
Right ØCRT
Zooplastic Tissue, Rapid Deployment Technique X2RF
**Replacement, hip**
Partial or total *see* Replacement, Lower Joints ØSR
Resurfacing only *see* Supplement, Lower Joints ØSU
**Replantation** *see* Reposition
**Replantation, scalp** *see* Reattachment, Skin, Scalp ØHMØ
**Reposition**
Acetabulum
Left ØQS5
Right ØQS4
Ampulla of Vater ØFSC
Anus ØDSQ
Aorta
Abdominal Ø4SØ
Thoracic
Ascending/Arch Ø2SXØZZ
Descending Ø2SWØZZ
Artery
Anterior Tibial
Left Ø4SQ
Right Ø4SP
Axillary
Left Ø3S6
Right Ø3S5
Brachial
Left Ø3S8
Right Ø3S7
Celiac Ø4S1
Colic
Left Ø4S7
Middle Ø4S8
Right Ø4S6
Common Carotid
Left Ø3SJ
Right Ø3SH
Common Iliac
Left Ø4SD
Right Ø4SC

**Reposition** — *continued*
Artery — *continued*
Coronary
One Artery Ø2SØØZZ
Two Arteries Ø2S1ØZZ
External Carotid
Left Ø3SN
Right Ø3SM
External Iliac
Left Ø4SJ
Right Ø4SH
Face Ø3SR
Femoral
Left Ø4SL
Right Ø4SK
Foot
Left Ø4SW
Right Ø4SV
Gastric Ø4S2
Hand
Left Ø3SF
Right Ø3SD
Hepatic Ø4S3
Inferior Mesenteric Ø4SB
Innominate Ø3S2
Internal Carotid
Left Ø3SL
Right Ø3SK
Internal Iliac
Left Ø4SF
Right Ø4SE
Internal Mammary
Left Ø3S1
Right Ø3SØ
Intracranial Ø3SG
Lower Ø4SY
Peroneal
Left Ø4SU
Right Ø4ST
Popliteal
Left Ø4SN
Right Ø4SM
Posterior Tibial
Left Ø4SS
Right Ø4SR
Pulmonary
Left Ø2SRØZZ
Right Ø2SQØZZ
Pulmonary Trunk Ø2SPØZZ
Radial
Left Ø3SC
Right Ø3SB
Renal
Left Ø4SA
Right Ø4S9
Splenic Ø4S4
Subclavian
Left Ø3S4
Right Ø3S3
Superior Mesenteric Ø4S5
Temporal
Left Ø3ST
Right Ø3SS
Thyroid
Left Ø3SV
Right Ø3SU
Ulnar
Left Ø3SA
Right Ø3S9
Upper Ø3SY
Vertebral
Left Ø3SQ
Right Ø3SP
Auditory Ossicle
Left Ø9SA
Right Ø9S9
Bladder ØTSB
Bladder Neck ØTSC
Bone
Ethmoid
Left ØNSG
Right ØNSF
Frontal ØNS1
Hyoid ØNSX
Lacrimal
Left ØNSJ
Right ØNSH
Nasal ØNSB
Occipital ØNS7

**Reposition** — *continued*
Bone — *continued*
Palatine
Left ØNSL
Right ØNSK
Parietal
Left ØNS4
Right ØNS3
Pelvic
Left ØQS3
Right ØQS2
Sphenoid ØNSC
Temporal
Left ØNS6
Right ØNS5
Zygomatic
Left ØNSN
Right ØNSM
Breast
Bilateral ØHSVØZZ
Left ØHSUØZZ
Right ØHSTØZZ
Bronchus
Lingula ØBS9ØZZ
Lower Lobe
Left ØBSBØZZ
Right ØBS6ØZZ
Main
Left ØBS7ØZZ
Right ØBS3ØZZ
Middle Lobe, Right ØBS5ØZZ
Upper Lobe
Left ØBS8ØZZ
Right ØBS4ØZZ
Bursa and Ligament
Abdomen
Left ØMSJ
Right ØMSH
Ankle
Left ØMSR
Right ØMSQ
Elbow
Left ØMS4
Right ØMS3
Foot
Left ØMST
Right ØMSS
Hand
Left ØMS8
Right ØMS7
Head and Neck ØMSØ
Hip
Left ØMSM
Right ØMSL
Knee
Left ØMSP
Right ØMSN
Lower Extremity
Left ØMSW
Right ØMSV
Perineum ØMSK
Rib(s) ØMSG
Shoulder
Left ØMS2
Right ØMS1
Spine
Lower ØMSD
Upper ØMSC
Sternum ØMSF
Upper Extremity
Left ØMSB
Right ØMS9
Wrist
Left ØMS6
Right ØMS5
Carina ØBS2ØZZ
Carpal
Left ØPSN
Right ØPSM
Cecum ØDSH
Cervix ØUSC
Clavicle
Left ØPSB
Right ØPS9
Coccyx ØQSS
Colon
Ascending ØDSK
Descending ØDSM
Sigmoid ØDSN

**Reposition** — *continued*
Colon — *continued*
Transverse ØDSL
Cord
Bilateral ØVSH
Left ØVSG
Right ØVSF
Cul-de-sac ØUSF
Diaphragm ØBSTØZZ
Duct
Common Bile ØFS9
Cystic ØFS8
Hepatic
Common ØFS7
Left ØFS6
Right ØFS5
Lacrimal
Left Ø8SY
Right Ø8SX
Pancreatic ØFSD
Accessory ØFSF
Parotid
Left ØCSC
Right ØCSB
Duodenum ØDS9
Ear
Bilateral Ø9S2
Left Ø9S1
Right Ø9SØ
Epiglottis ØCSR
Esophagus ØDS5
Eustachian Tube
Left Ø9SG
Right Ø9SF
Eyelid
Lower
Left Ø8SR
Right Ø8SQ
Upper
Left Ø8SP
Right Ø8SN
Fallopian Tube
Left ØUS6
Right ØUS5
Fallopian Tubes, Bilateral ØUS7
Femoral Shaft
Left ØQS9
Right ØQS8
Femur
Lower
Left ØQSC
Right ØQSB
Upper
Left ØQS7
Right ØQS6
Fibula
Left ØQSK
Right ØQSJ
Gallbladder ØFS4
Gland
Adrenal
Left ØGS2
Right ØGS3
Lacrimal
Left Ø8SW
Right Ø8SV
Glenoid Cavity
Left ØPS8
Right ØPS7
Hair ØHSSXZZ
Humeral Head
Left ØPSD
Right ØPSC
Humeral Shaft
Left ØPSG
Right ØPSF
Ileum ØDSB
Intestine
Large ØDSE
Small ØDS8
Iris
Left Ø8SD3ZZ
Right Ø8SC3ZZ
Jejunum ØDSA
Joint
Acromioclavicular
Left ØRSH
Right ØRSG

**Reposition** — *continued*
Joint — *continued*
Ankle
Left ØSSG
Right ØSSF
Carpal
Left ØRSR
Right ØRSQ
Carpometacarpal
Left ØRST
Right ØRSS
Cervical Vertebral ØRS1
Cervicothoracic Vertebral ØRS4
Coccygeal ØSS6
Elbow
Left ØRSM
Right ØRSL
Finger Phalangeal
Left ØRSX
Right ØRSW
Hip
Left ØSSB
Right ØSS9
Knee
Left ØSSD
Right ØSSC
Lumbar Vertebral ØSSØ
Lumbosacral ØSS3
Metacarpophalangeal
Left ØRSV
Right ØRSU
Metatarsal-Phalangeal
Left ØSSN
Right ØSSM
Occipital-cervical ØRSØ
Sacrococcygeal ØSS5
Sacroiliac
Left ØSS8
Right ØSS7
Shoulder
Left ØRSK
Right ØRSJ
Sternoclavicular
Left ØRSF
Right ØRSE
Tarsal
Left ØSSJ
Right ØSSH
Tarsometatarsal
Left ØSSL
Right ØSSK
Temporomandibular
Left ØRSD
Right ØRSC
Thoracic Vertebral ØRS6
Thoracolumbar Vertebral ØRSA
Toe Phalangeal
Left ØSSQ
Right ØSSP
Wrist
Left ØRSP
Right ØRSN
Kidney
Left ØTS1
Right ØTSØ
Kidney Pelvis
Left ØTS4
Right ØTS3
Kidneys, Bilateral ØTS2
Lens
Left Ø8SK3ZZ
Right Ø8SJ3ZZ
Lip
Lower ØCS1
Upper ØCSØ
Liver ØFSØ
Lung
Left ØBSLØZZ
Lower Lobe
Left ØBSJØZZ
Right ØBSFØZZ
Middle Lobe, Right ØBSDØZZ
Right ØBSKØZZ
Upper Lobe
Left ØBSGØZZ
Right ØBSCØZZ
Lung Lingula ØBSHØZZ
Mandible
Left ØNSV

**Reposition** — *continued*
Mandible — *continued*
Right ØNST
Maxilla ØNSR
Metacarpal
Left ØPSQ
Right ØPSP
Metatarsal
Left ØQSP
Right ØQSN
Muscle
Abdomen
Left ØKSL
Right ØKSK
Extraocular
Left Ø8SM
Right Ø8SL
Facial ØKS1
Foot
Left ØKSW
Right ØKSV
Hand
Left ØKSD
Right ØKSC
Head ØKSØ
Hip
Left ØKSP
Right ØKSN
Lower Arm and Wrist
Left ØKSB
Right ØKS9
Lower Leg
Left ØKST
Right ØKSS
Neck
Left ØKS3
Right ØKS2
Perineum ØKSM
Shoulder
Left ØKS6
Right ØKS5
Thorax
Left ØKSJ
Right ØKSH
Tongue, Palate, Pharynx ØKS4
Trunk
Left ØKSG
Right ØKSF
Upper Arm
Left ØKS8
Right ØKS7
Upper Leg
Left ØKSR
Right ØKSQ
Nasal Mucosa and Soft Tissue Ø9SK
Nerve
Abducens ØØSL
Accessory ØØSR
Acoustic ØØSN
Brachial Plexus Ø1S3
Cervical Ø1S1
Cervical Plexus Ø1SØ
Facial ØØSM
Femoral Ø1SD
Glossopharyngeal ØØSP
Hypoglossal ØØSS
Lumbar Ø1SB
Lumbar Plexus Ø1S9
Lumbosacral Plexus Ø1SA
Median Ø1S5
Oculomotor ØØSH
Olfactory ØØSF
Optic ØØSG
Peroneal Ø1SH
Phrenic Ø1S2
Pudendal Ø1SC
Radial Ø1S6
Sacral Ø1SR
Sacral Plexus Ø1SQ
Sciatic Ø1SF
Thoracic Ø1S8
Tibial Ø1SG
Trigeminal ØØSK
Trochlear ØØSJ
Ulnar Ø1S4
Vagus ØØSQ
Nipple
Left ØHSXXZZ
Right ØHSWXZZ

**Reposition** — *continued*
Orbit
Left ØNSQ
Right ØNSP
Ovary
Bilateral ØUS2
Left ØUS1
Right ØUSØ
Palate
Hard ØCS2
Soft ØCS3
Pancreas ØFSG
Parathyroid Gland ØGSR
Inferior
Left ØGSP
Right ØGSN
Multiple ØGSQ
Superior
Left ØGSM
Right ØGSL
Patella
Left ØQSF
Right ØQSD
Phalanx
Finger
Left ØPSV
Right ØPST
Thumb
Left ØPSS
Right ØPSR
Toe
Left ØQSR
Right ØQSQ
Products of Conception 1ØSØ
Ectopic 1ØS2
Radius
Left ØPSJ
Right ØPSH
Rectum ØDSP
Retinal Vessel
Left Ø8SH3ZZ
Right Ø8SG3ZZ
Ribs
1 to 2 ØPS1
3 or More ØPS2
Sacrum ØQS1
Scapula
Left ØPS6
Right ØPS5
Septum, Nasal Ø9SM
Sesamoid Bone(s) 1st Toe
*see* Reposition, Metatarsal, Left ØQSP
*see* Reposition, Metatarsal, Right ØQSN
Skull ØNSØ
Spinal Cord
Cervical ØØSW
Lumbar ØØSY
Thoracic ØØSX
Spleen Ø7SPØZZ
Sternum ØPSØ
Stomach ØDS6
Tarsal
Left ØQSM
Right ØQSL
Tendon
Abdomen
Left ØLSG
Right ØLSF
Ankle
Left ØLST
Right ØLSS
Foot
Left ØLSW
Right ØLSV
Hand
Left ØLS8
Right ØLS7
Head and Neck ØLSØ
Hip
Left ØLSK
Right ØLSJ
Knee
Left ØLSR
Right ØLSQ
Lower Arm and Wrist
Left ØLS6
Right ØLS5
Lower Leg
Left ØLSP

**Reposition** — *continued*
Tendon — *continued*
Lower Leg — *continued*
Right ØLSN
Perineum ØLSH
Shoulder
Left ØLS2
Right ØLS1
Thorax
Left ØLSD
Right ØLSC
Trunk
Left ØLSB
Right ØLS9
Upper Arm
Left ØLS4
Right ØLS3
Upper Leg
Left ØLSM
Right ØLSL
Testis
Bilateral ØVSC
Left ØVSB
Right ØVS9
Thymus Ø7SMØZZ
Thyroid Gland
Left Lobe ØGSG
Right Lobe ØGSH
Tibia
Left ØQSH
Right ØQSG
Tongue ØCS7
Tooth
Lower ØCSX
Upper ØCSW
Trachea ØBS1ØZZ
Turbinate, Nasal Ø9SL
Tympanic Membrane
Left Ø9S8
Right Ø9S7
Ulna
Left ØPSL
Right ØPSK
Ureter
Left ØTS7
Right ØTS6
Ureters, Bilateral ØTS8
Urethra ØTSD
Uterine Supporting Structure ØUS4
Uterus ØUS9
Uvula ØCSN
Vagina ØUSG
Vein
Axillary
Left Ø5S8
Right Ø5S7
Azygos Ø5SØ
Basilic
Left Ø5SC
Right Ø5SB
Brachial
Left Ø5SA
Right Ø5S9
Cephalic
Left Ø5SF
Right Ø5SD
Colic Ø6S7
Common Iliac
Left Ø6SD
Right Ø6SC
Esophageal Ø6S3
External Iliac
Left Ø6SG
Right Ø6SF
External Jugular
Left Ø5SQ
Right Ø5SP
Face
Left Ø5SV
Right Ø5ST
Femoral
Left Ø6SN
Right Ø6SM
Foot
Left Ø6SV
Right Ø6ST
Gastric Ø6S2
Hand
Left Ø5SH

**Reposition** — *continued*
Vein — *continued*
Hand — *continued*
Right Ø5SG
Hemiazygos Ø5S1
Hepatic Ø6S4
Hypogastric
Left Ø6SJ
Right Ø6SH
Inferior Mesenteric Ø6S6
Innominate
Left Ø5S4
Right Ø5S3
Internal Jugular
Left Ø5SN
Right Ø5SM
Intracranial Ø5SL
Lower Ø6SY
Portal Ø6S8
Pulmonary
Left Ø2STØZZ
Right Ø2SSØZZ
Renal
Left Ø6SB
Right Ø6S9
Saphenous
Left Ø6SQ
Right Ø6SP
Splenic Ø6S1
Subclavian
Left Ø5S6
Right Ø5S5
Superior Mesenteric Ø6S5
Upper Ø5SY
Vertebral
Left Ø5SS
Right Ø5SR
Vena Cava
Inferior Ø6SØ
Superior Ø2SVØZZ
Vertebra
Cervical ØPS3
Magnetically Controlled Growth Rod(s) XNS3
Lumbar ØQSØ
Magnetically Controlled Growth Rod(s) XNSØ
Thoracic ØPS4
Magnetically Controlled Growth Rod(s) XNS4
Vocal Cord
Left ØCSV
Right ØCST
**Resection**
Acetabulum
Left ØQT5ØZZ
Right ØQT4ØZZ
Adenoids ØCTQ
Ampulla of Vater ØFTC
Anal Sphincter ØDTR
Anus ØDTQ
Aortic Body ØGTD
Appendix ØDTJ
Auditory Ossicle
Left Ø9TA
Right Ø9T9
Bladder ØTTB
Bladder Neck ØTTC
Bone
Ethmoid
Left ØNTGØZZ
Right ØNTFØZZ
Frontal ØNT1ØZZ
Hyoid ØNTXØZZ
Lacrimal
Left ØNTJØZZ
Right ØNTHØZZ
Nasal ØNTBØZZ
Occipital ØNT7ØZZ
Palatine
Left ØNTLØZZ
Right ØNTKØZZ
Parietal
Left ØNT4ØZZ
Right ØNT3ØZZ
Pelvic
Left ØQT3ØZZ
Right ØQT2ØZZ
Sphenoid ØNTCØZZ
Temporal
Left ØNT6ØZZ
Right ØNT5ØZZ

**Resection** — *continued*
Bone — *continued*
Zygomatic
Left ØNTNØZZ
Right ØNTMØZZ
Breast
Bilateral ØHTVØZZ
Left ØHTUØZZ
Right ØHTTØZZ
Supernumerary ØHTYØZZ
Bronchus
Lingula ØBT9
Lower Lobe
Left ØBTB
Right ØBT6
Main
Left ØBT7
Right ØBT3
Middle Lobe, Right ØBT5
Upper Lobe
Left ØBT8
Right ØBT4
Bursa and Ligament
Abdomen
Left ØMTJ
Right ØMTH
Ankle
Left ØMTR
Right ØMTQ
Elbow
Left ØMT4
Right ØMT3
Foot
Left ØMTT
Right ØMTS
Hand
Left ØMT8
Right ØMT7
Head and Neck ØMTØ
Hip
Left ØMTM
Right ØMTL
Knee
Left ØMTP
Right ØMTN
Lower Extremity
Left ØMTW
Right ØMTV
Perineum ØMTK
Rib(s) ØMTG
Shoulder
Left ØMT2
Right ØMT1
Spine
Lower ØMTD
Upper ØMTC
Sternum ØMTF
Upper Extremity
Left ØMTB
Right ØMT9
Wrist
Left ØMT6
Right ØMT5
Carina ØBT2
Carotid Bodies, Bilateral ØGT8
Carotid Body
Left ØGT6
Right ØGT7
Carpal
Left ØPTNØZZ
Right ØPTMØZZ
Cecum ØDTH
Cerebral Hemisphere ØØT7
Cervix ØUTC
Chordae Tendineae Ø2T9
Cisterna Chyli Ø7TL
Clavicle
Left ØPTBØZZ
Right ØPT9ØZZ
Clitoris ØUTJ
Coccygeal Glomus ØGTB
Coccyx ØQTSØZZ
Colon
Ascending ØDTK
Descending ØDTM
Sigmoid ØDTN
Transverse ØDTL
Conduction Mechanism Ø2T8

Subterms under main terms may continue to next column or page

**Resection** — *continued*
Cord
Bilateral ØVTH
Left ØVTG
Right ØVTF
Cornea
Left Ø8T9XZZ
Right Ø8T8XZZ
Cul-de-sac ØUTF
Diaphragm ØBTT
Disc
Cervical Vertebral ØRT3ØZZ
Cervicothoracic Vertebral ØRT5ØZZ
Lumbar Vertebral ØST2ØZZ
Lumbosacral ØST4ØZZ
Thoracic Vertebral ØRT9ØZZ
Thoracolumbar Vertebral ØRTBØZZ
Duct
Common Bile ØFT9
Cystic ØFT8
Hepatic
Common ØFT7
Left ØFT6
Right ØFT5
Lacrimal
Left Ø8TY
Right Ø8TX
Pancreatic ØFTD
Accessory ØFTF
Parotid
Left ØCTCØZZ
Right ØCTBØZZ
Duodenum ØDT9
Ear
External
Left Ø9T1
Right Ø9TØ
Inner
Left Ø9TE
Right Ø9TD
Middle
Left Ø9T6
Right Ø9T5
Epididymis
Bilateral ØVTL
Left ØVTK
Right ØVTJ
Epiglottis ØCTR
Esophagogastric Junction ØDT4
Esophagus ØDT5
Lower ØDT3
Middle ØDT2
Upper ØDT1
Eustachian Tube
Left Ø9TG
Right Ø9TF
Eye
Left Ø8T1XZZ
Right Ø8TØXZZ
Eyelid
Lower
Left Ø8TR
Right Ø8TQ
Upper
Left Ø8TP
Right Ø8TN
Fallopian Tube
Left ØUT6
Right ØUT5
Fallopian Tubes, Bilateral ØUT7
Femoral Shaft
Left ØQT9ØZZ
Right ØQT8ØZZ
Femur
Lower
Left ØQTCØZZ
Right ØQTBØZZ
Upper
Left ØQT7ØZZ
Right ØQT6ØZZ
Fibula
Left ØQTKØZZ
Right ØQTJØZZ
Finger Nail ØHTQXZZ
Gallbladder ØFT4
Gland
Adrenal
Bilateral ØGT4
Left ØGT2

**Resection** — *continued*
Gland — *continued*
Adrenal — *continued*
Right ØGT3
Lacrimal
Left Ø8TW
Right Ø8TV
Minor Salivary ØCTJØZZ
Parotid
Left ØCT9ØZZ
Right ØCT8ØZZ
Pituitary ØGTØ
Sublingual
Left ØCTFØZZ
Right ØCTDØZZ
Submaxillary
Left ØCTHØZZ
Right ØCTGØZZ
Vestibular ØUTL
Glenoid Cavity
Left ØPT8ØZZ
Right ØPT7ØZZ
Glomus Jugulare ØGTC
Humeral Head
Left ØPTDØZZ
Right ØPTCØZZ
Humeral Shaft
Left ØPTGØZZ
Right ØPTFØZZ
Hymen ØUTK
Ileocecal Valve ØDTC
Ileum ØDTB
Intestine
Large ØDTE
Left ØDTG
Right ØDTF
Small ØDT8
Iris
Left Ø8TD3ZZ
Right Ø8TC3ZZ
Jejunum ØDTA
Joint
Acromioclavicular
Left ØRTHØZZ
Right ØRTGØZZ
Ankle
Left ØSTGØZZ
Right ØSTFØZZ
Carpal
Left ØRTRØZZ
Right ØRTQØZZ
Carpometacarpal
Left ØRTTØZZ
Right ØRTSØZZ
Cervicothoracic Vertebral ØRT4ØZZ
Coccygeal ØST6ØZZ
Elbow
Left ØRTMØZZ
Right ØRTLØZZ
Finger Phalangeal
Left ØRTXØZZ
Right ØRTWØZZ
Hip
Left ØSTBØZZ
Right ØST9ØZZ
Knee
Left ØSTDØZZ
Right ØSTCØZZ
Metacarpophalangeal
Left ØRTVØZZ
Right ØRTUØZZ
Metatarsal-Phalangeal
Left ØSTNØZZ
Right ØSTMØZZ
Sacrococcygeal ØST5ØZZ
Sacroiliac
Left ØST8ØZZ
Right ØST7ØZZ
Shoulder
Left ØRTKØZZ
Right ØRTJØZZ
Sternoclavicular
Left ØRTFØZZ
Right ØRTEØZZ
Tarsal
Left ØSTJØZZ
Right ØSTHØZZ
Tarsometatarsal
Left ØSTLØZZ

**Resection** — *continued*
Joint — *continued*
Tarsometatarsal — *continued*
Right ØSTKØZZ
Temporomandibular
Left ØRTDØZZ
Right ØRTCØZZ
Toe Phalangeal
Left ØSTQØZZ
Right ØSTPØZZ
Wrist
Left ØRTPØZZ
Right ØRTNØZZ
Kidney
Left ØTT1
Right ØTTØ
Kidney Pelvis
Left ØTT4
Right ØTT3
Kidneys, Bilateral ØTT2
Larynx ØCTS
Lens
Left Ø8TK3ZZ
Right Ø8TJ3ZZ
Lip
Lower ØCT1
Upper ØCTØ
Liver ØFTØ
Left Lobe ØFT2
Right Lobe ØFT1
Lung
Bilateral ØBTM
Left ØBTL
Lower Lobe
Left ØBTJ
Right ØBTF
Middle Lobe, Right ØBTD
Right ØBTK
Upper Lobe
Left ØBTG
Right ØBTC
Lung Lingula ØBTH
Lymphatic
Aortic Ø7TD
Axillary
Left Ø7T6
Right Ø7T5
Head Ø7TØ
Inguinal
Left Ø7TJ
Right Ø7TH
Internal Mammary
Left Ø7T9
Right Ø7T8
Lower Extremity
Left Ø7TG
Right Ø7TF
Mesenteric Ø7TB
Neck
Left Ø7T2
Right Ø7T1
Pelvis Ø7TC
Thoracic Duct Ø7TK
Thorax Ø7T7
Upper Extremity
Left Ø7T4
Right Ø7T3
Mandible
Left ØNTVØZZ
Right ØNTTØZZ
Maxilla ØNTRØZZ
Metacarpal
Left ØPTQØZZ
Right ØPTPØZZ
Metatarsal
Left ØQTPØZZ
Right ØQTNØZZ
Muscle
Abdomen
Left ØKTL
Right ØKTK
Extraocular
Left Ø8TM
Right Ø8TL
Facial ØKT1
Foot
Left ØKTW
Right ØKTV

**Resection** — *continued*
- Muscle — *continued*
  - Hand
    - Left ØKTD
    - Right ØKTC
  - Head ØKTØ
  - Hip
    - Left ØKTP
    - Right ØKTN
  - Lower Arm and Wrist
    - Left ØKTB
    - Right ØKT9
  - Lower Leg
    - Left ØKTT
    - Right ØKTS
  - Neck
    - Left ØKT3
    - Right ØKT2
  - Papillary Ø2TD
  - Perineum ØKTM
  - Shoulder
    - Left ØKT6
    - Right ØKT5
  - Thorax
    - Left ØKTJ
    - Right ØKTH
  - Tongue, Palate, Pharynx ØKT4
  - Trunk
    - Left ØKTG
    - Right ØKTF
  - Upper Arm
    - Left ØKT8
    - Right ØKT7
  - Upper Leg
    - Left ØKTR
    - Right ØKTQ
- Nasal Mucosa and Soft Tissue Ø9TK
- Nasopharynx Ø9TN
- Nipple
  - Left ØHTXXZZ
  - Right ØHTWXZZ
- Omentum ØDTU
- Orbit
  - Left ØNTQØZZ
  - Right ØNTPØZZ
- Ovary
  - Bilateral ØUT2
  - Left ØUT1
  - Right ØUTØ
- Palate
  - Hard ØCT2
  - Soft ØCT3
- Pancreas ØFTG
- Para-aortic Body ØGT9
- Paraganglion Extremity ØGTF
- Parathyroid Gland ØGTR
  - Inferior
    - Left ØGTP
    - Right ØGTN
  - Multiple ØGTQ
  - Superior
    - Left ØGTM
    - Right ØGTL
- Patella
  - Left ØQTFØZZ
  - Right ØQTDØZZ
- Penis ØVTS
- Pericardium Ø2TN
- Phalanx
  - Finger
    - Left ØPTVØZZ
    - Right ØPTTØZZ
  - Thumb
    - Left ØPTSØZZ
    - Right ØPTRØZZ
  - Toe
    - Left ØQTRØZZ
    - Right ØQTQØZZ
- Pharynx ØCTM
- Pineal Body ØGT1
- Prepuce ØVTT
- Products of Conception, Ectopic 1ØT2
- Prostate ØVTØ
- Radius
  - Left ØPTJØZZ
  - Right ØPTHØZZ
- Rectum ØDTP
- Ribs
  - 1 to 2 ØPT1ØZZ

**Resection** — *continued*
- Ribs — *continued*
  - 3 or More ØPT2ØZZ
- Scapula
  - Left ØPT6ØZZ
  - Right ØPT5ØZZ
- Scrotum ØVT5
- Septum
  - Atrial Ø2T5
  - Nasal Ø9TM
  - Ventricular Ø2TM
- Sinus
  - Accessory Ø9TP
  - Ethmoid
    - Left Ø9TV
    - Right Ø9TU
  - Frontal
    - Left Ø9TT
    - Right Ø9TS
  - Mastoid
    - Left Ø9TC
    - Right Ø9TB
  - Maxillary
    - Left Ø9TR
    - Right Ø9TQ
  - Sphenoid
    - Left Ø9TX
    - Right Ø9TW
- Spleen Ø7TP
- Sternum ØPTØØZZ
- Stomach ØDT6
  - Pylorus ØDT7
- Tarsal
  - Left ØQTMØZZ
  - Right ØQTLØZZ
- Tendon
  - Abdomen
    - Left ØLTG
    - Right ØLTF
  - Ankle
    - Left ØLTT
    - Right ØLTS
  - Foot
    - Left ØLTW
    - Right ØLTV
  - Hand
    - Left ØLT8
    - Right ØLT7
  - Head and Neck ØLTØ
  - Hip
    - Left ØLTK
    - Right ØLTJ
  - Knee
    - Left ØLTR
    - Right ØLTQ
  - Lower Arm and Wrist
    - Left ØLT6
    - Right ØLT5
  - Lower Leg
    - Left ØLTP
    - Right ØLTN
  - Perineum ØLTH
  - Shoulder
    - Left ØLT2
    - Right ØLT1
  - Thorax
    - Left ØLTD
    - Right ØLTC
  - Trunk
    - Left ØLTB
    - Right ØLT9
  - Upper Arm
    - Left ØLT4
    - Right ØLT3
  - Upper Leg
    - Left ØLTM
    - Right ØLTL
- Testis
  - Bilateral ØVTC
  - Left ØVTB
  - Right ØVT9
- Thymus Ø7TM
- Thyroid Gland ØGTK
  - Left Lobe ØGTG
  - Right Lobe ØGTH
- Thyroid Gland Isthmus ØGTJ
- Tibia
  - Left ØQTHØZZ
  - Right ØQTGØZZ

**Resection** — *continued*
- Toe Nail ØHTRXZZ
- Tongue ØCT7
- Tonsils ØCTP
- Tooth
  - Lower ØCTXØZ
  - Upper ØCTWØZ
- Trachea ØBT1
- Tunica Vaginalis
  - Left ØVT7
  - Right ØVT6
- Turbinate, Nasal Ø9TL
- Tympanic Membrane
  - Left Ø9T8
  - Right Ø9T7
- Ulna
  - Left ØPTLØZZ
  - Right ØPTKØZZ
- Ureter
  - Left ØTT7
  - Right ØTT6
- Urethra ØTTD
- Uterine Supporting Structure ØUT4
- Uterus ØUT9
- Uvula ØCTN
- Vagina ØUTG
- Valve, Pulmonary Ø2TH
- Vas Deferens
  - Bilateral ØVTQ
  - Left ØVTP
  - Right ØVTN
- Vesicle
  - Bilateral ØVT3
  - Left ØVT2
  - Right ØVT1
- Vitreous
  - Left Ø8T53ZZ
  - Right Ø8T43ZZ
- Vocal Cord
  - Left ØCTV
  - Right ØCTT
- Vulva ØUTM

**Resection, Left ventricular outflow tract obstruction (LVOT)** *see* Dilation, Ventricle, Left Ø27L

**Resection, Subaortic membrane (Left ventricular outflow tract obstruction)** *see* Dilation, Ventricle, Left Ø27L

**Restoration, Cardiac, Single, Rhythm** 5A2204Z

**RestoreAdvanced neurostimulator (SureScan) (MRI Safe)** *use* Stimulator Generator, Multiple Array Rechargeable in ØJH

**RestoreSensor neurostimulator (SureScan) (MRI Safe)** *use* Stimulator Generator, Multiple Array Rechargeable in ØJH

**RestoreUltra neurostimulator (SureScan) (MRI Safe)** *use* Simulator Generator, Multiple Array Rechargeable in ØJH

**Restriction**
- Ampulla of Vater ØFVC
- Anus ØDVQ
- Aorta
  - Abdominal Ø4VØ
    - Intraluminal Device, Branched or Fenestrated Ø4VØ
  - Thoracic
    - Ascending/Arch, Intraluminal Device, Branched or Fenestrated Ø2VX
    - Descending, Intraluminal Device, Branched or Fenestrated Ø2VW
- Artery
  - Anterior Tibial
    - Left Ø4VQ
    - Right Ø4VP
  - Axillary
    - Left Ø3V6
    - Right Ø3V5
  - Brachial
    - Left Ø3V8
    - Right Ø3V7
  - Celiac Ø4V1
  - Colic
    - Left Ø4V7
    - Middle Ø4V8
    - Right Ø4V6
  - Common Carotid
    - Left Ø3VJ
    - Right Ø3VH

**Restriction** — *continued*
Artery — *continued*
Common Iliac
Left Ø4VD
Right Ø4VC
External Carotid
Left Ø3VN
Right Ø3VM
External Iliac
Left Ø4VJ
Right Ø4VH
Face Ø3VR
Femoral
Left Ø4VL
Right Ø4VK
Foot
Left Ø4VW
Right Ø4VV
Gastric Ø4V2
Hand
Left Ø3VF
Right Ø3VD
Hepatic Ø4V3
Inferior Mesenteric Ø4VB
Innominate Ø3V2
Internal Carotid
Left Ø3VL
Right Ø3VK
Internal Iliac
Left Ø4VF
Right Ø4VE
Internal Mammary
Left Ø3V1
Right Ø3VØ
Intracranial Ø3VG
Lower Ø4VY
Peroneal
Left Ø4VU
Right Ø4VT
Popliteal
Left Ø4VN
Right Ø4VM
Posterior Tibial
Left Ø4VS
Right Ø4VR
Pulmonary
Left Ø2VR
Right Ø2VQ
Pulmonary Trunk Ø2VP
Radial
Left Ø3VC
Right Ø3VB
Renal
Left Ø4VA
Right Ø4V9
Splenic Ø4V4
Subclavian
Left Ø3V4
Right Ø3V3
Superior Mesenteric Ø4V5
Temporal
Left Ø3VT
Right Ø3VS
Thyroid
Left Ø3VV
Right Ø3VU
Ulnar
Left Ø3VA
Right Ø3V9
Upper Ø3VY
Vertebral
Left Ø3VQ
Right Ø3VP
Bladder ØTVB
Bladder Neck ØTVC
Bronchus
Lingula ØBV9
Lower Lobe
Left ØBVB
Right ØBV6
Main
Left ØBV7
Right ØBV3
Middle Lobe, Right ØBV5
Upper Lobe
Left ØBV8
Right ØBV4
Carina ØBV2
Cecum ØDVH

**Restriction** — *continued*
Cervix ØUVC
Cisterna Chyli Ø7VL
Colon
Ascending ØDVK
Descending ØDVM
Sigmoid ØDVN
Transverse ØDVL
Duct
Common Bile ØFV9
Cystic ØFV8
Hepatic
Common ØFV7
Left ØFV6
Right ØFV5
Lacrimal
Left Ø8VY
Right Ø8VX
Pancreatic ØFVD
Accessory ØFVF
Parotid
Left ØCVC
Right ØCVB
Duodenum ØDV9
Esophagogastric Junction ØDV4
Esophagus ØDV5
Lower ØDV3
Middle ØDV2
Upper ØDV1
Heart Ø2VA
Ileocecal Valve ØDVC
Ileum ØDVB
Intestine
Large ØDVE
Left ØDVG
Right ØDVF
Small ØDV8
Jejunum ØDVA
Kidney Pelvis
Left ØTV4
Right ØTV3
Lymphatic
Aortic Ø7VD
Axillary
Left Ø7V6
Right Ø7V5
Head Ø7VØ
Inguinal
Left Ø7VJ
Right Ø7VH
Internal Mammary
Left Ø7V9
Right Ø7V8
Lower Extremity
Left Ø7VG
Right Ø7VF
Mesenteric Ø7VB
Neck
Left Ø7V2
Right Ø7V1
Pelvis Ø7VC
Thoracic Duct Ø7VK
Thorax Ø7V7
Upper Extremity
Left Ø7V4
Right Ø7V3
Rectum ØDVP
Stomach ØDV6
Pylorus ØDV7
Trachea ØBV1
Ureter
Left ØTV7
Right ØTV6
Urethra ØTVD
Valve, Mitral Ø2VG
Vein
Axillary
Left Ø5V8
Right Ø5V7
Azygos Ø5VØ
Basilic
Left Ø5VC
Right Ø5VB
Brachial
Left Ø5VA
Right Ø5V9
Cephalic
Left Ø5VF
Right Ø5VD

**Restriction** — *continued*
Vein — *continued*
Colic Ø6V7
Common Iliac
Left Ø6VD
Right Ø6VC
Esophageal Ø6V3
External Iliac
Left Ø6VG
Right Ø6VF
External Jugular
Left Ø5VQ
Right Ø5VP
Face
Left Ø5VV
Right Ø5VT
Femoral
Left Ø6VN
Right Ø6VM
Foot
Left Ø6VV
Right Ø6VT
Gastric Ø6V2
Hand
Left Ø5VH
Right Ø5VG
Hemiazygos Ø5V1
Hepatic Ø6V4
Hypogastric
Left Ø6VJ
Right Ø6VH
Inferior Mesenteric Ø6V6
Innominate
Left Ø5V4
Right Ø5V3
Internal Jugular
Left Ø5VN
Right Ø5VM
Intracranial Ø5VL
Lower Ø6VY
Portal Ø6V8
Pulmonary
Left Ø2VT
Right Ø2VS
Renal
Left Ø6VB
Right Ø6V9
Saphenous
Left Ø6VQ
Right Ø6VP
Splenic Ø6V1
Subclavian
Left Ø5V6
Right Ø5V5
Superior Mesenteric Ø6V5
Upper Ø5VY
Vertebral
Left Ø5VS
Right Ø5VR
Vena Cava
Inferior Ø6VØ
Superior Ø2VV
**Resurfacing Device**
Removal of device from
Left ØSPBØBZ
Right ØSP9ØBZ
Revision of device in
Left ØSWBØBZ
Right ØSW9ØBZ
Supplement
Left ØSUBØBZ
Acetabular Surface ØSUEØBZ
Femoral Surface ØSUSØBZ
Right ØSU9ØBZ
Acetabular Surface ØSUAØBZ
Femoral Surface ØSURØBZ
**Resuscitation**
Cardiopulmonary *see* Assistance, Cardiac 5AØ2
Cardioversion 5A22Ø4Z
Defibrillation 5A22Ø4Z
Endotracheal intubation *see* Insertion of device in, Trachea ØBH1
External chest compression 5A12Ø12
Pulmonary 5A19Ø54

**Resuscitative endovascular balloon occlusion of the aorta (REBOA)**
Ø2LW3DJ
Ø4LØ3DJ
**Resuture, Heart valve prosthesis** *see* Revision of device in, Heart and Great Vessels Ø2W
**Retained placenta, manual removal** *see* Extraction, Products of Conception, Retained 1ØD1
**Retraining**
Cardiac *see* Motor Treatment, Rehabilitation FØ7
Vocational *see* Activities of Daily Living Treatment, Rehabilitation FØ8
**Retrogasserian rhizotomy** *see* Division, Nerve, Trigeminal ØØ8K
**Retroperitoneal lymph node** *use* Lymphatic, Aortic
**Retroperitoneal space** *use* Retroperitoneum
**Retropharyngeal lymph node**
*use* Lymphatic, Neck, Left
*use* Lymphatic, Neck, Right
**Retropubic space** *use* Pelvic Cavity
**Reveal (DX) (XT)** *use* Monitoring Device
**Reverse total shoulder replacement** *see* Replacement, Upper Joints ØRR
**Reverse® Shoulder Prosthesis** *use* Synthetic Substitute, Reverse Ball and Socket in ØRR
**Revision**
Correcting a portion of existing device *see* Revision of device in
Removal of device without replacement *see* Removal of device from
Replacement of existing device
*see* Removal of device from
*see* Root operation to place new device, e.g., Insertion, Replacement, Supplement
**Revision of device in**
Abdominal Wall ØWWF
Acetabulum
Left ØQW5
Right ØQW4
Anal Sphincter ØDWR
Anus ØDWQ
Artery
Lower Ø4WY
Upper Ø3WY
Auditory Ossicle
Left Ø9WA
Right Ø9W9
Back
Lower ØWWL
Upper ØWWK
Bladder ØTWB
Bone
Facial ØNWW
Lower ØQWY
Nasal ØNWB
Pelvic
Left ØQW3
Right ØQW2
Upper ØPWY
Bone Marrow Ø7WT
Brain ØØWØ
Breast
Left ØHWU
Right ØHWT
Bursa and Ligament
Lower ØMWY
Upper ØMWX
Carpal
Left ØPWN
Right ØPWM
Cavity, Cranial ØWW1
Cerebral Ventricle ØØW6
Chest Wall ØWW8
Cisterna Chyli Ø7WL
Clavicle
Left ØPWB
Right ØPW9
Coccyx ØQWS
Diaphragm ØBWT
Disc
Cervical Vertebral ØRW3
Cervicothoracic Vertebral ØRW5
Lumbar Vertebral ØSW2
Lumbosacral ØSW4
Thoracic Vertebral ØRW9
Thoracolumbar Vertebral ØRWB
Duct
Hepatobiliary ØFWB

**Revision of device in** — *continued*
Duct — *continued*
Pancreatic ØFWD
Ear
Inner
Left Ø9WE
Right Ø9WD
Left Ø9WJ
Right Ø9WH
Epididymis and Spermatic Cord ØVWM
Esophagus ØDW5
Extremity
Lower
Left ØYWB
Right ØYW9
Upper
Left ØXW7
Right ØXW6
Eye
Left Ø8W1
Right Ø8WØ
Face ØWW2
Fallopian Tube ØUW8
Femoral Shaft
Left ØQW9
Right ØQW8
Femur
Lower
Left ØQWC
Right ØQWB
Upper
Left ØQW7
Right ØQW6
Fibula
Left ØQWK
Right ØQWJ
Finger Nail ØHWQX
Gallbladder ØFW4
Gastrointestinal Tract ØWWP
Genitourinary Tract ØWWR
Gland
Adrenal ØGW5
Endocrine ØGWS
Pituitary ØGWØ
Salivary ØCWA
Glenoid Cavity
Left ØPW8
Right ØPW7
Great Vessel Ø2WY
Hair ØHWSX
Head ØWWØ
Heart Ø2WA
Humeral Head
Left ØPWD
Right ØPWC
Humeral Shaft
Left ØPWG
Right ØPWF
Intestinal Tract
Lower ØDWD
Upper ØDWØ
Intestine
Large ØDWE
Small ØDW8
Jaw
Lower ØWW5
Upper ØWW4
Joint
Acromioclavicular
Left ØRWH
Right ØRWG
Ankle
Left ØSWG
Right ØSWF
Carpal
Left ØRWR
Right ØRWQ
Carpometacarpal
Left ØRWT
Right ØRWS
Cervical Vertebral ØRW1
Cervicothoracic Vertebral ØRW4
Coccygeal ØSW6
Elbow
Left ØRWM
Right ØRWL
Finger Phalangeal
Left ØRWX
Right ØRWW

**Revision of device in** — *continued*
Joint — *continued*
Hip
Left ØSWB
Acetabular Surface ØSWE
Femoral Surface ØSWS
Right ØSW9
Acetabular Surface ØSWA
Femoral Surface ØSWR
Knee
Left ØSWD
Femoral Surface ØSWU
Tibial Surface ØSWW
Right ØSWC
Femoral Surface ØSWT
Tibial Surface ØSWV
Lumbar Vertebral ØSWØ
Lumbosacral ØSW3
Metacarpophalangeal
Left ØRWV
Right ØRWU
Metatarsal-Phalangeal
Left ØSWN
Right ØSWM
Occipital-cervical ØRWØ
Sacrococcygeal ØSW5
Sacroiliac
Left ØSW8
Right ØSW7
Shoulder
Left ØRWK
Right ØRWJ
Sternoclavicular
Left ØRWF
Right ØRWE
Tarsal
Left ØSWJ
Right ØSWH
Tarsometatarsal
Left ØSWL
Right ØSWK
Temporomandibular
Left ØRWD
Right ØRWC
Thoracic Vertebral ØRW6
Thoracolumbar Vertebral ØRWA
Toe Phalangeal
Left ØSWQ
Right ØSWP
Wrist
Left ØRWP
Right ØRWN
Kidney ØTW5
Larynx ØCWS
Lens
Left Ø8WK
Right Ø8WJ
Liver ØFWØ
Lung
Left ØBWL
Right ØBWK
Lymphatic Ø7WN
Thoracic Duct Ø7WK
Mediastinum ØWWC
Mesentery ØDWV
Metacarpal
Left ØPWQ
Right ØPWP
Metatarsal
Left ØQWP
Right ØQWN
Mouth and Throat ØCWY
Muscle
Extraocular
Left Ø8WM
Right Ø8WL
Lower ØKWY
Upper ØKWX
Nasal Mucosa and Soft Tissue Ø9WK
Neck ØWW6
Nerve
Cranial ØØWE
Peripheral Ø1WY
Omentum ØDWU
Ovary ØUW3
Pancreas ØFWG
Parathyroid Gland ØGWR
Patella
Left ØQWF

**Revision of device in** — *continued*
Patella — *continued*
Right ØQWD
Pelvic Cavity ØWWJ
Penis ØVWS
Pericardial Cavity ØWWD
Perineum
Female ØWWN
Male ØWWM
Peritoneal Cavity ØWWG
Peritoneum ØDWW
Phalanx
Finger
Left ØPWV
Right ØPWT
Thumb
Left ØPWS
Right ØPWR
Toe
Left ØQWR
Right ØQWQ
Pineal Body ØGW1
Pleura ØBWQ
Pleural Cavity
Left ØWWB
Right ØWW9
Prostate and Seminal Vesicles ØVW4
Radius
Left ØPWJ
Right ØPWH
Respiratory Tract ØWWQ
Retroperitoneum ØWWH
Ribs
1 to 2 ØPW1
3 or More ØPW2
Sacrum ØQW1
Scapula
Left ØPW6
Right ØPW5
Scrotum and Tunica Vaginalis ØVW8
Septum
Atrial Ø2W5
Ventricular Ø2WM
Sinus Ø9WY
Skin ØHWPX
Skull ØNWØ
Spinal Canal ØØWU
Spinal Cord ØØWV
Spleen Ø7WP
Sternum ØPWØ
Stomach ØDW6
Subcutaneous Tissue and Fascia
Head and Neck ØJWS
Lower Extremity ØJWW
Trunk ØJWT
Upper Extremity ØJWV
Tarsal
Left ØQWM
Right ØQWL
Tendon
Lower ØLWY
Upper ØLWX
Testis ØVWD
Thymus Ø7WM
Thyroid Gland ØGWK
Tibia
Left ØQWH
Right ØQWG
Toe Nail ØHWRX
Trachea ØBW1
Tracheobronchial Tree ØBWØ
Tympanic Membrane
Left Ø9W8
Right Ø9W7
Ulna
Left ØPWL
Right ØPWK
Ureter ØTW9
Urethra ØTWD
Uterus and Cervix ØUWD
Vagina and Cul-de-sac ØUWH
Valve
Aortic Ø2WF
Mitral Ø2WG
Pulmonary Ø2WH
Tricuspid Ø2WJ
Vas Deferens ØVWR
Vein
Azygos Ø5WØ

**Revision of device in** — *continued*
Vein — *continued*
Innominate
Left Ø5W4
Right Ø5W3
Lower Ø6WY
Upper Ø5WY
Vertebra
Cervical ØPW3
Lumbar ØQWØ
Thoracic ØPW4
Vulva ØUWM
**Revo MRI™ SureScan® pacemaker** *use* Pacemaker, Dual Chamber in ØJH
**rhBMP-2** *use* Recombinant Bone Morphogenetic Protein
**Rheos® System device** *use* Stimulator Generator in Subcutaneous Tissue and Fascia
**Rheos® System lead** *use* Stimulator Lead in Upper Arteries
**Rhinopharynx** *use* Nasopharynx
**Rhinoplasty**
*see* Alteration, Nasal Mucosa and Soft Tissue Ø9ØK
*see* Repair, Nasal Mucosa and Soft Tissue Ø9QK
*see* Replacement, Nasal Mucosa and Soft Tissue Ø9RK
*see* Supplement, Nasal Mucosa and Soft Tissue Ø9UK
**Rhinorrhaphy** *see* Repair, Nasal Mucosa and Soft Tissue Ø9QK
**Rhinoscopy** Ø9JKXZZ
**Rhizotomy**
*see* Division, Central Nervous System and Cranial Nerves ØØ8
*see* Division, Peripheral Nervous System Ø18
**Rhomboid major muscle**
*use* Muscle, Trunk, Left
*use* Muscle, Trunk, Right
**Rhomboid minor muscle**
*use* Muscle, Trunk, Left
*use* Muscle, Trunk, Right
**Rhythm electrocardiogram** *see* Measurement, Cardiac 4AØ2
**Rhytidectomy** *see* Face lift
**Right ascending lumbar vein** *use* Vein, Azygos
**Right atrioventricular valve** *use* Valve, Tricuspid
**Right auricular appendix** *use* Atrium, Right
**Right colic vein** *use* Vein, Colic
**Right coronary sulcus** *use* Heart, Right
**Right gastric artery** *use* Artery, Gastric
**Right gastroepiploic vein** *use* Vein, Superior Mesenteric
**Right inferior phrenic vein** *use* Vena Cava, Inferior
**Right inferior pulmonary vein** *use* Vein, Pulmonary, Right
**Right jugular trunk** *use* Lymphatic, Neck, Right
**Right lateral ventricle** *use* Cerebral Ventricle
**Right lymphatic duct** *use* Lymphatic, Neck, Right
**Right ovarian vein** *use* Vena Cava, Inferior
**Right second lumbar vein** *use* Vena Cava, Inferior
**Right subclavian trunk** *use* Lymphatic, Neck, Right
**Right subcostal vein** *use* Vein, Azygos
**Right superior pulmonary vein** *use* Vein, Pulmonary, Right
**Right suprarenal vein** *use* Vena Cava, Inferior
**Right testicular vein** *use* Vena Cava, Inferior
**Rima glottidis** *use* Larynx
**Risorius muscle** *use* Muscle, Facial
**RNS System lead** *use* Neurostimulator Lead in Central Nervous System and Cranial Nerves
**RNS system neurostimulator generator** *use* Neurostimulator Generator in Head and Facial Bones
**Robotic Assisted Procedure**
Extremity
Lower 8EØY
Upper 8EØX
Head and Neck Region 8EØ9
Trunk Region 8EØW
**Rotation of fetal head**
Forceps 1ØSØ7ZZ
Manual 1ØSØXZZ
**Round ligament of uterus** *use* Uterine Supporting Structure
**Round window**
*use* Ear, Inner, Left
*use* Ear, Inner, Right
**Roux-en-Y operation**
*see* Bypass, Gastrointestinal System ØD1
*see* Bypass, Hepatobiliary System and Pancreas ØF1
**Rupture**
Adhesions *see* Release

**Rupture** — *continued*
Fluid collection *see* Drainage

## S

**Sacral ganglion** *use* Nerve, Sacral Sympathetic
**Sacral lymph node** *use* Lymphatic, Pelvis
**Sacral nerve modulation (SNM) lead** *use* Stimulator Lead in Urinary System
**Sacral neuromodulation lead** *use* Stimulator Lead in Urinary System
**Sacral splanchnic nerve** *use* Nerve, Sacral Sympathetic
**Sacrectomy** *see* Excision, Lower Bones ØQB
**Sacrococcygeal ligament** *use* Lower Spine Bursa and Ligament
**Sacrococcygeal symphysis** *use* Joint, Sacrococcygeal
**Sacroiliac ligament** *use* Lower Spine Bursa and LIgament
**Sacrospinous ligament** *use* Lower Spine Bursa and Ligament
**Sacrotuberous ligament** *use* Lower Spine Bursa and Ligament
**Salpingectomy**
*see* Excision, Female Reproductive System ØUB
*see* Resection, Female Reproductive System ØUT
**Salpingolysis** *see* Release, Female Reproductive System ØUN
**Salpingopexy**
*see* Repair, Female Reproductive System ØUQ
*see* Reposition, Female Reproductive System ØUS
**Salpingopharyngeus muscle** *use* Muscle, Tongue, Palate, Pharynx
**Salpingoplasty**
*see* Repair, Female Reproductive System ØUQ
*see* Supplement, Female Reproductive System ØUU
**Salpingorrhaphy** *see* Repair, Female Reproductive System ØUQ
**Salpingoscopy** ØUJ88ZZ
**Salpingostomy** *see* Drainage, Female Reproductive System ØU9
**Salpingotomy** *see* Drainage, Female Reproductive System ØU9
**Salpinx**
*use* Fallopian Tube, Left
*use* Fallopian Tube, Right
**Saphenous nerve** *use* Nerve, Femoral
**SAPIEN transcatheter aortic valve** *use* Zooplastic Tissue in Heart and Great Vessels
**Sartorius muscle**
*use* Muscle, Upper Leg, Left
*use* Muscle, Upper Leg, Right
**Scalene muscle**
*use* Muscle, Neck, Left
*use* Muscle, Neck, Right
**Scan**
Computerized Tomography (CT) *see* Computerized Tomography (CT Scan)
Radioisotope *see* Planar Nuclear Medicine Imaging
**Scaphoid bone**
*use* Carpal, Left
*use* Carpal, Right
**Scapholunate ligament**
*use* Bursa and Ligament, Hand, Left
*use* Bursa and Ligament, Hand, Right
**Scaphotrapezium ligament**
*use* Bursa and Ligament, Hand, Left
*use* Bursa and Ligament, Hand, Right
**Scapulectomy**
*see* Excision, Upper Bones ØPB
*see* Resection, Upper Bones ØPT
**Scapulopexy**
*see* Repair, Upper Bones ØPQ
*see* Reposition, Upper Bones ØPS
**Scarpa's (vestibular) ganglion** *use* Nerve, Acoustic
**Sclerectomy** *see* Excision, Eye Ø8B
**Sclerotherapy, mechanical** *see* Destruction
**Sclerotomy** *see* Drainage, Eye Ø89
**Scrotectomy**
*see* Excision, Male Reproductive System ØVB
*see* Resection, Male Reproductive System ØVT
**Scrotoplasty**
*see* Repair, Male Reproductive System ØVQ
*see* Supplement, Male Reproductive System ØVU
**Scrotorrhaphy** *see* Repair, Male Reproductive System ØVQ
**Scrototomy** *see* Drainage, Male Reproductive System ØV9

**Sebaceous gland** *use* Skin
**Second cranial nerve** *use* Nerve, Optic
**Section, cesarean** *see* Extraction, Pregnancy 10D
**Secura (DR) (VR)** *use* Defibrillator Generator in 0JH
**Sella turcica** *use* Sphenoid Bone
**Semicircular canal**
*use* Ear, Inner, Left
*use* Ear, Inner, Right
**Semimembranosus muscle**
*use* Muscle, Upper Leg, Left
*use* Muscle, Upper Leg, Right
**Semitendinosus muscle**
*use* Muscle, Upper Leg, Left
*use* Muscle, Upper Leg, Right
**Seprafilm** *use* Adhesion Barrier
**Septal cartilage** *use* Septum, Nasal
**Septectomy**
*see* Excision, Ear, Nose, Sinus 09B
*see* Excision, Heart and Great Vessels 02B
*see* Resection, Ear, Nose, Sinus 09T
*see* Resection, Heart and Great Vessels 02T
**Septoplasty**
*see* Repair, Ear, Nose, Sinus 09Q
*see* Repair, Heart and Great Vessels 02Q
*see* Replacement, Ear, Nose, Sinus 09R
*see* Replacement, Heart and Great Vessels 02R
*see* Reposition, Ear, Nose, Sinus 09S
*see* Supplement, Ear, Nose, Sinus 09U
*see* Supplement, Heart and Great Vessels 02U
**Septostomy**, balloon atrial 02163Z7
**Septotomy** *see* Drainage, Ear, Nose, Sinus 099
**Sequestrectomy, bone** *see* Extirpation
**Serratus anterior muscle**
*use* Muscle, Thorax, Left
*use* Muscle, Thorax, Right
**Serratus posterior muscle**
*use* Muscle, Trunk, Left
*use* Muscle, Trunk, Right
**Seventh cranial nerve** *use* Nerve, Facial
**Sheffield hybrid external fixator**
*use* External Fixation Device, Hybrid in 0PH
*use* External Fixation Device, Hybrid in 0PS
*use* External Fixation Device, Hybrid in 0QH
*use* External Fixation Device, Hybrid in 0QS
**Sheffield ring external fixator**
*use* External Fixation Device, Ring in 0PH
*use* External Fixation Device, Ring in 0PS
*use* External Fixation Device, Ring in 0QH
*use* External Fixation Device, Ring in 0QS
**Shirodkar cervical cerclage** 0UVC7ZZ
**Shock Wave Therapy, Musculoskeletal** 6A93
**Short gastric artery** *use* Artery, Splenic
**Shortening**
*see* Excision
*see* Repair
*see* Reposition
**Shunt creation** *see* Bypass
**Sialoadenectomy**
Complete *see* Resection, Mouth and Throat 0CT
Partial *see* Excision, Mouth and Throat 0CB
**Sialodochoplasty**
*see* Repair, Mouth and Throat 0CQ
*see* Replacement, Mouth and Throat 0CR
*see* Supplement, Mouth and Throat 0CU
**Sialoectomy**
*see* Excision, Mouth and Throat 0CB
*see* Resection, Mouth and Throat 0CT
**Sialography** *see* Plain Radiography, Ear, Nose, Mouth and Throat B90
**Sialolithotomy** *see* Extirpation, Mouth and Throat 0CC
**Sigmoid artery** *use* Artery, Inferior Mesenteric
**Sigmoid flexure** *use* Colon, Sigmoid
**Sigmoid vein** *use* Vein, Inferior Mesenteric
**Sigmoidectomy**
*see* Excision, Gastrointestinal System 0DB
*see* Resection, Gastrointestinal System 0DT
**Sigmoidorrhaphy** *see* Repair, Gastrointestinal System 0DQ
**Sigmoidoscopy** 0DJD8ZZ
**Sigmoidotomy** *see* Drainage, Gastrointestinal System 0D9
**Single lead pacemaker (atrium) (ventricle)** *use* Pacemaker, Single Chamber in 0JH
**Single lead rate responsive pacemaker (atrium) (ventricle)** *use* Pacemaker, Single Chamber Rate Responsive in 0JH
**Sinoatrial node** *use* Conduction Mechanism
**Sinogram**
Abdominal Wall *see* Fluoroscopy, Abdomen and Pelvis BW11
Chest Wall *see* Plain Radiography, Chest BW03
Retroperitoneum *see* Fluoroscopy, Abdomen and Pelvis BW11
**Sinus venosus** *use* Atrium, Right
**Sinusectomy**
*see* Excision, Ear, Nose, Sinus 09B
*see* Resection, Ear, Nose, Sinus 09T
**Sinusoscopy** 09JY4ZZ
**Sinusotomy** *see* Drainage, Ear, Nose, Sinus 099
**Sirolimus-eluting coronary stent** *use* Intraluminal Device, Drug-eluting in Heart and Great Vessels
**Sixth cranial nerve** *use* Nerve, Abducens
**Size reduction, breast** *see* Excision, Skin and Breast 0HB
**SJM Biocor® Stented Valve System** *use* Zooplastic Tissue in Heart and Great Vessels
**Skene's (paraurethral) gland** *use* Gland, Vestibular
**Skin Substitute, Porcine Liver Derived, Replacement** XHRPXL2
**Sling**
Fascial, orbicularis muscle (mouth) *see* Supplement, Muscle, Facial 0KU1
Levator muscle, for urethral suspension *see* Reposition, Bladder Neck 0TSC
Pubococcygeal, for urethral suspension *see* Reposition, Bladder Neck 0TSC
Rectum *see* Reposition, Rectum 0DSP
**Small bowel series** *see* Fluoroscopy, Bowel, Small BD13
**Small saphenous vein**
*use* Saphenous Vein, Left
*use* Saphenous Vein, Right
**Snaring, polyp, colon** *see* Excision, Gastrointestinal System 0DB
**Solar (celiac) plexus** *use* Nerve, Abdominal Sympathetic
**Soletra® single-channel neurostimulator** *use* Stimulator Generator, Single Array in 0JH
**Soleus muscle**
*use* Muscle, Lower Leg, Left
*use* Muscle, Lower Leg, Right
**Spacer**
Insertion of device in
Disc
Lumbar Vertebral 0SH2
Lumbosacral 0SH4
Joint
Acromioclavicular
Left 0RHH
Right 0RHG
Ankle
Left 0SHG
Right 0SHF
Carpal
Left 0RHR
Right 0RHQ
Carpometacarpal
Left 0RHT
Right 0RHS
Cervical Vertebral 0RH1
Cervicothoracic Vertebral 0RH4
Coccygeal 0SH6
Elbow
Left 0RHM
Right 0RHL
Finger Phalangeal
Left 0RHX
Right 0RHW
Hip
Left 0SHB
Right 0SH9
Knee
Left 0SHD
Right 0SHC
Lumbar Vertebral 0SH0
Lumbosacral 0SH3
Metacarpophalangeal
Left 0RHV
Right 0RHU
Metatarsal-Phalangeal
Left 0SHN
Right 0SHM
Occipital-cervical 0RH0
Sacrococcygeal 0SH5
Sacroiliac
Left 0SH8
Right 0SH7
**Spacer** — *continued*
Insertion of device in — *continued*
Joint — *continued*
Shoulder
Left 0RHK
Right 0RHJ
Sternoclavicular
Left 0RHF
Right 0RHE
Tarsal
Left 0SHJ
Right 0SHH
Tarsometatarsal
Left 0SHL
Right 0SHK
Temporomandibular
Left 0RHD
Right 0RHC
Thoracic Vertebral 0RH6
Thoracolumbar Vertebral 0RHA
Toe Phalangeal
Left 0SHQ
Right 0SHP
Wrist
Left 0RHP
Right 0RHN
Removal of device from
Acromioclavicular
Left 0RPH
Right 0RPG
Ankle
Left 0SPG
Right 0SPF
Carpal
Left 0RPR
Right 0RPQ
Carpometacarpal
Left 0RPT
Right 0RPS
Cervical Vertebral 0RP1
Cervicothoracic Vertebral 0RP4
Coccygeal 0SP6
Elbow
Left 0RPM
Right 0RPL
Finger Phalangeal
Left 0RPX
Right 0RPW
Hip
Left 0SPB
Right 0SP9
Knee
Left 0SPD
Right 0SPC
Lumbar Vertebral 0SP0
Lumbosacral 0SP3
Metacarpophalangeal
Left 0RPV
Right 0RPU
Metatarsal-Phalangeal
Left 0SPN
Right 0SPM
Occipital-cervical 0RP0
Sacrococcygeal 0SP5
Sacroiliac
Left 0SP8
Right 0SP7
Shoulder
Left 0RPK
Right 0RPJ
Sternoclavicular
Left 0RPF
Right 0RPE
Tarsal
Left 0SPJ
Right 0SPH
Tarsometatarsal
Left 0SPL
Right 0SPK
Temporomandibular
Left 0RPD
Right 0RPC
Thoracic Vertebral 0RP6
Thoracolumbar Vertebral 0RPA
Toe Phalangeal
Left 0SPQ
Right 0SPP
Wrist
Left 0RPP

**Spacer** — *continued*
Removal of device from — *continued*
Wrist — *continued*
Right ØRPN
Revision of device in
Acromioclavicular
Left ØRWH
Right ØRWG
Ankle
Left ØSWG
Right ØSWF
Carpal
Left ØRWR
Right ØRWQ
Carpometacarpal
Left ØRWT
Right ØRWS
Cervical Vertebral ØRW1
Cervicothoracic Vertebral ØRW4
Coccygeal ØSW6
Elbow
Left ØRWM
Right ØRWL
Finger Phalangeal
Left ØRWX
Right ØRWW
Hip
Left ØSWB
Right ØSW9
Knee
Left ØSWD
Right ØSWC
Lumbar Vertebral ØSWØ
Lumbosacral ØSW3
Metacarpophalangeal
Left ØRWV
Right ØRWU
Metatarsal-Phalangeal
Left ØSWN
Right ØSWM
Occipital-cervical ØRWØ
Sacrococcygeal ØSW5
Sacroiliac
Left ØSW8
Right ØSW7
Shoulder
Left ØRWK
Right ØRWJ
Sternoclavicular
Left ØRWF
Right ØRWE
Tarsal
Left ØSWJ
Right ØSWH
Tarsometatarsal
Left ØSWL
Right ØSWK
Temporomandibular
Left ØRWD
Right ØRWC
Thoracic Vertebral ØRW6
Thoracolumbar Vertebral ØRWA
Toe Phalangeal
Left ØSWQ
Right ØSWP
Wrist
Left ØRWP
Right ØRWN
**Spectroscopy**
Intravascular 8EØ23DZ
Near infrared 8EØ23DZ
**Speech Assessment** FØØ
**Speech therapy** *see* Speech Treatment, Rehabilitation FØ6
**Speech Treatment** FØ6
**Sphenoidectomy**
*see* Excision, Ear, Nose, Sinus Ø9B
*see* Excision, Head and Facial Bones ØNB
*see* Resection, Ear, Nose, Sinus Ø9T
*see* Resection, Head and Facial Bones ØNT
**Sphenoidotomy** *see* Drainage, Ear, Nose, Sinus Ø99
**Sphenomandibular ligament** *use* Bursa and Ligament, Head and Neck
**Sphenopalatine (pterygopalatine) ganglion** *use* Nerve, Head and Neck Sympathetic
**Sphincterorrhaphy, anal** *see* Repair, Anal Sphincter ØDQR
**Sphincterotomy, anal**
*see* Division, Anal Sphincter ØD8R
*see* Drainage, Anal Sphincter ØD9R
**Spinal cord neurostimulator lead** *use* Neurostimulator Lead in Central Nervous System and Cranial Nerves
**Spinal growth rods, magnetically controlled** *use* Magnetically Controlled Growth Rod(s) in New Technology
**Spinal nerve, cervical** *use* Nerve, Cervical
**Spinal nerve, lumbar** *use* Nerve, Lumbar
**Spinal nerve, sacral** *use* Nerve, Sacral
**Spinal nerve, thoracic** *use* Nerve, Thoracic
**Spinal Stabilization Device**
Facet Replacement
Cervical Vertebral ØRH1
Cervicothoracic Vertebral ØRH4
Lumbar Vertebral ØSHØ
Lumbosacral ØSH3
Occipital-cervical ØRHØ
Thoracic Vertebral ØRH6
Thoracolumbar Vertebral ØRHA
Interspinous Process
Cervical Vertebral ØRH1
Cervicothoracic Vertebral ØRH4
Lumbar Vertebral ØSHØ
Lumbosacral ØSH3
Occipital-cervical ØRHØ
Thoracic Vertebral ØRH6
Thoracolumbar Vertebral ØRHA
Pedicle-Based
Cervical Vertebral ØRH1
Cervicothoracic Vertebral ØRH4
Lumbar Vertebral ØSHØ
Lumbosacral ØSH3
Occipital-cervical ØRHØ
Thoracic Vertebral ØRH6
Thoracolumbar Vertebral ØRHA
**Spinous process**
*use* Vertebra, Cervical
*use* Vertebra, Lumbar
*use* Vertebra, Thoracic
**Spiral ganglion** *use* Nerve, Acoustic
**Spiration IBV™ Valve System** *use* Intraluminal Device, Endobronchial Valve in Respiratory System
**Splenectomy**
*see* Excision, Lymphatic and Hemic Systems Ø7B
*see* Resection, Lymphatic and Hemic Systems Ø7T
**Splenic flexure** *use* Colon, Transverse
**Splenic plexus** *use* Nerve, Abdominal Sympathetic
**Splenius capitis muscle** *use* Muscle, Head
**Splenius cervicis muscle**
*use* Muscle, Neck, Left
*use* Muscle, Neck, Right
**Splenolysis** *see* Release, Lymphatic and Hemic Systems Ø7N
**Splenopexy**
*see* Repair, Lymphatic and Hemic Systems Ø7Q
*see* Reposition, Lymphatic and Hemic Systems Ø7S
**Splenoplasty** *see* Repair, Lymphatic and Hemic Systems Ø7Q
**Splenorrhaphy** *see* Repair, Lymphatic and Hemic Systems Ø7Q
**Splenotomy** *see* Drainage, Lymphatic and Hemic Systems Ø79
**Splinting, musculoskeletal** *see* Immobilization, Anatomical Regions 2W3
**SPY system intravascular fluorescence angiography** *see* Monitoring, Physiological Systems 4A1
**Stapedectomy**
*see* Excision, Ear, Nose, Sinus Ø9B
*see* Resection, Ear, Nose, Sinus Ø9T
**Stapediolysis** *see* Release, Ear, Nose, Sinus Ø9N
**Stapedioplasty**
*see* Repair, Ear, Nose, Sinus Ø9Q
*see* Replacement, Ear, Nose, Sinus Ø9R
*see* Supplement, Ear, Nose, Sinus Ø9U
**Stapedotomy** *see* Drainage, Ear, Nose, Sinus Ø99
**Stapes**
*use* Auditory Ossicle, Left
*use* Auditory Ossicle, Right
**STELARA®** *use* Other New Technology Therapeutic Substance
**Stellate ganglion** *use* Nerve, Head and Neck Sympathetic
**Stem cell transplant** *see* Transfusion, Circulatory 3Ø2
**Stensen's duct**
*use* Duct, Parotid, Left
*use* Duct, Parotid, Right
**Stent, intraluminal (cardiovascular) (gastrointestinal) (hepatobiliary) (urinary)** *use* Intraluminal Device
**Stented tissue valve** *use* Zooplastic Tissue in Heart and Great Vessels
**Stereotactic Radiosurgery**
Abdomen DW23
Adrenal Gland DG22
Bile Ducts DF22
Bladder DT22
Bone Marrow D72Ø
Brain DØ2Ø
Brain Stem DØ21
Breast
Left DM2Ø
Right DM21
Bronchus DB21
Cervix DU21
Chest DW22
Chest Wall DB27
Colon DD25
Diaphragm DB28
Duodenum DD22
Ear D92Ø
Esophagus DD2Ø
Eye D82Ø
Gallbladder DF21
Gamma Beam
Abdomen DW23JZZ
Adrenal Gland DG22JZZ
Bile Ducts DF22JZZ
Bladder DT22JZZ
Bone Marrow D72ØJZZ
Brain DØ2ØJZZ
Brain Stem DØ21JZZ
Breast
Left DM2ØJZZ
Right DM21JZZ
Bronchus DB21JZZ
Cervix DU21JZZ
Chest DW22JZZ
Chest Wall DB27JZZ
Colon DD25JZZ
Diaphragm DB28JZZ
Duodenum DD22JZZ
Ear D92ØJZZ
Esophagus DD2ØJZZ
Eye D82ØJZZ
Gallbladder DF21JZZ
Gland
Adrenal DG22JZZ
Parathyroid DG24JZZ
Pituitary DG2ØJZZ
Thyroid DG25JZZ
Glands, Salivary D926JZZ
Head and Neck DW21JZZ
Ileum DD24JZZ
Jejunum DD23JZZ
Kidney DT2ØJZZ
Larynx D92BJZZ
Liver DF2ØJZZ
Lung DB22JZZ
Lymphatics
Abdomen D726JZZ
Axillary D724JZZ
Inguinal D728JZZ
Neck D723JZZ
Pelvis D727JZZ
Thorax D725JZZ
Mediastinum DB26JZZ
Mouth D924JZZ
Nasopharynx D92DJZZ
Neck and Head DW21JZZ
Nerve, Peripheral DØ27JZZ
Nose D921JZZ
Ovary DU2ØJZZ
Palate
Hard D928JZZ
Soft D929JZZ
Pancreas DF23JZZ
Parathyroid Gland DG24JZZ
Pelvic Region DW26JZZ
Pharynx D92CJZZ
Pineal Body DG21JZZ
Pituitary Gland DG2ØJZZ
Pleura DB25JZZ
Prostate DV2ØJZZ
Rectum DD27JZZ
Sinuses D927JZZ

- **Stereotactic Radiosurgery** — *continued*
  - Gamma Beam — *continued*
    - Spinal Cord DØ26JZZ
    - Spleen D722JZZ
    - Stomach DD21JZZ
    - Testis DV21JZZ
    - Thymus D721JZZ
    - Thyroid Gland DG25JZZ
    - Tongue D925JZZ
    - Trachea DB2ØJZZ
    - Ureter DT21JZZ
    - Urethra DT23JZZ
    - Uterus DU22JZZ
  - Gland
    - Adrenal DG22
    - Parathyroid DG24
    - Pituitary DG2Ø
    - Thyroid DG25
  - Glands, Salivary D926
  - Head and Neck DW21
  - Ileum DD24
  - Jejunum DD23
  - Kidney DT2Ø
  - Larynx D92B
  - Liver DF2Ø
  - Lung DB22
  - Lymphatics
    - Abdomen D726
    - Axillary D724
    - Inguinal D728
    - Neck D723
    - Pelvis D727
    - Thorax D725
  - Mediastinum DB26
  - Mouth D924
  - Nasopharynx D92D
  - Neck and Head DW21
  - Nerve, Peripheral DØ27
  - Nose D921
  - Other Photon
    - Abdomen DW23DZZ
    - Adrenal Gland DG22DZZ
    - Bile Ducts DF22DZZ
    - Bladder DT22DZZ
    - Bone Marrow D72ØDZZ
    - Brain DØ2ØDZZ
    - Brain Stem DØ21DZZ
    - Breast
      - Left DM2ØDZZ
      - Right DM21DZZ
    - Bronchus DB21DZZ
    - Cervix DU21DZZ
    - Chest DW22DZZ
    - Chest Wall DB27DZZ
    - Colon DD25DZZ
    - Diaphragm DB28DZZ
    - Duodenum DD22DZZ
    - Ear D92ØDZZ
    - Esophagus DD2ØDZZ
    - Eye D82ØDZZ
    - Gallbladder DF21DZZ
    - Gland
      - Adrenal DG22DZZ
      - Parathyroid DG24DZZ
      - Pituitary DG2ØDZZ
      - Thyroid DG25DZZ
    - Glands, Salivary D926DZZ
    - Head and Neck DW21DZZ
    - Ileum DD24DZZ
    - Jejunum DD23DZZ
    - Kidney DT2ØDZZ
    - Larynx D92BDZZ
    - Liver DF2ØDZZ
    - Lung DB22DZZ
    - Lymphatics
      - Abdomen D726DZZ
      - Axillary D724DZZ
      - Inguinal D728DZZ
      - Neck D723DZZ
      - Pelvis D727DZZ
      - Thorax D725DZZ
    - Mediastinum DB26DZZ
    - Mouth D924DZZ
    - Nasopharynx D92DDZZ
    - Neck and Head DW21DZZ
    - Nerve, Peripheral DØ27DZZ
    - Nose D921DZZ
    - Ovary DU2ØDZZ

- **Stereotactic Radiosurgery** — *continued*
  - Other Photon — *continued*
    - Palate
      - Hard D928DZZ
      - Soft D929DZZ
    - Pancreas DF23DZZ
    - Parathyroid Gland DG24DZZ
    - Pelvic Region DW26DZZ
    - Pharynx D92CDZZ
    - Pineal Body DG21DZZ
    - Pituitary Gland DG2ØDZZ
    - Pleura DB25DZZ
    - Prostate DV2ØDZZ
    - Rectum DD27DZZ
    - Sinuses D927DZZ
    - Spinal Cord DØ26DZZ
    - Spleen D722DZZ
    - Stomach DD21DZZ
    - Testis DV21DZZ
    - Thymus D721DZZ
    - Thyroid Gland DG25DZZ
    - Tongue D925DZZ
    - Trachea DB2ØDZZ
    - Ureter DT21DZZ
    - Urethra DT23DZZ
    - Uterus DU22DZZ
  - Ovary DU2Ø
  - Palate
    - Hard D928
    - Soft D929
  - Pancreas DF23
  - Parathyroid Gland DG24
  - Particulate
    - Abdomen DW23HZZ
    - Adrenal Gland DG22HZZ
    - Bile Ducts DF22HZZ
    - Bladder DT22HZZ
    - Bone Marrow D72ØHZZ
    - Brain DØ2ØHZZ
    - Brain Stem DØ21HZZ
    - Breast
      - Left DM2ØHZZ
      - Right DM21HZZ
    - Bronchus DB21HZZ
    - Cervix DU21HZZ
    - Chest DW22HZZ
    - Chest Wall DB27HZZ
    - Colon DD25HZZ
    - Diaphragm DB28HZZ
    - Duodenum DD22HZZ
    - Ear D92ØHZZ
    - Esophagus DD2ØHZZ
    - Eye D82ØHZZ
    - Gallbladder DF21HZZ
    - Gland
      - Adrenal DG22HZZ
      - Parathyroid DG24HZZ
      - Pituitary DG2ØHZZ
      - Thyroid DG25HZZ
    - Glands, Salivary D926HZZ
    - Head and Neck DW21HZZ
    - Ileum DD24HZZ
    - Jejunum DD23HZZ
    - Kidney DT2ØHZZ
    - Larynx D92BHZZ
    - Liver DF2ØHZZ
    - Lung DB22HZZ
    - Lymphatics
      - Abdomen D726HZZ
      - Axillary D724HZZ
      - Inguinal D728HZZ
      - Neck D723HZZ
      - Pelvis D727HZZ
      - Thorax D725HZZ
    - Mediastinum DB26HZZ
    - Mouth D924HZZ
    - Nasopharynx D92DHZZ
    - Neck and Head DW21HZZ
    - Nerve, Peripheral DØ27HZZ
    - Nose D921HZZ
    - Ovary DU2ØHZZ
    - Palate
      - Hard D928HZZ
      - Soft D929HZZ
    - Pancreas DF23HZZ
    - Parathyroid Gland DG24HZZ
    - Pelvic Region DW26HZZ
    - Pharynx D92CHZZ
    - Pineal Body DG21HZZ

- **Stereotactic Radiosurgery** — *continued*
  - Particulate — *continued*
    - Pituitary Gland DG2ØHZZ
    - Pleura DB25HZZ
    - Prostate DV2ØHZZ
    - Rectum DD27HZZ
    - Sinuses D927HZZ
    - Spinal Cord DØ26HZZ
    - Spleen D722HZZ
    - Stomach DD21HZZ
    - Testis DV21HZZ
    - Thymus D721HZZ
    - Thyroid Gland DG25HZZ
    - Tongue D925HZZ
    - Trachea DB2ØHZZ
    - Ureter DT21HZZ
    - Urethra DT23HZZ
    - Uterus DU22HZZ
  - Pelvic Region DW26
  - Pharynx D92C
  - Pineal Body DG21
  - Pituitary Gland DG2Ø
  - Pleura DB25
  - Prostate DV2Ø
  - Rectum DD27
  - Sinuses D927
  - Spinal Cord DØ26
  - Spleen D722
  - Stomach DD21
  - Testis DV21
  - Thymus D721
  - Thyroid Gland DG25
  - Tongue D925
  - Trachea DB2Ø
  - Ureter DT21
  - Urethra DT23
  - Uterus DU22
- **Sternoclavicular ligament**
  - *use* Bursa and Ligament, Shoulder, Left
  - *use* Bursa and Ligament, Shoulder, Right
- **Sternocleidomastoid artery**
  - *use* Artery, Thyroid, Left
  - *use* Artery, Thyroid, Right
- **Sternocleidomastoid muscle**
  - *use* Muscle, Neck, Left
  - *use* Muscle, Neck, Right
- **Sternocostal ligament**
  - *use* Rib(s) Bursa and Ligament
  - *use* Sternum Bursa and Ligament
- **Sternotomy**
  - *see* Division, Sternum ØP8Ø
  - *see* Drainage, Sternum ØP9Ø
- **Stimulation, cardiac**
  - Cardioversion 5A22Ø4Z
  - Electrophysiologic testing *see* Measurement, Cardiac 4AØ2
- **Stimulator Generator**
  - Insertion of device in
    - Abdomen ØJH8
    - Back ØJH7
    - Chest ØJH6
  - Multiple Array
    - Abdomen ØJH8
    - Back ØJH7
    - Chest ØJH6
  - Multiple Array Rechargeable
    - Abdomen ØJH8
    - Back ØJH7
    - Chest ØJH6
  - Removal of device from, Subcutaneous Tissue and Fascia, Trunk ØJPT
  - Revision of device in, Subcutaneous Tissue and Fascia, Trunk ØJWT
  - Single Array
    - Abdomen ØJH8
    - Back ØJH7
    - Chest ØJH6
  - Single Array Rechargeable
    - Abdomen ØJH8
    - Back ØJH7
    - Chest ØJH6
- **Stimulator Lead**
  - Insertion of device in
    - Anal Sphincter ØDHR
    - Artery
      - Left Ø3HL
      - Right Ø3HK
    - Bladder ØTHB

**Stimulator Lead** — *continued*
Insertion of device in — *continued*
Muscle
Lower ØKHY
Upper ØKHX
Stomach ØDH6
Ureter ØTH9
Removal of device from
Anal Sphincter ØDPR
Artery, Upper Ø3PY
Bladder ØTPB
Muscle
Lower ØKPY
Upper ØKPX
Stomach ØDP6
Ureter ØTP9
Revision of device in
Anal Sphincter ØDWR
Artery, Upper Ø3WY
Bladder ØTWB
Muscle
Lower ØKWY
Upper ØKWX
Stomach ØDW6
Ureter ØTW9
**Stoma**
Excision
Abdominal Wall ØWBFXZ2
Neck ØWB6XZ2
Repair
Abdominal Wall ØWQFXZ2
Neck ØWQ6XZ2
**Stomatoplasty**
*see* Repair, Mouth and Throat ØCQ
*see* Replacement, Mouth and Throat ØCR
*see* Supplement, Mouth and Throat ØCU
**Stomatorrhaphy** *see* Repair, Mouth and Throat ØCQ
**Stratos LV** *use* Cardiac Resynchronization Pacemaker Pulse Generator in ØJH
**Stress test** 4A12XM4
**Stripping** *see* Extraction
**Study**
Electrophysiologic stimulation, cardiac *see* Measurement, Cardiac 4AØ2
Ocular motility 4AØ7X7Z
Pulmonary airway flow measurement *see* Measurement, Respiratory 4AØ9
Visual acuity 4AØ7XØZ
**Styloglossus muscle** *use* Muscle, Tongue, Palate, Pharynx
**Stylomandibular ligament** *use* Bursa and Ligament, Head and Neck
**Stylopharyngeus muscle** *use* Muscle, Tongue, Palate, Pharynx
**Subacromial bursa**
*use* Bursa and Ligament, Shoulder, Left
*use* Bursa and Ligament, Shoulder, Right
**Subaortic (common iliac) lymph node** *use* Lymphatic, Pelvis
**Subarachnoid space, spinal** *use* Spinal Canal
**Subclavicular (apical) lymph node**
*use* Lymphatic, Axillary, Left
*use* Lymphatic, Axillary, Right
**Subclavius muscle**
*use* Muscle, Thorax, Left
*use* Muscle, Thorax, Right
**Subclavius nerve** *use* Nerve, Brachial Plexus
**Subcostal artery** *use* Upper Artery
**Subcostal muscle**
*use* Muscle, Thorax, Left
*use* Muscle, Thorax, Right
**Subcostal nerve** *use* Nerve, Thoracic
**Subcutaneous injection reservoir, port** *use* Vascular Access Device, Totally Implantable in Subcutaneous Tissue and Fascia
**Subcutaneous injection reservoir, pump** *use* Infusion Device, Pump in Subcutaneous Tissue and Fascia
**Subdermal progesterone implant** *use* Contraceptive Device in Subcutaneous Tissue and Fascia
**Subdural space, spinal** *use* Spinal Canal
**Submandibular ganglion**
*use* Nerve, Facial
*use* Nerve, Head and Neck Sympathetic
**Submandibular gland**
*use* Gland, Submaxillary, Left
*use* Gland, Submaxillary, Right
**Submandibular lymph node** *use* Lymphatic, Head
**Submaxillary ganglion** *use* Nerve, Head and Neck Sympathetic
**Submaxillary lymph node** *use* Lymphatic, Head
**Submental artery** *use* Artery, Face
**Submental lymph node** *use* Lymphatic, Head
**Submucous (Meissner's) plexus** *use* Nerve, Abdominal Sympathetic
**Suboccipital nerve** *use* Nerve, Cervical
**Suboccipital venous plexus**
*use* Vein, Vertebral, Left
*use* Vein, Vertebral, Right
**Subparotid lymph node** *use* Lymphatic, Head
**Subscapular aponeurosis**
*use* Subcutaneous Tissue and Fascia, Upper Arm, Left
*use* Subcutaneous Tissue and Fascia, Upper Arm, Right
**Subscapular artery**
*use* Artery, Axillary, Left
*use* Artery, Axillary, Right
**Subscapular (posterior) lymph node**
*use* Lymphatic, Axillary, Left
*use* Lymphatic, Axillary, Right
**Subscapularis muscle**
*use* Muscle, Shoulder, Left
*use* Muscle, Shoulder, Right
**Substance Abuse Treatment**
Counseling
Family, for substance abuse, Other Family Counseling HZ63ZZZ
Group
12-Step HZ43ZZZ
Behavioral HZ41ZZZ
Cognitive HZ4ØZZZ
Cognitive-Behavioral HZ42ZZZ
Confrontational HZ48ZZZ
Continuing Care HZ49ZZZ
Infectious Disease
Post-Test HZ4CZZZ
Pre-Test HZ4CZZZ
Interpersonal HZ44ZZZ
Motivational Enhancement HZ47ZZZ
Psychoeducation HZ46ZZZ
Spiritual HZ4BZZZ
Vocational HZ45ZZZ
Individual
12-Step HZ33ZZZ
Behavioral HZ31ZZZ
Cognitive HZ3ØZZZ
Cognitive-Behavioral HZ32ZZZ
Confrontational HZ38ZZZ
Continuing Care HZ39ZZZ
Infectious Disease
Post-Test HZ3CZZZ
Pre-Test HZ3CZZZ
Interpersonal HZ34ZZZ
Motivational Enhancement HZ37ZZZ
Psychoeducation HZ36ZZZ
Spiritual HZ3BZZZ
Vocational HZ35ZZZ
Detoxification Services, for substance abuse HZ2ZZZZ
Medication Management
Antabuse HZ83ZZZ
Bupropion HZ87ZZZ
Clonidine HZ86ZZZ
Levo-alpha-acetyl-methadol (LAAM) HZ82ZZZ
Methadone Maintenance HZ81ZZZ
Naloxone HZ85ZZZ
Naltrexone HZ84ZZZ
Nicotine Replacement HZ8ØZZZ
Other Replacement Medication HZ89ZZZ
Psychiatric Medication HZ88ZZZ
Pharmacotherapy
Antabuse HZ93ZZZ
Bupropion HZ97ZZZ
Clonidine HZ96ZZZ
Levo-alpha-acetyl-methadol (LAAM) HZ92ZZZ
Methadone Maintenance HZ91ZZZ
Naloxone HZ95ZZZ
Naltrexone HZ94ZZZ
Nicotine Replacement HZ9ØZZZ
Psychiatric Medication HZ98ZZZ
Replacement Medication, Other HZ99ZZZ
Psychotherapy
12-Step HZ53ZZZ
Behavioral HZ51ZZZ
Cognitive HZ5ØZZZ
Cognitive-Behavioral HZ52ZZZ
Confrontational HZ58ZZZ
Interactive HZ55ZZZ
**Substance Abuse Treatment** — *continued*
Psychotherapy — *continued*
Interpersonal HZ54ZZZ
Motivational Enhancement HZ57ZZZ
Psychoanalysis HZ5BZZZ
Psychodynamic HZ5CZZZ
Psychoeducation HZ56ZZZ
Psychophysiological HZ5DZZZ
Supportive HZ59ZZZ
**Substantia nigra** *use* Basal Ganglia
**Subtalar (talocalcaneal) joint**
*use* Joint, Tarsal, Left
*use* Joint, Tarsal, Right
**Subtalar ligament**
*use* Bursa and Ligament, Foot, Left
*use* Bursa and Ligament, Foot, Right
**Subthalamic nucleus** *use* Basal Ganglia
**Suction curettage (D&C), nonobstetric** *see* Extraction, Endometrium ØUDB
**Suction curettage, obstetric post-delivery** *see* Extraction, Products of Conception, Retained 1ØD1
**Superficial circumflex iliac vein**
*use* Saphenous Vein, Left
*use* Saphenous Vein, Right
**Superficial epigastric artery**
*use* Artery, Femoral, Left
*use* Artery, Femoral, Right
**Superficial epigastric vein**
*use* Saphenous Vein, Left
*use* Saphenous Vein, Right
**Superficial Inferior Epigastric Artery Flap**
Replacement
Bilateral ØHRVØ78
Left ØHRUØ78
Right ØHRTØ78
Transfer
Left ØKXG
Right ØKXF
**Superficial palmar arch**
*use* Artery, Hand, Left
*use* Artery, Hand, Right
**Superficial palmar venous arch**
*use* Vein, Hand, Left
*use* Vein, Hand, Right
**Superficial temporal artery**
*use* Artery, Temporal, Left
*use* Artery, Temporal, Right
**Superficial transverse perineal muscle** *use* Muscle, Perineum
**Superior cardiac nerve** *use* Nerve, Thoracic Sympathetic
**Superior cerebellar vein** *use* Vein, Intracranial
**Superior cerebral vein** *use* Vein, Intracranial
**Superior clunic (cluneal) nerve** *use* Nerve, Lumbar
**Superior epigastric artery**
*use* Artery, Internal Mammary, Left
*use* Artery, Internal Mammary, Right
**Superior genicular artery**
*use* Artery, Popliteal, Left
*use* Artery, Popliteal, Right
**Superior gluteal artery**
*use* Artery, Internal Iliac, Left
*use* Artery, Internal Iliac, Right
**Superior gluteal nerve** *use* Nerve, Lumbar Plexus
**Superior hypogastric plexus** *use* Nerve, Abdominal Sympathetic
**Superior labial artery** *use* Artery, Face
**Superior laryngeal artery**
*use* Artery, Thyroid, Left
*use* Artery, Thyroid, Right
**Superior laryngeal nerve** *use* Nerve, Vagus
**Superior longitudinal muscle** *use* Muscle, Tongue, Palate, Pharynx
**Superior mesenteric ganglion** *use* Nerve, Abdominal Sympathetic
**Superior mesenteric lymph node** *use* Lymphatic, Mesenteric
**Superior mesenteric plexus** *use* Nerve, Abdominal Sympathetic
**Superior oblique muscle**
*use* Muscle, Extraocular, Left
*use* Muscle, Extraocular, Right
**Superior olivary nucleus** *use* Pons
**Superior rectal artery** *use* Artery, Inferior Mesenteric
**Superior rectal vein** *use* Vein, Inferior Mesenteric
**Superior rectus muscle**
*use* Muscle, Extraocular, Left
*use* Muscle, Extraocular, Right

**Superior tarsal plate**
*use* Eyelid, Upper, Left
*use* Eyelid, Upper, Right
**Superior thoracic artery**
*use* Artery, Axillary, Left
*use* Artery, Axillary, Right
**Superior thyroid artery**
*use* Artery, External Carotid, Left
*use* Artery, External Carotid, Right
*use* Artery, Thyroid, Left
*use* Artery, Thyroid, Right
**Superior turbinate** *use* Turbinate, Nasal
**Superior ulnar collateral artery**
*use* Artery, Brachial, Left
*use* Artery, Brachial, Right
**Supplement**
Abdominal Wall ØWUF
Acetabulum
Left ØQU5
Right ØQU4
Ampulla of Vater ØFUC
Anal Sphincter ØDUR
Ankle Region
Left ØYUL
Right ØYUK
Anus ØDUQ
Aorta
Abdominal Ø4UØ
Thoracic
Ascending/Arch Ø2UX
Descending Ø2UW
Arm
Lower
Left ØXUF
Right ØXUD
Upper
Left ØXU9
Right ØXU8
Artery
Anterior Tibial
Left Ø4UQ
Right Ø4UP
Axillary
Left Ø3U6
Right Ø3U5
Brachial
Left Ø3U8
Right Ø3U7
Celiac Ø4U1
Colic
Left Ø4U7
Middle Ø4U8
Right Ø4U6
Common Carotid
Left Ø3UJ
Right Ø3UH
Common Iliac
Left Ø4UD
Right Ø4UC
External Carotid
Left Ø3UN
Right Ø3UM
External Iliac
Left Ø4UJ
Right Ø4UH
Face Ø3UR
Femoral
Left Ø4UL
Right Ø4UK
Foot
Left Ø4UW
Right Ø4UV
Gastric Ø4U2
Hand
Left Ø3UF
Right Ø3UD
Hepatic Ø4U3
Inferior Mesenteric Ø4UB
Innominate Ø3U2
Internal Carotid
Left Ø3UL
Right Ø3UK
Internal Iliac
Left Ø4UF
Right Ø4UE
Internal Mammary
Left Ø3U1
Right Ø3UØ

**Supplement** — *continued*
Artery — *continued*
Intracranial Ø3UG
Lower Ø4UY
Peroneal
Left Ø4UU
Right Ø4UT
Popliteal
Left Ø4UN
Right Ø4UM
Posterior Tibial
Left Ø4US
Right Ø4UR
Pulmonary
Left Ø2UR
Right Ø2UQ
Pulmonary Trunk Ø2UP
Radial
Left Ø3UC
Right Ø3UB
Renal
Left Ø4UA
Right Ø4U9
Splenic Ø4U4
Subclavian
Left Ø3U4
Right Ø3U3
Superior Mesenteric Ø4U5
Temporal
Left Ø3UT
Right Ø3US
Thyroid
Left Ø3UV
Right Ø3UU
Ulnar
Left Ø3UA
Right Ø3U9
Upper Ø3UY
Vertebral
Left Ø3UQ
Right Ø3UP
Atrium
Left Ø2U7
Right Ø2U6
Auditory Ossicle
Left Ø9UA
Right Ø9U9
Axilla
Left ØXU5
Right ØXU4
Back
Lower ØWUL
Upper ØWUK
Bladder ØTUB
Bladder Neck ØTUC
Bone
Ethmoid
Left ØNUG
Right ØNUF
Frontal ØNU1
Hyoid ØNUX
Lacrimal
Left ØNUJ
Right ØNUH
Nasal ØNUB
Occipital ØNU7
Palatine
Left ØNUL
Right ØNUK
Parietal
Left ØNU4
Right ØNU3
Pelvic
Left ØQU3
Right ØQU2
Sphenoid ØNUC
Temporal
Left ØNU6
Right ØNU5
Zygomatic
Left ØNUN
Right ØNUM
Breast
Bilateral ØHUV
Left ØHUU
Right ØHUT
Bronchus
Lingula ØBU9

**Supplement** — *continued*
Bronchus — *continued*
Lower Lobe
Left ØBUB
Right ØBU6
Main
Left ØBU7
Right ØBU3
Middle Lobe, Right ØBU5
Upper Lobe
Left ØBU8
Right ØBU4
Buccal Mucosa ØCU4
Bursa and Ligament
Abdomen
Left ØMUJ
Right ØMUH
Ankle
Left ØMUR
Right ØMUQ
Elbow
Left ØMU4
Right ØMU3
Foot
Left ØMUT
Right ØMUS
Hand
Left ØMU8
Right ØMU7
Head and Neck ØMUØ
Hip
Left ØMUM
Right ØMUL
Knee
Left ØMUP
Right ØMUN
Lower Extremity
Left ØMUW
Right ØMUV
Perineum ØMUK
Rib(s) ØMUG
Shoulder
Left ØMU2
Right ØMU1
Spine
Lower ØMUD
Upper ØMUC
Sternum ØMUF
Upper Extremity
Left ØMUB
Right ØMU9
Wrist
Left ØMU6
Right ØMU5
Buttock
Left ØYU1
Right ØYUØ
Carina ØBU2
Carpal
Left ØPUN
Right ØPUM
Cecum ØDUH
Cerebral Meninges ØØU1
Cerebral Ventricle ØØU6
Chest Wall ØWU8
Chordae Tendineae Ø2U9
Cisterna Chyli Ø7UL
Clavicle
Left ØPUB
Right ØPU9
Clitoris ØUUJ
Coccyx ØQUS
Colon
Ascending ØDUK
Descending ØDUM
Sigmoid ØDUN
Transverse ØDUL
Cord
Bilateral ØVUH
Left ØVUG
Right ØVUF
Cornea
Left Ø8U9
Right Ø8U8
Cul-de-sac ØUUF
Diaphragm ØBUT
Disc
Cervical Vertebral ØRU3
Cervicothoracic Vertebral ØRU5

**Supplement** — *continued*
Disc — *continued*
Lumbar Vertebral ØSU2
Lumbosacral ØSU4
Thoracic Vertebral ØRU9
Thoracolumbar Vertebral ØRUB
Duct
Common Bile ØFU9
Cystic ØFU8
Hepatic
Common ØFU7
Left ØFU6
Right ØFU5
Lacrimal
Left Ø8UY
Right Ø8UX
Pancreatic ØFUD
Accessory ØFUF
Duodenum ØDU9
Dura Mater ØØU2
Ear
External
Bilateral Ø9U2
Left Ø9U1
Right Ø9UØ
Inner
Left Ø9UE
Right Ø9UD
Middle
Left Ø9U6
Right Ø9U5
Elbow Region
Left ØXUC
Right ØXUB
Epididymis
Bilateral ØVUL
Left ØVUK
Right ØVUJ
Epiglottis ØCUR
Esophagogastric Junction ØDU4
Esophagus ØDU5
Lower ØDU3
Middle ØDU2
Upper ØDU1
Extremity
Lower
Left ØYUB
Right ØYU9
Upper
Left ØXU7
Right ØXU6
Eye
Left Ø8U1
Right Ø8UØ
Eyelid
Lower
Left Ø8UR
Right Ø8UQ
Upper
Left Ø8UP
Right Ø8UN
Face ØWU2
Fallopian Tube
Left ØUU6
Right ØUU5
Fallopian Tubes, Bilateral ØUU7
Femoral Region
Bilateral ØYUE
Left ØYU8
Right ØYU7
Femoral Shaft
Left ØQU9
Right ØQU8
Femur
Lower
Left ØQUC
Right ØQUB
Upper
Left ØQU7
Right ØQU6
Fibula
Left ØQUK
Right ØQUJ
Finger
Index
Left ØXUP
Right ØXUN
Little
Left ØXUW

**Supplement** — *continued*
Finger — *continued*
Little — *continued*
Right ØXUV
Middle
Left ØXUR
Right ØXUQ
Ring
Left ØXUT
Right ØXUS
Foot
Left ØYUN
Right ØYUM
Gingiva
Lower ØCU6
Upper ØCU5
Glenoid Cavity
Left ØPU8
Right ØPU7
Hand
Left ØXUK
Right ØXUJ
Head ØWUØ
Heart Ø2UA
Humeral Head
Left ØPUD
Right ØPUC
Humeral Shaft
Left ØPUG
Right ØPUF
Hymen ØUUK
Ileocecal Valve ØDUC
Ileum ØDUB
Inguinal Region
Bilateral ØYUA
Left ØYU6
Right ØYU5
Intestine
Large ØDUE
Left ØDUG
Right ØDUF
Small ØDU8
Iris
Left Ø8UD
Right Ø8UC
Jaw
Lower ØWU5
Upper ØWU4
Jejunum ØDUA
Joint
Acromioclavicular
Left ØRUH
Right ØRUG
Ankle
Left ØSUG
Right ØSUF
Carpal
Left ØRUR
Right ØRUQ
Carpometacarpal
Left ØRUT
Right ØRUS
Cervical Vertebral ØRU1
Cervicothoracic Vertebral ØRU4
Coccygeal ØSU6
Elbow
Left ØRUM
Right ØRUL
Finger Phalangeal
Left ØRUX
Right ØRUW
Hip
Left ØSUB
Acetabular Surface ØSUE
Femoral Surface ØSUS
Right ØSU9
Acetabular Surface ØSUA
Femoral Surface ØSUR
Knee
Left ØSUD
Femoral Surface ØSUUØ9Z
Tibial Surface ØSUWØ9Z
Right ØSUC
Femoral Surface ØSUTØ9Z
Tibial Surface ØSUVØ9Z
Lumbar Vertebral ØSUØ
Lumbosacral ØSU3
Metacarpophalangeal
Left ØRUV

**Supplement** — *continued*
Joint — *continued*
Metacarpophalangeal — *continued*
Right ØRUU
Metatarsal-Phalangeal
Left ØSUN
Right ØSUM
Occipital-cervical ØRUØ
Sacrococcygeal ØSU5
Sacroiliac
Left ØSU8
Right ØSU7
Shoulder
Left ØRUK
Right ØRUJ
Sternoclavicular
Left ØRUF
Right ØRUE
Tarsal
Left ØSUJ
Right ØSUH
Tarsometatarsal
Left ØSUL
Right ØSUK
Temporomandibular
Left ØRUD
Right ØRUC
Thoracic Vertebral ØRU6
Thoracolumbar Vertebral ØRUA
Toe Phalangeal
Left ØSUQ
Right ØSUP
Wrist
Left ØRUP
Right ØRUN
Kidney Pelvis
Left ØTU4
Right ØTU3
Knee Region
Left ØYUG
Right ØYUF
Larynx ØCUS
Leg
Lower
Left ØYUJ
Right ØYUH
Upper
Left ØYUD
Right ØYUC
Lip
Lower ØCU1
Upper ØCUØ
Lymphatic
Aortic Ø7UD
Axillary
Left Ø7U6
Right Ø7U5
Head Ø7UØ
Inguinal
Left Ø7UJ
Right Ø7UH
Internal Mammary
Left Ø7U9
Right Ø7U8
Lower Extremity
Left Ø7UG
Right Ø7UF
Mesenteric Ø7UB
Neck
Left Ø7U2
Right Ø7U1
Pelvis Ø7UC
Thoracic Duct Ø7UK
Thorax Ø7U7
Upper Extremity
Left Ø7U4
Right Ø7U3
Mandible
Left ØNUV
Right ØNUT
Maxilla ØNUR
Mediastinum ØWUC
Mesentery ØDUV
Metacarpal
Left ØPUQ
Right ØPUP
Metatarsal
Left ØQUP
Right ØQUN

**Supplement** — *continued*
- Muscle
  - Abdomen
    - Left ØKUL
    - Right ØKUK
  - Extraocular
    - Left Ø8UM
    - Right Ø8UL
  - Facial ØKU1
  - Foot
    - Left ØKUW
    - Right ØKUV
  - Hand
    - Left ØKUD
    - Right ØKUC
  - Head ØKUØ
  - Hip
    - Left ØKUP
    - Right ØKUN
  - Lower Arm and Wrist
    - Left ØKUB
    - Right ØKU9
  - Lower Leg
    - Left ØKUT
    - Right ØKUS
  - Neck
    - Left ØKU3
    - Right ØKU2
  - Papillary Ø2UD
  - Perineum ØKUM
  - Shoulder
    - Left ØKU6
    - Right ØKU5
  - Thorax
    - Left ØKUJ
    - Right ØKUH
  - Tongue, Palate, Pharynx ØKU4
  - Trunk
    - Left ØKUG
    - Right ØKUF
  - Upper Arm
    - Left ØKU8
    - Right ØKU7
  - Upper Leg
    - Left ØKUR
    - Right ØKUQ
- Nasal Mucosa and Soft Tissue Ø9UK
- Nasopharynx Ø9UN
- Neck ØWU6
- Nerve
  - Abducens ØØUL
  - Accessory ØØUR
  - Acoustic ØØUN
  - Cervical Ø1U1
  - Facial ØØUM
  - Femoral Ø1UD
  - Glossopharyngeal ØØUP
  - Hypoglossal ØØUS
  - Lumbar Ø1UB
  - Median Ø1U5
  - Oculomotor ØØUH
  - Olfactory ØØUF
  - Optic ØØUG
  - Peroneal Ø1UH
  - Phrenic Ø1U2
  - Pudendal Ø1UC
  - Radial Ø1U6
  - Sacral Ø1UR
  - Sciatic Ø1UF
  - Thoracic Ø1U8
  - Tibial Ø1UG
  - Trigeminal ØØUK
  - Trochlear ØØUJ
  - Ulnar Ø1U4
  - Vagus ØØUQ
- Nipple
  - Left ØHUX
  - Right ØHUW
- Omentum ØDUU
- Orbit
  - Left ØNUQ
  - Right ØNUP
- Palate
  - Hard ØCU2
  - Soft ØCU3
- Patella
  - Left ØQUF
  - Right ØQUD
- Penis ØVUS

**Supplement** — *continued*
- Pericardium Ø2UN
- Perineum
  - Female ØWUN
  - Male ØWUM
- Peritoneum ØDUW
- Phalanx
  - Finger
    - Left ØPUV
    - Right ØPUT
  - Thumb
    - Left ØPUS
    - Right ØPUR
  - Toe
    - Left ØQUR
    - Right ØQUQ
- Pharynx ØCUM
- Prepuce ØVUT
- Radius
  - Left ØPUJ
  - Right ØPUH
- Rectum ØDUP
- Retina
  - Left Ø8UF
  - Right Ø8UE
- Retinal Vessel
  - Left Ø8UH
  - Right Ø8UG
- Ribs
  - 1 to 2 ØPU1
  - 3 or More ØPU2
- Sacrum ØQU1
- Scapula
  - Left ØPU6
  - Right ØPU5
- Scrotum ØVU5
- Septum
  - Atrial Ø2U5
  - Nasal Ø9UM
  - Ventricular Ø2UM
- Shoulder Region
  - Left ØXU3
  - Right ØXU2
- Skull ØNUØ
- Spinal Meninges ØØUT
- Sternum ØPUØ
- Stomach ØDU6
  - Pylorus ØDU7
- Subcutaneous Tissue and Fascia
  - Abdomen ØJU8
  - Back ØJU7
  - Buttock ØJU9
  - Chest ØJU6
  - Face ØJU1
  - Foot
    - Left ØJUR
    - Right ØJUQ
  - Hand
    - Left ØJUK
    - Right ØJUJ
  - Lower Arm
    - Left ØJUH
    - Right ØJUG
  - Lower Leg
    - Left ØJUP
    - Right ØJUN
  - Neck
    - Left ØJU5
    - Right ØJU4
  - Pelvic Region ØJUC
  - Perineum ØJUB
  - Scalp ØJUØ
  - Upper Arm
    - Left ØJUF
    - Right ØJUD
  - Upper Leg
    - Left ØJUM
    - Right ØJUL
- Tarsal
  - Left ØQUM
  - Right ØQUL
- Tendon
  - Abdomen
    - Left ØLUG
    - Right ØLUF
  - Ankle
    - Left ØLUT
    - Right ØLUS

**Supplement** — *continued*
- Tendon — *continued*
  - Foot
    - Left ØLUW
    - Right ØLUV
  - Hand
    - Left ØLU8
    - Right ØLU7
  - Head and Neck ØLUØ
  - Hip
    - Left ØLUK
    - Right ØLUJ
  - Knee
    - Left ØLUR
    - Right ØLUQ
  - Lower Arm and Wrist
    - Left ØLU6
    - Right ØLU5
  - Lower Leg
    - Left ØLUP
    - Right ØLUN
  - Perineum ØLUH
  - Shoulder
    - Left ØLU2
    - Right ØLU1
  - Thorax
    - Left ØLUD
    - Right ØLUC
  - Trunk
    - Left ØLUB
    - Right ØLU9
  - Upper Arm
    - Left ØLU4
    - Right ØLU3
  - Upper Leg
    - Left ØLUM
    - Right ØLUL
- Testis
  - Bilateral ØVUCØ
  - Left ØVUBØ
  - Right ØVU9Ø
- Thumb
  - Left ØXUM
  - Right ØXUL
- Tibia
  - Left ØQUH
  - Right ØQUG
- Toe
  - 1st
    - Left ØYUQ
    - Right ØYUP
  - 2nd
    - Left ØYUS
    - Right ØYUR
  - 3rd
    - Left ØYUU
    - Right ØYUT
  - 4th
    - Left ØYUW
    - Right ØYUV
  - 5th
    - Left ØYUY
    - Right ØYUX
- Tongue ØCU7
- Trachea ØBU1
- Tunica Vaginalis
  - Left ØVU7
  - Right ØVU6
- Turbinate, Nasal Ø9UL
- Tympanic Membrane
  - Left Ø9U8
  - Right Ø9U7
- Ulna
  - Left ØPUL
  - Right ØPUK
- Ureter
  - Left ØTU7
  - Right ØTU6
- Urethra ØTUD
- Uterine Supporting Structure ØUU4
- Uvula ØCUN
- Vagina ØUUG
- Valve
  - Aortic Ø2UF
  - Mitral Ø2UG
  - Pulmonary Ø2UH
  - Tricuspid Ø2UJ
- Vas Deferens
  - Bilateral ØVUQ

**Supplement** — *continued*
Vas Deferens — *continued*
Left ØVUP
Right ØVUN
Vein
Axillary
Left Ø5U8
Right Ø5U7
Azygos Ø5UØ
Basilic
Left Ø5UC
Right Ø5UB
Brachial
Left Ø5UA
Right Ø5U9
Cephalic
Left Ø5UF
Right Ø5UD
Colic Ø6U7
Common Iliac
Left Ø6UD
Right Ø6UC
Esophageal Ø6U3
External Iliac
Left Ø6UG
Right Ø6UF
External Jugular
Left Ø5UQ
Right Ø5UP
Face
Left Ø5UV
Right Ø5UT
Femoral
Left Ø6UN
Right Ø6UM
Foot
Left Ø6UV
Right Ø6UT
Gastric Ø6U2
Hand
Left Ø5UH
Right Ø5UG
Hemiazygos Ø5U1
Hepatic Ø6U4
Hypogastric
Left Ø6UJ
Right Ø6UH
Inferior Mesenteric Ø6U6
Innominate
Left Ø5U4
Right Ø5U3
Internal Jugular
Left Ø5UN
Right Ø5UM
Intracranial Ø5UL
Lower Ø6UY
Portal Ø6U8
Pulmonary
Left Ø2UT
Right Ø2US
Renal
Left Ø6UB
Right Ø6U9
Saphenous
Left Ø6UQ
Right Ø6UP
Splenic Ø6U1
Subclavian
Left Ø5U6
Right Ø5U5
Superior Mesenteric Ø6U5
Upper Ø5UY
Vertebral
Left Ø5US
Right Ø5UR
Vena Cava
Inferior Ø6UØ
Superior Ø2UV
Ventricle
Left Ø2UL
Right Ø2UK
Vertebra
Cervical ØPU3
Lumbar ØQUØ
Thoracic ØPU4
Vesicle
Bilateral ØVU3
Left ØVU2
Right ØVU1

**Supplement** — *continued*
Vocal Cord
Left ØCUV
Right ØCUT
Vulva ØUUM
Wrist Region
Left ØXUH
Right ØXUG
**Supraclavicular (Virchow's) lymph node**
*use* Lymphatic, Left Neck
*use* Lymphatic, Right Neck
**Supraclavicular nerve** *use* Nerve, Cervical Plexus
**Suprahyoid lymph node** *use* Lymphatic, Head
**Suprahyoid muscle**
*use* Nech Muscle, Right
*use* Neck Muscle, Left
**Suprainguinal lymph node** *use* Lymphatic, Pelvis
**Supraorbital vein**
*use* Face Vein, Left
*use* Face Vein, Right
**Suprarenal gland**
*use* Adrenal Gland
*use* Adrenal Gland, Bilateral
*use* Adrenal Gland, Left
*use* Adrenal Gland, Right
**Suprarenal plexus** *use* Abdominal Sympathetic Nerve
**Suprascapular nerve** *use* Brachial Plexus
**Supraspinatus fascia**
*use* Subcutaneous Tissue and Fascia, Left Upper Arm
*use* Subcutaneous Tissue and Fascia, Right Upper Arm
**Supraspinatus muscle**
*use* Shoulder Muscle, Left
*use* Shoulder Muscle, Right
**Supraspinous ligament**
*use* Lower Spine Bursa and Ligament
*use* Upper Spine Bursa and LIgament
**Suprasternal notch** *use* Sternum
**Supratrochlear lymph node**
*use* Lymphatic, Left Upper Extremity
*use* Lymphatic, Right Upper Extremity
**Sural artery**
*use* Popliteal Artery, Left
*use* Popliteal Artery, Right
**Suspension**
Bladder Neck *see* Reposition, Bladder Neck ØTSC
Kidney *see* Reposition, Urinary System ØTS
Urethra *see* Reposition, Urinary System ØTS
Urethrovesical *see* Reposition, Bladder Neck ØTSC
Uterus *see* Reposition, Uterus ØUS9
Vagina *see* Reposition, Vagina ØUSG
**Suture**
Laceration repair *see* Repair
Ligation *see* Occlusion
**Suture Removal**
Extremity
Lower 8EØYXY8
Upper 8EØXXY8
Head and Neck Region 8EØ9XY8
Trunk Region 8EØWXY8
**Sutureless valve, Perceval** *use* Zooplastic Tissue, Rapid Deployment Technique in New Technology
**Sweat gland** *use* Skin
**Sympathectomy** *see* Excision, Peripheral Nervous System Ø1B
**SynCardia Total Artificial Heart** *use* Synthetic Substitute
**Synchra CRT-P** *use* Cardiac Resynchronization Pacemaker Pulse Generator in ØJH
**SynchroMed pump** *use* Infusion Device, Pump in Subcutaneous Tissue and Fascia
**Synechiotomy, iris** *see* Release, Eye Ø8N
**Synovectomy**
Lower joint *see* Excision, Lower Joints ØSB
Upper joint *see* Excision, Upper Joints ØRB
**Systemic Nuclear Medicine Therapy**
Abdomen CW7Ø
Anatomical Regions, Multiple CW7YYZZ
Chest CW73
Thyroid CW7G
Whole Body CW7N

# T

**Takedown**
Arteriovenous shunt *see* Removal of device from, Upper Arteries Ø3P

**Takedown** — *continued*
Arteriovenous shunt, with creation of new shunt *see* Bypass, Upper Arteries Ø31
Stoma
*see* Excision
*see* Reposition
**Talent® Converter** *use* Intraluminal Device
**Talent® Occluder** *use* Intraluminal Device
**Talent® Stent Graft (abdominal) (thoracic)** *use* Intraluminal Device
**Talocalcaneal (subtalar) joint**
*use* Tarsal Joint, Left
*use* Tarsal Joint, Right
**Talocalcaneal ligament**
*use* Foot Bursa and Ligament, Left
*use* Foot Bursa and Ligament, Right
**Talocalcaneonavicular joint**
*use* Tarsal Joint, Left
*use* Tarsal Joint, Right
**Talocalcaneonavicular ligament**
*use* Foot Bursa and Ligament, Left
*use* Foot Bursa and Ligament, Right
**Talocrural joint**
*use* Ankle Joint, Left
*use* Joint, Ankle, Right
**Talofibular ligament**
*use* Ankle Bursa and Ligament, Left
*use* Ankle Bursa and Ligament, Right
**Talus bone**
*use* Tarsal, Left
*use* Tarsal, Right
**TandemHeart® System** *use* Short-term External Heart Assist System in Heart and Great Vessels
**Tarsectomy**
*see* Excision, Lower Bones ØQB
*see* Resection, Lower Bones ØQT
**Tarsometatarsal ligament**
*use* Foot Bursa and Ligament, Left
*use* Foot Bursa and Ligament, Right
**Tarsorrhaphy** *see* Repair, Eye Ø8Q
**Tattooing**
Cornea 3EØCXMZ
Skin *see* Introduction of substance in or on, Skin 3EØØ
**TAXUS® Liberté® Paclitaxel-eluting Coronary Stent System** *use* Intraluminal Device, Drug-eluting in Heart and Great Vessels
**TBNA (transbronchial needle aspiration)** *see* Drainage, Respiratory System ØB9
**Telemetry** 4A12X4Z
Ambulatory 4A12X45
**Temperature gradient study** 4AØZXKZ
**Temporal lobe** *use* Cerebral Hemisphere
**Temporalis muscle** *use* Head Muscle
**Temporoparietalis muscle** *use* Head Muscle
**Tendolysis** *see* Release, Tendons ØLN
**Tendonectomy**
*see* Excision, Tendons ØLB
*see* Resection, Tendons ØLT
**Tendonoplasty, tenoplasty**
*see* Repair, Tendons ØLQ
*see* Replacement, Tendons ØLR
*see* Supplement, Tendons ØLU
**Tendorrhaphy** *see* Repair, Tendons ØLQ
**Tendototomy**
*see* Division, Tendons ØL8
*see* Drainage, Tendons ØL9
**Tenectomy, tenonectomy**
*see* Excision, Tendons ØLB
*see* Resection, Tendons ØLT
**Tenolysis** *see* Release, Tendons ØLN
**Tenontorrhaphy** *see* Repair, Tendons ØLQ
**Tenontotomy**
*see* Division, Tendons ØL8
*see* Drainage, Tendons ØL9
**Tenorrhaphy** *see* Repair, Tendons ØLQ
**Tenosynovectomy**
*see* Excision, Tendons ØLB
*see* Resection, Tendons ØLT
**Tenotomy**
*see* Division, Tendons ØL8
*see* Drainage, Tendons ØL9
**Tensor fasciae latae muscle**
*use* Hip Muscle, Left
*use* Hip Muscle, Right
**Tensor veli palatini muscle** *use* Tongue, Palate, Pharynx Muscle

**Tenth cranial nerve** *use* Vagus Nerve
**Tentorium cerebelli** *use* Dura Mater
**Teres major muscle**
*use* Shoulder Muscle, Left
*use* Shoulder Muscle, Right
**Teres minor muscle**
*use* Shoulder Muscle, Left
*use* Shoulder Muscle, Right
**Termination of pregnancy**
Aspiration curettage 10A07ZZ
Dilation and curettage 10A07ZZ
Hysterotomy 10A00ZZ
Intra-amniotic injection 10A03ZZ
Laminaria 10A07ZW
Vacuum 10A07Z6
**Testectomy**
*see* Excision, Male Reproductive System 0VB
*see* Resection, Male Reproductive System 0VT
**Testicular artery** *use* Abdominal Aorta
**Testing**
Glaucoma 4A07XBZ
Hearing *see* Hearing Assessment, Diagnostic Audiology F13
Mental health *see* Psychological Tests
Muscle function, electromyography (EMG) *see* Measurement, Musculoskeletal 4A0F
Muscle function, manual *see* Motor Function Assessment, Rehabilitation F01
Neurophysiologic monitoring, intra-operative *see* Monitoring, Physiological Systems 4A1
Range of motion *see* Motor Function Assessment, Rehabilitation F01
Vestibular function *see* Vestibular Assessment, Diagnostic Audiology F15
**Thalamectomy** *see* Excision, Thalamus 00B9
**Thalamotomy** *see* Drainage, Thalamus 0099
**Thenar muscle**
*use* Hand Muscle, Left
*use* Hand Muscle, Right
**Therapeutic Massage**
Musculoskeletal System 8E0KX1Z
Reproductive System
Prostate 8E0VX1C
Rectum 8E0VX1D
**Therapeutic occlusion coil(s)** *use* Intraluminal Device
**Thermography** 4A0ZXKZ
**Thermotherapy, prostate** *see* Destruction, Prostate 0V50
**Third cranial nerve** *use* Nerve, Oculomotor
**Third occipital nerve** *use* Cervical Nerve
**Third ventricle** *use* Cerebral Ventricle
**Thoracectomy** *see* Excision, Anatomical Regions, General 0WB
**Thoracentesis** *see* Drainage, Anatomical Regions, General 0W9
**Thoracic aortic plexus** *use* Thoracic Sympathetic Nerve
**Thoracic esophagus** *use* Esophagus, Middle
**Thoracic facet joint** *use* Thoracic Vertebral Joint
**Thoracic ganglion** *use* Thoracic Sympathetic Nerve
**Thoracoacromial artery**
*use* Axillary Artery, Left
*use* Axillary Artery, Right
**Thoracocentesis** *see* Drainage, Anatomical Regions, General 0W9
**Thoracolumbar facet joint** *use* Thoracolumbar Vertebral Joint
**Thoracoplasty**
*see* Repair, Anatomical Regions, General 0WQ
*see* Supplement, Anatomical Regions, General 0WU
**Thoracostomy, for lung collapse** *see* Drainage, Respiratory System 0B9
**Thoracostomy tube** *use* Drainage Device
**Thoracotomy** *see* Drainage, Anatomical Regions, General 0W9
**Thoratec IVAD (Implantable Ventricular Assist Device)** *use* Implantable Heart Assist System in Heart and Great Vessels
**Thoratec Paracorporeal Ventricular Assist Device**
*use* Short-term External Heart Assist System in Heart and Great Vessels
**Thrombectomy** *see* Extirpation
**Thymectomy**
*see* Excision, Lymphatic and Hemic Systems 07B
*see* Resection, Lymphatic and Hemic Systems 07T
**Thymopexy**
*see* Repair, Lymphatic and Hemic Systems 07Q
*see* Reposition, Lymphatic and Hemic Systems 07S
**Thymus gland** *use* Thymus
**Thyroarytenoid muscle**
*use* Neck Muscle, Left
*use* Neck Muscle, Right
**Thyrocervical trunk**
*use* Thyroid Artery, Left
*use* Thyroid Artery, Right
**Thyroid cartilage** *use* Larynx
**Thyroidectomy**
*see* Excision, Endocrine System 0GB
*see* Resection, Endocrine System 0GT
**Thyroidorrhaphy** *see* Repair, Endocrine System 0GQ
**Thyroidoscopy** 0GJK4ZZ
**Thyroidotomy** *see* Drainage, Endocrine System 0G9
**Tibial insert** *use* Liner in Lower Joints
**Tibialis anterior muscle**
*use* Lower Leg Muscle, Left
*use* Lower Leg Muscle, Right
**Tibialis posterior muscle**
*use* Lower Leg Muscle, Left
*use* Lower Leg Muscle, Right
**Tibiofemoral joint**
*use* Knee Joint, Left
*use* Knee Joint, Right
*use* Knee Joint, Tibial Surface, Left
*use* Knee Joint, Tibial Surface, Right
**Tissue bank graft** *use* Nonautologous Tissue Substitute
**Tissue Expander**
Insertion of device in
Breast
Bilateral 0HHV
Left 0HHU
Right 0HHT
Nipple
Left 0HHX
Right 0HHW
Subcutaneous Tissue and Fascia
Abdomen 0JH8
Back 0JH7
Buttock 0JH9
Chest 0JH6
Face 0JH1
Foot
Left 0JHR
Right 0JHQ
Hand
Left 0JHK
Right 0JHJ
Lower Arm
Left 0JHH
Right 0JHG
Lower Leg
Left 0JHP
Right 0JHN
Neck
Left 0JH5
Right 0JH4
Pelvic Region 0JHC
Perineum 0JHB
Scalp 0JH0
Upper Arm
Left 0JHF
Right 0JHD
Upper Leg
Left 0JHM
Right 0JHL
Removal of device from
Breast
Left 0HPU
Right 0HPT
Subcutaneous Tissue and Fascia
Head and Neck 0JPS
Lower Extremity 0JPW
Trunk 0JPT
Upper Extremity 0JPV
Revision of device in
Breast
Left 0HWU
Right 0HWT
Subcutaneous Tissue and Fascia
Head and Neck 0JWS
Lower Extremity 0JWW
Trunk 0JWT
Upper Extremity 0JWV
**Tissue expander (inflatable) (injectable)**
*use* Tissue Expander in Skin and Breast
*use* Tissue Expander in Subcutaneous Tissue and Fascia
**Tissue Plasminogen Activator (tPA) (r-tPA)** *use* Thrombolytic, Other
**Titanium Sternal Fixation System (TSFS)**
*use* Internal Fixation Device, Rigid Plate in 0PS
*use* Internal Fixation Device, Rigid Plate in 0PH
**Tomographic (Tomo) Nuclear Medicine Imaging**
Abdomen CW20
Abdomen and Chest CW24
Abdomen and Pelvis CW21
Anatomical Regions, Multiple CW2YYZZ
Bladder, Kidneys and Ureters CT23
Brain C020
Breast CH2YYZZ
Bilateral CH22
Left CH21
Right CH20
Bronchi and Lungs CB22
Central Nervous System C02YYZZ
Cerebrospinal Fluid C025
Chest CW23
Chest and Abdomen CW24
Chest and Neck CW26
Digestive System CD2YYZZ
Endocrine System CG2YYZZ
Extremity
Lower CW2D
Bilateral CP2F
Left CP2D
Right CP2C
Upper CW2M
Bilateral CP2B
Left CP29
Right CP28
Gallbladder CF24
Gastrointestinal Tract CD27
Gland, Parathyroid CG21
Head and Neck CW2B
Heart C22YYZZ
Right and Left C226
Hepatobiliary System and Pancreas CF2YYZZ
Kidneys, Ureters and Bladder CT23
Liver CF25
Liver and Spleen CF26
Lungs and Bronchi CB22
Lymphatics and Hematologic System C72YYZZ
Musculoskeletal System, Other CP2YYZZ
Myocardium C22G
Neck and Chest CW26
Neck and Head CW2B
Pancreas and Hepatobiliary System CF2YYZZ
Pelvic Region CW2J
Pelvis CP26
Pelvis and Abdomen CW21
Pelvis and Spine CP27
Respiratory System CB2YYZZ
Skin CH2YYZZ
Skull CP21
Skull and Cervical Spine CP23
Spine
Cervical CP22
Cervical and Skull CP23
Lumbar CP2H
Thoracic CP2G
Thoracolumbar CP2J
Spine and Pelvis CP27
Spleen C722
Spleen and Liver CF26
Subcutaneous Tissue CH2YYZZ
Thorax CP24
Ureters, Kidneys and Bladder CT23
Urinary System CT2YYZZ
**Tomography, computerized** *see* Computerized Tomography (CT Scan)
**Tongue, base of** *use* Pharynx
**Tonometry** 4A07XBZ
**Tonsillectomy**
*see* Excision, Mouth and Throat 0CB
*see* Resection, Mouth and Throat 0CT
**Tonsillotomy** *see* Drainage, Mouth and Throat 0C9
**Total Anomalous Pulmonary Venous Return (TAPVR) repair**
*see* Bypass, Atrium, Left 0217
*see* Bypass, Vena Cava, Superior 021V
**Total artificial (replacement) heart** *use* Synthetic Substitute
**Total parenteral nutrition (TPN)** *see* Introduction of Nutritional Substance

**Transfer** — *continued*
Subcutaneous Tissue and Fascia — *continued*
Neck
Left ØJX5
Right ØJX4
Pelvic Region ØJXC
Perineum ØJXB
Scalp ØJXØ
Upper Arm
Left ØJXF
Right ØJXD
Upper Leg
Left ØJXM
Right ØJXL
Tendon
Abdomen
Left ØLXG
Right ØLXF
Ankle
Left ØLXT
Right ØLXS
Foot
Left ØLXW
Right ØLXV
Hand
Left ØLX8
Right ØLX7
Head and Neck ØLXØ
Hip
Left ØLXK
Right ØLXJ
Knee
Left ØLXR
Right ØLXQ
Lower Arm and Wrist
Left ØLX6
Right ØLX5
Lower Leg
Left ØLXP
Right ØLXN
Perineum ØLXH
Shoulder
Left ØLX2
Right ØLX1
Thorax
Left ØLXD
Right ØLXC
Trunk
Left ØLXB
Right ØLX9
Upper Arm
Left ØLX4
Right ØLX3
Upper Leg
Left ØLXM
Right ØLXL
Tongue ØCX7
**Transfusion**
Artery
Central
Antihemophilic Factors 3Ø26
Blood
Platelets 3Ø26
Red Cells 3Ø26
Frozen 3Ø26
White Cells 3Ø26
Whole 3Ø26
Bone Marrow 3Ø26
Factor IX 3Ø26
Fibrinogen 3Ø26
Globulin 3Ø26
Plasma
Fresh 3Ø26
Frozen 3Ø26
Plasma Cryoprecipitate 3Ø26
Serum Albumin 3Ø26
Stem Cells
Cord Blood 3Ø26
Hematopoietic 3Ø26
Peripheral
Antihemophilic Factors 3Ø25
Blood
Platelets 3Ø25
Red Cells 3Ø25
Frozen 3Ø25
White Cells 3Ø25
Whole 3Ø25
Bone Marrow 3Ø25
Factor IX 3Ø25
**Transfusion** — *continued*
Artery — *continued*
Peripheral — *continued*
Fibrinogen 3Ø25
Globulin 3Ø25
Plasma
Fresh 3Ø25
Frozen 3Ø25
Plasma Cryoprecipitate 3Ø25
Serum Albumin 3Ø25
Stem Cells
Cord Blood 3Ø25
Hematopoietic 3Ø25
Products of Conception
Antihemophilic Factors 3Ø27
Blood
Platelets 3Ø27
Red Cells 3Ø27
Frozen 3Ø27
White Cells 3Ø27
Whole 3Ø27
Factor IX 3Ø27
Fibrinogen 3Ø27
Globulin 3Ø27
Plasma
Fresh 3Ø27
Frozen 3Ø27
Plasma Cryoprecipitate 3Ø27
Serum Albumin 3Ø27
Vein
4-Factor Prothrombin Complex Concentrate 3Ø28ØB1
Central
Antihemophilic Factors 3Ø24
Blood
Platelets 3Ø24
Red Cells 3Ø24
Frozen 3Ø24
White Cells 3Ø24
Whole 3Ø24
Bone Marrow 3Ø24
Factor IX 3Ø24
Fibrinogen 3Ø24
Globulin 3Ø24
Plasma
Fresh 3Ø24
Frozen 3Ø24
Plasma Cryoprecipitate 3Ø24
Serum Albumin 3Ø24
Stem Cells
Cord Blood 3Ø24
Embryonic 3Ø24
Hematopoietic 3Ø24
Peripheral
Antihemophilic Factors 3Ø23
Blood
Platelets 3Ø23
Red Cells 3Ø23
Frozen 3Ø23
White Cells 3Ø23
Whole 3Ø23
Bone Marrow 3Ø23
Factor IX 3Ø23
Fibrinogen 3Ø23
Globulin 3Ø23
Plasma
Fresh 3Ø23
Frozen 3Ø23
Plasma Cryoprecipitate 3Ø23
Serum Albumin 3Ø23
Stem Cells
Cord Blood 3Ø23
Embryonic 3Ø23
Hematopoietic 3Ø23
**Transplant** *see* Transplantation
**Transplantation**
Bone marrow *see* Transfusion, Circulatory 3Ø2
Esophagus ØDY5ØZ
Face ØWY2ØZ
Hand
Left ØXYKØZ
Right ØXYJØZ
Heart Ø2YAØZ
Hematopoietic cell *see* Transfusion, Circulatory 3Ø2
Intestine
Large ØDYEØZ
Small ØDY8ØZ
Kidney
Left ØTY1ØZ
**Transplantation** — *continued*
Kidney — *continued*
Right ØTYØØZ
Liver ØFYØØZ
Lung
Bilateral ØBYMØZ
Left ØBYLØZ
Lower Lobe
Left ØBYJØZ
Right ØBYFØZ
Middle Lobe, Right ØBYDØZ
Right ØBYKØZ
Upper Lobe
Left ØBYGØZ
Right ØBYCØZ
Lung Lingula ØBYHØZ
Ovary
Left ØUY1ØZ
Right ØUYØØZ
Pancreas ØFYGØZ
Products of Conception 1ØYØ
Spleen Ø7YPØZ
Stem cell *see* Transfusion, Circulatory 3Ø2
Stomach ØDY6ØZ
Thymus Ø7YMØZ
**Transposition**
*see* Bypass
*see* Reposition
*see* Transfer
**Transversalis fascia** *use* Subcutaneous Tissue and Fascia, Trunk
**Transverse acetabular ligament**
*use* Hip Bursa and Ligament, Left
*use* Hip Bursa and Ligament, Right
**Transverse (cutaneous) cervical nerve** *use* Cervical Plexus
**Transverse facial artery**
*use* Temporal Artery, Left
*use* Temporal Artery, Right
**Transverse foramen** *use* Cervical Vertebra
**Transverse humeral ligament**
*use* Shoulder Bursa and Ligament, Left
*use* Shoulder Bursa and Ligament, Right
**Transverse ligament of atlas** *use* Bursa and Ligament, Head and Neck
**Transverse process**
*use* Cervical Vertebra
*use* Lumbar Vertebra
*use* Thoracic Vertebra
**Transverse Rectus Abdominis Myocutaneous Flap**
Replacement
Bilateral ØHRVØ76
Left ØHRUØ76
Right ØHRTØ76
Transfer
Left ØKXL
Right ØKXK
**Transverse scapular ligament**
*use* Shoulder Bursa and Ligament, Left
*use* Shoulder Bursa and Ligament, Right
**Transverse thoracis muscle**
*use* Thorax Muscle, Left
*use* Thorax Muscle, Right
**Transversospinalis muscle**
*use* Trunk Muscle, Left
*use* Trunk Muscle, Right
**Transversus abdominis muscle**
*use* Abdomen Muscle, Left
*use* Abdomen Muscle, Right
**Trapezium bone**
*use* Carpal, Left
*use* Carpal, Right
**Trapezius muscle**
*use* Trunk Muscle, Left
*use* Trunk Muscle, Right
**Trapezoid bone**
*use* Carpal, Left
*use* Carpal, Right
**Triceps brachii muscle**
*use* Upper Arm Muscle, Left
*use* Upper Arm Muscle, Right
**Tricuspid annulus** *use* Tricuspid Valve
**Trifacial nerve** *use* Nerve, Trigeminal
**Trifecta™ Valve (aortic)** *use* Zooplastic Tissue in Heart and Great Vessels
**Trigone of bladder** *use* Bladder
**Trimming, excisional** *see* Excision





Subterms under main terms may continue to next column or page

**Triquetral bone**
*use* Carpal, Left
*use* Carpal, Right
**Trochanteric bursa**
*use* Hip Bursa and Ligament, Left
*use* Hip Bursa and Ligament, Right
**TUMT (transurethral microwave thermotherapy of prostate)** ØV5Ø7ZZ
**TUNA (transurethral needle ablation of prostate)** ØV5Ø7ZZ
**Tunneled central venous catheter** *use* Vascular Access Device, Tunneled in Subcutaneous Tissue and Fascia
**Tunneled spinal (intrathecal) catheter** *use* Infusion Device
**Turbinectomy**
*see* Excision, Ear, Nose, Sinus Ø9B
*see* Resection, Ear, Nose, Sinus Ø9T
**Turbinoplasty**
*see* Repair, Ear, Nose, Sinus Ø9Q
*see* Replacement, Ear, Nose, Sinus Ø9R
*see* Supplement, Ear, Nose, Sinus Ø9U
**Turbinotomy**
*see* Division, Ear, Nose, Sinus Ø98
*see* Drainage, Ear, Nose, Sinus Ø99
**TURP (transurethral resection of prostate)** ØVBØ7ZZ
*see* Excision, Prostate ØVBØ
*see* Resection, Prostate ØVTØ
**Twelfth cranial nerve** *use* Nerve, Hypoglossal
**Two lead pacemaker** *use* Pacemaker, Dual Chamber in ØJH
**Tympanic cavity**
*use* Middle Ear, Left
*use* Middle Ear, Right
**Tympanic nerve** *use* Glossopharyngeal Nerve
**Tympanic part of temoporal bone**
*use* Temporal Bone, Left
*use* Temporal Bone, Right
**Tympanogram** *see* Hearing Assessment, Diagnostic Audiology F13
**Tympanoplasty**
*see* Repair, Ear, Nose, Sinus Ø9Q
*see* Replacement, Ear, Nose, Sinus Ø9R
*see* Supplement, Ear, Nose, Sinus Ø9U
**Tympanosympathectomy** *see* Excision, Nerve, Head and Neck Sympathetic Ø1BK
**Tympanotomy** *see* Drainage, Ear, Nose, Sinus Ø99

# U

**Ulnar collateral carpal ligament**
*use* Wrist Bursa and Ligament, Left
*use* Wrist Bursa and Ligament, Right
**Ulnar collateral ligament**
*use* Elbow Bursa and Ligament, Left
*use* Elbow Bursa and Ligament, Right
**Ulnar notch**
*use* Radius, Left
*use* Radius, Right
**Ulnar vein**
*use* Brachial Vein, Left
*use* Brachial Vein, Right
**Ultrafiltration**
Hemodialysis *see* Performance, Urinary 5A1D
Therapeutic plasmapheresis *see* Pheresis, Circulatory 6A55
**Ultraflex™ Precision Colonic Stent System** *use* Intraluminal Device
**ULTRAPRO Hernia System (UHS)** *use* Synthetic Substitute
**ULTRAPRO Partially Absorbable Lightweight Mesh** *use* Synthetic Substitute
**ULTRAPRO Plug** *use* Synthetic Substitute
**Ultrasonic osteogenic stimulator**
*use* Bone Growth Stimulator in Head and Facial Bones
*use* Bone Growth Stimulator in Lower Bones
*use* Bone Growth Stimulator in Upper Bones
**Ultrasonography**
Abdomen BW4ØZZZ
Abdomen and Pelvis BW41ZZZ
Abdominal Wall BH49ZZZ
Aorta
Abdominal, Intravascular B44ØZZ3
Thoracic, Intravascular B34ØZZ3
Appendix BD48ZZZ

**Ultrasonography** — *continued*
Artery
Brachiocephalic-Subclavian, Right, Intravascular B341ZZ3
Celiac and Mesenteric, Intravascular B44KZZ3
Common Carotid
Bilateral, Intravascular B345ZZ3
Left, Intravascular B344ZZ3
Right, Intravascular B343ZZ3
Coronary
Multiple B241YZZ
Intravascular B241ZZ3
Transesophageal B241ZZ4
Single B24ØYZZ
Intravascular B24ØZZ3
Transesophageal B24ØZZ4
Femoral, Intravascular B44LZZ3
Inferior Mesenteric, Intravascular B445ZZ3
Internal Carotid
Bilateral, Intravascular B348ZZ3
Left, Intravascular B347ZZ3
Right, Intravascular B346ZZ3
Intra-Abdominal, Other, Intravascular B44BZZ3
Intracranial, Intravascular B34RZZ3
Lower Extremity
Bilateral, Intravascular B44HZZ3
Left, Intravascular B44GZZ3
Right, Intravascular B44FZZ3
Mesenteric and Celiac, Intravascular B44KZZ3
Ophthalmic, Intravascular B34VZZ3
Penile, Intravascular B44NZZ3
Pulmonary
Left, Intravascular B34TZZ3
Right, Intravascular B34SZZ3
Renal
Bilateral, Intravascular B448ZZ3
Left, Intravascular B447ZZ3
Right, Intravascular B446ZZ3
Subclavian, Left, Intravascular B342ZZ3
Superior Mesenteric, Intravascular B444ZZ3
Upper Extremity
Bilateral, Intravascular B34KZZ3
Left, Intravascular B34JZZ3
Right, Intravascular B34HZZ3
Bile Duct BF4ØZZZ
Bile Duct and Gallbladder BF43ZZZ
Bladder BT4ØZZZ
and Kidney BT4JZZZ
Brain BØ4ØZZZ
Breast
Bilateral BH42ZZZ
Left BH41ZZZ
Right BH4ØZZZ
Chest Wall BH4BZZZ
Coccyx BR4FZZZ
Connective Tissue
Lower Extremity BL41ZZZ
Upper Extremity BL4ØZZZ
Duodenum BD49ZZZ
Elbow
Left, Densitometry BP4HZZ1
Right, Densitometry BP4GZZ1
Esophagus BD41ZZZ
Extremity
Lower BH48ZZZ
Upper BH47ZZZ
Eye
Bilateral B847ZZZ
Left B846ZZZ
Right B845ZZZ
Fallopian Tube
Bilateral BU42
Left BU41
Right BU4Ø
Fetal Umbilical Cord BY47ZZZ
Fetus
First Trimester, Multiple Gestation BY4BZZZ
Second Trimester, Multiple Gestation BY4DZZZ
Single
First Trimester BY49ZZZ
Second Trimester BY4CZZZ
Third Trimester BY4FZZZ
Third Trimester, Multiple Gestation BY4GZZZ
Gallbladder BF42ZZZ
Gallbladder and Bile Duct BF43ZZZ
Gastrointestinal Tract BD47ZZZ
Gland
Adrenal
Bilateral BG42ZZZ

**Ultrasonography** — *continued*
Gland — *continued*
Adrenal — *continued*
Left BG41ZZZ
Right BG4ØZZZ
Parathyroid BG43ZZZ
Thyroid BG44ZZZ
Hand
Left, Densitometry BP4PZZ1
Right, Densitometry BP4NZZ1
Head and Neck BH4CZZZ
Heart
Left B245YZZ
Intravascular B245ZZ3
Transesophageal B245ZZ4
Pediatric B24DYZZ
Intravascular B24DZZ3
Transesophageal B24DZZ4
Right B244YZZ
Intravascular B244ZZ3
Transesophageal B244ZZ4
Right and Left B246YZZ
Intravascular B246ZZ3
Transesophageal B246ZZ4
Heart with Aorta B24BYZZ
Intravascular B24BZZ3
Transesophageal B24BZZ4
Hepatobiliary System, All BF4CZZZ
Hip
Bilateral BQ42ZZZ
Left BQ41ZZZ
Right BQ4ØZZZ
Kidney
and Bladder BT4JZZZ
Bilateral BT43ZZZ
Left BT42ZZZ
Right BT41ZZZ
Transplant BT49ZZZ
Knee
Bilateral BQ49ZZZ
Left BQ48ZZZ
Right BQ47ZZZ
Liver BF45ZZZ
Liver and Spleen BF46ZZZ
Mediastinum BB4CZZZ
Neck BW4FZZZ
Ovary
Bilateral BU45
Left BU44
Right BU43
Ovary and Uterus BU4C
Pancreas BF47ZZZ
Pelvic Region BW4GZZZ
Pelvis and Abdomen BW41ZZZ
Penis BV4BZZZ
Pericardium B24CYZZ
Intravascular B24CZZ3
Transesophageal B24CZZ4
Placenta BY48ZZZ
Pleura BB4BZZZ
Prostate and Seminal Vesicle BV49ZZZ
Rectum BD4CZZZ
Sacrum BR4FZZZ
Scrotum BV44ZZZ
Seminal Vesicle and Prostate BV49ZZZ
Shoulder
Left, Densitometry BP49ZZ1
Right, Densitometry BP48ZZ1
Spinal Cord BØ4BZZZ
Spine
Cervical BR4ØZZZ
Lumbar BR49ZZZ
Thoracic BR47ZZZ
Spleen and Liver BF46ZZZ
Stomach BD42ZZZ
Tendon
Lower Extremity BL43ZZZ
Upper Extremity BL42ZZZ
Ureter
Bilateral BT48ZZZ
Left BT47ZZZ
Right BT46ZZZ
Urethra BT45ZZZ
Uterus BU46
Uterus and Ovary BU4C
Vein
Jugular
Left, Intravascular B544ZZ3
Right, Intravascular B543ZZ3

**Ultrasonography** — *continued*
Vein — *continued*
Lower Extremity
Bilateral, Intravascular B54DZZ3
Left, Intravascular B54CZZ3
Right, Intravascular B54BZZ3
Portal, Intravascular B54TZZ3
Renal
Bilateral, Intravascular B54LZZ3
Left, Intravascular B54KZZ3
Right, Intravascular B54JZZ3
Spanchnic, Intravascular B54TZZ3
Subclavian
Left, Intravascular B547ZZ3
Right, Intravascular B546ZZ3
Upper Extremity
Bilateral, Intravascular B54PZZ3
Left, Intravascular B54NZZ3
Right, Intravascular B54MZZ3
Vena Cava
Inferior, Intravascular B549ZZ3
Superior, Intravascular B548ZZ3
Wrist
Left, Densitometry BP4MZZ1
Right, Densitometry BP4LZZ1
**Ultrasound bone healing system**
*use* Bone Growth Stimulator in Head and Facial Bones
*use* Bone Growth Stimulator in Lower Bones
*use* Bone Growth Stimulator in Upper Bones
**Ultrasound Therapy**
Heart 6A75
No Qualifier 6A75
Vessels
Head and Neck 6A75
Other 6A75
Peripheral 6A75
**Ultraviolet Light Therapy, Skin** 6A8Ø
**Umbilical artery**
*use* Internal Iliac Artery, Left
*use* Internal Iliac Artery, Right
*use* Lower Artery
**Uniplanar external fixator**
*use* External Fixation Device, Monoplanar in ØPH
*use* External Fixation Device, Monoplanar in ØPS
*use* External Fixation Device, Monoplanar in ØQH
*use* External Fixation Device, Monoplanar in ØQS
**Upper GI series** *see* Fluoroscopy, Gastrointestinal, Upper BD15
**Ureteral orifice**
*use* Ureter
*use* Ureter, Left
*use* Ureter, Right
*use* Ureters, Bilateral
**Ureterectomy**
*see* Excision, Urinary System ØTB
*see* Resection, Urinary System ØTT
**Ureterocolostomy** *see* Bypass, Urinary System ØT1
**Ureterocystostomy** *see* Bypass, Urinary System ØT1
**Ureteroenterostomy** *see* Bypass, Urinary System ØT1
**Ureteroileostomy** *see* Bypass, Urinary System ØT1
**Ureterolithotomy** *see* Extirpation, Urinary System ØTC
**Ureterolysis** *see* Release, Urinary System ØTN
**Ureteroneocystostomy**
*see* Bypass, Urinary System ØT1
*see* Reposition, Urinary System ØTS
**Ureteropelvic junction (UPJ)**
*use* Kidney Pelvis, Left
*use* Kidney Pelvis, Right
**Ureteropexy**
*see* Repair, Urinary System ØTQ
*see* Reposition, Urinary System ØTS
**Ureteroplasty**
*see* Repair, Urinary System ØTQ
*see* Replacement, Urinary System ØTR
*see* Supplement, Urinary System ØTU
**Ureteroplication** *see* Restriction, Urinary System ØTV
**Ureteropyelography** *see* Fluoroscopy, Urinary System BT1
**Ureterorrhaphy** *see* Repair, Urinary System ØTQ
**Ureteroscopy** ØTJ98ZZ
**Ureterostomy**
*see* Bypass, Urinary System ØT1
*see* Drainage, Urinary System ØT9
**Ureterotomy** *see* Drainage, Urinary System ØT9
**Ureteroureterostomy** *see* Bypass, Urinary System ØT1
**Ureterovesical orifice**
*use* Ureter
**Ureterovesical orifice** — *continued*
*use* Ureter, Left
*use* Ureter, Right
*use* Ureters, Bilateral
**Urethral catheterization, indwelling** ØT9B7ØZ
**Urethrectomy**
*see* Excision, Urethra ØTBD
*see* Resection, Urethra ØTTD
**Urethrolithotomy** *see* Extirpation, Urethra ØTCD
**Urethrolysis** *see* Release, Urethra ØTND
**Urethropexy**
*see* Repair, Urethra ØTQD
*see* Reposition, Urethra ØTSD
**Urethroplasty**
*see* Repair, Urethra ØTQD
*see* Replacement, Urethra ØTRD
*see* Supplement, Urethra ØTUD
**Urethrorrhaphy** *see* Repair, Urethra ØTQD
**Urethroscopy** ØTJD8ZZ
**Urethrotomy** *see* Drainage, Urethra ØT9D
**Uridine Triacetate** XWØDX82
**Urinary incontinence stimulator lead** *use* Stimulator Lead in Urinary System
**Urography** *see* Fluoroscopy, Urinary System BT1
**Ustekinumab** *use* Other New Technology Therapeutic Substance
**Uterine Artery**
*use* Internal Iliac Artery, Left
*use* Internal Iliac Artery, Right
**Uterine artery embolization (UAE)** *see* Occlusion, Lower Arteries Ø4L
**Uterine cornu** *use* Uterus
**Uterine tube**
*use* Fallopian Tube, Left
*use* Fallopian Tube, Right
**Uterine vein**
*use* Hypogastric Vein, Left
*use* Hypogastric Vein, Right
**Uvulectomy**
*see* Excision, Uvula ØCBN
*see* Resection, Uvula ØCTN
**Uvulorrhaphy** *see* Repair, Uvula ØCQN
**Uvulotomy** *see* Drainage, Uvula ØC9N

## V

**Vaccination** *see* Introduction of Serum, Toxoid, and Vaccine
**Vacuum extraction, obstetric** 1ØDØ7Z6
**Vaginal artery**
*use* Internal Iliac Artery, Left
*use* Internal Iliac Artery, Right
**Vaginal pessary** *use* Intraluminal Device, Pessary in Female Reproductive System
**Vaginal vein**
*use* Hypogastric Vein, Left
*use* Hypogastric Vein, Right
**Vaginectomy**
*see* Excision, Vagina ØUBG
*see* Resection, Vagina ØUTG
**Vaginofixation**
*see* Repair, Vagina ØUQG
*see* Reposition, Vagina ØUSG
**Vaginoplasty**
*see* Repair, Vagina ØUQG
*see* Supplement, Vagina ØUUG
**Vaginorrhaphy** *see* Repair, Vagina ØUQG
**Vaginoscopy** ØUJH8ZZ
**Vaginotomy** *see* Drainage, Female Reproductive System ØU9
**Vagotomy** *see* Division, Nerve, Vagus ØØ8Q
**Valiant Thoracic Stent Graft** *use* Intraluminal Device
**Valvotomy, valvulotomy**
*see* Division, Heart and Great Vessels Ø28
*see* Release, Heart and Great Vessels Ø2N
**Valvuloplasty**
*see* Repair, Heart and Great Vessels Ø2Q
*see* Replacement, Heart and Great Vessels Ø2R
*see* Supplement, Heart and Great Vessels Ø2U
**Valvuloplasty, Alfieri Stitch** *see* Restriction, Valve, Mitral Ø2VG
**Vascular Access Device**
Totally Implantable
Insertion of device in
Abdomen ØJH8
Chest ØJH6
**Vascular Access Device** — *continued*
Totally Implantable — *continued*
Insertion of device in — *continued*
Lower Arm
Left ØJHH
Right ØJHG
Lower Leg
Left ØJHP
Right ØJHN
Upper Arm
Left ØJHF
Right ØJHD
Upper Leg
Left ØJHM
Right ØJHL
Removal of device from
Lower Extremity ØJPW
Trunk ØJPT
Upper Extremity ØJPV
Revision of device in
Lower Extremity ØJWW
Trunk ØJWT
Upper Extremity ØJWV
Tunneled
Insertion of device in
Abdomen ØJH8
Chest ØJH6
Lower Arm
Left ØJHH
Right ØJHG
Lower Leg
Left ØJHP
Right ØJHN
Upper Arm
Left ØJHF
Right ØJHD
Upper Leg
Left ØJHM
Right ØJHL
Removal of device from
Lower Extremity ØJPW
Trunk ØJPT
Upper Extremity ØJPV
Revision of device in
Lower Extremity ØJWW
Trunk ØJWT
Upper Extremity ØJWV
**Vasectomy** *see* Excision, Male Reproductive System ØVB
**Vasography**
*see* Fluoroscopy, Male Reproductive System BV1
*see* Plain Radiography, Male Reproductive System BVØ
**Vasoligation** *see* Occlusion, Male Reproductive System ØVL
**Vasorrhaphy** *see* Repair, Male Reproductive System ØVQ
**Vasostomy** *see* Bypass, Male Reproductive System ØV1
**Vasotomy**
With ligation *see* Occlusion, Male Reproductive System ØVL
Drainage *see* Drainage, Male Reproductive System ØV9
**Vasovasostomy** *see* Repair, Male Reproductive System ØVQ
**Vastus intermedius muscle**
*use* Upper Leg Muscle, Left
*use* Upper Leg Muscle, Right
**Vastus lateralis muscle**
*use* Upper Leg Muscle, Left
*use* Upper Leg Muscle, Right
**Vastus medialis muscle**
*use* Upper Leg Muscle, Left
*use* Upper Leg Muscle, Right
**VCG (vectorcardiogram)** *see* Measurement, Cardiac 4AØ2
**Vectra® Vascular Access Graft** *use* Vascular Access Device, Tunneled in Subcutaneous Tissue and Fascia
**Venectomy**
*see* Excision, Lower Veins Ø6B
*see* Excision, Upper Veins Ø5B
**Venography**
*see* Fluoroscopy, Veins B51
*see* Plain Radiography, Veins B5Ø
**Venorrhaphy**
*see* Repair, Lower Veins Ø6Q
*see* Repair, Upper Veins Ø5Q
**Venotripsy**
*see* Occlusion, Lower Veins Ø6L
*see* Occlusion, Upper Veins Ø5L
**Ventricular fold** *use* Larynx

**Ventriculoatriostomy** *see* Bypass, Central Nervous System and Cranial Nerves ØØ1
**Ventriculocisternostomy** *see* Bypass, Central Nervous System and Cranial Nerves ØØ1
**Ventriculogram, cardiac**
Combined left and right heart *see* Fluoroscopy, Heart, Right and Left B216
Left ventricle *see* Fluoroscopy, Heart, Left B215
Right ventricle *see* Fluoroscopy, Heart, Right B214
**Ventriculopuncture, through previously implanted catheter** 8CØ1X6J
**Ventriculoscopy** ØØJØ4ZZ
**Ventriculostomy**
External drainage *see* Drainage, Cerebral Ventricle ØØ96
Internal shunt *see* Bypass, Cerebral Ventricle ØØ16
**Ventriculovenostomy** *see* Bypass, Cerebral Ventricle ØØ16
**Ventrio™ Hernia Patch** *use* Synthetic Substitute
**VEP (visual evoked potential)** 4AØ7XØZ
**Vermiform appendix** *use* Appendix
**Vermilion border**
*use* Lower Lip
*use* Upper Lip
**Versa** *use* Pacemaker, Dual Chamber in ØJH
**Version, obstetric**
External 1ØSØXZZ
Internal 1ØSØ7ZZ
**Vertebral arch**
*use* Cervical Vertebra
*use* Lumbar Vertebra
*use* Thoracic Vertebra
**Vertebral body**
*use* Cervical Vertebra
*use* Lumbar Vertebra
*use* Thoracic Vertebra
**Vertebral canal** *use* Spinal Canal
**Vertebral foramen**
*use* Cervical Vertebra
*use* Lumbar Vertebra
*use* Thoracic Vertebra
**Vertebral lamina**
*use* Cervical Vertebra
*use* Lumbar Vertebra
*use* Thoracic Vertebra
**Vertebral pedicle**
*use* Cervical Vertebra
*use* Lumbar Vertebra
*use* Thoracic Vertebra
**Vesical vein**
*use* Hypogastric Vein, Left
*use* Hypogastric Vein, Right
**Vesicotomy** *see* Drainage, Urinary System ØT9
**Vesiculectomy**
*see* Excision, Male Reproductive System ØVB
*see* Resection, Male Reproductive System ØVT
**Vesiculogram, seminal** *see* Plain Radiography, Male Reproductive System BVØ
**Vesiculotomy** *see* Drainage, Male Reproductive System ØV9
**Vestibular Assessment** F15Z
**Vestibular (Scarpa's) ganglion** *use* Nerve, Acoustic
**Vestibular nerve** *use* Acoustic Nerve
**Vestibular Treatment** FØC
**Vestibulocochlear nerve** *use* Acoustic Nerve
**VH-IVUS (virtual histology intravascular ultrasound)** *see* Ultrasonography, Heart B24
**Virchow's (supraclavicular) lymph node**
*use* Lymphatic, Left Neck
*use* Lymphatic, Right Neck
**Virtuoso (II) (DR) (VR)** *use* Defibrillator Generator in ØJH
**Vistogard(R)** *use* Uridine Triacetate
**Vitrectomy**
*see* Excision, Eye Ø8B
*see* Resection, Eye Ø8T
**Vitreous body**
*use* Vitreous, Left
*use* Vitreous, Right
**Viva (XT) (S)** *use* Cardiac Resynchronization Defibrillator Pulse Generator in ØJH
**Vocal fold**
*use* Vocal Cord, Left
*use* Vocal Cord, Right
**Vocational**
Assessment *see* Activities of Daily Living Assessment, Rehabilitation FØ2
Retraining *see* Activities of Daily Living Treatment, Rehabilitation FØ8
**Volar (palmar) digital vein**
*use* Hand Vein, Left
*use* Hand Vein, Right
**Volar (palmar) metacarpal vein**
*use* Hand Vein, Left
*use* Hand Vein, Right
**Vomer bone** *use* Nasal Bone
**Vomer of nasal septum** *use* Nasal Bone
**Voraxaze** *use* Glucarpidase
**Vulvectomy**
*see* Excision, Female Reproductive System ØUB
*see* Resection, Female Reproductive System ØUT
**VYXEOS™** *use* Cytarabine and Daunorubicin Liposome Antineoplastic

# W

**WALLSTENT® Endoprosthesis** *use* Intraluminal Device
**Washing** *see* Irrigation
**Wedge resection, pulmonary** *see* Excision, Respiratory System ØBB
**Window** *see* Drainage
**Wiring, dental** 2W31X9Z

# X

**Xact Carotid Stent System** *use* Intraluminal Device
**Xenograft** *use* Zooplastic Tissue in Heart and Great Vessels
**XIENCE Everolimus Eluting Coronary Stent System** *use* Intraluminal Device, Drug-eluting in Heart and Great Vessels
**Xiphoid process** *use* Sternum
**XLIF® System** *use* Interbody Fusion Device in Lower Joints
**X-ray** *see* Plain Radiography
**X-STOP® Spacer**
*use* Spinal Stabilization Device, Interspinous Process in ØRH
*use* Spinal Stabilization Device, Interspinous Process in ØSH

# Y

**Yoga Therapy** 8EØZXY4

# Z

**Zenith AAA Endovascular Graft**
*use* Intraluminal Device
*use* Intraluminal Device, Branched or Fenestrated, One or Two Arteries in Ø4V
*use* Intraluminal Device, Branched or Fenestrated, Three or More Arteries in Ø4V
**Zenith Flex® AAA Endovascular Graft** *use* Intraluminal Device
**Zenith TX2® TAA Endovascular Graft** *use* Intraluminal Device
**Zenith® Renu™ AAA Ancillary Graft** *use* Intraluminal Device
**Zilver® PTX® (paclitaxel) Drug-Eluting Peripheral Stent**
*use* Intraluminal Device, Drug-eluting in Lower Arteries
*use* Intraluminal Device, Drug-eluting in Upper Arteries
**Zimmer® NexGen® LPS Mobile Bearing Knee** *use* Synthetic Substitute
**Zimmer® NexGen® LPS-Flex Mobile Knee** *use* Synthetic Substitute
**ZINPLAVA™** use Bezlotoxumab Monoclonal Antibody
**Zonule of Zinn**
*use* Lens, Left
*use* Lens, Right
**Zooplastic Tissue, Rapid Deployment Technique, Replacement** X2RF
**Zotarolimus-eluting Coronary Stent** *use* Intraluminal Device, Drug-eluting in Heart and Great Vessels
**Z-plasty, skin for scar contracture** *see* Release, Skin and Breast ØHN
**Zygomatic process of frontal bone** *use* Frontal Bone
**Zygomatic process of temporal bone**
*use* Temporal Bone, Left
*use* Temporal Bone, Right
**Zygomaticus muscle** *use* Facial Muscle
**Zyvox** *use* Oxazolidinones

# ICD-10-PCS Tables



## Central Nervous System and Cranial Nerves 001–00X

### Character Meanings

**This Character Meaning table is provided as a guide to assist the user in the identification of character members that may be found in this section of code tables. It SHOULD NOT be used to build a PCS code.**

| Operation–Character 3 | | Body Part–Character 4 | | Approach–Character 5 | | Device–Character 6 | | Qualifier–Character 7 | |
|---|---|---|---|---|---|---|---|---|---|
| 1 | Bypass | Ø | Brain | Ø | Open | Ø | Drainage Device | Ø | Nasopharynx |
| 2 | Change | 1 | Cerebral Meninges | 3 | Percutaneous | 2 | Monitoring Device | 1 | Mastoid Sinus |
| 5 | Destruction | 2 | Dura Mater | 4 | Percutaneous Endoscopic | 3 | Infusion Device | 2 | Atrium |
| 7 | Dilation | 3 | Epidural Space, Intracranial | X | External | 4 | Radioactive Element, Cesium-131 Collagen Implant | 3 | Blood Vessel |
| 8 | Division | 4 | Subdural Space, Intracranial | | | 7 | Autologous Tissue Substitute | 4 | Pleural Cavity |
| 9 | Drainage | 5 | Subarachnoid Space, Intracranial | | | J | Synthetic Substitute | 5 | Intestine |
| B | Excision | 6 | Cerebral Ventricle | | | K | Nonautologous Tissue Substitute | 6 | Peritoneal Cavity |
| C | Extirpation | 7 | Cerebral Hemisphere | | | M | Neurostimulator Lead | 7 | Urinary Tract |
| D | Extraction | 8 | Basal Ganglia | | | Y | Other Device | 8 | Bone Marrow |
| F | Fragmentation | 9 | Thalamus | | | Z | No Device | 9 | Fallopian Tube |
| H | Insertion | A | Hypothalamus | | | | | B | Cerebral Cisterns |
| J | Inspection | B | Pons | | | | | F | Olfactory Nerve |
| K | Map | C | Cerebellum | | | | | G | Optic Nerve |
| N | Release | D | Medulla Oblongata | | | | | H | Oculomotor Nerve |
| P | Removal | E | Cranial Nerve | | | | | J | Trochlear Nerve |
| Q | Repair | F | Olfactory Nerve | | | | | K | Trigeminal Nerve |
| R | Replacement | G | Optic Nerve | | | | | L | Abducens Nerve |
| S | Reposition | H | Oculomotor Nerve | | | | | M | Facial Nerve |
| T | Resection | J | Trochlear Nerve | | | | | N | Acoustic Nerve |
| U | Supplement | K | Trigeminal Nerve | | | | | P | Glossopharyngeal Nerve |
| W | Revision | L | Abducens Nerve | | | | | Q | Vagus Nerve |
| X | Transfer | M | Facial Nerve | | | | | R | Accessory Nerve |
| | | N | Acoustic Nerve | | | | | S | Hypoglossal Nerve |
| | | P | Glossopharyngeal Nerve | | | | | X | Diagnostic |
| | | Q | Vagus Nerve | | | | | Z | No Qualifier |
| | | R | Accessory Nerve | | | | | | |
| | | S | Hypoglossal Nerve | | | | | | |
| | | T | Spinal Meninges | | | | | | |
| | | U | Spinal Canal | | | | | | |
| | | V | Spinal Cord | | | | | | |
| | | W | Cervical Spinal Cord | | | | | | |
| | | X | Thoracic Spinal Cord | | | | | | |
| | | Y | Lumbar Spinal Cord | | | | | | |

**AHA Coding Clinic for table ØØ1**
**2015, 2Q, 9** Revision of ventriculoperitoneal (VP) shunt
**2013, 2Q, 36** Insertion of ventriculoperitoneal shunt with laparoscopic assistance

**AHA Coding Clinic for table ØØ9**
**2017, 1Q, 50** Failed lumbar puncture
**2015, 3Q, 10** Open evacuation of subdural hematoma
**2015, 3Q, 11** Percutaneous drainage of subdural hematoma
**2015, 3Q, 12** Subdural evacuation portal system (SEPS) placement
**2015, 3Q, 12** Placement of ventriculostomy catheter via burr hole
**2015, 2Q, 30** Drainage of syrinx
**2015, 1Q, 31** Intrathecal chemotherapy
**2014, 1Q, 8** Diagnostic lumbar tap
**2014, 1Q, 8** Lumbar drainage port aspiration

**AHA Coding Clinic for table ØØB**
**2016, 2Q, 12** Resection of malignant neoplasm of infratemporal fossa
**2016, 2Q, 18** Amygdalohippocampectomy
**2014, 4Q, 34** Resection of brain malignancy with implantation of chemotherapeutic wafer
**2014, 3Q, 24** Repair of lipomyelomeningocele and tethered cord

**AHA Coding Clinic for table ØØC**
**2016, 2Q, 29** Decompressive craniectomy with cryopreservation and storage of bone flap
**2015, 3Q, 10** Open evacuation of subdural hematoma
**2015, 3Q, 11** Percutaneous drainage of subdural hematoma
**2015, 3Q, 13** Evacuation of intracerebral hematoma

**AHA Coding Clinic for table ØØD**
**2015, 3Q, 13** Nonexcisional debridement of cranial wound with removal and replacement of hardware

**AHA Coding Clinic for table ØØH**
**2014, 3Q, 19** End of life replacement of Baclofen pump

**AHA Coding Clinic for table ØØJ**
**2017, 1Q, 50** Failed lumbar puncture

**AHA Coding Clinic for table ØØN**
**2017, 2Q, 23** Decompression of spinal cord and placement of instrumentation
**2016, 2Q, 29** Decompressive craniectomy with cryopreservation and storage of bone flap
**2015, 2Q, 20** Cervical laminoplasty
**2015, 2Q, 21** Multiple decompressive cervical laminectomies
**2015, 2Q, 34** Decompressive laminectomy
**2014, 3Q, 24** Repair of lipomyelomeningocele and tethered cord

**AHA Coding Clinic for table ØØP**
**2014, 3Q, 19** End of life replacement of Baclofen pump

**AHA Coding Clinic for table ØØQ**
**2014, 3Q, 7** Hemi-cranioplasty for repair of cranial defect
**2013, 3Q, 25** Fracture of frontal bone with repair and coagulation for hemostasis

**AHA Coding Clinic for table ØØS**
**2014, 4Q, 35** Reimplantation of buccal nerve

**AHA Coding Clinic for table ØØU**
**2015, 4Q, 39** Dural patch graft
**2014, 3Q, 24** Repair of lipomyelomeningocele and tethered cord

## Brain

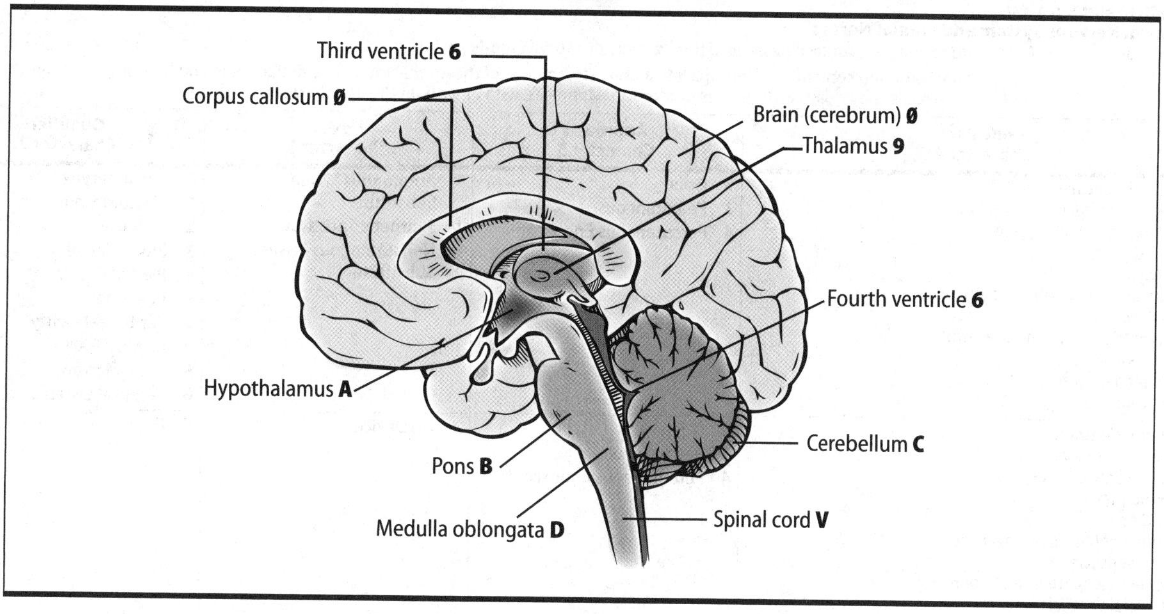
Third ventricle 6
Corpus callosum Ø
Brain (cerebrum) Ø
Thalamus 9
Fourth ventricle 6
Hypothalamus A
Cerebellum C
Pons B
Medulla oblongata D
Spinal cord V

## Cranial Nerves

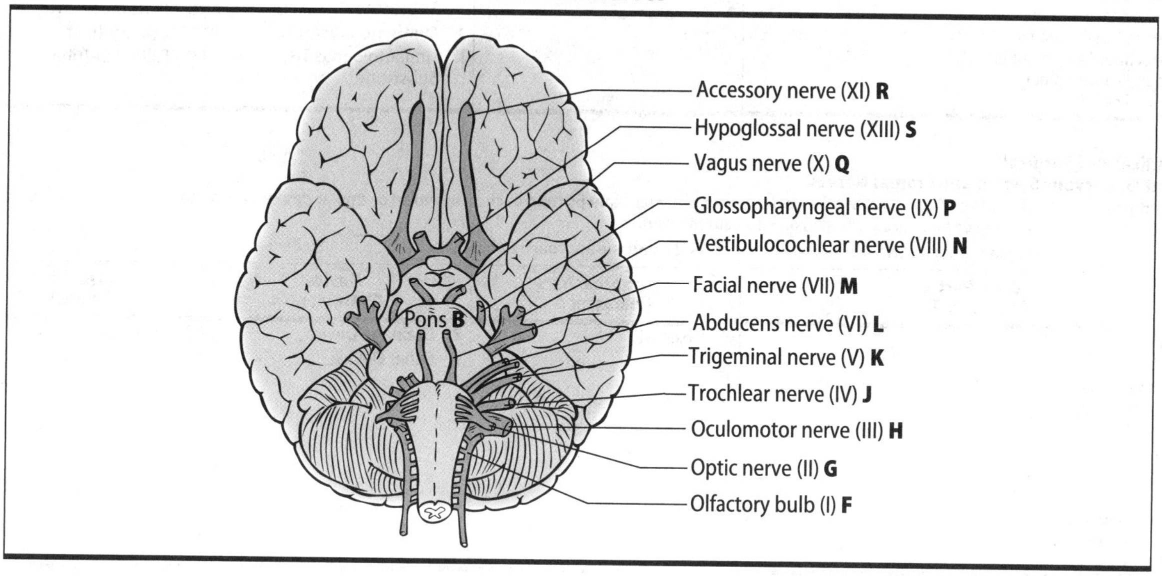
Accessory nerve (XI) R
Hypoglossal nerve (XIII) S
Vagus nerve (X) Q
Glossopharyngeal nerve (IX) P
Vestibulocochlear nerve (VIII) N
Facial nerve (VII) M
Pons B
Abducens nerve (VI) L
Trigeminal nerve (V) K
Trochlear nerve (IV) J
Oculomotor nerve (III) H
Optic nerve (II) G
Olfactory bulb (I) F

Central Nervous System and Cranial Nerves

**Ø Medical and Surgical**
**Ø Central Nervous System and Cranial Nerves**
**1 Bypass** Definition: Altering the route of passage of the contents of a tubular body part

Explanation: Rerouting contents of a body part to a downstream area of the normal route, to a similar route and body part, or to an abnormal route and dissimilar body part. Includes one or more anastomoses, with or without the use of a device.

| Body Part Character 4 | Approach Character 5 | Device Character 6 | Qualifier Character 7 |
|---|---|---|---|
| **6 Cerebral Ventricle**<br>Aqueduct of Sylvius<br>Cerebral aqueduct (Sylvius)<br>Choroid plexus<br>Ependyma<br>Foramen of Monro (intraventricular)<br>Fourth ventricle<br>Interventricular foramen (Monro)<br>Left lateral ventricle<br>Right lateral ventricle<br>Third ventricle | **Ø Open**<br>**3 Percutaneous**<br>4 Percutaneous Endoscopic | **7 Autologous Tissue Substitute**<br>**J Synthetic Substitute**<br>**K Nonautologous Tissue Substitute** | **Ø Nasopharynx**<br>**1 Mastoid Sinus**<br>**2 Atrium**<br>**3 Blood Vessel**<br>**4 Pleural Cavity**<br>**5 Intestine**<br>**6 Peritoneal Cavity**<br>**7 Urinary Tract**<br>**8 Bone Marrow**<br>**B Cerebral Cisterns** |
| 6 Cerebral Ventricle<br>Aqueduct of Sylvius<br>Cerebral aqueduct (Sylvius)<br>Choroid plexus<br>Ependyma<br>Foramen of Monro (intraventricular)<br>Fourth ventricle<br>Interventricular foramen (Monro)<br>Left lateral ventricle<br>Right lateral ventricle<br>Third ventricle | Ø Open<br>3 Percutaneous<br>4 Percutaneous Endoscopic | Z No Device | B Cerebral Cisterns |
| **U Spinal Canal**<br>Epidural space, spinal<br>Extradural space, spinal<br>Subarachnoid space, spinal<br>Subdural space, spinal<br>Vertebral canal | **Ø Open**<br>**3 Percutaneous** | **7 Autologous Tissue Substitute**<br>**J Synthetic Substitute**<br>**K Nonautologous Tissue Substitute** | **4 Pleural Cavity**<br>**6 Peritoneal Cavity**<br>**7 Urinary Tract**<br>**9 Fallopian Tube** |

**Ø Medical and Surgical**
**Ø Central Nervous System and Cranial Nerves**
**2 Change** Definition: Taking out or off a device from a body part and putting back an identical or similar device in or on the same body part without cutting or puncturing the skin or a mucous membrane

Explanation: All CHANGE procedures are coded using the approach EXTERNAL

| Body Part Character 4 | Approach Character 5 | Device Character 6 | Qualifier Character 7 |
|---|---|---|---|
| **Ø Brain**<br>Cerebrum<br>Corpus callosum<br>Encephalon<br>**E Cranial Nerve**<br>**U Spinal Canal**<br>Epidural space, spinal<br>Extradural space, spinal<br>Subarachnoid space, spinal<br>Subdural space, spinal<br>Vertebral canal | **X External** | **Ø Drainage Device**<br>**Y Other Device** | **Z No Qualifier** |

Non-OR All body part, approach, device, and qualifier values

**Ø Medical and Surgical**
**Ø Central Nervous System and Cranial Nerves**
**5 Destruction** Definition: Physical eradication of all or a portion of a body part by the direct use of energy, force, or a destructive agent
Explanation: None of the body part is physically taken out

| Body Part Character 4 | Body Part Character 4 | Approach Character 5 | Device Character 6 | Qualifier Character 7 |
|---|---|---|---|---|
| **Ø Brain**<br>Cerebrum<br>Corpus callosum<br>Encephalon<br>**1 Cerebral Meninges**<br>Arachnoid mater, intracranial<br>Leptomeninges, intracranial<br>Pia mater, intracranial<br>**2 Dura Mater**<br>Diaphragma sellae<br>Dura mater, intracranial<br>Falx cerebri<br>Tentorium cerebelli<br>**6 Cerebral Ventricle**<br>Aqueduct of Sylvius<br>Cerebral aqueduct (Sylvius)<br>Choroid plexus<br>Ependyma<br>Foramen of Monro (intraventricular)<br>Fourth ventricle<br>Interventricular foramen (Monro)<br>Left lateral ventricle<br>Right lateral ventricle<br>Third ventricle<br>**7 Cerebral Hemisphere**<br>Frontal lobe<br>Occipital lobe<br>Parietal lobe<br>Temporal lobe<br>**8 Basal Ganglia**<br>Basal nuclei<br>Claustrum<br>Corpus striatum<br>Globus pallidus<br>Substantia nigra<br>Subthalamic nucleus<br>**9 Thalamus**<br>Epithalamus<br>Geniculate nucleus<br>Metathalamus<br>Pulvinar<br>**A Hypothalamus**<br>Mammillary body<br>**B Pons**<br>Apneustic center<br>Basis pontis<br>Locus ceruleus<br>Pneumotaxic center<br>Pontine tegmentum<br>Superior olivary nucleus<br>**C Cerebellum**<br>Culmen<br>**D Medulla Oblongata**<br>Myelencephalon<br>**F Olfactory Nerve**<br>First cranial nerve<br>Olfactory bulb<br>**G Optic Nerve**<br>Optic chiasma<br>Second cranial nerve | **H Oculomotor Nerve**<br>Third cranial nerve<br>**J Trochlear Nerve**<br>Fourth cranial nerve<br>**K Trigeminal Nerve**<br>Fifth cranial nerve<br>Gasserian ganglion<br>Mandibular nerve<br>Maxillary nerve<br>Ophthalmic nerve<br>Trifacial nerve<br>**L Abducens Nerve**<br>Sixth cranial nerve<br>**M Facial Nerve**<br>Chorda tympani<br>Geniculate ganglion<br>Greater superficial petrosal nerve<br>Nerve to the stapedius<br>Parotid plexus<br>Posterior auricular nerve<br>Seventh cranial nerve<br>Submandibular ganglion<br>**N Acoustic Nerve**<br>Cochlear nerve<br>Eighth cranial nerve<br>Scarpa's (vestibular) ganglion<br>Spiral ganglion<br>Vestibular (Scarpa's) ganglion<br>Vestibular nerve<br>Vestibulocochlear nerve<br>**P Glossopharyngeal Nerve**<br>Carotid sinus nerve<br>Ninth cranial nerve<br>Tympanic nerve<br>**Q Vagus Nerve**<br>Anterior vagal trunk<br>Pharyngeal plexus<br>Pneumogastric nerve<br>Posterior vagal trunk<br>Pulmonary plexus<br>Recurrent laryngeal nerve<br>Superior laryngeal nerve<br>Tenth cranial nerve<br>**R Accessory Nerve**<br>Eleventh cranial nerve<br>**S Hypoglossal Nerve**<br>Twelfth cranial nerve<br>**T Spinal Meninges**<br>Arachnoid mater, spinal<br>Denticulate (dentate) ligament<br>Dura mater, spinal<br>Filum terminale<br>Leptomeninges, spinal<br>Pia mater, spinal<br>**W Cervical Spinal Cord**<br>**X Thoracic Spinal Cord**<br>**Y Lumbar Spinal Cord**<br>Cauda equina<br>Conus medullaris | **Ø Open**<br>**3 Percutaneous**<br>**4 Percutaneous Endoscopic** | **Z No Device** | **Z No Qualifier** |

**Non-OR** ØØ5[F,G,H,J,K,L,M,N,P,Q,R,S][Ø,3,4]ZZ

**Ø Medical and Surgical**
**Ø Central Nervous System and Cranial Nerves**
**7 Dilation** Definition: Expanding an orifice or the lumen of a tubular body part

Explanation: The orifice can be a natural orifice or an artificially created orifice. Accomplished by stretching a tubular body part using intraluminal pressure or by cutting part of the orifice or wall of the tubular body part.

| Body Part<br>Character 4 | Approach<br>Character 5 | Device<br>Character 6 | Qualifier<br>Character 7 |
|---|---|---|---|
| 6 Cerebral Ventricle<br>Aqueduct of Sylvius<br>Cerebral aqueduct (Sylvius)<br>Choroid plexus<br>Ependyma<br>Foramen of Monro (intraventricular)<br>Fourth ventricle<br>Interventricular foramen (Monro)<br>Left lateral ventricle<br>Right lateral ventricle<br>Third ventricle | Ø Open<br>3 Percutaneous<br>4 Percutaneous Endoscopic | Z No Device | Z No Qualifier |

**Ø Medical and Surgical**
**Ø Central Nervous System and Cranial Nerves**
**8 Division** Definition: Cutting into a body part, without draining fluids and/or gases from the body part, in order to separate or transect a body part

Explanation: All or a portion of the body part is separated into two or more portions

| Body Part<br>Character 4 | | Approach<br>Character 5 | Device<br>Character 6 | Qualifier<br>Character 7 |
|---|---|---|---|---|
| **Ø Brain**<br>Cerebrum<br>Corpus callosum<br>Encephalon<br>**7 Cerebral Hemisphere**<br>Frontal lobe<br>Occipital lobe<br>Parietal lobe<br>Temporal lobe<br>**8 Basal Ganglia**<br>Basal nuclei<br>Claustrum<br>Corpus striatum<br>Globus pallidus<br>Substantia nigra<br>Subthalamic nucleus<br>**F Olfactory Nerve**<br>First cranial nerve<br>Olfactory bulb<br>**G Optic Nerve**<br>Optic chiasma<br>Second cranial nerve<br>**H Oculomotor Nerve**<br>Third cranial nerve<br>**J Trochlear Nerve**<br>Fourth cranial nerve<br>**K Trigeminal Nerve**<br>Fifth cranial nerve<br>Gasserian ganglion<br>Mandibular nerve<br>Maxillary nerve<br>Ophthalmic nerve<br>Trifacial nerve<br>**L Abducens Nerve**<br>Sixth cranial nerve<br>**M Facial Nerve**<br>Chorda tympani<br>Geniculate ganglion<br>Greater superficial petrosal nerve<br>Nerve to the stapedius<br>Parotid plexus<br>Posterior auricular nerve<br>Seventh cranial nerve<br>Submandibular ganglion | **N Acoustic Nerve**<br>Cochlear nerve<br>Eighth cranial nerve<br>Scarpa's (vestibular) ganglion<br>Spiral ganglion<br>Vestibular (Scarpa's) ganglion<br>Vestibular nerve<br>Vestibulocochlear nerve<br>**P Glossopharyngeal Nerve**<br>Carotid sinus nerve<br>Ninth cranial nerve<br>Tympanic nerve<br>**Q Vagus Nerve**<br>Anterior vagal trunk<br>Pharyngeal plexus<br>Pneumogastric nerve<br>Posterior vagal trunk<br>Pulmonary plexus<br>Recurrent laryngeal nerve<br>Superior laryngeal nerve<br>Tenth cranial nerve<br>**R Accessory Nerve**<br>Eleventh cranial nerve<br>**S Hypoglossal Nerve**<br>Twelfth cranial nerve<br>**W Cervical Spinal Cord**<br>**X Thoracic Spinal Cord**<br>**Y Lumbar Spinal Cord**<br>Cauda equina<br>Conus medullaris | **Ø Open**<br>**3 Percutaneous**<br>**4 Percutaneous Endoscopic** | Z No Device | Z No Qualifier |

**0 Medical and Surgical**
**0 Central Nervous System and Cranial Nerves**
**9 Drainage** Definition: Taking or letting out fluids and/or gases from a body part
Explanation: The qualifier DIAGNOSTIC is used to identify drainage procedures that are biopsies

| Body Part Character 4 | Approach Character 5 | Device Character 6 | Qualifier Character 7 |
|---|---|---|---|
| **0 Brain** Cerebrum; Corpus callosum; Encephalon<br>**1 Cerebral Meninges** Arachnoid mater, intracranial; Leptomeninges, intracranial; Pia mater, intracranial<br>**2 Dura Mater** Diaphragma sellae; Dura mater, intracranial; Falx cerebri; Tentorium cerebelli<br>**3 Epidural Space, Intracranial** Extradural space, intracranial<br>**4 Subdural Space, Intracranial**<br>**5 Subarachnoid Space, Intracranial**<br>**6 Cerebral Ventricle** Aqueduct of Sylvius; Cerebral aqueduct (Sylvius); Choroid plexus; Ependyma; Foramen of Monro (intraventricular); Fourth ventricle; Interventricular foramen (Monro); Left lateral ventricle; Right lateral ventricle; Third ventricle<br>**7 Cerebral Hemisphere** Frontal lobe; Occipital lobe; Parietal lobe; Temporal lobe<br>**8 Basal Ganglia** Basal nuclei; Claustrum; Corpus striatum; Globus pallidus; Substantia nigra; Subthalamic nucleus<br>**9 Thalamus** Epithalamus; Geniculate nucleus; Metathalamus; Pulvinar<br>**A Hypothalamus** Mammillary body<br>**B Pons** Apneustic center; Basis pontis; Locus ceruleus; Pneumotaxic center; Pontine tegmentum; Superior olivary nucleus<br>**C Cerebellum** Culmen<br>**D Medulla Oblongata** Myelencephalon<br>**F Olfactory Nerve** First cranial nerve; Olfactory bulb<br>**G Optic Nerve** Optic chiasma; Second cranial nerve<br>**H Oculomotor Nerve** Third cranial nerve<br>**J Trochlear Nerve** Fourth cranial nerve<br>**K Trigeminal Nerve** Fifth cranial nerve; Gasserian ganglion; Mandibular nerve; Maxillary nerve; Ophthalmic nerve; Trifacial nerve<br>**L Abducens Nerve** Sixth cranial nerve<br>**M Facial Nerve** Chorda tympani; Geniculate ganglion; Greater superficial petrosal nerve; Nerve to the stapedius; Parotid plexus; Posterior auricular nerve; Seventh cranial nerve; Submandibular ganglion<br>**N Acoustic Nerve** Cochlear nerve; Eighth cranial nerve; Scarpa's (vestibular) ganglion; Spiral ganglion; Vestibular (Scarpa's) ganglion; Vestibular nerve; Vestibulocochlear nerve<br>**P Glossopharyngeal Nerve** Carotid sinus nerve; Ninth cranial nerve; Tympanic nerve<br>**Q Vagus Nerve** Anterior vagal trunk; Pharyngeal plexus; Pneumogastric nerve; Posterior vagal trunk; Pulmonary plexus; Recurrent laryngeal nerve; Superior laryngeal nerve; Tenth cranial nerve<br>**R Accessory Nerve** Eleventh cranial nerve<br>**S Hypoglossal Nerve** Twelfth cranial nerve<br>**T Spinal Meninges** Arachnoid mater, spinal; Denticulate (dentate) ligament; Dura mater, spinal; Filum terminale; Leptomeninges, spinal; Pia mater, spinal<br>**U Spinal Canal** Epidural space, spinal; Extradural space, spinal; Subarachnoid space, spinal; Subdural space, spinal; Vertebral canal<br>**W Cervical Spinal Cord**<br>**X Thoracic Spinal Cord**<br>**Y Lumbar Spinal Cord** Cauda equina; Conus medullaris | **0 Open**<br>**3 Percutaneous**<br>**4 Percutaneous Endoscopic** | **0 Drainage Device** | **Z No Qualifier** |

*009 Continued on next page*

**Non-OR** 009[3,T]30Z
**Non-OR** 009U[3,4]0Z
**Non-OR** 009[W,X,Y]30Z

**ØØ9 Continued**

**Ø Medical and Surgical**
**Ø Central Nervous System and Cranial Nerves**
**9 Drainage** Definition: Taking or letting out fluids and/or gases from a body part
Explanation: The qualifier DIAGNOSTIC is used to identify drainage procedures that are biopsies

| Body Part Character 4 | Approach Character 5 | Device Character 6 | Qualifier Character 7 |
|---|---|---|---|
| **Ø Brain**<br>Cerebrum<br>Corpus callosum<br>Encephalon<br>**1 Cerebral Meninges**<br>Arachnoid mater, intracranial<br>Leptomeninges, intracranial<br>Pia mater, intracranial<br>**2 Dura Mater**<br>Diaphragma sellae<br>Dura mater, intracranial<br>Falx cerebri<br>Tentorium cerebelli<br>**3 Epidural Space, Intracranial**<br>Extradural space, intracranial<br>**4 Subdural Space, Intracranial**<br>**5 Subarachnoid Space, Intracranial**<br>**6 Cerebral Ventricle**<br>Aqueduct of Sylvius<br>Cerebral aqueduct (Sylvius)<br>Choroid plexus<br>Ependyma<br>Foramen of Monro (intraventricular)<br>Fourth ventricle<br>Interventricular foramen (Monro)<br>Left lateral ventricle<br>Right lateral ventricle<br>Third ventricle<br>**7 Cerebral Hemisphere**<br>Frontal lobe<br>Occipital lobe<br>Parietal lobe<br>Temporal lobe<br>**8 Basal Ganglia**<br>Basal nuclei<br>Claustrum<br>Corpus striatum<br>Globus pallidus<br>Substantia nigra<br>Subthalamic nucleus<br>**9 Thalamus**<br>Epithalamus<br>Geniculate nucleus<br>Metathalamus<br>Pulvinar<br>**A Hypothalamus**<br>Mammillary body<br>**B Pons**<br>Apneustic center<br>Basis pontis<br>Locus ceruleus<br>Pneumotaxic center<br>Pontine tegmentum<br>Superior olivary nucleus<br>**C Cerebellum**<br>Culmen<br>**D Medulla Oblongata**<br>Myelencephalon<br>**F Olfactory Nerve**<br>First cranial nerve<br>Olfactory bulb<br>**G Optic Nerve**<br>Optic chiasma<br>Second cranial nerve<br>**H Oculomotor Nerve**<br>Third cranial nerve<br>**J Trochlear Nerve**<br>Fourth cranial nerve<br>**K Trigeminal Nerve**<br>Fifth cranial nerve<br>Gasserian ganglion<br>Mandibular nerve<br>Maxillary nerve<br>Ophthalmic nerve<br>Trifacial nerve<br>**L Abducens Nerve**<br>Sixth cranial nerve<br>**M Facial Nerve**<br>Chorda tympani<br>Geniculate ganglion<br>Greater superficial petrosal nerve<br>Nerve to the stapedius<br>Parotid plexus<br>Posterior auricular nerve<br>Seventh cranial nerve<br>Submandibular ganglion<br>**N Acoustic Nerve**<br>Cochlear nerve<br>Eighth cranial nerve<br>Scarpa's (vestibular) ganglion<br>Spiral ganglion<br>Vestibular (Scarpa's) ganglion<br>Vestibular nerve<br>Vestibulocochlear nerve<br>**P Glossopharyngeal Nerve**<br>Carotid sinus nerve<br>Ninth cranial nerve<br>Tympanic nerve<br>**Q Vagus Nerve**<br>Anterior vagal trunk<br>Pharyngeal plexus<br>Pneumogastric nerve<br>Posterior vagal trunk<br>Pulmonary plexus<br>Recurrent laryngeal nerve<br>Superior laryngeal nerve<br>Tenth cranial nerve<br>**R Accessory Nerve**<br>Eleventh cranial nerve<br>**S Hypoglossal Nerve**<br>Twelfth cranial nerve<br>**T Spinal Meninges**<br>Arachnoid mater, spinal<br>Denticulate (dentate) ligament<br>Dura mater, spinal<br>Filum terminale<br>Leptomeninges, spinal<br>Pia mater, spinal<br>**U Spinal Canal**<br>Epidural space, spinal<br>Extradural space, spinal<br>Subarachnoid space, spinal<br>Subdural space, spinal<br>Vertebral canal<br>**W Cervical Spinal Cord**<br>**X Thoracic Spinal Cord**<br>**Y Lumbar Spinal Cord**<br>Cauda equina<br>Conus medullaris | **Ø Open**<br>**3 Percutaneous**<br>**4 Percutaneous Endoscopic** | **Z No Device** | **X Diagnostic**<br>**Z No Qualifier** |

**Non-OR** ØØ9[Ø,1,2,3,4,5,6,7,8,9,A,B,C,D,F,G,H,J,K,L,M,N,P,Q,R,S][3,4]ZX
**Non-OR** ØØ933ZZ
**Non-OR** ØØ9T3Z[X,Z]
**Non-OR** ØØ9U[3,4]Z[X,Z]
**Non-OR** ØØ9[W,X,Y]3Z[X,Z]

**Ø Medical and Surgical**
**Ø Central Nervous System and Cranial Nerves**
**B Excision** Definition: Cutting out or off, without replacement, a portion of a body part
Explanation: The qualifier DIAGNOSTIC is used to identify excision procedures that are biopsies

| Body Part Character 4 | | Approach Character 5 | Device Character 6 | Qualifier Character 7 |
|---|---|---|---|---|
| **Ø Brain**<br>Cerebrum<br>Corpus callosum<br>Encephalon<br>**1 Cerebral Meninges**<br>Arachnoid mater, intracranial<br>Leptomeninges, intracranial<br>Pia mater, intracranial<br>**2 Dura Mater**<br>Diaphragma sellae<br>Dura mater, intracranial<br>Falx cerebri<br>Tentorium cerebelli<br>**6 Cerebral Ventricle**<br>Aqueduct of Sylvius<br>Cerebral aqueduct (Sylvius)<br>Choroid plexus<br>Ependyma<br>Foramen of Monro (intraventricular)<br>Fourth ventricle<br>Interventricular foramen (Monro)<br>Left lateral ventricle<br>Right lateral ventricle<br>Third ventricle<br>**7 Cerebral Hemisphere**<br>Frontal lobe<br>Occipital lobe<br>Parietal lobe<br>Temporal lobe<br>**8 Basal Ganglia**<br>Basal nuclei<br>Claustrum<br>Corpus striatum<br>Globus pallidus<br>Substantia nigra<br>Subthalamic nucleus<br>**9 Thalamus**<br>Epithalamus<br>Geniculate nucleus<br>Metathalamus<br>Pulvinar<br>**A Hypothalamus**<br>Mammillary body<br>**B Pons**<br>Apneustic center<br>Basis pontis<br>Locus ceruleus<br>Pneumotaxic center<br>Pontine tegmentum<br>Superior olivary nucleus<br>**C Cerebellum**<br>Culmen<br>**D Medulla Oblongata**<br>Myelencephalon<br>**F Olfactory Nerve**<br>First cranial nerve<br>Olfactory bulb<br>**G Optic Nerve**<br>Optic chiasma<br>Second cranial nerve | **H Oculomotor Nerve**<br>Third cranial nerve<br>**J Trochlear Nerve**<br>Fourth cranial nerve<br>**K Trigeminal Nerve**<br>Fifth cranial nerve<br>Gasserian ganglion<br>Mandibular nerve<br>Maxillary nerve<br>Ophthalmic nerve<br>Trifacial nerve<br>**L Abducens Nerve**<br>Sixth cranial nerve<br>**M Facial Nerve**<br>Chorda tympani<br>Geniculate ganglion<br>Greater superficial petrosal nerve<br>Nerve to the stapedius<br>Parotid plexus<br>Posterior auricular nerve<br>Seventh cranial nerve<br>Submandibular ganglion<br>**N Acoustic Nerve**<br>Cochlear nerve<br>Eighth cranial nerve<br>Scarpa's (vestibular) ganglion<br>Spiral ganglion<br>Vestibular (Scarpa's) ganglion<br>Vestibular nerve<br>Vestibulocochlear nerve<br>**P Glossopharyngeal Nerve**<br>Carotid sinus nerve<br>Ninth cranial nerve<br>Tympanic nerve<br>**Q Vagus Nerve**<br>Anterior vagal trunk<br>Pharyngeal plexus<br>Pneumogastric nerve<br>Posterior vagal trunk<br>Pulmonary plexus<br>Recurrent laryngeal nerve<br>Superior laryngeal nerve<br>Tenth cranial nerve<br>**R Accessory Nerve**<br>Eleventh cranial nerve<br>**S Hypoglossal Nerve**<br>Twelfth cranial nerve<br>**T Spinal Meninges**<br>Arachnoid mater, spinal<br>Denticulate (dentate) ligament<br>Dura mater, spinal<br>Filum terminale<br>Leptomeninges, spinal<br>Pia mater, spinal<br>**W Cervical Spinal Cord**<br>**X Thoracic Spinal Cord**<br>**Y Lumbar Spinal Cord**<br>Cauda equina<br>Conus medullaris | **Ø Open**<br>**3 Percutaneous**<br>**4 Percutaneous Endoscopic** | **Z No Device** | **X Diagnostic**<br>**Z No Qualifier** |

**Non-OR** ØØB[Ø,1,2,6,7,8,9,A,B,C,D,F,G,H,J,K,L,M,N,P,Q,R,S][3,4]ZX

**Ø Medical and Surgical**
**Ø Central Nervous System and Cranial Nerves**
**C Extirpation** Definition: Taking or cutting out solid matter from a body part

Explanation: The solid matter may be an abnormal byproduct of a biological function or a foreign body; it may be imbedded in a body part or in the lumen of a tubular body part. The solid matter may or may not have been previously broken into pieces.

| Body Part Character 4 | Approach Character 5 | Device Character 6 | Qualifier Character 7 |
|---|---|---|---|
| **Ø Brain**<br>Cerebrum<br>Corpus callosum<br>Encephalon<br>**1 Cerebral Meninges**<br>Arachnoid mater, intracranial<br>Leptomeninges, intracranial<br>Pia mater, intracranial<br>**2 Dura Mater**<br>Diaphragma sellae<br>Dura mater, intracranial<br>Falx cerebri<br>Tentorium cerebelli<br>**3 Epidural Space, Intracranial**<br>Extradural space, intracranial<br>**4 Subdural Space, Intracranial**<br>**5 Subarachnoid Space, Intracranial**<br>**6 Cerebral Ventricle**<br>Aqueduct of Sylvius<br>Cerebral aqueduct (Sylvius)<br>Choroid plexus<br>Ependyma<br>Foramen of Monro (intraventricular)<br>Fourth ventricle<br>Interventricular foramen (Monro)<br>Left lateral ventricle<br>Right lateral ventricle<br>Third ventricle<br>**7 Cerebral Hemisphere**<br>Frontal lobe<br>Occipital lobe<br>Parietal lobe<br>Temporal lobe<br>**8 Basal Ganglia**<br>Basal nuclei<br>Claustrum<br>Corpus striatum<br>Globus pallidus<br>Substantia nigra<br>Subthalamic nucleus<br>**9 Thalamus**<br>Epithalamus<br>Geniculate nucleus<br>Metathalamus<br>Pulvinar<br>**A Hypothalamus**<br>Mammillary body<br>**B Pons**<br>Apneustic center<br>Basis pontis<br>Locus ceruleus<br>Pneumotaxic center<br>Pontine tegmentum<br>Superior olivary nucleus<br>**C Cerebellum**<br>Culmen<br>**D Medulla Oblongata**<br>Myelencephalon<br>**F Olfactory Nerve**<br>First cranial nerve<br>Olfactory bulb<br>**G Optic Nerve**<br>Optic chiasma<br>Second cranial nerve<br>**H Oculomotor Nerve**<br>Third cranial nerve<br>**J Trochlear Nerve**<br>Fourth cranial nerve<br>**K Trigeminal Nerve**<br>Fifth cranial nerve<br>Gasserian ganglion<br>Mandibular nerve<br>Maxillary nerve<br>Ophthalmic nerve<br>Trifacial nerve<br>**L Abducens Nerve**<br>Sixth cranial nerve<br>**M Facial Nerve**<br>Chorda tympani<br>Geniculate ganglion<br>Greater superficial petrosal nerve<br>Nerve to the stapedius<br>Parotid plexus<br>Posterior auricular nerve<br>Seventh cranial nerve<br>Submandibular ganglion<br>**N Acoustic Nerve**<br>Cochlear nerve<br>Eighth cranial nerve<br>Scarpa's (vestibular) ganglion<br>Spiral ganglion<br>Vestibular (Scarpa's) ganglion<br>Vestibular nerve<br>Vestibulocochlear nerve<br>**P Glossopharyngeal Nerve**<br>Carotid sinus nerve<br>Ninth cranial nerve<br>Tympanic nerve<br>**Q Vagus Nerve**<br>Anterior vagal trunk<br>Pharyngeal plexus<br>Pneumogastric nerve<br>Posterior vagal trunk<br>Pulmonary plexus<br>Recurrent laryngeal nerve<br>Superior laryngeal nerve<br>Tenth cranial nerve<br>**R Accessory Nerve**<br>Eleventh cranial nerve<br>**S Hypoglossal Nerve**<br>Twelfth cranial nerve<br>**T Spinal Meninges**<br>Arachnoid mater, spinal<br>Denticulate (dentate) ligament<br>Dura mater, spinal<br>Filum terminale<br>Leptomeninges, spinal<br>Pia mater, spinal<br>**U Spinal Canal**<br>**W Cervical Spinal Cord**<br>**X Thoracic Spinal Cord**<br>**Y Lumbar Spinal Cord**<br>Cauda equina<br>Conus medullaris | **Ø Open**<br>**3 Percutaneous**<br>**4 Percutaneous Endoscopic** | **Z No Device** | **Z No Qualifier** |

**Ø Medical and Surgical**
**Ø Central Nervous System and Cranial Nerves**
**D Extraction** Definition: Pulling or stripping out or off all or a portion of a body part by the use of force
Explanation: The qualifier DIAGNOSTIC is used to identify extraction procedures that are biopsies

| Body Part Character 4 | | Approach Character 5 | Device Character 6 | Qualifier Character 7 |
|---|---|---|---|---|
| **1 Cerebral Meninges**<br>Arachnoid mater, intracranial<br>Leptomeninges, intracranial<br>Pia mater, intracranial<br>**2 Dura Mater**<br>Diaphragma sellae<br>Dura mater, intracranial<br>Falx cerebri<br>Tentorium cerebelli<br>**F Olfactory Nerve**<br>First cranial nerve<br>Olfactory bulb<br>**G Optic Nerve**<br>Optic chiasma<br>Second cranial nerve<br>**H Oculomotor Nerve**<br>Third cranial nerve<br>**J Trochlear Nerve**<br>Fourth cranial nerve<br>**K Trigeminal Nerve**<br>Fifth cranial nerve<br>Gasserian ganglion<br>Mandibular nerve<br>Maxillary nerve<br>Ophthalmic nerve<br>Trifacial nerve<br>**L Abducens Nerve**<br>Sixth cranial nerve<br>**M Facial Nerve**<br>Chorda tympani<br>Geniculate ganglion<br>Greater superficial petrosal nerve<br>Nerve to the stapedius<br>Parotid plexus<br>Posterior auricular nerve<br>Seventh cranial nerve<br>Submandibular ganglion | **N Acoustic Nerve**<br>Cochlear nerve<br>Eighth cranial nerve<br>Scarpa's (vestibular) ganglion<br>Spiral ganglion<br>Vestibular (Scarpa's) ganglion<br>Vestibular nerve<br>Vestibulocochlear nerve<br>**P Glossopharyngeal Nerve**<br>Carotid sinus nerve<br>Ninth cranial nerve<br>Tympanic nerve<br>**Q Vagus Nerve**<br>Anterior vagal trunk<br>Pharyngeal plexus<br>Pneumogastric nerve<br>Posterior vagal trunk<br>Pulmonary plexus<br>Recurrent laryngeal nerve<br>Superior laryngeal nerve<br>Tenth cranial nerve<br>**R Accessory Nerve**<br>Eleventh cranial nerve<br>**S Hypoglossal Nerve**<br>Twelfth cranial nerve<br>**T Spinal Meninges**<br>Arachnoid mater, spinal<br>Denticulate (dentate) ligament<br>Dura mater, spinal<br>Filum terminale<br>Leptomeninges, spinal<br>Pia mater, spinal | **Ø Open**<br>**3 Percutaneous**<br>**4 Percutaneous Endoscopic** | **Z No Device** | **Z No Qualifier** |

**Ø Medical and Surgical**
**Ø Central Nervous System and Cranial Nerves**
**F Fragmentation** Definition: Breaking solid matter in a body part into pieces
Explanation: Physical force (e.g., manual, ultrasonic) applied directly or indirectly is used to break the solid matter into pieces. The solid matter may be an abnormal byproduct of a biological function or a foreign body. The pieces of solid matter are not taken out.

| Body Part Character 4 | Approach Character 5 | Device Character 6 | Qualifier Character 7 |
|---|---|---|---|
| **3 Epidural Space, Intracranial** NC<br>Extradural space, intracranial<br>**4 Subdural Space, Intracranial** NC<br>**5 Subarachnoid Space, Intracranial** NC<br>**6 Cerebral Ventricle** NC<br>Aqueduct of Sylvius<br>Cerebral aqueduct (Sylvius)<br>Choroid plexus<br>Ependyma<br>Foramen of Monro (intraventricular)<br>Fourth ventricle<br>Interventricular foramen (Monro)<br>Left lateral ventricle<br>Right lateral ventricle<br>Third ventricle<br>**U Spinal Canal**<br>Epidural space, spinal<br>Extradural space, spinal<br>Subarachnoid space, spinal<br>Subdural space, spinal<br>Vertebral canal | **Ø Open**<br>**3 Percutaneous**<br>**4 Percutaneous Endoscopic**<br>**X External** | **Z No Device** | **Z No Qualifier** |

**Non-OR** ØØF[3,4,5,6]XZZ
NC ØØF[3,4,5,6]XZZ

**Ø Medical and Surgical**
**Ø Central Nervous System and Cranial Nerves**
**H Insertion** Definition: Putting in a nonbiological appliance that monitors, assists, performs, or prevents a physiological function but does not physically take the place of a body part
Explanation: None

| Body Part Character 4 | Approach Character 5 | Device Character 6 | Qualifier Character 7 |
|---|---|---|---|
| **Ø** Brain ⊞<br>Cerebrum<br>Corpus callosum<br>Encephalon | **Ø** Open | **2** Monitoring Device<br>**3** Infusion Device<br>**4** Radioactive Element, Cesium-131 Collagen Implant<br>**M** Neurostimulator Lead<br>**Y** Other Device | **Z** No Qualifier |
| **Ø** Brain ⊞<br>Cerebrum<br>Corpus callosum<br>Encephalon | **3** Percutaneous<br>**4** Percutaneous Endoscopic | **2** Monitoring Device<br>**3** Infusion Device<br>**M** Neurostimulator Lead<br>**Y** Other Device | **Z** No Qualifier |
| **6** Cerebral Ventricle ⊞<br>Aqueduct of Sylvius<br>Cerebral aqueduct (Sylvius)<br>Choroid plexus<br>Ependyma<br>Foramen of Monro (intraventricular)<br>Fourth ventricle Interventricular foramen (Monro)<br>Left lateral ventricle<br>Right lateral ventricle<br>Third ventricle<br>**E** Cranial Nerve ⊞<br>**U** Spinal Canal ⊞<br>Epidural space, spinal<br>Extradural space, spinal<br>Subarachnoid space, spinal<br>Subdural space, spinal<br>Vertebral canal<br>**V** Spinal Cord ⊞ | **Ø** Open<br>**3** Percutaneous<br>**4** Percutaneous Endoscopic | **2** Monitoring Device<br>**3** Infusion Device<br>**M** Neurostimulator Lead<br>**Y** Other Device | **Z** No Qualifier |

Non-OR ØØHØ32Z
Non-OR ØØHØ[3,4]YZ
Non-OR ØØH[6,E,U,V]32Z
Non-OR ØØH[6,E][3,4]YZ
Non-OR ØØH[U,V][Ø,3,4][3,Y]Z

**See Appendix L for Procedure Combinations**
⊞ ØØHØØMZ
⊞ ØØHØ[3,4]MZ
⊞ ØØH[6,E,U,V][Ø,3,4]MZ

**Ø Medical and Surgical**
**Ø Central Nervous System and Cranial Nerves**
**J Inspection** Definition: Visually and/or manually exploring a body part
Explanation: Visual exploration may be performed with or without optical instrumentation. Manual exploration may be performed directly or through intervening body layers.

| Body Part Character 4 | Approach Character 5 | Device Character 6 | Qualifier Character 7 |
|---|---|---|---|
| **Ø** Brain<br>Cerebrum<br>Corpus callosum<br>Encephalon<br>**E** Cranial Nerve<br>**U** Spinal Canal<br>Epidural space, spinal<br>Extradural space, spinal<br>Subarachnoid space, spinal<br>Subdural space, spinal<br>Vertebral canal<br>**V** Spinal Cord | **Ø** Open<br>**3** Percutaneous<br>**4** Percutaneous Endoscopic | **Z** No Device | **Z** No Qualifier |

DRG Non-OR ØØJ[Ø,U,V]3ZZ
Non-OR ØØJE3ZZ

**Ø Medical and Surgical**
**Ø Central Nervous System and Cranial Nerves**
**K Map** Definition: Locating the route of passage of electrical impulses and/or locating functional areas in a body part
Explanation: Applicable only to the cardiac conduction mechanism and the central nervous system

| Body Part Character 4 | Approach Character 5 | Device Character 6 | Qualifier Character 7 |
|---|---|---|---|
| **Ø** Brain<br>Cerebrum<br>Corpus callosum<br>Encephalon<br>**7** Cerebral Hemisphere<br>Frontal lobe<br>Occipital lobe<br>Parietal lobe<br>Temporal lobe<br>**8** Basal Ganglia<br>Basal nuclei<br>Claustrum<br>Corpus striatum<br>Globus pallidus<br>Substantia nigra<br>Subthalamic nucleus<br>**9** Thalamus<br>Epithalamus<br>Geniculate nucleus<br>Metathalamus<br>Pulvinar<br>**A** Hypothalamus<br>Mammillary body<br>**B** Pons<br>Apneustic center<br>Basis pontis<br>Locus ceruleus<br>Pneumotaxic center<br>Pontine tegmentum<br>Superior olivary nucleus<br>**C** Cerebellum<br>Culmen<br>**D** Medulla Oblongata<br>Myelencephalon | **Ø** Open<br>**3** Percutaneous<br>**4** Percutaneous Endoscopic | **Z** No Device | **Z** No Qualifier |

**Ø Medical and Surgical**
**Ø Central Nervous System and Cranial Nerves**
**N Release** Definition: Freeing a body part from an abnormal physical constraint by cutting or by the use of force
Explanation: Some of the restraining tissue may be taken out but none of the body part is taken out

| Body Part Character 4 | | Approach Character 5 | Device Character 6 | Qualifier Character 7 |
|---|---|---|---|---|
| **Ø Brain**<br>Cerebrum<br>Corpus callosum<br>Encephalon<br>**1 Cerebral Meninges**<br>Arachnoid mater, intracranial<br>Leptomeninges, intracranial<br>Pia mater, intracranial<br>**2 Dura Mater**<br>Diaphragma sellae<br>Dura mater, intracranial<br>Falx cerebri<br>Tentorium cerebelli<br>**6 Cerebral Ventricle**<br>Aqueduct of Sylvius<br>Cerebral aqueduct (Sylvius)<br>Choroid plexus<br>Ependyma<br>Foramen of Monro (intraventricular)<br>Fourth ventricle<br>Interventricular foramen (Monro)<br>Left lateral ventricle<br>Right lateral ventricle<br>Third ventricle<br>**7 Cerebral Hemisphere**<br>Frontal lobe<br>Occipital lobe<br>Parietal lobe<br>Temporal lobe<br>**8 Basal Ganglia**<br>Basal nuclei<br>Claustrum<br>Corpus striatum<br>Globus pallidus<br>Substantia nigra<br>Subthalamic nucleus<br>**9 Thalamus**<br>Epithalamus<br>Geniculate nucleus<br>Metathalamus<br>Pulvinar<br>**A Hypothalamus**<br>Mammillary body<br>**B Pons**<br>Apneustic center<br>Basis pontis<br>Locus ceruleus<br>Pneumotaxic center<br>Pontine tegmentum<br>Superior olivary nucleus<br>**C Cerebellum**<br>Culmen<br>**D Medulla Oblongata**<br>Myelencephalon<br>**F Olfactory Nerve**<br>First cranial nerve<br>Olfactory bulb<br>**G Optic Nerve**<br>Optic chiasma<br>Second cranial nerve | **H Oculomotor Nerve**<br>Third cranial nerve<br>**J Trochlear Nerve**<br>Fourth cranial nerve<br>**K Trigeminal Nerve**<br>Fifth cranial nerve<br>Gasserian ganglion<br>Mandibular nerve<br>Maxillary nerve<br>Ophthalmic nerve<br>Trifacial nerve<br>**L Abducens Nerve**<br>Sixth cranial nerve<br>**M Facial Nerve**<br>Chorda tympani<br>Geniculate ganglion<br>Greater superficial petrosal nerve<br>Nerve to the stapedius<br>Parotid plexus<br>Posterior auricular nerve<br>Seventh cranial nerve<br>Submandibular ganglion<br>**N Acoustic Nerve**<br>Cochlear nerve<br>Eighth cranial nerve<br>Scarpa's (vestibular) ganglion<br>Spiral ganglion<br>Vestibular (Scarpa's) ganglion<br>Vestibular nerve<br>Vestibulocochlear nerve<br>**P Glossopharyngeal Nerve**<br>Carotid sinus nerve<br>Ninth cranial nerve<br>Tympanic nerve<br>**Q Vagus Nerve**<br>Anterior vagal trunk<br>Pharyngeal plexus<br>Pneumogastric nerve<br>Posterior vagal trunk<br>Pulmonary plexus<br>Recurrent laryngeal nerve<br>Superior laryngeal nerve<br>Tenth cranial nerve<br>**R Accessory Nerve**<br>Eleventh cranial nerve<br>**S Hypoglossal Nerve**<br>Twelfth cranial nerve<br>**T Spinal Meninges**<br>Arachnoid mater, spinal<br>Denticulate (dentate) ligament<br>Dura mater, spinal<br>Filum terminale<br>Leptomeninges, spinal<br>Pia mater, spinal<br>**W Cervical Spinal Cord**<br>**X Thoracic Spinal Cord**<br>**Y Lumbar Spinal Cord**<br>Cauda equina<br>Conus medullaris | **Ø Open**<br>**3 Percutaneous**<br>**4 Percutaneous Endoscopic** | **Z No Device** | **Z No Qualifier** |

**Ø Medical and Surgical**
**Ø Central Nervous System and Cranial Nerves**
**P Removal** Definition: Taking out or off a device from a body part

Explanation: If a device is taken out and a similar device put in without cutting or puncturing the skin or mucous membrane, the procedure is coded to the root operation CHANGE. Otherwise, the procedure for taking out a device is coded to the root operation REMOVAL.

| Body Part Character 4 | Approach Character 5 | Device Character 6 | Qualifier Character 7 |
|---|---|---|---|
| Ø Brain<br>Cerebrum<br>Corpus callosum<br>Encephalon<br>V Spinal Cord | Ø Open<br>3 Percutaneous<br>4 Percutaneous Endoscopic | Ø Drainage Device<br>2 Monitoring Device<br>3 Infusion Device<br>7 Autologous Tissue Substitute<br>J Synthetic Substitute<br>K Nonautologous Tissue Substitute<br>M Neurostimulator Lead<br>Y Other Device | Z No Qualifier |
| Ø Brain<br>Cerebrum<br>Corpus callosum<br>Encephalon<br>V Spinal Cord | X External | Ø Drainage Device<br>2 Monitoring Device<br>3 Infusion Device<br>M Neurostimulator Lead | Z No Qualifier |
| 6 Cerebral Ventricle<br>Aqueduct of Sylvius<br>Cerebral aqueduct (Sylvius)<br>Choroid plexus<br>Ependyma<br>Foramen of Monro (intraventricular)<br>Fourth ventricle<br>Interventricular foramen (Monro)<br>Left lateral ventricle<br>Right lateral ventricle<br>Third ventricle<br>U Spinal Canal<br>Epidural space, spinal<br>Extradural space, spinal<br>Subarachnoid space, spinal<br>Subdural space, spinal<br>Vertebral canal | Ø Open<br>3 Percutaneous<br>4 Percutaneous Endoscopic | Ø Drainage Device<br>2 Monitoring Device<br>3 Infusion Device<br>J Synthetic Substitute<br>M Neurostimulator Lead<br>Y Other Device | Z No Qualifier |
| 6 Cerebral Ventricle<br>Aqueduct of Sylvius<br>Cerebral aqueduct (Sylvius)<br>Choroid plexus<br>Ependyma<br>Foramen of Monro (intraventricular)<br>Fourth ventricle<br>Interventricular foramen (Monro)<br>Left lateral ventricle<br>Right lateral ventricle<br>Third ventricle<br>U Spinal Canal<br>Epidural space, spinal<br>Extradural space, spinal<br>Subarachnoid space, spinal<br>Subdural space, spinal<br>Vertebral canal | X External | Ø Drainage Device<br>2 Monitoring Device<br>3 Infusion Device<br>M Neurostimulator Lead | Z No Qualifier |
| E Cranial Nerve | Ø Open<br>3 Percutaneous<br>4 Percutaneous Endoscopic | Ø Drainage Device<br>2 Monitoring Device<br>3 Infusion Device<br>7 Autologous Tissue Substitute<br>M Neurostimulator Lead<br>Y Other Device | Z No Qualifier |
| E Cranial Nerve | X External | Ø Drainage Device<br>2 Monitoring Device<br>3 Infusion Device<br>M Neurostimulator Lead | Z No Qualifier |

**Non-OR** ØØP[Ø,V]3[Ø,2,3]Z
**Non-OR** ØØP[Ø,V][3,4]YZ
**Non-OR** ØØP[Ø,V]X[Ø,2,3,M]Z
**Non-OR** ØØP[6,U]3[Ø,2,3]Z
**Non-OR** ØØP[6,U][3,4]YZ
**Non-OR** ØØP6X[Ø,2,3,M]Z
**Non-OR** ØØPUX[Ø,2,3,M]Z
**Non-OR** ØØPE3[Ø,2,3]Z
**Non-OR** ØØPE[3,4]YZ
**Non-OR** ØØPEX[Ø,2,3,M]Z

**Ø Medical and Surgical**
**Ø Central Nervous System and Cranial Nerves**
**Q Repair** Definition: Restoring, to the extent possible, a body part to its normal anatomic structure and function
Explanation: Used only when the method to accomplish the repair is not one of the other root operations

| Body Part Character 4 | | Approach Character 5 | Device Character 6 | Qualifier Character 7 |
|---|---|---|---|---|
| **Ø Brain**<br>Cerebrum<br>Corpus callosum<br>Encephalon<br>**1 Cerebral Meninges**<br>Arachnoid mater, intracranial<br>Leptomeninges, intracranial<br>Pia mater, intracranial<br>**2 Dura Mater**<br>Diaphragma sellae<br>Dura mater, intracranial<br>Falx cerebri<br>Tentorium cerebelli<br>**6 Cerebral Ventricle**<br>Aqueduct of Sylvius<br>Cerebral aqueduct (Sylvius)<br>Choroid plexus<br>Ependyma<br>Foramen of Monro (intraventricular)<br>Fourth ventricle<br>Interventricular foramen (Monro)<br>Left lateral ventricle<br>Right lateral ventricle<br>Third ventricle<br>**7 Cerebral Hemisphere**<br>Frontal lobe<br>Occipital lobe<br>Parietal lobe<br>Temporal lobe<br>**8 Basal Ganglia**<br>Basal nuclei<br>Claustrum<br>Corpus striatum<br>Globus pallidus<br>Substantia nigra<br>Subthalamic nucleus<br>**9 Thalamus**<br>Epithalamus<br>Geniculate nucleus<br>Metathalamus<br>Pulvinar<br>**A Hypothalamus**<br>Mammillary body<br>**B Pons**<br>Apneustic center<br>Basis pontis<br>Locus ceruleus<br>Pneumotaxic center<br>Pontine tegmentum<br>Superior olivary nucleus<br>**C Cerebellum**<br>Culmen<br>**D Medulla Oblongata**<br>Myelencephalon<br>**F Olfactory Nerve**<br>First cranial nerve<br>Olfactory bulb<br>**G Optic Nerve**<br>Optic chiasma<br>Second cranial nerve | **H Oculomotor Nerve**<br>Third cranial nerve<br>**J Trochlear Nerve**<br>Fourth cranial nerve<br>**K Trigeminal Nerve**<br>Fifth cranial nerve<br>Gasserian ganglion<br>Mandibular nerve<br>Maxillary nerve<br>Ophthalmic nerve<br>Trifacial nerve<br>**L Abducens Nerve**<br>Sixth cranial nerve<br>**M Facial Nerve**<br>Chorda tympani<br>Geniculate ganglion<br>Greater superficial petrosal nerve<br>Nerve to the stapedius<br>Parotid plexus<br>Posterior auricular nerve<br>Seventh cranial nerve<br>Submandibular ganglion<br>**N Acoustic Nerve**<br>Cochlear nerve<br>Eighth cranial nerve<br>Scarpa's (vestibular) ganglion<br>Spiral ganglion<br>Vestibular (Scarpa's) ganglion<br>Vestibular nerve<br>Vestibulocochlear nerve<br>**P Glossopharyngeal Nerve**<br>Carotid sinus nerve<br>Ninth cranial nerve<br>Tympanic nerve<br>**Q Vagus Nerve**<br>Anterior vagal trunk<br>Pharyngeal plexus<br>Pneumogastric nerve<br>Posterior vagal trunk<br>Pulmonary plexus<br>Recurrent laryngeal nerve<br>Superior laryngeal nerve<br>Tenth cranial nerve<br>**R Accessory Nerve**<br>Eleventh cranial nerve<br>**S Hypoglossal Nerve**<br>Twelfth cranial nerve<br>**T Spinal Meninges**<br>Arachnoid mater, spinal<br>Denticulate (dentate) ligament<br>Dura mater, spinal<br>Filum terminale<br>Leptomeninges, spinal<br>Pia mater, spinal<br>**W Cervical Spinal Cord**<br>**X Thoracic Spinal Cord**<br>**Y Lumbar Spinal Cord**<br>Cauda equina<br>Conus medullaris | **Ø Open**<br>**3 Percutaneous**<br>**4 Percutaneous Endoscopic** | **Z No Device** | **Z No Qualifier** |

**Ø Medical and Surgical**
**Ø Central Nervous System and Cranial Nerves**
**R Replacement** Definition: Putting in or on biological or synthetic material that physically takes the place and/or function of all or a portion of a body part

Explanation: The body part may have been taken out or replaced, or may be taken out, physically eradicated, or rendered nonfunctional during the REPLACEMENT procedure. A REMOVAL procedure is coded for taking out the device used in a previous replacement procedure.

| Body Part Character 4 | | Approach Character 5 | Device Character 6 | Qualifier Character 7 |
|---|---|---|---|---|
| 1 Cerebral Meninges<br>Arachnoid mater, intracranial<br>Leptomeninges, intracranial<br>Pia mater, intracranial<br>2 Dura Mater<br>Diaphragma sellae<br>Dura mater, intracranial<br>Falx cerebri<br>Tentorium cerebelli<br>6 Cerebral Ventricle<br>Aqueduct of Sylvius<br>Cerebral aqueduct (Sylvius)<br>Choroid plexus<br>Ependyma<br>Foramen of Monro (intraventricular)<br>Fourth ventricle<br>Interventricular foramen (Monro)<br>Left lateral ventricle<br>Right lateral ventricle<br>Third ventricle<br>F Olfactory Nerve<br>First cranial nerve<br>Olfactory bulb<br>G Optic Nerve<br>Optic chiasma<br>Second cranial nerve<br>H Oculomotor Nerve<br>Third cranial nerve<br>J Trochlear Nerve<br>Fourth cranial nerve<br>K Trigeminal Nerve<br>Fifth cranial nerve<br>Gasserian ganglion<br>Mandibular nerve<br>Maxillary nerve<br>Ophthalmic nerve<br>Trifacial nerve<br>L Abducens Nerve<br>Sixth cranial nerve | M Facial Nerve<br>Chorda tympani<br>Geniculate ganglion<br>Greater superficial petrosal nerve<br>Nerve to the stapedius<br>Parotid plexus<br>Posterior auricular nerve<br>Seventh cranial nerve<br>Submandibular ganglion<br>N Acoustic Nerve<br>Cochlear nerve<br>Eighth cranial nerve<br>Scarpa's (vestibular) ganglion<br>Spiral ganglion<br>Vestibular (Scarpa's) ganglion<br>Vestibular nerve<br>Vestibulocochlear nerve<br>P Glossopharyngeal Nerve<br>Carotid sinus nerve<br>Ninth cranial nerve<br>Tympanic nerve<br>Q Vagus Nerve<br>Anterior vagal trunk<br>Pharyngeal plexus<br>Pneumogastric nerve<br>Posterior vagal trunk<br>Pulmonary plexus<br>Recurrent laryngeal nerve<br>Superior laryngeal nerve<br>Tenth cranial nerve<br>R Accessory Nerve<br>Eleventh cranial nerve<br>S Hypoglossal Nerve<br>Twelfth cranial nerve<br>T Spinal Meninges<br>Arachnoid mater, spinal<br>Denticulate (dentate) ligament<br>Dura mater, spinal<br>Filum terminale<br>Leptomeninges, spinal<br>Pia mater, spinal | Ø Open<br>4 Percutaneous Endoscopic | 7 Autologous Tissue Substitute<br>J Synthetic Substitute<br>K Nonautologous Tissue Substitute | Z No Qualifier |

**Ø Medical and Surgical**
**Ø Central Nervous System and Cranial Nerves**
**S Reposition** Definition: Moving to its normal location, or other suitable location, all or a portion of a body part

Explanation: The body part is moved to a new location from an abnormal location, or from a normal location where it is not functioning correctly. The body part may or may not be cut out or off to be moved to the new location.

| Body Part Character 4 | | Approach Character 5 | Device Character 6 | Qualifier Character 7 |
|---|---|---|---|---|
| **F Olfactory Nerve**<br>First cranial nerve<br>Olfactory bulb<br>**G Optic Nerve**<br>Optic chiasma<br>Second cranial nerve<br>**H Oculomotor Nerve**<br>Third cranial nerve<br>**J Trochlear Nerve**<br>Fourth cranial nerve<br>**K Trigeminal Nerve**<br>Fifth cranial nerve<br>Gasserian ganglion<br>Mandibular nerve<br>Maxillary nerve<br>Ophthalmic nerve<br>Trifacial nerve<br>**L Abducens Nerve**<br>Sixth cranial nerve<br>**M Facial Nerve**<br>Chorda tympani<br>Geniculate ganglion<br>Greater superficial petrosal nerve<br>Nerve to the stapedius<br>Parotid plexus<br>Posterior auricular nerve<br>Seventh cranial nerve<br>Submandibular ganglion | **N Acoustic Nerve**<br>Cochlear nerve<br>Eighth cranial nerve<br>Scarpa's (vestibular) ganglion<br>Spiral ganglion<br>Vestibular (Scarpa's) ganglion<br>Vestibular nerve<br>Vestibulocochlear nerve<br>**P Glossopharyngeal Nerve**<br>Carotid sinus nerve<br>Ninth cranial nerve<br>Tympanic nerve<br>**Q Vagus Nerve**<br>Anterior vagal trunk<br>Pharyngeal plexus<br>Pneumogastric nerve<br>Posterior vagal trunk<br>Pulmonary plexus<br>Recurrent laryngeal nerve<br>Superior laryngeal nerve<br>Tenth cranial nerve<br>**R Accessory Nerve**<br>Eleventh cranial nerve<br>**S Hypoglossal Nerve**<br>Twelfth cranial nerve<br>**W Cervical Spinal Cord**<br>**X Thoracic Spinal Cord**<br>**Y Lumbar Spinal Cord**<br>Cauda equina<br>Conus medullaris | **Ø Open**<br>**3 Percutaneous**<br>**4 Percutaneous Endoscopic** | **Z No Device** | **Z No Qualifier** |

**Ø Medical and Surgical**
**Ø Central Nervous System and Cranial Nerves**
**T Resection** Definition: Cutting out or off, without replacement, all of a body part

Explanation: None

| Body Part Character 4 | Approach Character 5 | Device Character 6 | Qualifier Character 7 |
|---|---|---|---|
| **7 Cerebral Hemisphere**<br>Frontal lobe<br>Occipital lobe<br>Parietal lobe<br>Temporal lobe | **Ø Open**<br>**3 Percutaneous**<br>**4 Percutaneous Endoscopic** | **Z No Device** | **Z No Qualifier** |

**Ø Medical and Surgical**
**Ø Central Nervous System and Cranial Nerves**
**U Supplement** Definition: Putting in or on biological or synthetic material that physically reinforces and/or augments the function of a portion of a body part

Explanation: The biological material is non-living, or is living and from the same individual. The body part may have been previously replaced, and the SUPPLEMENT procedure is performed to physically reinforce and/or augment the function of the replaced body part.

| Body Part Character 4 | | Approach Character 5 | Device Character 6 | Qualifier Character 7 |
|---|---|---|---|---|
| **1 Cerebral Meninges** Arachnoid mater, intracranial; Leptomeninges, intracranial; Pia mater, intracranial<br>**2 Dura Mater** Diaphragma sellae; Dura mater, intracranial; Falx cerebri; Tentorium cerebelli<br>**6 Cerebral Ventricle** Aqueduct of Sylvius; Cerebral aqueduct (Sylvius); Choroid plexus; Ependyma; Foramen of Monro (intraventricular); Fourth ventricle; Interventricular foramen (Monro); Left lateral ventricle; Right lateral ventricle; Third ventricle<br>**F Olfactory Nerve** First cranial nerve; Olfactory bulb<br>**G Optic Nerve** Optic chiasma; Second cranial nerve<br>**H Oculomotor Nerve** Third cranial nerve<br>**J Trochlear Nerve** Fourth cranial nerve<br>**K Trigeminal Nerve** Fifth cranial nerve; Gasserian ganglion; Mandibular nerve; Maxillary nerve; Ophthalmic nerve; Trifacial nerve<br>**L Abducens Nerve** Sixth cranial nerve | **M Facial Nerve** Chorda tympani; Geniculate ganglion; Greater superficial petrosal nerve; Nerve to the stapedius; Parotid plexus; Posterior auricular nerve; Seventh cranial nerve; Submandibular ganglion<br>**N Acoustic Nerve** Cochlear nerve; Eighth cranial nerve; Scarpa's (vestibular) ganglion; Spiral ganglion; Vestibular (Scarpa's) ganglion; Vestibular nerve; Vestibulocochlear nerve<br>**P Glossopharyngeal Nerve** Carotid sinus nerve; Ninth cranial nerve; Tympanic nerve<br>**Q Vagus Nerve** Anterior vagal trunk; Pharyngeal plexus; Pneumogastric nerve; Posterior vagal trunk; Pulmonary plexus; Recurrent laryngeal nerve; Superior laryngeal nerve; Tenth cranial nerve<br>**R Accessory Nerve** Eleventh cranial nerve<br>**S Hypoglossal Nerve** Twelfth cranial nerve<br>**T Spinal Meninges** Arachnoid mater, spinal; Denticulate (dentate) ligament; Dura mater, spinal; Filum terminale; Leptomeninges, spinal; Pia mater, spinal | **Ø** Open<br>**3** Percutaneous<br>**4** Percutaneous Endoscopic | **7** Autologous Tissue Substitute<br>**J** Synthetic Substitute<br>**K** Nonautologous Tissue Substitute | **Z** No Qualifier |

**Ø Medical and Surgical**
**Ø Central Nervous System and Cranial Nerves**
**W Revision** Definition: Correcting, to the extent possible, a portion of a malfunctioning device or the position of a displaced device

Explanation: Revision can include correcting a malfunctioning or displaced device by taking out or putting in components of the device such as a screw or pin

| Body Part Character 4 | Approach Character 5 | Device Character 6 | Qualifier Character 7 |
|---|---|---|---|
| Ø Brain<br>Cerebrum<br>Corpus callosum<br>Encephalon<br>V Spinal Cord | Ø Open<br>3 Percutaneous<br>4 Percutaneous Endoscopic | Ø Drainage Device<br>2 Monitoring Device<br>3 Infusion Device<br>7 Autologous Tissue Substitute<br>J Synthetic Substitute<br>K Nonautologous Tissue Substitute<br>M Neurostimulator Lead<br>Y Other Device | Z No Qualifier |
| Ø Brain<br>Cerebrum<br>Corpus callosum<br>Encephalon<br>V Spinal Cord | X External | Ø Drainage Device<br>2 Monitoring Device<br>3 Infusion Device<br>7 Autologous Tissue Substitute<br>J Synthetic Substitute<br>K Nonautologous Tissue Substitute<br>M Neurostimulator Lead | Z No Qualifier |
| 6 Cerebral Ventricle<br>Aqueduct of Sylvius<br>Cerebral aqueduct (Sylvius)<br>Choroid plexus<br>Ependyma<br>Foramen of Monro (intraventricular)<br>Fourth ventricle<br>Interventricular foramen (Monro)<br>Left lateral ventricle<br>Right lateral ventricle<br>Third ventricle<br>U Spinal Canal<br>Epidural space, spinal<br>Extradural space, spinal<br>Subarachnoid space, spinal<br>Subdural space, spinal<br>Vertebral canal | Ø Open<br>3 Percutaneous<br>4 Percutaneous Endoscopic | Ø Drainage Device<br>2 Monitoring Device<br>3 Infusion Device<br>J Synthetic Substitute<br>M Neurostimulator Lead<br>Y Other Device | Z No Qualifier |
| 6 Cerebral Ventricle<br>Aqueduct of Sylvius<br>Cerebral aqueduct (Sylvius)<br>Choroid plexus<br>Ependyma<br>Foramen of Monro (intraventricular)<br>Fourth ventricle<br>Interventricular foramen (Monro)<br>Left lateral ventricle<br>Right lateral ventricle<br>Third ventricle<br>U Spinal Canal<br>Epidural space, spinal<br>Extradural space, spinal<br>Subarachnoid space, spinal<br>Subdural space, spinal<br>Vertebral canal | X External | Ø Drainage Device<br>2 Monitoring Device<br>3 Infusion Device<br>J Synthetic Substitute<br>M Neurostimulator Lead | Z No Qualifier |
| E Cranial Nerve | Ø Open<br>3 Percutaneous<br>4 Percutaneous Endoscopic | Ø Drainage Device<br>2 Monitoring Device<br>3 Infusion Device<br>7 Autologous Tissue Substitute<br>M Neurostimulator Lead<br>Y Other Device | Z No Qualifier |
| E Cranial Nerve | X External | Ø Drainage Device<br>2 Monitoring Device<br>3 Infusion Device<br>7 Autologous Tissue Substitute<br>M Neurostimulator Lead | Z No Qualifier |

Non-OR ØØW[Ø,V][3,4]YZ
Non-OR ØØW[Ø,V]X[Ø,2,3,7,J,K,M]Z
Non-OR ØØW[6,U][3,4]YZ
Non-OR ØØW[6,U]X[Ø,2,3,J,M]Z
Non-OR ØØWE[3,4]YZ
Non-OR ØØWEX[Ø,2,3,7,M]Z

**Ø Medical and Surgical**
**Ø Central Nervous System and Cranial Nerves**
**X Transfer** Definition: Moving, without taking out, all or a portion of a body part to another location to take over the function of all or a portion of a body part

Explanation: The body part transferred remains connected to its vascular and nervous supply

| Body Part Character 4 | Approach Character 5 | Device Character 6 | Qualifier Character 7 |
|---|---|---|---|
| **F Olfactory Nerve**<br>First cranial nerve<br>Olfactory bulb<br>**G Optic Nerve**<br>Optic chiasma<br>Second cranial nerve<br>**H Oculomotor Nerve**<br>Third cranial nerve<br>**J Trochlear Nerve**<br>Fourth cranial nerve<br>**K Trigeminal Nerve**<br>Fifth cranial nerve<br>Gasserian ganglion<br>Mandibular nerve<br>Maxillary nerve<br>Ophthalmic nerve<br>Trifacial nerve<br>**L Abducens Nerve**<br>Sixth cranial nerve<br>**M Facial Nerve**<br>Chorda tympani<br>Geniculate ganglion<br>Greater superficial petrosal nerve<br>Nerve to the stapedius<br>Parotid plexus<br>Posterior auricular nerve<br>Seventh cranial nerve<br>Submandibular ganglion<br>**N Acoustic Nerve**<br>Cochlear nerve<br>Eighth cranial nerve<br>Scarpa's (vestibular) ganglion<br>Spiral ganglion<br>Vestibular (Scarpa's) ganglion<br>Vestibular nerve<br>Vestibulocochlear nerve<br>**P Glossopharyngeal Nerve**<br>Carotid sinus nerve<br>Ninth cranial nerve<br>Tympanic nerve<br>**Q Vagus Nerve**<br>Anterior vagal trunk<br>Pharyngeal plexus<br>Pneumogastric nerve<br>Posterior vagal trunk<br>Pulmonary plexus<br>Recurrent laryngeal nerve<br>Superior laryngeal nerve<br>Tenth cranial nerve<br>**R Accessory Nerve**<br>Eleventh cranial nerve<br>**S Hypoglossal Nerve**<br>Twelfth cranial nerve | **Ø Open**<br>**4 Percutaneous Endoscopic** | **Z No Device** | **F Olfactory Nerve**<br>**G Optic Nerve**<br>**H Oculomotor Nerve**<br>**J Trochlear Nerve**<br>**K Trigeminal Nerve**<br>**L Abducens Nerve**<br>**M Facial Nerve**<br>**N Acoustic Nerve**<br>**P Glossopharyngeal Nerve**<br>**Q Vagus Nerve**<br>**R Accessory Nerve**<br>**S Hypoglossal Nerve** |

# Peripheral Nervous System Ø12–Ø1X



## Character Meanings

This Character Meaning table is provided as a guide to assist the user in the identification of character members that may be found in this section of code tables. It **SHOULD NOT** be used to build a PCS code.

| Operation–Character 3 | Body Part–Character 4 | Approach–Character 5 | Device–Character 6 | Qualifier–Character 7 |
|---|---|---|---|---|
| 2 Change | Ø Cervical Plexus | Ø Open | Ø Drainage Device | 1 Cervical Nerve |
| 5 Destruction | 1 Cervical Nerve | 3 Percutaneous | 2 Monitoring Device | 2 Phrenic Nerve |
| 8 Division | 2 Phrenic Nerve | 4 Percutaneous Endoscopic | 7 Autologous Tissue Substitute | 4 Ulnar Nerve |
| 9 Drainage | 3 Brachial Plexus | X External | M Neurostimulator Lead | 5 Median Nerve |
| B Excision | 4 Ulnar Nerve | | Y Other Device | 6 Radial Nerve |
| C Extirpation | 5 Median Nerve | | Z No Device | 8 Thoracic Nerve |
| D Extraction | 6 Radial Nerve | | | B Lumbar Nerve |
| H Insertion | 8 Thoracic Nerve | | | C Perineal Nerve |
| J Inspection | 9 Lumbar Plexus | | | D Femoral Nerve |
| N Release | A Lumbosacral Plexus | | | F Sciatic Nerve |
| P Removal | B Lumbar Nerve | | | G Tibial Nerve |
| Q Repair | C Pudendal Nerve | | | H Peroneal Nerve |
| R Replacement | D Femoral Nerve | | | X Diagnostic |
| S Reposition | F Sciatic Nerve | | | Z No Qualifier |
| U Supplement | G Tibial Nerve | | | |
| W Revision | H Peroneal Nerve | | | |
| X Transfer | K Head and Neck Sympathetic Nerve | | | |
| | L Thoracic Sympathetic Nerve | | | |
| | M Abdominal Sympathetic Nerve | | | |
| | N Lumbar Sympathetic Nerve | | | |
| | P Sacral Sympathetic Nerve | | | |
| | Q Sacral Plexus | | | |
| | R Sacral Nerve | | | |
| | Y Peripheral Nerve | | | |

**AHA Coding Clinic for table Ø1B**

**2017, 2Q, 19** Thoracic outlet decompression with sympathectomy

**AHA Coding Clinic for table Ø1N**

**2017, 2Q, 19** Thoracic outlet decompression with sympathectomy
**2016, 2Q, 16** Decompressive laminectomy/foraminotomy and lumbar discectomy
**2016, 2Q, 17** Removal of longitudinal ligament to decompress cervical nerve root
**2016, 2Q, 23** Thoracic outlet syndrome and release of brachial plexus
**2015, 2Q, 34** Decompressive laminectomy
**2014, 3Q, 33** Radial fracture treatment with open reduction internal fixation, and release of carpal ligament

### Median and Ulnar Nerves

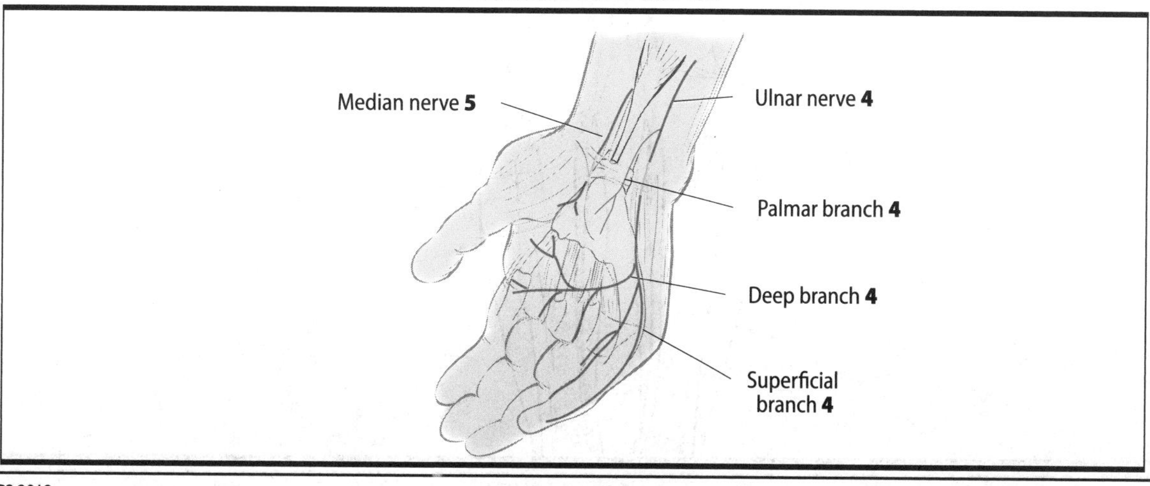
Median nerve 5
Ulnar nerve 4
Palmar branch 4
Deep branch 4
Superficial branch 4

## Peripheral Nervous System

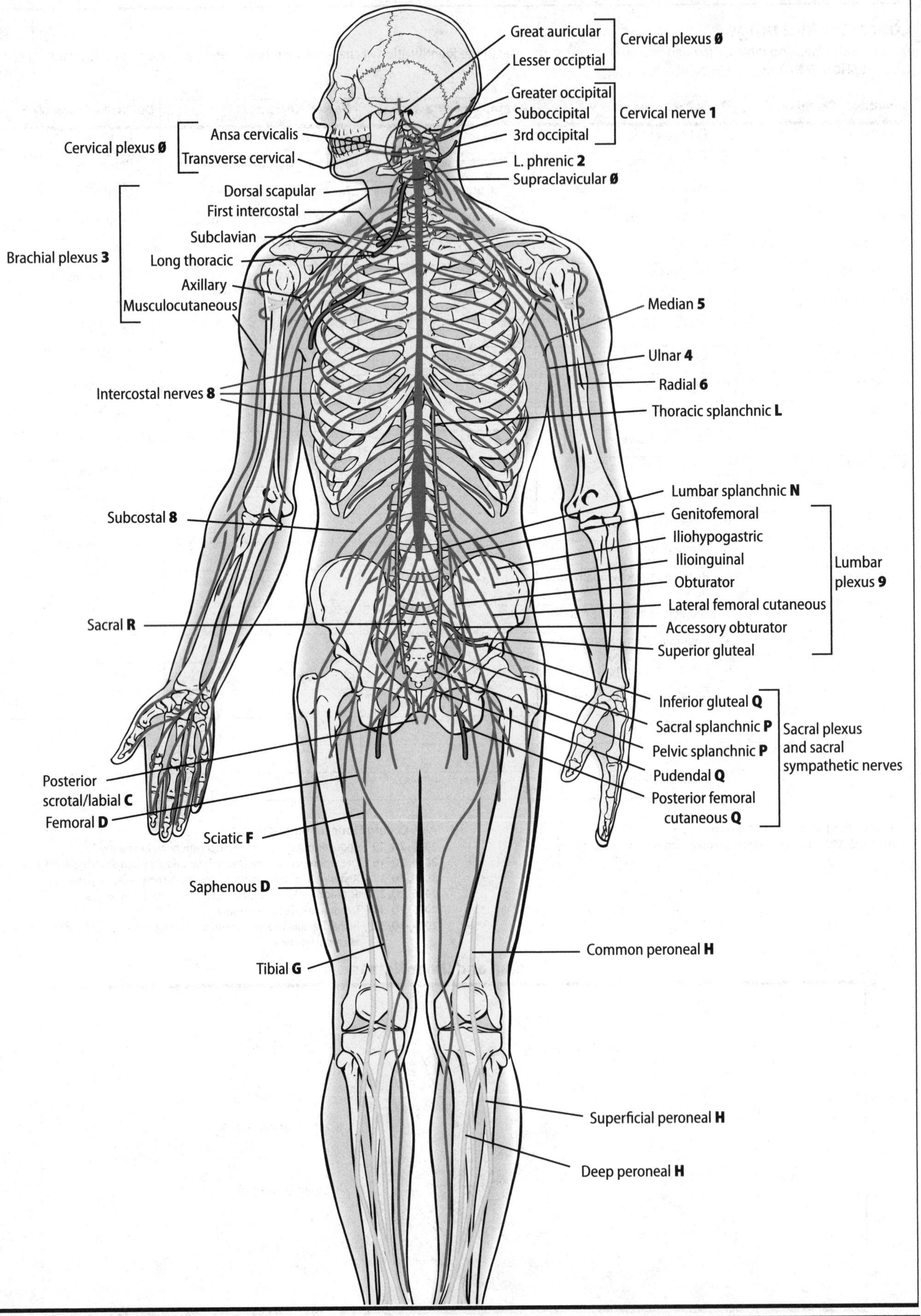
Great auricular
Lesser occiptial
Cervical plexus Ø
Greater occipital
Suboccipital
3rd occipital
Cervical nerve 1
Ansa cervicalis
Transverse cervical
Cervical plexus Ø
L. phrenic 2
Supraclavicular Ø
Dorsal scapular
First intercostal
Subclavian
Long thoracic
Axillary
Musculocutaneous
Brachial plexus 3
Median 5
Ulnar 4
Radial 6
Intercostal nerves 8
Thoracic splanchnic L
Lumbar splanchnic N
Genitofemoral
Iliohypogastric
Ilioinguinal
Obturator
Lateral femoral cutaneous
Accessory obturator
Superior gluteal
Lumbar plexus 9
Subcostal 8
Sacral R
Inferior gluteal Q
Sacral splanchnic P
Pelvic splanchnic P
Pudendal Q
Posterior femoral cutaneous Q
Sacral plexus and sacral sympathetic nerves
Posterior scrotal/labial C
Femoral D
Sciatic F
Saphenous D
Common peroneal H
Tibial G
Superficial peroneal H
Deep peroneal H

**Ø Medical and Surgical**
**1 Peripheral Nervous System**
**2 Change**

Definition: Taking out or off a device from a body part and putting back an identical or similar device in or on the same body part without cutting or puncturing the skin or a mucous membrane

Explanation: All CHANGE procedures are coded using the approach EXTERNAL

| Body Part Character 4 | Approach Character 5 | Device Character 6 | Qualifier Character 7 |
|---|---|---|---|
| Y Peripheral Nerve | X External | Ø Drainage Device<br>Y Other Device | Z No Qualifier |

**Non-OR** All body part, approach, device, and qualifier values

**Ø Medical and Surgical**
**1 Peripheral Nervous System**
**5 Destruction**

Definition: Physical eradication of all or a portion of a body part by the direct use of energy, force, or a destructive agent

Explanation: None of the body part is physically taken out

| Body Part Character 4 | Approach Character 5 | Device Character 6 | Qualifier Character 7 |
|---|---|---|---|
| **Ø Cervical Plexus**<br>Ansa cervicalis<br>Cutaneous (transverse) cervical nerve<br>Great auricular nerve<br>Lesser occipital nerve<br>Supraclavicular nerve<br>Transverse (cutaneous) cervical nerve<br>**1 Cervical Nerve**<br>Greater occipital nerve<br>Spinal nerve, cervical<br>Suboccipital nerve<br>Third occipital nerve<br>**2 Phrenic Nerve**<br>Accessory phrenic nerve<br>**3 Brachial Plexus**<br>Axillary nerve<br>Dorsal scapular nerve<br>First intercostal nerve<br>Long thoracic nerve<br>Musculocutaneous nerve<br>Subclavius nerve<br>Suprascapular nerve<br>**4 Ulnar Nerve**<br>Cubital nerve<br>**5 Median Nerve**<br>Anterior interosseous nerve<br>Palmar cutaneous nerve<br>**6 Radial Nerve**<br>Dorsal digital nerve<br>Musculospiral nerve<br>Palmar cutaneous nerve<br>Posterior interosseous nerve<br>**8 Thoracic Nerve**<br>Intercostal nerve<br>Intercostobrachial nerve<br>Spinal nerve, thoracic<br>Subcostal nerve<br>**9 Lumbar Plexus**<br>Accessory obturator nerve<br>Genitofemoral nerve<br>Iliohypogastric nerve<br>Ilioinguinal nerve<br>Lateral femoral cutaneous nerve<br>Obturator nerve<br>Superior gluteal nerve<br>**A Lumbosacral Plexus**<br>**B Lumbar Nerve**<br>Lumbosacral trunk<br>Spinal nerve, lumbar<br>Superior clunic (cluneal) nerve<br>**C Pudendal Nerve**<br>Posterior labial nerve<br>Posterior scrotal nerve<br>**D Femoral Nerve**<br>Anterior crural nerve<br>Saphenous nerve<br>**F Sciatic Nerve**<br>Ischiatic nerve<br>**G Tibial Nerve**<br>Lateral plantar nerve<br>Medial plantar nerve<br>Medial popliteal nerve<br>Medial sural cutaneous nerve<br>**H Peroneal Nerve**<br>Common fibular nerve<br>Common peroneal nerve<br>External popliteal nerve<br>Lateral sural cutaneous nerve<br>**K Head and Neck Sympathetic Nerve**<br>Cavernous plexus<br>Cervical ganglion<br>Ciliary ganglion<br>Internal carotid plexus<br>Otic ganglion<br>Pterygopalatine (sphenopalatine) ganglion<br>Sphenopalatine (pterygopalatine) ganglion<br>Stellate ganglion<br>Submandibular ganglion<br>Submaxillary ganglion<br>**L Thoracic Sympathetic Nerve**<br>Cardiac plexus<br>Esophageal plexus<br>Greater splanchnic nerve<br>Inferior cardiac nerve<br>Least splanchnic nerve<br>Lesser splanchnic nerve<br>Middle cardiac nerve<br>Pulmonary plexus<br>Superior cardiac nerve<br>Thoracic aortic plexus<br>Thoracic ganglion<br>**M Abdominal Sympathetic Nerve**<br>Abdominal aortic plexus<br>Auerbach's (myenteric) plexus<br>Celiac (solar) plexus<br>Celiac ganglion<br>Gastric plexus<br>Hepatic plexus<br>Inferior hypogastric plexus<br>Inferior mesenteric ganglion<br>Inferior mesenteric plexus<br>Meissner's (submucous) plexus<br>Myenteric (Auerbach's) plexus<br>Pancreatic plexus<br>Pelvic splanchnic nerve<br>Renal plexus<br>Solar (celiac) plexus<br>Splenic plexus<br>Submucous (Meissner's) plexus<br>Superior hypogastric plexus<br>Superior mesenteric ganglion<br>Superior mesenteric plexus<br>Suprarenal plexus<br>**N Lumbar Sympathetic Nerve**<br>Lumbar ganglion<br>Lumbar splanchnic nerve<br>**P Sacral Sympathetic Nerve**<br>Ganglion impar (ganglion of Walther)<br>Pelvic splanchnic nerve<br>Sacral ganglion<br>Sacral splanchnic nerve<br>**Q Sacral Plexus**<br>Inferior gluteal nerve<br>Posterior femoral cutaneous nerve<br>Pudendal nerve<br>**R Sacral Nerve**<br>Spinal nerve, sacral | Ø Open<br>3 Percutaneous<br>4 Percutaneous Endoscopic | Z No Device | Z No Qualifier |

**Non-OR** Ø15[Ø,2,3,4,5,6,9,A,C,D,F,G,H,Q][Ø,3,4]ZZ
**Non-OR** Ø15[1,8,B,R]3ZZ

**Ø Medical and Surgical**
**1 Peripheral Nervous System**
**8 Division**
Definition: Cutting into a body part, without draining fluids and/or gases from the body part, in order to separate or transect a body part
Explanation: All or a portion of the body part is separated into two or more portions

| Body Part Character 4 | Approach Character 5 | Device Character 6 | Qualifier Character 7 |
|---|---|---|---|
| **Ø Cervical Plexus**<br>Ansa cervicalis<br>Cutaneous (transverse) cervical nerve<br>Great auricular nerve<br>Lesser occipital nerve<br>Supraclavicular nerve<br>Transverse (cutaneous) cervical nerve | **Ø Open**<br>**3 Percutaneous**<br>**4 Percutaneous Endoscopic** | **Z No Device** | **Z No Qualifier** |
| **1 Cervical Nerve**<br>Greater occipital nerve<br>Spinal nerve, cervical<br>Suboccipital nerve<br>Third occipital nerve | | | |
| **2 Phrenic Nerve**<br>Accessory phrenic nerve | | | |
| **3 Brachial Plexus**<br>Axillary nerve<br>Dorsal scapular nerve<br>First intercostal nerve<br>Long thoracic nerve<br>Musculocutaneous nerve<br>Subclavius nerve<br>Suprascapular nerve | | | |
| **4 Ulnar Nerve**<br>Cubital nerve | | | |
| **5 Median Nerve**<br>Anterior interosseous nerve<br>Palmar cutaneous nerve | | | |
| **6 Radial Nerve**<br>Dorsal digital nerve<br>Musculospiral nerve<br>Palmar cutaneous nerve<br>Posterior interosseous nerve | | | |
| **8 Thoracic Nerve**<br>Intercostal nerve<br>Intercostobrachial nerve<br>Spinal nerve, thoracic<br>Subcostal nerve | | | |
| **9 Lumbar Plexus**<br>Accessory obturator nerve<br>Genitofemoral nerve<br>Iliohypogastric nerve<br>Ilioinguinal nerve<br>Lateral femoral cutaneous nerve<br>Obturator nerve<br>Superior gluteal nerve | | | |
| **A Lumbosacral Plexus** | | | |
| **B Lumbar Nerve**<br>Lumbosacral trunk<br>Spinal nerve, lumbar<br>Superior clunic (cluneal) nerve | | | |
| **C Pudendal Nerve**<br>Posterior labial nerve<br>Posterior scrotal nerve | | | |
| **D Femoral Nerve**<br>Anterior crural nerve<br>Saphenous nerve | | | |
| **F Sciatic Nerve**<br>Ischiatic nerve | | | |
| **G Tibial Nerve**<br>Lateral plantar nerve<br>Medial plantar nerve<br>Medial popliteal nerve<br>Medial sural cutaneous nerve | | | |
| **H Peroneal Nerve**<br>Common fibular nerve<br>Common peroneal nerve<br>External popliteal nerve<br>Lateral sural cutaneous nerve | | | |
| **K Head and Neck Sympathetic Nerve**<br>Cavernous plexus<br>Cervical ganglion<br>Ciliary ganglion<br>Internal carotid plexus<br>Otic ganglion<br>Pterygopalatine (sphenopalatine) ganglion<br>Sphenopalatine (pterygopalatine) ganglion<br>Stellate ganglion<br>Submandibular ganglion<br>Submaxillary ganglion | | | |
| **L Thoracic Sympathetic Nerve**<br>Cardiac plexus<br>Esophageal plexus<br>Greater splanchnic nerve<br>Inferior cardiac nerve<br>Least splanchnic nerve<br>Lesser splanchnic nerve<br>Middle cardiac nerve<br>Pulmonary plexus<br>Superior cardiac nerve<br>Thoracic aortic plexus<br>Thoracic ganglion | | | |
| **M Abdominal Sympathetic Nerve**<br>Abdominal aortic plexus<br>Auerbach's (myenteric) plexus<br>Celiac (solar) plexus<br>Celiac ganglion<br>Gastric plexus<br>Hepatic plexus<br>Inferior hypogastric plexus<br>Inferior mesenteric ganglion<br>Inferior mesenteric plexus<br>Meissner's (submucous) plexus<br>Myenteric (Auerbach's) plexus<br>Pancreatic plexus<br>Pelvic splanchnic nerve<br>Renal plexus<br>Solar (celiac) plexus<br>Splenic plexus<br>Submucous (Meissner's) plexus<br>Superior hypogastric plexus<br>Superior mesenteric ganglion<br>Superior mesenteric plexus<br>Suprarenal plexus | | | |
| **N Lumbar Sympathetic Nerve**<br>Lumbar ganglion<br>Lumbar splanchnic nerve | | | |
| **P Sacral Sympathetic Nerve**<br>Ganglion impar (ganglion of Walther)<br>Pelvic splanchnic nerve<br>Sacral ganglion<br>Sacral splanchnic nerve | | | |
| **Q Sacral Plexus**<br>Inferior gluteal nerve<br>Posterior femoral cutaneous nerve<br>Pudendal nerve | | | |
| **R Sacral Nerve**<br>Spinal nerve, sacral | | | |

**Ø Medical and Surgical**
**1 Peripheral Nervous System**
**9 Drainage** Definition: Taking or letting out fluids and/or gases from a body part
Explanation: The qualifier DIAGNOSTIC is used to identify drainage procedures that are biopsies

| Body Part Character 4 | | Approach Character 5 | Device Character 6 | Qualifier Character 7 |
|---|---|---|---|---|
| **Ø Cervical Plexus**<br>Ansa cervicalis<br>Cutaneous (transverse) cervical nerve<br>Great auricular nerve<br>Lesser occipital nerve<br>Supraclavicular nerve<br>Transverse (cutaneous) cervical nerve<br>**1 Cervical Nerve**<br>Greater occipital nerve<br>Spinal nerve, cervical<br>Suboccipital nerve<br>Third occipital nerve<br>**2 Phrenic Nerve**<br>Accessory phrenic nerve<br>**3 Brachial Plexus**<br>Axillary nerve<br>Dorsal scapular nerve<br>First intercostal nerve<br>Long thoracic nerve<br>Musculocutaneous nerve<br>Subclavius nerve<br>Suprascapular nerve<br>**4 Ulnar Nerve**<br>Cubital nerve<br>**5 Median Nerve**<br>Anterior interosseous nerve<br>Palmar cutaneous nerve<br>**6 Radial Nerve**<br>Dorsal digital nerve<br>Musculospiral nerve<br>Palmar cutaneous nerve<br>Posterior interosseous nerve<br>**8 Thoracic Nerve**<br>Intercostal nerve<br>Intercostobrachial nerve<br>Spinal nerve, thoracic<br>Subcostal nerve<br>**9 Lumbar Plexus**<br>Accessory obturator nerve<br>Genitofemoral nerve<br>Iliohypogastric nerve<br>Ilioinguinal nerve<br>Lateral femoral cutaneous nerve<br>Obturator nerve<br>Superior gluteal nerve<br>**A Lumbosacral Plexus**<br>**B Lumbar Nerve**<br>Lumbosacral trunk<br>Spinal nerve, lumbar<br>Superior clunic (cluneal) nerve<br>**C Pudendal Nerve**<br>Posterior labial nerve<br>Posterior scrotal nerve<br>**D Femoral Nerve**<br>Anterior crural nerve<br>Saphenous nerve<br>**F Sciatic Nerve**<br>Ischiatic nerve<br>**G Tibial Nerve**<br>Lateral plantar nerve<br>Medial plantar nerve<br>Medial popliteal nerve<br>Medial sural cutaneous nerve | **H Peroneal Nerve**<br>Common fibular nerve<br>Common peroneal nerve<br>External popliteal nerve<br>Lateral sural cutaneous nerve<br>**K Head and Neck Sympathetic Nerve**<br>Cavernous plexus<br>Cervical ganglion<br>Ciliary ganglion<br>Internal carotid plexus<br>Otic ganglion<br>Pterygopalatine (sphenopalatine) ganglion<br>Sphenopalatine (pterygopalatine) ganglion<br>Stellate ganglion<br>Submandibular ganglion<br>Submaxillary ganglion<br>**L Thoracic Sympathetic Nerve**<br>Cardiac plexus<br>Esophageal plexus<br>Greater splanchnic nerve<br>Inferior cardiac nerve<br>Least splanchnic nerve<br>Lesser splanchnic nerve<br>Middle cardiac nerve<br>Pulmonary plexus<br>Superior cardiac nerve<br>Thoracic aortic plexus<br>Thoracic ganglion<br>**M Abdominal Sympathetic Nerve**<br>Abdominal aortic plexus<br>Auerbach's (myenteric) plexus<br>Celiac (solar) plexus<br>Celiac ganglion<br>Gastric plexus<br>Hepatic plexus<br>Inferior hypogastric plexus<br>Inferior mesenteric ganglion<br>Inferior mesenteric plexus<br>Meissner's (submucous) plexus<br>Myenteric (Auerbach's) plexus<br>Pancreatic plexus<br>Pelvic splanchnic nerve<br>Renal plexus<br>Solar (celiac) plexus<br>Splenic plexus<br>Submucous (Meissner's) plexus<br>Superior hypogastric plexus<br>Superior mesenteric ganglion<br>Superior mesenteric plexus<br>Suprarenal plexus<br>**N Lumbar Sympathetic Nerve**<br>Lumbar ganglion<br>Lumbar splanchnic nerve<br>**P Sacral Sympathetic Nerve**<br>Ganglion impar (ganglion of Walther)<br>Pelvic splanchnic nerve<br>Sacral ganglion<br>Sacral splanchnic nerve<br>**Q Sacral Plexus**<br>Inferior gluteal nerve<br>Posterior femoral cutaneous nerve<br>Pudendal nerve<br>**R Sacral Nerve**<br>Spinal nerve, sacral | **Ø Open**<br>**3 Percutaneous**<br>**4 Percutaneous Endoscopic** | **Ø Drainage Device** | **Z No Qualifier** |

***Ø19 Continued on next page***

**Non-OR** Ø19[Ø,1,2,3,4,5,6,8,9,A,B,C,D,F,G,H,K,L,M,N,P,Q,R]3ØZ

**Ø19 Continued**

**Ø Medical and Surgical**
**1 Peripheral Nervous System**
**9 Drainage** Definition: Taking or letting out fluids and/or gases from a body part
Explanation: The qualifier DIAGNOSTIC is used to identify drainage procedures that are biopsies

| Body Part Character 4 | Approach Character 5 | Device Character 6 | Qualifier Character 7 |
|---|---|---|---|
| **Ø Cervical Plexus** Ansa cervicalis; Cutaneous (transverse) cervical nerve; Great auricular nerve; Lesser occipital nerve; Supraclavicular nerve; Transverse (cutaneous) cervical nerve<br>**1 Cervical Nerve** Greater occipital nerve; Spinal nerve, cervical; Suboccipital nerve; Third occipital nerve<br>**2 Phrenic Nerve** Accessory phrenic nerve<br>**3 Brachial Plexus** Axillary nerve; Dorsal scapular nerve; First intercostal nerve; Long thoracic nerve; Musculocutaneous nerve; Subclavius nerve; Suprascapular nerve<br>**4 Ulnar Nerve** Cubital nerve<br>**5 Median Nerve** Anterior interosseous nerve; Palmar cutaneous nerve<br>**6 Radial Nerve** Dorsal digital nerve; Musculospiral nerve; Palmar cutaneous nerve; Posterior interosseous nerve<br>**8 Thoracic Nerve** Intercostal nerve; Intercostobrachial nerve; Spinal nerve, thoracic; Subcostal nerve<br>**9 Lumbar Plexus** Accessory obturator nerve; Genitofemoral nerve; Iliohypogastric nerve; Ilioinguinal nerve; Lateral femoral cutaneous nerve; Obturator nerve; Superior gluteal nerve<br>**A Lumbosacral Plexus**<br>**B Lumbar Nerve** Lumbosacral trunk; Spinal nerve, lumbar; Superior clunic (cluneal) nerve<br>**C Pudendal Nerve** Posterior labial nerve; Posterior scrotal nerve<br>**D Femoral Nerve** Anterior crural nerve; Saphenous nerve<br>**F Sciatic Nerve** Ischiatic nerve<br>**G Tibial Nerve** Lateral plantar nerve; Medial plantar nerve; Medial popliteal nerve; Medial sural cutaneous nerve<br>**H Peroneal Nerve** Common fibular nerve; Common peroneal nerve; External popliteal nerve; Lateral sural cutaneous nerve<br>**K Head and Neck Sympathetic Nerve** Cavernous plexus; Cervical ganglion; Ciliary ganglion; Internal carotid plexus; Otic ganglion; Pterygopalatine (sphenopalatine) ganglion; Sphenopalatine (pterygopalatine) ganglion; Stellate ganglion; Submandibular ganglion; Submaxillary ganglion<br>**L Thoracic Sympathetic Nerve** Cardiac plexus; Esophageal plexus; Greater splanchnic nerve; Inferior cardiac nerve; Least splanchnic nerve; Lesser splanchnic nerve; Middle cardiac nerve; Pulmonary plexus; Superior cardiac nerve; Thoracic aortic plexus; Thoracic ganglion<br>**M Abdominal Sympathetic Nerve** Abdominal aortic plexus; Auerbach's (myenteric) plexus; Celiac (solar) plexus; Celiac ganglion; Gastric plexus; Hepatic plexus; Inferior hypogastric plexus; Inferior mesenteric ganglion; Inferior mesenteric plexus; Meissner's (submucous) plexus; Myenteric (Auerbach's) plexus; Pancreatic plexus; Pelvic splanchnic nerve; Renal plexus; Solar (celiac) plexus; Splenic plexus; Submucous (Meissner's) plexus; Superior hypogastric plexus; Superior mesenteric ganglion; Superior mesenteric plexus; Suprarenal plexus<br>**N Lumbar Sympathetic Nerve** Lumbar ganglion; Lumbar splanchnic nerve<br>**P Sacral Sympathetic Nerve** Ganglion impar (ganglion of Walther); Pelvic splanchnic nerve; Sacral ganglion; Sacral splanchnic nerve<br>**Q Sacral Plexus** Inferior gluteal nerve; Posterior femoral cutaneous nerve; Pudendal nerve<br>**R Sacral Nerve** Spinal nerve, sacral | **Ø Open**<br>**3 Percutaneous**<br>**4 Percutaneous Endoscopic** | **Z No Device** | **X Diagnostic**<br>**Z No Qualifier** |

Non-OR Ø19[Ø,1,2,3,4,5,6,8,9,A,B,C,D,F,G,H,Q,R][3,4]ZX
Non-OR Ø19[Ø,1,2,3,4,5,6,8,9,A,B,C,D,F,G,H,K,L,M,N,P,Q,R]3ZZ

**Ø Medical and Surgical**
**1 Peripheral Nervous System**
**B Excision** Definition: Cutting out or off, without replacement, a portion of a body part
Explanation: The qualifier DIAGNOSTIC is used to identify excision procedures that are biopsies

| Body Part Character 4 | Approach Character 5 | Device Character 6 | Qualifier Character 7 |
|---|---|---|---|
| **Ø Cervical Plexus**<br>Ansa cervicalis<br>Cutaneous (transverse) cervical nerve<br>Great auricular nerve<br>Lesser occipital nerve<br>Supraclavicular nerve<br>Transverse (cutaneous) cervical nerve<br>**1 Cervical Nerve**<br>Greater occipital nerve<br>Spinal nerve, cervical<br>Suboccipital nerve<br>Third occipital nerve<br>**2 Phrenic Nerve**<br>Accessory phrenic nerve<br>**3 Brachial Plexus**<br>Axillary nerve<br>Dorsal scapular nerve<br>First intercostal nerve<br>Long thoracic nerve<br>Musculocutaneous nerve<br>Subclavius nerve<br>Suprascapular nerve<br>**4 Ulnar Nerve**<br>Cubital nerve<br>**5 Median Nerve**<br>Anterior interosseous nerve<br>Palmar cutaneous nerve<br>**6 Radial Nerve**<br>Dorsal digital nerve<br>Musculospiral nerve<br>Palmar cutaneous nerve<br>Posterior interosseous nerve<br>**8 Thoracic Nerve**<br>Intercostal nerve<br>Intercostobrachial nerve<br>Spinal nerve, thoracic<br>Subcostal nerve<br>**9 Lumbar Plexus**<br>Accessory obturator nerve<br>Genitofemoral nerve<br>Iliohypogastric nerve<br>Ilioinguinal nerve<br>Lateral femoral cutaneous nerve<br>Obturator nerve<br>Superior gluteal nerve<br>**A Lumbosacral Plexus**<br>**B Lumbar Nerve**<br>Lumbosacral trunk<br>Spinal nerve, lumbar<br>Superior clunic (cluneal) nerve<br>**C Pudendal Nerve**<br>Posterior labial nerve<br>Posterior scrotal nerve<br>**D Femoral Nerve**<br>Anterior crural nerve<br>Saphenous nerve<br>**F Sciatic Nerve**<br>Ischiatic nerve<br>**G Tibial Nerve**<br>Lateral plantar nerve<br>Medial plantar nerve<br>Medial popliteal nerve<br>Medial sural cutaneous nerve<br>**H Peroneal Nerve**<br>Common fibular nerve<br>Common peroneal nerve<br>External popliteal nerve<br>Lateral sural cutaneous nerve<br>**K Head and Neck Sympathetic Nerve**<br>Cavernous plexus<br>Cervical ganglion<br>Ciliary ganglion<br>Internal carotid plexus<br>Otic ganglion<br>Pterygopalatine (sphenopalatine) ganglion<br>Sphenopalatine (pterygopalatine) ganglion<br>Stellate ganglion<br>Submandibular ganglion<br>Submaxillary ganglion<br>**L Thoracic Sympathetic Nerve**<br>Cardiac plexus<br>Esophageal plexus<br>Greater splanchnic nerve<br>Inferior cardiac nerve<br>Least splanchnic nerve<br>Lesser splanchnic nerve<br>Middle cardiac nerve<br>Pulmonary plexus<br>Superior cardiac nerve<br>Thoracic aortic plexus<br>Thoracic ganglion<br>**M Abdominal Sympathetic Nerve**<br>Abdominal aortic plexus<br>Auerbach's (myenteric) plexus<br>Celiac (solar) plexus<br>Celiac ganglion<br>Gastric plexus<br>Hepatic plexus<br>Inferior hypogastric plexus<br>Inferior mesenteric ganglion<br>Inferior mesenteric plexus<br>Meissner's (submucous) plexus<br>Myenteric (Auerbach's) plexus<br>Pancreatic plexus<br>Pelvic splanchnic nerve<br>Renal plexus<br>Solar (celiac) plexus<br>Splenic plexus<br>Submucous (Meissner's) plexus<br>Superior hypogastric plexus<br>Superior mesenteric ganglion<br>Superior mesenteric plexus<br>Suprarenal plexus<br>**N Lumbar Sympathetic Nerve**<br>Lumbar ganglion<br>Lumbar splanchnic nerve<br>**P Sacral Sympathetic Nerve**<br>Ganglion impar (ganglion of Walther)<br>Pelvic splanchnic nerve<br>Sacral ganglion<br>Sacral splanchnic nerve<br>**Q Sacral Plexus**<br>Inferior gluteal nerve<br>Posterior femoral cutaneous nerve<br>Pudendal nerve<br>**R Sacral Nerve**<br>Spinal nerve, sacral | **Ø Open**<br>**3 Percutaneous**<br>**4 Percutaneous Endoscopic** | **Z No Device** | **X Diagnostic**<br>**Z No Qualifier** |

**Non-OR** Ø1B[Ø,1,2,3,4,5,6,8,9,A,B,C,D,F,G,H,Q,R][3,4]ZX

**Ø Medical and Surgical**
**1 Peripheral Nervous System**
**C Extirpation** Definition: Taking or cutting out solid matter from a body part

Explanation: The solid matter may be an abnormal byproduct of a biological function or a foreign body; it may be imbedded in a body part or in the lumen of a tubular body part. The solid matter may or may not have been previously broken into pieces.

| Body Part Character 4 | Approach Character 5 | Device Character 6 | Qualifier Character 7 |
|---|---|---|---|
| **Ø Cervical Plexus**<br>Ansa cervicalis<br>Cutaneous (transverse) cervical nerve<br>Great auricular nerve<br>Lesser occipital nerve<br>Supraclavicular nerve<br>Transverse (cutaneous) cervical nerve<br>**1 Cervical Nerve**<br>Greater occipital nerve<br>Spinal nerve, cervical<br>Suboccipital nerve<br>Third occipital nerve<br>**2 Phrenic Nerve**<br>Accessory phrenic nerve<br>**3 Brachial Plexus**<br>Axillary nerve<br>Dorsal scapular nerve<br>First intercostal nerve<br>Long thoracic nerve<br>Musculocutaneous nerve<br>Subclavius nerve<br>Suprascapular nerve<br>**4 Ulnar Nerve**<br>Cubital nerve<br>**5 Median Nerve**<br>Anterior interosseous nerve<br>Palmar cutaneous nerve<br>**6 Radial Nerve**<br>Dorsal digital nerve<br>Musculospiral nerve<br>Palmar cutaneous nerve<br>Posterior interosseous nerve<br>**8 Thoracic Nerve**<br>Intercostal nerve<br>Intercostobrachial nerve<br>Spinal nerve, thoracic<br>Subcostal nerve<br>**9 Lumbar Plexus**<br>Accessory obturator nerve<br>Genitofemoral nerve<br>Iliohypogastric nerve<br>Ilioinguinal nerve<br>Lateral femoral cutaneous nerve<br>Obturator nerve<br>Superior gluteal nerve<br>**A Lumbosacral Plexus**<br>**B Lumbar Nerve**<br>Lumbosacral trunk<br>Spinal nerve, lumbar<br>Superior clunic (cluneal) nerve<br>**C Pudendal Nerve**<br>Posterior labial nerve<br>Posterior scrotal nerve<br>**D Femoral Nerve**<br>Anterior crural nerve<br>Saphenous nerve<br>**F Sciatic Nerve**<br>Ischiatic nerve<br>**G Tibial Nerve**<br>Lateral plantar nerve<br>Medial plantar nerve<br>Medial popliteal nerve<br>Medial sural cutaneous nerve<br>**H Peroneal Nerve**<br>Common fibular nerve<br>Common peroneal nerve<br>External popliteal nerve<br>Lateral sural cutaneous nerve<br>**K Head and Neck Sympathetic Nerve**<br>Cavernous plexus<br>Cervical ganglion<br>Ciliary ganglion<br>Internal carotid plexus<br>Otic ganglion<br>Pterygopalatine (sphenopalatine) ganglion<br>Sphenopalatine (pterygopalatine) ganglion<br>Stellate ganglion<br>Submandibular ganglion<br>Submaxillary ganglion<br>**L Thoracic Sympathetic Nerve**<br>Cardiac plexus<br>Esophageal plexus<br>Greater splanchnic nerve<br>Inferior cardiac nerve<br>Least splanchnic nerve<br>Lesser splanchnic nerve<br>Middle cardiac nerve<br>Pulmonary plexus<br>Superior cardiac nerve<br>Thoracic aortic plexus<br>Thoracic ganglion<br>**M Abdominal Sympathetic Nerve**<br>Abdominal aortic plexus<br>Auerbach's (myenteric) plexus<br>Celiac (solar) plexus<br>Celiac ganglion<br>Gastric plexus<br>Hepatic plexus<br>Inferior hypogastric plexus<br>Inferior mesenteric ganglion<br>Inferior mesenteric plexus<br>Meissner's (submucous) plexus<br>Myenteric (Auerbach's) plexus<br>Pancreatic plexus<br>Pelvic splanchnic nerve<br>Renal plexus<br>Solar (celiac) plexus<br>Splenic plexus<br>Submucous (Meissner's) plexus<br>Superior hypogastric plexus<br>Superior mesenteric ganglion<br>Superior mesenteric plexus<br>Suprarenal plexus<br>**N Lumbar Sympathetic Nerve**<br>Lumbar ganglion<br>Lumbar splanchnic nerve<br>**P Sacral Sympathetic Nerve**<br>Ganglion impar (ganglion of Walther)<br>Pelvic splanchnic nerve<br>Sacral ganglion<br>Sacral splanchnic nerve<br>**Q Sacral Plexus**<br>Inferior gluteal nerve<br>Posterior femoral cutaneous nerve<br>Pudendal nerve<br>**R Sacral Nerve**<br>Spinal nerve, sacral | **Ø Open**<br>**3 Percutaneous**<br>**4 Percutaneous Endoscopic** | **Z No Device** | **Z No Qualifier** |

**Ø Medical and Surgical**
**1 Peripheral Nervous System**
**D Extraction** Definition: Pulling or stripping out or off all or a portion of a body part by the use of force
Explanation: The qualifier DIAGNOSTIC is used to identify extraction procedures that are biopsies

| Body Part Character 4 | Approach Character 5 | Device Character 6 | Qualifier Character 7 |
|---|---|---|---|
| **Ø Cervical Plexus** Ansa cervicalis; Cutaneous (transverse) cervical nerve; Great auricular nerve; Lesser occipital nerve; Supraclavicular nerve; Transverse (cutaneous) cervical nerve<br>**1 Cervical Nerve** Greater occipital nerve; Spinal nerve, cervical; Suboccipital nerve; Third occipital nerve<br>**2 Phrenic Nerve** Accessory phrenic nerve<br>**3 Brachial Plexus** Axillary nerve; Dorsal scapular nerve; First intercostal nerve; Long thoracic nerve; Musculocutaneous nerve; Subclavius nerve; Suprascapular nerve<br>**4 Ulnar Nerve** Cubital nerve<br>**5 Median Nerve** Anterior interosseous nerve; Palmar cutaneous nerve<br>**6 Radial Nerve** Dorsal digital nerve; Musculospiral nerve; Palmar cutaneous nerve; Posterior interosseous nerve<br>**8 Thoracic Nerve** Intercostal nerve; Intercostobrachial nerve; Spinal nerve, thoracic; Subcostal nerve<br>**9 Lumbar Plexus** Accessory obturator nerve; Genitofemoral nerve; Iliohypogastric nerve; Ilioinguinal nerve; Lateral femoral cutaneous nerve; Obturator nerve; Superior gluteal nerve<br>**A Lumbosacral Plexus**<br>**B Lumbar Nerve** Lumbosacral trunk; Spinal nerve, lumbar; Superior clunic (cluneal) nerve<br>**C Pudendal Nerve]** Posterior labial nerve; Posterior scrotal nerve<br>**D Femoral Nerve** Anterior crural nerve; Saphenous nerve<br>**F Sciatic Nerve** Ischiatic nerve<br>**G Tibial Nerve** Lateral plantar nerve; Medial plantar nerve; Medial popliteal nerve; Medial sural cutaneous nerve<br>**H Peroneal Nerve** Common fibular nerve; Common peroneal nerve; External popliteal nerve; Lateral sural cutaneous nerve<br>**K Head and Neck Sympathetic Nerve** Cavernous plexus; Cervical ganglion; Ciliary ganglion; Internal carotid plexus; Otic ganglion; Pterygopalatine (sphenopalatine) ganglion; Sphenopalatine (pterygopalatine) ganglion; Stellate ganglion; Submandibular ganglion; Submaxillary ganglion<br>**L Thoracic Sympathetic Nerve** Cardiac plexus; Esophageal plexus; Greater splanchnic nerve; Inferior cardiac nerve; Least splanchnic nerve; Lesser splanchnic nerve; Middle cardiac nerve; Pulmonary plexus; Superior cardiac nerve; Thoracic aortic plexus; Thoracic ganglion<br>**M Abdominal Sympathetic Nerve** Abdominal aortic plexus; Auerbach's (myenteric) plexus; Celiac (solar) plexus; Celiac ganglion; Gastric plexus; Hepatic plexus; Inferior hypogastric plexus; Inferior mesenteric ganglion; Inferior mesenteric plexus; Meissner's (submucous) plexus; Myenteric (Auerbach's) plexus; Pancreatic plexus; Pelvic splanchnic nerve; Renal plexus; Solar (celiac) plexus; Splenic plexus; Submucous (Meissner's) plexus; Superior hypogastric plexus; Superior mesenteric ganglion; Superior mesenteric plexus; Suprarenal plexus<br>**N Lumbar Sympathetic Nerve** Lumbar ganglion; Lumbar splanchnic nerve<br>**P Sacral Sympathetic Nerve** Ganglion impar (ganglion of Walther); Pelvic splanchnic nerve; Sacral ganglion; Sacral splanchnic nerve<br>**Q Sacral Plexus** Inferior gluteal nerve; Posterior femoral cutaneous nerve; Pudendal nerve<br>**R Sacral Nerve** Spinal nerve, sacral | **Ø Open**<br>**3 Percutaneous**<br>**4 Percutaneous Endoscopic** | **Z No Device** | **Z No Qualifier** |

**Ø Medical and Surgical**
**1 Peripheral Nervous System**
**H Insertion** Definition: Putting in a nonbiological appliance that monitors, assists, performs, or prevents a physiological function but does not physically take the place of a body part

Explanation: None

| Body Part Character 4 | Approach Character 5 | Device Character 6 | Qualifier Character 7 |
|---|---|---|---|
| **Y** Peripheral Nerve ⊞ | **Ø** Open<br>**3** Percutaneous<br>**4** Percutaneous Endoscopic | **2** Monitoring Device<br>**M** Neurostimulator Lead<br>**Y** Other Device | **Z** No Qualifier |

Non-OR Ø1HY[3,4]YZ

See Appendix L for Procedure Combinations
⊞ Ø1HY[Ø,3,4]MZ

**Ø Medical and Surgical**
**1 Peripheral Nervous System**
**J Inspection** Definition: Visually and/or manually exploring a body part

Explanation: Visual exploration may be performed with or without optical instrumentation. Manual exploration may be performed directly or through intervening body layers.

| Body Part Character 4 | Approach Character 5 | Device Character 6 | Qualifier Character 7 |
|---|---|---|---|
| **Y** Peripheral Nerve | **Ø** Open<br>**3** Percutaneous<br>**4** Percutaneous Endoscopic | **Z** No Device | **Z** No Qualifier |

Non-OR Ø1JY3ZZ

**Ø Medical and Surgical**
**1 Peripheral Nervous System**
**N Release** Definition: Freeing a body part from an abnormal physical constraint by cutting or by the use of force
Explanation: Some of the restraining tissue may be taken out but none of the body part is taken out

| Body Part Character 4 | | Approach Character 5 | Device Character 6 | Qualifier Character 7 |
|---|---|---|---|---|
| **Ø Cervical Plexus**<br>Ansa cervicalis<br>Cutaneous (transverse) cervical nerve<br>Great auricular nerve<br>Lesser occipital nerve<br>Supraclavicular nerve<br>Transverse (cutaneous) cervical nerve<br>**1 Cervical Nerve**<br>Greater occipital nerve<br>Spinal nerve, cervical<br>Suboccipital nerve<br>Third occipital nerve<br>**2 Phrenic Nerve**<br>Accessory phrenic nerve<br>**3 Brachial Plexus**<br>Axillary nerve<br>Dorsal scapular nerve<br>First intercostal nerve<br>Long thoracic nerve<br>Musculocutaneous nerve<br>Subclavius nerve<br>Suprascapular nerve<br>**4 Ulnar Nerve**<br>Cubital nerve<br>**5 Median Nerve**<br>Anterior interosseous nerve<br>Palmar cutaneous nerve<br>**6 Radial Nerve**<br>Dorsal digital nerve<br>Musculospiral nerve<br>Palmar cutaneous nerve<br>Posterior interosseous nerve<br>**8 Thoracic Nerve**<br>Intercostal nerve<br>Intercostobrachial nerve<br>Spinal nerve, thoracic<br>Subcostal nerve<br>**9 Lumbar Plexus**<br>Accessory obturator nerve<br>Genitofemoral nerve<br>Iliohypogastric nerve<br>Ilioinguinal nerve<br>Lateral femoral cutaneous nerve<br>Obturator nerve<br>Superior gluteal nerve<br>**A Lumbosacral Plexus**<br>**B Lumbar Nerve**<br>Lumbosacral trunk<br>Spinal nerve, lumbar<br>Superior clunic (cluneal) nerve<br>**C Pudendal Nerve**<br>Posterior labial nerve<br>Posterior scrotal nerve<br>**D Femoral Nerve**<br>Anterior crural nerve<br>Saphenous nerve<br>**F Sciatic Nerve**<br>Ischiatic nerve<br>**G Tibial Nerve**<br>Lateral plantar nerve<br>Medial plantar nerve<br>Medial popliteal nerve<br>Medial sural cutaneous nerve | **H Peroneal Nerve**<br>Common fibular nerve<br>Common peroneal nerve<br>External popliteal nerve<br>Lateral sural cutaneous nerve<br>**K Head and Neck Sympathetic Nerve**<br>Cavernous plexus<br>Cervical ganglion<br>Ciliary ganglion<br>Internal carotid plexus<br>Otic ganglion<br>Pterygopalatine (sphenopalatine) ganglion<br>Sphenopalatine (pterygopalatine) ganglion<br>Stellate ganglion<br>Submandibular ganglion<br>Submaxillary ganglion<br>**L Thoracic Sympathetic Nerve**<br>Cardiac plexus<br>Esophageal plexus<br>Greater splanchnic nerve<br>Inferior cardiac nerve<br>Least splanchnic nerve<br>Lesser splanchnic nerve<br>Middle cardiac nerve<br>Pulmonary plexus<br>Superior cardiac nerve<br>Thoracic aortic plexus<br>Thoracic ganglion<br>**M Abdominal Sympathetic Nerve**<br>Abdominal aortic plexus<br>Auerbach's (myenteric) plexus<br>Celiac (solar) plexus<br>Celiac ganglion<br>Gastric plexus<br>Hepatic plexus<br>Inferior hypogastric plexus<br>Inferior mesenteric ganglion<br>Inferior mesenteric plexus<br>Meissner's (submucous) plexus<br>Myenteric (Auerbach's) plexus<br>Pancreatic plexus<br>Pelvic splanchnic nerve<br>Renal plexus<br>Solar (celiac) plexus<br>Splenic plexus<br>Submucous (Meissner's) plexus<br>Superior hypogastric plexus<br>Superior mesenteric ganglion<br>Superior mesenteric plexus<br>Suprarenal plexus<br>**N Lumbar Sympathetic Nerve**<br>Lumbar ganglion<br>Lumbar splanchnic nerve<br>**P Sacral Sympathetic Nerve**<br>Ganglion impar (ganglion of Walther)<br>Pelvic splanchnic nerve<br>Sacral ganglion<br>Sacral splanchnic nerve<br>**Q Sacral Plexus**<br>Inferior gluteal nerve<br>Posterior femoral cutaneous nerve<br>Pudendal nerve<br>**R Sacral Nerve**<br>Spinal nerve, sacral | **Ø Open**<br>**3 Percutaneous**<br>**4 Percutaneous Endoscopic** | **Z No Device** | **Z No Qualifier** |

**Ø Medical and Surgical**
**1 Peripheral Nervous System**
**P Removal** Definition: Taking out or off a device from a body part

Explanation: If a device is taken out and a similar device put in without cutting or puncturing the skin or mucous membrane, the procedure is coded to the root operation CHANGE. Otherwise, the procedure for taking out a device is coded to the root operation REMOVAL.

| Body Part Character 4 | Approach Character 5 | Device Character 6 | Qualifier Character 7 |
|---|---|---|---|
| Y Peripheral Nerve | Ø Open<br>3 Percutaneous<br>4 Percutaneous Endoscopic | Ø Drainage Device<br>2 Monitoring Device<br>7 Autologous Tissue Substitute<br>M Neurostimulator Lead<br>Y Other Device | Z No Qualifier |
| Y Peripheral Nerve | X External | Ø Drainage Device<br>2 Monitoring Device<br>M Neurostimulator Lead | Z No Qualifier |

Non-OR Ø1PY3[Ø,2]Z
Non-OR Ø1PY[3,4]YZ
Non-OR Ø1PYX[Ø,2,M]Z

**Ø Medical and Surgical**
**1 Peripheral Nervous System**
**Q Repair** Definition: Restoring, to the extent possible, a body part to its normal anatomic structure and function
Explanation: Used only when the method to accomplish the repair is not one of the other root operations

| Body Part Character 4 | | Approach Character 5 | Device Character 6 | Qualifier Character 7 |
|---|---|---|---|---|
| **Ø Cervical Plexus**<br>Ansa cervicalis<br>Cutaneous (transverse) cervical nerve<br>Great auricular nerve<br>Lesser occipital nerve<br>Supraclavicular nerve<br>Transverse (cutaneous) cervical nerve<br>**1 Cervical Nerve**<br>Greater occipital nerve<br>Spinal nerve, cervical<br>Suboccipital nerve<br>Third occipital nerve<br>**2 Phrenic Nerve**<br>Accessory phrenic nerve<br>**3 Brachial Plexus**<br>Axillary nerve<br>Dorsal scapular nerve<br>First intercostal nerve<br>Long thoracic nerve<br>Musculocutaneous nerve<br>Subclavius nerve<br>Suprascapular nerve<br>**4 Ulnar Nerve**<br>Cubital nerve<br>**5 Median Nerve**<br>Anterior interosseous nerve<br>Palmar cutaneous nerve<br>**6 Radial Nerve**<br>Dorsal digital nerve<br>Musculospiral nerve<br>Palmar cutaneous nerve<br>Posterior interosseous nerve<br>**8 Thoracic Nerve**<br>Intercostal nerve<br>Intercostobrachial nerve<br>Spinal nerve, thoracic<br>Subcostal nerve<br>**9 Lumbar Plexus**<br>Accessory obturator nerve<br>Genitofemoral nerve<br>Iliohypogastric nerve<br>Ilioinguinal nerve<br>Lateral femoral cutaneous nerve<br>Obturator nerve<br>Superior gluteal nerve<br>**A Lumbosacral Plexus**<br>**B Lumbar Nerve**<br>Lumbosacral trunk<br>Spinal nerve, lumbar<br>Superior clunic (cluneal) nerve<br>**C Pudendal Nerve**<br>Posterior labial nerve<br>Posterior scrotal nerve<br>**D Femoral Nerve**<br>Anterior crural nerve<br>Saphenous nerve<br>**F Sciatic Nerve**<br>Ischiatic nerve<br>**G Tibial Nerve**<br>Lateral plantar nerve<br>Medial plantar nerve<br>Medial popliteal nerve<br>Medial sural cutaneous nerve | **H Peroneal Nerve**<br>Common fibular nerve<br>Common peroneal nerve<br>External popliteal nerve<br>Lateral sural cutaneous nerve<br>**K Head and Neck Sympathetic Nerve**<br>Cavernous plexus<br>Cervical ganglion<br>Ciliary ganglion<br>Internal carotid plexus<br>Otic ganglion<br>Pterygopalatine (sphenopalatine) ganglion<br>Sphenopalatine (pterygopalatine) ganglion<br>Stellate ganglion<br>Submandibular ganglion<br>Submaxillary ganglion<br>**L Thoracic Sympathetic Nerve**<br>Cardiac plexus<br>Esophageal plexus<br>Greater splanchnic nerve<br>Inferior cardiac nerve<br>Least splanchnic nerve<br>Lesser splanchnic nerve<br>Middle cardiac nerve<br>Pulmonary plexus<br>Superior cardiac nerve<br>Thoracic aortic plexus<br>Thoracic ganglion<br>**M Abdominal Sympathetic Nerve**<br>Abdominal aortic plexus<br>Auerbach's (myenteric) plexus<br>Celiac (solar) plexus<br>Celiac ganglion<br>Gastric plexus<br>Hepatic plexus<br>Inferior hypogastric plexus<br>Inferior mesenteric ganglion<br>Inferior mesenteric plexus<br>Meissner's (submucous) plexus<br>Myenteric (Auerbach's) plexus<br>Pancreatic plexus<br>Pelvic splanchnic nerve<br>Renal plexus<br>Solar (celiac) plexus<br>Splenic plexus<br>Submucous (Meissner's) plexus<br>Superior hypogastric plexus<br>Superior mesenteric ganglion<br>Superior mesenteric plexus<br>Suprarenal plexus<br>**N Lumbar Sympathetic Nerve**<br>Lumbar ganglion<br>Lumbar splanchnic nerve<br>**P Sacral Sympathetic Nerve**<br>Ganglion impar (ganglion of Walther)<br>Pelvic splanchnic nerve<br>Sacral ganglion<br>Sacral splanchnic nerve<br>**Q Sacral Plexus**<br>Inferior gluteal nerve<br>Posterior femoral cutaneous nerve<br>Pudendal nerve<br>**R Sacral Nerve**<br>Spinal nerve, sacral | **Ø Open**<br>**3 Percutaneous**<br>**4 Percutaneous Endoscopic** | **Z No Device** | **Z No Qualifier** |

**Ø Medical and Surgical**
**1 Peripheral Nervous System**
**R Replacement** Definition: Putting in or on biological or synthetic material that physically takes the place and/or function of all or a portion of a body part

Explanation: The body part may have been taken out or replaced, or may be taken out, physically eradicated, or rendered nonfunctional during the REPLACEMENT procedure. A REMOVAL procedure is coded for taking out the device used in a previous replacement procedure.

| Body Part Character 4 | Approach Character 5 | Device Character 6 | Qualifier Character 7 |
|---|---|---|---|
| 1 Cervical Nerve<br>Greater occipital nerve<br>Spinal nerve, cervical<br>Suboccipital nerve<br>Third occipital nerve<br>2 Phrenic Nerve<br>Accessory phrenic nerve<br>4 Ulnar Nerve<br>Cubital nerve<br>5 Median Nerve<br>Anterior interosseous nerve<br>Palmar cutaneous nerve<br>6 Radial Nerve<br>Dorsal digital nerve<br>Musculospiral nerve<br>Palmar cutaneous nerve<br>Posterior interosseous nerve<br>8 Thoracic Nerve<br>Intercostal nerve<br>Intercostobrachial nerve<br>Spinal nerve, thoracic<br>Subcostal nerve<br>B Lumbar Nerve<br>Lumbosacral trunk<br>Spinal nerve, lumbar<br>Superior clunic (cluneal) nerve<br>C Pudendal Nerve<br>Posterior labial nerve<br>Posterior scrotal nerve<br>D Femoral Nerve<br>Anterior crural nerve<br>Saphenous nerve<br>F Sciatic Nerve<br>Ischiatic nerve<br>G Tibial Nerve<br>Lateral plantar nerve<br>Medial plantar nerve<br>Medial popliteal nerve<br>Medial sural cutaneous nerve<br>H Peroneal Nerve<br>Common fibular nerve<br>Common peroneal nerve<br>External popliteal nerve<br>Lateral sural cutaneous nerve<br>R Sacral Nerve<br>Spinal nerve, sacral | Ø Open<br>4 Percutaneous Endoscopic | 7 Autologous Tissue Substitute<br>J Synthetic Substitute<br>K Nonautologous Tissue Substitute | Z No Qualifier |

**Ø Medical and Surgical**
**1 Peripheral Nervous System**
**S Reposition** Definition: Moving to its normal location, or other suitable location, all or a portion of a body part

Explanation: The body part is moved to a new location from an abnormal location, or from a normal location where it is not functioning correctly. The body part may or may not be cut out or off to be moved to the new location.

| Body Part Character 4 | Approach Character 5 | Device Character 6 | Qualifier Character 7 |
|---|---|---|---|
| **Ø Cervical Plexus**<br>Ansa cervicalis<br>Cutaneous (transverse) cervical nerve<br>Great auricular nerve<br>Lesser occipital nerve<br>Supraclavicular nerve<br>Transverse (cutaneous) cervical nerve<br>**1 Cervical Nerve**<br>Greater occipital nerve<br>Spinal nerve, cervical<br>Suboccipital nerve<br>Third occipital nerve<br>**2 Phrenic Nerve**<br>Accessory phrenic nerve<br>**3 Brachial Plexus**<br>Axillary nerve<br>Dorsal scapular nerve<br>First intercostal nerve<br>Long thoracic nerve<br>Musculocutaneous nerve<br>Subclavius nerve<br>Suprascapular nerve<br>**4 Ulnar Nerve**<br>Cubital nerve<br>**5 Median Nerve**<br>Anterior interosseous nerve<br>Palmar cutaneous nerve<br>**6 Radial Nerve**<br>Dorsal digital nerve<br>Musculospiral nerve<br>Palmar cutaneous nerve<br>Posterior interosseous nerve<br>**8 Thoracic Nerve**<br>Intercostal nerve<br>Intercostobrachial nerve<br>Spinal nerve, thoracic<br>Subcostal nerve<br>**9 Lumbar Plexus**<br>Accessory obturator nerve<br>Genitofemoral nerve<br>Iliohypogastric nerve<br>Ilioinguinal nerve<br>Lateral femoral cutaneous nerve<br>Obturator nerve<br>Superior gluteal nerve<br>**A Lumbosacral Plexus**<br>**B Lumbar Nerve**<br>Lumbosacral trunk<br>Spinal nerve, lumbar<br>Superior clunic (cluneal) nerve<br>**C Pudendal Nerve**<br>Posterior labial nerve<br>Posterior scrotal nerve<br>**D Femoral Nerve**<br>Anterior crural nerve<br>Saphenous nerve<br>**F Sciatic Nerve**<br>Ischiatic nerve<br>**G Tibial Nerve**<br>Lateral plantar nerve<br>Medial plantar nerve<br>Medial popliteal nerve<br>Medial sural cutaneous nerve<br>**H Peroneal Nerve**<br>Common fibular nerve<br>Common peroneal nerve<br>External popliteal nerve<br>Lateral sural cutaneous nerve<br>**Q Sacral Plexus**<br>Inferior gluteal nerve<br>Posterior femoral cutaneous nerve<br>Pudendal nerve<br>**R Sacral Nerve**<br>Spinal nerve, sacral | **Ø Open**<br>**3 Percutaneous**<br>**4 Percutaneous Endoscopic** | **Z No Device** | **Z No Qualifier** |

**Ø Medical and Surgical**
**1 Peripheral Nervous System**
**U Supplement** Definition: Putting in or on biological or synthetic material that physically reinforces and/or augments the function of a portion of a body part

Explanation: The biological material is non-living, or is living and from the same individual. The body part may have been previously replaced, and the SUPPLEMENT procedure is performed to physically reinforce and/or augment the function of the replaced body part.

| Body Part Character 4 | Approach Character 5 | Device Character 6 | Qualifier Character 7 |
|---|---|---|---|
| **1 Cervical Nerve**<br>Greater occipital nerve<br>Spinal nerve, cervical<br>Suboccipital nerve<br>Third occipital nerve<br>**2 Phrenic Nerve**<br>Accessory phrenic nerve<br>**4 Ulnar Nerve**<br>Cubital nerve<br>**5 Median Nerve**<br>Anterior interosseous nerve<br>Palmar cutaneous nerve<br>**6 Radial Nerve**<br>Dorsal digital nerve<br>Musculospiral nerve<br>Palmar cutaneous nerve<br>Posterior interosseous nerve<br>**8 Thoracic Nerve**<br>Intercostal nerve<br>Intercostobrachial nerve<br>Spinal nerve, thoracic<br>Subcostal nerve<br>**B Lumbar Nerve**<br>Lumbosacral trunk<br>Spinal nerve, lumbar<br>Superior clunic (cluneal) nerve<br>**C Pudendal Nerve**<br>Posterior labial nerve<br>Posterior scrotal nerve<br>**D Femoral Nerve**<br>Anterior crural nerve<br>Saphenous nerve<br>**F Sciatic Nerve**<br>Ischiatic nerve<br>**G Tibial Nerve**<br>Lateral plantar nerve<br>Medial plantar nerve<br>Medial popliteal nerve<br>Medial sural cutaneous nerve<br>**H Peroneal Nerve**<br>Common fibular nerve<br>Common peroneal nerve<br>External popliteal nerve<br>Lateral sural cutaneous nerve<br>**R Sacral Nerve**<br>Spinal nerve, sacral | **Ø Open**<br>**3 Percutaneous**<br>**4 Percutaneous Endoscopic** | **7 Autologous Tissue Substitute**<br>**J Synthetic Substitute**<br>**K Nonautologous Tissue Substitute** | **Z No Qualifier** |

**Ø Medical and Surgical**
**1 Peripheral Nervous System**
**W Revision** Definition: Correcting, to the extent possible, a portion of a malfunctioning device or the position of a displaced device

Explanation: Revision can include correcting a malfunctioning or displaced device by taking out or putting in components of the device such as a screw or pin

| Body Part Character 4 | Approach Character 5 | Device Character 6 | Qualifier Character 7 |
|---|---|---|---|
| **Y Peripheral Nerve** | **Ø Open**<br>**3 Percutaneous**<br>**4 Percutaneous Endoscopic** | **Ø Drainage Device**<br>**2 Monitoring Device**<br>**7 Autologous Tissue Substitute**<br>**M Neurostimulator Lead**<br>**Y Other Device** | **Z No Qualifier** |
| **Y Peripheral Nerve** | **X External** | **Ø Drainage Device**<br>**2 Monitoring Device**<br>**7 Autologous Tissue Substitute**<br>**M Neurostimulator Lead** | **Z No Qualifier** |

**Non-OR** Ø1WY[3,4]YZ
**Non-OR** Ø1WYX[Ø,2,7,M]Z

**Ø Medical and Surgical**
**1 Peripheral Nervous System**
**X Transfer** Definition: Moving, without taking out, all or a portion of a body part to another location to take over the function of all or a portion of a body part
Explanation: The body part transferred remains connected to its vascular and nervous supply

| Body Part Character 4 | Approach Character 5 | Device Character 6 | Qualifier Character 7 |
|---|---|---|---|
| **1 Cervical Nerve**<br>Greater occipital nerve<br>Spinal nerve, cervical<br>Suboccipital nerve<br>Third occipital nerve<br>**2 Phrenic Nerve**<br>Accessory phrenic nerve | **Ø Open**<br>**4 Percutaneous Endoscopic** | **Z No Device** | **1 Cervical Nerve**<br>**2 Phrenic Nerve** |
| **4 Ulnar Nerve**<br>Cubital nerve<br>**5 Median Nerve**<br>Anterior interosseous nerve<br>Palmar cutaneous nerve<br>**6 Radial Nerve**<br>Dorsal digital nerve<br>Musculospiral nerve<br>Palmar cutaneous nerve<br>Posterior interosseous nerve | **Ø Open**<br>**4 Percutaneous Endoscopic** | **Z No Device** | **4 Ulnar Nerve**<br>**5 Median Nerve**<br>**6 Radial Nerve** |
| **8 Thoracic Nerve**<br>Intercostal nerve<br>Intercostobrachial nerve<br>Spinal nerve, thoracic<br>Subcostal nerve | **Ø Open**<br>**4 Percutaneous Endoscopic** | **Z No Device** | **8 Thoracic Nerve** |
| **B Lumbar Nerve**<br>Lumbosacral trunk<br>Spinal nerve, lumbar<br>Superior clunic (cluneal) nerve<br>**C Pudendal Nerve**<br>Posterior labial nerve<br>Posterior scrotal nerve | **Ø Open**<br>**4 Percutaneous Endoscopic** | **Z No Device** | **B Lumbar Nerve**<br>**C Perineal Nerve** |
| **D Femoral Nerve**<br>Anterior crural nerve<br>Saphenous nerve<br>**F Sciatic Nerve**<br>Ischiatic nerve<br>**G Tibial Nerve**<br>Lateral plantar nerve<br>Medial plantar nerve<br>Medial popliteal nerve<br>Medial sural cutaneous nerve<br>**H Peroneal Nerve**<br>Common fibular nerve<br>Common peroneal nerve<br>External popliteal nerve<br>Lateral sural cutaneous nerve | **Ø Open**<br>**4 Percutaneous Endoscopic** | **Z No Device** | **D Femoral Nerve**<br>**F Sciatic Nerve**<br>**G Tibial Nerve**<br>**H Peroneal Nerve** |

# Heart and Great Vessels Ø21–Ø2Y



This Character Meaning table is provided as a guide to assist the user in the identification of character members that may be found in this section of code tables. It **SHOULD NOT** be used to build a PCS code.

| Operation–Character 3 | Body Part–Character 4 | Approach–Character 5 | Device–Character 6 | Qualifier–Character 7 |
|---|---|---|---|---|
| 1 Bypass | Ø Coronary Artery, One Artery | Ø Open | Ø Monitoring Device, Pressure Sensor | Ø Allogeneic |
| 4 Creation | 1 Coronary Artery, Two Arteries | 3 Percutaneous | 2 Monitoring Device | 1 Syngeneic |
| 5 Destruction | 2 Coronary Artery, Three Arteries | 4 Percutaneous Endoscopic | 3 Infusion Device | 2 Zooplastic OR Common Atrioventricular Valve |
| 7 Dilation | 3 Coronary Artery, Four or More Arteries | X External | 4 Intraluminal Device, Drug-eluting | 3 Coronary Artery |
| 8 Division | 4 Coronary Vein | | 5 Intraluminal Device, Drug-eluting, Two | 4 Coronary Vein |
| B Excision | 5 Atrial Septum | | 6 Intraluminal Device, Drug-eluting, Three | 5 Coronary Circulation |
| C Extirpation | 6 Atrium, Right | | 7 Intraluminal Device, Drug-eluting, Four or More OR Autologous Tissue Substitute | 6 Bifurcation |
| F Fragmentation | 7 Atrium, Left | | 8 Zooplastic Tissue | 7 Atrium, Left |
| H Insertion | 8 Conduction Mechanism | | 9 Autologous Venous Tissue | 8 Internal Mammary, Right |
| J Inspection | 9 Chordae Tendineae | | A Autologous Arterial Tissue | 9 Internal Mammary, Left |
| K Map | A Heart | | C Extraluminal Device | A Innominate Artery |
| L Occlusion | B Heart, Right | | D Intraluminal Device | B Subclavian |
| N Release | C Heart, Left | | E Intraluminal Device, Two OR Intraluminal Device, Branched or Fenestrated, One or Two Arteries | C Thoracic Artery |
| P Removal | D Papillary Muscle | | F Intraluminal Device, Three OR Intraluminal Device, Branched or Fenestrated, Three or More Arteries | D Carotid |
| Q Repair | F Aortic Valve | | G Intraluminal Device, Four or More | E Atrioventricular Valve, Left |
| R Replacement | G Mitral Valve | | J Synthetic Substitute OR Cardiac Lead, Pacemaker | F Abdominal Artery |
| S Reposition | H Pulmonary Valve | | K Nonautologous Tissue Substitute OR Cardiac Lead, Defibrillator | G Atrioventricular Valve, Right OR Axillary Artery |
| T Resection | J Tricuspid Valve | | M Cardiac Lead | H Transapical OR Brachial Artery |
| U Supplement | K Ventricle, Right | | N Intracardiac Pacemaker | J Truncal Valve OR Temporary OR Intraoperative |
| V Restriction | L Ventricle, Left | | Q Implantable Heart Assist System | K Left Atrial Appendage |
| W Revision | M Ventricular Septum | | R Short-term External Heart Assist System | P Pulmonary Trunk |
| Y Transplantation | N Pericardium | | T Intraluminal Device, Radioactive | Q Pulmonary Artery, Right |
| | P Pulmonary Trunk | | Y Other Device | R Pulmonary Artery, Left |
| | Q Pulmonary Artery, Right | | Z No Device | S Pulmonary Vein, Right OR Biventricular |
| | R Pulmonary Artery, Left | | | T Pulmonary Vein, Left OR Ductus Arteriosus |
| | S Pulmonary Vein, Right | | | U Pulmonary Vein, Confluence |

***Continued on next page***

*Continued from previous page*

| Operation–Character 3 | Body Part–Character 4 | Approach–Character 5 | Device–Character 6 | Qualifier–Character 7 |
|---|---|---|---|---|
| | T Pulmonary Vein, Left | | | W Aorta |
| | V Superior Vena Cava | | | X Diagnostic |
| | W Thoracic Aorta, Descending | | | Z No Qualifier |
| | X Thoracic Aorta, Ascending/ Arch | | | |
| | Y Great Vessel | | | |

**AHA Coding Clinic for table Ø21**
**2017, 1Q, 19** Norwood Sano procedure
**2016, 4Q, 80-81** Thoracic aorta, ascending/arch and descending
**2016, 4Q, 82-83** Coronary artery, number of arteries
**2016, 4Q, 102-109** Correction of congenital heart defects
**2016, 4Q, 144** Repair of atrial septal defect and anomalous pulmonary venous return
**2016, 4Q, 145** Modified Warden procedure for repair of septal defect and right partial anomalous pulmonary venous return
**2016, 1Q, 27** Aortocoronary bypass graft utilizing Y-graft
**2015, 4Q, 22, 24** Congenital heart corrective procedures
**2015, 3Q, 16** Revision of previous truncus arteriosus surgery with ventricle to pulmonary artery conduit
**2014, 3Q, 3** Blalock-Taussig shunt procedure
**2014, 3Q, 8** Coronary artery bypass graft utilizing internal mammary as pedicle graft
**2014, 3Q, 20** MAZE procedure performed with coronary artery bypass graft
**2014, 3Q, 29** Fontan completion procedure stage II
**2014, 3Q, 30** Creation of conduit from right ventricle to pulmonary artery
**2014, 1Q, 10** Repair of thoracic aortic aneurysm & coronary artery bypass graft
**2013, 2Q, 37** Coronary artery release performed during coronary artery bypass graft

**AHA Coding Clinic for table Ø24**
**2016, 4Q, 101** Root operation Creation
**2016, 4Q, 102-109** Correction of congenital heart defects

**AHA Coding Clinic for table Ø25**
**2016, 4Q, 80-81** Thoracic aorta, ascending/arch and descending
**2016, 3Q, 43-44** Peri-pulmonary catheter ablation
**2016, 3Q, 44-45** Maze procedure
**2016, 2Q, 17** Photodynamic therapy for treatment of malignant mesothelioma
**2014, 4Q, 47** Catheter ablation of peripulmonary veins
**2014, 3Q, 19** Ablation of ventricular tachycardia with Impella® support
**2014, 3Q, 20** MAZE procedure performed with coronary artery bypass graft
**2013, 2Q, 38** Catheter ablation to treat atrial fibrillation

**AHA Coding Clinic for table Ø27**
**2016, 4Q, 80-81** Thoracic aorta, ascending/arch and descending
**2016, 4Q, 82-83** Coronary artery, number of arteries
**2016, 4Q, 84-85** Coronary Artery, number of stents
**2016, 4Q, 86-88** Coronary and peripheral artery bifurcation
**2016, 1Q, 16** Pulmonary valvotomy and dilation of annulus
**2015, 4Q, 13** New Section X codes—New Technology procedures
**2015, 3Q, 9** Failed attempt to treat coronary artery occlusion
**2015, 3Q, 10** Coronary angioplasty with unsuccessful stent insertion
**2015, 3Q, 16** Revision of previous truncus arteriosus surgery with ventricle to pulmonary artery conduit
**2015, 2Q, 3-5** Coronary artery intervention site
**2014, 2Q, 4** Coronary angioplasty of bypassed vessel

**AHA Coding Clinic for table Ø2B**
**2017, 1Q, 38** Mitral valve repair and chordae tendineae transfer
**2016, 4Q, 80-81** Thoracic aorta, ascending/arch and descending
**2015, 2Q, 23** Annuloplasty ring

**AHA Coding Clinic for table Ø2C**
**2017, 2Q, 23** Thrombectomy via Fogarty catheter
**2016, 4Q, 80-81** Thoracic aorta, ascending/arch and descending
**2016, 4Q, 82-83** Coronary artery, number of arteries
**2016, 4Q, 86-87** Coronary and peripheral artery bifurcation
**2016, 2Q, 24** Repair/decalcification of mitral valve
**2016, 2Q, 25** Aortic valve surgery with excision of calcium deposits

**AHA Coding Clinic for table Ø2H**
**2017, 2Q, 24** Tunneled catheter versus totally implantable catheter
**2017, 2Q, 26** Exchange of tunneled catheter
**2017, 1Q, 10-11** External heart assist device
**2016, 4Q, 80-81** Thoracic aorta, ascending/arch and descending
**2016, 4Q, 95** Intracardiac pacemaker
**2016, 4Q, 137-138** Heart assist device systems
**2016, 2Q, 15** Removal and replacement of tunneled internal jugular catheter
**2015, 4Q, 14** New Section X codes—New Technology procedures
**2015, 4Q, 26-31** Vascular access devices
**2015, 3Q, 35** Swan Ganz catheterization
**2015, 2Q, 31** Leadless pacemaker insertion
**2015, 2Q, 33** Totally implantable central venous access device (Port-a-Cath)
**2013, 3Q, 18** Placement of peripherally inserted central catheter (PICC)

**AHA Coding Clinic for table Ø2J**
**2015, 3Q, 9** Failed attempt to treat coronary artery occlusion

**AHA Coding Clinic for table Ø2L**
**2016, 4Q, 102-109** Correction of congenital heart defects
**2016, 2Q, 26** Embolization of pulmonary arteriovenous fistula
**2015, 4Q, 23** Congenital heart corrective procedures
**2014, 3Q, 20** MAZE procedure performed with coronary artery bypass graft

**AHA Coding Clinic for table Ø2N**
**2016, 4Q, 80-81** Thoracic aorta, ascending/arch and descending
**2014, 3Q, 16** Repair of Tetralogy of Fallot

**AHA Coding Clinic for table Ø2P**
**2017, 2Q, 24** Tunneled catheter versus totally implantable catheter
**2017, 2Q, 26** Exchange of tunneled catheter
**2017, 1Q, 11** External heart assist device
**2017, 1Q, 13** SynCardia total artificial heart
**2016, 4Q, 95-96** Intracardiac pacemaker
**2016, 4Q, 137-139** Heart assist device systems
**2016, 3Q, 19** Nonoperative removal of peripherally inserted central catheter
**2016, 2Q, 15** Removal and replacement of tunneled internal jugular catheter
**2015, 4Q, 31** Vascular access devices
**2015, 3Q, 33** Approach values for repositioning and removal of cardiac lead

**AHA Coding Clinic for table Ø2Q**
**2017, 1Q, 18** Sutureless repair of pulmonary vein stenosis
**2016, 4Q, 80-81** Thoracic aorta, ascending/arch and descending
**2016, 4Q, 82-83** Coronary artery, number of arteries
**2016, 4Q, 101** Root operation Creation
**2016, 4Q, 102-109** Correction of congenital heart defects
**2015, 4Q, 23** Congenital heart corrective procedures
**2015, 3Q, 16** Vascular ring surgery and double aortic arch
**2015, 2Q, 23** Annuloplasty ring
**2013, 3Q, 26** Transcatheter replacement of heart valve (TAVR) with measurements

**AHA Coding Clinic for table Ø2R**
**2017, 1Q, 13** SynCardia total artificial heart
**2016, 4Q, 80-81** Thoracic aorta, ascending/arch and descending
**2016, 3Q, 32** Transcatheter tricuspid valve replacement
**2014, 1Q, 10** Repair of thoracic aortic aneurysm & coronary artery bypass graft

**AHA Coding Clinic for table Ø2S**
**2016, 4Q, 80-81** Thoracic aorta, ascending/arch and descending
**2016, 4Q, 82-83** Coronary artery, number of arteries
**2016, 4Q, 102-109** Correction of congenital heart defects
**2015, 4Q, 23** Congenital heart corrective procedures

**AHA Coding Clinic for table Ø2U**
**2017, 1Q, 19** Norwood Sano procedure
**2016, 4Q, 80-81** Thoracic aorta, ascending/arch and descending
**2016, 4Q, 101** Root operation Creation
**2016, 4Q, 102-109** Correction of congenital heart defects
**2016, 2Q, 23** Repair of tetralogy of Fallot with autologous pericardial patch graft
**2016, 2Q, 26** Aortic valve replacement with aortic root enlargement
**2015, 4Q, 22-24** Congenital heart corrective procedures
**2015, 3Q, 16** Revision of previous truncus arteriosus surgery with ventricle to pulmonary artery conduit
**2015, 2Q, 23** Annuloplasty ring
**2014, 3Q, 16** Repair of Tetralogy of Fallot

**AHA Coding Clinic for table Ø2V**
**2016, 4Q, 80-81** Thoracic aorta, ascending/arch and descending
**2016, 4Q, 89-92** Branched and fenestrated endograft repair of aneurysms

**AHA Coding Clinic for table Ø2W**
**2016, 4Q, 85** Coronary Artery, number of stents
**2016, 4Q, 95-96** Intracardiac pacemaker
**2015, 3Q, 32** Approach values for repositioning and removal of cardiac lead
**2014, 3Q, 31** Closure of paravalvular leak using Amplatzer® vascular plug

**AHA Coding Clinic for table Ø2Y**
**2013, 3Q, 18** Heart transplant surgery

## Coronary Arteries

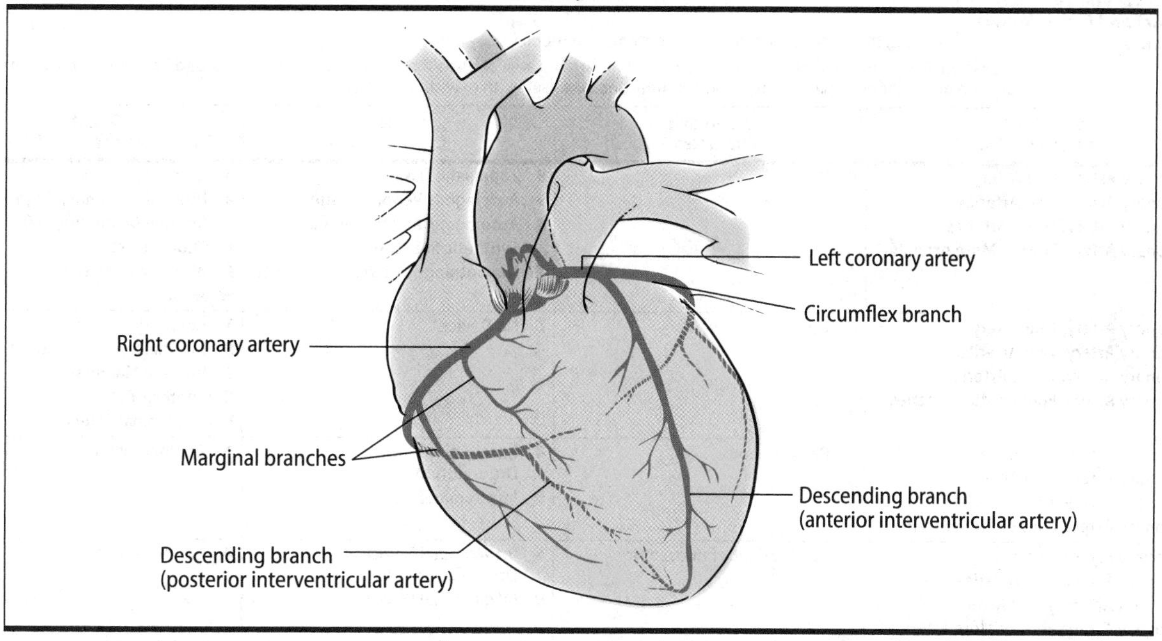
Left coronary artery
Circumflex branch
Right coronary artery
Marginal branches
Descending branch
(anterior interventricular artery)
Descending branch
(posterior interventricular artery)

## Heart Anatomy

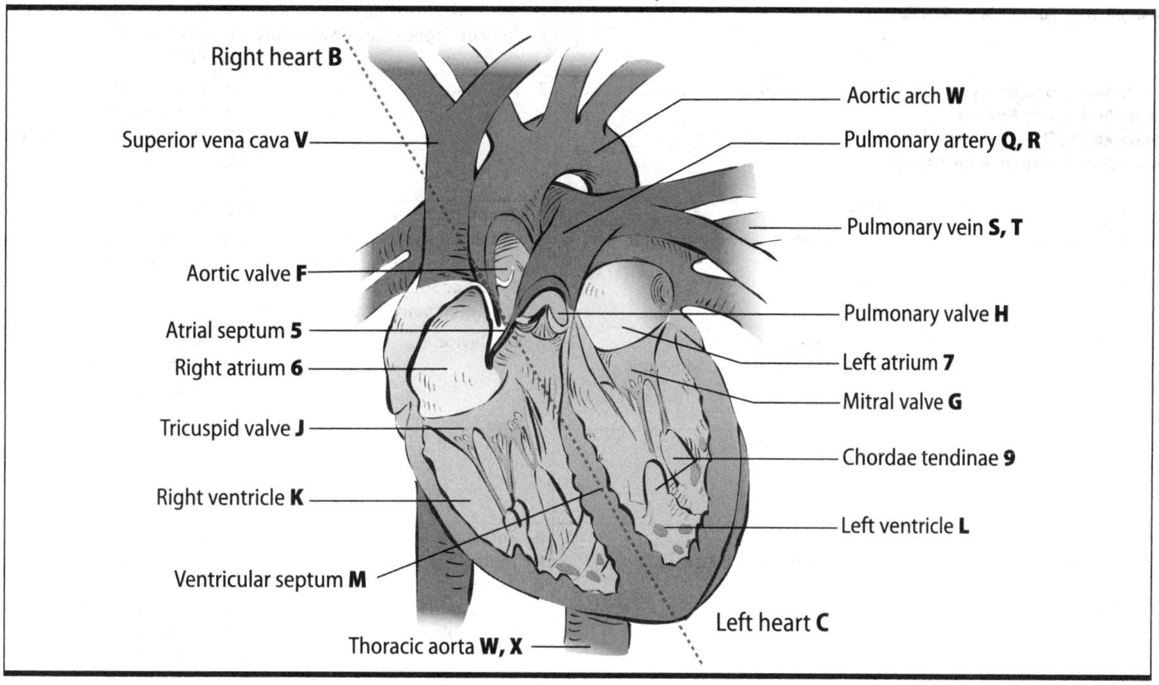
Right heart **B**
Superior vena cava **V**
Aortic arch **W**
Pulmonary artery **Q, R**
Pulmonary vein **S, T**
Aortic valve **F**
Pulmonary valve **H**
Atrial septum **5**
Right atrium **6**
Left atrium **7**
Mitral valve **G**
Tricuspid valve **J**
Chordae tendinae **9**
Right ventricle **K**
Left ventricle **L**
Ventricular septum **M**
Left heart **C**
Thoracic aorta **W, X**

**Ø Medical and Surgical**
**2 Heart and Great Vessels**
**1 Bypass** Definition: Altering the route of passage of the contents of a tubular body part

Explanation: Rerouting contents of a body part to a downstream area of the normal route, to a similar route and body part, or to an abnormal route and dissimilar body part. Includes one or more anastomoses, with or without the use of a device.

| Body Part Character 4 | Approach Character 5 | Device Character 6 | Qualifier Character 7 |
|---|---|---|---|
| Ø Coronary Artery, One Artery<br>1 Coronary Artery, Two Arteries<br>2 Coronary Artery, Three Arteries<br>3 Coronary Artery, Four or More Arteries | Ø Open | 8 Zooplastic Tissue<br>9 Autologous Venous Tissue<br>A Autologous Arterial Tissue<br>J Synthetic Substitute<br>K Nonautologous Tissue Substitute | 3 Coronary Artery<br>8 Internal Mammary, Right<br>9 Internal Mammary, Left<br>C Thoracic Artery<br>F Abdominal Artery<br>W Aorta |
| Ø Coronary Artery, One Artery<br>1 Coronary Artery, Two Arteries<br>2 Coronary Artery, Three Arteries<br>3 Coronary Artery, Four or More Arteries | Ø Open | Z No Device | 3 Coronary Artery<br>8 Internal Mammary, Right<br>9 Internal Mammary, Left<br>C Thoracic Artery<br>F Abdominal Artery |
| Ø Coronary Artery, One Artery<br>1 Coronary Artery, Two Arteries<br>2 Coronary Artery, Three Arteries<br>3 Coronary Artery, Four or More Arteries | 3 Percutaneous | 4 Intraluminal Device, Drug-eluting<br>D Intraluminal Device | 4 Coronary Vein |
| Ø Coronary Artery, One Artery<br>1 Coronary Artery, Two Arteries<br>2 Coronary Artery, Three Arteries<br>3 Coronary Artery, Four or More Arteries | 4 Percutaneous Endoscopic | 4 Intraluminal Device, Drug-eluting<br>D Intraluminal Device | 4 Coronary Vein |
| Ø Coronary Artery, One Artery<br>1 Coronary Artery, Two Arteries<br>2 Coronary Artery, Three Arteries<br>3 Coronary Artery, Four or More Arteries | 4 Percutaneous Endoscopic | 8 Zooplastic Tissue<br>9 Autologous Venous Tissue<br>A Autologous Arterial Tissue<br>J Synthetic Substitute<br>K Nonautologous Tissue Substitute | 3 Coronary Artery<br>8 Internal Mammary, Right<br>9 Internal Mammary, Left<br>C Thoracic Artery<br>F Abdominal Artery<br>W Aorta |
| Ø Coronary Artery, One Artery<br>1 Coronary Artery, Two Arteries<br>2 Coronary Artery, Three Arteries<br>3 Coronary Artery, Four or More Arteries | 4 Percutaneous Endoscopic | Z No Device | 3 Coronary Artery<br>8 Internal Mammary, Right<br>9 Internal Mammary, Left<br>C Thoracic Artery<br>F Abdominal Artery |
| 6 Atrium, Right<br>Atrium dextrum cordis<br>Right auricular appendix<br>Sinus venosus | Ø Open<br>4 Percutaneous Endoscopic | 8 Zooplastic Tissue<br>9 Autologous Venous Tissue<br>A Autologous Arterial Tissue<br>J Synthetic Substitute<br>K Nonautologous Tissue Substitute | P Pulmonary Trunk<br>Q Pulmonary Artery, Right<br>R Pulmonary Artery, Left |
| 6 Atrium, Right<br>Atrium dextrum cordis<br>Right auricular appendix<br>Sinus venosus | Ø Open<br>4 Percutaneous Endoscopic | Z No Device | 7 Atrium, Left<br>P Pulmonary Trunk<br>Q Pulmonary Artery, Right<br>R Pulmonary Artery, Left |
| 6 Atrium, Right<br>Atrium dextrum cordis<br>Right auricular appendix<br>Sinus venosus | 3 Percutaneous | Z No Device | 7 Atrium, Left |
| 7 Atrium, Left<br>Atrium pulmonale<br>Left auricular appendix<br>V Superior Vena Cava<br>Precava | Ø Open<br>4 Percutaneous Endoscopic | 8 Zooplastic Tissue<br>9 Autologous Venous Tissue<br>A Autologous Arterial Tissue<br>J Synthetic Substitute<br>K Nonautologous Tissue Substitute<br>Z No Device | P Pulmonary Trunk<br>Q Pulmonary Artery, Right<br>R Pulmonary Artery, Left<br>S Pulmonary Vein, Right<br>T Pulmonary Vein, Left<br>U Pulmonary Vein, Confluence |
| K Ventricle, Right<br>Conus arteriosus<br>L Ventricle, Left | Ø Open<br>4 Percutaneous Endoscopic | 8 Zooplastic Tissue<br>9 Autologous Venous Tissue<br>A Autologous Arterial Tissue<br>J Synthetic Substitute<br>K Nonautologous Tissue Substitute | P Pulmonary Trunk<br>Q Pulmonary Artery, Right<br>R Pulmonary Artery, Left |

*Ø21 Continued on next page*

**HAC** Ø21[Ø,1,2,3]Ø[8,9,A,J,K][3,8,9,C,F,W] when reported with SDx J98.51 or J98.59
**HAC** Ø21[Ø,1,2,3]ØZ[3,8,9,C,F] when reported with SDx J98.51 or J98.59
**HAC** Ø21[Ø,1,2,3]4[8,9,A,J,K][3,8,9,C,F,W] when reported with SDx J98.51 or J98.59
**HAC** Ø21[Ø,1,2,3]4Z[3,8,9,C,F] when reported with SDx J98.51 or J98.59=

**Ø Medical and Surgical**
**2 Heart and Great Vessels**
**1 Bypass** Definition: Altering the route of passage of the contents of a tubular body part

*Ø21 Continued*

Explanation: Rerouting contents of a body part to a downstream area of the normal route, to a similar route and body part, or to an abnormal route and dissimilar body part. Includes one or more anastomoses, with or without the use of a device.

| Body Part Character 4 | Approach Character 5 | Device Character 6 | Qualifier Character 7 |
|---|---|---|---|
| **K** Ventricle, Right<br>Conus arteriosus<br>**L** Ventricle, Left | **Ø** Open<br>**4** Percutaneous Endoscopic | **Z** No Device | **5** Coronary Circulation<br>**8** Internal Mammary, Right<br>**9** Internal Mammary, Left<br>**C** Thoracic Artery<br>**F** Abdominal Artery<br>**P** Pulmonary Trunk<br>**Q** Pulmonary Artery, Right<br>**R** Pulmonary Artery, Left<br>**W** Aorta |
| **P** Pulmonary Trunk<br>**Q** Pulmonary Artery, Right<br>**R** Pulmonary Artery, Left | **Ø** Open<br>**4** Percutaneous Endoscopic | **8** Zooplastic Tissue<br>**9** Autologous Venous Tissue<br>**A** Autologous Arterial Tissue<br>**J** Synthetic Substitute<br>**K** Nonautologous Tissue Substitute<br>**Z** No Device | **A** Innominate Artery<br>**B** Subclavian<br>**D** Carotid |
| **W** Thoracic Aorta, Descending | **Ø** Open | **8** Zooplastic Tissue<br>**9** Autologous Venous Tissue<br>**A** Autologous Arterial Tissue<br>**Z** No Device | **B** Subclavian<br>**D** Carotid<br>**P** Pulmonary Trunk<br>**Q** Pulmonary Artery, Right<br>**R** Pulmonary Artery, Left |
| **W** Thoracic Aorta, Descending | **Ø** Open | **J** Synthetic Substitute<br>**K** Nonautologous Tissue Substitute | **B** Subclavian<br>**D** Carotid<br>**G** Axillary Artery<br>**H** Brachial Artery<br>**P** Pulmonary Trunk<br>**Q** Pulmonary Artery, Right<br>**R** Pulmonary Artery, Left |
| **W** Thoracic Aorta, Descending | **4** Percutaneous Endoscopic | **8** Zooplastic Tissue<br>**9** Autologous Venous Tissue<br>**A** Autologous Arterial Tissue<br>**J** Synthetic Substitute<br>**K** Nonautologous Tissue Substitute<br>**Z** No Device | **B** Subclavian<br>**D** Carotid<br>**P** Pulmonary Trunk<br>**Q** Pulmonary Artery, Right<br>**R** Pulmonary Artery, Left |
| **X** Thoracic Aorta, Ascending/Arch<br>Aortic arch<br>Ascending aorta | **Ø** Open<br>**4** Percutaneous Endoscopic | **8** Zooplastic Tissue<br>**9** Autologous Venous Tissue<br>**A** Autologous Arterial Tissue<br>**J** Synthetic Substitute<br>**K** Nonautologous Tissue Substitute<br>**Z** No Device | **B** Subclavian<br>**D** Carotid<br>**P** Pulmonary Trunk<br>**Q** Pulmonary Artery, Right<br>**R** Pulmonary Artery, Left |

**Ø Medical and Surgical**
**2 Heart and Great Vessels**
**4 Creation** Definition: Putting in or on biological or synthetic material to form a new body part that to the extent possible replicates the anatomic structure or function of an absent body part

Explanation: Used for gender reassignment surgery and corrective procedures in individuals with congenital anomalies

| Body Part Character 4 | Approach Character 5 | Device Character 6 | Qualifier Character 7 |
|---|---|---|---|
| **F** Aortic Valve<br>Aortic annulus | **Ø** Open | **7** Autologous Tissue<br>**8** Zooplastic Tissue<br>**J** Synthetic Substitute<br>**K** Nonautologous Tissue Substitute | **J** Truncal Valve |
| **G** Mitral Valve<br>Bicuspid valve<br>Left atrioventricular valve<br>Mitral annulus<br>**J** Tricuspid Valve<br>Right atrioventricular valve<br>Tricuspid annulus | **Ø** Open | **7** Autologous Tissue<br>**8** Zooplastic Tissue<br>**J** Synthetic Substitute<br>**K** Nonautologous Tissue Substitute | **2** Common Atrioventricular Valve |

**Ø Medical and Surgical**
**2 Heart and Great Vessels**
**5 Destruction** Definition: Physical eradication of all or a portion of a body part by the direct use of energy, force, or a destructive agent
Explanation: None of the body part is physically taken out

| Body Part Character 4 | Approach Character 5 | Device Character 6 | Qualifier Character 7 |
|---|---|---|---|
| **4 Coronary Vein**<br>**5 Atrial Septum**<br>Interatrial septum<br>**6 Atrium, Right**<br>Atrium dextrum cordis<br>Right auricular appendix<br>Sinus venosus<br>**8 Conduction Mechanism**<br>Atrioventricular node<br>Bundle of His<br>Bundle of Kent<br>Sinoatrial node<br>**9 Chordae Tendineae**<br>**D Papillary Muscle**<br>**F Aortic Valve**<br>Aortic annulus<br>**G Mitral Valve**<br>Bicuspid valve<br>Left atrioventricular valve<br>Mitral annulus<br>**H Pulmonary Valve**<br>Pulmonary annulus<br>Pulmonic valve<br>**J Tricuspid Valve**<br>Right atrioventricular valve<br>Tricuspid annulus<br>**K Ventricle, Right**<br>Conus arteriosus<br>**L Ventricle, Left**<br>**M Ventricular Septum**<br>Interventricular septum<br>**N Pericardium**<br>**P Pulmonary Trunk**<br>**Q Pulmonary Artery, Right**<br>**R Pulmonary Artery, Left**<br>Arterial canal (duct)<br>Botallo's duct<br>Pulmoaortic canal<br>**S Pulmonary Vein, Right**<br>Right inferior pulmonary vein<br>Right superior pulmonary vein<br>**T Pulmonary Vein, Left**<br>Left inferior pulmonary vein<br>Left superior pulmonary vein<br>**V Superior Vena Cava**<br>Precava<br>**W Thoracic Aorta, Descending**<br>**X Thoracic Aorta, Ascending/Arch**<br>Aortic arch<br>Ascending aorta | **Ø Open**<br>**3 Percutaneous**<br>**4 Percutaneous Endoscopic** | **Z No Device** | **Z No Qualifier** |
| **7 Atrium, Left**<br>Atrium pulmonale<br>Left auricular appendix | **Ø Open**<br>**3 Percutaneous**<br>**4 Percutaneous Endoscopic** | **Z No Device** | **K Left Atrial Appendage**<br>**Z No Qualifier** |

DRG Non-OR Ø257[Ø,3,4]ZK

**Ø Medical and Surgical**
**2 Heart and Great Vessels**
**7 Dilation** Definition: Expanding an orifice or the lumen of a tubular body part

Explanation: The orifice can be a natural orifice or an artificially created orifice. Accomplished by stretching a tubular body part using intraluminal pressure or by cutting part of the orifice or wall of the tubular body part.

| Body Part Character 4 | Approach Character 5 | Device Character 6 | Qualifier Character 7 |
|---|---|---|---|
| **Ø** Coronary Artery, One Artery<br>**1** Coronary Artery, Two Arteries<br>**2** Coronary Artery, Three Arteries<br>**3** Coronary Artery, Four or More Arteries | **Ø** Open<br>**3** Percutaneous<br>**4** Percutaneous Endoscopic | **4** Intraluminal Device, Drug-eluting<br>**5** Intraluminal Device, Drug-eluting, Two<br>**6** Intraluminal Device, Drug-eluting, Three<br>**7** Intraluminal Device, Drug-eluting, Four or More<br>**D** Intraluminal Device<br>**E** Intraluminal Device, Two<br>**F** Intraluminal Device, Three<br>**G** Intraluminal Device, Four or More<br>**T** Intraluminal Device, Radioactive<br>**Z** No Device | **6** Bifurcation<br>**Z** No Qualifier |
| **F** Aortic Valve<br>Aortic annulus<br>**G** Mitral Valve<br>Bicuspid valve<br>Left atrioventricular valve<br>Mitral annulus<br>**H** Pulmonary Valve<br>Pulmonary annulus<br>Pulmonic valve<br>**J** Tricuspid Valve<br>Right atrioventricular valve<br>Tricuspid annulus<br>**K** Ventricle, Right<br>Conus arteriosus<br>**L** Ventricle, Left<br>**P** Pulmonary Trunk<br>**Q** Pulmonary Artery, Right<br>**S** Pulmonary Vein, Right<br>Right inferior pulmonary vein<br>Right superior pulmonary vein<br>**T** Pulmonary Vein, Left<br>Left inferior pulmonary vein<br>Left superior pulmonary vein<br>**V** Superior Vena Cava<br>Precava<br>**W** Thoracic Aorta, Descending<br>**X** Thoracic Aorta, Ascending/Arch<br>Aortic arch<br>Ascending aorta | **Ø** Open<br>**3** Percutaneous<br>**4** Percutaneous Endoscopic | **4** Intraluminal Device, Drug-eluting<br>**D** Intraluminal Device<br>**Z** No Device | **Z** No Qualifier |
| **R** Pulmonary Artery, Left<br>Arterial canal (duct)<br>Botallo's duct<br>Pulmoaortic canal | **Ø** Open<br>**3** Percutaneous<br>**4** Percutaneous Endoscopic | **4** Intraluminal Device, Drug-eluting<br>**D** Intraluminal Device<br>**Z** No Device | **T** Ductus Arteriosus<br>**Z** No Qualifier |

**Ø Medical and Surgical**
**2 Heart and Great Vessels**
**8 Division** Definition: Cutting into a body part, without draining fluids and/or gases from the body part, in order to separate or transect a body part

Explanation: All or a portion of the body part is separated into two or more portions

| Body Part Character 4 | Approach Character 5 | Device Character 6 | Qualifier Character 7 |
|---|---|---|---|
| **8** Conduction Mechanism<br>Atrioventricular node<br>Bundle of His<br>Bundle of Kent<br>Sinoatrial node<br>**9** Chordae Tendineae<br>**D** Papillary Muscle | **Ø** Open<br>**3** Percutaneous<br>**4** Percutaneous Endoscopic | **Z** No Device | **Z** No Qualifier |

**Ø Medical and Surgical**
**2 Heart and Great Vessels**
**B Excision** Definition: Cutting out or off, without replacement, a portion of a body part
Explanation: The qualifier DIAGNOSTIC is used to identify excision procedures that are biopsies

| Body Part Character 4 | Approach Character 5 | Device Character 6 | Qualifier Character 7 |
|---|---|---|---|
| **4 Coronary Vein**<br>**5 Atrial Septum**<br>Interatrial septum<br>**6 Atrium, Right**<br>Atrium dextrum cordis<br>Right auricular appendix<br>Sinus venosus<br>**8 Conduction Mechanism**<br>Atrioventricular node<br>Bundle of His<br>Bundle of Kent<br>Sinoatrial node<br>**9 Chordae Tendineae**<br>**D Papillary Muscle**<br>**F Aortic Valve**<br>Aortic annulus<br>**G Mitral Valve**<br>Bicuspid valve<br>Left atrioventricular valve<br>Mitral annulus<br>**H Pulmonary Valve**<br>Pulmonary annulus<br>Pulmonic valve<br>**J Tricuspid Valve**<br>Right atrioventricular valve<br>Tricuspid annulus<br>**K Ventricle, Right** NC<br>Conus arteriosus<br>**L Ventricle, Left** NC<br>**M Ventricular Septum**<br>Interventricular septum<br>**N Pericardium**<br>**P Pulmonary Trunk**<br>**Q Pulmonary Artery, Right**<br>**R Pulmonary Artery, Left**<br>Arterial canal (duct)<br>Botallo's duct<br>Pulmoaortic canal<br>**S Pulmonary Vein, Right**<br>Right inferior pulmonary vein<br>Right superior pulmonary vein<br>**T Pulmonary Vein, Left**<br>Left inferior pulmonary vein<br>Left superior pulmonary vein<br>**V Superior Vena Cava**<br>Precava<br>**W Thoracic Aorta, Descending**<br>**X Thoracic Aorta, Ascending/Arch**<br>Aortic arch<br>Ascending aorta | **Ø Open**<br>**3 Percutaneous**<br>**4 Percutaneous Endoscopic** | **Z No Device** | **X Diagnostic**<br>**Z No Qualifier** |
| **7 Atrium, Left**<br>Atrium pulmonale<br>Left auricular appendix | **Ø Open**<br>**3 Percutaneous**<br>**4 Percutaneous Endoscopic** | **Z No Device** | **K Left Atrial Appendage**<br>**X Diagnostic**<br>**Z No Qualifier** |

**DRG Non-OR** Ø2B7[Ø,3,4]ZK
**Non-OR** Ø2B[4,5,6,7,8,9,D,F,G,H,J,K,L,M][Ø,3,4]ZX
NC Ø2B[K,L][Ø,3,4]ZZ

**Ø Medical and Surgical**
**2 Heart and Great Vessels**
**C Extirpation** Definition: Taking or cutting out solid matter from a body part

Explanation: The solid matter may be an abnormal byproduct of a biological function or a foreign body; it may be imbedded in a body part or in the lumen of a tubular body part. The solid matter may or may not have been previously broken into pieces.

| Body Part Character 4 | Approach Character 5 | Device Character 6 | Qualifier Character 7 |
|---|---|---|---|
| **Ø Coronary Artery, One Artery**<br>**1 Coronary Artery, Two Arteries**<br>**2 Coronary Artery, Three Arteries**<br>**3 Coronary Artery, Four or More Arteries** | **Ø Open**<br>**3 Percutaneous**<br>**4 Percutaneous Endoscopic** | **Z No Device** | **6 Bifurcation**<br>**Z No Qualifier** |
| **4 Coronary Vein**<br>**5 Atrial Septum**<br>Interatrial septum<br>**6 Atrium, Right**<br>Atrium dextrum cordis<br>Right auricular appendix<br>Sinus venosus<br>**7 Atrium, Left**<br>Atrium pulmonale<br>Left auricular appendix<br>**8 Conduction Mechanism**<br>Atrioventricular node<br>Bundle of His<br>Bundle of Kent<br>Sinoatrial node<br>**9 Chordae Tendineae**<br>**D Papillary Muscle**<br>**F Aortic Valve**<br>Aortic annulus<br>**G Mitral Valve**<br>Bicuspid valve<br>Left atrioventricular valve<br>Mitral annulus<br>**H Pulmonary Valve**<br>Pulmonary annulus<br>Pulmonic valve<br>**J Tricuspid Valve**<br>Right atrioventricular valve<br>Tricuspid annulus<br>**K Ventricle, Right**<br>Conus arteriosus<br>**L Ventricle, Left**<br>**M Ventricular Septum**<br>Interventricular septum<br>**N Pericardium**<br>**P Pulmonary Trunk**<br>**Q Pulmonary Artery, Right**<br>**R Pulmonary Artery, Left**<br>Arterial canal (duct)<br>Botallo's duct<br>Pulmoaortic canal<br>**S Pulmonary Vein, Right**<br>Right inferior pulmonary vein<br>Right superior pulmonary vein<br>**T Pulmonary Vein, Left**<br>Left inferior pulmonary vein<br>Left superior pulmonary vein<br>**V Superior Vena Cava**<br>Precava<br>**W Thoracic Aorta, Descending**<br>**X Thoracic Aorta, Ascending/Arch**<br>Aortic arch<br>Ascending aorta | **Ø Open**<br>**3 Percutaneous**<br>**4 Percutaneous Endoscopic** | **Z No Device** | **Z No Qualifier** |

**Ø Medical and Surgical**
**2 Heart and Great Vessels**
**F Fragmentation** Definition: Breaking solid matter in a body part into pieces

Explanation: Physical force (e.g., manual, ultrasonic) applied directly or indirectly is used to break the solid matter into pieces. The solid matter may be an abnormal byproduct of a biological function or a foreign body. The pieces of solid matter are not taken out.

| Body Part Character 4 | Approach Character 5 | Device Character 6 | Qualifier Character 7 |
|---|---|---|---|
| **N Pericardium** NC | **Ø Open**<br>**3 Percutaneous**<br>**4 Percutaneous Endoscopic**<br>**X External** | **Z No Device** | **Z No Qualifier** |

Non-OR Ø2FNXZZ
NC Ø2FNXZZ

**Ø Medical and Surgical**
**2 Heart and Great Vessels**
**H Insertion** Definition: Putting in a nonbiological appliance that monitors, assists, performs, or prevents a physiological function but does not physically take the place of a body part

Explanation: None

| Body Part Character 4 | Approach Character 5 | Device Character 6 | Qualifier Character 7 |
|---|---|---|---|
| **4** Coronary Vein ⊞<br>**6** Atrium, Right ⊞<br>Atrium dextrum cordis<br>Right auricular appendix<br>Sinus venosus<br>**7** Atrium, Left ⊞<br>Atrium pulmonale<br>Left auricular appendix<br>**K** Ventricle, Right ⊞<br>Conus arteriosus<br>**L** Ventricle, Left ⊞ | **Ø** Open<br>**3** Percutaneous<br>**4** Percutaneous Endoscopic | **Ø** Monitoring Device, Pressure Sensor<br>**2** Monitoring Device<br>**3** Infusion Device<br>**D** Intraluminal Device<br>**J** Cardiac Lead, Pacemaker<br>**K** Cardiac Lead, Defibrillator<br>**M** Cardiac Lead<br>**N** Intracardiac Pacemaker<br>**Y** Other Device | **Z** No Qualifier |
| **A** Heart LC NC | **Ø** Open<br>**3** Percutaneous<br>**4** Percutaneous Endoscopic | **Q** Implantable Heart Assist System<br>**Y** Other Device | **Z** No Qualifier |
| **A** Heart ⊞ | **Ø** Open<br>**3** Percutaneous<br>**4** Percutaneous Endoscopic | **R** Short-term External Heart Assist System | **J** Intraoperative<br>**S** Biventricular<br>**Z** No Qualifier |
| **N** Pericardium ⊞ | **Ø** Open<br>**3** Percutaneous<br>**4** Percutaneous Endoscopic | **Ø** Monitoring Device, Pressure Sensor<br>**2** Monitoring Device<br>**J** Cardiac Lead, Pacemaker<br>**K** Cardiac Lead, Defibrillator<br>**M** Cardiac Lead<br>**Y** Other Device | **Z** No Qualifier |
| **P** Pulmonary Trunk<br>**Q** Pulmonary Artery, Right<br>**R** Pulmonary Artery, Left<br>Arterial canal (duct)<br>Botallo's duct<br>Pulmoaortic canal<br>**S** Pulmonary Vein, Right<br>Right inferior pulmonary vein<br>Right superior pulmonary vein<br>**T** Pulmonary Vein, Left<br>Left inferior pulmonary vein<br>Left superior pulmonary vein<br>**V** Superior Vena Cava<br>Precava<br>**W** Thoracic Aorta, Descending | **Ø** Open<br>**3** Percutaneous<br>**4** Percutaneous Endoscopic | **Ø** Monitoring Device, Pressure Sensor<br>**2** Monitoring Device<br>**3** Infusion Device<br>**D** Intraluminal Device<br>**Y** Other Device | **Z** No Qualifier |
| **X** Thoracic Aorta, Ascending/Arch<br>Aortic arch<br>Ascending aorta | **Ø** Open<br>**3** Percutaneous<br>**4** Percutaneous Endoscopic | **Ø** Monitoring Device, Pressure Sensor<br>**2** Monitoring Device<br>**3** Infusion Device<br>**D** Intraluminal Device | **Z** No Qualifier |

DRG Non-OR Ø2H[4,6,7][Ø,4][J,M]Z
DRG Non-OR Ø2H[6,7]3JZ
DRG Non-OR Ø2H[K,L][Ø,3,4][J,M]Z
DRG Non-OR Ø2HK32Z
DRG Non-OR Ø2HN32Z
Non-OR Ø2H[4,6,7,L]3[2,3,D]Z
Non-OR Ø2HK3[3,D]Z
Non-OR Ø2H[4,6,7,K,L][3,4]YZ
Non-OR Ø2HA[3,4]YZ
Non-OR Ø2HN[3,4]YZ
Non-OR Ø2HP[Ø,3,4][Ø,2,3,Y]Z
Non-OR Ø2HP3DZ
Non-OR Ø2H[Q,R][Ø,3,4][2,3]Z
Non-OR Ø2H[Q,R]3DZ
Non-OR Ø2H[Q,R][3,4]YZ
Non-OR Ø2H[S,T,V][Ø,4]3Z
Non-OR Ø2H[S,T,V]3[2,3,D]Z
Non-OR Ø2H[S,T,V][3,4]YZ
Non-OR Ø2HW[Ø,4][Ø,3]Z
Non-OR Ø2HW3[Ø,2,3,D]Z
Non-OR Ø2HW[Ø,3,4]YZ
Non-OR Ø2HX[Ø,3,4][Ø,3]Z

HAC Ø2H43[J,K,M]Z when reported with SDx K68.11 or T81.4XXA or T82.6XXA or T82.7XXA
HAC Ø2H[6,K]33Z when reported with SDx J95.811
HAC Ø2H[6,7]3[J,M]Z when reported with SDx K68.11 or T81.4XXA or T82.6XXA or T82.7XXA
HAC Ø2H[K,L]3JZ when reported with SDx K68.11 or T81.4XXA or T82.6XXA or T82.7XXA
HAC Ø2HN[Ø,3,4][J,M]Z when reported with SDx K68.11 or T81.4XXA or T82.6XXA or T82.7XXA
HAC Ø2H[S,T,V][3,4]3Z when reported with SDx J95.811
LC Ø2HAØQZ
NC Ø2HA[3,4]QZ

**See Appendix L for Procedure Combinations**

⊞ Ø2H[4,6,7,K,L][Ø,3,4]KZ
⊞ Ø2H43[J,M]Z
⊞ Ø2HA[Ø,4]R[S,Z]
⊞ Ø2HA3RS
⊞ Ø2HN[Ø,3,4][J,K,M]Z

**Ø Medical and Surgical**
**2 Heart and Great Vessels**
**J Inspection** Definition: Visually and/or manually exploring a body part

Explanation: Visual exploration may be performed with or without optical instrumentation. Manual exploration may be performed directly or through intervening body layers.

| Body Part Character 4 | Approach Character 5 | Device Character 6 | Qualifier Character 7 |
|---|---|---|---|
| **A** Heart<br>**Y** Great Vessel | **Ø** Open<br>**3** Percutaneous<br>**4** Percutaneous Endoscopic | **Z** No Device | **Z** No Qualifier |

Non-OR Ø2J[A,Y]3ZZ

**Ø Medical and Surgical**
**2 Heart and Great Vessels**
**K Map** Definition: Locating the route of passage of electrical impulses and/or locating functional areas in a body part

Explanation: Applicable only to the cardiac conduction mechanism and the central nervous system

| Body Part Character 4 | Approach Character 5 | Device Character 6 | Qualifier Character 7 |
|---|---|---|---|
| **8** Conduction Mechanism<br>Atrioventricular node<br>Bundle of His<br>Bundle of Kent<br>Sinoatrial node | **Ø** Open<br>**3** Percutaneous<br>**4** Percutaneous Endoscopic | **Z** No Device | **Z** No Qualifier |

DRG Non-OR Ø2K8[Ø,3,4]ZZ

**Ø Medical and Surgical**
**2 Heart and Great Vessels**
**L Occlusion** Definition: Completely closing an orifice or the lumen of a tubular body part

Explanation: The orifice can be a natural orifice or an artificially created orifice

| Body Part Character 4 | Approach Character 5 | Device Character 6 | Qualifier Character 7 |
|---|---|---|---|
| **7** Atrium, Left<br>Atrium pulmonale<br>Left auricular appendix | **Ø** Open<br>**3** Percutaneous<br>**4** Percutaneous Endoscopic | **C** Extraluminal Device<br>**D** Intraluminal Device<br>**Z** No Device | **K** Left Atrial Appendage |
| **H** Pulmonary Valve<br>Pulmonary annulus<br>Pulmonic valve<br>**P** Pulmonary Trunk<br>**Q** Pulmonary Artery, Right<br>**S** Pulmonary Vein, Right<br>Right inferior pulmonary vein<br>Right superior pulmonary vein<br>**T** Pulmonary Vein, Left<br>Left inferior pulmonary vein<br>Left superior pulmonary vein<br>**V** Superior Vena Cava<br>Precava | **Ø** Open<br>**3** Percutaneous<br>**4** Percutaneous Endoscopic | **C** Extraluminal Device<br>**D** Intraluminal Device<br>**Z** No Device | **Z** No Qualifier |
| **R** Pulmonary Artery, Left<br>Arterial canal (duct)<br>Botallo's duct<br>Pulmoaortic canal | **Ø** Open<br>**3** Percutaneous<br>**4** Percutaneous Endoscopic | **C** Extraluminal Device<br>**D** Intraluminal Device<br>**Z** No Device | **T** Ductus Arteriosus<br>**Z** No Qualifier |
| **W** Thoracic Aorta, Descending | **3** Percutaneous | **D** Intraluminal Device | **J** Temporary |

DRG Non-OR Ø2L7[Ø,3,4][C,D,Z]K

**Ø Medical and Surgical**
**2 Heart and Great Vessels**
**N Release** Definition: Freeing a body part from an abnormal physical constraint by cutting or by the use of force

Explanation: Some of the restraining tissue may be taken out but none of the body part is taken out

| Body Part Character 4 | Approach Character 5 | Device Character 6 | Qualifier Character 7 |
|---|---|---|---|
| Ø Coronary Artery, One Artery<br>1 Coronary Artery, Two Arteries<br>2 Coronary Artery, Three Arteries<br>3 Coronary Artery, Four or More Arteries<br>**4 Coronary Vein**<br>**5 Atrial Septum**<br>Interatrial septum<br>**6 Atrium, Right**<br>Atrium dextrum cordis<br>Right auricular appendix<br>Sinus venosus<br>**7 Atrium, Left**<br>Atrium pulmonale<br>Left auricular appendix<br>**8 Conduction Mechanism**<br>Atrioventricular node<br>Bundle of His<br>Bundle of Kent<br>Sinoatrial node<br>**9 Chordae Tendineae**<br>**D Papillary Muscle**<br>**F Aortic Valve**<br>Aortic annulus<br>**G Mitral Valve**<br>Bicuspid valve<br>Left atrioventricular valve<br>Mitral annulus<br>**H Pulmonary Valve**<br>Pulmonary annulus<br>Pulmonic valve<br>**J Tricuspid Valve**<br>Right atrioventricular valve<br>Tricuspid annulus<br>**K Ventricle, Right**<br>Conus arteriosus<br>**L Ventricle, Left**<br>**M Ventricular Septum**<br>Interventricular septum<br>**N Pericardium**<br>**P Pulmonary Trunk**<br>**Q Pulmonary Artery, Right**<br>**R Pulmonary Artery, Left**<br>Arterial canal (duct)<br>Botallo's duct<br>Pulmoaortic canal<br>**S Pulmonary Vein, Right**<br>Right inferior pulmonary vein<br>Right superior pulmonary vein<br>**T Pulmonary Vein, Left**<br>Left inferior pulmonary vein<br>Left superior pulmonary vein<br>**V Superior Vena Cava**<br>Precava<br>**W Thoracic Aorta, Descending**<br>**X Thoracic Aorta, Ascending/Arch**<br>Aortic arch<br>Ascending aorta | **Ø Open**<br>**3 Percutaneous**<br>**4 Percutaneous Endoscopic** | **Z No Device** | **Z No Qualifier** |

**Ø Medical and Surgical**
**2 Heart and Great Vessels**
**P Removal** Definition: Taking out or off a device from a body part

Explanation: If a device is taken out and a similar device put in without cutting or puncturing the skin or mucous membrane, the procedure is coded to the root operation CHANGE. Otherwise, the procedure for taking out a device is coded to the root operation REMOVAL.

| Body Part Character 4 | Approach Character 5 | Device Character 6 | Qualifier Character 7 |
|---|---|---|---|
| A Heart | Ø Open<br>3 Percutaneous<br>4 Percutaneous Endoscopic | 2 Monitoring Device<br>3 Infusion Device<br>7 Autologous Tissue Substitute<br>8 Zooplastic Tissue<br>C Extraluminal Device<br>D Intraluminal Device<br>J Synthetic Substitute<br>K Nonautologous Tissue Substitute<br>M Cardiac Lead<br>N Intracardiac Pacemaker<br>Q Implantable Heart Assist System<br>Y Other Device | Z No Qualifier |
| A Heart ⊞ | Ø Open<br>3 Percutaneous<br>4 Percutaneous Endoscopic | R Short-term External Heart Assist System | S Biventricular<br>Z No Qualifier |
| A Heart | X External | 2 Monitoring Device<br>3 Infusion Device<br>D Intraluminal Device<br>M Cardiac Lead | Z No Qualifier |
| Y Great Vessel | Ø Open<br>3 Percutaneous<br>4 Percutaneous Endoscopic | 2 Monitoring Device<br>3 Infusion Device<br>7 Autologous Tissue Substitute<br>8 Zooplastic Tissue<br>C Extraluminal Device<br>D Intraluminal Device<br>J Synthetic Substitute<br>K Nonautologous Tissue Substitute<br>Y Other Device | Z No Qualifier |
| Y Great Vessel | X External | 2 Monitoring Device<br>3 Infusion Device<br>D Intraluminal Device | Z No Qualifier |

Non-OR Ø2PA3[2,3,D]Z
Non-OR Ø2PA[3,4]YZ
Non-OR Ø2PAX[2,3,D,M]Z
Non-OR Ø2PY3[2,3,D]Z
Non-OR Ø2PY[3,4]YZ
Non-OR Ø2PYX[2,3,D]Z
HAC Ø2PA[Ø,3,4]MZ when reported with SDx K68.11 or T81.4XXA or T82.6XXA or T82.7XXA
HAC Ø2PAXMZ when reported with SDx K68.11 or T81.4XXA or T82.6XXA or T82.7XXA

**See Appendix L for Procedure Combinations**
⊞ Ø2PA[Ø,3,4]RZ

**Ø Medical and Surgical**
**2 Heart and Great Vessels**
**Q Repair** Definition: Restoring, to the extent possible, a body part to its normal anatomic structure and function
Explanation: Used only when the method to accomplish the repair is not one of the other root operations

| Body Part Character 4 | Approach Character 5 | Device Character 6 | Qualifier Character 7 |
|---|---|---|---|
| **Ø Coronary Artery, One Artery**<br>**1 Coronary Artery, Two Arteries**<br>**2 Coronary Artery, Three Arteries**<br>**3 Coronary Artery, Four or More Arteries**<br>**4 Coronary Vein**<br>**5 Atrial Septum**<br>Interatrial septum<br>**6 Atrium, Right**<br>Atrium dextrum cordis<br>Right auricular appendix<br>Sinus venosus<br>**7 Atrium, Left**<br>Atrium pulmonale<br>Left auricular appendix<br>**8 Conduction Mechanism**<br>Atrioventricular node<br>Bundle of His<br>Bundle of Kent<br>Sinoatrial node<br>**9 Chordae Tendineae**<br>**A Heart**<br>**B Heart, Right**<br>Right coronary sulcus<br>**C Heart, Left**<br>Left coronary sulcus<br>Obtuse margin<br>**D Papillary Muscle**<br>**H Pulmonary Valve**<br>Pulmonary annulus<br>Pulmonic valve<br>**K Ventricle, Right**<br>Conus arteriosus<br>**L Ventricle, Left**<br>**M Ventricular Septum**<br>Interventricular septum<br>**N Pericardium**<br>**P Pulmonary Trunk**<br>**Q Pulmonary Artery, Right**<br>**R Pulmonary Artery, Left**<br>Arterial canal (duct)<br>Botallo's duct<br>Pulmoaortic canal<br>**S Pulmonary Vein, Right**<br>Right inferior pulmonary vein<br>Right superior pulmonary vein<br>**T Pulmonary Vein, Left**<br>Left inferior pulmonary vein<br>Left superior pulmonary vein<br>**V Superior Vena Cava**<br>Precava<br>**W Thoracic Aorta, Descending**<br>**X Thoracic Aorta, Ascending/Arch**<br>Aortic arch<br>Ascending aorta | **Ø Open**<br>**3 Percutaneous**<br>**4 Percutaneous Endoscopic** | **Z No Device** | **Z No Qualifier** |
| **F Aortic Valve**<br>Aortic annulus | **Ø Open**<br>**3 Percutaneous**<br>**4 Percutaneous Endoscopic** | **Z No Device** | **J Truncal Valve**<br>**Z No Qualifier** |
| **G Mitral Valve**<br>Bicuspid valve<br>Left atrioventricular valve<br>Mitral annulus | **Ø Open**<br>**3 Percutaneous**<br>**4 Percutaneous Endoscopic** | **Z No Device** | **E Atrioventricular Valve, Left**<br>**Z No Qualifier** |
| **J Tricuspid Valve**<br>Right atrioventricular valve<br>Tricuspid annulus | **Ø Open**<br>**3 Percutaneous**<br>**4 Percutaneous Endoscopic** | **Z No Device** | **G Atrioventricular Valve, Right**<br>**Z No Qualifier** |

**Ø Medical and Surgical**
**2 Heart and Great Vessels**
**R Replacement** Definition: Putting in or on biological or synthetic material that physically takes the place and/or function of all or a portion of a body part

Explanation: The body part may have been taken out or replaced, or may be taken out, physically eradicated, or rendered nonfunctional during the REPLACEMENT procedure. A REMOVAL procedure is coded for taking out the device used in a previous replacement procedure.

| Body Part Character 4 | Approach Character 5 | Device Character 6 | Qualifier Character 7 |
|---|---|---|---|
| **5 Atrial Septum**<br>Interatrial septum<br>**6 Atrium, Right**<br>Atrium dextrum cordis<br>Right auricular appendix<br>Sinus venosus<br>**7 Atrium, Left**<br>Atrium pulmonale<br>Left auricular appendix<br>**9 Chordae Tendineae**<br>**D Papillary Muscle**<br>**K Ventricle, Right** ⊞ LC NC<br>Conus arteriosus<br>**L Ventricle, Left** ⊞ LC NC<br>**M Ventricular Septum**<br>Interventricular septum<br>**N Pericardium**<br>**P Pulmonary Trunk**<br>**Q Pulmonary Artery, Right**<br>**R Pulmonary Artery, Left**<br>Arterial canal (duct)<br>Botallo's duct<br>Pulmoaortic canal<br>**S Pulmonary Vein, Right**<br>Right inferior pulmonary vein<br>Right superior pulmonary vein<br>**T Pulmonary Vein, Left**<br>Left inferior pulmonary vein<br>Left superior pulmonary vein<br>**V Superior Vena Cava**<br>Precava<br>**W Thoracic Aorta, Descending**<br>**X Thoracic Aorta, Ascending/Arch**<br>Aortic arch<br>Ascending aorta | **Ø Open**<br>**4 Percutaneous Endoscopic** | **7 Autologous Tissue Substitute**<br>**8 Zooplastic Tissue**<br>**J Synthetic Substitute**<br>**K Nonautologous Tissue Substitute** | **Z No Qualifier** |
| **F Aortic Valve**<br>Aortic annulus<br>**G Mitral Valve**<br>Bicuspid valve<br>Left atrioventricular valve<br>Mitral annulus<br>**H Pulmonary Valve**<br>Pulmonary annulus<br>Pulmonic valve<br>**J Tricuspid Valve**<br>Right atrioventricular valve<br>Tricuspid annulus | **Ø Open**<br>**4 Percutaneous Endoscopic** | **7 Autologous Tissue Substitute**<br>**8 Zooplastic Tissue**<br>**J Synthetic Substitute**<br>**K Nonautologous Tissue Substitute** | **Z No Qualifier** |
| **F Aortic Valve**<br>Aortic annulus<br>**G Mitral Valve**<br>Bicuspid valve<br>Left atrioventricular valve<br>Mitral annulus<br>**H Pulmonary Valve**<br>Pulmonary annulus<br>Pulmonic valve<br>**J Tricuspid Valve**<br>Right atrioventricular valve<br>Tricuspid annulus | **3 Percutaneous** | **7 Autologous Tissue Substitute**<br>**8 Zooplastic Tissue**<br>**J Synthetic Substitute**<br>**K Nonautologous Tissue Substitute** | **H Transapical**<br>**Z No Qualifier** |

LC Ø2RKØJZ with Ø2RLØJZ with diagnosis code ZØØ.6
NC Ø2RKØJZ with Ø2RLØJZ without diagnosis code ZØØ.6

**See Appendix L for Procedure Combinations**
⊞ Ø2R[K,L]ØJZ

**Ø Medical and Surgical**
**2 Heart and Great Vessels**
**S Reposition** Definition: Moving to its normal location, or other suitable location, all or a portion of a body part

Explanation: The body part is moved to a new location from an abnormal location, or from a normal location where it is not functioning correctly. The body part may or may not be cut out or off to be moved to the new location.

| Body Part Character 4 | Approach Character 5 | Device Character 6 | Qualifier Character 7 |
|---|---|---|---|
| **Ø Coronary Artery, One Artery**<br>**1 Coronary Artery, Two Arteries**<br>**P Pulmonary Trunk**<br>**Q Pulmonary Artery, Right**<br>**R Pulmonary Artery, Left**<br>Arterial canal (duct)<br>Botallo's duct<br>Pulmoaortic canal<br>**S Pulmonary Vein, Right**<br>Right inferior pulmonary vein<br>Right superior pulmonary vein<br>**T Pulmonary Vein, Left**<br>Left inferior pulmonary vein<br>Left superior pulmonary vein<br>**V Superior Vena Cava**<br>Precava<br>**W Thoracic Aorta, Descending**<br>**X Thoracic Aorta, Ascending/Arch**<br>Aortic arch<br>Ascending aorta | **Ø Open** | **Z No Device** | **Z No Qualifier** |

**Ø Medical and Surgical**
**2 Heart and Great Vessels**
**T Resection** Definition: Cutting out or off, without replacement, all of a body part

Explanation: None

| Body Part Character 4 | Approach Character 5 | Device Character 6 | Qualifier Character 7 |
|---|---|---|---|
| **5 Atrial Septum**<br>Interatrial septum<br>**8 Conduction Mechanism**<br>Atrioventricular node<br>Bundle of His<br>Bundle of Kent<br>Sinoatrial node<br>**9 Chordae Tendineae**<br>**D Papillary Muscle**<br>**H Pulmonary Valve**<br>Pulmonary annulus<br>Pulmonic valve<br>**M Ventricular Septum**<br>Interventricular septum<br>**N Pericardium** | **Ø Open**<br>**3 Percutaneous**<br>**4 Percutaneous Endoscopic** | **Z No Device** | **Z No Qualifier** |

**Ø Medical and Surgical**
**2 Heart and Great Vessels**
**U Supplement** Definition: Putting in or on biological or synthetic material that physically reinforces and/or augments the function of a portion of a body part

Explanation: The biological material is non-living, or is living and from the same individual. The body part may have been previously replaced, and the SUPPLEMENT procedure is performed to physically reinforce and/or augment the function of the replaced body part.

| Body Part Character 4 | Approach Character 5 | Device Character 6 | Qualifier Character 7 |
|---|---|---|---|
| **5 Atrial Septum**<br>Interatrial septum<br>**6 Atrium, Right**<br>Atrium dextrum cordis<br>Right auricular appendix<br>Sinus venosus<br>**7 Atrium, Left**<br>Atrium pulmonale<br>Left auricular appendix<br>**9 Chordae Tendineae**<br>**A Heart**<br>**D Papillary Muscle**<br>**H Pulmonary Valve**<br>Pulmonary annulus<br>Pulmonic valve<br>**K Ventricle, Right**<br>Conus arteriosus<br>**L Ventricle, Left**<br>**M Ventricular Septum**<br>Interventricular septum<br>**N Pericardium**<br>**P Pulmonary Trunk**<br>**Q Pulmonary Artery, Right**<br>**R Pulmonary Artery, Left**<br>Arterial canal (duct)<br>Botallo's duct<br>Pulmoaortic canal<br>**S Pulmonary Vein, Right**<br>Right inferior pulmonary vein<br>Right superior pulmonary vein<br>**T Pulmonary Vein, Left**<br>Left inferior pulmonary vein<br>Left superior pulmonary vein<br>**V Superior Vena Cava**<br>Precava<br>**W Thoracic Aorta, Descending**<br>**X Thoracic Aorta, Ascending/Arch**<br>Aortic arch<br>Ascending aorta | **Ø Open**<br>**3 Percutaneous**<br>**4 Percutaneous Endoscopic** | **7 Autologous Tissue Substitute**<br>**8 Zooplastic Tissue**<br>**J Synthetic Substitute**<br>**K Nonautologous Tissue Substitute** | **Z No Qualifier** |
| **F Aortic Valve**<br>Aortic annulus | **Ø Open**<br>**3 Percutaneous**<br>**4 Percutaneous Endoscopic** | **7 Autologous Tissue Substitute**<br>**8 Zooplastic Tissue**<br>**J Synthetic Substitute**<br>**K Nonautologous Tissue Substitute** | **J Truncal Valve**<br>**Z No Qualifier** |
| **G Mitral Valve**<br>Bicuspid valve<br>Left atrioventricular valve<br>Mitral annulus | **Ø Open**<br>**3 Percutaneous**<br>**4 Percutaneous Endoscopic** | **7 Autologous Tissue Substitute**<br>**8 Zooplastic Tissue**<br>**J Synthetic Substitute**<br>**K Nonautologous Tissue Substitute** | **E Atrioventricular Valve, Left**<br>**Z No Qualifier** |
| **J Tricuspid Valve**<br>Right atrioventricular valve<br>Tricuspid annulus | **Ø Open**<br>**3 Percutaneous**<br>**4 Percutaneous Endoscopic** | **7 Autologous Tissue Substitute**<br>**8 Zooplastic Tissue**<br>**J Synthetic Substitute**<br>**K Nonautologous Tissue Substitute** | **G Atrioventricular Valve, Right**<br>**Z No Qualifier** |

DRG Non-OR Ø2U7[3,4]JZ

**Ø Medical and Surgical**
**2 Heart and Great Vessels**
**V Restriction** Definition: Partially closing an orifice or the lumen of a tubular body part
Explanation: The orifice can be a natural orifice or an artificially created orifice

| Body Part Character 4 | Approach Character 5 | Device Character 6 | Qualifier Character 7 |
|---|---|---|---|
| **A Heart** | **Ø Open**<br>**3 Percutaneous**<br>**4 Percutaneous Endoscopic** | **C Extraluminal Device**<br>**Z No Device** | **Z No Qualifier** |
| G Mitral Valve<br>Bicuspid valve<br>Left atrioventricular valve<br>Mitral annulus | Ø Open<br>3 Percutaneous<br>4 Percutaneous Endoscopic | Z No Device | Z No Qualifier |
| **P Pulmonary Trunk**<br>**Q Pulmonary Artery, Right**<br>**S Pulmonary Vein, Right**<br>Right inferior pulmonary vein<br>Right superior pulmonary vein<br>**T Pulmonary Vein, Left**<br>Left inferior pulmonary vein<br>Left superior pulmonary vein<br>**V Superior Vena Cava**<br>Precava | **Ø Open**<br>**3 Percutaneous**<br>**4 Percutaneous Endoscopic** | **C Extraluminal Device**<br>**D Intraluminal Device**<br>**Z No Device** | **Z No Qualifier** |
| **R Pulmonary Artery, Left**<br>Arterial canal (duct)<br>Botallo's duct<br>Pulmoaortic canal | **Ø Open**<br>**3 Percutaneous**<br>**4 Percutaneous Endoscopic** | **C Extraluminal Device**<br>**D Intraluminal Device**<br>**Z No Device** | **T Ductus Arteriosus**<br>**Z No Qualifier** |
| **W Thoracic Aorta, Descending**<br>**X Thoracic Aorta, Ascending/Arch**<br>Aortic arch<br>Ascending aorta | **Ø Open**<br>**3 Percutaneous**<br>**4 Percutaneous Endoscopic** | **C Extraluminal Device**<br>**D Intraluminal Device**<br>**E Intraluminal Device, Branched or Fenestrated, One or Two Arteries**<br>**F Intraluminal Device, Branched or Fenestrated, Three or More Arteries**<br>**Z No Device** | **Z No Qualifier** |

**Ø Medical and Surgical**
**2 Heart and Great Vessels**
**W Revision** Definition: Correcting, to the extent possible, a portion of a malfunctioning device or the position of a displaced device
Explanation: Revision can include correcting a malfunctioning or displaced device by taking out or putting in components of the device such as a screw or pin

| Body Part Character 4 | Approach Character 5 | Device Character 6 | Qualifier Character 7 |
|---|---|---|---|
| **5 Atrial Septum**<br>Interatrial septum<br>**M Ventricular Septum**<br>Interventricular septum | **Ø Open**<br>**4 Percutaneous Endoscopic** | **J Synthetic Substitute** | **Z No Qualifier** |
| **A Heart** ⊞ LC NC | **Ø Open**<br>**3 Percutaneous**<br>**4 Percutaneous Endoscopic** | **2 Monitoring Device**<br>**3 Infusion Device**<br>**7 Autologous Tissue Substitute**<br>**8 Zooplastic Tissue**<br>**C Extraluminal Device**<br>**D Intraluminal Device**<br>**J Synthetic Substitute**<br>**K Nonautologous Tissue Substitute**<br>**M Cardiac Lead**<br>**N Intracardiac Pacemaker**<br>**Q Implantable Heart Assist System**<br>Y Other Device | **Z No Qualifier** |
| A Heart ⊞ | Ø Open<br>3 Percutaneous<br>4 Percutaneous Endoscopic | R Short-term External Heart Assist System | S Biventricular<br>Z No Qualifier |
| **A Heart** | **X External** | **2 Monitoring Device**<br>**3 Infusion Device**<br>**7 Autologous Tissue Substitute**<br>**8 Zooplastic Tissue**<br>**C Extraluminal Device**<br>**D Intraluminal Device**<br>**J Synthetic Substitute**<br>**K Nonautologous Tissue Substitute**<br>**M Cardiac Lead**<br>**N Intracardiac Pacemaker**<br>**Q Implantable Heart Assist System** | **Z No Qualifier** |
| A Heart | X External | R Short-term External Heart Assist System | S Biventricular<br>Z No Qualifier |
| **F Aortic Valve**<br>Aortic annulus<br>**G Mitral Valve**<br>Bicuspid valve<br>Left atrioventricular valve<br>Mitral annulus<br>**H Pulmonary Valve**<br>Pulmonary annulus<br>Pulmonic valve<br>**J Tricuspid Valve**<br>Right atrioventricular valve<br>Tricuspid annulus | **Ø Open**<br>**3 Percutaneous**<br>**4 Percutaneous Endoscopic** | **7 Autologous Tissue Substitute**<br>**8 Zooplastic Tissue**<br>**J Synthetic Substitute**<br>**K Nonautologous Tissue Substitute** | **Z No Qualifier** |
| **Y Great Vessel** | **Ø Open**<br>**3 Percutaneous**<br>**4 Percutaneous Endoscopic** | **2 Monitoring Device**<br>**3 Infusion Device**<br>**7 Autologous Tissue Substitute**<br>**8 Zooplastic Tissue**<br>**C Extraluminal Device**<br>**D Intraluminal Device**<br>**J Synthetic Substitute**<br>**K Nonautologous Tissue Substitute**<br>Y Other Device | **Z No Qualifier** |
| **Y Great Vessel** | **X External** | **2 Monitoring Device**<br>**3 Infusion Device**<br>**7 Autologous Tissue Substitute**<br>**8 Zooplastic Tissue**<br>**C Extraluminal Device**<br>**D Intraluminal Device**<br>**J Synthetic Substitute**<br>**K Nonautologous Tissue Substitute** | **Z No Qualifier** |

**Non-OR** Ø2WA3[2,3,D]Z
**Non-OR** Ø2WA[3,4]YZ
**Non-OR** Ø2WAX[2,3,7,8,C,D,J,K,M,N,Q]Z
**Non-OR** Ø2WAXRZ
**Non-OR** Ø2WY3[2,3,D]Z
**Non-OR** Ø2WY[3,4]YZ
**Non-OR** Ø2WYX[2,3,7,8,C,D,J,K]Z

**HAC** Ø2WA[Ø,3,4]MZ when reported with SDx K68.11 or T81.4XXA or T82.6XXA or T82.7XXA
LC Ø2WAØ[J,Q]Z
NC Ø2WA[3,4]QZ

**See Appendix L for Procedure Combinations**
⊞ Ø2WA[Ø,3,4]QZ
⊞ Ø2WA[Ø,3,4]RZ

**Ø Medical and Surgical**
**2 Heart and Great Vessels**
**Y Transplantation** Definition: Putting in or on all or a portion of a living body part taken from another individual or animal to physically take the place and/or function of all or a portion of a similar body part

Explanation: The native body part may or may not be taken out, and the transplanted body part may take over all or a portion of its function

| Body Part Character 4 | Approach Character 5 | Device Character 6 | Qualifier Character 7 |
|---|---|---|---|
| A Heart LC | Ø Open | Z No Device | Ø Allogeneic<br>1 Syngeneic<br>2 Zooplastic |

LC Ø2YAØZ[Ø,1,2]

# Upper Arteries Ø31–Ø3W

## Character Meanings

This Character Meaning table is provided as a guide to assist the user in the identification of character members that may be found in this section of code tables. It **SHOULD NOT** be used to build a PCS code.

| Operation–Character 3 | Body Part–Character 4 | Approach–Character 5 | Device–Character 6 | Qualifier–Character 7 |
|---|---|---|---|---|
| 1 Bypass | Ø Internal Mammary Artery, Right | Ø Open | Ø Drainage Device | Ø Upper Arm Artery, Right |
| 5 Destruction | 1 Internal Mammary Artery, Left | 3 Percutaneous | 2 Monitoring Device | 1 Upper Arm Artery, Left |
| 7 Dilation | 2 Innominate Artery | 4 Percutaneous Endoscopic | 3 Infusion Device | 2 Upper Arm Artery, Bilateral |
| 9 Drainage | 3 Subclavian Artery, Right | X External | 4 Intraluminal Device, Drug-eluting | 3 Lower Arm Artery, Right |
| B Excision | 4 Subclavian Artery, Left | | 5 Intraluminal Device, Drug-eluting, Two | 4 Lower Arm Artery, Left |
| C Extirpation | 5 Axillary Artery, Right | | 6 Intraluminal Device, Drug-eluting, Three | 5 Lower Arm Artery, Bilateral |
| H Insertion | 6 Axillary Artery, Left | | 7 Intraluminal Device, Drug-eluting, Four or More OR Autologous Tissue Substitute | 6 Upper Leg Artery, Right OR Bifurcation |
| J Inspection | 7 Brachial Artery, Right | | 9 Autologous Venous Tissue | 7 Upper Leg Artery, Left |
| L Occlusion | 8 Brachial Artery, Left | | A Autologous Arterial Tissue | 8 Upper Leg Artery, Bilateral |
| N Release | 9 Ulnar Artery, Right | | B Intraluminal Device, Bioactive | 9 Lower Leg Artery, Right |
| P Removal | A Ulnar Artery, Left | | C Extraluminal Device | B Lower Leg Artery, Left |
| Q Repair | B Radial Artery, Right | | D Intraluminal Device | C Lower Leg Artery, Bilateral |
| R Replacement | C Radial Artery, Left | | E Intraluminal Device, Two | D Upper Arm Vein |
| S Reposition | D Hand Artery, Right | | F Intraluminal Device, Three | F Lower Arm Vein |
| U Supplement | F Hand Artery, Left | | G Intraluminal Device, Four or More | G Intracranial Artery |
| V Restriction | G Intracranial Artery | | J Synthetic Substitute | J Extracranial Artery, Right |
| W Revision | H Common Carotid Artery, Right | | K Nonautologous Tissue Substitute | K Extracranial Artery, Left |
| | J Common Carotid Artery, Left | | M Stimulator Lead | M Pulmonary Artery, Right |
| | K Internal Carotid Artery, Right | | Z No Device | N Pulmonary Artery, Left |
| | L Internal Carotid Artery, Left | | | V Superior Vena Cava |
| | M External Carotid Artery, Right | | | X Diagnostic |
| | N External Carotid Artery, Left | | | Z No Qualifier |
| | P Vertebral Artery, Right | | | |
| | Q Vertebral Artery, Left | | | |
| | R Face Artery | | | |
| | S Temporal Artery, Right | | | |
| | T Temporal Artery, Left | | | |
| | U Thyroid Artery, Right | | | |
| | V Thyroid Artery, Left | | | |
| | Y Upper Artery | | | |

**AHA Coding Clinic for table Ø31**

| | |
|---|---|
| **2017, 2Q, 22** | Carotid artery to subclavian artery transposition |
| **2017, 1Q, 31** | Left to right common carotid artery bypass |
| **2016, 3Q, 37** | Insertion of arteriovenous graft using HeRO device |
| **2016, 3Q, 39** | Revision of arteriovenous graft |
| **2013, 4Q, 125** | Stage II cephalic vein transposition (superficialization) of arteriovenous fistula |
| **2013, 1Q, 27** | Creation of radial artery fistula |

**AHA Coding Clinic for table Ø37**

| | |
|---|---|
| **2016, 4Q, 86** | Peripheral artery, number of stents |
| **2016, 4Q, 86-87** | Coronary and peripheral artery bifurcation |
| **2015, 1Q, 32** | Deployment of stent for herniated/migrated coil in basilar artery |

**AHA Coding Clinic for table Ø3B**

| | |
|---|---|
| **2016, 2Q, 12** | Resection of malignant neoplasm of infratemporal fossa |

**AHA Coding Clinic for table Ø3C**

| | |
|---|---|
| **2017, 2Q, 23** | Thrombectomy via Fogarty catheter |
| **2016, 4Q, 86-87** | Coronary and peripheral artery bifurcation |
| **2016, 2Q, 11** | Carotid endarterectomy with patch angioplasty |
| **2015, 1Q, 29** | Discontinued carotid endarterectomy |

**AHA Coding Clinic for table Ø3H**

| | |
|---|---|
| **2016, 2Q, 32** | Arterial catheter placement |

**AHA Coding Clinic for table Ø3J**

| | |
|---|---|
| **2015, 1Q, 29** | Discontinued carotid endarterectomy |

**AHA Coding Clinic for table Ø3L**

| | |
|---|---|
| **2016, 2Q, 30** | Clipping (occlusion) of cerebral artery, decompressive craniectomy and storage of bone flap in abdominal wall |
| **2014, 4Q, 20** | Control of epistaxis |
| **2014, 4Q, 37** | Endovascular embolization of arteriovenous malformation using Onyx-18 liquid |

**AHA Coding Clinic for table Ø3Q**

| | |
|---|---|
| **2017, 1Q, 31** | Left to right common carotid artery bypass |

**AHA Coding Clinic for table Ø3S**

| | |
|---|---|
| **2017, 2Q, 22** | Carotid artery to subclavian artery transposition |
| **2015, 3Q, 27** | Moyamoya disease and hemispheric pial synagiosis with craniotomy |

**AHA Coding Clinic for table Ø3U**

| | |
|---|---|
| **2016, 2Q, 11** | Carotid endarterectomy with patch angioplasty |

**AHA Coding Clinic for table Ø3V**

| | |
|---|---|
| **2016, 1Q, 19** | Embolization of superior hypophyseal aneurysm using stent-assisted coil |

**AHA Coding Clinic for table Ø3W**

| | |
|---|---|
| **2016, 3Q, 39** | Revision of arteriovenous graft |
| **2015, 1Q, 32** | Deployment of stent for herniated/migrated coil in basilar artery |

## Upper Arteries

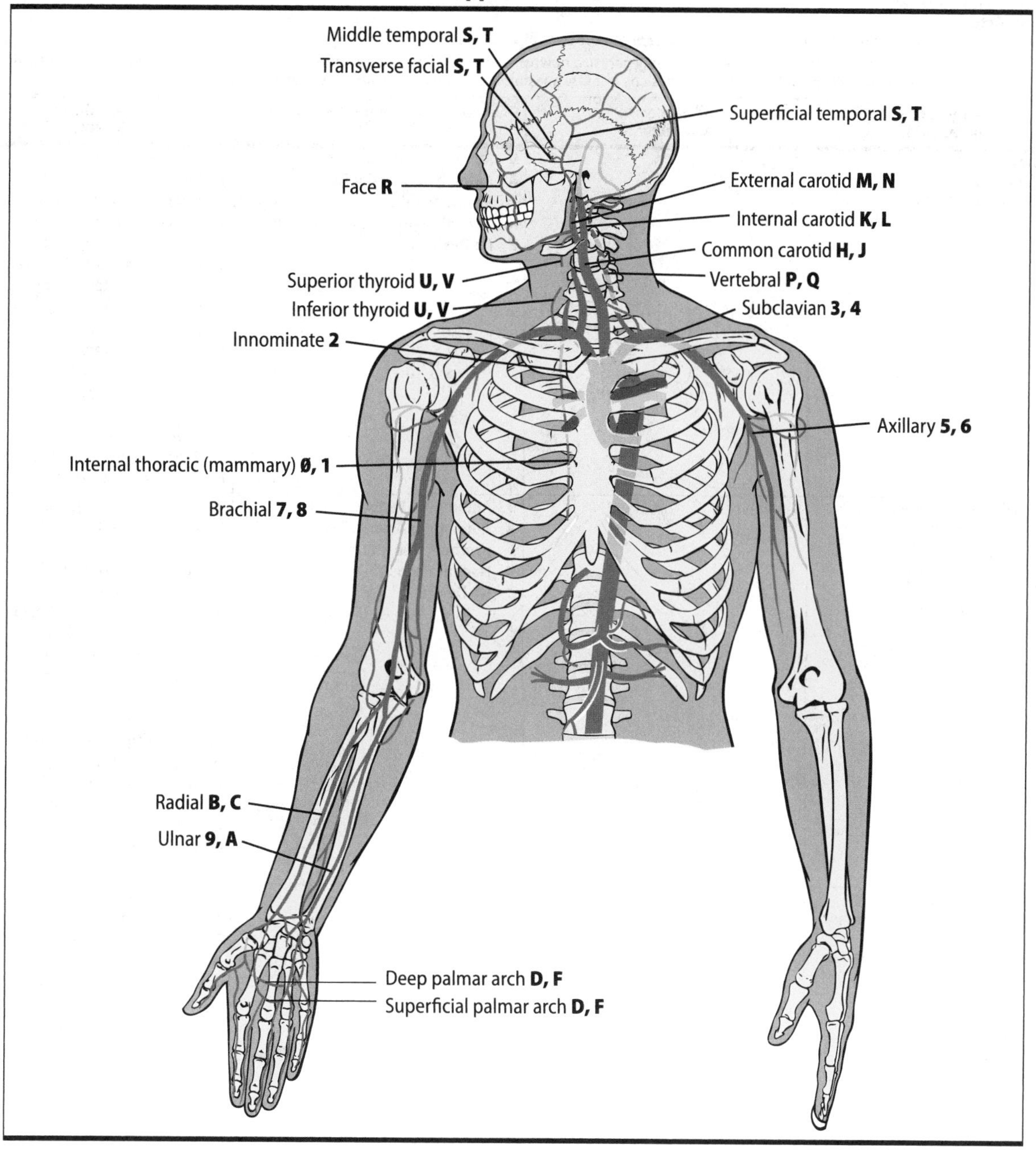
Middle temporal **S, T**
Transverse facial **S, T**
Superficial temporal **S, T**
Face **R**
External carotid **M, N**
Internal carotid **K, L**
Common carotid **H, J**
Superior thyroid **U, V**
Vertebral **P, Q**
Inferior thyroid **U, V**
Subclavian **3, 4**
Innominate **2**
Axillary **5, 6**
Internal thoracic (mammary) **Ø, 1**
Brachial **7, 8**
Radial **B, C**
Ulnar **9, A**
Deep palmar arch **D, F**
Superficial palmar arch **D, F**

## Head and Neck Arteries

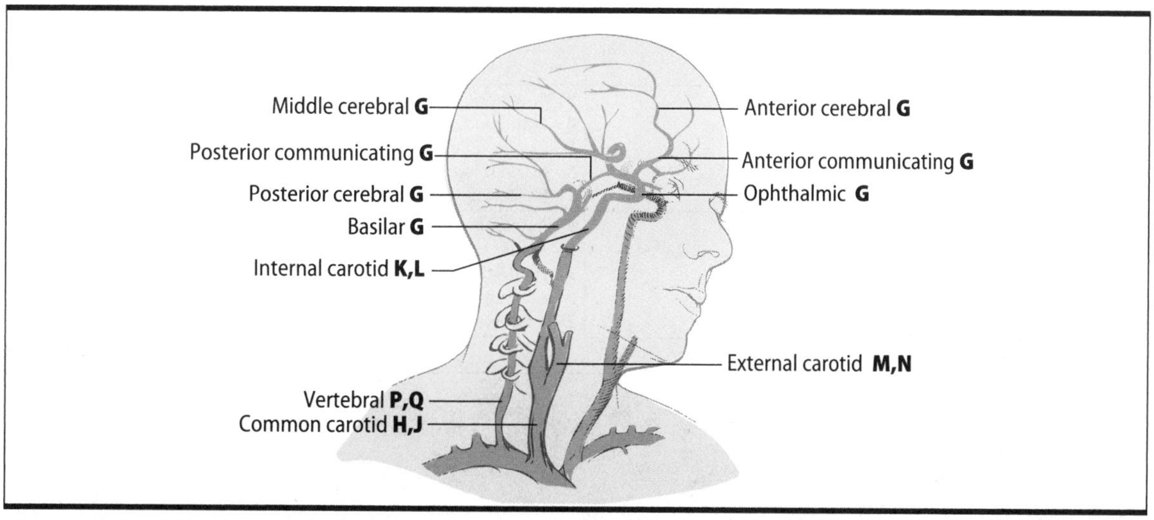
Middle cerebral **G**
Anterior cerebral **G**
Posterior communicating **G**
Anterior communicating **G**
Posterior cerebral **G**
Ophthalmic **G**
Basilar **G**
Internal carotid **K,L**
External carotid **M,N**
Vertebral **P,Q**
Common carotid **H,J**

**Ø Medical and Surgical**
**3 Upper Arteries**
**1 Bypass** Definition: Altering the route of passage of the contents of a tubular body part

Explanation: Rerouting contents of a body part to a downstream area of the normal route, to a similar route and body part, or to an abnormal route and dissimilar body part. Includes one or more anastomoses, with or without the use of a device.

| Body Part Character 4 | Approach Character 5 | Device Character 6 | Qualifier Character 7 |
|---|---|---|---|
| **2 Innominate Artery**<br>Brachiocephalic artery<br>Brachiocephalic trunk | **Ø Open** | **9 Autologous Venous Tissue**<br>**A Autologous Arterial Tissue**<br>**J Synthetic Substitute**<br>**K Nonautologous Tissue Substitute**<br>**Z No Device** | **Ø Upper Arm Artery, Right**<br>**1 Upper Arm Artery, Left**<br>**2 Upper Arm Artery, Bilateral**<br>**3 Lower Arm Artery, Right**<br>**4 Lower Arm Artery, Left**<br>**5 Lower Arm Artery, Bilateral**<br>**6 Upper Leg Artery, Right**<br>**7 Upper Leg Artery, Left**<br>**8 Upper Leg Artery, Bilateral**<br>**9 Lower Leg Artery, Right**<br>**B Lower Leg Artery, Left**<br>**C Lower Leg Artery, Bilateral**<br>**D Upper Arm Vein**<br>**F Lower Arm Vein**<br>**J Extracranial Artery, Right**<br>**K Extracranial Artery, Left** |
| **3 Subclavian Artery, Right**<br>Costocervical trunk<br>Dorsal scapular artery<br>Internal thoracic artery<br>**4 Subclavian Artery, Left**<br>*See 3 Subclavian Artery, Right* | **Ø Open** | **9 Autologous Venous Tissue**<br>**A Autologous Arterial Tissue**<br>**J Synthetic Substitute**<br>**K Nonautologous Tissue Substitute**<br>**Z No Device** | **Ø Upper Arm Artery, Right**<br>**1 Upper Arm Artery, Left**<br>**2 Upper Arm Artery, Bilateral**<br>**3 Lower Arm Artery, Right**<br>**4 Lower Arm Artery, Left**<br>**5 Lower Arm Artery, Bilateral**<br>**6 Upper Leg Artery, Right**<br>**7 Upper Leg Artery, Left**<br>**8 Upper Leg Artery, Bilateral**<br>**9 Lower Leg Artery, Right**<br>**B Lower Leg Artery, Left**<br>**C Lower Leg Artery, Bilateral**<br>**D Upper Arm Vein**<br>**F Lower Arm Vein**<br>**J Extracranial Artery, Right**<br>**K Extracranial Artery, Left**<br>**M Pulmonary Artery, Right**<br>**N Pulmonary Artery, Left** |
| **5 Axillary Artery, Right**<br>Anterior circumflex humeral artery<br>Lateral thoracic artery<br>Posterior circumflex humeral artery<br>Subscapular artery<br>Superior thoracic artery<br>Thoracoacromial artery<br>**6 Axillary Artery, Left**<br>*See 5 Axillary Artery, Right* | **Ø Open** | **9 Autologous Venous Tissue**<br>**A Autologous Arterial Tissue**<br>**J Synthetic Substitute**<br>**K Nonautologous Tissue Substitute**<br>**Z No Device** | **Ø Upper Arm Artery, Right**<br>**1 Upper Arm Artery, Left**<br>**2 Upper Arm Artery, Bilateral**<br>**3 Lower Arm Artery, Right**<br>**4 Lower Arm Artery, Left**<br>**5 Lower Arm Artery, Bilateral**<br>**6 Upper Leg Artery, Right**<br>**7 Upper Leg Artery, Left**<br>**8 Upper Leg Artery, Bilateral**<br>**9 Lower Leg Artery, Right**<br>**B Lower Leg Artery, Left**<br>**C Lower Leg Artery, Bilateral**<br>**D Upper Arm Vein**<br>**F Lower Arm Vein**<br>**J Extracranial Artery, Right**<br>**K Extracranial Artery, Left**<br>**V Superior Vena Cava** |
| **7 Brachial Artery, Right**<br>Inferior ulnar collateral artery<br>Profunda brachii<br>Superior ulnar collateral artery | **Ø Open** | **9 Autologous Venous Tissue**<br>**A Autologous Arterial Tissue**<br>**J Synthetic Substitute**<br>**K Nonautologous Tissue Substitute**<br>**Z No Device** | **Ø Upper Arm Artery, Right**<br>**3 Lower Arm Artery, Right**<br>**D Upper Arm Vein**<br>**F Lower Arm Vein**<br>**V Superior Vena Cava** |
| **8 Brachial Artery, Left**<br>Inferior ulnar collateral artery<br>Profunda brachii<br>Superior ulnar collateral artery | **Ø Open** | **9 Autologous Venous Tissue**<br>**A Autologous Arterial Tissue**<br>**J Synthetic Substitute**<br>**K Nonautologous Tissue Substitute**<br>**Z No Device** | **1 Upper Arm Artery, Left**<br>**4 Lower Arm Artery, Left**<br>**D Upper Arm Vein**<br>**F Lower Arm Vein**<br>**V Superior Vena Cava** |

***Ø31 Continued on next page***

**Ø Medical and Surgical**
**3 Upper Arteries**
**1 Bypass**

**Ø31 Continued**

Definition: Altering the route of passage of the contents of a tubular body part

Explanation: Rerouting contents of a body part to a downstream area of the normal route, to a similar route and body part, or to an abnormal route and dissimilar body part. Includes one or more anastomoses, with or without the use of a device.

| Body Part Character 4 | Approach Character 5 | Device Character 6 | Qualifier Character 7 |
|---|---|---|---|
| **9 Ulnar Artery, Right**<br>Anterior ulnar recurrent artery<br>Common interosseous artery<br>Posterior ulnar recurrent artery<br>**B Radial Artery, Right**<br>Radial recurrent artery | **Ø Open** | **9 Autologous Venous Tissue**<br>**A Autologous Arterial Tissue**<br>**J Synthetic Substitute**<br>**K Nonautologous Tissue Substitute**<br>**Z No Device** | **3 Lower Arm Artery, Right**<br>**F Lower Arm Vein** |
| **A Ulnar Artery, Left**<br>Anterior ulnar recurrent artery<br>Common interosseous artery<br>Posterior ulnar recurrent artery<br>**C Radial Artery, Left**<br>Radial recurrent artery | **Ø Open** | **9 Autologous Venous Tissue**<br>**A Autologous Arterial Tissue**<br>**J Synthetic Substitute**<br>**K Nonautologous Tissue Substitute**<br>**Z No Device** | **4 Lower Arm Artery, Left**<br>**F Lower Arm Vein** |
| **G Intracranial Artery**<br>Anterior cerebral artery<br>Anterior choroidal artery<br>Anterior communicating artery<br>Basilar artery<br>Circle of Willis<br>Internal carotid artery, intracranial portion<br>Middle cerebral artery<br>Ophthalmic artery<br>Posterior cerebral artery<br>Posterior communicating artery<br>Posterior inferior cerebellar artery (PICA)<br>**S Temporal Artery, Right** NC<br>Middle temporal artery<br>Superficial temporal artery<br>Transverse facial artery<br>**T Temporal Artery, Left** NC<br>*See S Temporal Artery, Right* | **Ø Open** | **9 Autologous Venous Tissue**<br>**A Autologous Arterial Tissue**<br>**J Synthetic Substitute**<br>**K Nonautologous Tissue Substitute**<br>**Z No Device** | **G Intracranial Artery** |
| **H Common Carotid Artery, Right** NC<br>**J Common Carotid Artery, Left** NC | **Ø Open** | **9 Autologous Venous Tissue**<br>**A Autologous Arterial Tissue**<br>**J Synthetic Substitute**<br>**K Nonautologous Tissue Substitute**<br>**Z No Device** | **G Intracranial Artery**<br>**J Extracranial Artery, Right**<br>**K Extracranial Artery, Left** |
| **K Internal Carotid Artery, Right**<br>Caroticotympanic artery<br>Carotid sinus<br>**L Internal Carotid Artery, Left**<br>Caroticotympanic artery<br>Carotid sinus<br>**M External Carotid Artery, Right**<br>Ascending pharyngeal artery<br>Internal maxillary artery<br>Lingual artery<br>Maxillary artery<br>Occipital artery<br>Posterior auricular artery<br>Superior thyroid artery<br>**N External Carotid Artery, Left**<br>Ascending pharyngeal artery<br>Internal maxillary artery<br>Lingual artery<br>Maxillary artery<br>Occipital artery<br>Posterior auricular artery<br>Superior thyroid artery | **Ø Open** | **9 Autologous Venous Tissue**<br>**A Autologous Arterial Tissue**<br>**J Synthetic Substitute**<br>**K Nonautologous Tissue Substitute**<br>**Z No Device** | **J Extracranial Artery, Right**<br>**K Extracranial Artery, Left** |

NC Ø31SØ[9,A,J,K,Z]G
NC Ø31TØ[9,A,J,K,Z]G
NC Ø31HØ[9,A,J,K,Z]G
NC Ø31JØ[9,A,J,K,Z]G

**Ø Medical and Surgical**
**3 Upper Arteries**
**5 Destruction** Definition: Physical eradication of all or a portion of a body part by the direct use of energy, force, or a destructive agent
Explanation: None of the body part is physically taken out

| Body Part Character 4 | Approach Character 5 | Device Character 6 | Qualifier Character 7 |
|---|---|---|---|
| **Ø Internal Mammary Artery, Right**<br>Anterior intercostal artery<br>Internal thoracic artery<br>Musculophrenic artery<br>Pericardiophrenic artery<br>Superior epigastric artery<br>**1 Internal Mammary Artery, Left**<br>*See Ø Internal Mammary Artery, Right*<br>**2 Innominate Artery**<br>Brachiocephalic artery<br>Brachiocephalic trunk<br>**3 Subclavian Artery, Right**<br>Costocervical trunk<br>Dorsal scapular artery<br>Internal thoracic artery<br>**4 Subclavian Artery, Left**<br>*See 3 Subclavian Artery, Right*<br>**5 Axillary Artery, Right**<br>Anterior circumflex humeral artery<br>Lateral thoracic artery<br>Posterior circumflex humeral artery<br>Subscapular artery<br>Superior thoracic artery<br>Thoracoacromial artery<br>**6 Axillary Artery, Left**<br>*See 5 Axillary Artery, Right*<br>**7 Brachial Artery, Right**<br>Inferior ulnar collateral artery<br>Profunda brachii<br>Superior ulnar collateral artery<br>**8 Brachial Artery, Left**<br>*See 7 Brachial Artery, Right*<br>**9 Ulnar Artery, Right**<br>Anterior ulnar recurrent artery<br>Common interosseous artery<br>Posterior ulnar recurrent artery<br>**A Ulnar Artery, Left**<br>*See 9 Ulnar Artery, Right*<br>**B Radial Artery, Right**<br>Radial recurrent artery<br>**C Radial Artery, Left**<br>*See B Radial Artery, Right*<br>**D Hand Artery, Right**<br>Deep palmar arch<br>Princeps pollicis artery<br>Radialis indicis<br>Superficial palmar arch<br>**F Hand Artery, Left**<br>*See D Hand Artery, Right*<br>**G Intracranial Artery**<br>Anterior cerebral artery<br>Anterior choroidal artery<br>Anterior communicating artery<br>Basilar artery<br>Circle of Willis<br>Internal carotid artery, intracranial portion<br>Middle cerebral artery<br>Ophthalmic artery<br>Posterior cerebral artery<br>Posterior communicating artery<br>Posterior inferior cerebellar artery (PICA)<br>**H Common Carotid Artery, Right**<br>**J Common Carotid Artery, Left**<br>**K Internal Carotid Artery, Right**<br>Caroticotympanic artery<br>Carotid sinus<br>**L Internal Carotid Artery, Left**<br>*See K Internal Carotid Artery, Right*<br>**M External Carotid Artery, Right**<br>Ascending pharyngeal artery<br>Internal maxillary artery<br>Lingual artery<br>Maxillary artery<br>Occipital artery<br>Posterior auricular artery<br>Superior thyroid artery<br>**N External Carotid Artery, Left**<br>*See M External Carotid Artery, Right*<br>**P Vertebral Artery, Right**<br>Anterior spinal artery<br>Posterior spinal artery<br>**Q Vertebral Artery, Left**<br>*See P Vertebral Artery, Right*<br>**R Face Artery**<br>Angular artery<br>Ascending palatine artery<br>External maxillary artery<br>Facial artery<br>Inferior labial artery<br>Submental artery<br>Superior labial artery<br>**S Temporal Artery, Right**<br>Middle temporal artery<br>Superficial temporal artery<br>Transverse facial artery<br>**T Temporal Artery, Left**<br>*See S Temporal Artery, Right*<br>**U Thyroid Artery, Right**<br>Cricothyroid artery<br>Hyoid artery<br>Sternocleidomastoid artery<br>Superior laryngeal artery<br>Superior thyroid artery<br>Thyrocervical trunk<br>**V Thyroid Artery, Left**<br>*See U Thyroid Artery, Right*<br>**Y Upper Artery**<br>Aortic intercostal artery<br>Bronchial artery<br>Esophageal artery<br>Subcostal artery | **Ø Open**<br>**3 Percutaneous**<br>**4 Percutaneous Endoscopic** | **Z No Device** | **Z No Qualifier** |

**Ø Medical and Surgical**
**3 Upper Arteries**
**7 Dilation**

Definition: Expanding an orifice or the lumen of a tubular body part

Explanation: The orifice can be a natural orifice or an artificially created orifice. Accomplished by stretching a tubular body part using intraluminal pressure or by cutting part of the orifice or wall of the tubular body part.

| Body Part Character 4 | Approach Character 5 | Device Character 6 | Qualifier Character 7 |
|---|---|---|---|
| **Ø Internal Mammary Artery, Right**<br>Anterior intercostal artery<br>Internal thoracic artery<br>Musculophrenic artery<br>Pericardiophrenic artery<br>Superior epigastric artery<br>**1 Internal Mammary Artery, Left**<br>*See Ø Internal Mammary Artery, Right*<br>**2 Innominate Artery**<br>Brachiocephalic artery<br>Brachiocephalic trunk<br>**3 Subclavian Artery, Right**<br>Costocervical trunk<br>Dorsal scapular artery<br>Internal thoracic artery<br>**4 Subclavian Artery, Left**<br>*See 3 Subclavian Artery, Right*<br>**5 Axillary Artery, Right**<br>Anterior circumflex humeral artery<br>Lateral thoracic artery<br>Posterior circumflex humeral artery<br>Subscapular artery<br>Superior thoracic artery<br>Thoracoacromial artery<br>**6 Axillary Artery, Left**<br>*See 5 Axillary Artery, Right*<br>**7 Brachial Artery, Right**<br>Inferior ulnar collateral artery<br>Profunda brachii<br>Superior ulnar collateral artery<br>**8 Brachial Artery, Left**<br>*See 7 Brachial Artery, Right*<br>**9 Ulnar Artery, Right**<br>Anterior ulnar recurrent artery<br>Common interosseous artery<br>Posterior ulnar recurrent artery<br>**A Ulnar Artery, Left**<br>*See 9 Ulnar Artery, Right*<br>**B Radial Artery, Right**<br>Radial recurrent artery<br>**C Radial Artery, Left**<br>*See B Radial Artery, Right*<br>**D Hand Artery, Right**<br>Deep palmar arch<br>Princeps pollicis artery<br>Radialis indicis<br>Superficial palmar arch<br>**F Hand Artery, Left**<br>*See D Hand Artery, Right*<br>**G Intracranial Artery** NC<br>Anterior cerebral artery<br>Anterior choroidal artery<br>Anterior communicating artery<br>Basilar artery<br>Circle of Willis<br>Internal carotid artery, intracranial portion<br>Middle cerebral artery<br>Ophthalmic artery<br>Posterior cerebral artery<br>Posterior communicating artery<br>Posterior inferior cerebellar artery (PICA)<br>**H Common Carotid Artery, Right**<br>**J Common Carotid Artery, Left**<br>**K Internal Carotid Artery, Right**<br>Caroticotympanic artery<br>Carotid sinus<br>**L Internal Carotid Artery, Left**<br>*See K Internal Carotid Artery, Right*<br>**M External Carotid Artery, Right**<br>Ascending pharyngeal artery<br>Internal maxillary artery<br>Lingual artery<br>Maxillary artery<br>Occipital artery<br>Posterior auricular artery<br>Superior thyroid artery<br>**N External Carotid Artery, Left**<br>*See M External Carotid Artery, Right*<br>**P Vertebral Artery, Right**<br>Anterior spinal artery<br>Posterior spinal artery<br>**Q Vertebral Artery, Left**<br>*See P Vertebral Artery, Right*<br>**R Face Artery**<br>Angular artery<br>Ascending palatine artery<br>External maxillary artery<br>Facial artery<br>Inferior labial artery<br>Submental artery<br>Superior labial artery<br>**S Temporal Artery, Right**<br>Middle temporal artery<br>Superficial temporal artery<br>Transverse facial artery<br>**T Temporal Artery, Left**<br>*See S Temporal Artery, Right*<br>**U Thyroid Artery, Right**<br>Cricothyroid artery<br>Hyoid artery<br>Sternocleidomastoid artery<br>Superior laryngeal artery<br>Superior thyroid artery<br>Thyrocervical trunk<br>**V Thyroid Artery, Left**<br>*See U Thyroid Artery, Right*<br>**Y Upper Artery**<br>Aortic intercostal artery<br>Bronchial artery<br>Esophageal artery<br>Subcostal artery | **Ø Open**<br>**3 Percutaneous**<br>**4 Percutaneous Endoscopic** | **4 Intraluminal Device, Drug-eluting**<br>**5 Intraluminal Device, Drug-eluting, Two**<br>**6 Intraluminal Device, Drug-eluting, Three**<br>**7 Intraluminal Device, Drug-eluting, Four or More**<br>**D Intraluminal Device**<br>**E Intraluminal Device, Two**<br>**F Intraluminal Device, Three**<br>**G Intraluminal Device, Four or More**<br>**Z No Device** | **6 Bifurcation**<br>**Z No Qualifier** |

NC 037G[3,4]Z[6,Z]

**Ø Medical and Surgical**
**3 Upper Arteries**
**9 Drainage** Definition: Taking or letting out fluids and/or gases from a body part
Explanation: The qualifier DIAGNOSTIC is used to identify drainage procedures that are biopsies

| Body Part<br>Character 4 | Approach<br>Character 5 | Device<br>Character 6 | Qualifier<br>Character 7 |
|---|---|---|---|
| **Ø Internal Mammary Artery, Right**<br>Anterior intercostal artery<br>Internal thoracic artery<br>Musculophrenic artery<br>Pericardiophrenic artery<br>Superior epigastric artery<br>**1 Internal Mammary Artery, Left**<br>*See Ø Internal Mammary Artery, Right above*<br>**2 Innominate Artery**<br>Brachiocephalic artery<br>Brachiocephalic trunk<br>**3 Subclavian Artery, Right**<br>Costocervical trunk<br>Dorsal scapular artery<br>Internal thoracic artery<br>**4 Subclavian Artery, Left**<br>*See 3 Subclavian Artery, Right*<br>**5 Axillary Artery, Right**<br>Anterior circumflex humeral artery<br>Lateral thoracic artery<br>Posterior circumflex humeral artery<br>Subscapular artery<br>Superior thoracic artery<br>Thoracoacromial artery<br>**6 Axillary Artery, Left**<br>*See 5 Axillary Artery, Right*<br>**7 Brachial Artery, Right**<br>Inferior ulnar collateral artery<br>Profunda brachii<br>Superior ulnar collateral artery<br>**8 Brachial Artery, Left**<br>*See 7 Brachial Artery, Right*<br>**9 Ulnar Artery, Right**<br>Anterior ulnar recurrent artery<br>Common interosseous artery<br>Posterior ulnar recurrent artery<br>**A Ulnar Artery, Left**<br>*See 9 Ulnar Artery, Right*<br>**B Radial Artery, Right**<br>Radial recurrent artery<br>**C Radial Artery, Left**<br>*See B Radial Artery, Right*<br>**D Hand Artery, Right**<br>Deep palmar arch<br>Princeps pollicis artery<br>Radialis indicis<br>Superficial palmar arch<br>**F Hand Artery, Left**<br>*See D Hand Artery, Right*<br>**G Intracranial Artery**<br>Anterior cerebral artery<br>Anterior choroidal artery<br>Anterior communicating artery<br>Basilar artery<br>Circle of Willis<br>Internal carotid artery, intracranial portion<br>Middle cerebral artery<br>Ophthalmic artery<br>Posterior cerebral artery<br>Posterior communicating artery<br>Posterior inferior cerebellar artery (PICA)<br>**H Common Carotid Artery, Right**<br>**J Common Carotid Artery, Left**<br>**K Internal Carotid Artery, Right**<br>Caroticotympanic artery<br>Carotid sinus<br>**L Internal Carotid Artery, Left**<br>*See K Internal Carotid Artery, Right*<br>**M External Carotid Artery, Right**<br>Ascending pharyngeal artery<br>Internal maxillary artery<br>Lingual artery<br>Maxillary artery<br>Occipital artery<br>Posterior auricular artery<br>Superior thyroid artery<br>**N External Carotid Artery, Left**<br>*See M External Carotid Artery, Right*<br>**P Vertebral Artery, Right**<br>Anterior spinal artery<br>Posterior spinal artery<br>**Q Vertebral Artery, Left**<br>*See P Vertebral Artery, Right*<br>**R Face Artery**<br>Angular artery<br>Ascending palatine artery<br>External maxillary artery<br>Facial artery<br>Inferior labial artery<br>Submental artery<br>Superior labial artery<br>**S Temporal Artery, Right**<br>Middle temporal artery<br>Superficial temporal artery<br>Transverse facial artery<br>**T Temporal Artery, Left**<br>*See S Temporal Artery, Right*<br>**U Thyroid Artery, Right**<br>Cricothyroid artery<br>Hyoid artery<br>Sternocleidomastoid artery<br>Superior laryngeal artery<br>Superior thyroid artery<br>Thyrocervical trunk<br>**V Thyroid Artery, Left**<br>*See U Thyroid Artery, Right*<br>**Y Upper Artery**<br>Aortic intercostal artery<br>Bronchial artery<br>Esophageal artery<br>Subcostal artery | **Ø Open**<br>**3 Percutaneous**<br>**4 Percutaneous Endoscopic** | **Ø Drainage Device** | **Z No Qualifier** |

***Ø39 Continued on next page***

**Non-OR** Ø39[Ø,1,2,3,4,5,6,7,8,9,A,B,C,D,F,G,H,J,K,L,M,N,P,Q,R,S,T,U,V,Y][Ø,3,4]ØZ

**Ø Medical and Surgical**
**3 Upper Arteries**
**9 Drainage** Definition: Taking or letting out fluids and/or gases from a body part
Explanation: The qualifier DIAGNOSTIC is used to identify drainage procedures that are biopsies

**Ø39 Continued**

| Body Part Character 4 | Approach Character 5 | Device Character 6 | Qualifier Character 7 |
|---|---|---|---|
| **Ø Internal Mammary Artery, Right**<br>Anterior intercostal artery<br>Internal thoracic artery<br>Musculophrenic artery<br>Pericardiophrenic artery<br>Superior epigastric artery<br>**1 Internal Mammary Artery, Left**<br>*See Ø Internal Mammary Artery, Right*<br>**2 Innominate Artery**<br>Brachiocephalic artery<br>Brachiocephalic trunk<br>**3 Subclavian Artery, Right**<br>Costocervical trunk<br>Dorsal scapular artery<br>Internal thoracic artery<br>**4 Subclavian Artery, Left**<br>*See 3 Subclavian Artery, Right*<br>**5 Axillary Artery, Right**<br>Anterior circumflex humeral artery<br>Lateral thoracic artery<br>Posterior circumflex humeral artery<br>Subscapular artery<br>Superior thoracic artery<br>Thoracoacromial artery<br>**6 Axillary Artery, Left**<br>*See 5 Axillary Artery, Right*<br>**7 Brachial Artery, Right**<br>Inferior ulnar collateral artery<br>Profunda brachii<br>Superior ulnar collateral artery<br>**8 Brachial Artery, Left**<br>*See 7 Brachial Artery, Right*<br>**9 Ulnar Artery, Right**<br>Anterior ulnar recurrent artery<br>Common interosseous artery<br>Posterior ulnar recurrent artery<br>**A Ulnar Artery, Left**<br>*See 9 Ulnar Artery, Right*<br>**B Radial Artery, Right**<br>Radial recurrent artery<br>**C Radial Artery, Left**<br>*See B Radial Artery, Right*<br>**D Hand Artery, Right**<br>Deep palmar arch<br>Princeps pollicis artery<br>Radialis indicis<br>Superficial palmar arch<br>**F Hand Artery, Left**<br>*See D Hand Artery, Right*<br>**G Intracranial Artery**<br>Anterior cerebral artery<br>Anterior choroidal artery<br>Anterior communicating artery<br>Basilar artery<br>Circle of Willis<br>Internal carotid artery, intracranial portion<br>Middle cerebral artery<br>Ophthalmic artery<br>Posterior cerebral artery<br>Posterior communicating artery<br>Posterior inferior cerebellar artery (PICA)<br>**H Common Carotid Artery, Right**<br>**J Common Carotid Artery, Left**<br>**K Internal Carotid Artery, Right**<br>Caroticotympanic artery<br>Carotid sinus<br>**L Internal Carotid Artery, Left**<br>*See K Internal Carotid Artery, Right*<br>**M External Carotid Artery, Right**<br>Ascending pharyngeal artery<br>Internal maxillary artery<br>Lingual artery<br>Maxillary artery<br>Occipital artery<br>Posterior auricular artery<br>Superior thyroid artery<br>**N External Carotid Artery, Left**<br>*See M External Carotid Artery, Right*<br>**P Vertebral Artery, Right**<br>Anterior spinal artery<br>Posterior spinal artery<br>**Q Vertebral Artery, Left**<br>*See P Vertebral Artery, Right*<br>**R Face Artery**<br>Angular artery<br>Ascending palatine artery<br>External maxillary artery<br>Facial artery<br>Inferior labial artery<br>Submental artery<br>Superior labial artery<br>**S Temporal Artery, Right**<br>Middle temporal artery<br>Superficial temporal artery<br>Transverse facial artery<br>**T Temporal Artery, Left**<br>*See S Temporal Artery, Right*<br>**U Thyroid Artery, Right**<br>Cricothyroid artery<br>Hyoid artery<br>Sternocleidomastoid artery<br>Superior laryngeal artery<br>Superior thyroid artery<br>Thyrocervical trunk<br>**V Thyroid Artery, Left**<br>*See U Thyroid Artery, Right*<br>**Y Upper Artery**<br>Aortic intercostal artery<br>Bronchial artery<br>Esophageal artery<br>Subcostal artery | **Ø Open**<br>**3 Percutaneous**<br>**4 Percutaneous Endoscopic** | **Z No Device** | **X Diagnostic**<br>**Z No Qualifier** |

**Non-OR** Ø39[Ø,1,2,3,4,5,6,7,8,9,A,B,C,D,F,G,H,J,K,L,M,N,P,Q,R,S,T,U,V,Y]3ZX
**Non-OR** Ø39[Ø,1,2,3,4,5,6,7,8,9,A,B,C,D,F,G,H,J,K,L,M,N,P,Q,R,S,T,U,V,Y][Ø,3,4]ZZ

**Ø Medical and Surgical**
**3 Upper Arteries**
**B Excision** Definition: Cutting out or off, without replacement, a portion of a body part
Explanation: The qualifier DIAGNOSTIC is used to identify excision procedures that are biopsies

| Body Part Character 4 | Approach Character 5 | Device Character 6 | Qualifier Character 7 |
|---|---|---|---|
| **Ø Internal Mammary Artery, Right**<br>Anterior intercostal artery<br>Internal thoracic artery<br>Musculophrenic artery<br>Pericardiophrenic artery<br>Superior epigastric artery<br>**1 Internal Mammary Artery, Left**<br>*See Ø Internal Mammary Artery, Right*<br>**2 Innominate Artery**<br>Brachiocephalic artery<br>Brachiocephalic trunk<br>**3 Subclavian Artery, Right**<br>Costocervical trunk<br>Dorsal scapular artery<br>Internal thoracic artery<br>**4 Subclavian Artery, Left**<br>*See 3 Subclavian Artery, Right*<br>**5 Axillary Artery, Right**<br>Anterior circumflex humeral artery<br>Lateral thoracic artery<br>Posterior circumflex humeral artery<br>Subscapular artery<br>Superior thoracic artery<br>Thoracoacromial artery<br>**6 Axillary Artery, Left**<br>*See 5 Axillary Artery, Right*<br>**7 Brachial Artery, Right**<br>Inferior ulnar collateral artery<br>Profunda brachii<br>Superior ulnar collateral artery<br>**8 Brachial Artery, Left**<br>*See 7 Brachial Artery, Right*<br>**9 Ulnar Artery, Right**<br>Anterior ulnar recurrent artery<br>Common interosseous artery<br>Posterior ulnar recurrent artery<br>**A Ulnar Artery, Left**<br>*See 9 Ulnar Artery, Right*<br>**B Radial Artery, Right**<br>Radial recurrent artery<br>**C Radial Artery, Left**<br>*See B Radial Artery, Right*<br>**D Hand Artery, Right**<br>Deep palmar arch<br>Princeps pollicis artery<br>Radialis indicis<br>Superficial palmar arch<br>**F Hand Artery, Left**<br>*See D Hand Artery, Right*<br>**G Intracranial Artery**<br>Anterior cerebral artery<br>Anterior choroidal artery<br>Anterior communicating artery<br>Basilar artery<br>Circle of Willis<br>Internal carotid artery, intracranial portion<br>Middle cerebral artery<br>Ophthalmic artery<br>Posterior cerebral artery<br>Posterior communicating artery<br>Posterior inferior cerebellar artery (PICA)<br>**H Common Carotid Artery, Right**<br>**J Common Carotid Artery, Left**<br>**K Internal Carotid Artery, Right**<br>Caroticotympanic artery<br>Carotid sinus<br>**L Internal Carotid Artery, Left**<br>*See K Internal Carotid Artery, Right*<br>**M External Carotid Artery, Right**<br>Ascending pharyngeal artery<br>Internal maxillary artery<br>Lingual artery<br>Maxillary artery<br>Occipital artery<br>Posterior auricular artery<br>Superior thyroid artery<br>**N External Carotid Artery, Left**<br>*See M External Carotid Artery, Right*<br>**P Vertebral Artery, Right**<br>Anterior spinal artery<br>Posterior spinal artery<br>**Q Vertebral Artery, Left**<br>*See P Vertebral Artery, Right*<br>**R Face Artery**<br>Angular artery<br>Ascending palatine artery<br>External maxillary artery<br>Facial artery<br>Inferior labial artery<br>Submental artery<br>Superior labial artery<br>**S Temporal Artery, Right**<br>Middle temporal artery<br>Superficial temporal artery<br>Transverse facial artery<br>**T Temporal Artery, Left**<br>*See S Temporal Artery, Right*<br>**U Thyroid Artery, Right**<br>Cricothyroid artery<br>Hyoid artery<br>Sternocleidomastoid artery<br>Superior laryngeal artery<br>Superior thyroid artery<br>Thyrocervical trunk<br>**V Thyroid Artery, Left**<br>*See U Thyroid Artery, Right*<br>**Y Upper Artery**<br>Aortic intercostal artery<br>Bronchial artery<br>Esophageal artery<br>Subcostal artery | **Ø Open**<br>**3 Percutaneous**<br>**4 Percutaneous Endoscopic** | **Z No Device** | **X Diagnostic**<br>**Z No Qualifier** |

**Ø Medical and Surgical**
**3 Upper Arteries**
**C Extirpation** Definition: Taking or cutting out solid matter from a body part

Explanation: The solid matter may be an abnormal byproduct of a biological function or a foreign body; it may be imbedded in a body part or in the lumen of a tubular body part. The solid matter may or may not have been previously broken into pieces.

| Body Part Character 4 | Approach Character 5 | Device Character 6 | Qualifier Character 7 |
|---|---|---|---|
| **Ø Internal Mammary Artery, Right**<br>Anterior intercostal artery<br>Internal thoracic artery<br>Musculophrenic artery<br>Pericardiophrenic artery<br>Superior epigastric artery<br>**1 Internal Mammary Artery, Left**<br>**See** *Ø Internal Mammary Artery, Right*<br>**2 Innominate Artery**<br>Brachiocephalic artery<br>Brachiocephalic trunk<br>**3 Subclavian Artery, Right**<br>Costocervical trunk<br>Dorsal scapular artery<br>Internal thoracic artery<br>**4 Subclavian Artery, Left**<br>**See** *3 Subclavian Artery, Right*<br>**5 Axillary Artery, Right**<br>Anterior circumflex humeral artery<br>Lateral thoracic artery<br>Posterior circumflex humeral artery<br>Subscapular artery<br>Superior thoracic artery<br>Thoracoacromial artery<br>**6 Axillary Artery, Left**<br>**See** *5 Axillary Artery, Right*<br>**7 Brachial Artery, Right**<br>Inferior ulnar collateral artery<br>Profunda brachii<br>Superior ulnar collateral artery<br>**8 Brachial Artery, Left**<br>**See** *7 Brachial Artery, Right*<br>**9 Ulnar Artery, Right**<br>Anterior ulnar recurrent artery<br>Common interosseous artery<br>Posterior ulnar recurrent artery<br>**A Ulnar Artery, Left**<br>**See** *9 Ulnar Artery, Right*<br>**B Radial Artery, Right**<br>Radial recurrent artery<br>**C Radial Artery, Left**<br>**See** *B Radial Artery, Right*<br>**D Hand Artery, Right**<br>Deep palmar arch<br>Princeps pollicis artery<br>Radialis indicis<br>Superficial palmar arch<br>**F Hand Artery, Left**<br>**See** *D Hand Artery, Right*<br>**G Intracranial Artery**<br>Anterior cerebral artery<br>Anterior choroidal artery<br>Anterior communicating artery<br>Basilar artery<br>Circle of Willis<br>Internal carotid artery, intracranial portion<br>Middle cerebral artery<br>Ophthalmic artery<br>Posterior cerebral artery<br>Posterior communicating artery<br>Posterior inferior cerebellar artery (PICA)<br>**H Common Carotid Artery, Right**<br>**J Common Carotid Artery, Left**<br>**K Internal Carotid Artery, Right**<br>Caroticotympanic artery<br>Carotid sinus<br>**L Internal Carotid Artery, Left**<br>**See** *K Internal Carotid Artery, Right*<br>**M External Carotid Artery, Right**<br>Ascending pharyngeal artery<br>Internal maxillary artery<br>Lingual artery<br>Maxillary artery<br>Occipital artery<br>Posterior auricular artery<br>Superior thyroid artery<br>**N External Carotid Artery, Left**<br>**See** *M External Carotid Artery, Right*<br>**P Vertebral Artery, Right**<br>Anterior spinal artery<br>Posterior spinal artery<br>**Q Vertebral Artery, Left**<br>**See** *P Vertebral Artery, Right*<br>**R Face Artery**<br>Angular artery<br>Ascending palatine artery<br>External maxillary artery<br>Facial artery<br>Inferior labial artery<br>Submental artery<br>Superior labial artery<br>**S Temporal Artery, Right**<br>Middle temporal artery<br>Superficial temporal artery<br>Transverse facial artery<br>**T Temporal Artery, Left**<br>**See** *S Temporal Artery, Right*<br>**U Thyroid Artery, Right**<br>Cricothyroid artery<br>Hyoid artery<br>Sternocleidomastoid artery<br>Superior laryngeal artery<br>Superior thyroid artery<br>Thyrocervical trunk<br>**V Thyroid Artery, Left**<br>**See** *U Thyroid Artery, Right*<br>**Y Upper Artery**<br>Aortic intercostal artery<br>Bronchial artery<br>Esophageal artery<br>Subcostal artery | **Ø Open**<br>**3 Percutaneous**<br>**4 Percutaneous Endoscopic** | **Z No Device** | **6 Bifurcation**<br>**Z No Qualifier** |

**Ø Medical and Surgical**
**3 Upper Arteries**
**H Insertion** Definition: Putting in a nonbiological appliance that monitors, assists, performs, or prevents a physiological function but does not physically take the place of a body part

Explanation: None

| Body Part Character 4 | Approach Character 5 | Device Character 6 | Qualifier Character 7 |
|---|---|---|---|
| **Ø Internal Mammary Artery, Right**<br>Anterior intercostal artery<br>Internal thoracic artery<br>Musculophrenic artery<br>Pericardiophrenic artery<br>Superior epigastric artery<br>**1 Internal Mammary Artery, Left**<br>*See Ø Internal Mammary Artery, Right*<br>**2 Innominate Artery**<br>Brachiocephalic artery<br>Brachiocephalic trunk<br>**3 Subclavian Artery, Right**<br>Costocervical trunk<br>Dorsal scapular artery<br>Internal thoracic artery<br>**4 Subclavian Artery, Left**<br>*See 3 Subclavian Artery, Right*<br>**5 Axillary Artery, Right**<br>Anterior circumflex humeral artery<br>Lateral thoracic artery<br>Posterior circumflex humeral artery<br>Subscapular artery<br>Superior thoracic artery<br>Thoracoacromial artery<br>**6 Axillary Artery, Left**<br>*See 5 Axillary Artery, Right*<br>**7 Brachial Artery, Right**<br>Inferior ulnar collateral artery<br>Profunda brachii<br>Superior ulnar collateral artery<br>**8 Brachial Artery, Left**<br>*See 7 Brachial Artery, Right*<br>**9 Ulnar Artery, Right**<br>Anterior ulnar recurrent artery<br>Common interosseous artery<br>Posterior ulnar recurrent artery<br>**A Ulnar Artery, Left**<br>*See 9 Ulnar Artery, Right*<br>**B Radial Artery, Right**<br>Radial recurrent artery<br>**C Radial Artery, Left**<br>*See B Radial Artery, Right*<br>**D Hand Artery, Right**<br>Deep palmar arch<br>Princeps pollicis artery<br>Radialis indicis<br>Superficial palmar arch<br>**F Hand Artery, Left**<br>*See D Hand Artery, Right*<br>**G Intracranial Artery**<br>Anterior cerebral artery<br>Anterior choroidal artery<br>Anterior communicating artery<br>Basilar artery<br>Circle of Willis<br>Internal carotid artery, intracranial portion<br>Middle cerebral artery<br>Ophthalmic artery<br>Posterior cerebral artery<br>Posterior communicating artery<br>Posterior inferior cerebellar artery (PICA)<br>**H Common Carotid Artery, Right**<br>**J Common Carotid Artery, Left**<br>**M External Carotid Artery, Right**<br>Ascending pharyngeal artery<br>Internal maxillary artery<br>Lingual artery<br>Maxillary artery<br>Occipital artery<br>Posterior auricular artery<br>Superior thyroid artery<br>**N External Carotid Artery, Left**<br>*See M External Carotid Artery, Right*<br>**P Vertebral Artery, Right**<br>Anterior spinal artery<br>Posterior spinal artery<br>**Q Vertebral Artery, Left**<br>*See P Vertebral Artery, Right*<br>**R Face Artery**<br>Angular artery<br>Ascending palatine artery<br>External maxillary artery<br>Facial artery<br>Inferior labial artery<br>Submental artery<br>Superior labial artery<br>**S Temporal Artery, Right**<br>Middle temporal artery<br>Superficial temporal artery<br>Transverse facial artery<br>**T Temporal Artery, Left**<br>*See S Temporal Artery, Right*<br>**U Thyroid Artery, Right**<br>Cricothyroid artery<br>Hyoid artery<br>Sternocleidomastoid artery<br>Superior laryngeal artery<br>Superior thyroid artery<br>Thyrocervical trunk<br>**V Thyroid Artery, Left**<br>*See U Thyroid Artery, Right* | **Ø Open**<br>**3 Percutaneous**<br>**4 Percutaneous Endoscopic** | **3 Infusion Device**<br>**D Intraluminal Device** | **Z No Qualifier** |
| **K Internal Carotid Artery, Right**<br>Caroticotympanic artery<br>Carotid sinus<br>**L Internal Carotid Artery, Left**<br>*See K Internal Carotid Artery, Right* | **Ø Open**<br>**3 Percutaneous**<br>**4 Percutaneous Endoscope** | **3 Infusion Device**<br>**D Intraluminal Device**<br>**M Stimulator Lead** | **Z No Qualifier** |
| **Y Upper Artery**<br>Aortic intercostal artery<br>Bronchial artery<br>Esophageal artery<br>Subcostal artery | **Ø Open**<br>**3 Percutaneous**<br>**4 Percutaneous Endoscopic** | **2 Monitoring Device**<br>**3 Infusion Device**<br>**D Intraluminal Device**<br>**Y Other Device** | **Z No Qualifier** |

| | |
|---|---|
| **Non-OR** | Ø3H[Ø,1,2,3,4,5,6,7,8,9,A,B,C,D,F,G,H,J,M,N,P,Q,R,S,T,U,V][Ø,3,4]3Z |
| **Non-OR** | Ø3H[K,L][Ø,3,4]3Z |
| **Non-OR** | Ø3HY[Ø,3,4]3Z |
| **Non-OR** | Ø3HY32Z |
| **Non-OR** | Ø3HY[3,4]YZ |

**Ø Medical and Surgical**
**3 Upper Arteries**
**J Inspection** Definition: Visually and/or manually exploring a body part

Explanation: Visual exploration may be performed with or without optical instrumentation. Manual exploration may be performed directly or through intervening body layers.

| Body Part Character 4 | Approach Character 5 | Device Character 6 | Qualifier Character 7 |
|---|---|---|---|
| **Y Upper Artery**<br>Aortic intercostal artery<br>Bronchial artery<br>Esophageal artery<br>Subcostal artery | **Ø Open**<br>**3 Percutaneous**<br>**4 Percutaneous Endoscopic**<br>**X External** | **Z No Device** | **Z No Qualifier** |

**Non-OR** Ø3JY[3,4,X]ZZ

**Ø Medical and Surgical**
**3 Upper Arteries**
**L Occlusion** Definition: Completely closing an orifice or the lumen of a tubular body part
Explanation: The orifice can be a natural orifice or an artificially created orifice

| Body Part Character 4 | | Approach Character 5 | Device Character 6 | Qualifier Character 7 |
|---|---|---|---|---|
| **Ø Internal Mammary Artery, Right**<br>Anterior intercostal artery<br>Internal thoracic artery<br>Musculophrenic artery<br>Pericardiophrenic artery<br>Superior epigastric artery<br>**1 Internal Mammary Artery, Left**<br>*See Ø Internal Mammary Artery, Left*<br>**2 Innominate Artery**<br>Brachiocephalic artery<br>Brachiocephalic trunk<br>**3 Subclavian Artery, Right**<br>Costocervical trunk<br>Dorsal scapular artery<br>Internal thoracic artery<br>**4 Subclavian Artery, Left**<br>*See 3 Subclavian Artery, Right*<br>**5 Axillary Artery, Right**<br>Anterior circumflex humeral artery<br>Lateral thoracic artery<br>Posterior circumflex humeral artery<br>Subscapular artery<br>Superior thoracic artery<br>Thoracoacromial artery<br>**6 Axillary Artery, Left**<br>*See 5 Axillary Artery, Right*<br>**7 Brachial Artery, Right**<br>Inferior ulnar collateral artery<br>Profunda brachii<br>Superior ulnar collateral artery<br>**8 Brachial Artery, Left**<br>*See 7 Brachial Artery, Right*<br>**9 Ulnar Artery, Right**<br>Anterior ulnar recurrent artery<br>Common interosseous artery<br>Posterior ulnar recurrent artery | **A Ulnar Artery, Left**<br>*See 9 Ulnar Artery, Right*<br>**B Radial Artery, Right**<br>Radial recurrent artery<br>**C Radial Artery, Left**<br>*See B Radial Artery, Right*<br>**D Hand Artery, Right**<br>Deep palmar arch<br>Princeps pollicis artery<br>Radialis indicis<br>Superficial palmar arch<br>**F Hand Artery, Left**<br>*See D Hand Artery, Right*<br>**R Face Artery**<br>Angular artery<br>Ascending palatine artery<br>External maxillary artery<br>Facial artery<br>Inferior labial artery<br>Submental artery<br>Superior labial artery<br>**S Temporal Artery, Right**<br>Middle temporal artery<br>Superficial temporal artery<br>Transverse facial artery<br>**T Temporal Artery, Left**<br>*See S Temporal Artery, Right*<br>**U Thyroid Artery, Right**<br>Cricothyroid artery<br>Hyoid artery<br>Sternocleidomastoid artery<br>Superior laryngeal artery<br>Superior thyroid artery<br>Thyrocervical trunk<br>**V Thyroid Artery, Left**<br>*See U Thyroid Artery, Right*<br>**Y Upper Artery**<br>Aortic intercostal artery<br>Bronchial artery<br>Esophageal artery<br>Subcostal artery | **Ø Open**<br>**3 Percutaneous**<br>**4 Percutaneous Endoscopic** | **C Extraluminal Device**<br>**D Intraluminal Device**<br>**Z No Device** | **Z No Qualifier** |
| **G Intracranial Artery**<br>Anterior cerebral artery<br>Anterior choroidal artery<br>Anterior communicating artery<br>Basilar artery<br>Circle of Willis<br>Internal carotid artery, intracranial portion<br>Middle cerebral artery<br>Ophthalmic artery<br>Posterior cerebral artery<br>Posterior communicating artery<br>Posterior inferior cerebellar artery (PICA)<br>**H Common Carotid Artery, Right**<br>**J Common Carotid Artery, Left**<br>**K Internal Carotid Artery, Right**<br>Caroticotympanic artery<br>Carotid sinus | **L Internal Carotid Artery, Left**<br>*See K Internal Carotid Artery, Right*<br>**M External Carotid Artery, Right**<br>Ascending pharyngeal artery<br>Internal maxillary artery<br>Lingual artery<br>Maxillary artery<br>Occipital artery<br>Posterior auricular artery<br>Superior thyroid artery<br>**N External Carotid Artery, Left**<br>*See M External Carotid Artery, Right*<br>**P Vertebral Artery, Right**<br>Anterior spinal artery<br>Posterior spinal artery<br>**Q Vertebral Artery, Left**<br>*See P Vertebral Artery, Right* | **Ø Open**<br>**3 Percutaneous**<br>**4 Percutaneous Endoscopic** | **B Intraluminal Device, Bioactive**<br>**C Extraluminal Device**<br>**D Intraluminal Device**<br>**Z No Device** | **Z No Qualifier** |

**Ø Medical and Surgical**
**3 Upper Arteries**
**N Release**

Definition: Freeing a body part from an abnormal physical constraint by cutting or by the use of force
Explanation: Some of the restraining tissue may be taken out but none of the body part is taken out

| Body Part Character 4 | Approach Character 5 | Device Character 6 | Qualifier Character 7 |
|---|---|---|---|
| **Ø Internal Mammary Artery, Right**<br>Anterior intercostal artery<br>Internal thoracic artery<br>Musculophrenic artery<br>Pericardiophrenic artery<br>Superior epigastric artery<br>**1 Internal Mammary Artery, Left**<br>*See Ø Internal Mammary Artery, Right*<br>**2 Innominate Artery**<br>Brachiocephalic artery<br>Brachiocephalic trunk<br>**3 Subclavian Artery, Right**<br>Costocervical trunk<br>Dorsal scapular artery<br>Internal thoracic artery<br>**4 Subclavian Artery, Left**<br>*See 3 Subclavian Artery, Right*<br>**5 Axillary Artery, Right**<br>Anterior circumflex humeral artery<br>Lateral thoracic artery<br>Posterior circumflex humeral artery<br>Subscapular artery<br>Superior thoracic artery<br>Thoracoacromial artery<br>**6 Axillary Artery, Left**<br>*See 5 Axillary Artery, Right*<br>**7 Brachial Artery, Right**<br>Inferior ulnar collateral artery<br>Profunda brachii<br>Superior ulnar collateral artery<br>**8 Brachial Artery, Left**<br>*See 7 Brachial Artery, Right*<br>**9 Ulnar Artery, Right**<br>Anterior ulnar recurrent artery<br>Common interosseous artery<br>Posterior ulnar recurrent artery<br>**A Ulnar Artery, Left**<br>*See 9 Ulnar Artery, Right*<br>**B Radial Artery, Right**<br>Radial recurrent artery<br>**C Radial Artery, Left**<br>*See B Radial Artery, Right*<br>**D Hand Artery, Right**<br>Deep palmar arch<br>Princeps pollicis artery<br>Radialis indicis<br>Superficial palmar arch<br>**F Hand Artery, Left**<br>*See D Hand Artery, Right*<br>**G Intracranial Artery**<br>Anterior cerebral artery<br>Anterior choroidal artery<br>Anterior communicating artery<br>Basilar artery<br>Circle of Willis<br>Internal carotid artery, intracranial portion<br>Middle cerebral artery<br>Ophthalmic artery<br>Posterior cerebral artery<br>Posterior communicating artery<br>Posterior inferior cerebellar artery (PICA)<br>**H Common Carotid Artery, Right**<br>**J Common Carotid Artery, Left**<br>**K Internal Carotid Artery, Right**<br>Caroticotympanic artery<br>Carotid sinus<br>**L Internal Carotid Artery, Left**<br>*See K Internal Carotid Artery, Right*<br>**M External Carotid Artery, Right**<br>Ascending pharyngeal artery<br>Internal maxillary artery<br>Lingual artery<br>Maxillary artery<br>Occipital artery<br>Posterior auricular artery<br>Superior thyroid artery<br>**N External Carotid Artery, Left**<br>*See M External Carotid Artery, Right*<br>**P Vertebral Artery, Right**<br>Anterior spinal artery<br>Posterior spinal artery<br>**Q Vertebral Artery, Left**<br>*See P Vertebral Artery, Right*<br>**R Face Artery**<br>Angular artery<br>Ascending palatine artery<br>External maxillary artery<br>Facial artery<br>Inferior labial artery<br>Submental artery<br>Superior labial artery<br>**S Temporal Artery, Right**<br>Middle temporal artery<br>Superficial temporal artery<br>Transverse facial artery<br>**T Temporal Artery, Left**<br>*See S Temporal Artery, Right*<br>**U Thyroid Artery, Right**<br>Cricothyroid artery<br>Hyoid artery<br>Sternocleidomastoid artery<br>Superior laryngeal artery<br>Superior thyroid artery<br>Thyrocervical trunk<br>**V Thyroid Artery, Left**<br>*See U Thyroid Artery, Right*<br>**Y Upper Artery**<br>Aortic intercostal artery<br>Bronchial artery<br>Esophageal artery<br>Subcostal artery | **Ø Open**<br>**3 Percutaneous**<br>**4 Percutaneous Endoscopic** | **Z No Device** | **Z No Qualifier** |

**Ø Medical and Surgical**
**3 Upper Arteries**
**P Removal** Definition: Taking out or off a device from a body part

Explanation: If a device is taken out and a similar device put in without cutting or puncturing the skin or mucous membrane, the procedure is coded to the root operation CHANGE. Otherwise, the procedure for taking out a device is coded to the root operation REMOVAL.

| Body Part Character 4 | Approach Character 5 | Device Character 6 | Qualifier Character 7 |
|---|---|---|---|
| **Y Upper Artery**<br>Aortic intercostal artery<br>Bronchial artery<br>Esophageal artery<br>Subcostal artery | **Ø Open**<br>**3 Percutaneous**<br>**4 Percutaneous Endoscopic** | **Ø Drainage Device**<br>**2 Monitoring Device**<br>**3 Infusion Device**<br>**7 Autologous Tissue Substitute**<br>**C Extraluminal Device**<br>**D Intraluminal Device**<br>**J Synthetic Substitute**<br>**K Nonautologous Tissue Substitute**<br>**M Stimulator Lead**<br>**Y Other Device** | **Z No Qualifier** |
| **Y Upper Artery**<br>Aortic intercostal artery<br>Bronchial artery<br>Esophageal artery<br>Subcostal artery | **X External** | **Ø Drainage Device**<br>**2 Monitoring Device**<br>**3 Infusion Device**<br>**D Intraluminal Device**<br>**M Stimulator Lead** | **Z No Qualifier** |

**Non-OR** Ø3PY3[Ø,2,3,D]Z
**Non-OR** Ø3PY[3,4]YZ
**Non-OR** Ø3PYX[Ø,2,3,D,M]Z

**Ø Medical and Surgical**
**3 Upper Arteries**
**Q Repair** Definition: Restoring, to the extent possible, a body part to its normal anatomic structure and function
Explanation: Used only when the method to accomplish the repair is not one of the other root operations

| Body Part Character 4 | Approach Character 5 | Device Character 6 | Qualifier Character 7 |
|---|---|---|---|
| **Ø Internal Mammary Artery, Right**<br>Anterior intercostal artery<br>Internal thoracic artery<br>Musculophrenic artery<br>Pericardiophrenic artery<br>Superior epigastric artery<br>**1 Internal Mammary Artery, Left**<br>*See Ø Internal Mammary Artery, Right*<br>**2 Innominate Artery**<br>Brachiocephalic artery<br>Brachiocephalic trunk<br>**3 Subclavian Artery, Right**<br>Costocervical trunk<br>Dorsal scapular artery<br>Internal thoracic artery<br>**4 Subclavian Artery, Left**<br>*See 3 Subclavian Artery, Right*<br>**5 Axillary Artery, Right**<br>Anterior circumflex humeral artery<br>Lateral thoracic artery<br>Posterior circumflex humeral artery<br>Subscapular artery<br>Superior thoracic artery<br>Thoracoacromial artery<br>**6 Axillary Artery, Left**<br>*See 5 Axillary Artery, Right*<br>**7 Brachial Artery, Right**<br>Inferior ulnar collateral artery<br>Profunda brachii<br>Superior ulnar collateral artery<br>**8 Brachial Artery, Left**<br>*See 7 Brachial Artery, Right*<br>**9 Ulnar Artery, Right**<br>Anterior ulnar recurrent artery<br>Common interosseous artery<br>Posterior ulnar recurrent artery<br>**A Ulnar Artery, Left**<br>*See 9 Ulnar Artery, Right*<br>**B Radial Artery, Right**<br>Radial recurrent artery<br>**C Radial Artery, Left**<br>*See B Radial Artery, Right*<br>**D Hand Artery, Right**<br>Deep palmar arch<br>Princeps pollicis artery<br>Radialis indicis<br>Superficial palmar arch<br>**F Hand Artery, Left**<br>*See D Hand Artery, Right*<br>**G Intracranial Artery**<br>Anterior cerebral artery<br>Anterior choroidal artery<br>Anterior communicating artery<br>Basilar artery<br>Circle of Willis<br>Internal carotid artery, intracranial portion<br>Middle cerebral artery<br>Ophthalmic artery<br>Posterior cerebral artery<br>Posterior communicating artery<br>Posterior inferior cerebellar artery (PICA)<br>**H Common Carotid Artery, Right**<br>**J Common Carotid Artery, Left**<br>**K Internal Carotid Artery, Right**<br>Caroticotympanic artery<br>Carotid sinus<br>**L Internal Carotid Artery, Left**<br>*See K Internal Carotid Artery, Right*<br>**M External Carotid Artery, Right**<br>Ascending pharyngeal artery<br>Internal maxillary artery<br>Lingual artery<br>Maxillary artery<br>Occipital artery<br>Posterior auricular artery<br>Superior thyroid artery<br>**N External Carotid Artery, Left**<br>*See M External Carotid Artery, Right*<br>**P Vertebral Artery, Right**<br>Anterior spinal artery<br>Posterior spinal artery<br>**Q Vertebral Artery, Left**<br>*See P Vertebral Artery, Right*<br>**R Face Artery**<br>Angular artery<br>Ascending palatine artery<br>External maxillary artery<br>Facial artery<br>Inferior labial artery<br>Submental artery<br>Superior labial artery<br>**S Temporal Artery, Right**<br>Middle temporal artery<br>Superficial temporal artery<br>Transverse facial artery<br>**T Temporal Artery, Left**<br>*See S Temporal Artery, Right*<br>**U Thyroid Artery, Right**<br>Cricothyroid artery<br>Hyoid artery<br>Sternocleidomastoid artery<br>Superior laryngeal artery<br>Superior thyroid artery<br>Thyrocervical trunk<br>**V Thyroid Artery, Left**<br>*See U Thyroid Artery, Right*<br>**Y Upper Artery**<br>Aortic intercostal artery<br>Bronchial artery<br>Esophageal artery<br>Subcostal artery | **Ø Open**<br>**3 Percutaneous**<br>**4 Percutaneous Endoscopic** | **Z No Device** | **Z No Qualifier** |

**Ø Medical and Surgical**
**3 Upper Arteries**
**R Replacement** Definition: Putting in or on biological or synthetic material that physically takes the place and/or function of all or a portion of a body part

Explanation: The body part may have been taken out or replaced, or may be taken out, physically eradicated, or rendered nonfunctional during the REPLACEMENT procedure. A REMOVAL procedure is coded for taking out the device used in a previous replacement procedure.

| Body Part Character 4 | | Approach Character 5 | Device Character 6 | Qualifier Character 7 |
|---|---|---|---|---|
| **Ø Internal Mammary Artery, Right**<br>Anterior intercostal artery<br>Internal thoracic artery<br>Musculophrenic artery<br>Pericardiophrenic artery<br>Superior epigastric artery<br>**1 Internal Mammary Artery, Left**<br>***See*** *Ø Internal Mammary Artery, Right*<br>**2 Innominate Artery**<br>Brachiocephalic artery<br>Brachiocephalic trunk<br>**3 Subclavian Artery, Right**<br>Costocervical trunk<br>Dorsal scapular artery<br>Internal thoracic artery<br>**4 Subclavian Artery, Left**<br>***See*** *3 Subclavian Artery, Right*<br>**5 Axillary Artery, Right**<br>Anterior circumflex humeral artery<br>Lateral thoracic artery<br>Posterior circumflex humeral artery<br>Subscapular artery<br>Superior thoracic artery<br>Thoracoacromial artery<br>**6 Axillary Artery, Left**<br>***See*** *5 Axillary Artery, Right*<br>**7 Brachial Artery, Right**<br>Inferior ulnar collateral artery<br>Profunda brachii<br>Superior ulnar collateral artery<br>**8 Brachial Artery, Left**<br>***See*** *7 Brachial Artery, Right*<br>**9 Ulnar Artery, Right**<br>Anterior ulnar recurrent artery<br>Common interosseous artery<br>Posterior ulnar recurrent artery<br>**A Ulnar Artery, Left**<br>***See*** *9 Ulnar Artery, Right*<br>**B Radial Artery, Right**<br>Radial recurrent artery<br>**C Radial Artery, Left**<br>***See*** *B Radial Artery, Right*<br>**D Hand Artery, Right**<br>Deep palmar arch<br>Princeps pollicis artery<br>Radialis indicis<br>Superficial palmar arch<br>**F Hand Artery, Left**<br>***See*** *D Hand Artery, Right*<br>**G Intracranial Artery**<br>Anterior cerebral artery<br>Anterior choroidal artery<br>Anterior communicating artery<br>Basilar artery<br>Circle of Willis<br>Internal carotid artery, intracranial portion<br>Middle cerebral artery<br>Ophthalmic artery<br>Posterior cerebral artery<br>Posterior communicating artery<br>Posterior inferior cerebellar artery (PICA) | **H Common Carotid Artery, Right**<br>**J Common Carotid Artery, Left**<br>**K Internal Carotid Artery, Right**<br>Caroticotympanic artery<br>Carotid sinus<br>**L Internal Carotid Artery, Left**<br>***See*** *K Internal Carotid Artery, Right*<br>**M External Carotid Artery, Right**<br>Ascending pharyngeal artery<br>Internal maxillary artery<br>Lingual artery<br>Maxillary artery<br>Occipital artery<br>Posterior auricular artery<br>Superior thyroid artery<br>**N External Carotid Artery, Left**<br>***See*** *M External Carotid Artery, Right*<br>**P Vertebral Artery, Right**<br>Anterior spinal artery<br>Posterior spinal artery<br>**Q Vertebral Artery, Left**<br>***See*** *P Vertebral Artery, Right*<br>**R Face Artery**<br>Angular artery<br>Ascending palatine artery<br>External maxillary artery<br>Facial artery<br>Inferior labial artery<br>Submental artery<br>Superior labial artery<br>**S Temporal Artery, Right**<br>Middle temporal artery<br>Superficial temporal artery<br>Transverse facial artery<br>**T Temporal Artery, Left**<br>***See*** *S Temporal Artery, Right*<br>**U Thyroid Artery, Right**<br>Cricothyroid artery<br>Hyoid artery<br>Sternocleidomastoid artery<br>Superior laryngeal artery<br>Superior thyroid artery<br>Thyrocervical trunk<br>**V Thyroid Artery, Left**<br>***See*** *U Thyroid Artery, Right*<br>**Y Upper Artery**<br>Aortic intercostal artery<br>Bronchial artery<br>Esophageal artery<br>Subcostal artery | **Ø Open**<br>**4 Percutaneous Endoscopic** | **7 Autologous Tissue Substitute**<br>**J Synthetic Substitute**<br>**K Nonautologous Tissue Substitute** | **Z No Qualifier** |

**Ø Medical and Surgical**
**3 Upper Arteries**
**S Reposition**

Definition: Moving to its normal location, or other suitable location, all or a portion of a body part

Explanation: The body part is moved to a new location from an abnormal location, or from a normal location where it is not functioning correctly. The body part may or may not be cut out or off to be moved to the new location.

| Body Part Character 4 | Approach Character 5 | Device Character 6 | Qualifier Character 7 |
|---|---|---|---|
| **Ø Internal Mammary Artery, Right**<br>Anterior intercostal artery<br>Internal thoracic artery<br>Musculophrenic artery<br>Pericardiophrenic artery<br>Superior epigastric artery<br>**1 Internal Mammary Artery, Left**<br>*See Ø Internal Mammary Artery, Right*<br>**2 Innominate Artery**<br>Brachiocephalic artery<br>Brachiocephalic trunk<br>**3 Subclavian Artery, Right**<br>Costocervical trunk<br>Dorsal scapular artery<br>Internal thoracic artery<br>**4 Subclavian Artery, Left**<br>*See 3 Subclavian Artery, Right*<br>**5 Axillary Artery, Right**<br>Anterior circumflex humeral artery<br>Lateral thoracic artery<br>Posterior circumflex humeral artery<br>Subscapular artery<br>Superior thoracic artery<br>Thoracoacromial artery<br>**6 Axillary Artery, Left**<br>*See 5 Axillary Artery, Right*<br>**7 Brachial Artery, Right**<br>Inferior ulnar collateral artery<br>Profunda brachii<br>Superior ulnar collateral artery<br>**8 Brachial Artery, Left**<br>*See 7 Brachial Artery, Right*<br>**9 Ulnar Artery, Right**<br>Anterior ulnar recurrent artery<br>Common interosseous artery<br>Posterior ulnar recurrent artery<br>**A Ulnar Artery, Left**<br>*See 9 Ulnar Artery, Right*<br>**B Radial Artery, Right**<br>Radial recurrent artery<br>**C Radial Artery, Left**<br>*See B Radial Artery, Right*<br>**D Hand Artery, Right**<br>Deep palmar arch<br>Princeps pollicis artery<br>Radialis indicis<br>Superficial palmar arch<br>**F Hand Artery, Left**<br>*See D Hand Artery, Right*<br>**G Intracranial Artery**<br>Anterior cerebral artery<br>Anterior choroidal artery<br>Anterior communicating artery<br>Basilar artery<br>Circle of Willis<br>Internal carotid artery, intracranial portion<br>Middle cerebral artery<br>Ophthalmic artery<br>Posterior cerebral artery<br>Posterior communicating artery<br>Posterior inferior cerebellar artery (PICA)<br>**H Common Carotid Artery, Right**<br>**J Common Carotid Artery, Left**<br>**K Internal Carotid Artery, Right**<br>Caroticotympanic artery<br>Carotid sinus<br>**L Internal Carotid Artery, Left**<br>*See K Internal Carotid Artery, Right*<br>**M External Carotid Artery, Right**<br>Ascending pharyngeal artery<br>Internal maxillary artery<br>Lingual artery<br>Maxillary artery<br>Occipital artery<br>Posterior auricular artery<br>Superior thyroid artery<br>**N External Carotid Artery, Left**<br>*See M External Carotid Artery, Right*<br>**P Vertebral Artery, Right**<br>Anterior spinal artery<br>Posterior spinal artery<br>**Q Vertebral Artery, Left**<br>*See P Vertebral Artery, Right*<br>**R Face Artery**<br>Angular artery<br>Ascending palatine artery<br>External maxillary artery<br>Facial artery<br>Inferior labial artery<br>Submental artery<br>Superior labial artery<br>**S Temporal Artery, Right**<br>Middle temporal artery<br>Superficial temporal artery<br>Transverse facial artery<br>**T Temporal Artery, Left**<br>*See S Temporal Artery, Right*<br>**U Thyroid Artery, Right**<br>Cricothyroid artery<br>Hyoid artery<br>Sternocleidomastoid artery<br>Superior laryngeal artery<br>Superior thyroid artery<br>Thyrocervical trunk<br>**V Thyroid Artery, Left**<br>*See U Thyroid Artery, Right*<br>**Y Upper Artery**<br>Aortic intercostal artery<br>Bronchial artery<br>Esophageal artery<br>Subcostal artery | **Ø Open**<br>**3 Percutaneous**<br>**4 Percutaneous Endoscopic** | **Z No Device** | **Z No Qualifier** |

**Ø Medical and Surgical**
**3 Upper Arteries**
**U Supplement** Definition: Putting in or on biological or synthetic material that physically reinforces and/or augments the function of a portion of a body part

Explanation: The biological material is non-living, or is living and from the same individual. The body part may have been previously replaced, and the SUPPLEMENT procedure is performed to physically reinforce and/or augment the function of the replaced body part.

| Body Part Character 4 | Approach Character 5 | Device Character 6 | Qualifier Character 7 |
|---|---|---|---|
| **Ø Internal Mammary Artery, Right**<br>Anterior intercostal artery<br>Internal thoracic artery<br>Musculophrenic artery<br>Pericardiophrenic artery<br>Superior epigastric artery<br>**1 Internal Mammary Artery, Left**<br>*See Ø Internal Mammary Artery, Right*<br>**2 Innominate Artery**<br>Brachiocephalic artery<br>Brachiocephalic trunk<br>**3 Subclavian Artery, Right**<br>Costocervical trunk<br>Dorsal scapular artery<br>Internal thoracic artery<br>**4 Subclavian Artery, Left**<br>*See 3 Subclavian Artery, Right*<br>**5 Axillary Artery, Right**<br>Anterior circumflex humeral artery<br>Lateral thoracic artery<br>Posterior circumflex humeral artery<br>Subscapular artery<br>Superior thoracic artery<br>Thoracoacromial artery<br>**6 Axillary Artery, Left**<br>*See 5 Axillary Artery, Right*<br>**7 Brachial Artery, Right**<br>Inferior ulnar collateral artery<br>Profunda brachii<br>Superior ulnar collateral artery<br>**8 Brachial Artery, Left**<br>*See 7 Brachial Artery, Right*<br>**9 Ulnar Artery, Right**<br>Anterior ulnar recurrent artery<br>Common interosseous artery<br>Posterior ulnar recurrent artery<br>**A Ulnar Artery, Left**<br>*See 9 Ulnar Artery, Right*<br>**B Radial Artery, Right**<br>Radial recurrent artery<br>**C Radial Artery, Left**<br>*See B Radial Artery, Right*<br>**D Hand Artery, Right**<br>Deep palmar arch<br>Princeps pollicis artery<br>Radialis indicis<br>Superficial palmar arch<br>**F Hand Artery, Left**<br>*See D Hand Artery, Right*<br>**G Intracranial Artery**<br>Anterior cerebral artery<br>Anterior choroidal artery<br>Anterior communicating artery<br>Basilar artery<br>Circle of Willis<br>Internal carotid artery, intracranial portion<br>Middle cerebral artery<br>Ophthalmic artery<br>Posterior cerebral artery<br>Posterior communicating artery<br>Posterior inferior cerebellar artery (PICA)<br>**H Common Carotid Artery, Right**<br>**J Common Carotid Artery, Left**<br>**K Internal Carotid Artery, Right**<br>Caroticotympanic artery<br>Carotid sinus<br>**L Internal Carotid Artery, Left**<br>*See K Internal Carotid Artery, Right*<br>**M External Carotid Artery, Right**<br>Ascending pharyngeal artery<br>Internal maxillary artery<br>Lingual artery<br>Maxillary artery<br>Occipital artery<br>Posterior auricular artery<br>Superior thyroid artery<br>**N External Carotid Artery, Left**<br>*See M External Carotid Artery, Right*<br>**P Vertebral Artery, Right**<br>Anterior spinal artery<br>Posterior spinal artery<br>**Q Vertebral Artery, Left**<br>*See P Vertebral Artery, Right*<br>**R Face Artery**<br>Angular artery<br>Ascending palatine artery<br>External maxillary artery<br>Facial artery<br>Inferior labial artery<br>Submental artery<br>Superior labial artery<br>**S Temporal Artery, Right**<br>Middle temporal artery<br>Superficial temporal artery<br>Transverse facial artery<br>**T Temporal Artery, Left**<br>*See S Temporal Artery, Right*<br>**U Thyroid Artery, Right**<br>Cricothyroid artery<br>Hyoid artery<br>Sternocleidomastoid artery<br>Superior laryngeal artery<br>Superior thyroid artery<br>Thyrocervical trunk<br>**V Thyroid Artery, Left**<br>*See U Thyroid Artery, Right*<br>**Y Upper Artery**<br>Aortic intercostal artery<br>Bronchial artery<br>Esophageal artery<br>Subcostal artery | **Ø Open**<br>**3 Percutaneous**<br>**4 Percutaneous Endoscopic** | **7 Autologous Tissue Substitute**<br>**J Synthetic Substitute**<br>**K Nonautologous Tissue Substitute** | **Z No Qualifier** |

**Ø Medical and Surgical**
**3 Upper Arteries**
**V Restriction** Definition: Partially closing an orifice or the lumen of a tubular body part
Explanation: The orifice can be a natural orifice or an artificially created orifice

| Body Part Character 4 | Approach Character 5 | Device Character 6 | Qualifier Character 7 |
|---|---|---|---|
| **Ø Internal Mammary Artery, Right**<br>Anterior intercostal artery<br>Internal thoracic artery<br>Musculophrenic artery<br>Pericardiophrenic artery<br>Superior epigastric artery<br>**1 Internal Mammary Artery, Left**<br>*See Ø Internal Mammary Artery, Right*<br>**2 Innominate Artery**<br>Brachiocephalic artery<br>Brachiocephalic trunk<br>**3 Subclavian Artery, Right**<br>Costocervical trunk<br>Dorsal scapular artery<br>Internal thoracic artery<br>**4 Subclavian Artery, Left**<br>*See 3 Subclavian Artery, Right*<br>**5 Axillary Artery, Right**<br>Anterior circumflex humeral artery<br>Lateral thoracic artery<br>Posterior circumflex humeral artery<br>Subscapular artery<br>Superior thoracic artery<br>Thoracoacromial artery<br>**6 Axillary Artery, Left**<br>*See 5 Axillary Artery, Right*<br>**7 Brachial Artery, Right**<br>Inferior ulnar collateral artery<br>Profunda brachii<br>Superior ulnar collateral artery<br>**8 Brachial Artery, Left**<br>*See 7 Brachial Artery, Right*<br>**9 Ulnar Artery, Right**<br>Anterior ulnar recurrent artery<br>Common interosseous artery<br>Posterior ulnar recurrent artery<br>**A Ulnar Artery, Left**<br>*See 9 Ulnar Artery, Right*<br>**B Radial Artery, Right**<br>Radial recurrent artery<br>**C Radial Artery, Left**<br>*See B Radial Artery, Right*<br>**D Hand Artery, Right**<br>Deep palmar arch<br>Princeps pollicis artery<br>Radialis indicis<br>Superficial palmar arch<br>**F Hand Artery, Left**<br>*See D Hand Artery, Right*<br>**R Face Artery**<br>Angular artery<br>Ascending palatine artery<br>External maxillary artery<br>Facial artery<br>Inferior labial artery<br>Submental artery<br>Superior labial artery<br>**S Temporal Artery, Right**<br>Middle temporal artery<br>Superficial temporal artery<br>Transverse facial artery<br>**T Temporal Artery, Left**<br>*See S Temporal Artery, Right*<br>**U Thyroid Artery, Right**<br>Cricothyroid artery<br>Hyoid artery<br>Sternocleidomastoid artery<br>Superior laryngeal artery<br>Superior thyroid artery<br>Thyrocervical trunk<br>**V Thyroid Artery, Left**<br>*See U Thyroid Artery, Right*<br>**Y Upper Artery**<br>Aortic intercostal artery<br>Bronchial artery<br>Esophageal artery<br>Subcostal artery | **Ø Open**<br>**3 Percutaneous**<br>**4 Percutaneous Endoscopic** | **C Extraluminal Device**<br>**D Intraluminal Device**<br>**Z No Device** | **Z No Qualifier** |
| **G Intracranial Artery**<br>Anterior cerebral artery<br>Anterior choroidal artery<br>Anterior communicating artery<br>Basilar artery<br>Circle of Willis<br>Internal carotid artery, intracranial portion<br>Middle cerebral artery<br>Ophthalmic artery<br>Posterior cerebral artery<br>Posterior communicating artery<br>Posterior inferior cerebellar artery (PICA)<br>**H Common Carotid Artery, Right**<br>**J Common Carotid Artery, Left**<br>**K Internal Carotid Artery, Right**<br>Caroticotympanic artery<br>Carotid sinus<br>**L Internal Carotid Artery, Left**<br>*See K Internal Carotid Artery, Right*<br>**M External Carotid Artery, Right**<br>Ascending pharyngeal artery<br>Internal maxillary artery<br>Lingual artery<br>Maxillary artery<br>Occipital artery<br>Posterior auricular artery<br>Superior thyroid artery<br>**N External Carotid Artery, Left**<br>*See M External Carotid Artery, Right*<br>**P Vertebral Artery, Right**<br>Anterior spinal artery<br>Posterior spinal artery<br>**Q Vertebral Artery, Left**<br>*See P Vertebral Artery, Right* | **Ø Open**<br>**3 Percutaneous**<br>**4 Percutaneous Endoscopic** | **B Intraluminal Device, Bioactive**<br>**C Extraluminal Device**<br>**D Intraluminal Device**<br>**Z No Device** | **Z No Qualifier** |

**Ø Medical and Surgical**
**3 Upper Arteries**
**W Revision**

Definition: Correcting, to the extent possible, a portion of a malfunctioning device or the position of a displaced device

Explanation: Revision can include correcting a malfunctioning or displaced device by taking out or putting in components of the device such as a screw or pin

| Body Part Character 4 | Approach Character 5 | Device Character 6 | Qualifier Character 7 |
|---|---|---|---|
| **Y** Upper Artery<br>Aortic intercostal artery<br>Bronchial artery<br>Esophageal artery<br>Subcostal artery | **Ø** Open<br>**3** Percutaneous<br>**4** Percutaneous Endoscopic | **Ø** Drainage Device<br>**2** Monitoring Device<br>**3** Infusion Device<br>**7** Autologous Tissue Substitute<br>**C** Extraluminal Device<br>**D** Intraluminal Device<br>**J** Synthetic Substitute<br>**K** Nonautologous Tissue Substitute<br>**M** Stimulator Lead<br>**Y** Other Device | **Z** No Qualifier |
| **Y** Upper Artery<br>Aortic intercostal artery<br>Bronchial artery<br>Esophageal artery<br>Subcostal artery | **X** External | **Ø** Drainage Device<br>**2** Monitoring Device<br>**3** Infusion Device<br>**7** Autologous Tissue Substitute<br>**C** Extraluminal Device<br>**D** Intraluminal Device<br>**J** Synthetic Substitute<br>**K** Nonautologous Tissue Substitute<br>**M** Stimulator Lead | **Z** No Qualifier |

Non-OR Ø3WY3[Ø,2,3,D]Z
Non-OR Ø3WY[3,4]YZ
Non-OR Ø3WYX[Ø,2,3,7,C,D,J,K,M]Z

# Lower Arteries Ø41–Ø4W



## Character Meanings

This Character Meaning table is provided as a guide to assist the user in the identification of character members that may be found in this section of code tables. It **SHOULD NOT** be used to build a PCS code.

| Operation–Character 3 | Body Part–Character 4 | Approach–Character 5 | Device–Character 6 | Qualifier–Character 7 |
|---|---|---|---|---|
| 1 Bypass | Ø Abdominal Aorta | Ø Open | Ø Drainage Device | Ø Abdominal Aorta |
| 5 Destruction | 1 Celiac Artery | 3 Percutaneous | 1 Radioactive Element | 1 Celiac Artery OR Drug-coated Balloon |
| 7 Dilation | 2 Gastric Artery | 4 Percutaneous Endoscopic | 2 Monitoring Device | 2 Mesenteric Artery |
| 9 Drainage | 3 Hepatic Artery | X External | 3 Infusion Device | 3 Renal Artery, Right |
| B Excision | 4 Splenic Artery | | 4 Intraluminal Device, Drug-eluting | 4 Renal Artery, Left |
| C Extirpation | 5 Superior Mesenteric Artery | | 5 Intraluminal Device, Drug-eluting, Two | 5 Renal Artery, Bilateral |
| H Insertion | 6 Colic Artery, Right | | 6 Intraluminal Device, Drug-eluting, Three | 6 Common Iliac Artery, Right OR Bifurcation |
| J Inspection | 7 Colic Artery, Left | | 7 Intraluminal Device, Drug-eluting, Four or More OR Autologous Tissue Substitute | 7 Common Iliac Artery, Left |
| L Occlusion | 8 Colic Artery, Middle | | 9 Autologous Venous Tissue | 8 Common Iliac Arteries, Bilateral |
| N Release | 9 Renal Artery, Right | | A Autologous Arterial Tissue | 9 Internal Iliac Artery, Right |
| P Removal | A Renal Artery, Left | | C Extraluminal Device | B Internal Iliac Artery, Left |
| Q Repair | B Inferior Mesenteric Artery | | D Intraluminal Device | C Internal Iliac Arteries, Bilateral |
| R Replacement | C Common Iliac Artery, Right | | E Intraluminal Device, Two OR Intraluminal Device, Branched or Fenestrated, One or Two Arteries | D External Iliac Artery, Right |
| S Reposition | D Common Iliac Artery, Left | | F Intraluminal Device, Three OR Intraluminal Device, Branched or Fenestrated, Three or More Arteries | F External Iliac Artery, Left |
| U Supplement | E Internal Iliac Artery, Right | | G Intraluminal Device, Four or More | G External Iliac Arteries, Bilateral |
| V Restriction | F Internal Iliac Artery, Left | | J Synthetic Substitute | H Femoral Artery, Right |
| W Revision | H External Iliac Artery, Right | | K Nonautologous Tissue Substitute | J Femoral Artery, Left OR Temporary |
| | J External Iliac Artery, Left | | Y Other Device | K Femoral Arteries, Bilateral |
| | K Femoral Artery, Right | | Z No Device | L Popliteal Artery |
| | L Femoral Artery, Left | | | M Peroneal Artery |
| | M Popliteal Artery, Right | | | N Posterior Tibial Artery |
| | N Popliteal Artery, Left | | | P Foot Artery |
| | P Anterior Tibial Artery, Right | | | Q Lower Extremity Artery |
| | Q Anterior Tibial Artery, Left | | | R Lower Artery |
| | R Posterior Tibial Artery, Right | | | S Lower Extremity Vein |
| | S Posterior Tibial Artery, Left | | | T Uterine Artery, Right |
| | T Peroneal Artery, Right | | | U Uterine Artery, Left |
| | U Peroneal Artery, Left | | | X Diagnostic |
| | V Foot Artery, Right | | | Z No Qualifier |
| | W Foot Artery, Left | | | |
| | Y Lower Artery | | | |

**AHA Coding Clinic for table Ø41**
**2017, 1Q, 32** Peroneal artery to dorsalis pedis artery bypass using saphenous vein graft
**2016, 2Q, 18** Femoral-tibial artery bypass and saphenous vein graft
**2015, 3Q, 28** Bilateral renal artery bypass

**AHA Coding Clinic for table Ø47**
**2016, 4Q, 86** Peripheral artery, number of stents
**2016, 4Q, 86-88** Coronary and peripheral artery bifurcation
**2016, 3Q, 39** Infrarenal abdominal aortic aneurysm repair with iliac graft extension
**2015, 4Q, 4-7, 15** Drug-coated balloon angioplasty in peripheral vessels
**2015, 3Q, 9** Aborted endovascular stenting of superficial femoral artery

**AHA Coding Clinic for table Ø4C**
**2017, 2Q, 23** Thrombectomy via Fogarty catheter
**2016, 4Q, 86-88** Coronary and peripheral artery bifurcation
**2016, 1Q, 31** Iliofemoral endarterectomy with patch repair
**2015, 1Q, 29** Discontinued carotid endarterectomy
**2015, 1Q, 36** Percutaneous mechanical thrombectomy of femoropopliteal bypass graft

**AHA Coding Clinic for table Ø4H**
**2017, 1Q, 30** Insertion of umbilical artery catheter

**AHA Coding Clinic for table Ø4L**
**2015, 2Q, 27** Uterine artery embolization using Gelfoam
**2014, 3Q, 26** Coil embolization of gastroduodenal artery with chemoembolization of hepatic artery
**2014, 1Q, 24** Endovascular embolization for gastrointestinal bleeding

**AHA Coding Clinic for table Ø4N**
**2015, 2Q, 28** Release and replacement of celiac artery

**AHA Coding Clinic for table Ø4Q**
**2014, 1Q, 21** Repair of femoral artery pseudoaneurysm

**AHA Coding Clinic for table Ø4R**
**2015, 2Q, 28** Release and replacement of celiac artery

**AHA Coding Clinic for table Ø4U**
**2016, 2Q, 18** Femoral-tibial artery bypass and saphenous vein graft
**2016, 1Q, 31** Iliofemoral endarterectomy with patch repair
**2014, 4Q, 37** Bovine patch arterioplasty
**2014, 1Q, 22** Repair of pseudoaneurysm of femoral-popliteal bypass graft

**AHA Coding Clinic for table Ø4V**
**2016, 4Q, 86-87** Coronary and peripheral artery bifurcation
**2016, 4Q, 89-93** Branched and fenestrated endograft repair of aneurysms
**2016, 3Q, 39** Infrarenal abdominal aortic aneurysm repair with iliac graft extension
**2014, 1Q, 9** Endovascular repair of abdominal aortic aneurysm

**AHA Coding Clinic for table Ø4W**
**2015, 1Q, 36** Revision of femoropopliteal bypass graft
**2014, 1Q, 9** Endovascular repair of endoleak
**2014, 1Q, 22** Repair of pseudoaneurysm of femoral-popliteal bypass graft

## Lower Arteries

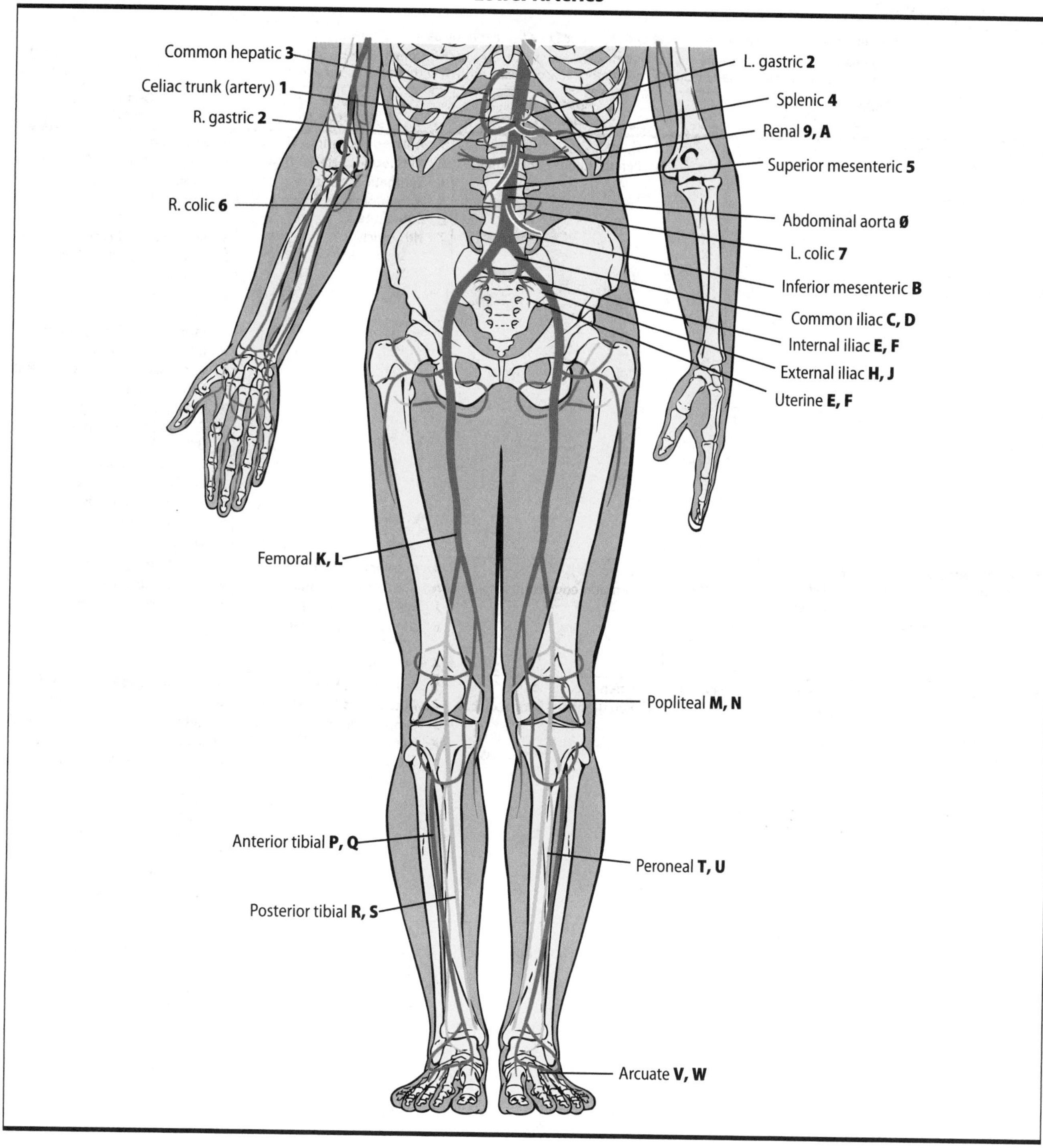
Common hepatic **3**
Celiac trunk (artery) **1**
R. gastric **2**
R. colic **6**
L. gastric **2**
Splenic **4**
Renal **9, A**
Superior mesenteric **5**
Abdominal aorta **Ø**
L. colic **7**
Inferior mesenteric **B**
Common iliac **C, D**
Internal iliac **E, F**
External iliac **H, J**
Uterine **E, F**
Femoral **K, L**
Popliteal **M, N**
Anterior tibial **P, Q**
Peroneal **T, U**
Posterior tibial **R, S**
Arcuate **V, W**

**Ø Medical and Surgical**
**4 Lower Arteries**
**1 Bypass**

Definition: Altering the route of passage of the contents of a tubular body part

Explanation: Rerouting contents of a body part to a downstream area of the normal route, to a similar route and body part, or to an abnormal route and dissimilar body part. Includes one or more anastomoses, with or without the use of a device.

| Body Part Character 4 | Approach Character 5 | Device Character 6 | Qualifier Character 7 |
|---|---|---|---|
| **Ø Abdominal Aorta**<br>Inferior phrenic artery<br>Lumbar artery<br>Median sacral artery<br>Middle suprarenal artery<br>Ovarian artery<br>Testicular artery<br>**C Common Iliac Artery, Right**<br>**D Common Iliac Artery, Left** | **Ø Open**<br>**4 Percutaneous Endoscopic** | **9 Autologous Venous Tissue**<br>**A Autologous Arterial Tissue**<br>**J Synthetic Substitute**<br>**K Nonautologous Tissue Substitute**<br>**Z No Device** | **Ø Abdominal Aorta**<br>**1 Celiac Artery**<br>**2 Mesenteric Artery**<br>**3 Renal Artery, Right**<br>**4 Renal Artery, Left**<br>**5 Renal Artery, Bilateral**<br>**6 Common Iliac Artery, Right**<br>**7 Common Iliac Artery, Left**<br>**8 Common Iliac Arteries, Bilateral**<br>**9 Internal Iliac Artery, Right**<br>**B Internal Iliac Artery, Left**<br>**C Internal Iliac Arteries, Bilateral**<br>**D External Iliac Artery, Right**<br>**F External Iliac Artery, Left**<br>**G External Iliac Arteries, Bilateral**<br>**H Femoral Artery, Right**<br>**J Femoral Artery, Left**<br>**K Femoral Arteries, Bilateral**<br>**Q Lower Extremity Artery**<br>**R Lower Artery** |
| **3 Hepatic Artery**<br>Common hepatic artery<br>Gastroduodenal artery<br>Hepatic artery proper<br>**4 Splenic Artery**<br>Left gastroepiploic artery<br>Pancreatic artery<br>Short gastric artery | **Ø Open**<br>**4 Percutaneous Endoscopic** | **9 Autologous Venous Tissue**<br>**A Autologous Arterial Tissue**<br>**J Synthetic Substitute**<br>**K Nonautologous Tissue Substitute**<br>**Z No Device** | **3 Renal Artery, Right**<br>**4 Renal Artery, Left**<br>**5 Renal Artery, Bilateral** |
| **E Internal Iliac Artery, Right**<br>Deferential artery<br>Hypogastric artery<br>Iliolumbar artery<br>Inferior gluteal artery<br>Inferior vesical artery<br>Internal pudendal artery<br>Lateral sacral artery<br>Middle rectal artery<br>Obturator artery<br>Superior gluteal artery<br>Umbilical artery<br>Uterine artery<br>Vaginal artery<br>**F Internal Iliac Artery, Left**<br>*See E Internal Iliac Artery, Right*<br>**H External Iliac Artery, Right**<br>Deep circumflex iliac artery<br>Inferior epigastric artery<br>**J External Iliac Artery, Left**<br>*See H External Iliac Artery, Right* | **Ø Open**<br>**4 Percutaneous Endoscopic** | **9 Autologous Venous Tissue**<br>**A Autologous Arterial Tissue**<br>**J Synthetic Substitute**<br>**K Nonautologous Tissue Substitute**<br>**Z No Device** | **9 Internal Iliac Artery, Right**<br>**B Internal Iliac Artery, Left**<br>**C Internal Iliac Arteries, Bilateral**<br>**D External Iliac Artery, Right**<br>**F External Iliac Artery, Left**<br>**G External Iliac Arteries, Bilateral**<br>**H Femoral Artery, Right**<br>**J Femoral Artery, Left**<br>**K Femoral Arteries, Bilateral**<br>**P Foot Artery**<br>**Q Lower Extremity Artery** |
| **K Femoral Artery, Right**<br>Circumflex iliac artery<br>Deep femoral artery<br>Descending genicular artery<br>External pudendal artery<br>Superficial epigastric artery<br>**L Femoral Artery, Left**<br>*See K Femoral Artery, Right* | **Ø Open**<br>**4 Percutaneous Endoscopic** | **9 Autologous Venous Tissue**<br>**A Autologous Arterial Tissue**<br>**J Synthetic Substitute**<br>**K Nonautologous Tissue Substitute**<br>**Z No Device** | **H Femoral Artery, Right**<br>**J Femoral Artery, Left**<br>**K Femoral Arteries, Bilateral**<br>**L Popliteal Artery**<br>**M Peroneal Artery**<br>**N Posterior Tibial Artery**<br>**P Foot Artery**<br>**Q Lower Extremity Artery**<br>**S Lower Extremity Vein** |
| **M Popliteal Artery, Right**<br>Inferior genicular artery<br>Middle genicular artery<br>Superior genicular artery<br>Sural artery<br>**N Popliteal Artery, Left**<br>*See M Popliteal Artery, Right* | **Ø Open**<br>**4 Percutaneous Endoscopic** | **9 Autologous Venous Tissue**<br>**A Autologous Arterial Tissue**<br>**J Synthetic Substitute**<br>**K Nonautologous Tissue Substitute**<br>**Z No Device** | **L Popliteal Artery**<br>**M Peroneal Artery**<br>**P Foot Artery**<br>**Q Lower Extremity Artery**<br>**S Lower Extremity Vein** |
| **T Peroneal Artery, Right**<br>Fibular artery<br>**U Peroneal Artery, Left**<br>*See T Peroneal Artery, Right*<br>**V Foot Artery, Right**<br>Arcuate artery<br>Dorsal metatarsal artery<br>Lateral plantar artery<br>Lateral tarsal artery<br>Medial plantar artery<br>**W Foot Artery, Left**<br>*See V Foot Artery, Right* | **Ø Open**<br>**4 Percutaneous Endoscopic** | **9 Autologous Venous Tissue**<br>**A Autologous Arterial Tissue**<br>**J Synthetic Substitute**<br>**K Nonautologous Tissue Substitute**<br>**Z No Device** | **P Foot Artery**<br>**Q Lower Extremity Artery**<br>**S Lower Extremity Vein** |

**Ø Medical and Surgical**
**4 Lower Arteries**
**5 Destruction** Definition: Physical eradication of all or a portion of a body part by the direct use of energy, force, or a destructive agent
Explanation: None of the body part is physically taken out

| Body Part Character 4 | Approach Character 5 | Device Character 6 | Qualifier Character 7 |
|---|---|---|---|
| **Ø Abdominal Aorta**<br>Inferior phrenic artery<br>Lumbar artery<br>Median sacral artery<br>Middle suprarenal artery<br>Ovarian artery<br>Testicular artery<br>**1 Celiac Artery**<br>Celiac trunk<br>**2 Gastric Artery**<br>Left gastric artery<br>Right gastric artery<br>**3 Hepatic Artery**<br>Common hepatic artery<br>Gastroduodenal artery<br>Hepatic artery proper<br>**4 Splenic Artery**<br>Left gastroepiploic artery<br>Pancreatic artery<br>Short gastric artery<br>**5 Superior Mesenteric Artery**<br>Ileal artery<br>Ileocolic artery<br>Inferior pancreaticoduodenal artery<br>Jejunal artery<br>**6 Colic Artery, Right**<br>**7 Colic Artery, Left**<br>**8 Colic Artery, Middle**<br>**9 Renal Artery, Right**<br>Inferior suprarenal artery<br>Renal segmental artery<br>**A Renal Artery, Left**<br>***See*** *9 Renal Artery, Right*<br>**B Inferior Mesenteric Artery**<br>Sigmoid artery<br>Superior rectal artery<br>**C Common Iliac Artery, Right**<br>**D Common Iliac Artery, Left**<br>**E Internal Iliac Artery, Right**<br>Deferential artery<br>Hypogastric artery<br>Iliolumbar artery<br>Inferior gluteal artery<br>Inferior vesical artery<br>Internal pudendal artery<br>Lateral sacral artery<br>Middle rectal artery<br>Obturator artery<br>Superior gluteal artery<br>Umbilical artery<br>Uterine artery<br>Vaginal artery<br>**F Internal Iliac Artery, Left**<br>***See*** *E Internal Iliac Artery, Right*<br>**H External Iliac Artery, Right**<br>Deep circumflex iliac artery<br>Inferior epigastric artery<br>**J External Iliac Artery, Left**<br>***See*** *H External Iliac Artery, Right*<br>**K Femoral Artery, Right**<br>Circumflex iliac artery<br>Deep femoral artery<br>Descending genicular artery<br>External pudendal artery<br>Superficial epigastric artery<br>**L Femoral Artery, Left**<br>***See*** *K Femoral Artery, Right*<br>**M Popliteal Artery, Right**<br>Inferior genicular artery<br>Middle genicular artery<br>Superior genicular artery<br>Sural artery<br>**N Popliteal Artery, Left**<br>***See*** *M Popliteal Artery, Right*<br>**P Anterior Tibial Artery, Right**<br>Anterior lateral malleolar artery<br>Anterior medial malleolar artery<br>Anterior tibial recurrent artery<br>Dorsalis pedis artery<br>Posterior tibial recurrent artery<br>**Q Anterior Tibial Artery, Left**<br>***See*** *P Anterior Tibial Artery, Right*<br>**R Posterior Tibial Artery, Right**<br>**S Posterior Tibial Artery, Left**<br>**T Peroneal Artery, Right**<br>Fibular artery<br>**U Peroneal Artery, Left**<br>***See*** *T Peroneal Artery, Right*<br>**V Foot Artery, Right**<br>Arcuate artery<br>Dorsal metatarsal artery<br>Lateral plantar artery<br>Lateral tarsal artery<br>Medial plantar artery<br>**W Foot Artery, Left**<br>***See*** *V Foot Artery, Right*<br>**Y Lower Artery**<br>Umbilical artery | **Ø Open**<br>**3 Percutaneous**<br>**4 Percutaneous Endoscopic** | **Z No Device** | **Z No Qualifier** |

**Ø Medical and Surgical**
**4 Lower Arteries**
**7 Dilation** Definition: Expanding an orifice or the lumen of a tubular body part

Explanation: The orifice can be a natural orifice or an artificially created orifice. Accomplished by stretching a tubular body part using intraluminal pressure or by cutting part of the orifice or wall of the tubular body part.

| Body Part Character 4 | Approach Character 5 | Device Character 6 | Qualifier Character 7 |
|---|---|---|---|
| **Ø Abdominal Aorta**<br>Inferior phrenic artery<br>Lumbar artery<br>Median sacral artery<br>Middle suprarenal artery<br>Ovarian artery<br>Testicular artery<br>**1 Celiac Artery**<br>Celiac trunk<br>**2 Gastric Artery**<br>Left gastric artery<br>Right gastric artery<br>**3 Hepatic Artery**<br>Common hepatic artery<br>Gastroduodenal artery<br>Hepatic artery proper<br>**4 Splenic Artery**<br>Left gastroepiploic artery<br>Pancreatic artery<br>Short gastric artery<br>**5 Superior Mesenteric Artery**<br>Ileal artery<br>Ileocolic artery<br>Inferior pancreaticoduodenal artery<br>Jejunal artery<br>**6 Colic Artery, Right**<br>**7 Colic Artery, Left**<br>**8 Colic Artery, Middle**<br>**9 Renal Artery, Right**<br>Inferior suprarenal artery<br>Renal segmental artery<br>**A Renal Artery, Left**<br>*See 9 Renal Artery, Right*<br>**B Inferior Mesenteric Artery**<br>Sigmoid artery<br>Superior rectal artery<br>**C Common Iliac Artery, Right**<br>**D Common Iliac Artery, Left**<br>**E Internal Iliac Artery, Right**<br>Deferential artery<br>Hypogastric artery<br>Iliolumbar artery<br>Inferior gluteal artery<br>Inferior vesical artery<br>Internal pudendal artery<br>Lateral sacral artery<br>Middle rectal artery<br>Obturator artery<br>Superior gluteal artery<br>Umbilical artery<br>Uterine artery<br>Vaginal artery<br>**F Internal Iliac Artery, Left**<br>*See E Internal Iliac Artery, Right*<br>**H External Iliac Artery, Right**<br>Deep circumflex iliac artery<br>Inferior epigastric artery<br>**J External Iliac Artery, Left**<br>*See H External Iliac Artery, Right*<br>**K Femoral Artery, Right**<br>Circumflex iliac artery<br>Deep femoral artery<br>Descending genicular artery<br>External pudendal artery<br>Superficial epigastric artery<br>**L Femoral Artery, Left**<br>*See K Femoral Artery, Right*<br>**M Popliteal Artery, Right**<br>Inferior genicular artery<br>Middle genicular artery<br>Superior genicular artery<br>Sural artery<br>**N Popliteal Artery, Left**<br>*See M Popliteal Artery, Right*<br>**P Anterior Tibial Artery, Right**<br>Anterior lateral malleolar artery<br>Anterior medial malleolar artery<br>Anterior tibial recurrent artery<br>Dorsalis pedis artery<br>Posterior tibial recurrent artery<br>**Q Anterior Tibial Artery, Left**<br>*See P Anterior Tibial Artery, Right*<br>**R Posterior Tibial Artery, Right**<br>**S Posterior Tibial Artery, Left**<br>**T Peroneal Artery, Right**<br>Fibular artery<br>**U Peroneal Artery, Left**<br>*See T Peroneal Artery, Right*<br>**V Foot Artery, Right**<br>Arcuate artery<br>Dorsal metatarsal artery<br>Lateral plantar artery<br>Lateral tarsal artery<br>Medial plantar artery<br>**W Foot Artery, Left**<br>*See V Foot Artery, Right*<br>**Y Lower Artery**<br>Umbilical artery | **Ø Open**<br>**3 Percutaneous**<br>**4 Percutaneous Endoscopic** | **4 Intraluminal Device, Drug-eluting**<br>**D Intraluminal Device**<br>**Z No Device** | **1 Drug-coated Balloon**<br>**6 Bifurcation**<br>**Z No Qualifier** |

**Ø47 Continued on next page**

**Ø Medical and Surgical**
**4 Lower Arteries**
**7 Dilation** Definition: Expanding an orifice or the lumen of a tubular body part

Explanation: The orifice can be a natural orifice or an artificially created orifice. Accomplished by stretching a tubular body part using intraluminal pressure or by cutting part of the orifice or wall of the tubular body part.

*Ø47 Continued*

| Body Part Character 4 | | Approach Character 5 | Device Character 6 | Qualifier Character 7 |
|---|---|---|---|---|
| **Ø Abdominal Aorta**<br>Inferior phrenic artery<br>Lumbar artery<br>Median sacral artery<br>Middle suprarenal artery<br>Ovarian artery<br>Testicular artery<br>**1 Celiac Artery**<br>Celiac trunk<br>**2 Gastric Artery**<br>Left gastric artery<br>Right gastric artery<br>**3 Hepatic Artery**<br>Common hepatic artery<br>Gastroduodenal artery<br>Hepatic artery proper<br>**4 Splenic Artery**<br>Left gastroepiploic artery<br>Pancreatic artery<br>Short gastric artery<br>**5 Superior Mesenteric Artery**<br>Ileal artery<br>Ileocolic artery<br>Inferior pancreaticoduodenal artery<br>Jejunal artery<br>**6 Colic Artery, Right**<br>**7 Colic Artery, Left**<br>**8 Colic Artery, Middle**<br>**9 Renal Artery, Right**<br>Inferior suprarenal artery<br>Renal segmental artery<br>**A Renal Artery, Left**<br>*See 9 Renal Artery, Right*<br>**B Inferior Mesenteric Artery**<br>Sigmoid artery<br>Superior rectal artery<br>**C Common Iliac Artery, Right**<br>**D Common Iliac Artery, Left**<br>**E Internal Iliac Artery, Right**<br>Deferential artery<br>Hypogastric artery<br>Iliolumbar artery<br>Inferior gluteal artery<br>Inferior vesical artery<br>Internal pudendal artery<br>Lateral sacral artery<br>Middle rectal artery<br>Obturator artery<br>Superior gluteal artery<br>Umbilical artery<br>Uterine artery<br>Vaginal artery | **F Internal Iliac Artery, Left**<br>*See E Internal Iliac Artery, Right*<br>**H External Iliac Artery, Right**<br>Deep circumflex iliac artery<br>Inferior epigastric artery<br>**J External Iliac Artery, Left**<br>*See H External Iliac Artery, Right*<br>**K Femoral Artery, Right**<br>Circumflex iliac artery<br>Deep femoral artery<br>Descending genicular artery<br>External pudendal artery<br>Superficial epigastric artery<br>**L Femoral Artery, Left**<br>*See K Femoral Artery, Right*<br>**M Popliteal Artery, Right**<br>Inferior genicular artery<br>Middle genicular artery<br>Superior genicular artery<br>Sural artery<br>**N Popliteal Artery, Left**<br>*See M Popliteal Artery, Right*<br>**P Anterior Tibial Artery, Right**<br>Anterior lateral malleolar artery<br>Anterior medial malleolar artery<br>Anterior tibial recurrent artery<br>Dorsalis pedis artery<br>Posterior tibial recurrent artery<br>**Q Anterior Tibial Artery, Left**<br>*See P Anterior Tibial Artery, Right*<br>**R Posterior Tibial Artery, Right**<br>**S Posterior Tibial Artery, Left**<br>**T Peroneal Artery, Right**<br>Fibular artery<br>**U Peroneal Artery, Left**<br>*See T Peroneal Artery, Right*<br>**V Foot Artery, Right**<br>Arcuate artery<br>Dorsal metatarsal artery<br>Lateral plantar artery<br>Lateral tarsal artery<br>Medial plantar artery<br>**W Foot Artery, Left**<br>*See V Foot Artery, Right*<br>**Y Lower Artery**<br>Umbilical artery | **Ø Open**<br>**3 Percutaneous**<br>**4 Percutaneous Endoscopic** | **5 Intraluminal Device, Drug-eluting, Two**<br>**6 Intraluminal Device, Drug-eluting, Three**<br>**7 Intraluminal Device, Drug-eluting, Four or More**<br>**E Intraluminal Device, Two**<br>**F Intraluminal Device, Three**<br>**G Intraluminal Device, Four or More** | **6 Bifurcation**<br>**Z No Qualifier** |

**0 Medical and Surgical**
**4 Lower Arteries**
**9 Drainage** Definition: Taking or letting out fluids and/or gases from a body part
Explanation: The qualifier DIAGNOSTIC is used to identify drainage procedures that are biopsies

| Body Part Character 4 | Approach Character 5 | Device Character 6 | Qualifier Character 7 |
|---|---|---|---|
| **0 Abdominal Aorta**<br>Inferior phrenic artery<br>Lumbar artery<br>Median sacral artery<br>Middle suprarenal artery<br>Ovarian artery<br>Testicular artery<br>**1 Celiac Artery**<br>Celiac trunk<br>**2 Gastric Artery**<br>Left gastric artery<br>Right gastric artery<br>**3 Hepatic Artery**<br>Common hepatic artery<br>Gastroduodenal artery<br>Hepatic artery proper<br>**4 Splenic Artery**<br>Left gastroepiploic artery<br>Pancreatic artery<br>Short gastric artery<br>**5 Superior Mesenteric Artery**<br>Ileal artery<br>Ileocolic artery<br>Inferior pancreaticoduodenal artery<br>Jejunal artery<br>**6 Colic Artery, Right**<br>**7 Colic Artery, Left**<br>**8 Colic Artery, Middle**<br>**9 Renal Artery, Right**<br>Inferior suprarenal artery<br>Renal segmental artery<br>**A Renal Artery, Left**<br>*See 9 Renal Artery, Right*<br>**B Inferior Mesenteric Artery**<br>Sigmoid artery<br>Superior rectal artery<br>**C Common Iliac Artery, Right**<br>**D Common Iliac Artery, Left**<br>**E Internal Iliac Artery, Right**<br>Deferential artery<br>Hypogastric artery<br>Iliolumbar artery<br>Inferior gluteal artery<br>Inferior vesical artery<br>Internal pudendal artery<br>Lateral sacral artery<br>Middle rectal artery<br>Obturator artery<br>Superior gluteal artery<br>Umbilical artery<br>Uterine artery<br>Vaginal artery<br>**F Internal Iliac Artery, Left**<br>*See E Internal Iliac Artery, Right*<br>**H External Iliac Artery, Right**<br>Deep circumflex iliac artery<br>Inferior epigastric artery<br>**J External Iliac Artery, Left**<br>*See H External Iliac Artery, Right*<br>**K Femoral Artery, Right**<br>Circumflex iliac artery<br>Deep femoral artery<br>Descending genicular artery<br>External pudendal artery<br>Superficial epigastric artery<br>**L Femoral Artery, Left**<br>*See K Femoral Artery, Right*<br>**M Popliteal Artery, Right**<br>Inferior genicular artery<br>Middle genicular artery<br>Superior genicular artery<br>Sural artery<br>**N Popliteal Artery, Left**<br>*See M Popliteal Artery, Right*<br>**P Anterior Tibial Artery, Right**<br>Anterior lateral malleolar artery<br>Anterior medial malleolar artery<br>Anterior tibial recurrent artery<br>Dorsalis pedis artery<br>Posterior tibial recurrent artery<br>**Q Anterior Tibial Artery, Left**<br>*See P Anterior Tibial Artery, Right*<br>**R Posterior Tibial Artery, Right**<br>**S Posterior Tibial Artery, Left**<br>**T Peroneal Artery, Right**<br>Fibular artery<br>**U Peroneal Artery, Left**<br>*See T Peroneal Artery, Right*<br>**V Foot Artery, Right**<br>Arcuate artery<br>Dorsal metatarsal artery<br>Lateral plantar artery<br>Lateral tarsal artery<br>Medial plantar artery<br>**W Foot Artery, Left**<br>*See V Foot Artery, Right*<br>**Y Lower Artery**<br>Umbilical artery | **0** Open<br>**3** Percutaneous<br>**4** Percutaneous Endoscopic | **0** Drainage Device | **Z** No Qualifier |

**049 Continued on next page**

**Non-OR** 049[0,1,2,3,4,5,6,7,8,9,A,B,C,D,E,F,H,J,K,L,M,N,P,Q,R,S,T,U,V,W,Y][0,3,4]0Z

Ø49 Continued

**Ø Medical and Surgical**
**4 Lower Arteries**
**9 Drainage** Definition: Taking or letting out fluids and/or gases from a body part
Explanation: The qualifier DIAGNOSTIC is used to identify drainage procedures that are biopsies

| Body Part Character 4 | | Approach Character 5 | Device Character 6 | Qualifier Character 7 |
|---|---|---|---|---|
| **Ø Abdominal Aorta**<br>Inferior phrenic artery<br>Lumbar artery<br>Median sacral artery<br>Middle suprarenal artery<br>Ovarian artery<br>Testicular artery<br>**1 Celiac Artery**<br>Celiac trunk<br>**2 Gastric Artery**<br>Left gastric artery<br>Right gastric artery<br>**3 Hepatic Artery**<br>Common hepatic artery<br>Gastroduodenal artery<br>Hepatic artery proper<br>**4 Splenic Artery**<br>Left gastroepiploic artery<br>Pancreatic artery<br>Short gastric artery<br>**5 Superior Mesenteric Artery**<br>Ileal artery<br>Ileocolic artery<br>Inferior pancreaticoduodenal artery<br>Jejunal artery<br>**6 Colic Artery, Right**<br>**7 Colic Artery, Left**<br>**8 Colic Artery, Middle**<br>**9 Renal Artery, Right**<br>Inferior suprarenal artery<br>Renal segmental artery<br>**A Renal Artery, Left**<br>*See 9 Renal Artery, Right*<br>**B Inferior Mesenteric Artery**<br>Sigmoid artery<br>Superior rectal artery<br>**C Common Iliac Artery, Right**<br>**D Common Iliac Artery, Left**<br>**E Internal Iliac Artery, Right**<br>Deferential artery<br>Hypogastric artery<br>Iliolumbar artery<br>Inferior gluteal artery<br>Inferior vesical artery<br>Internal pudendal artery<br>Lateral sacral artery<br>Middle rectal artery<br>Obturator artery<br>Superior gluteal artery<br>Umbilical artery<br>Uterine artery<br>Vaginal artery | **F Internal Iliac Artery, Left**<br>*See E Internal Iliac Artery, Right*<br>**H External Iliac Artery, Right**<br>Deep circumflex iliac artery<br>Inferior epigastric artery<br>**J External Iliac Artery, Left**<br>*See H External Iliac Artery, Right*<br>**K Femoral Artery, Right**<br>Circumflex iliac artery<br>Deep femoral artery<br>Descending genicular artery<br>External pudendal artery<br>Superficial epigastric artery<br>**L Femoral Artery, Left**<br>*See K Femoral Artery, Right*<br>**M Popliteal Artery, Right**<br>Inferior genicular artery<br>Middle genicular artery<br>Superior genicular artery<br>Sural artery<br>**N Popliteal Artery, Left**<br>*See M Popliteal Artery, Right*<br>**P Anterior Tibial Artery, Right**<br>Anterior lateral malleolar artery<br>Anterior medial malleolar artery<br>Anterior tibial recurrent artery<br>Dorsalis pedis artery<br>Posterior tibial recurrent artery<br>**Q Anterior Tibial Artery, Left**<br>*See P Anterior Tibial Artery, Right*<br>**R Posterior Tibial Artery, Right**<br>**S Posterior Tibial Artery, Left**<br>**T Peroneal Artery, Right**<br>Fibular artery<br>**U Peroneal Artery, Left**<br>*See T Peroneal Artery, Right*<br>**V Foot Artery, Right**<br>Arcuate artery<br>Dorsal metatarsal artery<br>Lateral plantar artery<br>Lateral tarsal artery<br>Medial plantar artery<br>**W Foot Artery, Left**<br>*See V Foot Artery, Right*<br>**Y Lower Artery**<br>Umbilical artery | **Ø** Open<br>**3** Percutaneous<br>**4** Percutaneous Endoscopic | **Z** No Device | **X** Diagnostic<br>**Z** No Qualifier |

**Non-OR** Ø49[Ø,1,2,3,4,5,6,7,8,9,A,B,C,D,E,F,H,J,K,L,M,N,P,Q,R,S,T,U,V,W,Y]3ZX
**Non-OR** Ø49[Ø,1,2,3,4,5,6,7,8,9,A,B,C,D,E,F,H,J,K,L,M,N,P,Q,R,S,T,U,V,W,Y][Ø,3,4]ZZ

**0 Medical and Surgical**
**4 Lower Arteries**
**B Excision** Definition: Cutting out or off, without replacement, a portion of a body part
Explanation: The qualifier DIAGNOSTIC is used to identify excision procedures that are biopsies

| Body Part Character 4 | Approach Character 5 | Device Character 6 | Qualifier Character 7 |
|---|---|---|---|
| **0 Abdominal Aorta**<br>Inferior phrenic artery<br>Lumbar artery<br>Median sacral artery<br>Middle suprarenal artery<br>Ovarian artery<br>Testicular artery<br>**1 Celiac Artery**<br>Celiac trunk<br>**2 Gastric Artery**<br>Left gastric artery<br>Right gastric artery<br>**3 Hepatic Artery**<br>Common hepatic artery<br>Gastroduodenal artery<br>Hepatic artery proper<br>**4 Splenic Artery**<br>Left gastroepiploic artery<br>Pancreatic artery<br>Short gastric artery<br>**5 Superior Mesenteric Artery**<br>Ileal artery<br>Ileocolic artery<br>Inferior pancreaticoduodenal artery<br>Jejunal artery<br>**6 Colic Artery, Right**<br>**7 Colic Artery, Left**<br>**8 Colic Artery, Middle**<br>**9 Renal Artery, Right**<br>Inferior suprarenal artery<br>Renal segmental artery<br>**A Renal Artery, Left**<br>*See 9 Renal Artery, Right*<br>**B Inferior Mesenteric Artery**<br>Sigmoid artery<br>Superior rectal artery<br>**C Common Iliac Artery, Right**<br>**D Common Iliac Artery, Left**<br>**E Internal Iliac Artery, Right**<br>Deferential artery<br>Hypogastric artery<br>Iliolumbar artery<br>Inferior gluteal artery<br>Inferior vesical artery<br>Internal pudendal artery<br>Lateral sacral artery<br>Middle rectal artery<br>Obturator artery<br>Superior gluteal artery<br>Umbilical artery<br>Uterine artery<br>Vaginal artery<br>**F Internal Iliac Artery, Left**<br>*See E Internal Iliac Artery, Right*<br>**H External Iliac Artery, Right**<br>Deep circumflex iliac artery<br>Inferior epigastric artery<br>**J External Iliac Artery, Left**<br>*See H External Iliac Artery, Right*<br>**K Femoral Artery, Right**<br>Circumflex iliac artery<br>Deep femoral artery<br>Descending genicular artery<br>External pudendal artery<br>Superficial epigastric artery<br>**L Femoral Artery, Left**<br>*See K Femoral Artery, Right*<br>**M Popliteal Artery, Right**<br>Inferior genicular artery<br>Middle genicular artery<br>Superior genicular artery<br>Sural artery<br>**N Popliteal Artery, Left**<br>*See M Popliteal Artery, Right*<br>**P Anterior Tibial Artery, Right**<br>Anterior lateral malleolar artery<br>Anterior medial malleolar artery<br>Anterior tibial recurrent artery<br>Dorsalis pedis artery<br>Posterior tibial recurrent artery<br>**Q Anterior Tibial Artery, Left**<br>*See P Anterior Tibial Artery, Right*<br>**R Posterior Tibial Artery, Right**<br>**S Posterior Tibial Artery, Left**<br>**T Peroneal Artery, Right**<br>Fibular artery<br>**U Peroneal Artery, Left**<br>*See T Peroneal Artery, Right*<br>**V Foot Artery, Right**<br>Arcuate artery<br>Dorsal metatarsal artery<br>Lateral plantar artery<br>Lateral tarsal artery<br>Medial plantar artery<br>**W Foot Artery, Left**<br>*See V Foot Artery, Right*<br>**Y Lower Artery**<br>Umbilical artery | **0 Open**<br>**3 Percutaneous**<br>**4 Percutaneous Endoscopic** | **Z No Device** | **X Diagnostic**<br>**Z No Qualifier** |

**Ø Medical and Surgical**
**4 Lower Arteries**
**C Extirpation** Definition: Taking or cutting out solid matter from a body part

Explanation: The solid matter may be an abnormal byproduct of a biological function or a foreign body; it may be imbedded in a body part or in the lumen of a tubular body part. The solid matter may or may not have been previously broken into pieces.

| Body Part Character 4 | Approach Character 5 | Device Character 6 | Qualifier Character 7 |
|---|---|---|---|
| **Ø Abdominal Aorta**<br>Inferior phrenic artery<br>Lumbar artery<br>Median sacral artery<br>Middle suprarenal artery<br>Ovarian artery<br>Testicular artery<br>**1 Celiac Artery**<br>Celiac trunk<br>**2 Gastric Artery**<br>Left gastric artery<br>Right gastric artery<br>**3 Hepatic Artery**<br>Common hepatic artery<br>Gastroduodenal artery<br>Hepatic artery proper<br>**4 Splenic Artery**<br>Left gastroepiploic artery<br>Pancreatic artery<br>Short gastric artery<br>**5 Superior Mesenteric Artery**<br>Ileal artery<br>Ileocolic artery<br>Inferior pancreaticoduodenal artery<br>Jejunal artery<br>**6 Colic Artery, Right**<br>**7 Colic Artery, Left**<br>**8 Colic Artery, Middle**<br>**9 Renal Artery, Right**<br>Inferior suprarenal artery<br>Renal segmental artery<br>**A Renal Artery, Left**<br>***See*** *9 Renal Artery, Right*<br>**B Inferior Mesenteric Artery**<br>Sigmoid artery<br>Superior rectal artery<br>**C Common Iliac Artery, Right**<br>**D Common Iliac Artery, Left**<br>**E Internal Iliac Artery, Right**<br>Deferential artery<br>Hypogastric artery<br>Iliolumbar artery<br>Inferior gluteal artery<br>Inferior vesical artery<br>Internal pudendal artery<br>Lateral sacral artery<br>Middle rectal artery<br>Obturator artery<br>Superior gluteal artery<br>Umbilical artery<br>Uterine artery<br>Vaginal artery<br>**F Internal Iliac Artery, Left**<br>***See*** *E Internal Iliac Artery, Right*<br>**H External Iliac Artery, Right**<br>Deep circumflex iliac artery<br>Inferior epigastric artery<br>**J External Iliac Artery, Left**<br>***See*** *H External Iliac Artery, Right*<br>**K Femoral Artery, Right**<br>Circumflex iliac artery<br>Deep femoral artery<br>Descending genicular artery<br>External pudendal artery<br>Superficial epigastric artery<br>**L Femoral Artery, Left**<br>***See*** *K Femoral Artery, Right*<br>**M Popliteal Artery, Right**<br>Inferior genicular artery<br>Middle genicular artery<br>Superior genicular artery<br>Sural artery<br>**N Popliteal Artery, Left**<br>***See*** *M Popliteal Artery, Right*<br>**P Anterior Tibial Artery, Right**<br>Anterior lateral malleolar artery<br>Anterior medial malleolar artery<br>Anterior tibial recurrent artery<br>Dorsalis pedis artery<br>Posterior tibial recurrent artery<br>**Q Anterior Tibial Artery, Left**<br>***See*** *P Anterior Tibial Artery, Right*<br>**R Posterior Tibial Artery, Right**<br>**S Posterior Tibial Artery, Left**<br>**T Peroneal Artery, Right**<br>Fibular artery<br>**U Peroneal Artery, Left**<br>***See*** *T Peroneal Artery, Right*<br>**V Foot Artery, Right**<br>Arcuate artery<br>Dorsal metatarsal artery<br>Lateral plantar artery<br>Lateral tarsal artery<br>Medial plantar artery<br>**W Foot Artery, Left**<br>***See*** *V Foot Artery, Right*<br>**Y Lower Artery**<br>Umbilical artery | **Ø Open**<br>**3 Percutaneous**<br>**4 Percutaneous Endoscopic** | **Z No Device** | **6 Bifurcation**<br>**Z No Qualifier** |

**Ø Medical and Surgical**
**4 Lower Arteries**
**H Insertion** Definition: Putting in a nonbiological appliance that monitors, assists, performs, or prevents a physiological function but does not physically take the place of a body part
Explanation: None

| Body Part Character 4 | Approach Character 5 | Device Character 6 | Qualifier Character 7 |
|---|---|---|---|
| **Ø Abdominal Aorta**<br>Inferior phrenic artery<br>Lumbar artery<br>Median sacral artery<br>Middle suprarenal artery<br>Ovarian artery<br>Testicular artery | Ø Open<br>3 Percutaneous<br>4 Percutaneous Endoscopic | 2 Monitoring Device<br>3 Infusion Device<br>D Intraluminal Device | Z No Qualifier |
| **1 Celiac Artery**<br>Celiac trunk<br>**2 Gastric Artery**<br>Left gastric artery<br>Right gastric artery<br>**3 Hepatic Artery**<br>Common hepatic artery<br>Gastroduodenal artery<br>Hepatic artery proper<br>**4 Splenic Artery**<br>Left gastroepiploic artery<br>Pancreatic artery<br>Short gastric artery<br>**5 Superior Mesenteric Artery**<br>Ileal artery<br>Ileocolic artery<br>Inferior pancreaticoduodenal artery<br>Jejunal artery<br>**6 Colic Artery, Right**<br>**7 Colic Artery, Left**<br>**8 Colic Artery, Middle**<br>**9 Renal Artery, Right**<br>Inferior suprarenal artery<br>Renal segmental artery<br>**A Renal Artery, Left**<br>*See 9 Renal Artery, Right*<br>**B Inferior Mesenteric Artery**<br>Sigmoid artery<br>Superior rectal artery<br>**C Common Iliac Artery, Right**<br>**D Common Iliac Artery, Left**<br>**E Internal Iliac Artery, Right**<br>Deferential artery<br>Hypogastric artery<br>Iliolumbar artery<br>Inferior gluteal artery<br>Inferior vesical artery<br>Internal pudendal artery<br>Lateral sacral artery<br>Middle rectal artery<br>Obturator artery<br>Superior gluteal artery<br>Umbilical artery<br>Uterine artery<br>Vaginal artery<br>**F Internal Iliac Artery, Left**<br>*See E Internal Iliac Artery, Right*<br>**H External Iliac Artery, Right**<br>Deep circumflex iliac artery<br>Inferior epigastric artery<br>**J External Iliac Artery, Left**<br>*See H External Iliac Artery, Right*<br>**K Femoral Artery, Right**<br>Circumflex iliac artery<br>Deep femoral artery<br>Descending genicular artery<br>External pudendal artery<br>Superficial epigastric artery<br>**L Femoral Artery, Left**<br>*See K Femoral Artery, Right*<br>**M Popliteal Artery, Right**<br>Inferior genicular artery<br>Middle genicular artery<br>Superior genicular artery<br>Sural artery<br>**N Popliteal Artery, Left**<br>*See M Popliteal Artery, Right*<br>**P Anterior Tibial Artery, Right**<br>Anterior lateral malleolar artery<br>Anterior medial malleolar artery<br>Anterior tibial recurrent artery<br>Dorsalis pedis artery<br>Posterior tibial recurrent artery<br>**Q Anterior Tibial Artery, Left**<br>*See P Anterior Tibial Artery, Right*<br>**R Posterior Tibial Artery, Right**<br>**S Posterior Tibial Artery, Left**<br>**T Peroneal Artery, Right**<br>Fibular artery<br>**U Peroneal Artery, Left**<br>*See T Peroneal Artery, Right*<br>**V Foot Artery, Right**<br>Arcuate artery<br>Dorsal metatarsal artery<br>Lateral plantar artery<br>Lateral tarsal artery<br>Medial plantar artery<br>**W Foot Artery, Left**<br>*See V Foot Artery, Right* | Ø Open<br>3 Percutaneous<br>4 Percutaneous Endoscopic | 3 Infusion Device<br>D Intraluminal Device | Z No Qualifier |
| **Y Lower Artery**<br>Umbilical artery | Ø Open<br>3 Percutaneous<br>4 Percutaneous Endoscopic | 2 Monitoring Device<br>3 Infusion Device<br>D Intraluminal Device<br>Y Other Device | Z No Qualifier |

| | |
|---|---|
| DRG Non-OR | Ø4HY32Z |
| Non-OR | Ø4HØ[Ø,3,4][2,3]Z |
| Non-OR | Ø4H[1,2,3,4,5,6,7,8,9,A,B,C,D,E,F,H,J,K,L,M,N,P,Q,R,S,T,U,V,W][Ø,3,4]3Z |
| Non-OR | Ø4HY[Ø,3,4]3Z |
| Non-OR | Ø4HY[3,4]YZ |

**0 Medical and Surgical**
**4 Lower Arteries**
**J Inspection** Definition: Visually and/or manually exploring a body part

Explanation: Visual exploration may be performed with or without optical instrumentation. Manual exploration may be performed directly or through intervening body layers.

| Body Part Character 4 | Approach Character 5 | Device Character 6 | Qualifier Character 7 |
|---|---|---|---|
| Y Lower Artery<br>Umbilical artery | 0 Open<br>3 Percutaneous<br>4 Percutaneous Endoscopic<br>X External | Z No Device | Z No Qualifier |

Non-OR 04JY[3,4,X]ZZ

**0 Medical and Surgical**
**4 Lower Arteries**
**L Occlusion** Definition: Completely closing an orifice or the lumen of a tubular body part

Explanation: The orifice can be a natural orifice or an artificially created orifice

| Body Part Character 4 | Approach Character 5 | Device Character 6 | Qualifier Character 7 |
|---|---|---|---|
| 0 Abdominal Aorta<br>Inferior phrenic artery<br>Lumbar artery<br>Median sacral artery<br>Middle suprarenal artery<br>Ovarian artery<br>Testicular artery | 0 Open<br>4 Percutaneous Endoscopic | C Extraluminal Device<br>D Intraluminal Device<br>Z No Device | Z No Qualifier |
| 0 Abdominal Aorta<br>Inferior phrenic artery<br>Lumbar artery<br>Median sacral artery<br>Middle suprarenal artery<br>Ovarian artery<br>Testicular artery | 3 Percutaneous | C Extraluminal Device<br>Z No Device | Z No Qualifier |
| 0 Abdominal Aorta<br>Inferior phrenic artery<br>Lumbar artery<br>Median sacral artery<br>Middle suprarenal artery<br>Ovarian artery<br>Testicular artery | 3 Percutaneous | D Intraluminal Device | J Temporary<br>Z No Qualifier |

*04L Continued on next page*

**Ø4L Continued**

**Ø Medical and Surgical**
**4 Lower Arteries**
**L Occlusion** Definition: Completely closing an orifice or the lumen of a tubular body part
Explanation: The orifice can be a natural orifice or an artificially created orifice

| Body Part Character 4 | Approach Character 5 | Device Character 6 | Qualifier Character 7 |
|---|---|---|---|
| **1 Celiac Artery**<br>Celiac trunk<br>**2 Gastric Artery**<br>Left gastric artery<br>Right gastric artery<br>**3 Hepatic Artery**<br>Common hepatic artery<br>Gastroduodenal artery<br>Hepatic artery proper<br>**4 Splenic Artery**<br>Left gastroepiploic artery<br>Pancreatic artery<br>Short gastric artery<br>**5 Superior Mesenteric Artery**<br>Ileal artery<br>Ileocolic artery<br>Inferior pancreaticoduodenal artery<br>Jejunal artery<br>**6 Colic Artery, Right**<br>**7 Colic Artery, Left**<br>**8 Colic Artery, Middle**<br>**9 Renal Artery, Right**<br>Inferior suprarenal artery<br>Renal segmental artery<br>**A Renal Artery, Left**<br>*See 9 Renal Artery, Right*<br>**B Inferior Mesenteric Artery**<br>Sigmoid artery<br>Superior rectal artery<br>**C Common Iliac Artery, Right**<br>**D Common Iliac Artery, Left**<br>**H External Iliac Artery, Right**<br>Deep circumflex iliac artery<br>Inferior epigastric artery<br>**J External Iliac Artery, Left**<br>*See H External Iliac Artery, Right*<br>**K Femoral Artery, Right**<br>Circumflex iliac artery<br>Deep femoral artery<br>Descending genicular artery<br>External pudendal artery<br>Superficial epigastric artery<br>**L Femoral Artery, Left**<br>*See K Femoral Artery, Right*<br>**M Popliteal Artery, Right**<br>Inferior genicular artery<br>Middle genicular artery<br>Superior genicular artery<br>Sural artery<br>**N Popliteal Artery, Left**<br>*See M Popliteal Artery, Right*<br>**P Anterior Tibial Artery, Right**<br>Anterior lateral malleolar artery<br>Anterior medial malleolar artery<br>Anterior tibial recurrent artery<br>Dorsalis pedis artery<br>Posterior tibial recurrent artery<br>**Q Anterior Tibial Artery, Left**<br>*See P Anterior Tibial Artery, Right*<br>**R Posterior Tibial Artery, Right**<br>**S Posterior Tibial Artery, Left**<br>**T Peroneal Artery, Right**<br>Fibular artery<br>**U Peroneal Artery, Left**<br>*See T Peroneal Artery, Right*<br>**V Foot Artery, Right**<br>Arcuate artery<br>Dorsal metatarsal artery<br>Lateral plantar artery<br>Lateral tarsal artery<br>Medial plantar artery<br>**W Foot Artery, Left**<br>*See V Foot Artery, Right*<br>**Y Lower Artery**<br>Umbilical artery | **Ø Open**<br>**3 Percutaneous**<br>**4 Percutaneous Endoscopic** | **C Extraluminal Device**<br>**D Intraluminal Device**<br>**Z No Device** | **Z No Qualifier** |
| **E Internal Iliac Artery, Right**<br>Deferential artery<br>Hypogastric artery<br>Iliolumbar artery<br>Inferior gluteal artery<br>Inferior vesical artery<br>Internal pudendal artery<br>Lateral sacral artery<br>Middle rectal artery<br>Obturator artery<br>Superior gluteal artery<br>Umbilical artery<br>Uterine artery<br>Vaginal artery | **Ø Open**<br>**3 Percutaneous**<br>**4 Percutaneous Endoscopic** | **C Extraluminal Device**<br>**D Intraluminal Device**<br>**Z No Device** | **T Uterine Artery, Right** ♀<br>**Z No Qualifier** |
| **F Internal Iliac Artery, Left**<br>Deferential artery<br>Hypogastric artery<br>Iliolumbar artery<br>Inferior gluteal artery<br>Inferior vesical artery<br>Internal pudendal artery<br>Lateral sacral artery<br>Middle rectal artery<br>Obturator artery<br>Superior gluteal artery<br>Umbilical artery<br>Uterine Artery<br>Vaginal artery | **Ø Open**<br>**3 Percutaneous**<br>**4 Percutaneous Endoscopic** | **C Extraluminal Device**<br>**D Intraluminal Device**<br>**Z No Device** | **U Uterine Artery, Left** ♀<br>**Z No Qualifier** |

**Non-OR** Ø4L23DZ
♀ Ø4LE[Ø,3,4][C,D,Z]T
♀ Ø4LF[Ø,3,4][C,D,Z]U

**Ø Medical and Surgical**
**4 Lower Arteries**
**N Release** Definition: Freeing a body part from an abnormal physical constraint by cutting or by the use of force
Explanation: Some of the restraining tissue may be taken out but none of the body part is taken out

| Body Part Character 4 | Approach Character 5 | Device Character 6 | Qualifier Character 7 |
|---|---|---|---|
| **Ø Abdominal Aorta**<br>Inferior phrenic artery<br>Lumbar artery<br>Median sacral artery<br>Middle suprarenal artery<br>Ovarian artery<br>Testicular artery<br>**1 Celiac Artery**<br>Celiac trunk<br>**2 Gastric Artery**<br>Left gastric artery<br>Right gastric artery<br>**3 Hepatic Artery**<br>Common hepatic artery<br>Gastroduodenal artery<br>Hepatic artery proper<br>**4 Splenic Artery**<br>Left gastroepiploic artery<br>Pancreatic artery<br>Short gastric artery<br>**5 Superior Mesenteric Artery**<br>Ileal artery<br>Ileocolic artery<br>Inferior pancreaticoduodenal artery<br>Jejunal artery<br>**6 Colic Artery, Right**<br>**7 Colic Artery, Left**<br>**8 Colic Artery, Middle**<br>**9 Renal Artery, Right**<br>Inferior suprarenal artery<br>Renal segmental artery<br>**A Renal Artery, Left**<br>*See 9 Renal Artery, Right*<br>**B Inferior Mesenteric Artery**<br>Sigmoid artery<br>Superior rectal artery<br>**C Common Iliac Artery, Right**<br>**D Common Iliac Artery, Left**<br>**E Internal Iliac Artery, Right**<br>Deferential artery<br>Hypogastric artery<br>Iliolumbar artery<br>Inferior gluteal artery<br>Inferior vesical artery<br>Internal pudendal artery<br>Lateral sacral artery<br>Middle rectal artery<br>Obturator artery<br>Superior gluteal artery<br>Umbilical artery<br>Uterine artery<br>Vaginal artery<br>**F Internal Iliac Artery, Left**<br>*See E Internal Iliac Artery, Right*<br>**H External Iliac Artery, Right**<br>Deep circumflex iliac artery<br>Inferior epigastric artery<br>**J External Iliac Artery, Left**<br>*See H External Iliac Artery, Right*<br>**K Femoral Artery, Right**<br>Circumflex iliac artery<br>Deep femoral artery<br>Descending genicular artery<br>External pudendal artery<br>Superficial epigastric artery<br>**L Femoral Artery, Left**<br>*See K Femoral Artery, Right*<br>**M Popliteal Artery, Right**<br>Inferior genicular artery<br>Middle genicular artery<br>Superior genicular artery<br>Sural artery<br>**N Popliteal Artery, Left**<br>*See M Popliteal Artery, Right*<br>**P Anterior Tibial Artery, Right**<br>Anterior lateral malleolar artery<br>Anterior medial malleolar artery<br>Anterior tibial recurrent artery<br>Dorsalis pedis artery<br>Posterior tibial recurrent artery<br>**Q Anterior Tibial Artery, Left**<br>*See P Anterior Tibial Artery, Right*<br>**R Posterior Tibial Artery, Right**<br>**S Posterior Tibial Artery, Left**<br>**T Peroneal Artery, Right**<br>Fibular artery<br>**U Peroneal Artery, Left**<br>*See T Peroneal Artery, Right*<br>**V Foot Artery, Right**<br>Arcuate artery<br>Dorsal metatarsal artery<br>Lateral plantar artery<br>Lateral tarsal artery<br>Medial plantar artery<br>**W Foot Artery, Left**<br>*See V Foot Artery, Right*<br>**Y Lower Artery**<br>Umbilical artery | **Ø Open**<br>**3 Percutaneous**<br>**4 Percutaneous Endoscopic** | **Z No Device** | **Z No Qualifier** |

**Ø Medical and Surgical**
**4 Lower Arteries**
**P Removal** Definition: Taking out or off a device from a body part

Explanation: If a device is taken out and a similar device put in without cutting or puncturing the skin or mucous membrane, the procedure is coded to the root operation CHANGE. Otherwise, the procedure for taking out a device is coded to the root operation REMOVAL.

| Body Part Character 4 | Approach Character 5 | Device Character 6 | Qualifier Character 7 |
|---|---|---|---|
| **Y Lower Artery**<br>Umbilical artery | **Ø Open**<br>**3 Percutaneous**<br>**4 Percutaneous Endoscopic** | **Ø Drainage Device**<br>**2 Monitoring Device**<br>**3 Infusion Device**<br>**7 Autologous Tissue Substitute**<br>**C Extraluminal Device**<br>**D Intraluminal Device**<br>**J Synthetic Substitute**<br>**K Nonautologous Tissue Substitute**<br>**Y Other Device** | **Z No Qualifier** |
| **Y Lower Artery**<br>Umbilical artery | **X External** | **Ø Drainage Device**<br>**1 Radioactive Element**<br>**2 Monitoring Device**<br>**3 Infusion Device**<br>**D Intraluminal Device** | **Z No Qualifier** |

**DRG Non-OR** Ø4PY3[Ø,2,3]Z
**Non-OR** Ø4PY3DZ
**Non-OR** Ø4PY[3,4]YZ
**Non-OR** Ø4PYX[Ø,1,2,3,D]Z

**Ø Medical and Surgical**
**4 Lower Arteries**
**Q Repair** Definition: Restoring, to the extent possible, a body part to its normal anatomic structure and function
Explanation: Used only when the method to accomplish the repair is not one of the other root operations

| Body Part Character 4 | | Approach Character 5 | Device Character 6 | Qualifier Character 7 |
|---|---|---|---|---|
| **Ø Abdominal Aorta**<br>Inferior phrenic artery<br>Lumbar artery<br>Median sacral artery<br>Middle suprarenal artery<br>Ovarian artery<br>Testicular artery<br>**1 Celiac Artery**<br>Celiac trunk<br>**2 Gastric Artery**<br>Left gastric artery<br>Right gastric artery<br>**3 Hepatic Artery**<br>Common hepatic artery<br>Gastroduodenal artery<br>Hepatic artery proper<br>**4 Splenic Artery**<br>Left gastroepiploic artery<br>Pancreatic artery<br>Short gastric artery<br>**5 Superior Mesenteric Artery**<br>Ileal artery<br>Ileocolic artery<br>Inferior pancreaticoduodenal artery<br>Jejunal artery<br>**6 Colic Artery, Right**<br>**7 Colic Artery, Left**<br>**8 Colic Artery, Middle**<br>**9 Renal Artery, Right**<br>Inferior suprarenal artery<br>Renal segmental artery<br>**A Renal Artery, Left**<br>***See*** *9 Renal Artery, Right*<br>**B Inferior Mesenteric Artery**<br>Sigmoid artery<br>Superior rectal artery<br>**C Common Iliac Artery, Right**<br>**D Common Iliac Artery, Left**<br>**E Internal Iliac Artery, Right**<br>Deferential artery<br>Hypogastric artery<br>Iliolumbar artery<br>Inferior gluteal artery<br>Inferior vesical artery<br>Internal pudendal artery<br>Lateral sacral artery<br>Middle rectal artery<br>Obturator artery<br>Superior gluteal artery<br>Umbilical artery<br>Uterine artery<br>Vaginal artery | **F Internal Iliac Artery, Left**<br>***See*** *E Internal Iliac Artery, Right*<br>**H External Iliac Artery, Right**<br>Deep circumflex iliac artery<br>Inferior epigastric artery<br>**J External Iliac Artery, Left**<br>***See*** *H External Iliac Artery, Right*<br>**K Femoral Artery, Right**<br>Circumflex iliac artery<br>Deep femoral artery<br>Descending genicular artery<br>External pudendal artery<br>Superficial epigastric artery<br>**L Femoral Artery, Left**<br>***See*** *K Femoral Artery, Right*<br>**M Popliteal Artery, Right**<br>Inferior genicular artery<br>Middle genicular artery<br>Superior genicular artery<br>Sural artery<br>**N Popliteal Artery, Left**<br>***See*** *M Popliteal Artery, Right*<br>**P Anterior Tibial Artery, Right**<br>Anterior lateral malleolar artery<br>Anterior medial malleolar artery<br>Anterior tibial recurrent artery<br>Dorsalis pedis artery<br>Posterior tibial recurrent artery<br>**Q Anterior Tibial Artery, Left**<br>***See*** *P Anterior Tibial Artery, Right*<br>**R Posterior Tibial Artery, Right**<br>**S Posterior Tibial Artery, Left**<br>**T Peroneal Artery, Right**<br>Fibular artery<br>**U Peroneal Artery, Left**<br>***See*** *T Peroneal Artery, Right*<br>**V Foot Artery, Right**<br>Arcuate artery<br>Dorsal metatarsal artery<br>Lateral plantar artery<br>Lateral tarsal artery<br>Medial plantar artery<br>**W Foot Artery, Left**<br>***See*** *V Foot Artery, Right*<br>**Y Lower Artery**<br>Umbilical artery | **Ø Open**<br>**3 Percutaneous**<br>**4 Percutaneous Endoscopic** | **Z No Device** | **Z No Qualifier** |

**Ø Medical and Surgical**
**4 Lower Arteries**
**R Replacement** Definition: Putting in or on biological or synthetic material that physically takes the place and/or function of all or a portion of a body part

Explanation: The body part may have been taken out or replaced, or may be taken out, physically eradicated, or rendered nonfunctional during the REPLACEMENT procedure. A REMOVAL procedure is coded for taking out the device used in a previous replacement procedure.

| Body Part Character 4 | Approach Character 5 | Device Character 6 | Qualifier Character 7 |
|---|---|---|---|
| **Ø Abdominal Aorta**<br>Inferior phrenic artery<br>Lumbar artery<br>Median sacral artery<br>Middle suprarenal artery<br>Ovarian artery<br>Testicular artery<br>**1 Celiac Artery**<br>Celiac trunk<br>**2 Gastric Artery**<br>Left gastric artery<br>Right gastric artery<br>**3 Hepatic Artery**<br>Common hepatic artery<br>Gastroduodenal artery<br>Hepatic artery proper<br>**4 Splenic Artery**<br>Left gastroepiploic artery<br>Pancreatic artery<br>Short gastric artery<br>**5 Superior Mesenteric Artery**<br>Ileal artery<br>Ileocolic artery<br>Inferior pancreaticoduodenal artery<br>Jejunal artery<br>**6 Colic Artery, Right**<br>**7 Colic Artery, Left**<br>**8 Colic Artery, Middle**<br>**9 Renal Artery, Right**<br>Inferior suprarenal artery<br>Renal segmental artery<br>**A Renal Artery, Left**<br>***See*** *9 Renal Artery, Right*<br>**B Inferior Mesenteric Artery**<br>Sigmoid artery<br>Superior rectal artery<br>**C Common Iliac Artery, Right**<br>**D Common Iliac Artery, Left**<br>**E Internal Iliac Artery, Right**<br>Deferential artery<br>Hypogastric artery<br>Iliolumbar artery<br>Inferior gluteal artery<br>Inferior vesical artery<br>Internal pudendal artery<br>Lateral sacral artery<br>Middle rectal artery<br>Obturator artery<br>Superior gluteal artery<br>Umbilical artery<br>Uterine artery<br>Vaginal artery<br>**F Internal Iliac Artery, Left**<br>***See*** *E Internal Iliac Artery, Right*<br>**H External Iliac Artery, Right**<br>Deep circumflex iliac artery<br>Inferior epigastric artery<br>**J External Iliac Artery, Left**<br>***See*** *H External Iliac Artery, Right*<br>**K Femoral Artery, Right**<br>Circumflex iliac artery<br>Deep femoral artery<br>Descending genicular artery<br>External pudendal artery<br>Superficial epigastric artery<br>**L Femoral Artery, Left**<br>***See*** *K Femoral Artery, Right*<br>**M Popliteal Artery, Right**<br>Inferior genicular artery<br>Middle genicular artery<br>Superior genicular artery<br>Sural artery<br>**N Popliteal Artery, Left**<br>***See*** *M Popliteal Artery, Right*<br>**P Anterior Tibial Artery, Right**<br>Anterior lateral malleolar artery<br>Anterior medial malleolar artery<br>Anterior tibial recurrent artery<br>Dorsalis pedis artery<br>Posterior tibial recurrent artery<br>**Q Anterior Tibial Artery, Left**<br>***See*** *P Anterior Tibial Artery, Right*<br>**R Posterior Tibial Artery, Right**<br>**S Posterior Tibial Artery, Left**<br>**T Peroneal Artery, Right**<br>Fibular artery<br>**U Peroneal Artery, Left**<br>***See*** *T Peroneal Artery, Right*<br>**V Foot Artery, Right**<br>Arcuate artery<br>Dorsal metatarsal artery<br>Lateral plantar artery<br>Lateral tarsal artery<br>Medial plantar artery<br>**W Foot Artery, Left**<br>***See*** *V Foot Artery, Right*<br>**Y Lower Artery**<br>Umbilical artery | **Ø Open**<br>**4 Percutaneous Endoscopic** | **7 Autologous Tissue Substitute**<br>**J Synthetic Substitute**<br>**K Nonautologous Tissue Substitute** | **Z No Qualifier** |

**Ø Medical and Surgical**
**4 Lower Arteries**
**S Reposition** Definition: Moving to its normal location, or other suitable location, all or a portion of a body part

Explanation: The body part is moved to a new location from an abnormal location, or from a normal location where it is not functioning correctly. The body part may or may not be cut out or off to be moved to the new location.

| Body Part Character 4 | | Approach Character 5 | Device Character 6 | Qualifier Character 7 |
|---|---|---|---|---|
| **Ø Abdominal Aorta**<br>Inferior phrenic artery<br>Lumbar artery<br>Median sacral artery<br>Middle suprarenal artery<br>Ovarian artery<br>Testicular artery<br>**1 Celiac Artery**<br>Celiac trunk<br>**2 Gastric Artery**<br>Left gastric artery<br>Right gastric artery<br>**3 Hepatic Artery**<br>Common hepatic artery<br>Gastroduodenal artery<br>Hepatic artery proper<br>**4 Splenic Artery**<br>Left gastroepiploic artery<br>Pancreatic artery<br>Short gastric artery<br>**5 Superior Mesenteric Artery**<br>Ileal artery<br>Ileocolic artery<br>Inferior pancreaticoduodenal artery<br>Jejunal artery<br>**6 Colic Artery, Right**<br>**7 Colic Artery, Left**<br>**8 Colic Artery, Middle**<br>**9 Renal Artery, Right**<br>Inferior suprarenal artery<br>Renal segmental artery<br>**A Renal Artery, Left**<br>*See 9 Renal Artery, Right*<br>**B Inferior Mesenteric Artery**<br>Sigmoid artery<br>Superior rectal artery<br>**C Common Iliac Artery, Right**<br>**D Common Iliac Artery, Left**<br>**E Internal Iliac Artery, Right**<br>Deferential artery<br>Hypogastric artery<br>Iliolumbar artery<br>Inferior gluteal artery<br>Inferior vesical artery<br>Internal pudendal artery<br>Lateral sacral artery<br>Middle rectal artery<br>Obturator artery<br>Superior gluteal artery<br>Umbilical artery<br>Uterine artery<br>Vaginal artery | **F Internal Iliac Artery, Left**<br>*See E Internal Iliac Artery, Right*<br>**H External Iliac Artery, Right**<br>Deep circumflex iliac artery<br>Inferior epigastric artery<br>**J External Iliac Artery, Left**<br>*See H External Iliac Artery, Right*<br>**K Femoral Artery, Right**<br>Circumflex iliac artery<br>Deep femoral artery<br>Descending genicular artery<br>External pudendal artery<br>Superficial epigastric artery<br>**L Femoral Artery, Left**<br>*See K Femoral Artery, Right*<br>**M Popliteal Artery, Right**<br>Inferior genicular artery<br>Middle genicular artery<br>Superior genicular artery<br>Sural artery<br>**N Popliteal Artery, Left**<br>*See M Popliteal Artery, Right*<br>**P Anterior Tibial Artery, Right**<br>Anterior lateral malleolar artery<br>Anterior medial malleolar artery<br>Anterior tibial recurrent artery<br>Dorsalis pedis artery<br>Posterior tibial recurrent artery<br>**Q Anterior Tibial Artery, Left**<br>*See P Anterior Tibial Artery, Right*<br>**R Posterior Tibial Artery, Right**<br>**S Posterior Tibial Artery, Left**<br>**T Peroneal Artery, Right**<br>Fibular artery<br>**U Peroneal Artery, Left**<br>*See T Peroneal Artery, Right*<br>**V Foot Artery, Right**<br>Arcuate artery<br>Dorsal metatarsal artery<br>Lateral plantar artery<br>Lateral tarsal artery<br>Medial plantar artery<br>**W Foot Artery, Left**<br>*See V Foot Artery, Right*<br>**Y Lower Artery**<br>Umbilical artery | **Ø Open**<br>**3 Percutaneous**<br>**4 Percutaneous Endoscopic** | **Z No Device** | **Z No Qualifier** |

**Ø Medical and Surgical**
**4 Lower Arteries**
**U Supplement** Definition: Putting in or on biological or synthetic material that physically reinforces and/or augments the function of a portion of a body part

Explanation: The biological material is non-living, or is living and from the same individual. The body part may have been previously replaced, and the SUPPLEMENT procedure is performed to physically reinforce and/or augment the function of the replaced body part.

| Body Part<br>Character 4 | | Approach<br>Character 5 | Device<br>Character 6 | Qualifier<br>Character 7 |
|---|---|---|---|---|
| **Ø Abdominal Aorta**<br>Inferior phrenic artery<br>Lumbar artery<br>Median sacral artery<br>Middle suprarenal artery<br>Ovarian artery<br>Testicular artery<br>**1 Celiac Artery**<br>Celiac trunk<br>**2 Gastric Artery**<br>Left gastric artery<br>Right gastric artery<br>**3 Hepatic Artery**<br>Common hepatic artery<br>Gastroduodenal artery<br>Hepatic artery proper<br>**4 Splenic Artery**<br>Left gastroepiploic artery<br>Pancreatic artery<br>Short gastric artery<br>**5 Superior Mesenteric Artery**<br>Ileal artery<br>Ileocolic artery<br>Inferior pancreaticoduodenal artery<br>Jejunal artery<br>**6 Colic Artery, Right**<br>**7 Colic Artery, Left**<br>**8 Colic Artery, Middle**<br>**9 Renal Artery, Right**<br>Inferior suprarenal artery<br>Renal segmental artery<br>**A Renal Artery, Left**<br>***See*** *9 Renal Artery, Right*<br>**B Inferior Mesenteric Artery**<br>Sigmoid artery<br>Superior rectal artery<br>**C Common Iliac Artery, Right**<br>**D Common Iliac Artery, Left**<br>**E Internal Iliac Artery, Right**<br>Deferential artery<br>Hypogastric artery<br>Iliolumbar artery<br>Inferior gluteal artery<br>Inferior vesical artery<br>Internal pudendal artery<br>Lateral sacral artery<br>Middle rectal artery<br>Obturator artery<br>Superior gluteal artery<br>Umbilical artery<br>Uterine artery<br>Vaginal artery | **F Internal Iliac Artery, Left**<br>***See*** *E Internal Iliac Artery, Right*<br>**H External Iliac Artery, Right**<br>Deep circumflex iliac artery<br>Inferior epigastric artery<br>**J External Iliac Artery, Left**<br>***See*** *H External Iliac Artery, Right*<br>**K Femoral Artery, Right**<br>Circumflex iliac artery<br>Deep femoral artery<br>Descending genicular artery<br>External pudendal artery<br>Superficial epigastric artery<br>**L Femoral Artery, Left**<br>***See*** *K Femoral Artery, Right*<br>**M Popliteal Artery, Right**<br>Inferior genicular artery<br>Middle genicular artery<br>Superior genicular artery<br>Sural artery<br>**N Popliteal Artery, Left**<br>***See*** *M Popliteal Artery, Right*<br>**P Anterior Tibial Artery, Right**<br>Anterior lateral malleolar artery<br>Anterior medial malleolar artery<br>Anterior tibial recurrent artery<br>Dorsalis pedis artery<br>Posterior tibial recurrent artery<br>**Q Anterior Tibial Artery, Left**<br>***See*** *P Anterior Tibial Artery, Right*<br>**R Posterior Tibial Artery, Right**<br>**S Posterior Tibial Artery, Left**<br>**T Peroneal Artery, Right**<br>Fibular artery<br>**U Peroneal Artery, Left**<br>***See*** *T Peroneal Artery, Right*<br>**V Foot Artery, Right**<br>Arcuate artery<br>Dorsal metatarsal artery<br>Lateral plantar artery<br>Lateral tarsal artery<br>Medial plantar artery<br>**W Foot Artery, Left**<br>***See*** *V Foot Artery, Right*<br>**Y Lower Artery**<br>Umbilical artery | **Ø Open**<br>**3 Percutaneous**<br>**4 Percutaneous Endoscopic** | **7 Autologous Tissue Substitute**<br>**J Synthetic Substitute**<br>**K Nonautologous Tissue Substitute** | **Z No Qualifier** |

**Ø Medical and Surgical**
**4 Lower Arteries**
**V Restriction** Definition: Partially closing an orifice or the lumen of a tubular body part
Explanation: The orifice can be a natural orifice or an artificially created orifice

| Body Part<br>Character 4 | Approach<br>Character 5 | Device<br>Character 6 | Qualifier<br>Character 7 |
|---|---|---|---|
| **Ø Abdominal Aorta**<br>Inferior phrenic artery<br>Lumbar artery<br>Median sacral artery<br>Middle suprarenal artery<br>Ovarian artery<br>Testicular artery | **Ø Open**<br>**3 Percutaneous**<br>**4 Percutaneous Endoscopic** | **C Extraluminal Device**<br>**E Intraluminal Device, Branched or Fenestrated, One or Two Arteries**<br>**F Intraluminal Device, Branched or Fenestrated, Three or More Arteries**<br>**Z No Device** | **6 Bifurcation**<br>**Z No Qualifier** |
| **Ø Abdominal Aorta**<br>Inferior phrenic artery<br>Lumbar artery<br>Median sacral artery<br>Middle suprarenal artery<br>Ovarian artery<br>Testicular artery | **Ø Open**<br>**3 Percutaneous**<br>**4 Percutaneous Endoscopic** | **D Intraluminal Device** | **6 Bifurcation**<br>**J Temporary**<br>**Z No Qualifier** |
| **1 Celiac Artery**<br>Celiac trunk<br>**2 Gastric Artery**<br>Left gastric artery<br>Right gastric artery<br>**3 Hepatic Artery**<br>Common hepatic artery<br>Gastroduodenal artery<br>Hepatic artery proper<br>**4 Splenic Artery**<br>Left gastroepiploic artery<br>Pancreatic artery<br>Short gastric artery<br>**5 Superior Mesenteric Artery**<br>Ileal artery<br>Ileocolic artery<br>Inferior pancreaticoduodenal artery<br>Jejunal artery<br>**6 Colic Artery, Right**<br>**7 Colic Artery, Left**<br>**8 Colic Artery, Middle**<br>**9 Renal Artery, Right**<br>Inferior suprarenal artery<br>Renal segmental artery<br>**A Renal Artery, Left**<br>*See 9 Renal Artery, Right*<br>**B Inferior Mesenteric Artery**<br>Sigmoid artery<br>Superior rectal artery<br>**E Internal Iliac Artery, Right**<br>Deferential artery<br>Hypogastric artery<br>Iliolumbar artery<br>Inferior gluteal artery<br>Inferior vesical artery<br>Internal pudendal artery<br>Lateral sacral artery<br>Middle rectal artery<br>Obturator artery<br>Superior gluteal artery<br>Umbilical artery<br>Uterine artery<br>Vaginal artery<br>**F Internal Iliac Artery, Left**<br>*See E Internal Iliac Artery, Right*<br>**H External Iliac Artery, Right**<br>Deep circumflex iliac artery<br>Inferior epigastric artery<br>**J External Iliac Artery, Left**<br>*See H External Iliac Artery, Right*<br>**K Femoral Artery, Right**<br>Circumflex iliac artery<br>Deep femoral artery<br>Descending genicular artery<br>External pudendal artery<br>Superficial epigastric artery<br>**L Femoral Artery, Left**<br>*See K Femoral Artery, Right*<br>**M Popliteal Artery, Right**<br>Inferior genicular artery<br>Middle genicular artery<br>Superior genicular artery<br>Sural artery<br>**N Popliteal Artery, Left**<br>*See M Popliteal Artery, Right*<br>**P Anterior Tibial Artery, Right**<br>Anterior lateral malleolar artery<br>Anterior medial malleolar artery<br>Anterior tibial recurrent artery<br>Dorsalis pedis artery<br>Posterior tibial recurrent artery<br>**Q Anterior Tibial Artery, Left**<br>*See P Anterior Tibial Artery, Right*<br>**R Posterior Tibial Artery, Right**<br>**S Posterior Tibial Artery, Left**<br>**T Peroneal Artery, Right**<br>Fibular artery<br>**U Peroneal Artery, Left**<br>*See T Peroneal Artery, Right*<br>**V Foot Artery, Right**<br>Arcuate artery<br>Dorsal metatarsal artery<br>Lateral plantar artery<br>Lateral tarsal artery<br>Medial plantar artery<br>**W Foot Artery, Left**<br>*See V Foot Artery, Right*<br>**Y Lower Artery**<br>Umbilical artery | **Ø Open**<br>**3 Percutaneous**<br>**4 Percutaneous Endoscopic** | **C Extraluminal Device**<br>**D Intraluminal Device**<br>**Z No Device** | **Z No Qualifier** |
| **C Common Iliac Artery, Right**<br>**D Common Iliac Artery, Left** | **Ø Open**<br>**3 Percutaneous**<br>**4 Percutaneous Endoscopic** | **C Extraluminal Device**<br>**D Intraluminal Device**<br>**E Intraluminal Device, Branched or Fenestrated, One or Two Arteries**<br>**Z No Device** | **Z No Qualifier** |

**Ø Medical and Surgical**
**4 Lower Arteries**
**W Revision**

Definition: Correcting, to the extent possible, a portion of a malfunctioning device or the position of a displaced device

Explanation: Revision can include correcting a malfunctioning or displaced device by taking out or putting in components of the device such as a screw or pin

| Body Part Character 4 | Approach Character 5 | Device Character 6 | Qualifier Character 7 |
|---|---|---|---|
| **Y** Lower Artery<br>Umbilical artery | **Ø** Open<br>**3** Percutaneous<br>**4** Percutaneous Endoscopic | **Ø** Drainage Device<br>**2** Monitoring Device<br>**3** Infusion Device<br>**7** Autologous Tissue Substitute<br>**C** Extraluminal Device<br>**D** Intraluminal Device<br>**J** Synthetic Substitute<br>**K** Nonautologous Tissue Substitute<br>**Y** Other Device | **Z** No Qualifier |
| **Y** Lower Artery<br>Umbilical artery | **X** External | **Ø** Drainage Device<br>**2** Monitoring Device<br>**3** Infusion Device<br>**7** Autologous Tissue Substitute<br>**C** Extraluminal Device<br>**D** Intraluminal Device<br>**J** Synthetic Substitute<br>**K** Nonautologous Tissue Substitute | **Z** No Qualifier |

Non-OR Ø4WY3[Ø,2,3,D]Z
Non-OR Ø4WY[3,4]YZ
Non-OR Ø4WYX[Ø,2,3,7,C,D,J,K]Z

# Upper Veins Ø51–Ø5W



## Character Meanings

This Character Meaning table is provided as a guide to assist the user in the identification of character members that may be found in this section of code tables. It **SHOULD NOT** be used to build a PCS code.

| Operation–Character 3 | Body Part–Character 4 | Approach–Character 5 | Device–Character 6 | Qualifier–Character 7 |
|---|---|---|---|---|
| 1 Bypass | Ø Azygos Vein | Ø Open | Ø Drainage Device | X Diagnostic |
| 5 Destruction | 1 Hemiazygos Vein | 3 Percutaneous | 2 Monitoring Device | Y Upper Vein |
| 7 Dilation | 3 Innominate Vein, Right | 4 Percutaneous Endoscopic | 3 Infusion Device | Z No Qualifier |
| 9 Drainage | 4 Innominate Vein, Left | X External | 7 Autologous Tissue Substitute | |
| B Excision | 5 Subclavian Vein, Right | | 9 Autologous Venous Tissue | |
| C Extirpation | 6 Subclavian Vein, Left | | A Autologous Arterial Tissue | |
| D Extraction | 7 Axillary Vein, Right | | C Extraluminal Device | |
| H Insertion | 8 Axillary Vein, Left | | D Intraluminal Device | |
| J Inspection | 9 Brachial Vein, Right | | J Synthetic Substitute | |
| L Occlusion | A Brachial Vein, Left | | K Nonautologous Tissue Substitute | |
| N Release | B Basilic Vein, Right | | M Neurostimulator Lead | |
| P Removal | C Basilic Vein, Left | | Y Other Device | |
| Q Repair | D Cephalic Vein, Right | | Z No Device | |
| R Replacement | F Cephalic Vein, Left | | | |
| S Reposition | G Hand Vein, Right | | | |
| U Supplement | H Hand Vein, Left | | | |
| V Restriction | L Intracranial Vein | | | |
| W Revision | M Internal Jugular Vein, Right | | | |
| | N Internal Jugular Vein, Left | | | |
| | P External Jugular Vein, Right | | | |
| | Q External Jugular Vein, Left | | | |
| | R Vertebral Vein, Right | | | |
| | S Vertebral Vein, Left | | | |
| | T Face Vein, Right | | | |
| | V Face Vein, Left | | | |
| | Y Upper Vein | | | |

**AHA Coding Clinic for table Ø5B**
**2016, 2Q, 12** Resection of malignant neoplasm of infratemporal fossa

**AHA Coding Clinic for table Ø5H**
**2016, 4Q, 97-98** Phrenic neurostimulator

**AHA Coding Clinic for table Ø5P**
**2016, 4Q, 97-98** Phrenic neurostimulator

**AHA Coding Clinic for table Ø5S**
**2013, 4Q, 125** Stage II cephalic vein transposition (superficialization) of arteriovenous fistula

**AHA Coding Clinic for table Ø5W**
**2016, 4Q, 97-98** Phrenic neurostimulator

## Head and Neck Veins

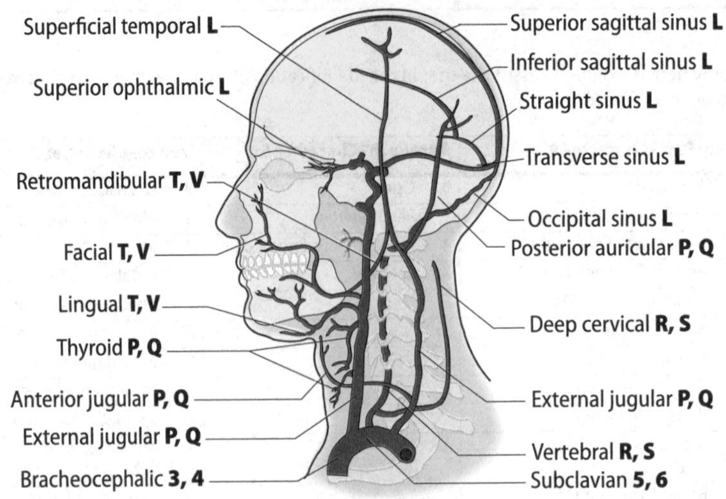
Superficial temporal **L**
Superior ophthalmic **L**
Retromandibular **T, V**
Facial **T, V**
Lingual **T, V**
Thyroid **P, Q**
Anterior jugular **P, Q**
External jugular **P, Q**
Bracheocephalic **3, 4**
Superior sagittal sinus **L**
Inferior sagittal sinus **L**
Straight sinus **L**
Transverse sinus **L**
Occipital sinus **L**
Posterior auricular **P, Q**
Deep cervical **R, S**
External jugular **P, Q**
Vertebral **R, S**
Subclavian **5, 6**

## Upper Veins

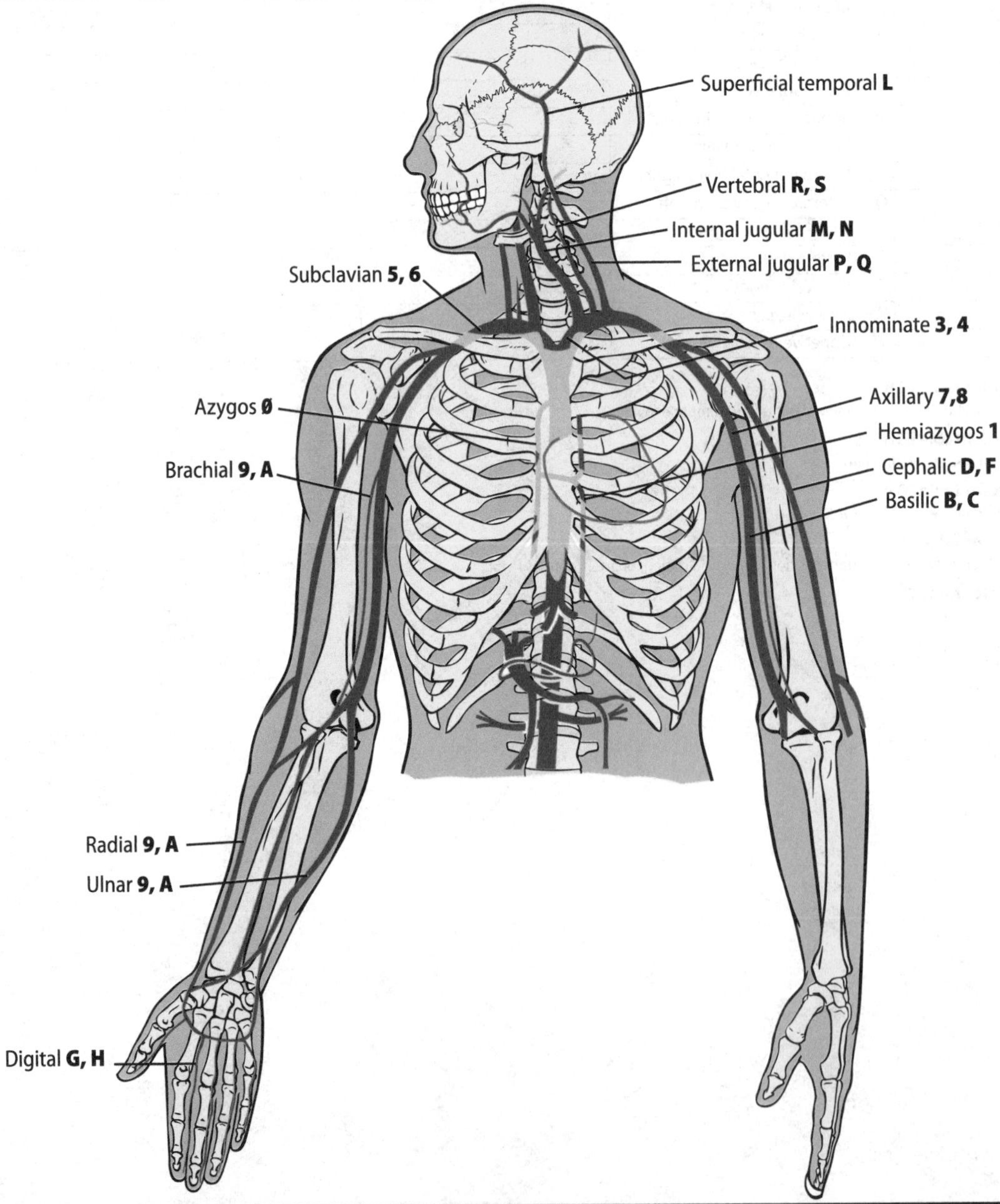
Superficial temporal **L**
Vertebral **R, S**
Internal jugular **M, N**
External jugular **P, Q**
Subclavian **5, 6**
Innominate **3, 4**
Azygos **Ø**
Axillary **7,8**
Hemiazygos **1**
Brachial **9, A**
Cephalic **D, F**
Basilic **B, C**
Radial **9, A**
Ulnar **9, A**
Digital **G, H**

**Ø Medical and Surgical**
**5 Upper Veins**
**1 Bypass** Definition: Altering the route of passage of the contents of a tubular body part

Explanation: Rerouting contents of a body part to a downstream area of the normal route, to a similar route and body part, or to an abnormal route and dissimilar body part. Includes one or more anastomoses, with or without the use of a device.

| Body Part Character 4 | Approach Character 5 | Device Character 6 | Qualifier Character 7 |
|---|---|---|---|
| **Ø Azygos Vein**<br>Right ascending lumbar vein<br>Right subcostal vein<br>**1 Hemiazygos Vein**<br>Left ascending lumbar vein<br>Left subcostal vein<br>**3 Innominate Vein, Right**<br>Brachiocephalic vein<br>Inferior thyroid vein<br>**4 Innominate Vein, Left**<br>*See 3 Innominate Vein, Right*<br>**5 Subclavian Vein, Right**<br>**6 Subclavian Vein, Left**<br>**7 Axillary Vein, Right**<br>**8 Axillary Vein, Left**<br>**9 Brachial Vein, Right**<br>Radial vein<br>Ulnar vein<br>**A Brachial Vein, Left**<br>*See 9 Brachial Vein, Right*<br>**B Basilic Vein, Right**<br>Median antebrachial vein<br>Median cubital vein<br>**C Basilic Vein, Left**<br>*See B Basilic Vein, Right*<br>**D Cephalic Vein, Right**<br>Accessory cephalic vein<br>**F Cephalic Vein, Left**<br>*See D Cephalic Vein, Right*<br>**G Hand Vein, Right**<br>Dorsal metacarpal vein<br>Palmar (volar) digital vein<br>Palmar (volar) metacarpal vein<br>Superficial palmar venous arch<br>Volar (palmar) digital vein<br>Volar (palmar) metacarpal vein<br>**H Hand Vein, Left**<br>*See G Hand Vein, Right*<br>**L Intracranial Vein**<br>Anterior cerebral vein<br>Basal (internal) cerebral vein<br>Dural venous sinus<br>Great cerebral vein<br>Inferior cerebellar vein<br>Inferior cerebral vein<br>Internal (basal) cerebral vein<br>Middle cerebral vein<br>Ophthalmic vein<br>Superior cerebellar vein<br>Superior cerebral vein<br>**M Internal Jugular Vein, Right**<br>**N Internal Jugular Vein, Left**<br>**P External Jugular Vein, Right**<br>Posterior auricular vein<br>**Q External Jugular Vein, Left**<br>*See P External Jugular Vein, Right*<br>**R Vertebral Vein, Right**<br>Deep cervical vein<br>Suboccipital venous plexus<br>**S Vertebral Vein, Left**<br>*See R Vertebral Vein, Right*<br>**T Face Vein, Right**<br>Angular vein<br>Anterior facial vein<br>Common facial vein<br>Deep facial vein<br>Frontal vein<br>Posterior facial (retromandibular) vein<br>Supraorbital vein<br>**V Face Vein, Left**<br>*See T Face Vein, Right* | **Ø Open**<br>**4 Percutaneous Endoscopic** | **7 Autologous Tissue Substitute**<br>**9 Autologous Venous Tissue**<br>**A Autologous Arterial Tissue**<br>**J Synthetic Substitute**<br>**K Nonautologous Tissue Substitute**<br>**Z No Device** | **Y Upper Vein** |

**0 Medical and Surgical**
**5 Upper Veins**
**5 Destruction** Definition: Physical eradication of all or a portion of a body part by the direct use of energy, force, or a destructive agent
Explanation: None of the body part is physically taken out

| Body Part Character 4 | Approach Character 5 | Device Character 6 | Qualifier Character 7 |
|---|---|---|---|
| **0 Azygos Vein**<br>Right ascending lumbar vein<br>Right subcostal vein<br>**1 Hemiazygos Vein**<br>Left ascending lumbar vein<br>Left subcostal vein<br>**3 Innominate Vein, Right**<br>Brachiocephalic vein<br>Inferior thyroid vein<br>**4 Innominate Vein, Left**<br>*See 3 Innominate Vein, Right*<br>**5 Subclavian Vein, Right**<br>**6 Subclavian Vein, Left**<br>**7 Axillary Vein, Right**<br>**8 Axillary Vein, Left**<br>**9 Brachial Vein, Right**<br>Radial vein<br>Ulnar vein<br>**A Brachial Vein, Left**<br>*See 9 Brachial Vein, Right*<br>**B Basilic Vein, Right**<br>Median antebrachial vein<br>Median cubital vein<br>**C Basilic Vein, Left**<br>*See B Basilic Vein, Right*<br>**D Cephalic Vein, Right**<br>Accessory cephalic vein<br>**F Cephalic Vein, Left**<br>*See D Cephalic Vein, Right*<br>**G Hand Vein, Right**<br>Dorsal metacarpal vein<br>Palmar (volar) digital vein<br>Palmar (volar) metacarpal vein<br>Superficial palmar venous arch<br>Volar (palmar) digital vein<br>Volar (palmar) metacarpal vein<br>**H Hand Vein, Left**<br>*See G Hand Vein, Right*<br>**L Intracranial Vein**<br>Anterior cerebral vein<br>Basal (internal) cerebral vein<br>Dural venous sinus<br>Great cerebral vein<br>Inferior cerebellar vein<br>Inferior cerebral vein<br>Internal (basal) cerebral vein<br>Middle cerebral vein<br>Ophthalmic vein<br>Superior cerebellar vein<br>Superior cerebral vein<br>**M Internal Jugular Vein, Right**<br>**N Internal Jugular Vein, Left**<br>**P External Jugular Vein, Right**<br>Posterior auricular vein<br>**Q External Jugular Vein, Left**<br>*See P External Jugular Vein, Right*<br>**R Vertebral Vein, Right**<br>Deep cervical vein<br>Suboccipital venous plexus<br>**S Vertebral Vein, Left**<br>*See R Vertebral Vein, Right*<br>**T Face Vein, Right**<br>Angular vein<br>Anterior facial vein<br>Common facial vein<br>Deep facial vein<br>Frontal vein<br>Posterior facial (retromandibular) vein<br>Supraorbital vein<br>**V Face Vein, Left**<br>*See T Face Vein, Right*<br>**Y Upper Vein** | **0 Open**<br>**3 Percutaneous**<br>**4 Percutaneous Endoscopic** | **Z No Device** | **Z No Qualifier** |

**Ø Medical and Surgical**
**5 Upper Veins**
**7 Dilation**

Definition: Expanding an orifice or the lumen of a tubular body part

Explanation: The orifice can be a natural orifice or an artificially created orifice. Accomplished by stretching a tubular body part using intraluminal pressure or by cutting part of the orifice or wall of the tubular body part.

| Body Part Character 4 | Approach Character 5 | Device Character 6 | Qualifier Character 7 |
|---|---|---|---|
| **Ø Azygos Vein**<br>Right ascending lumbar vein<br>Right subcostal vein<br>**1 Hemiazygos Vein**<br>Left ascending lumbar vein<br>Left subcostal vein<br>**3 Innominate Vein, Right**<br>Brachiocephalic vein<br>Inferior thyroid vein<br>**4 Innominate Vein, Left**<br>*See 3 Innominate Vein, Right*<br>**5 Subclavian Vein, Right**<br>**6 Subclavian Vein, Left**<br>**7 Axillary Vein, Right**<br>**8 Axillary Vein, Left**<br>**9 Brachial Vein, Right**<br>Radial vein<br>Ulnar vein<br>**A Brachial Vein, Left**<br>*See 9 Brachial Vein, Right*<br>**B Basilic Vein, Right**<br>Median antebrachial vein<br>Median cubital vein<br>**C Basilic Vein, Left**<br>*See B Basilic Vein, Right*<br>**D Cephalic Vein, Right**<br>Accessory cephalic vein<br>**F Cephalic Vein, Left**<br>*See D Cephalic Vein, Right*<br>**G Hand Vein, Right**<br>Dorsal metacarpal vein<br>Palmar (volar) digital vein<br>Palmar (volar) metacarpal vein<br>Superficial palmar venous arch<br>Volar (palmar) digital vein<br>Volar (palmar) metacarpal vein<br>**H Hand Vein, Left**<br>*See G Hand Vein, Right*<br>**L Intracranial Vein** NC<br>Anterior cerebral vein<br>Basal (internal) cerebral vein<br>Dural venous sinus<br>Great cerebral vein<br>Inferior cerebellar vein<br>Inferior cerebral vein<br>Internal (basal) cerebral vein<br>Middle cerebral vein<br>Ophthalmic vein<br>Superior cerebellar vein<br>Superior cerebral vein<br>**M Internal Jugular Vein, Right**<br>**N Internal Jugular Vein, Left**<br>**P External Jugular Vein, Right**<br>Posterior auricular vein<br>**Q External Jugular Vein, Left**<br>*See P External Jugular Vein, Right*<br>**R Vertebral Vein, Right**<br>Deep cervical vein<br>Suboccipital venous plexus<br>**S Vertebral Vein, Left**<br>*See R Vertebral Vein, Right*<br>**T Face Vein, Right**<br>Angular vein<br>Anterior facial vein<br>Common facial vein<br>Deep facial vein<br>Frontal vein<br>Posterior facial (retromandibular) vein<br>Supraorbital vein<br>**V Face Vein, Left**<br>*See T Face Vein, Right*<br>**Y Upper Vein** | **Ø Open**<br>**3 Percutaneous**<br>**4 Percutaneous Endoscopic** | **D Intraluminal Device**<br>**Z No Device** | **Z No Qualifier** |

NC Ø57L[3,4]ZZ

**Ø Medical and Surgical**
**5 Upper Veins**
**9 Drainage** Definition: Taking or letting out fluids and/or gases from a body part
Explanation: The qualifier DIAGNOSTIC is used to identify drainage procedures that are biopsies

| Body Part<br>Character 4 | Approach<br>Character 5 | Device<br>Character 6 | Qualifier<br>Character 7 |
|---|---|---|---|
| **Ø Azygos Vein**<br>Right ascending lumbar vein<br>Right subcostal vein<br>**1 Hemiazygos Vein**<br>Left ascending lumbar vein<br>Left subcostal vein<br>**3 Innominate Vein, Right**<br>Brachiocephalic vein<br>Inferior thyroid vein<br>**4 Innominate Vein, Left**<br>*See 3 Innominate Vein, Right*<br>**5 Subclavian Vein, Right**<br>**6 Subclavian Vein, Left**<br>**7 Axillary Vein, Right**<br>**8 Axillary Vein, Left**<br>**9 Brachial Vein, Right**<br>Radial vein<br>Ulnar vein<br>**A Brachial Vein, Left**<br>*See 9 Brachial Vein, Right*<br>**B Basilic Vein, Right**<br>Median antebrachial vein<br>Median cubital vein<br>**C Basilic Vein, Left**<br>*See B Basilic Vein, Right*<br>**D Cephalic Vein, Right**<br>Accessory cephalic vein<br>**F Cephalic Vein, Left**<br>*See D Cephalic Vein, Right*<br>**G Hand Vein, Right**<br>Dorsal metacarpal vein<br>Palmar (volar) digital vein<br>Palmar (volar) metacarpal vein<br>Superficial palmar venous arch<br>Volar (palmar) digital vein<br>Volar (palmar) metacarpal vein<br>**H Hand Vein, Left**<br>*See G Hand Vein, Right*<br>**L Intracranial Vein**<br>Anterior cerebral vein<br>Basal (internal) cerebral vein<br>Dural venous sinus<br>Great cerebral vein<br>Inferior cerebellar vein<br>Inferior cerebral vein<br>Internal (basal) cerebral vein<br>Middle cerebral vein<br>Ophthalmic vein<br>Superior cerebellar vein<br>Superior cerebral vein<br>**M Internal Jugular Vein, Right**<br>**N Internal Jugular Vein, Left**<br>**P External Jugular Vein, Right**<br>Posterior auricular vein<br>**Q External Jugular Vein, Left**<br>*See P External Jugular Vein, Right*<br>**R Vertebral Vein, Right**<br>Deep cervical vein<br>Suboccipital venous plexus<br>**S Vertebral Vein, Left**<br>*See R Vertebral Vein, Right*<br>**T Face Vein, Right**<br>Angular vein<br>Anterior facial vein<br>Common facial vein<br>Deep facial vein<br>Frontal vein<br>Posterior facial (retromandibular) vein<br>Supraorbital vein<br>**V Face Vein, Left**<br>*See T Face Vein, Right*<br>**Y Upper Vein** | **Ø Open**<br>**3 Percutaneous**<br>**4 Percutaneous Endoscopic** | **Ø Drainage Device** | **Z No Qualifier** |
| **Ø Azygos Vein**<br>Right ascending lumbar vein<br>Right subcostal vein<br>**1 Hemiazygos Vein**<br>Left ascending lumbar vein<br>Left subcostal vein<br>**3 Innominate Vein, Right**<br>Brachiocephalic vein<br>Inferior thyroid vein<br>**4 Innominate Vein, Left**<br>*See 3 Innominate Vein, Right*<br>**5 Subclavian Vein, Right**<br>**6 Subclavian Vein, Left**<br>**7 Axillary Vein, Right**<br>**8 Axillary Vein, Left**<br>**9 Brachial Vein, Right**<br>Radial vein<br>Ulnar vein<br>**A Brachial Vein, Left**<br>*See 9 Brachial Vein, Right*<br>**B Basilic Vein, Right**<br>Median antebrachial vein<br>Median cubital vein<br>**C Basilic Vein, Left**<br>*See B Basilic Vein, Right*<br>**D Cephalic Vein, Right**<br>Accessory cephalic vein<br>**F Cephalic Vein, Left**<br>*See D Cephalic Vein, Right*<br>**G Hand Vein, Right**<br>Dorsal metacarpal vein<br>Palmar (volar) digital vein<br>Palmar (volar) metacarpal vein<br>Superficial palmar venous arch<br>Volar (palmar) digital vein<br>Volar (palmar) metacarpal vein<br>**H Hand Vein, Left**<br>*See G Hand Vein, Right*<br>**L Intracranial Vein**<br>Anterior cerebral vein<br>Basal (internal) cerebral vein<br>Dural venous sinus<br>Great cerebral vein<br>Inferior cerebellar vein<br>Inferior cerebral vein<br>Internal (basal) cerebral vein<br>Middle cerebral vein<br>Ophthalmic vein<br>Superior cerebellar vein<br>Superior cerebral vein<br>**M Internal Jugular Vein, Right**<br>**N Internal Jugular Vein, Left**<br>**P External Jugular Vein, Right**<br>Posterior auricular vein<br>**Q External Jugular Vein, Left**<br>*See P External Jugular Vein, Right*<br>**R Vertebral Vein, Right**<br>Deep cervical vein<br>Suboccipital venous plexus<br>**S Vertebral Vein, Left**<br>*See R Vertebral Vein, Right*<br>**T Face Vein, Right**<br>Angular vein<br>Anterior facial vein<br>Common facial vein<br>Deep facial vein<br>Frontal vein<br>Posterior facial (retromandibular) vein<br>Supraorbital vein<br>**V Face Vein, Left**<br>*See T Face Vein, Right*<br>**Y Upper Vein** | **Ø Open**<br>**3 Percutaneous**<br>**4 Percutaneous Endoscopic** | **Z No Device** | **X Diagnostic**<br>**Z No Qualifier** |

**Non-OR** Ø59[Ø,1,3,4,5,6,7,8,9,A,B,C,D,F,G,H,L,M,N,P,Q,R,S,T,V,Y][Ø,3,4]ØZ
**Non-OR** Ø59[Ø,1,3,4,5,6,7,8,9,A,B,C,D,F,G,H,L,M,N,P,Q,R,S,T,V,Y]3ZX
**Non-OR** Ø59[Ø,1,3,4,5,6,7,8,9,A,B,C,D,F,G,H,L,M,N,P,Q,R,S,T,V,Y][Ø,3,4]ZZ

**Ø Medical and Surgical**
**5 Upper Veins**
**B Excision** Definition: Cutting out or off, without replacement, a portion of a body part
Explanation: The qualifier DIAGNOSTIC is used to identify excision procedures that are biopsies

| Body Part Character 4 | Approach Character 5 | Device Character 6 | Qualifier Character 7 |
|---|---|---|---|
| **Ø Azygos Vein**<br>Right ascending lumbar vein<br>Right subcostal vein<br>**1 Hemiazygos Vein**<br>Left ascending lumbar vein<br>Left subcostal vein<br>**3 Innominate Vein, Right**<br>Brachiocephalic vein<br>Inferior thyroid vein<br>**4 Innominate Vein, Left**<br>*See 3 Innominate Vein, Right*<br>**5 Subclavian Vein, Right**<br>**6 Subclavian Vein, Left**<br>**7 Axillary Vein, Right**<br>**8 Axillary Vein, Left**<br>**9 Brachial Vein, Right**<br>Radial vein<br>Ulnar vein<br>**A Brachial Vein, Left**<br>*See 9 Brachial Vein, Right*<br>**B Basilic Vein, Right**<br>Median antebrachial vein<br>Median cubital vein<br>**C Basilic Vein, Left**<br>*See B Basilic Vein, Right*<br>**D Cephalic Vein, Right**<br>Accessory cephalic vein<br>**F Cephalic Vein, Left**<br>*See D Cephalic Vein, Right*<br>**G Hand Vein, Right**<br>Dorsal metacarpal vein<br>Palmar (volar) digital vein<br>Palmar (volar) metacarpal vein<br>Superficial palmar venous arch<br>Volar (palmar) digital vein<br>Volar (palmar) metacarpal vein<br>**H Hand Vein, Left**<br>*See G Hand Vein, Right*<br>**L Intracranial Vein**<br>Anterior cerebral vein<br>Basal (internal) cerebral vein<br>Dural venous sinus<br>Great cerebral vein<br>Inferior cerebellar vein<br>Inferior cerebral vein<br>Internal (basal) cerebral vein<br>Middle cerebral vein<br>Ophthalmic vein<br>Superior cerebellar vein<br>Superior cerebral vein<br>**M Internal Jugular Vein, Right**<br>**N Internal Jugular Vein, Left**<br>**P External Jugular Vein, Right**<br>Posterior auricular vein<br>**Q External Jugular Vein, Left**<br>*See P External Jugular Vein, Right*<br>**R Vertebral Vein, Right**<br>Deep cervical vein<br>Suboccipital venous plexus<br>**S Vertebral Vein, Left**<br>*See R Vertebral Vein, Right*<br>**T Face Vein, Right**<br>Angular vein<br>Anterior facial vein<br>Common facial vein<br>Deep facial vein<br>Frontal vein<br>Posterior facial (retromandibular) vein<br>Supraorbital vein<br>**V Face Vein, Left**<br>*See T Face Vein, Right*<br>**Y Upper Vein** | **Ø Open**<br>**3 Percutaneous**<br>**4 Percutaneous Endoscopic** | **Z No Device** | **X Diagnostic**<br>**Z No Qualifier** |

**Ø Medical and Surgical**
**5 Upper Veins**
**C Extirpation** Definition: Taking or cutting out solid matter from a body part

Explanation: The solid matter may be an abnormal byproduct of a biological function or a foreign body; it may be imbedded in a body part or in the lumen of a tubular body part. The solid matter may or may not have been previously broken into pieces.

| Body Part Character 4 | | Approach Character 5 | Device Character 6 | Qualifier Character 7 |
|---|---|---|---|---|
| **Ø Azygos Vein** Right ascending lumbar vein Right subcostal vein<br>**1 Hemiazygos Vein** Left ascending lumbar vein Left subcostal vein<br>**3 Innominate Vein, Right** Brachiocephalic vein Inferior thyroid vein<br>**4 Innominate Vein, Left** *See 3 Innominate Vein, Right*<br>**5 Subclavian Vein, Right**<br>**6 Subclavian Vein, Left**<br>**7 Axillary Vein, Right**<br>**8 Axillary Vein, Left**<br>**9 Brachial Vein, Right** Radial vein Ulnar vein<br>**A Brachial Vein, Left** *See 9 Brachial Vein, Right*<br>**B Basilic Vein, Right** Median antebrachial vein Median cubital vein<br>**C Basilic Vein, Left** *See B Basilic Vein, Right*<br>**D Cephalic Vein, Right** Accessory cephalic vein<br>**F Cephalic Vein, Left** *See D Cephalic Vein, Right*<br>**G Hand Vein, Right** Dorsal metacarpal vein Palmar (volar) digital vein Palmar (volar) metacarpal vein Superficial palmar venous arch Volar (palmar) digital vein Volar (palmar) metacarpal vein | **H Hand Vein, Left** *See G Hand Vein, Right*<br>**L Intracranial Vein** Anterior cerebral vein Basal (internal) cerebral vein Dural venous sinus Great cerebral vein Inferior cerebellar vein Inferior cerebral vein Internal (basal) cerebral vein Middle cerebral vein Ophthalmic vein Superior cerebellar vein Superior cerebral vein<br>**M Internal Jugular Vein, Right**<br>**N Internal Jugular Vein, Left**<br>**P External Jugular Vein, Right** Posterior auricular vein<br>**Q External Jugular Vein, Left** *See P External Jugular Vein, Right*<br>**R Vertebral Vein, Right** Deep cervical vein Suboccipital venous plexus<br>**S Vertebral Vein, Left** *See R Vertebral Vein, Right*<br>**T Face Vein, Right** Angular vein Anterior facial vein Common facial vein Deep facial vein Frontal vein Posterior facial (retromandibular) vein Supraorbital vein<br>**V Face Vein, Left** *See T Face Vein, Right*<br>**Y Upper Vein** | **Ø Open**<br>**3 Percutaneous**<br>**4 Percutaneous Endoscopic** | **Z No Device** | **Z No Qualifier** |

**Ø Medical and Surgical**
**5 Upper Veins**
**D Extraction** Definition: Pulling or stripping out or off all or a portion of a body part by the use of force

Explanation: The qualifier DIAGNOSTIC is used to identify extraction procedures that are biopsies

| Body Part Character 4 | | Approach Character 5 | Device Character 6 | Qualifier Character 7 |
|---|---|---|---|---|
| **9 Brachial Vein, Right** Radial vein Ulnar vein<br>**A Brachial Vein, Left** *See 9 Brachial Vein, Right*<br>**B Basilic Vein, Right** Median antebrachial vein Median cubital vein<br>**C Basilic Vein, Left** *See B Basilic Vein, Right*<br>**D Cephalic Vein, Right** Accessory cephalic vein | **F Cephalic Vein, Left** *See D Cephalic Vein, Right*<br>**G Hand Vein, Right** Dorsal metacarpal vein Palmar (volar) digital vein Palmar (volar) metacarpal vein Superficial palmar venous arch Volar (palmar) digital vein Volar (palmar) metacarpal vein<br>**H Hand Vein, Left** *See G Hand Vein, Right*<br>**Y Upper Vein** | **Ø Open**<br>**3 Percutaneous** | **Z No Device** | **Z No Qualifier** |

**Ø Medical and Surgical**
**5 Upper Veins**
**H Insertion** Definition: Putting in a nonbiological appliance that monitors, assists, performs, or prevents a physiological function but does not physically take the place of a body part
Explanation: None

| Body Part Character 4 | Approach Character 5 | Device Character 6 | Qualifier Character 7 |
|---|---|---|---|
| **Ø Azygos Vein** ⊞<br>Right ascending lumbar vein<br>Right subcostal vein | **Ø** Open<br>**3** Percutaneous<br>**4** Percutaneous Endoscopic | **2** Monitoring Device<br>**3** Infusion Device<br>**D** Intraluminal Device<br>**M** Neurostimulator Lead | **Z** No Qualifier |
| **1 Hemiazygos Vein**<br>Left ascending lumbar vein<br>Left subcostal vein<br>**5 Subclavian Vein, Right**<br>**6 Subclavian Vein, Left**<br>**7 Axillary Vein, Right**<br>**8 Axillary Vein, Left**<br>**9 Brachial Vein, Right**<br>Radial vein<br>Ulnar vein<br>**A Brachial Vein, Left**<br>*See 9 Brachial Vein, Right*<br>**B Basilic Vein, Right**<br>Median antebrachial vein<br>Median cubital vein<br>**C Basilic Vein, Left**<br>*See B Basilic Vein, Right*<br>**D Cephalic Vein, Right**<br>Accessory cephalic vein<br>**F Cephalic Vein, Left**<br>*See D Cephalic Vein, Right*<br>**G Hand Vein, Right**<br>Dorsal metacarpal vein<br>Palmar (volar) digital vein<br>Palmar (volar) metacarpal vein<br>Superficial palmar venous arch<br>Volar (palmar) digital vein<br>Volar (palmar) metacarpal vein<br>**H Hand Vein, Left**<br>*See G Hand Vein, Right*<br>**L Intracranial Vein**<br>Anterior cerebral vein<br>Basal (internal) cerebral vein<br>Dural venous sinus<br>Great cerebral vein<br>Inferior cerebellar vein<br>Inferior cerebral vein<br>Internal (basal) cerebral vein<br>Middle cerebral vein<br>Ophthalmic vein<br>Superior cerebellar vein<br>Superior cerebral vein<br>**M Internal Jugular Vein, Right**<br>**N Internal Jugular Vein, Left**<br>**P External Jugular Vein, Right**<br>Posterior auricular vein<br>**Q External Jugular Vein, Left**<br>*See P External Jugular Vein, Right*<br>**R Vertebral Vein, Right**<br>Deep cervical vein<br>Suboccipital venous plexus<br>**S Vertebral Vein, Left**<br>*See R Vertebral Vein, Right*<br>**T Face Vein, Right**<br>Angular vein<br>Anterior facial vein<br>Common facial vein<br>Deep facial vein<br>Frontal vein<br>Posterior facial (retromandibular) vein<br>Supraorbital vein<br>**V Face Vein, Left**<br>*See T Face Vein, Right* | **Ø** Open<br>**3** Percutaneous<br>**4** Percutaneous Endoscopic | **3** Infusion Device<br>**D** Intraluminal Device | **Z** No Qualifier |
| **3 Innominate Vein, Right** ⊞<br>Brachiocephalic vein<br>Inferior thyroid vein<br>**4 Innominate Vein, Left** ⊞<br>*See 3 Innominate Vein, Right* | **Ø** Open<br>**3** Percutaneous<br>**4** Percutaneous Endoscopic | **3** Infusion Device<br>**D** Intraluminal Device<br>**M** Neurostimulator Lead | **Z** No Qualifier |
| **Y Upper Vein** | **Ø** Open<br>**3** Percutaneous<br>**4** Percutaneous Endoscopic | **2** Monitoring Device<br>**3** Infusion Device<br>**D** Intraluminal Device<br>**Y** Other Device | **Z** No Qualifier |

**Non-OR** Ø5HØ[Ø,3,4]3Z
**Non-OR** Ø5H[1,5,6,7,8,9,A,B,C,D,F,G,H,L,M,N,P,Q,R,S,T,V][Ø,3,4]3Z
**Non-OR** Ø5H[3,4][Ø,3,4]3Z
**Non-OR** Ø5HY[Ø,3,4]3Z
**Non-OR** Ø5HY32Z
**Non-OR** Ø5HY[3,4]YZ
**HAC** Ø5HØ[3,4]3Z when reported with SDx J95.811
**HAC** Ø5H[1,5,6][3,4]3Z when reported with SDx J95.811
**HAC** Ø5H[M,N,P,Q]33Z when reported with SDx J95.811
**HAC** Ø5H[3,4][3,4]3Z when reported with SDx J95.811

**See Appendix L for Procedure Combinations**
⊞ Ø5HØ[Ø,3,4]MZ
⊞ Ø5H[3,4][Ø,3,4]MZ

**Ø Medical and Surgical**
**5 Upper Veins**
**J Inspection** Definition: Visually and/or manually exploring a body part

Explanation: Visual exploration may be performed with or without optical instrumentation. Manual exploration may be performed directly or through intervening body layers.

| Body Part Character 4 | Approach Character 5 | Device Character 6 | Qualifier Character 7 |
|---|---|---|---|
| Y Upper Vein | Ø Open<br>3 Percutaneous<br>4 Percutaneous Endoscopic<br>X External | Z No Device | Z No Qualifier |

Non-OR Ø5JY[3,X]ZZ

**Ø Medical and Surgical**
**5 Upper Veins**
**L Occlusion** Definition: Completely closing an orifice or the lumen of a tubular body part

Explanation: The orifice can be a natural orifice or an artificially created orifice

| Body Part Character 4 | Body Part Character 4 | Approach Character 5 | Device Character 6 | Qualifier Character 7 |
|---|---|---|---|---|
| **Ø Azygos Vein**<br>Right ascending lumbar vein<br>Right subcostal vein<br>**1 Hemiazygos Vein**<br>Left ascending lumbar vein<br>Left subcostal vein<br>**3 Innominate Vein, Right**<br>Brachiocephalic vein<br>Inferior thyroid vein<br>**4 Innominate Vein, Left**<br>*See 3 Innominate Vein, Right*<br>**5 Subclavian Vein, Right**<br>**6 Subclavian Vein, Left**<br>**7 Axillary Vein, Right**<br>**8 Axillary Vein, Left**<br>**9 Brachial Vein, Right**<br>Radial vein<br>Ulnar vein<br>**A Brachial Vein, Left**<br>*See 9 Brachial Vein, Right*<br>**B Basilic Vein, Right**<br>Median antebrachial vein<br>Median cubital vein<br>**C Basilic Vein, Left**<br>*See B Basilic Vein, Right*<br>**D Cephalic Vein, Right**<br>Accessory cephalic vein<br>**F Cephalic Vein, Left**<br>*See D Cephalic Vein, Right*<br>**G Hand Vein, Right**<br>Dorsal metacarpal vein<br>Palmar (volar) digital vein<br>Palmar (volar) metacarpal vein<br>Superficial palmar venous arch<br>Volar (palmar) digital vein<br>Volar (palmar) metacarpal vein | **H Hand Vein, Left**<br>*See G Hand Vein, Right*<br>**L Intracranial Vein**<br>Anterior cerebral vein<br>Basal (internal) cerebral vein<br>Dural venous sinus<br>Great cerebral vein<br>Inferior cerebellar vein<br>Inferior cerebral vein<br>Internal (basal) cerebral vein<br>Middle cerebral vein<br>Ophthalmic vein<br>Superior cerebellar vein<br>Superior cerebral vein<br>**M Internal Jugular Vein, Right**<br>**N Internal Jugular Vein, Left**<br>**P External Jugular Vein, Right**<br>Posterior auricular vein<br>**Q External Jugular Vein, Left**<br>*See P External Jugular Vein, Right*<br>**R Vertebral Vein, Right**<br>Deep cervical vein<br>Suboccipital venous plexus<br>**S Vertebral Vein, Left**<br>*See R Vertebral Vein, Right*<br>**T Face Vein, Right**<br>Angular vein<br>Anterior facial vein<br>Common facial vein<br>Deep facial vein<br>Frontal vein<br>Posterior facial (retromandibular) vein<br>Supraorbital vein<br>**V Face Vein, Left**<br>*See T Face Vein, Right*<br>**Y Upper Vein** | Ø Open<br>3 Percutaneous<br>4 Percutaneous Endoscopic | C Extraluminal Device<br>D Intraluminal Device<br>Z No Device | Z No Qualifier |

**Ø Medical and Surgical**
**5 Upper Veins**
**N Release** Definition: Freeing a body part from an abnormal physical constraint by cutting or by the use of force
Explanation: Some of the restraining tissue may be taken out but none of the body part is taken out

| Body Part Character 4 | | Approach Character 5 | Device Character 6 | Qualifier Character 7 |
|---|---|---|---|---|
| **Ø Azygos Vein**<br>Right ascending lumbar vein<br>Right subcostal vein<br>**1 Hemiazygos Vein**<br>Left ascending lumbar vein<br>Left subcostal vein<br>**3 Innominate Vein, Right**<br>Brachiocephalic vein<br>Inferior thyroid vein<br>**4 Innominate Vein, Left**<br>*See 3 Innominate Vein, Right*<br>**5 Subclavian Vein, Right**<br>**6 Subclavian Vein, Left**<br>**7 Axillary Vein, Right**<br>**8 Axillary Vein, Left**<br>**9 Brachial Vein, Right**<br>Radial vein<br>Ulnar vein<br>**A Brachial Vein, Left**<br>*See 9 Brachial Vein, Right*<br>**B Basilic Vein, Right**<br>Median antebrachial vein<br>Median cubital vein<br>**C Basilic Vein, Left**<br>*See B Basilic Vein, Right*<br>**D Cephalic Vein, Right**<br>Accessory cephalic vein<br>**F Cephalic Vein, Left**<br>*See D Cephalic Vein, Right*<br>**G Hand Vein, Right**<br>Dorsal metacarpal vein<br>Palmar (volar) digital vein<br>Palmar (volar) metacarpal vein<br>Superficial palmar venous arch<br>Volar (palmar) digital vein<br>Volar (palmar) metacarpal vein | **H Hand Vein, Left**<br>*See G Hand Vein, Right*<br>**L Intracranial Vein**<br>Anterior cerebral vein<br>Basal (internal) cerebral vein<br>Dural venous sinus<br>Great cerebral vein<br>Inferior cerebellar vein<br>Inferior cerebral vein<br>Internal (basal) cerebral vein<br>Middle cerebral vein<br>Ophthalmic vein<br>Superior cerebellar vein<br>Superior cerebral vein<br>**M Internal Jugular Vein, Right**<br>**N Internal Jugular Vein, Left**<br>**P External Jugular Vein, Right**<br>Posterior auricular vein<br>**Q External Jugular Vein, Left**<br>*See P External Jugular Vein, Right*<br>**R Vertebral Vein, Right**<br>Deep cervical vein<br>Suboccipital venous plexus<br>**S Vertebral Vein, Left**<br>*See R Vertebral Vein, Right*<br>**T Face Vein, Right**<br>Angular vein<br>Anterior facial vein<br>Common facial vein<br>Deep facial vein<br>Frontal vein<br>Posterior facial (retromandibular) vein<br>Supraorbital vein<br>**V Face Vein, Left**<br>*See T Face Vein, Right*<br>**Y Upper Vein** | **Ø Open**<br>**3 Percutaneous**<br>**4 Percutaneous Endoscopic** | **Z No Device** | **Z No Qualifier** |

**Ø Medical and Surgical**
**5 Upper Veins**
**P Removal** Definition: Taking out or off a device from a body part

Explanation: If a device is taken out and a similar device put in without cutting or puncturing the skin or mucous membrane, the procedure is coded to the root operation CHANGE. Otherwise, the procedure for taking out a device is coded to the root operation REMOVAL.

| Body Part Character 4 | Approach Character 5 | Device Character 6 | Qualifier Character 7 |
|---|---|---|---|
| **Ø Azygos Vein**<br>Right ascending lumbar vein<br>Right subcostal vein | **Ø Open**<br>**3 Percutaneous**<br>**4 Percutaneous Endoscopic**<br>**X External** | **2 Monitoring Device**<br>**M Neurostimulator Lead** | **Z No Qualifier** |
| **3 Innominate Vein, Right**<br>Brachiocephalic vein<br>Inferior thyroid vein<br>**4 Innominate Vein, Left**<br>*See 3 Innominate Vein, Right* | **Ø Open**<br>**3 Percutaneous**<br>**4 Percutaneous Endoscopic**<br>**X External** | **M Neurostimulator Lead** | **Z No Qualifier** |
| **Y Upper Vein** | **Ø Open**<br>**3 Percutaneous**<br>**4 Percutaneous Endoscopic** | **Ø Drainage Device**<br>**2 Monitoring Device**<br>**3 Infusion Device**<br>**7 Autologous Tissue Substitute**<br>**C Extraluminal Device**<br>**D Intraluminal Device**<br>**J Synthetic Substitute**<br>**K Nonautologous Tissue Substitute**<br>**Y Other Device** | **Z No Qualifier** |
| **Y Upper Vein** | **X External** | **Ø Drainage Device**<br>**2 Monitoring Device**<br>**3 Infusion Device**<br>**D Intraluminal Device** | **Z No Qualifier** |

**Non-OR** Ø5PØ[Ø,3,4,X]2Z
**Non-OR** Ø5PY3[Ø,2,3]Z
**Non-OR** Ø5PY[3,4]YZ
**Non-OR** Ø5PYX[Ø,2,3,D]Z

**Ø Medical and Surgical**
**5 Upper Veins**
**Q Repair**

Definition: Restoring, to the extent possible, a body part to its normal anatomic structure and function
Explanation: Used only when the method to accomplish the repair is not one of the other root operations

| Body Part Character 4 | Approach Character 5 | Device Character 6 | Qualifier Character 7 |
|---|---|---|---|
| **Ø Azygos Vein**<br>Right ascending lumbar vein<br>Right subcostal vein<br>**1 Hemiazygos Vein**<br>Left ascending lumbar vein<br>Left subcostal vein<br>**3 Innominate Vein, Right**<br>Brachiocephalic vein<br>Inferior thyroid vein<br>**4 Innominate Vein, Left**<br>*See 3 Innominate Vein, Right*<br>**5 Subclavian Vein, Right**<br>**6 Subclavian Vein, Left**<br>**7 Axillary Vein, Right**<br>**8 Axillary Vein, Left**<br>**9 Brachial Vein, Right**<br>Radial vein<br>Ulnar vein<br>**A Brachial Vein, Left**<br>*See 9 Brachial Vein, Right*<br>**B Basilic Vein, Right**<br>Median antebrachial vein<br>Median cubital vein<br>**C Basilic Vein, Left**<br>*See B Basilic Vein, Right*<br>**D Cephalic Vein, Right**<br>Accessory cephalic vein<br>**F Cephalic Vein, Left**<br>*See D Cephalic Vein, Right*<br>**G Hand Vein, Right**<br>Dorsal metacarpal vein<br>Palmar (volar) digital vein<br>Palmar (volar) metacarpal vein<br>Superficial palmar venous arch<br>Volar (palmar) digital vein<br>Volar (palmar) metacarpal vein<br>**H Hand Vein, Left**<br>*See G Hand Vein, Right*<br>**L Intracranial Vein**<br>Anterior cerebral vein<br>Basal (internal) cerebral vein<br>Dural venous sinus<br>Great cerebral vein<br>Inferior cerebellar vein<br>Inferior cerebral vein<br>Internal (basal) cerebral vein<br>Middle cerebral vein<br>Ophthalmic vein<br>Superior cerebellar vein<br>Superior cerebral vein<br>**M Internal Jugular Vein, Right**<br>**N Internal Jugular Vein, Left**<br>**P External Jugular Vein, Right**<br>Posterior auricular vein<br>**Q External Jugular Vein, Left**<br>*See P External Jugular Vein, Right*<br>**R Vertebral Vein, Right**<br>Deep cervical vein<br>Suboccipital venous plexus<br>**S Vertebral Vein, Left**<br>*See R Vertebral Vein, Right*<br>**T Face Vein, Right**<br>Angular vein<br>Anterior facial vein<br>Common facial vein<br>Deep facial vein<br>Frontal vein<br>Posterior facial (retromandibular) vein<br>Supraorbital vein<br>**V Face Vein, Left**<br>*See T Face Vein, Right*<br>**Y Upper Vein** | **Ø Open**<br>**3 Percutaneous**<br>**4 Percutaneous Endoscopic** | **Z No Device** | **Z No Qualifier** |

**Ø Medical and Surgical**
**5 Upper Veins**
**R Replacement** Definition: Putting in or on biological or synthetic material that physically takes the place and/or function of all or a portion of a body part

Explanation: The body part may have been taken out or replaced, or may be taken out, physically eradicated, or rendered nonfunctional during the REPLACEMENT procedure. A REMOVAL procedure is coded for taking out the device used in a previous replacement procedure.

| Body Part Character 4 | Approach Character 5 | Device Character 6 | Qualifier Character 7 |
|---|---|---|---|
| **Ø Azygos Vein**<br>Right ascending lumbar vein<br>Right subcostal vein<br>**1 Hemiazygos Vein**<br>Left ascending lumbar vein<br>Left subcostal vein<br>**3 Innominate Vein, Right**<br>Brachiocephalic vein<br>Inferior thyroid vein<br>**4 Innominate Vein, Left**<br>*See 3 Innominate Vein, Right*<br>**5 Subclavian Vein, Right**<br>**6 Subclavian Vein, Left**<br>**7 Axillary Vein, Right**<br>**8 Axillary Vein, Left**<br>**9 Brachial Vein, Right**<br>Radial vein<br>Ulnar vein<br>**A Brachial Vein, Left**<br>*See 9 Brachial Vein, Right*<br>**B Basilic Vein, Right**<br>Median antebrachial vein<br>Median cubital vein<br>**C Basilic Vein, Left**<br>*See B Basilic Vein, Right*<br>**D Cephalic Vein, Right**<br>Accessory cephalic vein<br>**F Cephalic Vein, Left**<br>*See D Cephalic Vein, Right*<br>**G Hand Vein, Right**<br>Dorsal metacarpal vein<br>Palmar (volar) digital vein<br>Palmar (volar) metacarpal vein<br>Superficial palmar venous arch<br>Volar (palmar) digital vein<br>Volar (palmar) metacarpal vein<br>**H Hand Vein, Left**<br>*See G Hand Vein, Right*<br>**L Intracranial Vein**<br>Anterior cerebral vein<br>Basal (internal) cerebral vein<br>Dural venous sinus<br>Great cerebral vein<br>Inferior cerebellar vein<br>Inferior cerebral vein<br>Internal (basal) cerebral vein<br>Middle cerebral vein<br>Ophthalmic vein<br>Superior cerebellar vein<br>Superior cerebral vein<br>**M Internal Jugular Vein, Right**<br>**N Internal Jugular Vein, Left**<br>**P External Jugular Vein, Right**<br>Posterior auricular vein<br>**Q External Jugular Vein, Left**<br>*See P External Jugular Vein, Right*<br>**R Vertebral Vein, Right**<br>Deep cervical vein<br>Suboccipital venous plexus<br>**S Vertebral Vein, Left**<br>*See R Vertebral Vein, Right*<br>**T Face Vein, Right**<br>Angular vein<br>Anterior facial vein<br>Common facial vein<br>Deep facial vein<br>Frontal vein<br>Posterior facial (retromandibular) vein<br>Supraorbital vein<br>**V Face Vein, Left**<br>*See T Face Vein, Right*<br>**Y Upper Vein** | **Ø Open**<br>**4 Percutaneous Endoscopic** | **7 Autologous Tissue Substitute**<br>**J Synthetic Substitute**<br>**K Nonautologous Tissue Substitute** | **Z No Qualifier** |

**Ø Medical and Surgical**
**5 Upper Veins**
**S Reposition**

Definition: Moving to its normal location, or other suitable location, all or a portion of a body part

Explanation: The body part is moved to a new location from an abnormal location, or from a normal location where it is not functioning correctly. The body part may or may not be cut out or off to be moved to the new location.

| Body Part Character 4 | Approach Character 5 | Device Character 6 | Qualifier Character 7 |
|---|---|---|---|
| **Ø Azygos Vein**<br>Right ascending lumbar vein<br>Right subcostal vein<br>**1 Hemiazygos Vein**<br>Left ascending lumbar vein<br>Left subcostal vein<br>**3 Innominate Vein, Right**<br>Brachiocephalic vein<br>Inferior thyroid vein<br>**4 Innominate Vein, Left**<br>*See 3 Innominate Vein, Right*<br>**5 Subclavian Vein, Right**<br>**6 Subclavian Vein, Left**<br>**7 Axillary Vein, Right**<br>**8 Axillary Vein, Left**<br>**9 Brachial Vein, Right**<br>Radial vein<br>Ulnar vein<br>**A Brachial Vein, Left**<br>*See 9 Brachial Vein, Right*<br>**B Basilic Vein, Right**<br>Median antebrachial vein<br>Median cubital vein<br>**C Basilic Vein, Left**<br>*See B Basilic Vein, Right*<br>**D Cephalic Vein, Right**<br>Accessory cephalic vein<br>**F Cephalic Vein, Left**<br>*See D Cephalic Vein, Right*<br>**G Hand Vein, Right**<br>Dorsal metacarpal vein<br>Palmar (volar) digital vein<br>Palmar (volar) metacarpal vein<br>Superficial palmar venous arch<br>Volar (palmar) digital vein<br>Volar (palmar) metacarpal vein<br>**H Hand Vein, Left**<br>*See G Hand Vein, Right*<br>**L Intracranial Vein**<br>Anterior cerebral vein<br>Basal (internal) cerebral vein<br>Dural venous sinus<br>Great cerebral vein<br>Inferior cerebellar vein<br>Inferior cerebral vein<br>Internal (basal) cerebral vein<br>Middle cerebral vein<br>Ophthalmic vein<br>Superior cerebellar vein<br>Superior cerebral vein<br>**M Internal Jugular Vein, Right**<br>**N Internal Jugular Vein, Left**<br>**P External Jugular Vein, Right**<br>Posterior auricular vein<br>**Q External Jugular Vein, Left**<br>*See P External Jugular Vein, Right*<br>**R Vertebral Vein, Right**<br>Deep cervical vein<br>Suboccipital venous plexus<br>**S Vertebral Vein, Left**<br>*See R Vertebral Vein, Right*<br>**T Face Vein, Right**<br>Angular vein<br>Anterior facial vein<br>Common facial vein<br>Deep facial vein<br>Frontal vein<br>Posterior facial (retromandibular) vein<br>Supraorbital vein<br>**V Face Vein, Left**<br>*See T Face Vein, Right*<br>**Y Upper Vein** | **Ø Open**<br>**3 Percutaneous**<br>**4 Percutaneous Endoscopic** | **Z No Device** | **Z No Qualifier** |

**Ø Medical and Surgical**
**5 Upper Veins**
**U Supplement**

Definition: Putting in or on biological or synthetic material that physically reinforces and/or augments the function of a portion of a body part

Explanation: The biological material is non-living, or is living and from the same individual. The body part may have been previously replaced, and the SUPPLEMENT procedure is performed to physically reinforce and/or augment the function of the replaced body part.

| Body Part Character 4 | Approach Character 5 | Device Character 6 | Qualifier Character 7 |
|---|---|---|---|
| **Ø Azygos Vein**<br>Right ascending lumbar vein<br>Right subcostal vein<br>**1 Hemiazygos Vein**<br>Left ascending lumbar vein<br>Left subcostal vein<br>**3 Innominate Vein, Right**<br>Brachiocephalic vein<br>Inferior thyroid vein<br>**4 Innominate Vein, Left**<br>*See 3 Innominate Vein, Right*<br>**5 Subclavian Vein, Right**<br>**6 Subclavian Vein, Left**<br>**7 Axillary Vein, Right**<br>**8 Axillary Vein, Left**<br>**9 Brachial Vein, Right**<br>Radial vein<br>Ulnar vein<br>**A Brachial Vein, Left**<br>*See 9 Brachial Vein, Right*<br>**B Basilic Vein, Right**<br>Median antebrachial vein<br>Median cubital vein<br>**C Basilic Vein, Left**<br>*See B Basilic Vein, Right*<br>**D Cephalic Vein, Right**<br>Accessory cephalic vein<br>**F Cephalic Vein, Left**<br>*See D Cephalic Vein, Right*<br>**G Hand Vein, Right**<br>Dorsal metacarpal vein<br>Palmar (volar) digital vein<br>Palmar (volar) metacarpal vein<br>Superficial palmar venous arch<br>Volar (palmar) digital vein<br>Volar (palmar) metacarpal vein<br>**H Hand Vein, Left**<br>*See G Hand Vein, Right*<br>**L Intracranial Vein**<br>Anterior cerebral vein<br>Basal (internal) cerebral vein<br>Dural venous sinus<br>Great cerebral vein<br>Inferior cerebellar vein<br>Inferior cerebral vein<br>Internal (basal) cerebral vein<br>Middle cerebral vein<br>Ophthalmic vein<br>Superior cerebellar vein<br>Superior cerebral vein<br>**M Internal Jugular Vein, Right**<br>**N Internal Jugular Vein, Left**<br>**P External Jugular Vein, Right**<br>Posterior auricular vein<br>**Q External Jugular Vein, Left**<br>*See P External Jugular Vein, Right*<br>**R Vertebral Vein, Right**<br>Deep cervical vein<br>Suboccipital venous plexus<br>**S Vertebral Vein, Left**<br>*See R Vertebral Vein, Right*<br>**T Face Vein, Right**<br>Angular vein<br>Anterior facial vein<br>Common facial vein<br>Deep facial vein<br>Frontal vein<br>Posterior facial (retromandibular) vein<br>Supraorbital vein<br>**V Face Vein, Left**<br>*See T Face Vein, Right*<br>**Y Upper Vein** | **Ø Open**<br>**3 Percutaneous**<br>**4 Percutaneous Endoscopic** | **7 Autologous Tissue Substitute**<br>**J Synthetic Substitute**<br>**K Nonautologous Tissue Substitute** | **Z No Qualifier** |

**Ø Medical and Surgical**
**5 Upper Veins**
**V Restriction** Definition: Partially closing an orifice or the lumen of a tubular body part
Explanation: The orifice can be a natural orifice or an artificially created orifice

| Body Part Character 4 | | Approach Character 5 | Device Character 6 | Qualifier Character 7 |
|---|---|---|---|---|
| **Ø Azygos Vein**<br>Right ascending lumbar vein<br>Right subcostal vein<br>**1 Hemiazygos Vein**<br>Left ascending lumbar vein<br>Left subcostal vein<br>**3 Innominate Vein, Right**<br>Brachiocephalic vein<br>Inferior thyroid vein<br>**4 Innominate Vein, Left**<br>***See*** *3 Innominate Vein, Right*<br>**5 Subclavian Vein, Right**<br>**6 Subclavian Vein, Left**<br>**7 Axillary Vein, Right**<br>**8 Axillary Vein, Left**<br>**9 Brachial Vein, Right**<br>Radial vein<br>Ulnar vein<br>**A Brachial Vein, Left**<br>***See*** *9 Brachial Vein, Right*<br>**B Basilic Vein, Right**<br>Median antebrachial vein<br>Median cubital vein<br>**C Basilic Vein, Left**<br>***See*** *B Basilic Vein, Right*<br>**D Cephalic Vein, Right**<br>Accessory cephalic vein<br>**F Cephalic Vein, Left**<br>***See*** *D Cephalic Vein, Right*<br>**G Hand Vein, Right**<br>Dorsal metacarpal vein<br>Palmar (volar) digital vein<br>Palmar (volar) metacarpal vein<br>Superficial palmar venous arch<br>Volar (palmar) digital vein<br>Volar (palmar) metacarpal vein | **H Hand Vein, Left**<br>***See*** *G Hand Vein, Right*<br>**L Intracranial Vein**<br>Anterior cerebral vein<br>Basal (internal) cerebral vein<br>Dural venous sinus<br>Great cerebral vein<br>Inferior cerebellar vein<br>Inferior cerebral vein<br>Internal (basal) cerebral vein<br>Middle cerebral vein<br>Ophthalmic vein<br>Superior cerebellar vein<br>Superior cerebral vein<br>**M Internal Jugular Vein, Right**<br>**N Internal Jugular Vein, Left**<br>**P External Jugular Vein, Right**<br>Posterior auricular vein<br>**Q External Jugular Vein, Left**<br>***See*** *P External Jugular Vein, Right*<br>**R Vertebral Vein, Right**<br>Deep cervical vein<br>Suboccipital venous plexus<br>**S Vertebral Vein, Left**<br>***See*** *R Vertebral Vein, Right*<br>**T Face Vein, Right**<br>Angular vein<br>Anterior facial vein<br>Common facial vein<br>Deep facial vein<br>Frontal vein<br>Posterior facial (retromandibular) vein<br>Supraorbital vein<br>**V Face Vein, Left**<br>***See*** *T Face Vein, Right*<br>**Y Upper Vein** | **Ø** Open<br>**3** Percutaneous<br>**4** Percutaneous Endoscopic | **C** Extraluminal Device<br>**D** Intraluminal Device<br>**Z** No Device | **Z** No Qualifier |

**Ø Medical and Surgical**
**5 Upper Veins**
**W Revision**

Definition: Correcting, to the extent possible, a portion of a malfunctioning device or the position of a displaced device

Explanation: Revision can include correcting a malfunctioning or displaced device by taking out or putting in components of the device such as a screw or pin

| Body Part Character 4 | Approach Character 5 | Device Character 6 | Qualifier Character 7 |
|---|---|---|---|
| **Ø Azygos Vein**<br>Right ascending lumbar vein<br>Right subcostal vein | **Ø Open**<br>**3 Percutaneous**<br>**4 Percutaneous Endoscopic**<br>**X External** | **2 Monitoring Device**<br>**M Neurostimulator Lead** | **Z No Qualifier** |
| **3 Innominate Vein, Right**<br>Brachiocephalic vein<br>Inferior thyroid vein<br>**4 Innominate Vein, Left**<br>*See 3 Innominate Vein, Right* | **Ø Open**<br>**3 Percutaneous**<br>**4 Percutaneous Endoscopic**<br>**X External** | **M Neurostimulator Lead** | **Z No Qualifier** |
| **Y Upper Vein** | **Ø Open**<br>**3 Percutaneous**<br>**4 Percutaneous Endoscopic** | **Ø Drainage Device**<br>**2 Monitoring Device**<br>**3 Infusion Device**<br>**7 Autologous Tissue Substitute**<br>**C Extraluminal Device**<br>**D Intraluminal Device**<br>**J Synthetic Substitute**<br>**K Nonautologous Tissue Substitute**<br>**Y Other Device** | **Z No Qualifier** |
| **Y Upper Vein** | **X External** | **Ø Drainage Device**<br>**2 Monitoring Device**<br>**3 Infusion Device**<br>**7 Autologous Tissue Substitute**<br>**C Extraluminal Device**<br>**D Intraluminal Device**<br>**J Synthetic Substitute**<br>**K Nonautologous Tissue Substitute** | **Z No Qualifier** |

**Non-OR** Ø5WØXMZ
**Non-OR** Ø5W[3,4]XMZ
**Non-OR** Ø5WY3[Ø,2,3,D]Z
**Non-OR** Ø5WY[3,4]YZ
**Non-OR** Ø5WYX[Ø,2,3,7,C,D,J,K]Z

# Lower Veins Ø61–Ø6W



## Character Meanings

This Character Meaning table is provided as a guide to assist the user in the identification of character members that may be found in this section of code tables. It **SHOULD NOT** be used to build a PCS code.

| Operation–Character 3 | Body Part–Character 4 | Approach–Character 5 | Device–Character 6 | Qualifier–Character 7 |
|---|---|---|---|---|
| 1 Bypass | Ø Inferior Vena Cava | Ø Open | Ø Drainage Device | 4 Hepatic Vein |
| 5 Destruction | 1 Splenic Vein | 3 Percutaneous | 2 Monitoring Device | 5 Superior Mesenteric Vein |
| 7 Dilation | 2 Gastric Vein | 4 Percutaneous Endoscopic | 3 Infusion Device | 6 Inferior Mesenteric Vein |
| 9 Drainage | 3 Esophageal Vein | 7 Via Natural or Artificial Opening | 7 Autologous Tissue Substitute | 9 Renal Vein, Right |
| B Excision | 4 Hepatic Vein | 8 Via Natural or Artificial Opening Endoscopic | 9 Autologous Venous Tissue | B Renal Vein, Left |
| C Extirpation | 5 Superior Mesenteric Vein | X External | A Autologous Arterial Tissue | C Hemorrhoidal Plexus |
| D Extraction | 6 Inferior Mesenteric Vein | | C Extraluminal Device | P Pulmonary Trunk |
| H Insertion | 7 Colic Vein | | D Intraluminal Device | Q Pulmonary Artery, Right |
| J Inspection | 8 Portal Vein | | J Synthetic Substitute | R Pulmonary Artery, Left |
| L Occlusion | 9 Renal Vein, Right | | K Nonautologous Tissue Substitute | T Via Umbilical Vein |
| N Release | B Renal Vein, Left | | Z No Device | X Diagnostic |
| P Removal | C Common Iliac Vein, Right | | | Y Lower Vein |
| Q Repair | D Common Iliac Vein, Left | | | Z No Qualifier |
| R Replacement | F External Iliac Vein, Right | | | |
| S Reposition | G External Iliac Vein, Left | | | |
| U Supplement | H Hypogastric Vein, Right | | | |
| V Restriction | J Hypogastric Vein, Left | | | |
| W Revision | M Femoral Vein, Right | | | |
| | N Femoral Vein, Left | | | |
| | P Saphenous Vein, Right | | | |
| | Q Saphenous Vein, Left | | | |
| | T Foot Vein, Right | | | |
| | V Foot Vein, Left | | | |
| | Y Lower Vein | | | |

**AHA Coding Clinic for table Ø6B**

**2017, 1Q, 31** Left to right common carotid artery bypass
**2017, 1Q, 32** Peroneal artery to dorsalis pedis artery bypass using saphenous vein graft
**2016, 3Q, 31** Femoral to peroneal artery bypass with in-situ saphenous vein graft and lysis of valves
**2016, 2Q, 18** Femoral-tibial artery bypass and saphenous vein graft
**2016, 1Q, 27** Aortocoronary bypass graft utilizing Y-graft
**2014, 3Q, 8** Excision of saphenous vein for coronary artery bypass graft
**2014, 3Q, 20** MAZE procedure performed with coronary artery bypass graft
**2014, 1Q, 10** Repair of thoracic aortic aneurysm & coronary artery bypass graft

**AHA Coding Clinic for table Ø6H**

**2017, 1Q, 31** Umbilical vein catheterization
**2017, 1Q, 31** Central catheter placement in femoral vein
**2013, 3Q, 18** Heart transplant surgery

**AHA Coding Clinic for table Ø6L**

**2013, 4Q, 112** Endoscopic banding of esophageal varices

**AHA Coding Clinic for table Ø6W**

**2014, 3Q, 25** Revision of transjugular intrahepatic portosystemic shunt (TIPS)

## Lower Veins

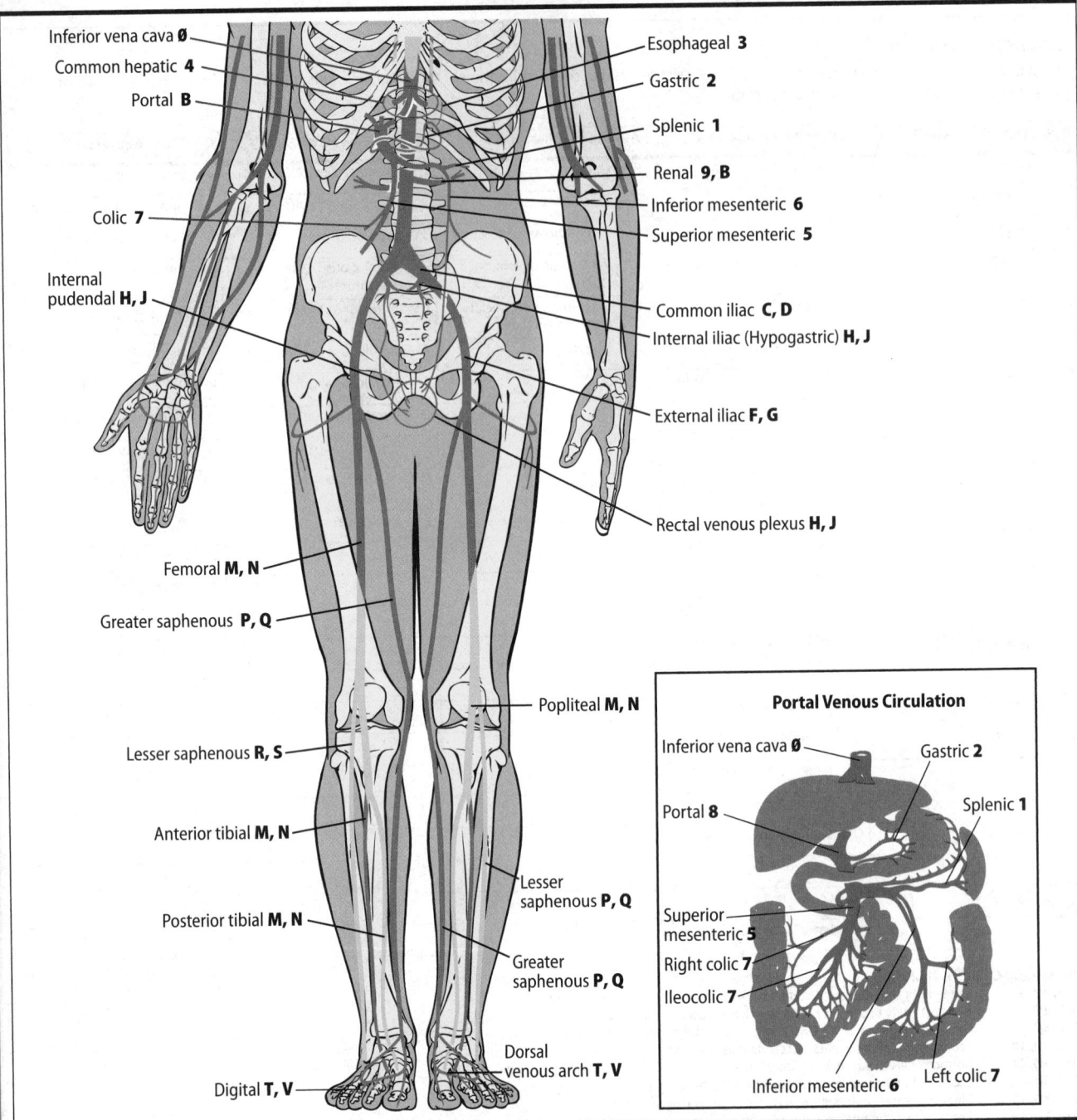

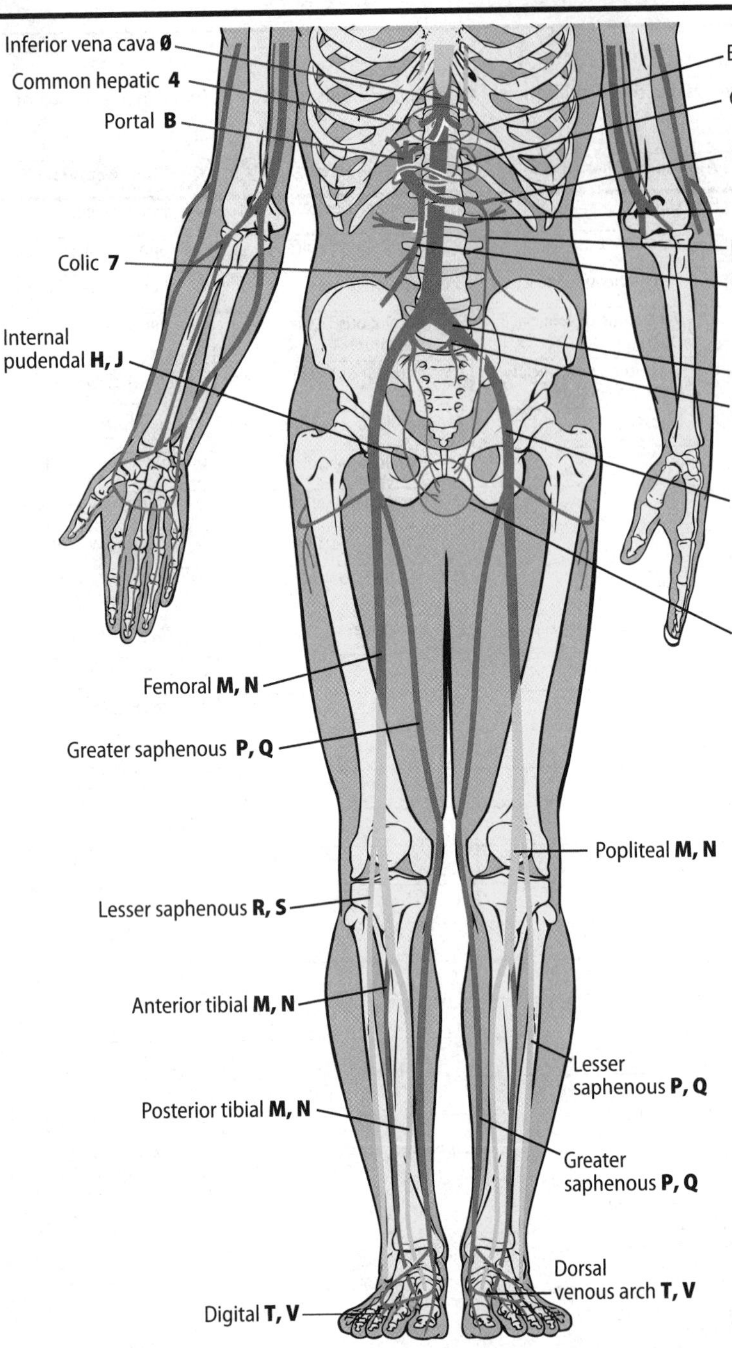
Inferior vena cava Ø
Common hepatic 4
Portal B
Colic 7
Internal pudendal H, J
Esophageal 3
Gastric 2
Splenic 1
Renal 9, B
Inferior mesenteric 6
Superior mesenteric 5
Common iliac C, D
Internal iliac (Hypogastric) H, J
External iliac F, G
Rectal venous plexus H, J
Femoral M, N
Greater saphenous P, Q
Popliteal M, N
Lesser saphenous R, S
Anterior tibial M, N
Lesser saphenous P, Q
Posterior tibial M, N
Greater saphenous P, Q
Dorsal venous arch T, V
Digital T, V

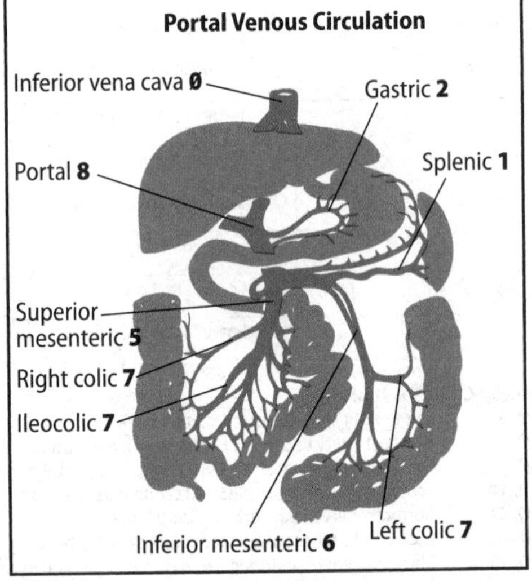
Portal Venous Circulation
Inferior vena cava Ø
Gastric 2
Splenic 1
Portal 8
Superior mesenteric 5
Right colic 7
Ileocolic 7
Inferior mesenteric 6
Left colic 7

**Ø Medical and Surgical**
**6 Lower Veins**
**1 Bypass**

Definition: Altering the route of passage of the contents of a tubular body part

Explanation: Rerouting contents of a body part to a downstream area of the normal route, to a similar route and body part, or to an abnormal route and dissimilar body part. Includes one or more anastomoses, with or without the use of a device.

| Body Part Character 4 | Approach Character 5 | Device Character 6 | Qualifier Character 7 |
|---|---|---|---|
| **Ø Inferior Vena Cava**<br>Postcava<br>Right inferior phrenic vein<br>Right ovarian vein<br>Right second lumbar vein<br>Right suprarenal vein<br>Right testicular vein | **Ø Open**<br>**4 Percutaneous Endoscopic** | **7 Autologous Tissue Substitute**<br>**9 Autologous Venous Tissue**<br>**A Autologous Arterial Tissue**<br>**J Synthetic Substitute**<br>**K Nonautologous Tissue Substitute**<br>**Z No Device** | **5 Superior Mesenteric Vein**<br>**6 Inferior Mesenteric Vein**<br>**P Pulmonary Trunk**<br>**Q Pulmonary Artery, Right**<br>**R Pulmonary Artery, Left**<br>**Y Lower Vein** |
| **1 Splenic Vein**<br>Left gastroepiploic vein<br>Pancreatic vein | **Ø Open**<br>**4 Percutaneous Endoscopic** | **7 Autologous Tissue Substitute**<br>**9 Autologous Venous Tissue**<br>**A Autologous Arterial Tissue**<br>**J Synthetic Substitute**<br>**K Nonautologous Tissue Substitute**<br>**Z No Device** | **9 Renal Vein, Right**<br>**B Renal Vein, Left**<br>**Y Lower Vein** |
| **2 Gastric Vein**<br>**3 Esophageal Vein**<br>**4 Hepatic Vein**<br>**5 Superior Mesenteric Vein**<br>Right gastroepiploic vein<br>**6 Inferior Mesenteric Vein**<br>Sigmoid vein<br>Superior rectal vein<br>**7 Colic Vein**<br>Ileocolic vein<br>Left colic vein<br>Middle colic vein<br>Right colic vein<br>**9 Renal Vein, Right**<br>**B Renal Vein, Left**<br>Left inferior phrenic vein<br>Left ovarian vein<br>Left second lumbar vein<br>Left suprarenal vein<br>Left testicular vein<br>**C Common Iliac Vein, Right**<br>**D Common Iliac Vein, Left**<br>**F External Iliac Vein, Right**<br>**G External Iliac Vein, Left**<br>**H Hypogastric Vein, Right**<br>Gluteal vein<br>Internal iliac vein<br>Internal pudendal vein<br>Lateral sacral vein<br>Middle hemorrhoidal vein<br>Obturator vein<br>Uterine vein<br>Vaginal vein<br>Vesical vein<br>**J Hypogastric Vein, Left**<br>*See H Hypogastric Vein, Right*<br>**M Femoral Vein, Right**<br>Deep femoral (profunda femoris) vein<br>Popliteal vein<br>Profunda femoris (deep femoral) vein<br>**N Femoral Vein, Left**<br>*See M Femoral Vein, Right*<br>**P Saphenous Vein, Right**<br>External pudendal vein<br>Great(er) saphenous vein<br>Lesser saphenous vein<br>Small saphenous vein<br>Superficial circumflex iliac vein<br>Superficial epigastric vein<br>**Q Saphenous Vein, Left**<br>*See P Saphenous Vein, Right*<br>**T Foot Vein, Right**<br>Common digital vein<br>Dorsal metatarsal vein<br>Dorsal venous arch<br>Plantar digital vein<br>Plantar metatarsal vein<br>Plantar venous arch<br>**V Foot Vein, Left**<br>*See T Foot Vein, Right* | **Ø Open**<br>**4 Percutaneous Endoscopic** | **7 Autologous Tissue Substitute**<br>**9 Autologous Venous Tissue**<br>**A Autologous Arterial Tissue**<br>**J Synthetic Substitute**<br>**K Nonautologous Tissue Substitute**<br>**Z No Device** | **Y Lower Vein** |
| **8 Portal Vein**<br>Hepatic portal vein | **Ø Open** | **7 Autologous Tissue Substitute**<br>**9 Autologous Venous Tissue**<br>**A Autologous Arterial Tissue**<br>**J Synthetic Substitute**<br>**K Nonautologous Tissue Substitute**<br>**Z No Device** | **9 Renal Vein, Right**<br>**B Renal Vein, Left**<br>**Y Lower Vein** |
| **8 Portal Vein**<br>Hepatic portal vein | **3 Percutaneous** | **J Synthetic Substitute** | **4 Hepatic Vein**<br>**Y Lower Vein** |
| **8 Portal Vein**<br>Hepatic portal vein | **4 Percutaneous Endoscopic** | **7 Autologous Tissue Substitute**<br>**9 Autologous Venous Tissue**<br>**A Autologous Arterial Tissue**<br>**K Nonautologous Tissue Substitute**<br>**Z No Device** | **9 Renal Vein, Right**<br>**B Renal Vein, Left**<br>**Y Lower Vein** |
| **8 Portal Vein**<br>Hepatic portal vein | **4 Percutaneous Endoscopic** | **J Synthetic Substitute** | **4 Hepatic Vein**<br>**9 Renal Vein, Right**<br>**B Renal Vein, Left**<br>**Y Lower Vein** |

Lower Veins Ø61–Ø61

**Ø Medical and Surgical**
**6 Lower Veins**
**5 Destruction** Definition: Physical eradication of all or a portion of a body part by the direct use of energy, force, or a destructive agent
Explanation: None of the body part is physically taken out

| Body Part Character 4 | Approach Character 5 | Device Character 6 | Qualifier Character 7 |
|---|---|---|---|
| **Ø Inferior Vena Cava**<br>Postcava<br>Right inferior phrenic vein<br>Right ovarian vein<br>Right second lumbar vein<br>Right suprarenal vein<br>Right testicular vein<br>**1 Splenic Vein**<br>Left gastroepiploic vein<br>Pancreatic vein<br>**2 Gastric Vein**<br>**3 Esophageal Vein**<br>**4 Hepatic Vein**<br>**5 Superior Mesenteric Vein**<br>Right gastroepiploic vein<br>**6 Inferior Mesenteric Vein**<br>Sigmoid vein<br>Superior rectal vein<br>**7 Colic Vein**<br>Ileocolic vein<br>Left colic vein<br>Middle colic vein<br>Right colic vein<br>**8 Portal Vein**<br>Hepatic portal vein<br>**9 Renal Vein, Right**<br>**B Renal Vein, Left**<br>Left inferior phrenic vein<br>Left ovarian vein<br>Left second lumbar vein<br>Left suprarenal vein<br>Left testicular vein<br>**C Common Iliac Vein, Right**<br>**D Common Iliac Vein, Left**<br>**F External Iliac Vein, Right**<br>**G External Iliac Vein, Left**<br>**H Hypogastric Vein, Right**<br>Gluteal vein<br>Internal iliac vein<br>Internal pudendal vein<br>Lateral sacral vein<br>Middle hemorrhoidal vein<br>Obturator vein<br>Uterine vein<br>Vaginal vein<br>Vesical vein<br>**J Hypogastric Vein, Left**<br>*See H Hypogastric Vein, Right*<br>**M Femoral Vein, Right**<br>Deep femoral (profunda femoris) vein<br>Popliteal vein<br>Profunda femoris (deep femoral) vein<br>**N Femoral Vein, Left**<br>*See M Femoral Vein, Right*<br>**P Saphenous Vein, Right**<br>External pudendal vein<br>Great(er) saphenous vein<br>Lesser saphenous vein<br>Small saphenous vein<br>Superficial circumflex iliac vein<br>Superficial epigastric vein<br>**Q Saphenous Vein, Left**<br>*See P Saphenous Vein, Right*<br>**T Foot Vein, Right**<br>Common digital vein<br>Dorsal metatarsal vein<br>Dorsal venous arch<br>Plantar digital vein<br>Plantar metatarsal vein<br>Plantar venous arch<br>**V Foot Vein, Left**<br>*See T Foot Vein, Right* | **Ø Open**<br>**3 Percutaneous**<br>**4 Percutaneous Endoscopic** | **Z No Device** | **Z No Qualifier** |
| **Y Lower Vein** | **Ø Open**<br>**3 Percutaneous**<br>**4 Percutaneous Endoscopic** | **Z No Device** | **C Hemorrhoidal Plexus**<br>**Z No Qualifier** |

**Ø Medical and Surgical**
**6 Lower Veins**
**7 Dilation** Definition: Expanding an orifice or the lumen of a tubular body part

Explanation: The orifice can be a natural orifice or an artificially created orifice. Accomplished by stretching a tubular body part using intraluminal pressure or by cutting part of the orifice or wall of the tubular body part.

| Body Part Character 4 | Approach Character 5 | Device Character 6 | Qualifier Character 7 |
|---|---|---|---|
| **Ø Inferior Vena Cava**<br>Postcava<br>Right inferior phrenic vein<br>Right ovarian vein<br>Right second lumbar vein<br>Right suprarenal vein<br>Right testicular vein<br>**1 Splenic Vein**<br>Left gastroepiploic vein<br>Pancreatic vein<br>**2 Gastric Vein**<br>**3 Esophageal Vein**<br>**4 Hepatic Vein**<br>**5 Superior Mesenteric Vein**<br>Right gastroepiploic vein<br>**6 Inferior Mesenteric Vein**<br>Sigmoid vein<br>Superior rectal vein<br>**7 Colic Vein**<br>Ileocolic vein<br>Left colic vein<br>Middle colic vein<br>Right colic vein<br>**8 Portal Vein**<br>Hepatic portal vein<br>**9 Renal Vein, Right**<br>**B Renal Vein, Left**<br>Left inferior phrenic vein<br>Left ovarian vein<br>Left second lumbar vein<br>Left suprarenal vein<br>Left testicular vein<br>**C Common Iliac Vein, Right**<br>**D Common Iliac Vein, Left**<br>**F External Iliac Vein, Right**<br>**G External Iliac Vein, Left**<br>**H Hypogastric Vein, Right**<br>Gluteal vein<br>Internal iliac vein<br>Internal pudendal vein<br>Lateral sacral vein<br>Middle hemorrhoidal vein<br>Obturator vein<br>Uterine vein<br>Vaginal vein<br>Vesical vein<br>**J Hypogastric Vein, Left**<br>*See H Hypogastric Vein, Right*<br>**M Femoral Vein, Right**<br>Deep femoral (profunda femoris) vein<br>Popliteal vein<br>Profunda femoris (deep femoral) vein<br>**N Femoral Vein, Left**<br>*See M Femoral Vein, Right*<br>**P Saphenous Vein, Right**<br>External pudendal vein<br>Great(er) saphenous vein<br>Lesser saphenous vein<br>Small saphenous vein<br>Superficial circumflex iliac vein<br>Superficial epigastric vein<br>**Q Saphenous Vein, Left**<br>*See P Saphenous Vein, Right*<br>**T Foot Vein, Right**<br>Common digital vein<br>Dorsal metatarsal vein<br>Dorsal venous arch<br>Plantar digital vein<br>Plantar metatarsal vein<br>Plantar venous arch<br>**V Foot Vein, Left**<br>*See T Foot Vein, Right*<br>**Y Lower Vein** | **Ø Open**<br>**3 Percutaneous**<br>**4 Percutaneous Endoscopic** | **D Intraluminal Device**<br>**Z No Device** | **Z No Qualifier** |

**Ø Medical and Surgical**
**6 Lower Veins**
**9 Drainage**

Definition: Taking or letting out fluids and/or gases from a body part

Explanation: The qualifier DIAGNOSTIC is used to identify drainage procedures that are biopsies

| Body Part Character 4 | | Approach Character 5 | Device Character 6 | Qualifier Character 7 |
|---|---|---|---|---|
| **Ø Inferior Vena Cava**<br>Postcava<br>Right inferior phrenic vein<br>Right ovarian vein<br>Right second lumbar vein<br>Right suprarenal vein<br>Right testicular vein<br>**1 Splenic Vein**<br>Left gastroepiploic vein<br>Pancreatic vein<br>**2 Gastric Vein**<br>**3 Esophageal Vein**<br>**4 Hepatic Vein**<br>**5 Superior Mesenteric Vein**<br>Right gastroepiploic vein<br>**6 Inferior Mesenteric Vein**<br>Sigmoid vein<br>Superior rectal vein<br>**7 Colic Vein**<br>Ileocolic vein<br>Left colic vein<br>Middle colic vein<br>Right colic vein<br>**8 Portal Vein**<br>Hepatic portal vein<br>**9 Renal Vein, Right**<br>**B Renal Vein, Left**<br>Left inferior phrenic vein<br>Left ovarian vein<br>Left second lumbar vein<br>Left suprarenal vein<br>Left testicular vein<br>**C Common Iliac Vein, Right**<br>**D Common Iliac Vein, Left**<br>**F External Iliac Vein, Right**<br>**G External Iliac Vein, Left** | **H Hypogastric Vein, Right**<br>Gluteal vein<br>Internal iliac vein<br>Internal pudendal vein<br>Lateral sacral vein<br>Middle hemorrhoidal vein<br>Obturator vein<br>Uterine vein<br>Vaginal vein<br>Vesical vein<br>**J Hypogastric Vein, Left**<br>***See*** *H Hypogastric Vein, Right*<br>**M Femoral Vein, Right**<br>Deep femoral (profunda femoris) vein<br>Popliteal vein<br>Profunda femoris (deep femoral) vein<br>**N Femoral Vein, Left**<br>***See*** *M Femoral Vein, Right*<br>**P Saphenous Vein, Right**<br>External pudendal vein<br>Great(er) saphenous vein<br>Lesser saphenous vein<br>Small saphenous vein<br>Superficial circumflex iliac vein<br>Superficial epigastric vein<br>**Q Saphenous Vein, Left**<br>***See*** *P Saphenous Vein, Right*<br>**T Foot Vein, Right**<br>Common digital vein<br>Dorsal metatarsal vein<br>Dorsal venous arch<br>Plantar digital vein<br>Plantar metatarsal vein<br>Plantar venous arch<br>**V Foot Vein, Left**<br>***See*** *T Foot Vein, Right*<br>**Y Lower Vein** | **Ø Open**<br>**3 Percutaneous**<br>**4 Percutaneous Endoscopic** | **Ø Drainage Device** | **Z No Qualifier** |

***Ø69 Continued on next page***

**Non-OR** Ø69[Ø,1,2,4,5,6,7,8,9,B,C,D,F,G,H,J,M,N,P,Q,T,V,Y][Ø,3,4]ØZ
**Non-OR** Ø6933ØZ

Ø Medical and Surgical
6 Lower Veins
9 Drainage

Definition: Taking or letting out fluids and/or gases from a body part

Explanation: The qualifier DIAGNOSTIC is used to identify drainage procedures that are biopsies

*Ø69 Continued*

| Body Part Character 4 | Approach Character 5 | Device Character 6 | Qualifier Character 7 |
|---|---|---|---|
| Ø Inferior Vena Cava<br>Postcava<br>Right inferior phrenic vein<br>Right ovarian vein<br>Right second lumbar vein<br>Right suprarenal vein<br>Right testicular vein<br>1 Splenic Vein<br>Left gastroepiploic vein<br>Pancreatic vein<br>2 Gastric Vein<br>3 Esophageal Vein<br>4 Hepatic Vein<br>5 Superior Mesenteric Vein<br>Right gastroepiploic vein<br>6 Inferior Mesenteric Vein<br>Sigmoid vein<br>Superior rectal vein<br>7 Colic Vein<br>Ileocolic vein<br>Left colic vein<br>Middle colic vein<br>Right colic vein<br>8 Portal Vein<br>Hepatic portal vein<br>9 Renal Vein, Right<br>B Renal Vein, Left<br>Left inferior phrenic vein<br>Left ovarian vein<br>Left second lumbar vein<br>Left suprarenal vein<br>Left testicular vein<br>C Common Iliac Vein, Right<br>D Common Iliac Vein, Left<br>F External Iliac Vein, Right<br>G External Iliac Vein, Left<br>H Hypogastric Vein, Right<br>Gluteal vein<br>Internal iliac vein<br>Internal pudendal vein<br>Lateral sacral vein<br>Middle hemorrhoidal vein<br>Obturator vein<br>Uterine vein<br>Vaginal vein<br>Vesical vein<br>J Hypogastric Vein, Left<br>*See H Hypogastric Vein, Right*<br>M Femoral Vein, Right<br>Deep femoral (profunda femoris) vein<br>Popliteal vein<br>Profunda femoris (deep femoral) vein<br>N Femoral Vein, Left<br>*See M Femoral Vein, Right*<br>P Saphenous Vein, Right<br>External pudendal vein<br>Great(er) saphenous vein<br>Lesser saphenous vein<br>Small saphenous vein<br>Superficial circumflex iliac vein<br>Superficial epigastric vein<br>Q Saphenous Vein, Left<br>*See P Saphenous Vein, Right*<br>T Foot Vein, Right<br>Common digital vein<br>Dorsal metatarsal vein<br>Dorsal venous arch<br>Plantar digital vein<br>Plantar metatarsal vein<br>Plantar venous arch<br>V Foot Vein, Left<br>*See T Foot Vein, Right*<br>Y Lower Vein | Ø Open<br>3 Percutaneous<br>4 Percutaneous Endoscopic | Z No Device | X Diagnostic<br>Z No Qualifier |

Non-OR Ø69[Ø,1,2,3,4,5,6,7,8,9,B,C,D,F,G,H,J,M,N,P,Q,T,V,Y]3ZX
Non-OR Ø69[Ø,1,2,4,5,6,7,8,9,B,C,D,F,G,H,J,M,N,P,Q,T,V,Y][Ø,3,4]ZZ
Non-OR Ø6933ZZ

**Ø Medical and Surgical**
**6 Lower Veins**
**B Excision**

Definition: Cutting out or off, without replacement, a portion of a body part

Explanation: The qualifier DIAGNOSTIC is used to identify excision procedures that are biopsies

| Body Part Character 4 | | Approach Character 5 | Device Character 6 | Qualifier Character 7 |
|---|---|---|---|---|
| **Ø Inferior Vena Cava**<br>Postcava<br>Right inferior phrenic vein<br>Right ovarian vein<br>Right second lumbar vein<br>Right suprarenal vein<br>Right testicular vein<br>**1 Splenic Vein**<br>Left gastroepiploic vein<br>Pancreatic vein<br>**2 Gastric Vein**<br>**3 Esophageal Vein**<br>**4 Hepatic Vein**<br>**5 Superior Mesenteric Vein**<br>Right gastroepiploic vein<br>**6 Inferior Mesenteric Vein**<br>Sigmoid vein<br>Superior rectal vein<br>**7 Colic Vein**<br>Ileocolic vein<br>Left colic vein<br>Middle colic vein<br>Right colic vein<br>**8 Portal Vein**<br>Hepatic portal vein<br>**9 Renal Vein, Right**<br>**B Renal Vein, Left**<br>Left inferior phrenic vein<br>Left ovarian vein<br>Left second lumbar vein<br>Left suprarenal vein<br>Left testicular vein<br>**C Common Iliac Vein, Right**<br>**D Common Iliac Vein, Left** | **F External Iliac Vein, Right**<br>**G External Iliac Vein, Left**<br>**H Hypogastric Vein, Right**<br>Gluteal vein<br>Internal iliac vein<br>Internal pudendal vein<br>Lateral sacral vein<br>Middle hemorrhoidal vein<br>Obturator vein<br>Uterine vein<br>Vaginal vein<br>Vesical vein<br>**J Hypogastric Vein, Left**<br>***See*** *H Hypogastric Vein, Right*<br>**M Femoral Vein, Right**<br>Deep femoral (profunda femoris) vein<br>Popliteal vein<br>Profunda femoris (deep femoral) vein<br>**N Femoral Vein, Left**<br>***See*** *M Femoral Vein, Right*<br>**P Saphenous Vein, Right**<br>External pudendal vein<br>Great(er) saphenous vein<br>Lesser saphenous vein<br>Small saphenous vein<br>Superficial circumflex iliac vein<br>Superficial epigastric vein<br>**Q Saphenous Vein, Left**<br>***See*** *P Saphenous Vein, Right*<br>**T Foot Vein, Right**<br>Common digital vein<br>Dorsal metatarsal vein<br>Dorsal venous arch<br>Plantar digital vein<br>Plantar metatarsal vein<br>Plantar venous arch<br>**V Foot Vein, Left**<br>***See*** *T Foot Vein, Right* | **Ø Open**<br>**3 Percutaneous**<br>**4 Percutaneous Endoscopic** | **Z No Device** | **X Diagnostic**<br>**Z No Qualifier** |
| **Y Lower Vein** | | **Ø Open**<br>**3 Percutaneous**<br>**4 Percutaneous Endoscopic** | **Z No Device** | **C Hemorrhoidal Plexus**<br>**X Diagnostic**<br>**Z No Qualifier** |

**Ø Medical and Surgical**
**6 Lower Veins**
**C Extirpation**

Definition: Taking or cutting out solid matter from a body part

Explanation: The solid matter may be an abnormal byproduct of a biological function or a foreign body; it may be imbedded in a body part or in the lumen of a tubular body part. The solid matter may or may not have been previously broken into pieces.

| Body Part Character 4 | | Approach Character 5 | Device Character 6 | Qualifier Character 7 |
|---|---|---|---|---|
| **Ø Inferior Vena Cava**<br>Postcava<br>Right inferior phrenic vein<br>Right ovarian vein<br>Right second lumbar vein<br>Right suprarenal vein<br>Right testicular vein<br>**1 Splenic Vein**<br>Left gastroepiploic vein<br>Pancreatic vein<br>**2 Gastric Vein**<br>**3 Esophageal Vein**<br>**4 Hepatic Vein**<br>**5 Superior Mesenteric Vein**<br>Right gastroepiploic vein<br>**6 Inferior Mesenteric Vein**<br>Sigmoid vein<br>Superior rectal vein<br>**7 Colic Vein**<br>Ileocolic vein<br>Left colic vein<br>Middle colic vein<br>Right colic vein<br>**8 Portal Vein**<br>Hepatic portal vein<br>**9 Renal Vein, Right**<br>**B Renal Vein, Left**<br>Left inferior phrenic vein<br>Left ovarian vein<br>Left second lumbar vein<br>Left suprarenal vein<br>Left testicular vein<br>**C Common Iliac Vein, Right**<br>**D Common Iliac Vein, Left** | **F External Iliac Vein, Right**<br>**G External Iliac Vein, Left**<br>**H Hypogastric Vein, Right**<br>Gluteal vein<br>Internal iliac vein<br>Internal pudendal vein<br>Lateral sacral vein<br>Middle hemorrhoidal vein<br>Obturator vein<br>Uterine vein<br>Vaginal vein<br>Vesical vein<br>**J Hypogastric Vein, Left**<br>*See H Hypogastric Vein, Right*<br>**M Femoral Vein, Right**<br>Deep femoral (profunda femoris) vein<br>Popliteal vein<br>Profunda femoris (deep femoral) vein<br>**N Femoral Vein, Left**<br>*See M Femoral Vein, Right*<br>**P Saphenous Vein, Right**<br>External pudendal vein<br>Great(er) saphenous vein<br>Lesser saphenous vein<br>Small saphenous vein<br>Superficial circumflex iliac vein<br>Superficial epigastric vein<br>**Q Saphenous Vein, Left**<br>*See P Saphenous Vein, Right*<br>**T Foot Vein, Right**<br>Common digital vein<br>Dorsal metatarsal vein<br>Dorsal venous arch<br>Plantar digital vein<br>Plantar metatarsal vein<br>Plantar venous arch<br>**V Foot Vein, Left**<br>*See T Foot Vein, Right*<br>**Y Lower Vein** | **Ø Open**<br>**3 Percutaneous**<br>**4 Percutaneous Endoscopic** | **Z No Device** | **Z No Qualifier** |

**Ø Medical and Surgical**
**6 Lower Veins**
**D Extraction**

Definition: Pulling or stripping out or off all or a portion of a body part by the use of force

Explanation: The qualifier DIAGNOSTIC is used to identify extraction procedures that are biopsies

| Body Part Character 4 | | Approach Character 5 | Device Character 6 | Qualifier Character 7 |
|---|---|---|---|---|
| **M Femoral Vein, Right**<br>Deep femoral (profunda femoris) vein<br>Popliteal vein<br>Profunda femoris (deep femoral) vein<br>**N Femoral Vein, Left**<br>*See M Femoral Vein, Right*<br>**P Saphenous Vein, Right**<br>External pudendal vein<br>Great(er) saphenous vein<br>Lesser saphenous vein<br>Small saphenous vein<br>Superficial circumflex iliac vein<br>Superficial epigastric vein<br>**Q Saphenous Vein, Left**<br>*See P Saphenous Vein, Right* | **T Foot Vein, Right**<br>Common digital vein<br>Dorsal metatarsal vein<br>Dorsal venous arch<br>Plantar digital vein<br>Plantar metatarsal vein<br>Plantar venous arch<br>**V Foot Vein, Left**<br>*See T Foot Vein, Right*<br>**Y Lower Vein** | **Ø Open**<br>**3 Percutaneous**<br>**4 Percutaneous Endoscopic** | **Z No Device** | **Z No Qualifier** |

**Ø Medical and Surgical**
**6 Lower Veins**
**H Insertion**

Definition: Putting in a nonbiological appliance that monitors, assists, performs, or prevents a physiological function but does not physically take the place of a body part

Explanation: None

| Body Part Character 4 | Approach Character 5 | Device Character 6 | Qualifier Character 7 |
|---|---|---|---|
| **Ø Inferior Vena Cava**<br>Postcava<br>Right inferior phrenic vein<br>Right ovarian vein<br>Right second lumbar vein<br>Right suprarenal vein<br>Right testicular vein | **Ø Open**<br>**3 Percutaneous** | **3 Infusion Device** | **T Via Umbilical Vein**<br>**Z No Qualifier** |
| **Ø Inferior Vena Cava**<br>Postcava<br>Right inferior phrenic vein<br>Right ovarian vein<br>Right second lumbar vein<br>Right suprarenal vein<br>Right testicular vein | **Ø Open**<br>**3 Percutaneous** | **D Intraluminal Device** | **Z No Qualifier** |
| **Ø Inferior Vena Cava**<br>Postcava<br>Right inferior phrenic vein<br>Right ovarian vein<br>Right second lumbar vein<br>Right suprarenal vein<br>Right testicular vein | **4 Percutaneous Endoscopic** | **3 Infusion Device**<br>**D Intraluminal Device** | **Z No Qualifier** |
| **1 Splenic Vein**<br>Left gastroepiploic vein<br>Pancreatic vein<br>**2 Gastric Vein**<br>**3 Esophageal Vein**<br>**4 Hepatic Vein**<br>**5 Superior Mesenteric Vein**<br>Right gastroepiploic vein<br>**6 Inferior Mesenteric Vein**<br>Sigmoid vein<br>Superior rectal vein<br>**7 Colic Vein**<br>Ileocolic vein<br>Left colic vein<br>Middle colic vein<br>Right colic vein<br>**8 Portal Vein**<br>Hepatic portal vein<br>**9 Renal Vein, Right**<br>**B Renal Vein, Left**<br>Left inferior phrenic vein<br>Left ovarian vein<br>Left second lumbar vein<br>Left suprarenal vein<br>Left testicular vein<br>**C Common Iliac Vein, Right**<br>**D Common Iliac Vein, Left**<br>**F External Iliac Vein, Right**<br>**G External Iliac Vein, Left**<br>**H Hypogastric Vein, Right**<br>Gluteal vein<br>Internal iliac vein<br>Internal pudendal vein<br>Lateral sacral vein<br>Middle hemorrhoidal vein<br>Obturator vein<br>Uterine vein<br>Vaginal vein<br>Vesical vein<br>**J Hypogastric Vein, Left**<br>*See H Hypogastric Vein, Right*<br>**M Femoral Vein, Right**<br>Deep femoral (profunda femoris) vein<br>Popliteal vein<br>Profunda femoris (deep femoral) vein<br>**N Femoral Vein, Left**<br>*See M Femoral Vein, Right*<br>**P Saphenous Vein, Right**<br>External pudendal vein<br>Great(er) saphenous vein<br>Lesser saphenous vein<br>Small saphenous vein<br>Superficial circumflex iliac vein<br>Superficial epigastric vein<br>**Q Saphenous Vein, Left**<br>*See P Saphenous Vein, Right*<br>**T Foot Vein, Right**<br>Common digital vein<br>Dorsal metatarsal vein<br>Dorsal venous arch<br>Plantar digital vein<br>Plantar metatarsal vein<br>Plantar venous arch<br>**V Foot Vein, Left**<br>*See T Foot Vein, Right* | **Ø Open**<br>**3 Percutaneous**<br>**4 Percutaneous Endoscopic** | **3 Infusion Device**<br>**D Intraluminal Device** | **Z No Qualifier** |
| **Y Lower Vein** | **Ø Open**<br>**3 Percutaneous**<br>**4 Percutaneous Endoscopic** | **2 Monitoring Device**<br>**3 Infusion Device**<br>**D Intraluminal Device**<br>Y Other Device | **Z No Qualifier** |

| | |
|---|---|
| **Non-OR** | Ø6HØ[Ø,3]3[T,Z] |
| **Non-OR** | Ø6HØ3DZ |
| **Non-OR** | Ø6HØ43Z |
| **Non-OR** | Ø6H[1,2,3,4,5,6,7,8,9,B,C,D,F,G,H,J,M,N,P,Q,T,V][Ø,3,4]3Z |
| **Non-OR** | Ø6HY[Ø,3,4]3Z |
| **Non-OR** | Ø6HY32Z |
| **Non-OR** | Ø6HY[3,4]YZ |

**Ø Medical and Surgical**
**6 Lower Veins**
**J Inspection**

Definition: Visually and/or manually exploring a body part

Explanation: Visual exploration may be performed with or without optical instrumentation. Manual exploration may be performed directly or through intervening body layers.

| Body Part Character 4 | Approach Character 5 | Device Character 6 | Qualifier Character 7 |
|---|---|---|---|
| **Y** Lower Vein | **Ø** Open<br>**3** Percutaneous<br>**4** Percutaneous Endoscopic<br>**X** External | **Z** No Device | **Z** No Qualifier |

Non-OR Ø6JY[3,X]ZZ

**Ø Medical and Surgical**
**6 Lower Veins**
**L Occlusion**

Definition: Completely closing an orifice or the lumen of a tubular body part

Explanation: The orifice can be a natural orifice or an artificially created orifice

| Body Part Character 4 | | Approach Character 5 | Device Character 6 | Qualifier Character 7 |
|---|---|---|---|---|
| **Ø Inferior Vena Cava**<br>Postcava<br>Right inferior phrenic vein<br>Right ovarian vein<br>Right second lumbar vein<br>Right suprarenal vein<br>Right testicular vein<br>**1 Splenic Vein**<br>Left gastroepiploic vein<br>Pancreatic vein<br>**2 Gastric Vein**<br>**4 Hepatic Vein**<br>**5 Superior Mesenteric Vein**<br>Right gastroepiploic vein<br>**6 Inferior Mesenteric Vein**<br>Sigmoid vein<br>Superior rectal vein<br>**7 Colic Vein**<br>Ileocolic vein<br>Left colic vein<br>Middle colic vein<br>Right colic vein<br>**8 Portal Vein**<br>Hepatic portal vein<br>**9 Renal Vein, Right**<br>**B Renal Vein, Left**<br>Left inferior phrenic vein<br>Left ovarian vein<br>Left second lumbar vein<br>Left suprarenal vein<br>Left testicular vein<br>**C Common Iliac Vein, Right**<br>**D Common Iliac Vein, Left**<br>**F External Iliac Vein, Right**<br>**G External Iliac Vein, Left** | **H Hypogastric Vein, Right**<br>Gluteal vein<br>Internal iliac vein<br>Internal pudendal vein<br>Lateral sacral vein<br>Middle hemorrhoidal vein<br>Obturator vein<br>Uterine vein<br>Vaginal vein<br>Vesical vein<br>**J Hypogastric Vein, Left**<br>*See H Hypogastric Vein, Right*<br>**M Femoral Vein, Right**<br>Deep femoral (profunda femoris) vein<br>Popliteal vein<br>Profunda femoris (deep femoral) vein<br>**N Femoral Vein, Left**<br>*See M Femoral Vein, Right*<br>P Saphenous Vein, Right<br>External pudendal vein<br>Great(er) saphenous vein<br>Lesser saphenous vein<br>Small saphenous vein<br>Superficial circumflex iliac vein<br>Superficial epigastric vein<br>Q Saphenous Vein, Left<br>*See P Saphenous Vein, Right*<br>**T Foot Vein, Right**<br>Common digital vein<br>Dorsal metatarsal vein<br>Dorsal venous arch<br>Plantar digital vein<br>Plantar metatarsal vein<br>Plantar venous arch<br>**V Foot Vein, Left**<br>*See T Foot Vein, Right* | **Ø** Open<br>**3** Percutaneous<br>**4** Percutaneous Endoscopic | **C** Extraluminal Device<br>**D** Intraluminal Device<br>**Z** No Device | **Z** No Qualifier |
| **3** Esophageal Vein | | **Ø** Open<br>**3** Percutaneous<br>**4** Percutaneous Endoscopic<br>7 Via Natural or Artificial Opening<br>8 Via Natural or Artificial Opening Endoscopic | **C** Extraluminal Device<br>**D** Intraluminal Device<br>**Z** No Device | **Z** No Qualifier |
| **Y** Lower Vein | | **Ø** Open<br>**3** Percutaneous<br>**4** Percutaneous Endoscopic | **C** Extraluminal Device<br>**D** Intraluminal Device<br>**Z** No Device | **C** Hemorrhoidal Plexus<br>**Z** No Qualifier |

Non-OR Ø6L3[3,4,7,8][C,D,Z]Z

**Ø Medical and Surgical**
**6 Lower Veins**
**N Release**

Definition: Freeing a body part from an abnormal physical constraint by cutting or by the use of force
Explanation: Some of the restraining tissue may be taken out but none of the body part is taken out

| Body Part Character 4 | Approach Character 5 | Device Character 6 | Qualifier Character 7 |
|---|---|---|---|
| **Ø Inferior Vena Cava**<br>Postcava<br>Right inferior phrenic vein<br>Right ovarian vein<br>Right second lumbar vein<br>Right suprarenal vein<br>Right testicular vein<br>**1 Splenic Vein**<br>Left gastroepiploic vein<br>Pancreatic vein<br>**2 Gastric Vein**<br>**3 Esophageal Vein**<br>**4 Hepatic Vein**<br>**5 Superior Mesenteric Vein**<br>Right gastroepiploic vein<br>**6 Inferior Mesenteric Vein**<br>Sigmoid vein<br>Superior rectal vein<br>**7 Colic Vein**<br>Ileocolic vein<br>Left colic vein<br>Middle colic vein<br>Right colic vein<br>**8 Portal Vein**<br>Hepatic portal vein<br>**9 Renal Vein, Right**<br>**B Renal Vein, Left**<br>Left inferior phrenic vein<br>Left ovarian vein<br>Left second lumbar vein<br>Left suprarenal vein<br>Left testicular vein<br>**C Common Iliac Vein, Right**<br>**D Common Iliac Vein, Left**<br>**F External Iliac Vein, Right**<br>**G External Iliac Vein, Left**<br>**H Hypogastric Vein, Right**<br>Gluteal vein<br>Internal iliac vein<br>Internal pudendal vein<br>Lateral sacral vein<br>Middle hemorrhoidal vein<br>Obturator vein<br>Uterine vein<br>Vaginal vein<br>Vesical vein<br>**J Hypogastric Vein, Left**<br>*See H Hypogastric Vein, Right*<br>**M Femoral Vein, Right**<br>Deep femoral (profunda femoris) vein<br>Popliteal vein<br>Profunda femoris (deep femoral) vein<br>**N Femoral Vein, Left**<br>*See M Femoral Vein, Right*<br>**P Saphenous Vein, Right**<br>External pudendal vein<br>Great(er) saphenous vein<br>Lesser saphenous vein<br>Small saphenous vein<br>Superficial circumflex iliac vein<br>Superficial epigastric vein<br>**Q Saphenous Vein, Left**<br>*See P Saphenous Vein, Right*<br>**T Foot Vein, Right**<br>Common digital vein<br>Dorsal metatarsal vein<br>Dorsal venous arch<br>Plantar digital vein<br>Plantar metatarsal vein<br>Plantar venous arch<br>**V Foot Vein, Left**<br>*See T Foot Vein, Right*<br>**Y Lower Vein** | **Ø Open**<br>**3 Percutaneous**<br>**4 Percutaneous Endoscopic** | **Z No Device** | **Z No Qualifier** |

**Ø Medical and Surgical**
**6 Lower Veins**
**P Removal**

Definition: Taking out or off a device from a body part
Explanation: If a device is taken out and a similar device put in without cutting or puncturing the skin or mucous membrane, the procedure is coded to the root operation CHANGE. Otherwise, the procedure for taking out a device is coded to the root operation REMOVAL.

| Body Part Character 4 | Approach Character 5 | Device Character 6 | Qualifier Character 7 |
|---|---|---|---|
| **Y Lower Vein** | **Ø Open**<br>**3 Percutaneous**<br>**4 Percutaneous Endoscopic** | **Ø Drainage Device**<br>**2 Monitoring Device**<br>**3 Infusion Device**<br>**7 Autologous Tissue Substitute**<br>**C Extraluminal Device**<br>**D Intraluminal Device**<br>**J Synthetic Substitute**<br>**K Nonautologous Tissue Substitute**<br>**Y Other Device** | **Z No Qualifier** |
| **Y Lower Vein** | **X External** | **Ø Drainage Device**<br>**2 Monitoring Device**<br>**3 Infusion Device**<br>**D Intraluminal Device** | **Z No Qualifier** |

Non-OR Ø6PY3[Ø,2,3]Z
Non-OR Ø6PY[3,4]YZ
Non-OR Ø6PYX[Ø,2,3,D]Z

**Ø Medical and Surgical**
**6 Lower Veins**
**Q Repair** Definition: Restoring, to the extent possible, a body part to its normal anatomic structure and function
Explanation: Used only when the method to accomplish the repair is not one of the other root operations

| Body Part Character 4 | Approach Character 5 | Device Character 6 | Qualifier Character 7 |
|---|---|---|---|
| **Ø Inferior Vena Cava**<br>Postcava<br>Right inferior phrenic vein<br>Right ovarian vein<br>Right second lumbar vein<br>Right suprarenal vein<br>Right testicular vein<br>**1 Splenic Vein**<br>Left gastroepiploic vein<br>Pancreatic vein<br>**2 Gastric Vein**<br>**3 Esophageal Vein**<br>**4 Hepatic Vein**<br>**5 Superior Mesenteric Vein**<br>Right gastroepiploic vein<br>**6 Inferior Mesenteric Vein**<br>Sigmoid vein<br>Superior rectal vein<br>**7 Colic Vein**<br>Ileocolic vein<br>Left colic vein<br>Middle colic vein<br>Right colic vein<br>**8 Portal Vein**<br>Hepatic portal vein<br>**9 Renal Vein, Right**<br>**B Renal Vein, Left**<br>Left inferior phrenic vein<br>Left ovarian vein<br>Left second lumbar vein<br>Left suprarenal vein<br>Left testicular vein<br>**C Common Iliac Vein, Right**<br>**D Common Iliac Vein, Left**<br>**F External Iliac Vein, Right**<br>**G External Iliac Vein, Left**<br>**H Hypogastric Vein, Right**<br>Gluteal vein<br>Internal iliac vein<br>Internal pudendal vein<br>Lateral sacral vein<br>Middle hemorrhoidal vein<br>Obturator vein<br>Uterine vein<br>Vaginal vein<br>Vesical vein<br>**J Hypogastric Vein, Left**<br>*See H Hypogastric Vein, Right*<br>**M Femoral Vein, Right**<br>Deep femoral (profunda femoris) vein<br>Popliteal vein<br>Profunda femoris (deep femoral) vein<br>**N Femoral Vein, Left**<br>*See M Femoral Vein, Right*<br>**P Saphenous Vein, Right**<br>External pudendal vein<br>Great(er) saphenous vein<br>Lesser saphenous vein<br>Small saphenous vein<br>Superficial circumflex iliac vein<br>Superficial epigastric vein<br>**Q Saphenous Vein, Left**<br>*See P Saphenous Vein, Right*<br>**T Foot Vein, Right**<br>Common digital vein<br>Dorsal metatarsal vein<br>Dorsal venous arch<br>Plantar digital vein<br>Plantar metatarsal vein<br>Plantar venous arch<br>**V Foot Vein, Left**<br>*See T Foot Vein, Right*<br>**Y Lower Vein** | **Ø Open**<br>**3 Percutaneous**<br>**4 Percutaneous Endoscopic** | **Z No Device** | **Z No Qualifier** |

**Ø Medical and Surgical**
**6 Lower Veins**
**R Replacement** Definition: Putting in or on biological or synthetic material that physically takes the place and/or function of all or a portion of a body part

Explanation: The body part may have been taken out or replaced, or may be taken out, physically eradicated, or rendered nonfunctional during the REPLACEMENT procedure. A REMOVAL procedure is coded for taking out the device used in a previous replacement procedure.

| Body Part Character 4 | Approach Character 5 | Device Character 6 | Qualifier Character 7 |
|---|---|---|---|
| **Ø Inferior Vena Cava**<br>Postcava<br>Right inferior phrenic vein<br>Right ovarian vein<br>Right second lumbar vein<br>Right suprarenal vein<br>Right testicular vein<br>**1 Splenic Vein**<br>Left gastroepiploic vein<br>Pancreatic vein<br>**2 Gastric Vein**<br>**3 Esophageal Vein**<br>**4 Hepatic Vein**<br>**5 Superior Mesenteric Vein**<br>Right gastroepiploic vein<br>**6 Inferior Mesenteric Vein**<br>Sigmoid vein<br>Superior rectal vein<br>**7 Colic Vein**<br>Ileocolic vein<br>Left colic vein<br>Middle colic vein<br>Right colic vein<br>**8 Portal Vein**<br>Hepatic portal vein<br>**9 Renal Vein, Right**<br>**B Renal Vein, Left**<br>Left inferior phrenic vein<br>Left ovarian vein<br>Left second lumbar vein<br>Left suprarenal vein<br>Left testicular vein<br>**C Common Iliac Vein, Right**<br>**D Common Iliac Vein, Left**<br>**F External Iliac Vein, Right**<br>**G External Iliac Vein, Left**<br>**H Hypogastric Vein, Right**<br>Gluteal vein<br>Internal iliac vein<br>Internal pudendal vein<br>Lateral sacral vein<br>Middle hemorrhoidal vein<br>Obturator vein<br>Uterine vein<br>Vaginal vein<br>Vesical vein<br>**J Hypogastric Vein, Left**<br>*See H Hypogastric Vein, Right*<br>**M Femoral Vein, Right**<br>Deep femoral (profunda femoris) vein<br>Popliteal vein<br>Profunda femoris (deep femoral) vein<br>**N Femoral Vein, Left**<br>*See M Femoral Vein, Right*<br>**P Saphenous Vein, Right**<br>External pudendal vein<br>Great(er) saphenous vein<br>Lesser saphenous vein<br>Small saphenous vein<br>Superficial circumflex iliac vein<br>Superficial epigastric vein<br>**Q Saphenous Vein, Left**<br>*See P Saphenous Vein, Right*<br>**T Foot Vein, Right**<br>Common digital vein<br>Dorsal metatarsal vein<br>Dorsal venous arch<br>Plantar digital vein<br>Plantar metatarsal vein<br>Plantar venous arch<br>**V Foot Vein, Left**<br>*See T Foot Vein, Right*<br>**Y Lower Vein** | **Ø Open**<br>**4 Percutaneous Endoscopic** | **7 Autologous Tissue Substitute**<br>**J Synthetic Substitute**<br>**K Nonautologous Tissue Substitute** | **Z No Qualifier** |

**Ø Medical and Surgical**
**6 Lower Veins**
**S Reposition** Definition: Moving to its normal location, or other suitable location, all or a portion of a body part

Explanation: The body part is moved to a new location from an abnormal location, or from a normal location where it is not functioning correctly. The body part may or may not be cut out or off to be moved to the new location.

| Body Part Character 4 | Approach Character 5 | Device Character 6 | Qualifier Character 7 |
|---|---|---|---|
| **Ø Inferior Vena Cava**<br>Postcava<br>Right inferior phrenic vein<br>Right ovarian vein<br>Right second lumbar vein<br>Right suprarenal vein<br>Right testicular vein<br>**1 Splenic Vein**<br>Left gastroepiploic vein<br>Pancreatic vein<br>**2 Gastric Vein**<br>**3 Esophageal Vein**<br>**4 Hepatic Vein**<br>**5 Superior Mesenteric Vein**<br>Right gastroepiploic vein<br>**6 Inferior Mesenteric Vein**<br>Sigmoid vein<br>Superior rectal vein<br>**7 Colic Vein**<br>Ileocolic vein<br>Left colic vein<br>Middle colic vein<br>Right colic vein<br>**8 Portal Vein**<br>Hepatic portal vein<br>**9 Renal Vein, Right**<br>**B Renal Vein, Left**<br>Left inferior phrenic vein<br>Left ovarian vein<br>Left second lumbar vein<br>Left suprarenal vein<br>Left testicular vein<br>**C Common Iliac Vein, Right**<br>**D Common Iliac Vein, Left**<br>**F External Iliac Vein, Right**<br>**G External Iliac Vein, Left**<br>**H Hypogastric Vein, Right**<br>Gluteal vein<br>Internal iliac vein<br>Internal pudendal vein<br>Lateral sacral vein<br>Middle hemorrhoidal vein<br>Obturator vein<br>Uterine vein<br>Vaginal vein<br>Vesical vein<br>**J Hypogastric Vein, Left**<br>*See H Hypogastric Vein, Right*<br>**M Femoral Vein, Right**<br>Deep femoral (profunda femoris) vein<br>Popliteal vein<br>Profunda femoris (deep femoral) vein<br>**N Femoral Vein, Left**<br>*See M Femoral Vein, Right*<br>**P Saphenous Vein, Right**<br>External pudendal vein<br>Great(er) saphenous vein<br>Lesser saphenous vein<br>Small saphenous vein<br>Superficial circumflex iliac vein<br>Superficial epigastric vein<br>**Q Saphenous Vein, Left**<br>*See P Saphenous Vein, Right*<br>**T Foot Vein, Right**<br>Common digital vein<br>Dorsal metatarsal vein<br>Dorsal venous arch<br>Plantar digital vein<br>Plantar metatarsal vein<br>Plantar venous arch<br>**V Foot Vein, Left**<br>*See T Foot Vein, Right*<br>**Y Lower Vein** | **Ø Open**<br>**3 Percutaneous**<br>**4 Percutaneous Endoscopic** | **Z No Device** | **Z No Qualifier** |

**Ø Medical and Surgical**
**6 Lower Veins**
**U Supplement**

Definition: Putting in or on biological or synthetic material that physically reinforces and/or augments the function of a portion of a body part

Explanation: The biological material is non-living, or is living and from the same individual. The body part may have been previously replaced, and the SUPPLEMENT procedure is performed to physically reinforce and/or augment the function of the replaced body part.

| Body Part Character 4 | Approach Character 5 | Device Character 6 | Qualifier Character 7 |
|---|---|---|---|
| **Ø Inferior Vena Cava**<br>Postcava<br>Right inferior phrenic vein<br>Right ovarian vein<br>Right second lumbar vein<br>Right suprarenal vein<br>Right testicular vein<br>**1 Splenic Vein**<br>Left gastroepiploic vein<br>Pancreatic vein<br>**2 Gastric Vein**<br>**3 Esophageal Vein**<br>**4 Hepatic Vein**<br>**5 Superior Mesenteric Vein**<br>Right gastroepiploic vein<br>**6 Inferior Mesenteric Vein**<br>Sigmoid vein<br>Superior rectal vein<br>**7 Colic Vein**<br>Ileocolic vein<br>Left colic vein<br>Middle colic vein<br>Right colic vein<br>**8 Portal Vein**<br>Hepatic portal vein<br>**9 Renal Vein, Right**<br>**B Renal Vein, Left**<br>Left inferior phrenic vein<br>Left ovarian vein<br>Left second lumbar vein<br>Left suprarenal vein<br>Left testicular vein<br>**C Common Iliac Vein, Right**<br>**D Common Iliac Vein, Left**<br>**F External Iliac Vein, Right**<br>**G External Iliac Vein, Left**<br>**H Hypogastric Vein, Right**<br>Gluteal vein<br>Internal iliac vein<br>Internal pudendal vein<br>Lateral sacral vein<br>Middle hemorrhoidal vein<br>Obturator vein<br>Uterine vein<br>Vaginal vein<br>Vesical vein<br>**J Hypogastric Vein, Left**<br>*See H Hypogastric Vein, Right*<br>**M Femoral Vein, Right**<br>Deep femoral (profunda femoris) vein<br>Popliteal vein<br>Profunda femoris (deep femoral) vein<br>**N Femoral Vein, Left**<br>*See M Femoral Vein, Right*<br>**P Saphenous Vein, Right**<br>External pudendal vein<br>Great(er) saphenous vein<br>Lesser saphenous vein<br>Small saphenous vein<br>Superficial circumflex iliac vein<br>Superficial epigastric vein<br>**Q Saphenous Vein, Left**<br>*See P Saphenous Vein, Right*<br>**T Foot Vein, Right**<br>Common digital vein<br>Dorsal metatarsal vein<br>Dorsal venous arch<br>Plantar digital vein<br>Plantar metatarsal vein<br>Plantar venous arch<br>**V Foot Vein, Left**<br>*See T Foot Vein, Right*<br>**Y Lower Vein** | **Ø Open**<br>**3 Percutaneous**<br>**4 Percutaneous Endoscopic** | **7 Autologous Tissue Substitute**<br>**J Synthetic Substitute**<br>**K Nonautologous Tissue Substitute** | **Z No Qualifier** |

**Ø Medical and Surgical**
**6 Lower Veins**
**V Restriction** Definition: Partially closing an orifice or the lumen of a tubular body part
Explanation: The orifice can be a natural orifice or an artificially created orifice

| Body Part Character 4 | Approach Character 5 | Device Character 6 | Qualifier Character 7 |
|---|---|---|---|
| **Ø Inferior Vena Cava**<br>Postcava<br>Right inferior phrenic vein<br>Right ovarian vein<br>Right second lumbar vein<br>Right suprarenal vein<br>Right testicular vein<br>**1 Splenic Vein**<br>Left gastroepiploic vein<br>Pancreatic vein<br>**2 Gastric Vein**<br>**3 Esophageal Vein**<br>**4 Hepatic Vein**<br>**5 Superior Mesenteric Vein**<br>Right gastroepiploic vein<br>**6 Inferior Mesenteric Vein**<br>Sigmoid vein<br>Superior rectal vein<br>**7 Colic Vein**<br>Ileocolic vein<br>Left colic vein<br>Middle colic vein<br>Right colic vein<br>**8 Portal Vein**<br>Hepatic portal vein<br>**9 Renal Vein, Right**<br>**B Renal Vein, Left**<br>Left inferior phrenic vein<br>Left ovarian vein<br>Left second lumbar vein<br>Left suprarenal vein<br>Left testicular vein<br>**C Common Iliac Vein, Right**<br>**D Common Iliac Vein, Left**<br>**F External Iliac Vein, Right**<br>**G External Iliac Vein, Left**<br>**H Hypogastric Vein, Right**<br>Gluteal vein<br>Internal iliac vein<br>Internal pudendal vein<br>Lateral sacral vein<br>Middle hemorrhoidal vein<br>Obturator vein<br>Uterine vein<br>Vaginal vein<br>Vesical vein<br>**J Hypogastric Vein, Left**<br>*See H Hypogastric Vein, Right*<br>**M Femoral Vein, Right**<br>Deep femoral (profunda femoris) vein<br>Popliteal vein<br>Profunda femoris (deep femoral) vein<br>**N Femoral Vein, Left**<br>*See M Femoral Vein, Right*<br>**P Saphenous Vein, Right**<br>External pudendal vein<br>Great(er) saphenous vein<br>Lesser saphenous vein<br>Small saphenous vein<br>Superficial circumflex iliac vein<br>Superficial epigastric vein<br>**Q Saphenous Vein, Left**<br>*See P Saphenous Vein, Right*<br>**T Foot Vein, Right**<br>Common digital vein<br>Dorsal metatarsal vein<br>Dorsal venous arch<br>Plantar digital vein<br>Plantar metatarsal vein<br>Plantar venous arch<br>**V Foot Vein, Left**<br>*See T Foot Vein, Right*<br>**Y Lower Vein** | **Ø Open**<br>**3 Percutaneous**<br>**4 Percutaneous Endoscopic** | **C Extraluminal Device**<br>**D Intraluminal Device**<br>**Z No Device** | **Z No Qualifier** |

**Ø Medical and Surgical**
**6 Lower Veins**
**W Revision**

Definition: Correcting, to the extent possible, a portion of a malfunctioning device or the position of a displaced device

Explanation: Revision can include correcting a malfunctioning or displaced device by taking out or putting in components of the device such as a screw or pin

| Body Part Character 4 | Approach Character 5 | Device Character 6 | Qualifier Character 7 |
|---|---|---|---|
| Y Lower Vein | Ø Open<br>3 Percutaneous<br>4 Percutaneous Endoscopic | Ø Drainage Device<br>2 Monitoring Device<br>3 Infusion Device<br>7 Autologous Tissue Substitute<br>C Extraluminal Device<br>D Intraluminal Device<br>J Synthetic Substitute<br>K Nonautologous Tissue Substitute<br>Y Other Device | Z No Qualifier |
| Y Lower Vein | X External | Ø Drainage Device<br>2 Monitoring Device<br>3 Infusion Device<br>7 Autologous Tissue Substitute<br>C Extraluminal Device<br>D Intraluminal Device<br>J Synthetic Substitute<br>K Nonautologous Tissue Substitute | Z No Qualifier |

Non-OR Ø6WY3[Ø,2,3,D]Z
Non-OR Ø6WY[3,4]YZ
Non-OR Ø6WYX[Ø,2,3,7,C,D,J,K]Z

# Lymphatic and Hemic Systems Ø72–Ø7Y



## Character Meanings*

This Character Meaning table is provided as a guide to assist the user in the identification of character members that may be found in this section of code tables. It **SHOULD NOT** be used to build a PCS code.

| Operation–Character 3 | Body Part–Character 4 | Approach–Character 5 | Device–Character 6 | Qualifier–Character 7 |
|---|---|---|---|---|
| 2 Change | Ø Lymphatic, Head | Ø Open | Ø Drainage Device | Ø Allogeneic |
| 5 Destruction | 1 Lymphatic, Right Neck | 3 Percutaneous | 3 Infusion Device | 1 Syngeneic |
| 9 Drainage | 2 Lymphatic, Left Neck | 4 Percutaneous Endoscopic | 7 Autologous Tissue Substitute | 2 Zooplastic |
| B Excision | 3 Lymphatic, Right Upper Extremity | 8 Via Natural or Artificial Opening Endoscopic | C Extraluminal Device | X Diagnostic |
| C Extirpation | 4 Lymphatic, Left Upper Extremity | X External | D Intraluminal Device | Z No Qualifier |
| D Extraction | 5 Lymphatic, Right Axillary | | J Synthetic Substitute | |
| H Insertion | 6 Lymphatic, Left Axillary | | K Nonautologous Tissue Substitute | |
| J Inspection | 7 Lymphatic, Thorax | | Y Other Device | |
| L Occlusion | 8 Lymphatic, Internal Mammary, Right | | Z No Device | |
| N Release | 9 Lymphatic, Internal Mammary, Left | | | |
| P Removal | B Lymphatic, Mesenteric | | | |
| Q Repair | C Lymphatic, Pelvis | | | |
| S Reposition | D Lymphatic, Aortic | | | |
| T Resection | F Lymphatic, Right Lower Extremity | | | |
| U Supplement | G Lymphatic, Left Lower Extremity | | | |
| V Restriction | H Lymphatic, Right Inguinal | | | |
| W Revision | J Lymphatic, Left Inguinal | | | |
| Y Transplantation | K Thoracic Duct | | | |
| | L Cisterna Chyli | | | |
| | M Thymus | | | |
| | N Lymphatic | | | |
| | P Spleen | | | |
| | Q Bone Marrow, Sternum | | | |
| | R Bone Marrow, Iliac | | | |
| | S Bone Marrow, Vertebral | | | |
| | T Bone Marrow | | | |

* Includes lymph vessels and lymph nodes.

**AHA Coding Clinic for table Ø79**
**2017, 1Q, 34** Lymphovenous bypass following mastectomy
**2014, 1Q, 26** Transbronchial needle aspiration lymph node biopsy
**2013, 4Q, 111** Transbronchial needle aspiration lymph node biopsy

**AHA Coding Clinic for table Ø7B**
**2016, 1Q, 30** Axillary lymph node resection with modified radical mastectomy
**2014, 3Q, 10** Selective excision of paratracheal lymph nodes
**2014, 1Q, 20** Fiducial marker placement
**2014, 1Q, 26** Transbronchial endoscopic lymph node aspiration biopsy

**AHA Coding Clinic for table Ø7D**
**2013, 4Q, 111** Root operation for bone marrow biopsy

**AHA Coding Clinic for table Ø7Q**
**2017, 1Q, 34** Lymphovenous bypass following mastectomy

**AHA Coding Clinic for table Ø7T**
**2016, 2Q, 12** Resection of malignant neoplasm of infratemporal fossa
**2016, 1Q, 30** Axillary lymph node resection with modified radical mastectomy
**2015, 4Q, 13** New Section X codes—New Technology procedures
**2014, 3Q, 9** Radical resection of level I lymph nodes
**2014, 3Q, 16** Repair of Tetralogy of Fallot

## Lymphatic System

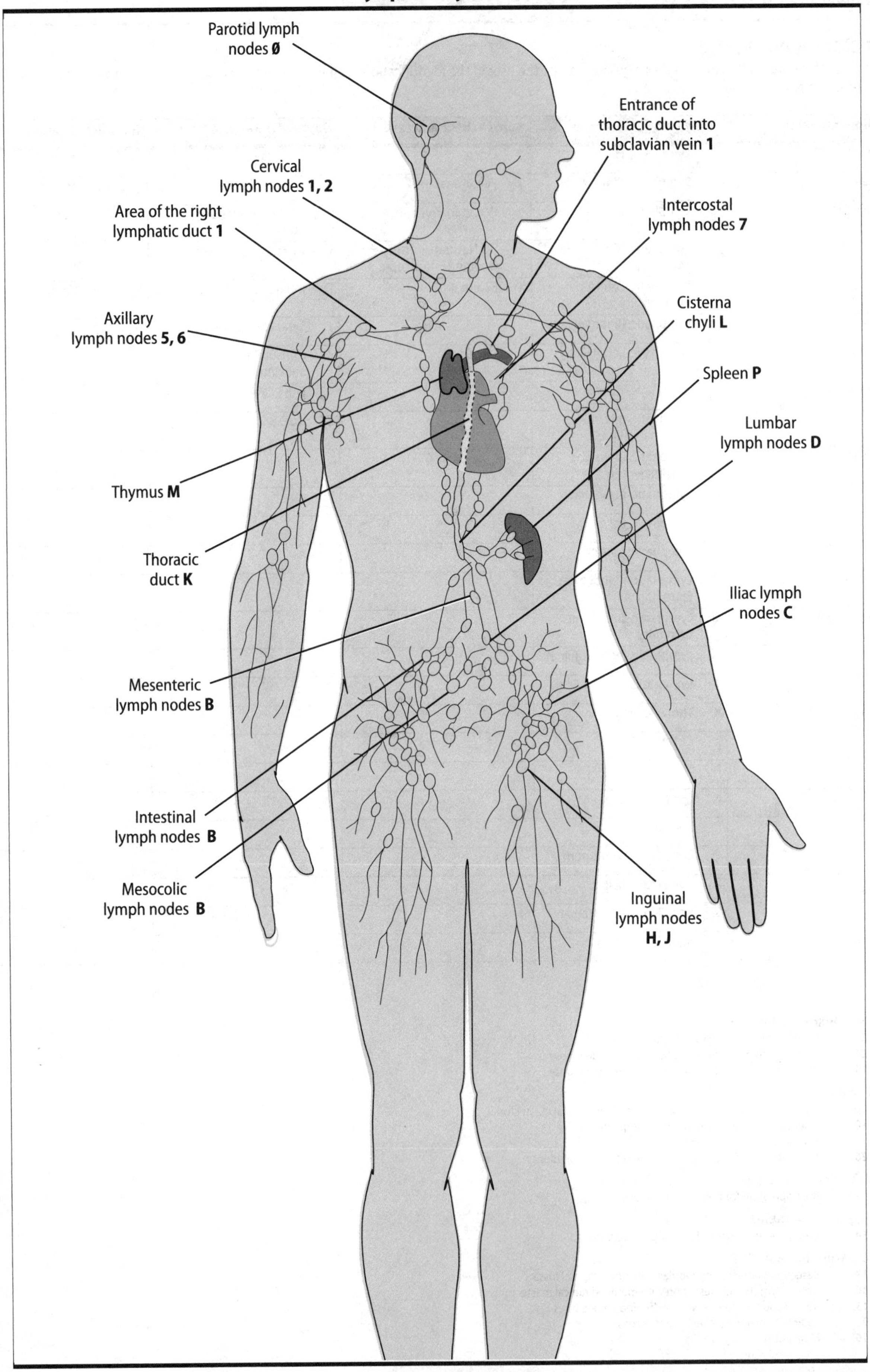
Parotid lymph nodes **Ø**
Entrance of thoracic duct into subclavian vein **1**
Cervical lymph nodes **1, 2**
Area of the right lymphatic duct **1**
Intercostal lymph nodes **7**
Cisterna chyli **L**
Axillary lymph nodes **5, 6**
Spleen **P**
Lumbar lymph nodes **D**
Thymus **M**
Thoracic duct **K**
Iliac lymph nodes **C**
Mesenteric lymph nodes **B**
Intestinal lymph nodes **B**
Mesocolic lymph nodes **B**
Inguinal lymph nodes **H, J**

**Ø Medical and Surgical**
**7 Lymphatic and Hemic Systems**
**2 Change** Definition: Taking out or off a device from a body part and putting back an identical or similar device in or on the same body part without cutting or puncturing the skin or a mucous membrane

Explanation: All CHANGE procedures are coded using the approach EXTERNAL

| Body Part Character 4 | | Approach Character 5 | Device Character 6 | Qualifier Character 7 |
|---|---|---|---|---|
| **K Thoracic Duct**<br>Left jugular trunk<br>Left subclavian trunk<br>**L Cisterna Chyli**<br>Intestinal lymphatic trunk<br>Lumbar lymphatic trunk | **M Thymus**<br>Thymus gland<br>**N Lymphatic**<br>**P Spleen**<br>Accessory spleen<br>**T Bone Marrow** | **X External** | **Ø Drainage Device**<br>**Y Other Device** | **Z No Qualifier** |

**Non-OR** All body part, approach, device, and qualifier values

**Ø Medical and Surgical**
**7 Lymphatic and Hemic Systems**
**5 Destruction** Definition: Physical eradication of all or a portion of a body part by the direct use of energy, force, or a destructive agent

Explanation: None of the body part is physically taken out

| Body Part Character 4 | | Approach Character 5 | Device Character 6 | Qualifier Character 7 |
|---|---|---|---|---|
| **Ø Lymphatic, Head**<br>Buccinator lymph node<br>Infraauricular lymph node<br>Infraparotid lymph node<br>Parotid lymph node<br>Preauricular lymph node<br>Submandibular lymph node<br>Submaxillary lymph node<br>Submental lymph node<br>Subparotid lymph node<br>Suprahyoid lymph node<br>**1 Lymphatic, Right Neck**<br>Cervical lymph node<br>Jugular lymph node<br>Mastoid (postauricular) lymph node<br>Occipital lymph node<br>Postauricular (mastoid) lymph node<br>Retropharyngeal lymph node<br>Right jugular trunk<br>Right lymphatic duct<br>Right subclavian trunk<br>Supraclavicular (Virchow's) lymph node<br>Virchow's (supraclavicular) lymph node<br>**2 Lymphatic, Left Neck**<br>Cervical lymph node<br>Jugular lymph node<br>Mastoid (postauricular) lymph node<br>Occipital lymph node<br>Postauricular (mastoid) lymph node<br>Retropharyngeal lymph node<br>Supraclavicular (Virchow's) lymph node<br>Virchow's (supraclavicular) lymph node<br>**3 Lymphatic, Right Upper Extremity**<br>Cubital lymph node<br>Deltopectoral (infraclavicular) lymph node<br>Epitrochlear lymph node<br>Infraclavicular (deltopectoral) lymph node<br>Supratrochlear lymph node<br>**4 Lymphatic, Left Upper Extremity**<br>*See 3 Lymphatic, Right Upper Extremity*<br>**5 Lymphatic, Right Axillary**<br>Anterior (pectoral) lymph node<br>Apical (subclavicular) lymph node<br>Brachial (lateral) lymph node<br>Central axillary lymph node<br>Lateral (brachial) lymph node<br>Pectoral (anterior) lymph node<br>Posterior (subscapular) lymph node<br>Subclavicular (apical) lymph node<br>Subscapular (posterior) lymph node | **6 Lymphatic, Left Axillary**<br>*See 5 Lymphatic, Right Axillary*<br>**7 Lymphatic, Thorax**<br>Intercostal lymph node<br>Mediastinal lymph node<br>Parasternal lymph node<br>Paratracheal lymph node<br>Tracheobronchial lymph node<br>**8 Lymphatic, Internal Mammary, Right**<br>**9 Lymphatic, Internal Mammary, Left**<br>**B Lymphatic, Mesenteric**<br>Inferior mesenteric lymph node<br>Pararectal lymph node<br>Superior mesenteric lymph node<br>**C Lymphatic, Pelvis**<br>Common iliac (subaortic) lymph node<br>Gluteal lymph node<br>Iliac lymph node<br>Inferior epigastric lymph node<br>Obturator lymph node<br>Sacral lymph node<br>Subaortic (common iliac) lymph node<br>Suprainguinal lymph node<br>**D Lymphatic, Aortic**<br>Celiac lymph node<br>Gastric lymph node<br>Hepatic lymph node<br>Lumbar lymph node<br>Pancreaticosplenic lymph node<br>Paraaortic lymph node<br>Retroperitoneal lymph node<br>**F Lymphatic, Right Lower Extremity**<br>Femoral lymph node<br>Popliteal lymph node<br>**G Lymphatic, Left Lower Extremity**<br>*See F Lymphatic, Right Lower Extremity*<br>**H Lymphatic, Right Inguinal**<br>**J Lymphatic, Left Inguinal**<br>**K Thoracic Duct**<br>Left jugular trunk<br>Left subclavian trunk<br>**L Cisterna Chyli**<br>Intestinal lymphatic trunk<br>Lumbar lymphatic trunk<br>**M Thymus**<br>Thymus gland<br>**P Spleen**<br>Accessory spleen | **Ø Open**<br>**3 Percutaneous**<br>**4 Percutaneous Endoscopic** | **Z No Device** | **Z No Qualifier** |

**Ø Medical and Surgical**
**7 Lymphatic and Hemic Systems**
**9 Drainage** Definition: Taking or letting out fluids and/or gases from a body part
Explanation: The qualifier DIAGNOSTIC is used to identify drainage procedures that are biopsies

| Body Part Character 4 | Approach Character 5 | Device Character 6 | Qualifier Character 7 |
|---|---|---|---|
| **Ø Lymphatic, Head**<br>Buccinator lymph node<br>Infraauricular lymph node<br>Infraparotid lymph node<br>Parotid lymph node<br>Preauricular lymph node<br>Submandibular lymph node<br>Submaxillary lymph node<br>Submental lymph node<br>Subparotid lymph node<br>Suprahyoid lymph node<br>**1 Lymphatic, Right Neck**<br>Cervical lymph node<br>Jugular lymph node<br>Mastoid (postauricular) lymph node<br>Occipital lymph node<br>Postauricular (mastoid) lymph node<br>Retropharyngeal lymph node<br>Right jugular trunk<br>Right lymphatic duct<br>Right subclavian trunk<br>Supraclavicular (Virchow's) lymph node<br>Virchow's (supraclavicular) lymph node<br>**2 Lymphatic, Left Neck**<br>Cervical lymph node<br>Jugular lymph node<br>Mastoid (postauricular) lymph node<br>Occipital lymph node<br>Postauricular (mastoid) lymph node<br>Retropharyngeal lymph node<br>Supraclavicular (Virchow's) lymph node<br>Virchow's (supraclavicular) lymph node<br>**3 Lymphatic, Right Upper Extremity**<br>Cubital lymph node<br>Deltopectoral (infraclavicular) lymph node<br>Epitrochlear lymph node<br>Infraclavicular (deltopectoral) lymph node<br>Supratrochlear lymph node<br>**4 Lymphatic, Left Upper Extremity**<br>*See 3 Lymphatic, Right Upper Extremity*<br>**5 Lymphatic, Right Axillary**<br>Anterior (pectoral) lymph node<br>Apical (subclavicular) lymph node<br>Brachial (lateral) lymph node<br>Central axillary lymph node<br>Lateral (brachial) lymph node<br>Pectoral (anterior) lymph node<br>Posterior (subscapular) lymph node<br>Subclavicular (apical) lymph node<br>Subscapular (posterior) lymph node<br>**6 Lymphatic, Left Axillary**<br>*See 5 Lymphatic, Right Axillary*<br>**7 Lymphatic, Thorax**<br>Intercostal lymph node<br>Mediastinal lymph node<br>Parasternal lymph node<br>Paratracheal lymph node<br>Tracheobronchial lymph node<br>**8 Lymphatic, Internal Mammary, Right**<br>**9 Lymphatic, Internal Mammary, Left**<br>**B Lymphatic, Mesenteric**<br>Inferior mesenteric lymph node<br>Pararectal lymph node<br>Superior mesenteric lymph node<br>**C Lymphatic, Pelvis**<br>Common iliac (subaortic) lymph node<br>Gluteal lymph node<br>Iliac lymph node<br>Inferior epigastric lymph node<br>Obturator lymph node<br>Sacral lymph node<br>Subaortic (common iliac) lymph node<br>Suprainguinal lymph node<br>**D Lymphatic, Aortic**<br>Celiac lymph node<br>Gastric lymph node<br>Hepatic lymph node<br>Lumbar lymph node<br>Pancreaticosplenic lymph node<br>Paraaortic lymph node<br>Retroperitoneal lymph node<br>**F Lymphatic, Right Lower Extremity**<br>Femoral lymph node<br>Popliteal lymph node<br>**G Lymphatic, Left Lower Extremity**<br>*See F Lymphatic, Right Lower Extremity*<br>**H Lymphatic, Right Inguinal**<br>**J Lymphatic, Left Inguinal**<br>**K Thoracic Duct**<br>Left jugular trunk<br>Left subclavian trunk<br>**L Cisterna Chyli**<br>Intestinal lymphatic trunk<br>Lumbar lymphatic trunk | **Ø Open**<br>**3 Percutaneous**<br>**4 Percutaneous Endoscopic**<br>**8 Via Natural or Artificial Opening Endoscopic** | **Ø Drainage Device** | **Z No Qualifier** |

*Ø79 Continued on next page*

| | |
|---|---|
| Non-OR | Ø79[Ø,1,2,3,4,5,6,7,8,9,B,C,D,F,G,H,J,K,L][3,8]ØZ |

**Ø Medical and Surgical**
**7 Lymphatic and Hemic Systems**
**9 Drainage** Definition: Taking or letting out fluids and/or gases from a body part
Explanation: The qualifier DIAGNOSTIC is used to identify drainage procedures that are biopsies

Ø79 Continued

| Body Part Character 4 | Approach Character 5 | Device Character 6 | Qualifier Character 7 |
|---|---|---|---|
| **Ø Lymphatic, Head**<br>Buccinator lymph node<br>Infraauricular lymph node<br>Infraparotid lymph node<br>Parotid lymph node<br>Preauricular lymph node<br>Submandibular lymph node<br>Submaxillary lymph node<br>Submental lymph node<br>Subparotid lymph node<br>Suprahyoid lymph node<br>**1 Lymphatic, Right Neck**<br>Cervical lymph node<br>Jugular lymph node<br>Mastoid (postauricular) lymph node<br>Occipital lymph node<br>Postauricular (mastoid) lymph node<br>Retropharyngeal lymph node<br>Right jugular trunk<br>Right lymphatic duct<br>Right subclavian trunk<br>Supraclavicular (Virchow's) lymph node<br>Virchow's (supraclavicular) lymph node<br>**2 Lymphatic, Left Neck**<br>Cervical lymph node<br>Jugular lymph node<br>Mastoid (postauricular) lymph node<br>Occipital lymph node<br>Postauricular (mastoid) lymph node<br>Retropharyngeal lymph node<br>Supraclavicular (Virchow's) lymph node<br>Virchow's (supraclavicular) lymph node<br>**3 Lymphatic, Right Upper Extremity**<br>Cubital lymph node<br>Deltopectoral (infraclavicular) lymph node<br>Epitrochlear lymph node<br>Infraclavicular (deltopectoral) lymph node<br>Supratrochlear lymph node<br>**4 Lymphatic, Left Upper Extremity**<br>*See 3 Lymphatic, Right Upper Extremity*<br>**5 Lymphatic, Right Axillary**<br>Anterior (pectoral) lymph node<br>Apical (subclavicular) lymph node<br>Brachial (lateral) lymph node<br>Central axillary lymph node<br>Lateral (brachial) lymph node<br>Pectoral (anterior) lymph node<br>Posterior (subscapular) lymph node<br>Subclavicular (apical) lymph node<br>Subscapular (posterior) lymph node<br>**6 Lymphatic, Left Axillary**<br>*See 5 Lymphatic, Right Axillary*<br>**7 Lymphatic, Thorax**<br>Intercostal lymph node<br>Mediastinal lymph node<br>Parasternal lymph node<br>Paratracheal lymph node<br>Tracheobronchial lymph node<br>**8 Lymphatic, Internal Mammary, Right**<br>**9 Lymphatic, Internal Mammary, Left**<br>**B Lymphatic, Mesenteric**<br>Inferior mesenteric lymph node<br>Pararectal lymph node<br>Superior mesenteric lymph node<br>**C Lymphatic, Pelvis**<br>Common iliac (subaortic) lymph node<br>Gluteal lymph node<br>Iliac lymph node<br>Inferior epigastric lymph node<br>Obturator lymph node<br>Sacral lymph node<br>Subaortic (common iliac) lymph node<br>Suprainguinal lymph node<br>**D Lymphatic, Aortic**<br>Celiac lymph node<br>Gastric lymph node<br>Hepatic lymph node<br>Lumbar lymph node<br>Pancreaticosplenic lymph node<br>Paraaortic lymph node<br>Retroperitoneal lymph node<br>**F Lymphatic, Right Lower Extremity**<br>Femoral lymph node<br>Popliteal lymph node<br>**G Lymphatic, Left Lower Extremity**<br>*See F Lymphatic, Right Lower Extremity*<br>**H Lymphatic, Right Inguinal**<br>**J Lymphatic, Left Inguinal**<br>**K Thoracic Duct**<br>Left jugular trunk<br>Left subclavian trunk<br>**L Cisterna Chyli**<br>Intestinal lymphatic trunk<br>Lumbar lymphatic trunk | **Ø Open**<br>**3 Percutaneous**<br>**4 Percutaneous Endoscopic**<br>8 Via Natural or Artificial Opening Endoscopic | **Z No Device** | **X Diagnostic**<br>**Z No Qualifier** |
| **M Thymus**<br>Thymus gland<br>**P Spleen**<br>Accessory spleen<br>**T Bone Marrow** | **Ø Open**<br>**3 Percutaneous**<br>**4 Percutaneous Endoscopic** | **Ø Drainage Device** | **Z No Qualifier** |
| **M Thymus**<br>Thymus gland<br>**P Spleen**<br>Accessory spleen<br>**T Bone Marrow** | **Ø Open**<br>**3 Percutaneous**<br>**4 Percutaneous Endoscopic** | **Z No Device** | **X Diagnostic**<br>**Z No Qualifier** |

**DRG Non-OR** Ø79M3ØZ
**DRG Non-OR** Ø79M3ZZ
**Non-OR** Ø79[Ø,1,2,3,4,5,6,7,8,9,B,C,D,F,G,H,J,K,L]8ZX
**Non-OR** Ø79[Ø,1,2,3,4,5,6,7,8,9,B,C,D,F,G,H,J,K,L][3,8]ZZ
**Non-OR** Ø79P[3,4]ØZ
**Non-OR** Ø79T[Ø,3,4]ØZ
**Non-OR** Ø79P[3,4]Z[X,Z]
**Non-OR** Ø79T[Ø,3,4]Z[X,Z]

**Ø Medical and Surgical**
**7 Lymphatic and Hemic Systems**
**B Excision** Definition: Cutting out or off, without replacement, a portion of a body part
Explanation: The qualifier DIAGNOSTIC is used to identify excision procedures that are biopsies

| Body Part Character 4 | Approach Character 5 | Device Character 6 | Qualifier Character 7 |
|---|---|---|---|
| **Ø Lymphatic, Head**<br>Buccinator lymph node<br>Infraauricular lymph node<br>Infraparotid lymph node<br>Parotid lymph node<br>Preauricular lymph node<br>Submandibular lymph node<br>Submaxillary lymph node<br>Submental lymph node<br>Subparotid lymph node<br>Suprahyoid lymph node<br>**1 Lymphatic, Right Neck**<br>Cervical lymph node<br>Jugular lymph node<br>Mastoid (postauricular) lymph node<br>Occipital lymph node<br>Postauricular (mastoid) lymph node<br>Retropharyngeal lymph node<br>Right jugular trunk<br>Right lymphatic duct<br>Right subclavian trunk<br>Supraclavicular (Virchow's) lymph node<br>Virchow's (supraclavicular) lymph node<br>**2 Lymphatic, Left Neck**<br>Cervical lymph node<br>Jugular lymph node<br>Mastoid (postauricular) lymph node<br>Occipital lymph node<br>Postauricular (mastoid) lymph node<br>Retropharyngeal lymph node<br>Supraclavicular (Virchow's) lymph node<br>Virchow's (supraclavicular) lymph node<br>**3 Lymphatic, Right Upper Extremity**<br>Cubital lymph node<br>Deltopectoral (infraclavicular) lymph node<br>Epitrochlear lymph node<br>Infraclavicular (deltopectoral) lymph node<br>Supratrochlear lymph node<br>**4 Lymphatic, Left Upper Extremity**<br>*See 3 Lymphatic, Right Upper Extremity*<br>**5 Lymphatic, Right Axillary**<br>Anterior (pectoral) lymph node<br>Apical (subclavicular) lymph node<br>Brachial (lateral) lymph node<br>Central axillary lymph node<br>Lateral (brachial) lymph node<br>Pectoral (anterior) lymph node<br>Posterior (subscapular) lymph node<br>Subclavicular (apical) lymph node<br>Subscapular (posterior) lymph node<br>**6 Lymphatic, Left Axillary**<br>*See 5 Lymphatic, Right Axillary*<br>**7 Lymphatic, Thorax**<br>Intercostal lymph node<br>Mediastinal lymph node<br>Parasternal lymph node<br>Paratracheal lymph node<br>Tracheobronchial lymph node<br>**8 Lymphatic, Internal Mammary, Right**<br>**9 Lymphatic, Internal Mammary, Left**<br>**B Lymphatic, Mesenteric**<br>Inferior mesenteric lymph node<br>Pararectal lymph node<br>Superior mesenteric lymph node<br>**C Lymphatic, Pelvis**<br>Common iliac (subaortic) lymph node<br>Gluteal lymph node<br>Iliac lymph node<br>Inferior epigastric lymph node<br>Obturator lymph node<br>Sacral lymph node<br>Subaortic (common iliac) lymph node<br>Suprainguinal lymph node<br>**D Lymphatic, Aortic**<br>Celiac lymph node<br>Gastric lymph node<br>Hepatic lymph node<br>Lumbar lymph node<br>Pancreaticosplenic lymph node<br>Paraaortic lymph node<br>Retroperitoneal lymph node<br>**F Lymphatic, Right Lower Extremity**<br>Femoral lymph node<br>Popliteal lymph node<br>**G Lymphatic, Left Lower Extremity**<br>*See F Lymphatic, Right Lower Extremity*<br>**H Lymphatic, Right Inguinal** ⊞<br>**J Lymphatic, Left Inguinal** ⊞<br>**K Thoracic Duct**<br>Left jugular trunk<br>Left subclavian trunk<br>**L Cisterna Chyli**<br>Intestinal lymphatic trunk<br>Lumbar lymphatic trunk<br>**M Thymus**<br>Thymus gland<br>**P Spleen**<br>Accessory spleen | **Ø Open**<br>**3 Percutaneous**<br>**4 Percutaneous Endoscopic** | **Z No Device** | **X Diagnostic**<br>**Z No Qualifier** |

Non-OR Ø7BP[3,4]ZX

**See Appendix L for Procedure Combinations**
⊞ Ø7B[H,J][Ø,4]ZZ

**0 Medical and Surgical**
**7 Lymphatic and Hemic Systems**
**C Extirpation** Definition: Taking or cutting out solid matter from a body part

Explanation: The solid matter may be an abnormal byproduct of a biological function or a foreign body; it may be imbedded in a body part or in the lumen of a tubular body part. The solid matter may or may not have been previously broken into pieces.

| Body Part Character 4 | Approach Character 5 | Device Character 6 | Qualifier Character 7 |
|---|---|---|---|
| **0 Lymphatic, Head**<br>Buccinator lymph node<br>Infraauricular lymph node<br>Infraparotid lymph node<br>Parotid lymph node<br>Preauricular lymph node<br>Submandibular lymph node<br>Submaxillary lymph node<br>Submental lymph node<br>Subparotid lymph node<br>Suprahyoid lymph node<br>**1 Lymphatic, Right Neck**<br>Cervical lymph node<br>Jugular lymph node<br>Mastoid (postauricular) lymph node<br>Occipital lymph node<br>Postauricular (mastoid) lymph node<br>Retropharyngeal lymph node<br>Right jugular trunk<br>Right lymphatic duct<br>Right subclavian trunk<br>Supraclavicular (Virchow's) lymph node<br>Virchow's (supraclavicular) lymph node<br>**2 Lymphatic, Left Neck**<br>Cervical lymph node<br>Jugular lymph node<br>Mastoid (postauricular) lymph node<br>Occipital lymph node<br>Postauricular (mastoid) lymph node<br>Retropharyngeal lymph node<br>Supraclavicular (Virchow's) lymph node<br>Virchow's (supraclavicular) lymph node<br>**3 Lymphatic, Right Upper Extremity**<br>Cubital lymph node<br>Deltopectoral (infraclavicular) lymph node<br>Epitrochlear lymph node<br>Infraclavicular (deltopectoral) lymph node<br>Supratrochlear lymph node<br>**4 Lymphatic, Left Upper Extremity**<br>*See 3 Lymphatic, Right Upper Extremity*<br>**5 Lymphatic, Right Axillary**<br>Anterior (pectoral) lymph node<br>Apical (subclavicular) lymph node<br>Brachial (lateral) lymph node<br>Central axillary lymph node<br>Lateral (brachial) lymph node<br>Pectoral (anterior) lymph node<br>Posterior (subscapular) lymph node<br>Subclavicular (apical) lymph node<br>Subscapular (posterior) lymph node<br>**6 Lymphatic, Left Axillary**<br>*See 5 Lymphatic, Right Axillary*<br>**7 Lymphatic, Thorax**<br>Intercostal lymph node<br>Mediastinal lymph node<br>Parasternal lymph node<br>Paratracheal lymph node<br>Tracheobronchial lymph node<br>**8 Lymphatic, Internal Mammary, Right**<br>**9 Lymphatic, Internal Mammary, Left**<br>**B Lymphatic, Mesenteric**<br>Inferior mesenteric lymph node<br>Pararectal lymph node<br>Superior mesenteric lymph node<br>**C Lymphatic, Pelvis**<br>Common iliac (subaortic) lymph node<br>Gluteal lymph node<br>Iliac lymph node<br>Inferior epigastric lymph node<br>Obturator lymph node<br>Sacral lymph node<br>Subaortic (common iliac) lymph node<br>Suprainguinal lymph node<br>**D Lymphatic, Aortic**<br>Celiac lymph node<br>Gastric lymph node<br>Hepatic lymph node<br>Lumbar lymph node<br>Pancreaticosplenic lymph node<br>Paraaortic lymph node<br>Retroperitoneal lymph node<br>**F Lymphatic, Right Lower Extremity**<br>Femoral lymph node<br>Popliteal lymph node<br>**G Lymphatic, Left Lower Extremity**<br>*See F Lymphatic, Right Lower Extremity*<br>**H Lymphatic, Right Inguinal**<br>**J Lymphatic, Left Inguinal**<br>**K Thoracic Duct**<br>Left jugular trunk<br>Left subclavian trunk<br>**L Cisterna Chyli**<br>Intestinal lymphatic trunk<br>Lumbar lymphatic trunk<br>**M Thymus**<br>Thymus gland<br>**P Spleen**<br>Accessory spleen | **0 Open**<br>**3 Percutaneous**<br>**4 Percutaneous Endoscopic** | **Z No Device** | **Z No Qualifier** |

**Non-OR** 07CP[3,4]ZZ

**0 Medical and Surgical**
**7 Lymphatic and Hemic Systems**
**D Extraction** Definition: Pulling or stripping out or off all or a portion of a body part by the use of force

Explanation: The qualifier DIAGNOSTIC is used to identify extraction procedures that are biopsies

| Body Part Character 4 | Approach Character 5 | Device Character 6 | Qualifier Character 7 |
|---|---|---|---|
| 0 Lymphatic, Head<br>Buccinator lymph node<br>Infraauricular lymph node<br>Infraparotid lymph node<br>Parotid lymph node<br>Preauricular lymph node<br>Submandibular lymph node<br>Submaxillary lymph node<br>Submental lymph node<br>Subparotid lymph node<br>Suprahyoid lymph node<br>1 Lymphatic, Right Neck<br>Cervical lymph node<br>Jugular lymph node<br>Mastoid (postauricular) lymph node<br>Occipital lymph node<br>Postauricular (mastoid) lymph node<br>Retropharyngeal lymph node<br>Right jugular trunk<br>Right lymphatic duct<br>Right subclavian trunk<br>Supraclavicular (Virchow's) lymph node<br>Virchow's (supraclavicular) lymph node<br>2 Lymphatic, Left Neck<br>Cervical lymph node<br>Jugular lymph node<br>Mastoid (postauricular) lymph node<br>Occipital lymph node<br>Postauricular (mastoid) lymph node<br>Retropharyngeal lymph node<br>Supraclavicular (Virchow's) lymph node<br>Virchow's (supraclavicular) lymph node<br>3 Lymphatic, Right Upper Extremity<br>Cubital lymph node<br>Deltopectoral (infraclavicular) lymph node<br>Epitrochlear lymph node<br>Infraclavicular (deltopectoral) lymph node<br>Supratrochlear lymph node<br>4 Lymphatic, Left Upper Extremity<br>*See 3 Lymphatic, Right Upper Extremity*<br>5 Lymphatic, Right Axillary<br>Anterior (pectoral) lymph node<br>Apical (subclavicular) lymph node<br>Brachial (lateral) lymph node<br>Central axillary lymph node<br>Lateral (brachial) lymph node<br>Pectoral (anterior) lymph node<br>Posterior (subscapular) lymph node<br>Subclavicular (apical) lymph node<br>Subscapular (posterior) lymph node<br>6 Lymphatic, Left Axillary<br>*See 5 Lymphatic, Right Axillary*<br>7 Lymphatic, Thorax<br>Intercostal lymph node<br>Mediastinal lymph node<br>Parasternal lymph node<br>Paratracheal lymph node<br>Tracheobronchial lymph node<br>8 Lymphatic, Internal Mammary, Right<br>9 Lymphatic, Internal Mammary, Left<br>B Lymphatic, Mesenteric<br>Inferior mesenteric lymph node<br>Pararectal lymph node<br>Superior mesenteric lymph node<br>C Lymphatic, Pelvis<br>Common iliac (subaortic) lymph node<br>Gluteal lymph node<br>Iliac lymph node<br>Inferior epigastric lymph node<br>Obturator lymph node<br>Sacral lymph node<br>Subaortic (common iliac) lymph node<br>Suprainguinal lymph node<br>D Lymphatic, Aortic<br>Celiac lymph node<br>Gastric lymph node<br>Hepatic lymph node<br>Lumbar lymph node<br>Pancreaticosplenic lymph node<br>Paraaortic lymph node<br>Retroperitoneal lymph node<br>F Lymphatic, Right Lower Extremity<br>Femoral lymph node<br>Popliteal lymph node<br>G Lymphatic, Left Lower Extremity<br>*See F Lymphatic, Right Lower Extremity*<br>H Lymphatic, Right Inguinal<br>J Lymphatic, Left Inguinal<br>K Thoracic Duct<br>Left jugular trunk<br>Left subclavian trunk<br>L Cisterna Chyli<br>Intestinal lymphatic trunk<br>Lumbar lymphatic trunk | 3 Percutaneous<br>4 Percutaneous Endoscopic<br>8 Via Natural or Artificial Opening Endoscopic | Z No Device | X Diagnostic |
| M Thymus<br>Thymus gland<br>P Spleen<br>Accessory spleen | 3 Percutaneous<br>4 Percutaneous Endoscopic | Z No Device | X Diagnostic |
| Q Bone Marrow, Sternum<br>R Bone Marrow, Iliac<br>S Bone Marrow, Vertebral | 0 Open<br>3 Percutaneous | Z No Device | X Diagnostic<br>Z No Qualifier |

Non-OR All body part, approach, device, and qualifier values

**Ø Medical and Surgical**
**7 Lymphatic and Hemic Systems**
**H Insertion** Definition: Putting in a nonbiological appliance that monitors, assists, performs, or prevents a physiological function but does not physically take the place of a body part

Explanation: None

| Body Part Character 4 | Approach Character 5 | Device Character 6 | Qualifier Character 7 |
|---|---|---|---|
| **K** Thoracic Duct<br>Left jugular trunk<br>Left subclavian trunk<br>**L** Cisterna Chyli<br>Intestinal lymphatic trunk<br>Lumbar lymphatic trunk<br>**M** Thymus<br>Thymus gland<br>**N** Lymphatic<br>**P** Spleen<br>Accessory spleen | **Ø** Open<br>**3** Percutaneous<br>**4** Percutaneous Endoscopic | **3** Infusion Device<br>**Y** Other Device | **Z** No Qualifier |

Non-OR All body part, approach, device, and qualifier values

**Ø Medical and Surgical**
**7 Lymphatic and Hemic Systems**
**J Inspection** Definition: Visually and/or manually exploring a body part

Explanation: Visual exploration may be performed with or without optical instrumentation. Manual exploration may be performed directly or through intervening body layers.

| Body Part Character 4 | Approach Character 5 | Device Character 6 | Qualifier Character 7 |
|---|---|---|---|
| **K** Thoracic Duct<br>Left jugular trunk<br>Left subclavian trunk<br>**L** Cisterna Chyli<br>Intestinal lymphatic trunk<br>Lumbar lymphatic trunk<br>**M** Thymus<br>Thymus gland<br>**T** Bone Marrow | **Ø** Open<br>**3** Percutaneous<br>**4** Percutaneous Endoscopic | **Z** No Device | **Z** No Qualifier |
| **N** Lymphatic | **Ø** Open<br>**3** Percutaneous<br>**4** Percutaneous Endoscopic<br>**8** Via Natural or Artificial Opening Endoscopic<br>**X** External | **Z** No Device | **Z** No Qualifier |
| **P** Spleen<br>Accessory spleen | **Ø** Open<br>**3** Percutaneous<br>**4** Percutaneous Endoscopic<br>**X** External | **Z** No Device | **Z** No Qualifier |

Non-OR Ø7J[K,L,M]3ZZ
Non-OR Ø7JT[Ø,3,4]ZZ
Non-OR Ø7JN[3,8,X]ZZ
Non-OR Ø7JP[3,4,X]ZZ

**Ø Medical and Surgical**
**7 Lymphatic and Hemic Systems**
**L Occlusion** Definition: Completely closing an orifice or the lumen of a tubular body part
Explanation: The orifice can be a natural orifice or an artificially created orifice

| Body Part Character 4 | Approach Character 5 | Device Character 6 | Qualifier Character 7 |
|---|---|---|---|
| **Ø Lymphatic, Head**<br>Buccinator lymph node<br>Infraauricular lymph node<br>Infraparotid lymph node<br>Parotid lymph node<br>Preauricular lymph node<br>Submandibular lymph node<br>Submaxillary lymph node<br>Submental lymph node<br>Subparotid lymph node<br>Suprahyoid lymph node<br>**1 Lymphatic, Right Neck**<br>Cervical lymph node<br>Jugular lymph node<br>Mastoid (postauricular) lymph node<br>Occipital lymph node<br>Postauricular (mastoid) lymph node<br>Retropharyngeal lymph node<br>Right jugular trunk<br>Right lymphatic duct<br>Right subclavian trunk<br>Supraclavicular (Virchow's) lymph node<br>Virchow's (supraclavicular) lymph node<br>**2 Lymphatic, Left Neck**<br>Cervical lymph node<br>Jugular lymph node<br>Mastoid (postauricular) lymph node<br>Occipital lymph node<br>Postauricular (mastoid) lymph node<br>Retropharyngeal lymph node<br>Supraclavicular (Virchow's) lymph node<br>Virchow's (supraclavicular) lymph node<br>**3 Lymphatic, Right Upper Extremity**<br>Cubital lymph node<br>Deltopectoral (infraclavicular) lymph node<br>Epitrochlear lymph node<br>Infraclavicular (deltopectoral) lymph node<br>Supratrochlear lymph node<br>**4 Lymphatic, Left Upper Extremity**<br>***See*** *3 Lymphatic, Right Upper Extremity*<br>**5 Lymphatic, Right Axillary**<br>Anterior (pectoral) lymph node<br>Apical (subclavicular) lymph node<br>Brachial (lateral) lymph node<br>Central axillary lymph node<br>Lateral (brachial) lymph node<br>Pectoral (anterior) lymph node<br>Posterior (subscapular) lymph node<br>Subclavicular (apical) lymph node<br>Subscapular (posterior) lymph node<br>**6 Lymphatic, Left Axillary**<br>***See*** *5 Lymphatic, Right Axillary*<br>**7 Lymphatic, Thorax**<br>Intercostal lymph node<br>Mediastinal lymph node<br>Parasternal lymph node<br>Paratracheal lymph node<br>Tracheobronchial lymph node<br>**8 Lymphatic, Internal Mammary, Right**<br>**9 Lymphatic, Internal Mammary, Left**<br>**B Lymphatic, Mesenteric**<br>Inferior mesenteric lymph node<br>Pararectal lymph node<br>Superior mesenteric lymph node<br>**C Lymphatic, Pelvis**<br>Common iliac (subaortic) lymph node<br>Gluteal lymph node<br>Iliac lymph node<br>Inferior epigastric lymph node<br>Obturator lymph node<br>Sacral lymph node<br>Subaortic (common iliac) lymph node<br>Suprainguinal lymph node<br>**D Lymphatic, Aortic**<br>Celiac lymph node<br>Gastric lymph node<br>Hepatic lymph node<br>Lumbar lymph node<br>Pancreaticosplenic lymph node<br>Paraaortic lymph node<br>Retroperitoneal lymph node<br>**F Lymphatic, Right Lower Extremity**<br>Femoral lymph node<br>Popliteal lymph node<br>**G Lymphatic, Left Lower Extremity**<br>***See*** *F Lymphatic, Right Lower Extremity*<br>**H Lymphatic, Right Inguinal**<br>**J Lymphatic, Left Inguinal**<br>**K Thoracic Duct**<br>Left jugular trunk<br>Left subclavian trunk<br>**L Cisterna Chyli**<br>Intestinal lymphatic trunk<br>Lumbar lymphatic trunk | **Ø Open**<br>**3 Percutaneous**<br>**4 Percutaneous Endoscopic** | **C Extraluminal Device**<br>**D Intraluminal Device**<br>**Z No Device** | **Z No Qualifier** |

**Ø Medical and Surgical**
**7 Lymphatic and Hemic Systems**
**N Release** Definition: Freeing a body part from an abnormal physical constraint by cutting or by the use of force
Explanation: Some of the restraining tissue may be taken out but none of the body part is taken out

| Body Part Character 4 | Approach Character 5 | Device Character 6 | Qualifier Character 7 |
|---|---|---|---|
| **Ø Lymphatic, Head**<br>Buccinator lymph node<br>Infraauricular lymph node<br>Infraparotid lymph node<br>Parotid lymph node<br>Preauricular lymph node<br>Submandibular lymph node<br>Submaxillary lymph node<br>Submental lymph node<br>Subparotid lymph node<br>Suprahyoid lymph node<br>**1 Lymphatic, Right Neck**<br>Cervical lymph node<br>Jugular lymph node<br>Mastoid (postauricular) lymph node<br>Occipital lymph node<br>Postauricular (mastoid) lymph node<br>Retropharyngeal lymph node<br>Right jugular trunk<br>Right lymphatic duct<br>Right subclavian trunk<br>Supraclavicular (Virchow's) lymph node<br>Virchow's (supraclavicular) lymph node<br>**2 Lymphatic, Left Neck**<br>Cervical lymph node<br>Jugular lymph node<br>Mastoid (postauricular) lymph node<br>Occipital lymph node<br>Postauricular (mastoid) lymph node<br>Retropharyngeal lymph node<br>Supraclavicular (Virchow's) lymph node<br>Virchow's (supraclavicular) lymph node<br>**3 Lymphatic, Right Upper Extremity**<br>Cubital lymph node<br>Deltopectoral (infraclavicular) lymph node<br>Epitrochlear lymph node<br>Infraclavicular (deltopectoral) lymph node<br>Supratrochlear lymph node<br>**4 Lymphatic, Left Upper Extremity**<br>**See** *3 Lymphatic, Right Upper Extremity*<br>**5 Lymphatic, Right Axillary**<br>Anterior (pectoral) lymph node<br>Apical (subclavicular) lymph node<br>Brachial (lateral) lymph node<br>Central axillary lymph node<br>Lateral (brachial) lymph node<br>Pectoral (anterior) lymph node<br>Posterior (subscapular) lymph node<br>Subclavicular (apical) lymph node<br>Subscapular (posterior) lymph node<br>**6 Lymphatic, Left Axillary**<br>**See** *5 Lymphatic, Right Axillary*<br>**7 Lymphatic, Thorax**<br>Intercostal lymph node<br>Mediastinal lymph node<br>Parasternal lymph node<br>Paratracheal lymph node<br>Tracheobronchial lymph node<br>**8 Lymphatic, Internal Mammary, Right**<br>**9 Lymphatic, Internal Mammary, Left**<br>**B Lymphatic, Mesenteric**<br>Inferior mesenteric lymph node<br>Pararectal lymph node<br>Superior mesenteric lymph node<br>**C Lymphatic, Pelvis**<br>Common iliac (subaortic) lymph node<br>Gluteal lymph node<br>Iliac lymph node<br>Inferior epigastric lymph node<br>Obturator lymph node<br>Sacral lymph node<br>Subaortic (common iliac) lymph node<br>Suprainguinal lymph node<br>**D Lymphatic, Aortic**<br>Celiac lymph node<br>Gastric lymph node<br>Hepatic lymph node<br>Lumbar lymph node<br>Pancreaticosplenic lymph node<br>Paraaortic lymph node<br>Retroperitoneal lymph node<br>**F Lymphatic, Right Lower Extremity**<br>Femoral lymph node<br>Popliteal lymph node<br>**G Lymphatic, Left Lower Extremity**<br>**See** *F Lymphatic, Right Lower Extremity*<br>**H Lymphatic, Right Inguinal**<br>**J Lymphatic, Left Inguinal**<br>**K Thoracic Duct**<br>Left jugular trunk<br>Left subclavian trunk<br>**L Cisterna Chyli**<br>Intestinal lymphatic trunk<br>Lumbar lymphatic trunk<br>**M Thymus**<br>Thymus gland<br>**P Spleen**<br>Accessory spleen | **Ø Open**<br>**3 Percutaneous**<br>**4 Percutaneous Endoscopic** | **Z No Device** | **Z No Qualifier** |

**Ø Medical and Surgical**
**7 Lymphatic and Hemic Systems**
**P Removal** Definition: Taking out or off a device from a body part

Explanation: If a device is taken out and a similar device put in without cutting or puncturing the skin or mucous membrane, the procedure is coded to the root operation CHANGE. Otherwise, the procedure for taking out a device is coded to the root operation REMOVAL.

| Body Part Character 4 | Approach Character 5 | Device Character 6 | Qualifier Character 7 |
|---|---|---|---|
| K Thoracic Duct<br>Left jugular trunk<br>Left subclavian trunk<br>L Cisterna Chyli<br>Intestinal lymphatic trunk<br>Lumbar lymphatic trunk<br>N Lymphatic | Ø Open<br>3 Percutaneous<br>4 Percutaneous Endoscopic | Ø Drainage Device<br>3 Infusion Device<br>7 Autologous Tissue Substitute<br>C Extraluminal Device<br>D Intraluminal Device<br>J Synthetic Substitute<br>K Nonautologous Tissue Substitute<br>Y Other Device | Z No Qualifier |
| K Thoracic Duct<br>Left jugular trunk<br>Left subclavian trunk<br>L Cisterna Chyli<br>Intestinal lymphatic trunk<br>Lumbar lymphatic trunk<br>N Lymphatic | X External | Ø Drainage Device<br>3 Infusion Device<br>D Intraluminal Device | Z No Qualifier |
| M Thymus<br>Thymus gland<br>P Spleen<br>Accessory spleen | Ø Open<br>3 Percutaneous<br>4 Percutaneous Endoscopic | Ø Drainage Device<br>3 Infusion Device<br>Y Other Device | Z No Qualifier |
| M Thymus<br>Thymus gland<br>P Spleen<br>Accessory spleen | X External | Ø Drainage Device<br>3 Infusion Device | Z No Qualifier |
| T Bone Marrow | Ø Open<br>3 Percutaneous<br>4 Percutaneous Endoscopic<br>X External | Ø Drainage Device | Z No Qualifier |

Non-OR Ø7P[K,L,N][3,4]YZ
Non-OR Ø7P[K,L,N]X[Ø,3,D]Z
Non-OR Ø7P[M,P][3,4]YZ
Non-OR Ø7P[M,P]X[Ø,3]Z
Non-OR Ø7PT[Ø,3,4,X]ØZ

**Ø Medical and Surgical**
**7 Lymphatic and Hemic Systems**
**Q Repair** Definition: Restoring, to the extent possible, a body part to its normal anatomic structure and function
Explanation: Used only when the method to accomplish the repair is not one of the other root operations

| Body Part Character 4 | Approach Character 5 | Device Character 6 | Qualifier Character 7 |
|---|---|---|---|
| **Ø Lymphatic, Head**<br>Buccinator lymph node<br>Infraauricular lymph node<br>Infraparotid lymph node<br>Parotid lymph node<br>Preauricular lymph node<br>Submandibular lymph node<br>Submaxillary lymph node<br>Submental lymph node<br>Subparotid lymph node<br>Suprahyoid lymph node<br>**1 Lymphatic, Right Neck**<br>Cervical lymph node<br>Jugular lymph node<br>Mastoid (postauricular) lymph node<br>Occipital lymph node<br>Postauricular (mastoid) lymph node<br>Retropharyngeal lymph node<br>Right jugular trunk<br>Right lymphatic duct<br>Right subclavian trunk<br>Supraclavicular (Virchow's) lymph node<br>Virchow's (supraclavicular) lymph node<br>**2 Lymphatic, Left Neck**<br>Cervical lymph node<br>Jugular lymph node<br>Mastoid (postauricular) lymph node<br>Occipital lymph node<br>Postauricular (mastoid) lymph node<br>Retropharyngeal lymph node<br>Supraclavicular (Virchow's) lymph node<br>Virchow's (supraclavicular) lymph node<br>**3 Lymphatic, Right Upper Extremity**<br>Cubital lymph node<br>Deltopectoral (infraclavicular) lymph node<br>Epitrochlear lymph node<br>Infraclavicular (deltopectoral) lymph node<br>Supratrochlear lymph node<br>**4 Lymphatic, Left Upper Extremity**<br>*See 3 Lymphatic, Right Upper Extremity*<br>**5 Lymphatic, Right Axillary**<br>Anterior (pectoral) lymph node<br>Apical (subclavicular) lymph node<br>Brachial (lateral) lymph node<br>Central axillary lymph node<br>Lateral (brachial) lymph node<br>Pectoral (anterior) lymph node<br>Posterior (subscapular) lymph node<br>Subclavicular (apical) lymph node<br>Subscapular (posterior) lymph node<br>**6 Lymphatic, Left Axillary**<br>*See 5 Lymphatic, Right Axillary*<br>**7 Lymphatic, Thorax**<br>Intercostal lymph node<br>Mediastinal lymph node<br>Parasternal lymph node<br>Paratracheal lymph node<br>Tracheobronchial lymph node<br>**8 Lymphatic, Internal Mammary, Right**<br>**9 Lymphatic, Internal Mammary, Left**<br>**B Lymphatic, Mesenteric**<br>Inferior mesenteric lymph node<br>Pararectal lymph node<br>Superior mesenteric lymph node<br>**C Lymphatic, Pelvis**<br>Common iliac (subaortic) lymph node<br>Gluteal lymph node<br>Iliac lymph node<br>Inferior epigastric lymph node<br>Obturator lymph node<br>Sacral lymph node<br>Subaortic (common iliac) lymph node<br>Suprainguinal lymph node<br>**D Lymphatic, Aortic**<br>Celiac lymph node<br>Gastric lymph node<br>Hepatic lymph node<br>Lumbar lymph node<br>Pancreaticosplenic lymph node<br>Paraaortic lymph node<br>Retroperitoneal lymph node<br>**F Lymphatic, Right Lower Extremity**<br>Femoral lymph node<br>Popliteal lymph node<br>**G Lymphatic, Left Lower Extremity**<br>*See F Lymphatic, Right Lower Extremity*<br>**H Lymphatic, Right Inguinal**<br>**J Lymphatic, Left Inguinal**<br>**K Thoracic Duct**<br>Left jugular trunk<br>Left subclavian trunk<br>**L Cisterna Chyli**<br>Intestinal lymphatic trunk<br>Lumbar lymphatic trunk | **Ø Open**<br>**3 Percutaneous**<br>**4 Percutaneous Endoscopic**<br>8 Via Natural or Artificial Opening Endoscopic | **Z No Device** | **Z No Qualifier** |
| **M Thymus**<br>Thymus gland<br>**P Spleen**<br>Accessory spleen | **Ø Open**<br>**3 Percutaneous**<br>**4 Percutaneous Endoscopic** | **Z No Device** | **Z No Qualifier** |

**Ø Medical and Surgical**
**7 Lymphatic and Hemic Systems**
**S Reposition** Definition: Moving to its normal location, or other suitable location, all or a portion of a body part

Explanation: The body part is moved to a new location from an abnormal location, or from a normal location where it is not functioning correctly. The body part may or may not be cut out or off to be moved to the new location.

| Body Part Character 4 | Approach Character 5 | Device Character 6 | Qualifier Character 7 |
|---|---|---|---|
| **M Thymus**<br>Thymus gland<br>**P Spleen**<br>Accessory spleen | **Ø Open** | **Z No Device** | **Z No Qualifier** |

**Ø Medical and Surgical**
**7 Lymphatic and Hemic Systems**
**T Resection** Definition: Cutting out or off, without replacement, all of a body part

Explanation: None

| Body Part Character 4 | Approach Character 5 | Device Character 6 | Qualifier Character 7 |
|---|---|---|---|
| **Ø Lymphatic, Head**<br>Buccinator lymph node<br>Infraauricular lymph node<br>Infraparotid lymph node<br>Parotid lymph node<br>Preauricular lymph node<br>Submandibular lymph node<br>Submaxillary lymph node<br>Submental lymph node<br>Subparotid lymph node<br>Suprahyoid lymph node<br>**1 Lymphatic, Right Neck**<br>Cervical lymph node<br>Jugular lymph node<br>Mastoid (postauricular) lymph node<br>Occipital lymph node<br>Postauricular (mastoid) lymph node<br>Retropharyngeal lymph node<br>Right jugular trunk<br>Right lymphatic duct<br>Right subclavian trunk<br>Supraclavicular (Virchow's) lymph node<br>Virchow's (supraclavicular) lymph node<br>**2 Lymphatic, Left Neck**<br>Cervical lymph node<br>Jugular lymph node<br>Mastoid (postauricular) lymph node<br>Occipital lymph node<br>Postauricular (mastoid) lymph node<br>Retropharyngeal lymph node<br>Supraclavicular (Virchow's) lymph node<br>Virchow's (supraclavicular) lymph node<br>**3 Lymphatic, Right Upper Extremity**<br>Cubital lymph node<br>Deltopectoral (infraclavicular) lymph node<br>Epitrochlear lymph node<br>Infraclavicular (deltopectoral) lymph node<br>Supratrochlear lymph node<br>**4 Lymphatic, Left Upper Extremity**<br>*See 3 Lymphatic, Right Upper Extremity*<br>**5 Lymphatic, Right Axillary** ⊞<br>Anterior (pectoral) lymph node<br>Apical (subclavicular) lymph node<br>Brachial (lateral) lymph node<br>Central axillary lymph node<br>Lateral (brachial) lymph node<br>Pectoral (anterior) lymph node<br>Posterior (subscapular) lymph node<br>Subclavicular (apical) lymph node<br>Subscapular (posterior) lymph node<br>**6 Lymphatic, Left Axillary** ⊞<br>*See 5 Lymphatic, Right Axillary*<br>**7 Lymphatic, Thorax** ⊞<br>Intercostal lymph node<br>Mediastinal lymph node<br>Parasternal lymph node<br>Paratracheal lymph node<br>Tracheobronchial lymph node<br>**8 Lymphatic, Internal Mammary, Right** ⊞<br>**9 Lymphatic, Internal Mammary, Left** ⊞<br>**B Lymphatic, Mesenteric**<br>Inferior mesenteric lymph node<br>Pararectal lymph node<br>Superior mesenteric lymph node<br>**C Lymphatic, Pelvis**<br>Common iliac (subaortic) lymph node<br>Gluteal lymph node<br>Iliac lymph node<br>Inferior epigastric lymph node<br>Obturator lymph node<br>Sacral lymph node<br>Subaortic (common iliac) lymph node<br>Suprainguinal lymph node<br>**D Lymphatic, Aortic**<br>Celiac lymph node<br>Gastric lymph node<br>Hepatic lymph node<br>Lumbar lymph node<br>Pancreaticosplenic lymph node<br>Paraaortic lymph node<br>Retroperitoneal lymph node<br>**F Lymphatic, Right Lower Extremity**<br>Femoral lymph node<br>Popliteal lymph node<br>**G Lymphatic, Left Lower Extremity**<br>*See F Lymphatic, Right Lower Extremity*<br>**H Lymphatic, Right Inguinal**<br>**J Lymphatic, Left Inguinal**<br>**K Thoracic Duct**<br>Left jugular trunk<br>Left subclavian trunk<br>**L Cisterna Chyli**<br>Intestinal lymphatic trunk<br>Lumbar lymphatic trunk<br>**M Thymus**<br>Thymus gland<br>**P Spleen**<br>Accessory spleen | **Ø Open**<br>**4 Percutaneous Endoscopic** | **Z No Device** | **Z No Qualifier** |

**See Appendix L for Procedure Combinations**

⊞ Ø7T[5,6,7,8,9]ØZZ

**Ø Medical and Surgical**
**7 Lymphatic and Hemic Systems**
**U Supplement** Definition: Putting in or on biological or synthetic material that physically reinforces and/or augments the function of a portion of a body part
Explanation: The biological material is non-living, or is living and from the same individual. The body part may have been previously replaced, and the SUPPLEMENT procedure is performed to physically reinforce and/or augment the function of the replaced body part.

| Body Part Character 4 | Approach Character 5 | Device Character 6 | Qualifier Character 7 |
|---|---|---|---|
| **Ø Lymphatic, Head**<br>Buccinator lymph node<br>Infraauricular lymph node<br>Infraparotid lymph node<br>Parotid lymph node<br>Preauricular lymph node<br>Submandibular lymph node<br>Submaxillary lymph node<br>Submental lymph node<br>Subparotid lymph node<br>Suprahyoid lymph node<br>**1 Lymphatic, Right Neck**<br>Cervical lymph node<br>Jugular lymph node<br>Mastoid (postauricular) lymph node<br>Occipital lymph node<br>Postauricular (mastoid) lymph node<br>Retropharyngeal lymph node<br>Right jugular trunk<br>Right lymphatic duct<br>Right subclavian trunk<br>Supraclavicular (Virchow's) lymph node<br>Virchow's (supraclavicular) lymph node<br>**2 Lymphatic, Left Neck**<br>Cervical lymph node<br>Jugular lymph node<br>Mastoid (postauricular) lymph node<br>Occipital lymph node<br>Postauricular (mastoid) lymph node<br>Retropharyngeal lymph node<br>Supraclavicular (Virchow's) lymph node<br>Virchow's (supraclavicular) lymph node<br>**3 Lymphatic, Right Upper Extremity**<br>Cubital lymph node<br>Deltopectoral (infraclavicular) lymph node<br>Epitrochlear lymph node<br>Infraclavicular (deltopectoral) lymph node<br>Supratrochlear lymph node<br>**4 Lymphatic, Left Upper Extremity**<br>*See 3 Lymphatic, Right Upper Extremity*<br>**5 Lymphatic, Right Axillary**<br>Anterior (pectoral) lymph node<br>Apical (subclavicular) lymph node<br>Brachial (lateral) lymph node<br>Central axillary lymph node<br>Lateral (brachial) lymph node<br>Pectoral (anterior) lymph node<br>Posterior (subscapular) lymph node<br>Subclavicular (apical) lymph node<br>Subscapular (posterior) lymph node<br>**6 Lymphatic, Left Axillary**<br>*See 5 Lymphatic, Right Axillary*<br>**7 Lymphatic, Thorax**<br>Intercostal lymph node<br>Mediastinal lymph node<br>Parasternal lymph node<br>Paratracheal lymph node<br>Tracheobronchial lymph node<br>**8 Lymphatic, Internal Mammary, Right**<br>**9 Lymphatic, Internal Mammary, Left**<br>**B Lymphatic, Mesenteric**<br>Inferior mesenteric lymph node<br>Pararectal lymph node<br>Superior mesenteric lymph node<br>**C Lymphatic, Pelvis**<br>Common iliac (subaortic) lymph node<br>Gluteal lymph node<br>Iliac lymph node<br>Inferior epigastric lymph node<br>Obturator lymph node<br>Sacral lymph node<br>Subaortic (common iliac) lymph node<br>Suprainguinal lymph node<br>**D Lymphatic, Aortic**<br>Celiac lymph node<br>Gastric lymph node<br>Hepatic lymph node<br>Lumbar lymph node<br>Pancreaticosplenic lymph node<br>Paraaortic lymph node<br>Retroperitoneal lymph node<br>**F Lymphatic, Right Lower Extremity**<br>Femoral lymph node<br>Popliteal lymph node<br>**G Lymphatic, Left Lower Extremity**<br>*See F Lymphatic, Right Lower Extremity*<br>**H Lymphatic, Right Inguinal**<br>**J Lymphatic, Left Inguinal**<br>**K Thoracic Duct**<br>Left jugular trunk<br>Left subclavian trunk<br>**L Cisterna Chyli**<br>Intestinal lymphatic trunk<br>Lumbar lymphatic trunk | **Ø Open**<br>**4 Percutaneous Endoscopic** | **7 Autologous Tissue Substitute**<br>**J Synthetic Substitute**<br>**K Nonautologous Tissue Substitute** | **Z No Qualifier** |

**Ø Medical and Surgical**
**7 Lymphatic and Hemic Systems**
**V Restriction** Definition: Partially closing an orifice or the lumen of a tubular body part
Explanation: The orifice can be a natural orifice or an artificially created orifice

| Body Part Character 4 | Approach Character 5 | Device Character 6 | Qualifier Character 7 |
|---|---|---|---|
| **Ø Lymphatic, Head**<br>Buccinator lymph node<br>Infraauricular lymph node<br>Infraparotid lymph node<br>Parotid lymph node<br>Preauricular lymph node<br>Submandibular lymph node<br>Submaxillary lymph node<br>Submental lymph node<br>Subparotid lymph node<br>Suprahyoid lymph node<br>**1 Lymphatic, Right Neck**<br>Cervical lymph node<br>Jugular lymph node<br>Mastoid (postauricular) lymph node<br>Occipital lymph node<br>Postauricular (mastoid) lymph node<br>Retropharyngeal lymph node<br>Right jugular trunk<br>Right lymphatic duct<br>Right subclavian trunk<br>Supraclavicular (Virchow's) lymph node<br>Virchow's (supraclavicular) lymph node<br>**2 Lymphatic, Left Neck**<br>Cervical lymph node<br>Jugular lymph node<br>Mastoid (postauricular) lymph node<br>Occipital lymph node<br>Postauricular (mastoid) lymph node<br>Retropharyngeal lymph node<br>Supraclavicular (Virchow's) lymph node<br>Virchow's (supraclavicular) lymph node<br>**3 Lymphatic, Right Upper Extremity**<br>Cubital lymph node<br>Deltopectoral (infraclavicular) lymph node<br>Epitrochlear lymph node<br>Infraclavicular (deltopectoral) lymph node<br>Supratrochlear lymph node<br>**4 Lymphatic, Left Upper Extremity**<br>***See** 3 Lymphatic, Right Upper Extremity*<br>**5 Lymphatic, Right Axillary**<br>Anterior (pectoral) lymph node<br>Apical (subclavicular) lymph node<br>Brachial (lateral) lymph node<br>Central axillary lymph node<br>Lateral (brachial) lymph node<br>Pectoral (anterior) lymph node<br>Posterior (subscapular) lymph node<br>Subclavicular (apical) lymph node<br>Subscapular (posterior) lymph node<br>**6 Lymphatic, Left Axillary**<br>***See** 5 Lymphatic, Right Axillary*<br>**7 Lymphatic, Thorax**<br>Intercostal lymph node<br>Mediastinal lymph node<br>Parasternal lymph node<br>Paratracheal lymph node<br>Tracheobronchial lymph node<br>**8 Lymphatic, Internal Mammary, Right**<br>**9 Lymphatic, Internal Mammary, Left**<br>**B Lymphatic, Mesenteric**<br>Inferior mesenteric lymph node<br>Pararectal lymph node<br>Superior mesenteric lymph node<br>**C Lymphatic, Pelvis**<br>Common iliac (subaortic) lymph node<br>Gluteal lymph node<br>Iliac lymph node<br>Inferior epigastric lymph node<br>Obturator lymph node<br>Sacral lymph node<br>Subaortic (common iliac) lymph node<br>Suprainguinal lymph node<br>**D Lymphatic, Aortic**<br>Celiac lymph node<br>Gastric lymph node<br>Hepatic lymph node<br>Lumbar lymph node<br>Pancreaticosplenic lymph node<br>Paraaortic lymph node<br>Retroperitoneal lymph node<br>**F Lymphatic, Right Lower Extremity**<br>Femoral lymph node<br>Popliteal lymph node<br>**G Lymphatic, Left Lower Extremity**<br>***See** F Lymphatic, Right Lower Extremity*<br>**H Lymphatic, Right Inguinal**<br>**J Lymphatic, Left Inguinal**<br>**K Thoracic Duct**<br>Left jugular trunk<br>Left subclavian trunk<br>**L Cisterna Chyli**<br>Intestinal lymphatic trunk<br>Lumbar lymphatic trunk | **Ø Open**<br>**3 Percutaneous**<br>**4 Percutaneous Endoscopic** | **C Extraluminal Device**<br>**D Intraluminal Device**<br>**Z No Device** | **Z No Qualifier** |

**Ø Medical and Surgical**
**7 Lymphatic and Hemic Systems**
**W Revision** Definition: Correcting, to the extent possible, a portion of a malfunctioning device or the position of a displaced device

Explanation: Revision can include correcting a malfunctioning or displaced device by taking out or putting in components of the device such as a screw or pin

| Body Part Character 4 | Approach Character 5 | Device Character 6 | Qualifier Character 7 |
|---|---|---|---|
| **K** Thoracic Duct<br>Left jugular trunk<br>Left subclavian trunk<br>**L** Cisterna Chyli<br>Intestinal lymphatic trunk<br>Lumbar lymphatic trunk<br>**N** Lymphatic | **Ø** Open<br>**3** Percutaneous<br>**4** Percutaneous Endoscopic | **Ø** Drainage Device<br>**3** Infusion Device<br>**7** Autologous Tissue Substitute<br>**C** Extraluminal Device<br>**D** Intraluminal Device<br>**J** Synthetic Substitute<br>**K** Nonautologous Tissue Substitute<br>**Y** Other Device | **Z** No Qualifier |
| **K** Thoracic Duct<br>Left jugular trunk<br>Left subclavian trunk<br>**L** Cisterna Chyli<br>Intestinal lymphatic trunk<br>Lumbar lymphatic trunk<br>**N** Lymphatic | **X** External | **Ø** Drainage Device<br>**3** Infusion Device<br>**7** Autologous Tissue Substitute<br>**C** Extraluminal Device<br>**D** Intraluminal Device<br>**J** Synthetic Substitute<br>**K** Nonautologous Tissue Substitute | **Z** No Qualifier |
| **M** Thymus<br>Thymus gland<br>**P** Spleen<br>Accessory spleen | **Ø** Open<br>**3** Percutaneous<br>**4** Percutaneous Endoscopic | **Ø** Drainage Device<br>**3** Infusion Device<br>**Y** Other Device | **Z** No Qualifier |
| **M** Thymus<br>Thymus gland<br>**P** Spleen<br>Accessory spleen | **X** External | **Ø** Drainage Device<br>**3** Infusion Device | **Z** No Qualifier |
| **T** Bone Marrow | **Ø** Open<br>**3** Percutaneous<br>**4** Percutaneous Endoscopic<br>**X** External | **Ø** Drainage Device | **Z** No Qualifier |

Non-OR Ø7W[K,L,N][3,4]YZ
Non-OR Ø7W[K,L,N]X[Ø,3,7,C,D,J,K]Z
Non-OR Ø7W[M,P][3,4]YZ
Non-OR Ø7W[M,P]X[Ø,3]Z
Non-OR Ø7WT[Ø,3,4,X]ØZ

**Ø Medical and Surgical**
**7 Lymphatic and Hemic Systems**
**Y Transplantation** Definition: Putting in or on all or a portion of a living body part taken from another individual or animal to physically take the place and/or function of all or a portion of a similar body part

Explanation: The native body part may or may not be taken out, and the transplanted body part may take over all or a portion of its function

| Body Part Character 4 | Approach Character 5 | Device Character 6 | Qualifier Character 7 |
|---|---|---|---|
| **M** Thymus<br>Thymus gland<br>**P** Spleen<br>Accessory spleen | **Ø** Open | **Z** No Device | **Ø** Allogeneic<br>**1** Syngeneic<br>**2** Zooplastic |

# Eye Ø8Ø–Ø8X

## Character Meanings

This Character Meaning table is provided as a guide to assist the user in the identification of character members that may be found in this section of code tables. It **SHOULD NOT** be used to build a PCS code.

| Operation–Character 3 | Body Part–Character 4 | Approach–Character 5 | Device–Character 6 | Qualifier–Character 7 |
|---|---|---|---|---|
| Ø Alteration | Ø Eye, Right | Ø Open | Ø Drainage Device OR Synthetic Substitute, Intraocular Telescope | 3 Nasal Cavity |
| 1 Bypass | 1 Eye, Left | 3 Percutaneous | 1 Radioactive Element | 4 Sclera |
| 2 Change | 2 Anterior Chamber, Right | 7 Via Natural or Artificial Opening | 3 Infusion Device | X Diagnostic |
| 5 Destruction | 3 Anterior Chamber, Left | 8 Via Natural or Artificial Opening Endoscopic | 5 Epiretinal Visual Prosthesis | Z No Qualifier |
| 7 Dilation | 4 Vitreous, Right | X External | 7 Autologous Tissue Substitute | |
| 9 Drainage | 5 Vitreous, Left | | C Extraluminal Device | |
| B Excision | 6 Sclera, Right | | D Intraluminal Device | |
| C Extirpation | 7 Sclera, Left | | J Synthetic Substitute | |
| D Extraction | 8 Cornea, Right | | K Nonautologous Tissue Substitute | |
| F Fragmentation | 9 Cornea, Left | | Y Other Device | |
| H Insertion | A Choroid, Right | | Z No Device | |
| J Inspection | B Choroid, Left | | | |
| L Occlusion | C Iris, Right | | | |
| M Reattachment | D Iris, Left | | | |
| N Release | E Retina, Right | | | |
| P Removal | F Retina, Left | | | |
| Q Repair | G Retinal Vessel, Right | | | |
| R Replacement | H Retinal Vessel, Left | | | |
| S Reposition | J Lens, Right | | | |
| T Resection | K Lens, Left | | | |
| U Supplement | L Extraocular Muscle, Right | | | |
| V Restriction | M Extraocular Muscle, Left | | | |
| W Revision | N Upper Eyelid, Right | | | |
| X Transfer | P Upper Eyelid, Left | | | |
| | Q Lower Eyelid, Right | | | |
| | R Lower Eyelid, Left | | | |
| | S Conjunctiva, Right | | | |
| | T Conjunctiva, Left | | | |
| | V Lacrimal Gland, Right | | | |
| | W Lacrimal Gland, Left | | | |
| | X Lacrimal Duct, Right | | | |
| | Y Lacrimal Duct, Left | | | |

**AHA Coding Clinic for table Ø89**
**2016, 2Q, 21** Laser trabeculoplasty

**AHA Coding Clinic for table Ø8B**
**2014, 4Q, 35** Vitrectomy with air/fluid exchange
**2014, 4Q, 36** Pars plans vitrectomy without mention of instillation of oil, air or fluid

**AHA Coding Clinic for table Ø8J**
**2015, 1Q, 35** Attempted removal of foreign body from cornea

**AHA Coding Clinic for table Ø8N**
**2015, 2Q, 24** Penetrating keratoplasty and anterior segment reconstruction

**AHA Coding Clinic for table Ø8R**
**2015, 2Q, 24** Penetrating keratoplasty and anterior segment reconstruction
**2015, 2Q, 25** Penetrating keratoplasty and placement of viscoelastic eye with paracentesis

**AHA Coding Clinic for table Ø8T**
**2015, 2Q, 12** Orbital exenteration

**AHA Coding Clinic for table Ø8U**
**2014, 3Q, 31** Corneal amniotic membrane transplantation

## Eye

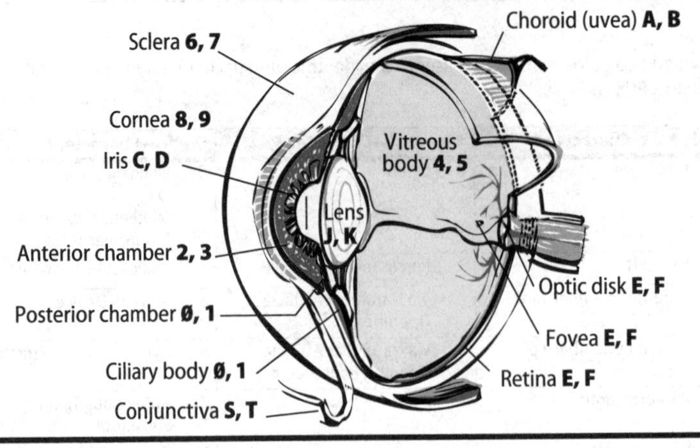
Sclera 6, 7
Choroid (uvea) A, B
Cornea 8, 9
Iris C, D
Vitreous body 4, 5
Lens J, K
Anterior chamber 2, 3
Optic disk E, F
Posterior chamber Ø, 1
Fovea E, F
Ciliary body Ø, 1
Retina E, F
Conjunctiva S, T

## Eye Musculature

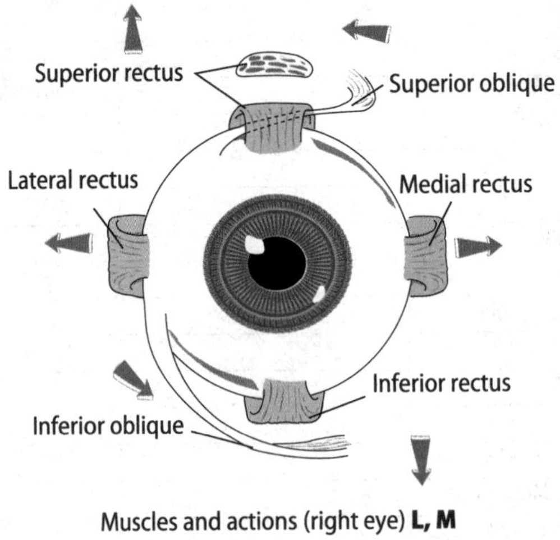
Superior rectus
Superior oblique
Lateral rectus
Medial rectus
Inferior rectus
Inferior oblique
Muscles and actions (right eye) L, M

## Lacrimal System

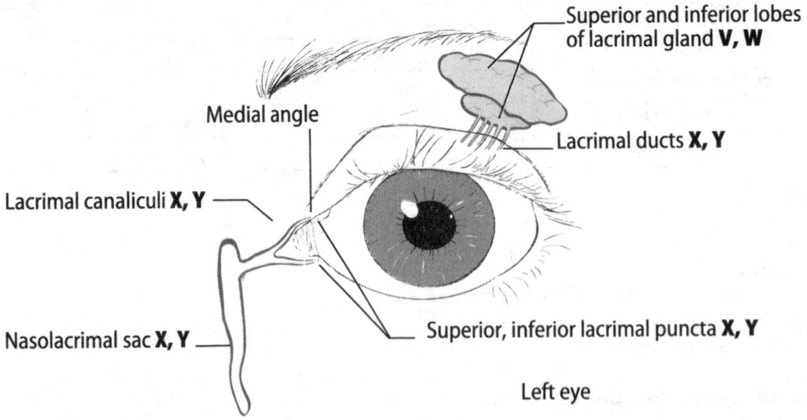
Superior and inferior lobes of lacrimal gland V, W
Medial angle
Lacrimal ducts X, Y
Lacrimal canaliculi X, Y
Nasolacrimal sac X, Y
Superior, inferior lacrimal puncta X, Y
Left eye

**Ø Medical and Surgical**
**8 Eye**
**Ø Alteration** Definition: Modifying the anatomic structure of a body part without affecting the function of the body part
Explanation: Principal purpose is to improve appearance

| Body Part Character 4 | Approach Character 5 | Device Character 6 | Qualifier Character 7 |
|---|---|---|---|
| **N Upper Eyelid, Right**<br>Lateral canthus<br>Levator palpebrae superioris muscle<br>Orbicularis oculi muscle<br>Superior tarsal plate<br>**P Upper Eyelid, Left**<br>*See N Upper Eyelid, Right*<br>**Q Lower Eyelid, Right**<br>Inferior tarsal plate<br>Medial canthus<br>**R Lower Eyelid, Left**<br>*See Q Lower Eyelid, Right* | **Ø** Open<br>**3** Percutaneous<br>**X** External | **7** Autologous Tissue Substitute<br>**J** Synthetic Substitute<br>**K** Nonautologous Tissue Substitute<br>**Z** No Device | **Z** No Qualifier |

Non-OR All body part, approach, device, and qualifier values

**Ø Medical and Surgical**
**8 Eye**
**1 Bypass** Definition: Altering the route of passage of the contents of a tubular body part
Explanation: Rerouting contents of a body part to a downstream area of the normal route, to a similar route and body part, or to an abnormal route and dissimilar body part. Includes one or more anastomoses, with or without the use of a device.

| Body Part Character 4 | Approach Character 5 | Device Character 6 | Qualifier Character 7 |
|---|---|---|---|
| **2 Anterior Chamber, Right**<br>Aqueous humour<br>**3 Anterior Chamber, Left**<br>*See 2 Anterior Chamber, Right* | **3** Percutaneous | **J** Synthetic Substitute<br>**K** Nonautologous Tissue Substitute<br>**Z** No Device | **4** Sclera |
| **X Lacrimal Duct, Right**<br>Lacrimal canaliculus<br>Lacrimal punctum<br>Lacrimal sac<br>Nasolacrimal duct<br>**Y Lacrimal Duct, Left**<br>*See X Lacrimal Duct, Right* | **Ø** Open<br>**3** Percutaneous | **J** Synthetic Substitute<br>**K** Nonautologous Tissue Substitute<br>**Z** No Device | **3** Nasal Cavity |

**Ø Medical and Surgical**
**8 Eye**
**2 Change** Definition: Taking out or off a device from a body part and putting back an identical or similar device in or on the same body part without cutting or puncturing the skin or a mucous membrane
Explanation: All CHANGE procedures are coded using the approach EXTERNAL

| Body Part Character 4 | Approach Character 5 | Device Character 6 | Qualifier Character 7 |
|---|---|---|---|
| **Ø Eye, Right**<br>Ciliary body<br>Posterior chamber<br>**1 Eye, Left**<br>*See Ø Eye, Right* | **X** External | **Ø** Drainage Device<br>**Y** Other Device | **Z** No Qualifier |

Non-OR All body part, approach, device, and qualifier values

**Ø Medical and Surgical**
**8 Eye**
**5 Destruction** Definition: Physical eradication of all or a portion of a body part by the direct use of energy, force, or a destructive agent

Explanation: None of the body part is physically taken out

| Body Part Character 4 | | Approach Character 5 | Device Character 6 | Qualifier Character 7 |
|---|---|---|---|---|
| **Ø Eye, Right**<br>Ciliary body<br>Posterior chamber<br>**1 Eye, Left**<br>*See Ø Eye, Right*<br>**6 Sclera, Right**<br>**7 Sclera, Left** | **8 Cornea, Right**<br>**9 Cornea, Left**<br>**S Conjunctiva, Right**<br>Plica semilunaris<br>**T Conjunctiva, Left**<br>*See S Conjunctiva, Right* | **X External** | **Z No Device** | **Z No Qualifier** |
| **2 Anterior Chamber, Right**<br>Aqueous humour<br>**3 Anterior Chamber, Left**<br>*See 2 Anterior Chamber, Right*<br>**4 Vitreous, Right**<br>Vitreous body<br>**5 Vitreous, Left**<br>*See 4 Vitreous, Right*<br>**C Iris, Right**<br>**D Iris, Left** | **E Retina, Right**<br>Fovea<br>Macula<br>Optic disc<br>**F Retina, Left**<br>*See E Retina, Right*<br>**G Retinal Vessel, Right**<br>**H Retinal Vessel, Left**<br>**J Lens, Right**<br>Zonule of Zinn<br>**K Lens, Left**<br>*See J Lens, Right* | **3 Percutaneous** | **Z No Device** | **Z No Qualifier** |
| **A Choroid, Right**<br>**B Choroid, Left**<br>**L Extraocular Muscle, Right**<br>Inferior oblique muscle<br>Inferior rectus muscle<br>Lateral rectus muscle<br>Medial rectus muscle<br>Superior oblique muscle<br>Superior rectus muscle | **M Extraocular Muscle, Left**<br>*See L Extraocular Muscle, Right*<br>**V Lacrimal Gland, Right**<br>**W Lacrimal Gland, Left** | **Ø Open**<br>**3 Percutaneous** | **Z No Device** | **Z No Qualifier** |
| **N Upper Eyelid, Right**<br>Lateral canthus<br>Levator palpebrae superioris muscle<br>Orbicularis oculi muscle<br>Superior tarsal plate<br>**P Upper Eyelid, Left**<br>*See N Upper Eyelid, Right* | **Q Lower Eyelid, Right**<br>Inferior tarsal plate<br>Medial canthus<br>**R Lower Eyelid, Left**<br>*See Q Lower Eyelid, Right* | **Ø Open**<br>**3 Percutaneous**<br>**X External** | **Z No Device** | **Z No Qualifier** |
| **X Lacrimal Duct, Right**<br>Lacrimal canaliculus<br>Lacrimal punctum<br>Lacrimal sac<br>Nasolacrimal duct | **Y Lacrimal Duct, Left**<br>*See X Lacrimal Duct, Right* | **Ø Open**<br>**3 Percutaneous**<br>**7 Via Natural or Artificial Opening**<br>**8 Via Natural or Artificial Opening Endoscopic** | **Z No Device** | **Z No Qualifier** |

Non-OR Ø85[E,F]3ZZ

**Ø Medical and Surgical**
**8 Eye**
**7 Dilation** Definition: Expanding an orifice or the lumen of a tubular body part

Explanation: The orifice can be a natural orifice or an artificially created orifice. Accomplished by stretching a tubular body part using intraluminal pressure or by cutting part of the orifice or wall of the tubular body part.

| Body Part Character 4 | Approach Character 5 | Device Character 6 | Qualifier Character 7 |
|---|---|---|---|
| **X Lacrimal Duct, Right**<br>Lacrimal canaliculus<br>Lacrimal punctum<br>Lacrimal sac<br>Nasolacrimal duct<br>**Y Lacrimal Duct, Left**<br>*See X Lacrimal Duct, Right* | **Ø Open**<br>**3 Percutaneous**<br>**7 Via Natural or Artificial Opening**<br>**8 Via Natural or Artificial Opening Endoscopic** | **D Intraluminal Device**<br>**Z No Device** | **Z No Qualifier** |

**Ø Medical and Surgical**
**8 Eye**
**9 Drainage** Definition: Taking or letting out fluids and/or gases from a body part
Explanation: The qualifier DIAGNOSTIC is used to identify drainage procedures that are biopsies

| Body Part Character 4 | | Approach Character 5 | Device Character 6 | Qualifier Character 7 |
|---|---|---|---|---|
| **Ø Eye, Right**<br>Ciliary body<br>Posterior chamber<br>**1 Eye, Left**<br>*See Ø Eye, Right*<br>**6 Sclera, Right**<br>**7 Sclera, Left** | **8 Cornea, Right**<br>**9 Cornea, Left**<br>**S Conjunctiva, Right**<br>Plica semilunaris<br>**T Conjunctiva, Left**<br>*See S Conjunctiva, Right* | **X External** | **Ø Drainage Device** | **Z No Qualifier** |
| **Ø Eye, Right**<br>Ciliary body<br>Posterior chamber<br>**1 Eye, Left**<br>*See Ø Eye, Right*<br>**6 Sclera, Right**<br>**7 Sclera, Left** | **8 Cornea, Right**<br>**9 Cornea, Left**<br>**S Conjunctiva, Right**<br>Plica semilunaris<br>**T Conjunctiva, Left**<br>*See S Conjunctiva, Right* | **X External** | **Z No Device** | **X Diagnostic**<br>**Z No Qualifier** |
| **2 Anterior Chamber, Right**<br>Aqueous humour<br>**3 Anterior Chamber, Left**<br>*See 2 Anterior Chamber, Right*<br>**4 Vitreous, Right**<br>Vitreous body<br>**5 Vitreous, Left**<br>*See 4 Vitreous, Right*<br>**C Iris, Right**<br>**D Iris, Left** | **E Retina, Right**<br>Fovea<br>Macula<br>Optic disc<br>**F Retina, Left**<br>*See E Retina, Right*<br>**G Retinal Vessel, Right**<br>**H Retinal Vessel, Left**<br>**J Lens, Right**<br>Zonule of Zinn<br>**K Lens, Left**<br>*See J Lens, Right* | **3 Percutaneous** | **Ø Drainage Device** | **Z No Qualifier** |
| **2 Anterior Chamber, Right**<br>Aqueous humour<br>**3 Anterior Chamber, Left**<br>*See 2 Anterior Chamber, Right*<br>**4 Vitreous, Right**<br>Vitreous body<br>**5 Vitreous, Left**<br>*See 4 Vitreous, Right*<br>**C Iris, Right**<br>**D Iris, Left** | **E Retina, Right**<br>Fovea<br>Macula<br>Optic disc<br>**F Retina, Left**<br>*See E Retina, Right*<br>**G Retinal Vessel, Right**<br>**H Retinal Vessel, Left**<br>**J Lens, Right**<br>Zonule of Zinn<br>**K Lens, Left**<br>*See J Lens, Right* | **3 Percutaneous** | **Z No Device** | **X Diagnostic**<br>**Z No Qualifier** |
| **A Choroid, Right**<br>**B Choroid, Left**<br>**L Extraocular Muscle, Right**<br>Inferior oblique muscle<br>Inferior rectus muscle<br>Lateral rectus muscle<br>Medial rectus muscle<br>Superior oblique muscle<br>Superior rectus muscle | **M Extraocular Muscle, Left**<br>*See L Extraocular Muscle, Right*<br>**V Lacrimal Gland, Right**<br>**W Lacrimal Gland, Left** | **Ø Open**<br>**3 Percutaneous** | **Ø Drainage Device** | **Z No Qualifier** |
| **A Choroid, Right**<br>**B Choroid, Left**<br>**L Extraocular Muscle, Right**<br>Inferior oblique muscle<br>Inferior rectus muscle<br>Lateral rectus muscle<br>Medial rectus muscle<br>Superior oblique muscle<br>Superior rectus muscle | **M Extraocular Muscle, Left**<br>*See L Extraocular Muscle, Right*<br>**V Lacrimal Gland, Right**<br>**W Lacrimal Gland, Left** | **Ø Open**<br>**3 Percutaneous** | **Z No Device** | **X Diagnostic**<br>**Z No Qualifier** |
| **N Upper Eyelid, Right**<br>Lateral canthus<br>Levator palpebrae superioris muscle<br>Orbicularis oculi muscle<br>Superior tarsal plate<br>**P Upper Eyelid, Left**<br>*See N Upper Eyelid, Right* | **Q Lower Eyelid, Right**<br>Inferior tarsal plate<br>Medial canthus<br>**R Lower Eyelid, Left**<br>*See Q Lower Eyelid, Right* | **Ø Open**<br>**3 Percutaneous**<br>**X External** | **Ø Drainage Device** | **Z No Qualifier** |

Ø89 Continued on next page

Non-OR Ø89[Ø,1,6,7,8,9,S,T]XZ[X,Z]
Non-OR Ø89[N,P,Q,R][Ø,3,X]ØZ

**Ø89 Continued**

**Ø Medical and Surgical**
**8 Eye**
**9 Drainage** Definition: Taking or letting out fluids and/or gases from a body part
Explanation: The qualifier DIAGNOSTIC is used to identify drainage procedures that are biopsies

| Body Part Character 4 | | Approach Character 5 | Device Character 6 | Qualifier Character 7 |
|---|---|---|---|---|
| **N Upper Eyelid, Right**<br>Lateral canthus<br>Levator palpebrae superioris muscle<br>Orbicularis oculi muscle<br>Superior tarsal plate<br>**P Upper Eyelid, Left**<br>*See N Upper Eyelid, Right* | **Q Lower Eyelid, Right**<br>Inferior tarsal plate<br>Medial canthus<br>**R Lower Eyelid, Left**<br>*See Q Lower Eyelid, Right* | **Ø Open**<br>**3 Percutaneous**<br>**X External** | **Z No Device** | **X Diagnostic**<br>**Z No Qualifier** |
| **X Lacrimal Duct, Right**<br>Lacrimal canaliculus<br>Lacrimal punctum<br>Lacrimal sac<br>Nasolacrimal duct | **Y Lacrimal Duct, Left**<br>*See X Lacrimal Duct, Right* | **Ø Open**<br>**3 Percutaneous**<br>**7 Via Natural or Artificial Opening**<br>**8 Via Natural or Artificial Opening Endoscopic** | **Ø Drainage Device** | **Z No Qualifier** |
| **X Lacrimal Duct, Right**<br>Lacrimal canaliculus<br>Lacrimal punctum<br>Lacrimal sac<br>Nasolacrimal duct | **Y Lacrimal Duct, Left**<br>*See X Lacrimal Duct, Right* | **Ø Open**<br>**3 Percutaneous**<br>**7 Via Natural or Artificial Opening**<br>**8 Via Natural or Artificial Opening Endoscopic** | **Z No Device** | **X Diagnostic**<br>**Z No Qualifier** |

Non-OR Ø89[N,P,Q,R]ØZZ
Non-OR Ø89[N,P,Q,R][3,X]Z[X,Z]

**Ø Medical and Surgical**
**8 Eye**
**B Excision** Definition: Cutting out or off, without replacement, a portion of a body part
Explanation: The qualifier DIAGNOSTIC is used to identify excision procedures that are biopsies

| Body Part Character 4 | | Approach Character 5 | Device Character 6 | Qualifier Character 7 |
|---|---|---|---|---|
| **Ø Eye, Right**<br>Ciliary body<br>Posterior chamber<br>**1 Eye, Left**<br>*See Ø Eye, Right*<br>**N Upper Eyelid, Right**<br>Lateral canthus<br>Levator palpebrae superioris muscle<br>Orbicularis oculi muscle<br>Superior tarsal plate | **P Upper Eyelid, Left**<br>*See N Upper Eyelid, Right*<br>**Q Lower Eyelid, Right**<br>Inferior tarsal plate<br>Medial canthus<br>**R Lower Eyelid, Left**<br>*See Q Lower Eyelid, Right* | **Ø Open**<br>**3 Percutaneous**<br>**X External** | **Z No Device** | **X Diagnostic**<br>**Z No Qualifier** |
| **4 Vitreous, Right**<br>Vitreous body<br>**5 Vitreous, Left**<br>*See 4 Vitreous, Right*<br>**C Iris, Right**<br>**D Iris, Left**<br>**E Retina, Right**<br>Fovea<br>Macula<br>Optic disc | **F Retina, Left**<br>*See E Retina, Right*<br>**J Lens, Right**<br>Zonule of Zinn<br>**K Lens, Left**<br>*See J Lens, Right* | **3 Percutaneous** | **Z No Device** | **X Diagnostic**<br>**Z No Qualifier** |
| **6 Sclera, Right**<br>**7 Sclera, Left**<br>**8 Cornea, Right**<br>**9 Cornea, Left** | **S Conjunctiva, Right**<br>Plica semilunaris<br>**T Conjunctiva, Left**<br>*See S Conjunctiva, Right* | **X External** | **Z No Device** | **X Diagnostic**<br>**Z No Qualifier** |
| **A Choroid, Right**<br>**B Choroid, Left**<br>**L Extraocular Muscle, Right**<br>Inferior oblique muscle<br>Inferior rectus muscle<br>Lateral rectus muscle<br>Medial rectus muscle<br>Superior oblique muscle<br>Superior rectus muscle | **M Extraocular Muscle, Left**<br>*See L Extraocular Muscle, Right*<br>**V Lacrimal Gland, Right**<br>**W Lacrimal Gland, Left** | **Ø Open**<br>**3 Percutaneous** | **Z No Device** | **X Diagnostic**<br>**Z No Qualifier** |
| **X Lacrimal Duct, Right**<br>Lacrimal canaliculus<br>Lacrimal punctum<br>Lacrimal sac<br>Nasolacrimal duct | **Y Lacrimal Duct, Left**<br>*See X Lacrimal Duct, Right* | **Ø Open**<br>**3 Percutaneous**<br>**7 Via Natural or Artificial Opening**<br>**8 Via Natural or Artificial Opening Endoscopic** | **Z No Device** | **X Diagnostic**<br>**Z No Qualifier** |

**Ø Medical and Surgical**
**8 Eye**
**C Extirpation** Definition: Taking or cutting out solid matter from a body part

Explanation: The solid matter may be an abnormal byproduct of a biological function or a foreign body; it may be imbedded in a body part or in the lumen of a tubular body part. The solid matter may or may not have been previously broken into pieces.

| Body Part Character 4 | Approach Character 5 | Device Character 6 | Qualifier Character 7 |
|---|---|---|---|
| **Ø Eye, Right**<br>Ciliary body<br>Posterior chamber<br>**1 Eye, Left**<br>*See Ø Eye, Right*<br>**6 Sclera, Right**<br>**7 Sclera, Left**<br>**8 Cornea, Right**<br>**9 Cornea, Left**<br>**S Conjunctiva, Right**<br>Plica semilunaris<br>**T Conjunctiva, Left**<br>*See S Conjunctiva, Right* | **X External** | **Z No Device** | **Z No Qualifier** |
| **2 Anterior Chamber, Right**<br>Aqueous humour<br>**3 Anterior Chamber, Left**<br>*See 2 Anterior Chamber, Right*<br>**4 Vitreous, Right**<br>Vitreous body<br>**5 Vitreous, Left**<br>*See 4 Vitreous, Right*<br>**C Iris, Right**<br>**D Iris, Left**<br>**E Retina, Right**<br>Fovea<br>Macula<br>Optic disc<br>**F Retina, Left**<br>*See* E Retina, Right<br>**G Retinal Vessel, Right**<br>**H Retinal Vessel, Left**<br>**J Lens, Right**<br>Zonule of Zinn<br>**K Lens, Left**<br>*See J Lens, Right* | **3 Percutaneous**<br>**X External** | **Z No Device** | **Z No Qualifier** |
| **A Choroid, Right**<br>**B Choroid, Left**<br>**L Extraocular Muscle, Right**<br>Inferior oblique muscle<br>Inferior rectus muscle<br>Lateral rectus muscle<br>Medial rectus muscle<br>Superior oblique muscle<br>Superior rectus muscle<br>**M Extraocular Muscle, Left**<br>*See L Extraocular Muscle, Right*<br>**N Upper Eyelid, Right**<br>Lateral canthus<br>Levator palpebrae superioris muscle<br>Orbicularis oculi muscle<br>Superior tarsal plate<br>**P Upper Eyelid, Left**<br>*See N Upper Eyelid, Right*<br>**Q Lower Eyelid, Right**<br>Inferior tarsal plate<br>Medial canthus<br>**R Lower Eyelid, Left**<br>*See Q Lower Eyelid, Right*<br>**V Lacrimal Gland, Right**<br>**W Lacrimal Gland, Left** | **Ø Open**<br>**3 Percutaneous**<br>**X External** | **Z No Device** | **Z No Qualifier** |
| **X Lacrimal Duct, Right**<br>Lacrimal canaliculus<br>Lacrimal punctum<br>Lacrimal sac<br>Nasolacrimal duct<br>**Y Lacrimal Duct, Left**<br>*See X Lacrimal Duct, Right* | **Ø Open**<br>**3 Percutaneous**<br>**7 Via Natural or Artificial Opening**<br>**8 Via Natural or Artificial Opening Endoscopic** | **Z No Device** | **Z No Qualifier** |

**Non-OR** Ø8C[Ø,1,6,7,S,T]XZZ
**Non-OR** Ø8C[2,3]XZZ
**Non-OR** Ø8C[N,P,Q,R][Ø,3,X]ZZ

**Ø Medical and Surgical**
**8 Eye**
**D Extraction** Definition: Pulling or stripping out or off all or a portion of a body part by the use of force

Explanation: The qualifier DIAGNOSTIC is used to identify extraction procedures that are biopsies

| Body Part Character 4 | Approach Character 5 | Device Character 6 | Qualifier Character 7 |
|---|---|---|---|
| **8 Cornea, Right**<br>**9 Cornea, Left** | **X External** | **Z No Device** | **X Diagnostic**<br>**Z No Qualifier** |
| **J Lens, Right**<br>Zonule of Zinn<br>**K Lens, Left**<br>*See J Lens, Right* | **3 Percutaneous** | **Z No Device** | **Z No Qualifier** |

**Ø Medical and Surgical**
**8 Eye**
**F Fragmentation** Definition: Breaking solid matter in a body part into pieces

Explanation: Physical force (e.g., manual, ultrasonic) applied directly or indirectly is used to break the solid matter into pieces. The solid matter may be an abnormal byproduct of a biological function or a foreign body. The pieces of solid matter are not taken out.

| Body Part Character 4 | Approach Character 5 | Device Character 6 | Qualifier Character 7 |
|---|---|---|---|
| **4 Vitreous, Right** NC<br>Vitreous body<br>**5 Vitreous, Left** NC<br>*See 4 Vitreous, Right* | **3 Percutaneous**<br>**X External** | **Z No Device** | **Z No Qualifier** |

**Non-OR** Ø8F[4,5]XZZ
NC Ø8F[4,5]XZZ

**Ø Medical and Surgical**
**8 Eye**
**H Insertion** Definition: Putting in a nonbiological appliance that monitors, assists, performs, or prevents a physiological function but does not physically take the place of a body part

Explanation: None

| Body Part Character 4 | Approach Character 5 | Device Character 6 | Qualifier Character 7 |
|---|---|---|---|
| **Ø Eye, Right**<br>Ciliary body<br>Posterior chamber<br>**1 Eye, Left**<br>*See Ø Eye, Right* | **Ø Open** | **5 Epiretinal Visual Prosthesis**<br>Y Other Device | **Z No Qualifier** |
| **Ø Eye, Right**<br>Ciliary body<br>Posterior chamber<br>**1 Eye, Left**<br>*See Ø Eye, Right* | **3 Percutaneous** | **1 Radioactive Element**<br>**3 Infusion Device**<br>Y Other Device | **Z No Qualifier** |
| Ø Eye, Right<br>Ciliary body<br>Posterior chamber<br>1 Eye, Left<br>*See Ø Eye, Right* | 7 Via Natural or Artificial Opening<br>8 Via Natural or Artificial Opening Endoscopic | Y Other Device | Z No Qualifier |
| **Ø Eye, Right**<br>Ciliary body<br>Posterior chamber<br>**1 Eye, Left**<br>*See Ø Eye, Right* | **X External** | **1 Radioactive Element**<br>**3 Infusion Device** | **Z No Qualifier** |

**Non-OR** Ø8H[Ø,1]3YZ
**Non-OR** Ø8H[Ø,1][7,8]YZ

**Ø Medical and Surgical**
**8 Eye**
**J Inspection** Definition: Visually and/or manually exploring a body part

Explanation: Visual exploration may be performed with or without optical instrumentation. Manual exploration may be performed directly or through intervening body layers.

| Body Part Character 4 | Approach Character 5 | Device Character 6 | Qualifier Character 7 |
|---|---|---|---|
| **Ø Eye, Right**<br>Ciliary body<br>Posterior chamber<br>**1 Eye, Left**<br>*See Ø Eye, Right*<br>**J Lens, Right**<br>Zonule of Zinn<br>**K Lens, Left**<br>*See J Lens, Right* | **X External** | **Z No Device** | **Z No Qualifier** |
| **L Extraocular Muscle, Right**<br>Inferior oblique muscle<br>Inferior rectus muscle<br>Lateral rectus muscle<br>Medial rectus muscle<br>Superior oblique muscle<br>Superior rectus muscle<br>**M Extraocular Muscle, Left**<br>*See L Extraocular Muscle, Right* | **Ø Open**<br>**X External** | **Z No Device** | **Z No Qualifier** |

Non-OR Ø8J[Ø,1,J,K]XZZ
Non-OR Ø8J[L,M]XZZ

**Ø Medical and Surgical**
**8 Eye**
**L Occlusion** Definition: Completely closing an orifice or the lumen of a tubular body part

Explanation: The orifice can be a natural orifice or an artificially created orifice

| Body Part Character 4 | Approach Character 5 | Device Character 6 | Qualifier Character 7 |
|---|---|---|---|
| **X Lacrimal Duct, Right**<br>Lacrimal canaliculus<br>Lacrimal punctum<br>Lacrimal sac<br>Nasolacrimal duct<br>**Y Lacrimal Duct, Left**<br>*See X Lacrimal Duct, Right* | **Ø Open**<br>**3 Percutaneous** | **C Extraluminal Device**<br>**D Intraluminal Device**<br>**Z No Device** | **Z No Qualifier** |
| **X Lacrimal Duct, Right**<br>Lacrimal canaliculus<br>Lacrimal punctum<br>Lacrimal sac<br>Nasolacrimal duct<br>**Y Lacrimal Duct, Left**<br>*See X Lacrimal Duct, Right* | **7 Via Natural or Artificial Opening**<br>**8 Via Natural or Artificial Opening Endoscopic** | **D Intraluminal Device**<br>**Z No Device** | **Z No Qualifier** |

**Ø Medical and Surgical**
**8 Eye**
**M Reattachment** Definition: Putting back in or on all or a portion of a separated body part to its normal location or other suitable location

Explanation: Vascular circulation and nervous pathways may or may not be reestablished

| Body Part Character 4 | Approach Character 5 | Device Character 6 | Qualifier Character 7 |
|---|---|---|---|
| **N Upper Eyelid, Right**<br>Lateral canthus<br>Levator palpebrae superioris muscle<br>Orbicularis oculi muscle<br>Superior tarsal plate<br>**P Upper Eyelid, Left**<br>*See N Upper Eyelid, Right*<br>**Q Lower Eyelid, Right**<br>Inferior tarsal plate<br>Medial canthus<br>**R Lower Eyelid, Left**<br>*See Q Lower Eyelid, Right* | **X External** | **Z No Device** | **Z No Qualifier** |

**Ø Medical and Surgical**
**8 Eye**
**N Release** Definition: Freeing a body part from an abnormal physical constraint by cutting or by the use of force
Explanation: Some of the restraining tissue may be taken out but none of the body part is taken out

| Body Part Character 4 | Approach Character 5 | Device Character 6 | Qualifier Character 7 |
|---|---|---|---|
| **Ø Eye, Right**<br>Ciliary body<br>Posterior chamber<br>**1 Eye, Left**<br>*See Ø Eye, Right*<br>**6 Sclera, Right**<br>**7 Sclera, Left**<br>**8 Cornea, Right**<br>**9 Cornea, Left**<br>**S Conjunctiva, Right**<br>Plica semilunaris<br>**T Conjunctiva, Left**<br>*See S Conjunctiva, Right* | **X External** | **Z No Device** | **Z No Qualifier** |
| **2 Anterior Chamber, Right**<br>Aqueous humour<br>**3 Anterior Chamber, Left**<br>*See 2 Anterior Chamber, Right*<br>**4 Vitreous, Right**<br>Vitreous body<br>**5 Vitreous, Left**<br>*See 4 Vitreous, Right*<br>**C Iris, Right**<br>**D Iris, Left**<br>**E Retina, Right**<br>Fovea<br>Macula<br>Optic disc<br>**F Retina, Left**<br>*See E Retina, Right*<br>**G Retinal Vessel, Right**<br>**H Retinal Vessel, Left**<br>**J Lens, Right**<br>Zonule of Zinn<br>**K Lens, Left**<br>*See J Lens, Right* | **3 Percutaneous** | **Z No Device** | **Z No Qualifier** |
| **A Choroid, Right**<br>**B Choroid, Left**<br>**L Extraocular Muscle, Right**<br>Inferior oblique muscle<br>Inferior rectus muscle<br>Lateral rectus muscle<br>Medial rectus muscle<br>Superior oblique muscle<br>Superior rectus muscle<br>**M Extraocular Muscle, Left**<br>*See L Extraocular Muscle, Right*<br>**V Lacrimal Gland, Right**<br>**W Lacrimal Gland, Left** | **Ø Open**<br>**3 Percutaneous** | **Z No Device** | **Z No Qualifier** |
| **N Upper Eyelid, Right**<br>Lateral canthus<br>Levator palpebrae superioris muscle<br>Orbicularis oculi muscle<br>Superior tarsal plate<br>**P Upper Eyelid, Left**<br>*See N Upper Eyelid, Right*<br>**Q Lower Eyelid, Right**<br>Inferior tarsal plate<br>Medial canthus<br>**R Lower Eyelid, Left**<br>*See Q Lower Eyelid, Right* | **Ø Open**<br>**3 Percutaneous**<br>**X External** | **Z No Device** | **Z No Qualifier** |
| **X Lacrimal Duct, Right**<br>Lacrimal canaliculus<br>Lacrimal punctum<br>Lacrimal sac<br>Nasolacrimal duct<br>**Y Lacrimal Duct, Left**<br>*See X Lacrimal Duct, Right* | **Ø Open**<br>**3 Percutaneous**<br>**7 Via Natural or Artificial Opening**<br>**8 Via Natural or Artificial Opening Endoscopic** | **Z No Device** | **Z No Qualifier** |

**Ø Medical and Surgical**
**8 Eye**
**P Removal**

Definition: Taking out or off a device from a body part

Explanation: If a device is taken out and a similar device put in without cutting or puncturing the skin or mucous membrane, the procedure is coded to the root operation CHANGE. Otherwise, the procedure for taking out a device is coded to the root operation REMOVAL.

| Body Part Character 4 | Approach Character 5 | Device Character 6 | Qualifier Character 7 |
|---|---|---|---|
| **Ø Eye, Right**<br>Ciliary body<br>Posterior chamber<br>**1 Eye, Left**<br>*See Ø Eye, Right* | **Ø Open**<br>**3 Percutaneous**<br>**7 Via Natural or Artificial Opening**<br>**8 Via Natural or Artificial Opening Endoscopic** | **Ø Drainage Device**<br>**1 Radioactive Element**<br>**3 Infusion Device**<br>**7 Autologous Tissue Substitute**<br>**C Extraluminal Device**<br>**D Intraluminal Device**<br>**J Synthetic Substitute**<br>**K Nonautologous Tissue Substitute**<br>Y Other Device | **Z No Qualifier** |
| **Ø Eye, Right**<br>Ciliary body<br>Posterior chamber<br>**1 Eye, Left**<br>*See Ø Eye, Right* | **X External** | **Ø Drainage Device**<br>**1 Radioactive Element**<br>**3 Infusion Device**<br>**7 Autologous Tissue Substitute**<br>**C Extraluminal Device**<br>**D Intraluminal Device**<br>**J Synthetic Substitute**<br>**K Nonautologous Tissue Substitute** | **Z No Qualifier** |
| **J Lens, Right**<br>Zonule of Zinn<br>**K Lens, Left**<br>*See J Lens, Right* | **3 Percutaneous** | **J Synthetic Substitute**<br>Y Other Device | **Z No Qualifier** |
| **L Extraocular Muscle, Right**<br>Inferior oblique muscle<br>Inferior rectus muscle<br>Lateral rectus muscle<br>Medial rectus muscle<br>Superior oblique muscle<br>Superior rectus muscle<br>**M Extraocular Muscle, Left**<br>*See L Extraocular Muscle, Right* | **Ø Open**<br>**3 Percutaneous** | **Ø Drainage Device**<br>**7 Autologous Tissue Substitute**<br>**J Synthetic Substitute**<br>**K Nonautologous Tissue Substitute**<br>Y Other Device | **Z No Qualifier** |

**Non-OR** Ø8PØ[Ø,1]3YZ
**Non-OR** Ø8PØ[Ø,1][7,8][Ø,3,D,Y]Z
**Non-OR** Ø8P[Ø,1]X[Ø,1,3,C,D,J]Z
**Non-OR** Ø8P[J,K]3YZ
**Non-OR** Ø8P[L,M]3YZ

**Ø Medical and Surgical**
**8 Eye**
**Q Repair** Definition: Restoring, to the extent possible, a body part to its normal anatomic structure and function
Explanation: Used only when the method to accomplish the repair is not one of the other root operations

| Body Part Character 4 | Approach Character 5 | Device Character 6 | Qualifier Character 7 |
|---|---|---|---|
| **Ø Eye, Right**<br>Ciliary body<br>Posterior chamber<br>**1 Eye, Left**<br>*See Ø Eye, Right*<br>**6 Sclera, Right**<br>**7 Sclera, Left**<br>**8 Cornea, Right** NC<br>**9 Cornea, Left** NC<br>**S Conjunctiva, Right**<br>Plica semilunaris<br>**T Conjunctiva, Left**<br>*See S Conjunctiva, Right* | **X External** | **Z No Device** | **Z No Qualifier** |
| **2 Anterior Chamber, Right**<br>Aqueous humour<br>**3 Anterior Chamber, Left**<br>*See 2 Anterior Chamber, Right*<br>**4 Vitreous, Right**<br>Vitreous body<br>**5 Vitreous, Left**<br>*See 4 Vitreous, Right*<br>**C Iris, Right**<br>**D Iris, Left**<br>**E Retina, Right**<br>Fovea<br>Macula<br>Optic disc<br>**F Retina, Left**<br>*See E Retina, Right*<br>**G Retinal Vessel, Right**<br>**H Retinal Vessel, Left**<br>**J Lens, Right**<br>Zonule of Zinn<br>**K Lens, Left**<br>*See J Lens, Right* | **3 Percutaneous** | **Z No Device** | **Z No Qualifier** |
| **A Choroid, Right**<br>**B Choroid, Left**<br>**L Extraocular Muscle, Right**<br>Inferior oblique muscle<br>Inferior rectus muscle<br>Lateral rectus muscle<br>Medial rectus muscle<br>Superior oblique muscle<br>Superior rectus muscle<br>**M Extraocular Muscle, Left**<br>*See L Extraocular Muscle, Right*<br>**V Lacrimal Gland, Right**<br>**W Lacrimal Gland, Left** | **Ø Open**<br>**3 Percutaneous** | **Z No Device** | **Z No Qualifier** |
| **N Upper Eyelid, Right**<br>Lateral canthus<br>Levator palpebrae superioris muscle<br>Orbicularis oculi muscle<br>Superior tarsal plate<br>**P Upper Eyelid, Left**<br>*See N Upper Eyelid, Right*<br>**Q Lower Eyelid, Right**<br>Inferior tarsal plate<br>Medial canthus<br>**R Lower Eyelid, Left**<br>*See Q Lower Eyelid, Right* | **Ø Open**<br>**3 Percutaneous**<br>**X External** | **Z No Device** | **Z No Qualifier** |
| **X Lacrimal Duct, Right**<br>Lacrimal canaliculus<br>Lacrimal punctum<br>Lacrimal sac<br>Nasolacrimal duct<br>**Y Lacrimal Duct, Left**<br>*See X Lacrimal Duct, Right* | **Ø Open**<br>**3 Percutaneous**<br>**7 Via Natural or Artificial Opening**<br>**8 Via Natural or Artificial Opening Endoscopic** | **Z No Device** | **Z No Qualifier** |

Non-OR Ø8Q[N,P,Q,R][Ø,3,X]ZZ
NC Ø8Q[8,9]XZZ

**Ø Medical and Surgical**
**8 Eye**
**R Replacement** Definition: Putting in or on biological or synthetic material that physically takes the place and/or function of all or a portion of a body part

Explanation: The body part may have been taken out or replaced, or may be taken out, physically eradicated, or rendered nonfunctional during the REPLACEMENT procedure. A REMOVAL procedure is coded for taking out the device used in a previous replacement procedure.

| Body Part Character 4 | Approach Character 5 | Device Character 6 | Qualifier Character 7 |
|---|---|---|---|
| **Ø Eye, Right**<br>Ciliary body<br>Posterior chamber<br>**1 Eye, Left**<br>*See Ø Eye, Right*<br>**A Choroid, Right**<br>**B Choroid, Left** | **Ø Open**<br>**3 Percutaneous** | **7 Autologous Tissue Substitute**<br>**J Synthetic Substitute**<br>**K Nonautologous Tissue Substitute** | **Z No Qualifier** |
| **4 Vitreous, Right**<br>Vitreous body<br>**5 Vitreous, Left**<br>*See 4 Vitreous, Right*<br>**C Iris, Right**<br>**D Iris, Left**<br>**G Retinal Vessel, Right**<br>**H Retinal Vessel, Left** | **3 Percutaneous** | **7 Autologous Tissue Substitute**<br>**J Synthetic Substitute**<br>**K Nonautologous Tissue Substitute** | **Z No Qualifier** |
| **6 Sclera, Right**<br>**7 Sclera, Left**<br>**S Conjunctiva, Right**<br>Plica semilunaris<br>**T Conjunctiva, Left**<br>*See S Conjunctiva, Right* | **X External** | **7 Autologous Tissue Substitute**<br>**J Synthetic Substitute**<br>**K Nonautologous Tissue Substitute** | **Z No Qualifier** |
| **8 Cornea, Right**<br>**9 Cornea, Left** | **3 Percutaneous**<br>**X External** | **7 Autologous Tissue Substitute**<br>**J Synthetic Substitute**<br>**K Nonautologous Tissue Substitute** | **Z No Qualifier** |
| **J Lens, Right**<br>Zonule of Zinn<br>**K Lens, Left**<br>*See J Lens, Right* | **3 Percutaneous** | **Ø Synthetic Substitute, Intraocular Telescope**<br>**7 Autologous Tissue Substitute**<br>**J Synthetic Substitute**<br>**K Nonautologous Tissue Substitute** | **Z No Qualifier** |
| **N Upper Eyelid, Right**<br>Lateral canthus<br>Levator palpebrae superioris muscle<br>Orbicularis oculi muscle<br>Superior tarsal plate<br>**P Upper Eyelid, Left**<br>*See N Upper Eyelid, Right*<br>**Q Lower Eyelid, Right**<br>Inferior tarsal plate<br>Medial canthus<br>**R Lower Eyelid, Left**<br>*See Q Lower Eyelid, Right* | **Ø Open**<br>**3 Percutaneous**<br>**X External** | **7 Autologous Tissue Substitute**<br>**J Synthetic Substitute**<br>**K Nonautologous Tissue Substitute** | **Z No Qualifier** |
| **X Lacrimal Duct, Right**<br>Lacrimal canaliculus<br>Lacrimal punctum<br>Lacrimal sac<br>Nasolacrimal duct<br>**Y Lacrimal Duct, Left**<br>*See X Lacrimal Duct, Right* | **Ø Open**<br>**3 Percutaneous**<br>**7 Via Natural or Artificial Opening**<br>**8 Via Natural or Artificial Opening Endoscopic** | **7 Autologous Tissue Substitute**<br>**J Synthetic Substitute**<br>**K Nonautologous Tissue Substitute** | **Z No Qualifier** |

**Ø Medical and Surgical**
**8 Eye**
**S Reposition**

Definition: Moving to its normal location, or other suitable location, all or a portion of a body part

Explanation: The body part is moved to a new location from an abnormal location, or from a normal location where it is not functioning correctly. The body part may or may not be cut out or off to be moved to the new location.

| Body Part Character 4 | Approach Character 5 | Device Character 6 | Qualifier Character 7 |
|---|---|---|---|
| **C Iris, Right**<br>**D Iris, Left**<br>**G Retinal Vessel, Right**<br>**H Retinal Vessel, Left**<br>**J Lens, Right**<br>Zonule of Zinn<br>**K Lens, Left**<br>*See J Lens, Right* | **3 Percutaneous** | **Z No Device** | **Z No Qualifier** |
| **L Extraocular Muscle, Right**<br>Inferior oblique muscle<br>Inferior rectus muscle<br>Lateral rectus muscle<br>Medial rectus muscle<br>Superior oblique muscle<br>Superior rectus muscle<br>**M Extraocular Muscle, Left**<br>*See L Extraocular Muscle, Right*<br>**V Lacrimal Gland, Right**<br>**W Lacrimal Gland, Left** | **Ø Open**<br>**3 Percutaneous** | **Z No Device** | **Z No Qualifier** |
| **N Upper Eyelid, Right**<br>Lateral canthus<br>Levator palpebrae superioris muscle<br>Orbicularis oculi muscle<br>Superior tarsal plate<br>**P Upper Eyelid, Left**<br>*See N Upper Eyelid, Right*<br>**Q Lower Eyelid, Right**<br>Inferior tarsal plate<br>Medial canthus<br>**R Lower Eyelid, Left**<br>*See Q Lower Eyelid, Right* | **Ø Open**<br>**3 Percutaneous**<br>**X External** | **Z No Device** | **Z No Qualifier** |
| **X Lacrimal Duct, Right**<br>Lacrimal canaliculus<br>Lacrimal punctum<br>Lacrimal sac<br>Nasolacrimal duct<br>**Y Lacrimal Duct, Left**<br>*See X Lacrimal Duct, Right* | **Ø Open**<br>**3 Percutaneous**<br>**7 Via Natural or Artificial Opening**<br>**8 Via Natural or Artificial Opening Endoscopic** | **Z No Device** | **Z No Qualifier** |

**Ø Medical and Surgical**
**8 Eye**
**T Resection** Definition: Cutting out or off, without replacement, all of a body part

Explanation: None

| Body Part Character 4 | Approach Character 5 | Device Character 6 | Qualifier Character 7 |
|---|---|---|---|
| **Ø Eye, Right**<br>Ciliary body<br>Posterior chamber<br>**1 Eye, Left**<br>*See Ø Eye, Right*<br>**8 Cornea, Right**<br>**9 Cornea, Left** | **X External** | **Z No Device** | **Z No Qualifier** |
| **4 Vitreous, Right**<br>Vitreous body<br>**5 Vitreous, Left**<br>*See 4 Vitreous, Right*<br>**C Iris, Right**<br>**D Iris, Left**<br>**J Lens, Right**<br>Zonule of Zinn<br>**K Lens, Left**<br>*See J Lens, Right* | **3 Percutaneous** | **Z No Device** | **Z No Qualifier** |
| **L Extraocular Muscle, Right**<br>Inferior oblique muscle<br>Inferior rectus muscle<br>Lateral rectus muscle<br>Medial rectus muscle<br>Superior oblique muscle<br>Superior rectus muscle<br>**M Extraocular Muscle, Left**<br>*See L Extraocular Muscle, Right*<br>**V Lacrimal Gland, Right**<br>**W Lacrimal Gland, Left** | **Ø Open**<br>**3 Percutaneous** | **Z No Device** | **Z No Qualifier** |
| **N Upper Eyelid, Right**<br>Lateral canthus<br>Levator palpebrae superioris muscle<br>Orbicularis oculi muscle<br>Superior tarsal plate<br>**P Upper Eyelid, Left**<br>*See N Upper Eyelid, Right*<br>**Q Lower Eyelid, Right**<br>Inferior tarsal plate<br>Medial canthus<br>**R Lower Eyelid, Left**<br>*See Q Lower Eyelid, Right* | **Ø Open**<br>**X External** | **Z No Device** | **Z No Qualifier** |
| **X Lacrimal Duct, Right**<br>Lacrimal canaliculus<br>Lacrimal punctum<br>Lacrimal sac<br>Nasolacrimal duct<br>**Y Lacrimal Duct, Left**<br>*See X Lacrimal Duct, Right* | **Ø Open**<br>**3 Percutaneous**<br>**7 Via Natural or Artificial Opening**<br>**8 Via Natural or Artificial Opening Endoscopic** | **Z No Device** | **Z No Qualifier** |

**Ø Medical and Surgical**
**8 Eye**
**U Supplement**

Definition: Putting in or on biological or synthetic material that physically reinforces and/or augments the function of a portion of a body part

Explanation: The biological material is non-living, or is living and from the same individual. The body part may have been previously replaced, and the SUPPLEMENT procedure is performed to physically reinforce and/or augment the function of the replaced body part.

| Body Part Character 4 | Approach Character 5 | Device Character 6 | Qualifier Character 7 |
|---|---|---|---|
| **Ø Eye, Right**<br>Ciliary body<br>Posterior chamber<br>**1 Eye, Left**<br>*See Ø Eye, Right*<br>**C Iris, Right**<br>**D Iris, Left**<br>**E Retina, Right**<br>Fovea<br>Macula<br>Optic disc<br>**F Retina, Left**<br>*See E Retina, Right*<br>**G Retinal Vessel, Right**<br>**H Retinal Vessel, Left**<br>**L Extraocular Muscle, Right**<br>Inferior oblique muscle<br>Inferior rectus muscle<br>Lateral rectus muscle<br>Medial rectus muscle<br>Superior oblique muscle<br>Superior rectus muscle<br>**M Extraocular Muscle, Left**<br>*See L Extraocular Muscle, Right* | **Ø Open**<br>**3 Percutaneous** | **7 Autologous Tissue Substitute**<br>**J Synthetic Substitute**<br>**K Nonautologous Tissue Substitute** | **Z No Qualifier** |
| **8 Cornea, Right** NC<br>**9 Cornea, Left** NC<br>**N Upper Eyelid, Right**<br>Lateral canthus<br>Levator palpebrae superioris muscle<br>Orbicularis oculi muscle<br>Superior tarsal plate<br>**P Upper Eyelid, Left**<br>*See N Upper Eyelid, Right*<br>**Q Lower Eyelid, Right**<br>Inferior tarsal plate<br>Medial canthus<br>**R Lower Eyelid, Left**<br>*See Q Lower Eyelid, Right* | **Ø Open**<br>**3 Percutaneous**<br>**X External** | **7 Autologous Tissue Substitute**<br>**J Synthetic Substitute**<br>**K Nonautologous Tissue Substitute** | **Z No Qualifier** |
| **X Lacrimal Duct, Right**<br>Lacrimal canaliculus<br>Lacrimal punctum<br>Lacrimal sac<br>Nasolacrimal duct<br>**Y Lacrimal Duct, Left**<br>*See X Lacrimal Duct, Right* | **Ø Open**<br>**3 Percutaneous**<br>**7 Via Natural or Artificial Opening**<br>**8 Via Natural or Artificial Opening Endoscopic** | **7 Autologous Tissue Substitute**<br>**J Synthetic Substitute**<br>**K Nonautologous Tissue Substitute** | **Z No Qualifier** |

NC Ø8U[8,9][Ø,3,X]KZ

**Ø Medical and Surgical**
**8 Eye**
**V Restriction**

Definition: Partially closing an orifice or the lumen of a tubular body part

Explanation: The orifice can be a natural orifice or an artificially created orifice

| Body Part Character 4 | Approach Character 5 | Device Character 6 | Qualifier Character 7 |
|---|---|---|---|
| **X Lacrimal Duct, Right**<br>Lacrimal canaliculus<br>Lacrimal punctum<br>Lacrimal sac<br>Nasolacrimal duct<br>**Y Lacrimal Duct, Left**<br>*See X Lacrimal Duct, Right* | **Ø Open**<br>**3 Percutaneous** | **C Extraluminal Device**<br>**D Intraluminal Device**<br>**Z No Device** | **Z No Qualifier** |
| **X Lacrimal Duct, Right**<br>Lacrimal canaliculus<br>Lacrimal punctum<br>Lacrimal sac<br>Nasolacrimal duct<br>**Y Lacrimal Duct, Left**<br>*See X Lacrimal Duct, Right* | **7 Via Natural or Artificial Opening**<br>**8 Via Natural or Artificial Opening Endoscopic** | **D Intraluminal Device**<br>**Z No Device** | **Z No Qualifier** |

**Ø Medical and Surgical**
**8 Eye**
**W Revision**

Definition: Correcting, to the extent possible, a portion of a malfunctioning device or the position of a displaced device

Explanation: Revision can include correcting a malfunctioning or displaced device by taking out or putting in components of the device such as a screw or pin

| Body Part Character 4 | Approach Character 5 | Device Character 6 | Qualifier Character 7 |
|---|---|---|---|
| **Ø Eye, Right**<br>Ciliary body<br>Posterior chamber<br>**1 Eye, Left**<br>*See Ø Eye, Right* | **Ø Open**<br>**3 Percutaneous**<br>**7 Via Natural or Artificial Opening**<br>**8 Via Natural or Artificial Opening Endoscopic** | **Ø Drainage Device**<br>**3 Infusion Device**<br>**7 Autologous Tissue Substitute**<br>**C Extraluminal Device**<br>**D Intraluminal Device**<br>**J Synthetic Substitute**<br>**K Nonautologous Tissue Substitute**<br>Y Other Device | **Z No Qualifier** |
| **Ø Eye, Right**<br>Ciliary body<br>Posterior chamber<br>**1 Eye, Left**<br>*See Ø Eye, Right* | **X External** | **Ø Drainage Device**<br>**3 Infusion Device**<br>**7 Autologous Tissue Substitute**<br>**C Extraluminal Device**<br>**D Intraluminal Device**<br>**J Synthetic Substitute**<br>**K Nonautologous Tissue Substitute** | **Z No Qualifier** |
| **J Lens, Right**<br>Zonule of Zinn<br>**K Lens, Left**<br>*See J Lens, Right* | **3 Percutaneous** | **J Synthetic Substitute**<br>Y Other Device | **Z No Qualifier** |
| **J Lens, Right**<br>Zonule of Zinn<br>**K Lens, Left**<br>*See J Lens, Right* | **X External** | **J Synthetic Substitute** | **Z No Qualifier** |
| **L Extraocular Muscle, Right**<br>Inferior oblique muscle<br>Inferior rectus muscle<br>Lateral rectus muscle<br>Medial rectus muscle<br>Superior oblique muscle<br>Superior rectus muscle<br>**M Extraocular Muscle, Left**<br>*See L Extraocular Muscle, Right* | **Ø Open**<br>**3 Percutaneous** | **Ø Drainage Device**<br>**7 Autologous Tissue Substitute**<br>**J Synthetic Substitute**<br>**K Nonautologous Tissue Substitute**<br>Y Other Device | **Z No Qualifier** |

**Non-OR** Ø8W[Ø,1][3,7,8]YZ
**Non-OR** Ø8W[Ø,1]X[Ø,3,7,C,D,J,K]Z
**Non-OR** Ø8W[J,K]3YZ
**Non-OR** Ø8W[J,K]XJZ
**Non-OR** Ø8W[L,M]3YZ

**Ø Medical and Surgical**
**8 Eye**
**X Transfer**

Definition: Moving, without taking out, all or a portion of a body part to another location to take over the function of all or a portion of a body part

Explanation: The body part transferred remains connected to its vascular and nervous supply

| Body Part Character 4 | Approach Character 5 | Device Character 6 | Qualifier Character 7 |
|---|---|---|---|
| **L Extraocular Muscle, Right**<br>Inferior oblique muscle<br>Inferior rectus muscle<br>Lateral rectus muscle<br>Medial rectus muscle<br>Superior oblique muscle<br>Superior rectus muscle<br>**M Extraocular Muscle, Left**<br>*See L Extraocular Muscle, Right* | **Ø Open**<br>**3 Percutaneous** | **Z No Device** | **Z No Qualifier** |

# Ear, Nose, Sinus Ø9Ø–Ø9W



## Character Meanings*

This Character Meaning table is provided as a guide to assist the user in the identification of character members that may be found in this section of code tables. It **SHOULD NOT** be used to build a PCS code.

| Operation–Character 3 | | Body Part–Character 4 | | Approach–Character 5 | | Device–Character 6 | | Qualifier–Character 7 | |
|---|---|---|---|---|---|---|---|---|---|
| Ø | Alteration | Ø | External Ear, Right | Ø | Open | Ø | Drainage Device | Ø | Endolymphatic |
| 1 | Bypass | 1 | External Ear, Left | 3 | Percutaneous | 4 | Hearing Device, Bone Conduction | X | Diagnostic |
| 2 | Change | 2 | External Ear, Bilateral | 4 | Percutaneous Endoscopic | 5 | Hearing Device, Single Channel Cochlear Prosthesis | Z | No Qualifier |
| 5 | Destruction | 3 | External Auditory Canal, Right | 7 | Via Natural or Artificial Opening | 6 | Hearing Device, Multiple Channel Cochlear Prosthesis | | |
| 7 | Dilation | 4 | External Auditory Canal, Left | 8 | Via Natural or Artificial Opening Endoscopic | 7 | Autologous Tissue Substitute | | |
| 8 | Division | 5 | Middle Ear, Right | X | External | B | Intraluminal Device, Airway | | |
| 9 | Drainage | 6 | Middle Ear, Left | | | D | Intraluminal Device | | |
| B | Excision | 7 | Tympanic Membrane, Right | | | J | Synthetic Substitute | | |
| C | Extirpation | 8 | Tympanic Membrane, Left | | | K | Nonautologous Tissue Substitute | | |
| D | Extraction | 9 | Auditory Ossicle, Right | | | S | Hearing Device | | |
| H | Insertion | A | Auditory Ossicle, Left | | | Y | Other Device | | |
| J | Inspection | B | Mastoid Sinus, Right | | | Z | No Device | | |
| M | Reattachment | C | Mastoid Sinus, Left | | | | | | |
| N | Release | D | Inner Ear, Right | | | | | | |
| P | Removal | E | Inner Ear, Left | | | | | | |
| Q | Repair | F | Eustachian Tube, Right | | | | | | |
| R | Replacement | G | Eustachian Tube, Left | | | | | | |
| S | Reposition | H | Ear, Right | | | | | | |
| T | Resection | J | Ear, Left | | | | | | |
| U | Supplement | K | Nasal Mucosa and Soft Tissue | | | | | | |
| W | Revision | L | Nasal Turbinate | | | | | | |
| | | M | Nasal Septum | | | | | | |
| | | N | Nasopharynx | | | | | | |
| | | P | Accessory Sinus | | | | | | |
| | | Q | Maxillary Sinus, Right | | | | | | |
| | | R | Maxillary Sinus, Left | | | | | | |
| | | S | Frontal Sinus, Right | | | | | | |
| | | T | Frontal Sinus, Left | | | | | | |
| | | U | Ethmoid Sinus, Right | | | | | | |
| | | V | Ethmoid Sinus, Left | | | | | | |
| | | W | Sphenoid Sinus, Right | | | | | | |
| | | X | Sphenoid Sinus, Left | | | | | | |
| | | Y | Sinus | | | | | | |

* Includes sinus ducts.

**AHA Coding Clinic for table Ø9Q**

**2014, 4Q, 20** Control of epistaxis
**2014, 3Q, 22** Transsphenoidal removal of pituitary tumor and fat graft placement
**2013, 4Q, 114** Balloon sinuplasty

## Ear Anatomy

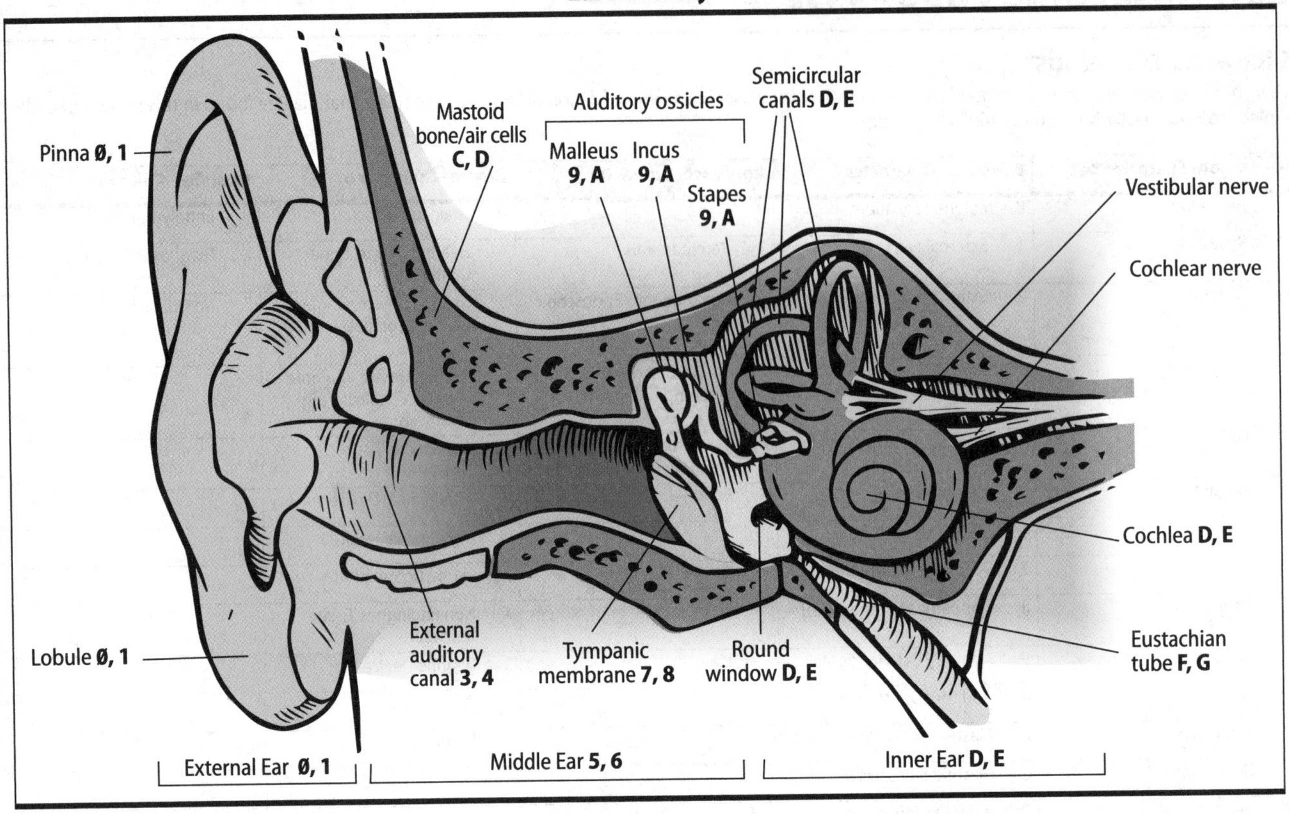
Pinna Ø, 1
Mastoid bone/air cells C, D
Auditory ossicles
Malleus 9, A
Incus 9, A
Stapes 9, A
Semicircular canals D, E
Vestibular nerve
Cochlear nerve
Cochlea D, E
Eustachian tube F, G
Round window D, E
Tympanic membrane 7, 8
External auditory canal 3, 4
Lobule Ø, 1
External Ear Ø, 1
Middle Ear 5, 6
Inner Ear D, E

## Nasal Turbinates

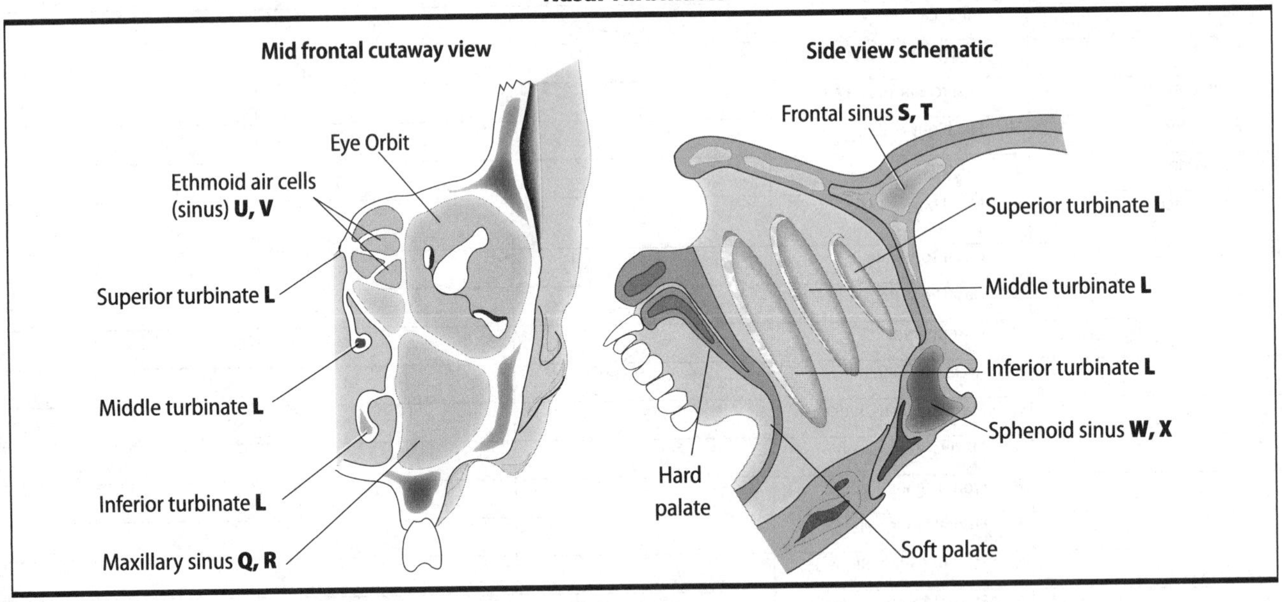
Mid frontal cutaway view
Eye Orbit
Ethmoid air cells (sinus) U, V
Superior turbinate L
Middle turbinate L
Inferior turbinate L
Maxillary sinus Q, R
Side view schematic
Frontal sinus S, T
Superior turbinate L
Middle turbinate L
Inferior turbinate L
Sphenoid sinus W, X
Hard palate
Soft palate

## Paranasal Sinuses

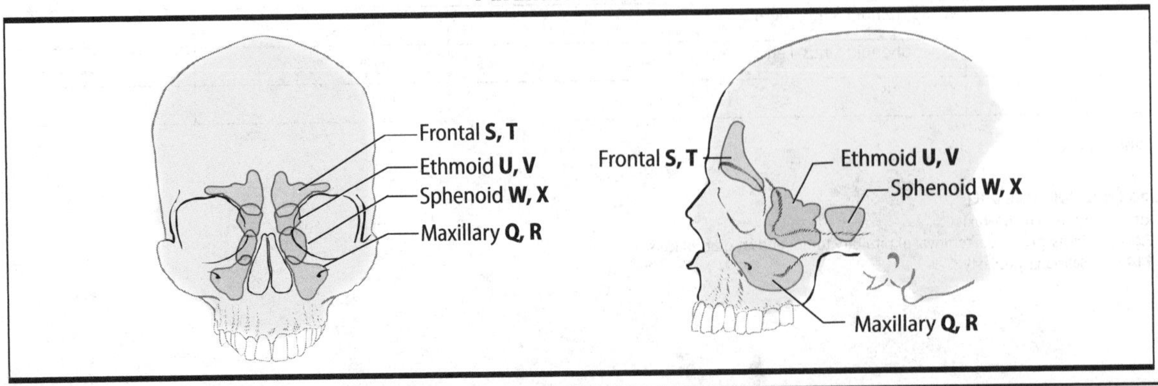
Frontal S, T
Ethmoid U, V
Sphenoid W, X
Maxillary Q, R
Frontal S, T
Ethmoid U, V
Sphenoid W, X
Maxillary Q, R

**Ø Medical and Surgical**
**9 Ear, Nose, Sinus**
**Ø Alteration** Definition: Modifying the anatomic structure of a body part without affecting the function of the body part
Explanation: Principal purpose is to improve appearance

| Body Part Character 4 | Approach Character 5 | Device Character 6 | Qualifier Character 7 |
|---|---|---|---|
| **Ø External Ear, Right**<br>Antihelix<br>Antitragus<br>Auricle<br>Earlobe<br>Helix<br>Pinna<br>Tragus<br>**1 External Ear, Left**<br>*See Ø External Ear, Right*<br>**2 External Ear, Bilateral**<br>*See Ø External Ear, Right*<br>K Nasal Mucosa and Soft Tissue<br>Columella<br>External naris<br>Greater alar cartilage<br>Internal naris<br>Lateral nasal cartilage<br>Lesser alar cartilage<br>Nasal cavity<br>Nostril | **Ø Open**<br>**3 Percutaneous**<br>**4 Percutaneous Endoscopic**<br>**X External** | **7 Autologous Tissue Substitute**<br>**J Synthetic Substitute**<br>**K Nonautologous Tissue Substitute**<br>**Z No Device** | **Z No Qualifier** |

**Ø Medical and Surgical**
**9 Ear, Nose, Sinus**
**1 Bypass** Definition: Altering the route of passage of the contents of a tubular body part
Explanation: Rerouting contents of a body part to a downstream area of the normal route, to a similar route and body part, or to an abnormal route and dissimilar body part. Includes one or more anastomoses, with or without the use of a device.

| Body Part Character 4 | Approach Character 5 | Device Character 6 | Qualifier Character 7 |
|---|---|---|---|
| **D Inner Ear, Right**<br>Bony labyrinth<br>Bony vestibule<br>Cochlea<br>Round window<br>Semicircular canal<br>**E Inner Ear, Left**<br>*See D Inner Ear, Right* | **Ø Open** | **7 Autologous Tissue Substitute**<br>**J Synthetic Substitute**<br>**K Nonautologous Tissue Substitute**<br>**Z No Device** | **Ø Endolymphatic** |

**Ø Medical and Surgical**
**9 Ear, Nose, Sinus**
**2 Change** Definition: Taking out or off a device from a body part and putting back an identical or similar device in or on the same body part without cutting or puncturing the skin or a mucous membrane
Explanation: All CHANGE procedures are coded using the approach EXTERNAL

| Body Part Character 4 | Approach Character 5 | Device Character 6 | Qualifier Character 7 |
|---|---|---|---|
| **H Ear, Right**<br>**J Ear, Left**<br>K Nasal Mucosa and Soft Tissue<br>Columella<br>External naris<br>Greater alar cartilage<br>Internal naris<br>Lateral nasal cartilage<br>Lesser alar cartilage<br>Nasal cavity<br>Nostril<br>**Y Sinus** | **X External** | **Ø Drainage Device**<br>**Y Other Device** | **Z No Qualifier** |

**Non-OR** All body part, approach, device, and qualifier values

Ear, Nose, Sinus

090–092

**Ø Medical and Surgical**
**9 Ear, Nose, Sinus**
**5 Destruction** Definition: Physical eradication of all or a portion of a body part by the direct use of energy, force, or a destructive agent
Explanation: None of the body part is physically taken out

| Body Part Character 4 | | Approach Character 5 | Device Character 6 | Qualifier Character 7 |
|---|---|---|---|---|
| **Ø External Ear, Right**<br>Antihelix<br>Antitragus<br>Auricle<br>Earlobe<br>Helix<br>Pinna<br>Tragus | **1 External Ear, Left**<br>*See Ø External Ear, Right* | **Ø Open**<br>**3 Percutaneous**<br>**4 Percutaneous Endoscopic**<br>**X External** | **Z No Device** | **Z No Qualifier** |
| **3 External Auditory Canal, Right**<br>External auditory meatus | **4 External Auditory Canal, Left**<br>*See 3 External Auditory Canal, Right* | **Ø Open**<br>**3 Percutaneous**<br>**4 Percutaneous Endoscopic**<br>**7 Via Natural or Artificial Opening**<br>**8 Via Natural or Artificial Opening Endoscopic**<br>**X External** | **Z No Device** | **Z No Qualifier** |
| **5 Middle Ear, Right**<br>Oval window<br>Tympanic cavity<br>**6 Middle Ear, Left**<br>*See 5 Middle Ear, Right*<br>**9 Auditory Ossicle, Right**<br>Incus<br>Malleus<br>Stapes<br>**A Auditory Ossicle, Left**<br>*See 9 Auditory Ossicle, Right* | **D Inner Ear, Right**<br>Bony labyrinth<br>Bony vestibule<br>Cochlea<br>Round window<br>Semicircular canal<br>**E Inner Ear, Left**<br>*See D Inner Ear, Right* | **Ø Open**<br>**8 Via Natural or Artificial Opening Endoscopic** | **Z No Device** | **Z No Qualifier** |
| **7 Tympanic Membrane, Right**<br>Pars flaccida<br>**8 Tympanic Membrane, Left**<br>*See 7 Tympanic Membrane, Right*<br>**F Eustachian Tube, Right**<br>Auditory tube<br>Pharyngotympanic tube<br>**G Eustachian Tube, Left**<br>*See F Eustachian Tube, Right* | **L Nasal Turbinate**<br>Inferior turbinate<br>Middle turbinate<br>Nasal concha<br>Superior turbinate<br>**N Nasopharynx**<br>Choana<br>Fossa of Rosenmuller<br>Pharyngeal recess<br>Rhinopharynx | **Ø Open**<br>**3 Percutaneous**<br>**4 Percutaneous Endoscopic**<br>**7 Via Natural or Artificial Opening**<br>**8 Via Natural or Artificial Opening Endoscopic** | **Z No Device** | **Z No Qualifier** |
| **B Mastoid Sinus, Right**<br>Mastoid air cells<br>**C Mastoid Sinus, Left**<br>*See B Mastoid Sinus, Right*<br>**M Nasal Septum**<br>Quadrangular cartilage<br>Septal cartilage<br>Vomer bone<br>**P Accessory Sinus**<br>**Q Maxillary Sinus, Right**<br>Antrum of Highmore | **R Maxillary Sinus, Left**<br>*See Q Maxillary Sinus, Right*<br>**S Frontal Sinus, Right**<br>**T Frontal Sinus, Left**<br>**U Ethmoid Sinus, Right**<br>Ethmoidal air cell<br>**V Ethmoid Sinus, Left**<br>*See U Ethmoid Sinus, Right*<br>**W Sphenoid Sinus, Right**<br>**X Sphenoid Sinus, Left** | **Ø Open**<br>**3 Percutaneous**<br>**4 Percutaneous Endoscopic**<br>**8 Via Natural or Artificial Opening Endoscopic** | **Z No Device** | **Z No Qualifier** |
| **K Nasal Mucosa and Soft Tissue**<br>Columella<br>External naris<br>Greater alar cartilage<br>Internal naris<br>Lateral nasal cartilage<br>Lesser alar cartilage<br>Nasal cavity<br>Nostril | | **Ø Open**<br>**3 Percutaneous**<br>**4 Percutaneous Endoscopic**<br>**8 Via Natural or Artificial Opening Endoscopic**<br>**X External** | **Z No Device** | **Z No Qualifier** |

**Non-OR** Ø95[Ø,1][Ø,3,4,X]ZZ
**Non-OR** Ø95[3,4][Ø,3,4,7,8,X]ZZ
**Non-OR** Ø95[F,G][Ø,3,4,7,8]ZZ
**Non-OR** Ø95M[Ø,3,4,8]ZZ
**Non-OR** Ø95K[Ø,3,4,8,X]ZZ

**Ø Medical and Surgical**
**9 Ear, Nose, Sinus**
**7 Dilation** Definition: Expanding an orifice or the lumen of a tubular body part

Explanation: The orifice can be a natural orifice or an artificially created orifice. Accomplished by stretching a tubular body part using intraluminal pressure or by cutting part of the orifice or wall of the tubular body part.

| Body Part Character 4 | Approach Character 5 | Device Character 6 | Qualifier Character 7 |
|---|---|---|---|
| **F** Eustachian Tube, Right<br>Auditory tube<br>Pharyngotympanic tube<br>**G** Eustachian Tube, Left<br>*See F Eustachian Tube, Right* | **Ø** Open<br>**7** Via Natural or Artificial Opening<br>**8** Via Natural or Artificial Opening Endoscopic | **D** Intraluminal Device<br>**Z** No Device | **Z** No Qualifier |
| **F** Eustachian Tube, Right<br>Auditory tube<br>Pharyngotympanic tube<br>**G** Eustachian Tube, Left<br>*See F Eustachian Tube, Right* | **3** Percutaneous<br>**4** Percutaneous Endoscopic | **Z** No Device | **Z** No Qualifier |

Non-OR All body part, approach, device, and qualifier values

**Ø Medical and Surgical**
**9 Ear, Nose, Sinus**
**8 Division** Definition: Cutting into a body part, without draining fluids and/or gases from the body part, in order to separate or transect a body part

Explanation: All or a portion of the body part is separated into two or more portions

| Body Part Character 4 | Approach Character 5 | Device Character 6 | Qualifier Character 7 |
|---|---|---|---|
| **L** Nasal Turbinate<br>Inferior turbinate<br>Middle turbinate<br>Nasal concha<br>Superior turbinate | **Ø** Open<br>**3** Percutaneous<br>**4** Percutaneous Endoscopic<br>**7** Via Natural or Artificial Opening<br>**8** Via Natural or Artificial Opening Endoscopic | **Z** No Device | **Z** No Qualifier |

**Ø Medical and Surgical**
**9 Ear, Nose, Sinus**
**9 Drainage** Definition: Taking or letting out fluids and/or gases from a body part
Explanation: The qualifier DIAGNOSTIC is used to identify drainage procedures that are biopsies

| Body Part Character 4 | | Approach Character 5 | Device Character 6 | Qualifier Character 7 |
|---|---|---|---|---|
| **Ø External Ear, Right**<br>Antihelix<br>Antitragus<br>Auricle<br>Earlobe<br>Helix<br>Pinna<br>Tragus | **1 External Ear, Left**<br>*See Ø External Ear, Right* | **Ø Open**<br>**3 Percutaneous**<br>**4 Percutaneous Endoscopic**<br>**X External** | **Ø Drainage Device** | **Z No Qualifier** |
| **Ø External Ear, Right**<br>Antihelix<br>Antitragus<br>Auricle<br>Earlobe<br>Helix<br>Pinna<br>Tragus | **1 External Ear, Left**<br>*See Ø External Ear, Right* | **Ø Open**<br>**3 Percutaneous**<br>**4 Percutaneous Endoscopic**<br>**X External** | **Z No Device** | **X Diagnostic**<br>**Z No Qualifier** |
| **3 External Auditory Canal, Right**<br>External auditory meatus<br>**4 External Auditory Canal, Left**<br>*See 3 External Auditory Canal, Right* | **K Nasal Mucosa and Soft Tissue**<br>Columella<br>External naris<br>Greater alar cartilage<br>Internal naris<br>Lateral nasal cartilage<br>Lesser alar cartilage<br>Nasal cavity<br>Nostril | **Ø Open**<br>**3 Percutaneous**<br>**4 Percutaneous Endoscopic**<br>**7 Via Natural or Artificial Opening**<br>**8 Via Natural or Artificial Opening Endoscopic**<br>**X External** | **Ø Drainage Device** | **Z No Qualifier** |
| **3 External Auditory Canal, Right**<br>External auditory meatus<br>**4 External Auditory Canal, Left**<br>*See 3 External Auditory Canal, Right* | **K Nasal Mucosa and Soft Tissue**<br>Columella<br>External naris<br>Greater alar cartilage<br>Internal naris<br>Lateral nasal cartilage<br>Lesser alar cartilage<br>Nasal cavity<br>Nostril | **Ø Open**<br>**3 Percutaneous**<br>**4 Percutaneous Endoscopic**<br>**7 Via Natural or Artificial Opening**<br>**8 Via Natural or Artificial Opening Endoscopic**<br>**X External** | **Z No Device** | **X Diagnostic**<br>**Z No Qualifier** |
| **5 Middle Ear, Right**<br>Oval window<br>Tympanic cavity<br>**6 Middle Ear, Left**<br>*See 5 Middle Ear, Right*<br>**9 Auditory Ossicle, Right**<br>Incus<br>Malleus<br>Stapes | **A Auditory Ossicle, Left**<br>*See 9 Auditory Ossicle, Right*<br>**D Inner Ear, Right**<br>Bony labyrinth<br>Bony vestibule<br>Cochlea<br>Round window<br>Semicircular canal<br>**E Inner Ear, Left**<br>*See D Inner Ear, Right* | **Ø Open**<br>**7 Via Natural or Artificial Opening**<br>**8 Via Natural or Artificial Opening Endoscopic** | **Ø Drainage Device** | **Z No Qualifier** |
| **5 Middle Ear, Right**<br>Oval window<br>Tympanic cavity<br>**6 Middle Ear, Left**<br>*See 5 Middle Ear, Right*<br>**9 Auditory Ossicle, Right**<br>Incus<br>Malleus<br>Stapes | **A Auditory Ossicle, Left**<br>*See 9 Auditory Ossicle, Right*<br>**D Inner Ear, Right**<br>Bony labyrinth<br>Bony vestibule<br>Cochlea<br>Round window<br>Semicircular canal<br>**E Inner Ear, Left**<br>*See D Inner Ear, Right* | **Ø Open**<br>**7 Via Natural or Artificial Opening**<br>**8 Via Natural or Artificial Opening Endoscopic** | **Z No Device** | **X Diagnostic**<br>**Z No Qualifier** |

***Ø99 Continued on next page***

**Non-OR** Ø99[Ø,1][Ø,3,4,X]ØZ
**Non-OR** Ø99[Ø,1][Ø,3,4,X]Z[X,Z]
**Non-OR** Ø99[3,4,K][Ø,3,4,7,8,X]ØZ
**Non-OR** Ø99[3,4,K][Ø,3,4,7,8,X]Z[X,Z]
**Non-OR** Ø9958ØZ
**Non-OR** Ø99[6,9,A,D,E][7,8]ØZ
**Non-OR** Ø99[5,6]ØZZ
**Non-OR** Ø99[5,6,9,A,D,E][7,8]Z[X,Z]

**Ø Medical and Surgical**
**9 Ear, Nose, Sinus**
**9 Drainage** Definition: Taking or letting out fluids and/or gases from a body part
Explanation: The qualifier DIAGNOSTIC is used to identify drainage procedures that are biopsies

*Ø99 Continued*

| Body Part Character 4 | | Approach Character 5 | Device Character 6 | Qualifier Character 7 |
|---|---|---|---|---|
| **7 Tympanic Membrane, Right**<br>Pars flaccida<br>**8 Tympanic Membrane, Left**<br>*See 7 Tympanic Membrane, Right*<br>**B Mastoid Sinus, Right**<br>Mastoid air cells<br>**C Mastoid Sinus, Left**<br>*See B Mastoid Sinus, Right*<br>**F Eustachian Tube, Right**<br>Auditory tube<br>Pharyngotympanic tube<br>**G Eustachian Tube, Left**<br>*See F Eustachian Tube, Right*<br>**L Nasal Turbinate**<br>Inferior turbinate<br>Middle turbinate<br>Nasal concha<br>Superior turbinate<br>**M Nasal Septum**<br>Quadrangular cartilage<br>Septal cartilage<br>Vomer bone | **N Nasopharynx**<br>Choana<br>Fossa of Rosenmuller<br>Pharyngeal recess<br>Rhinopharynx<br>**P Accessory Sinus**<br>**Q Maxillary Sinus, Right**<br>Antrum of Highmore<br>**R Maxillary Sinus, Left**<br>*See Q Maxillary Sinus, Right*<br>**S Frontal Sinus, Right**<br>**T Frontal Sinus, Left**<br>**U Ethmoid Sinus, Right**<br>Ethmoidal air cell<br>**V Ethmoid Sinus, Left**<br>*See U Ethmoid Sinus, Right*<br>**W Sphenoid Sinus, Right**<br>**X Sphenoid Sinus, Left** | **Ø Open**<br>**3 Percutaneous**<br>**4 Percutaneous Endoscopic**<br>**7 Via Natural or Artificial Opening**<br>**8 Via Natural or Artificial Opening Endoscopic** | **Ø Drainage Device** | **Z No Qualifier** |
| **7 Tympanic Membrane, Right**<br>Pars flaccida<br>**8 Tympanic Membrane, Left**<br>*See 7 Tympanic Membrane, Right*<br>**B Mastoid Sinus, Right**<br>Mastoid air cells<br>**C Mastoid Sinus, Left**<br>*See B Mastoid Sinus, Right*<br>**F Eustachian Tube, Right**<br>Auditory tube<br>Pharyngotympanic tube<br>**G Eustachian Tube, Left**<br>*See F Eustachian Tube, Right*<br>**L Nasal Turbinate**<br>Inferior turbinate<br>Middle turbinate<br>Nasal concha<br>Superior turbinate<br>**M Nasal Septum**<br>Quadrangular cartilage<br>Septal cartilage<br>Vomer bone | **N Nasopharynx**<br>Choana<br>Fossa of Rosenmuller<br>Pharyngeal recess<br>Rhinopharynx<br>**P Accessory Sinus**<br>**Q Maxillary Sinus, Right**<br>Antrum of Highmore<br>**R Maxillary Sinus, Left**<br>*See Q Maxillary Sinus, Right*<br>**S Frontal Sinus, Right**<br>**T Frontal Sinus, Left**<br>**U Ethmoid Sinus, Right**<br>Ethmoidal air cell<br>**V Ethmoid Sinus, Left**<br>*See U Ethmoid Sinus, Right*<br>**W Sphenoid Sinus, Right**<br>**X Sphenoid Sinus, Left** | **Ø Open**<br>**3 Percutaneous**<br>**4 Percutaneous Endoscopic**<br>**7 Via Natural or Artificial Opening**<br>**8 Via Natural or Artificial Opening Endoscopic** | **Z No Device** | **X Diagnostic**<br>**Z No Qualifier** |

**Non-OR** Ø99[B,C][3,7,8]ØZ
**Non-OR** Ø99[F,G,L,M][Ø,3,4,7,8]ØZ
**Non-OR** Ø99N3ØZ
**Non-OR** Ø99[P,Q,R,S,T,U,V,W,X][3,4,7,8]ØZ
**Non-OR** Ø99[7,8][Ø,3,4,7,8]ZZ
**Non-OR** Ø99[7,8][7,8]ZX
**Non-OR** Ø99[B,C]3ZZ
**Non-OR** Ø99[B,C][7,8]Z[X,Z]
**Non-OR** Ø99[F,G][Ø,3,4,7,8]ZZ
**Non-OR** Ø99[F,G][7,8]ZX
**Non-OR** Ø99[L,M][Ø,3,4,7,8]Z[X,Z]
**Non-OR** Ø99N[Ø,3,4,7,8]ZX
**Non-OR** Ø99N3ZZ
**Non-OR** Ø99[P,Q,R,S,T,U,V,W,X][3,4,7,8]Z[X,Z]

**Ø Medical and Surgical**
**9 Ear, Nose, Sinus**
**B Excision** Definition: Cutting out or off, without replacement, a portion of a body part

Explanation: The qualifier DIAGNOSTIC is used to identify excision procedures that are biopsies

| Body Part Character 4 | | Approach Character 5 | Device Character 6 | Qualifier Character 7 |
|---|---|---|---|---|
| **Ø External Ear, Right**<br>Antihelix<br>Antitragus<br>Auricle<br>Earlobe<br>Helix<br>Pinna<br>Tragus | **1 External Ear, Left**<br>*See Ø External Ear, Right* | **Ø Open**<br>**3 Percutaneous**<br>**4 Percutaneous Endoscopic**<br>**X External** | **Z No Device** | **X Diagnostic**<br>**Z No Qualifier** |
| **3 External Auditory Canal, Right**<br>External auditory meatus | **4 External Auditory Canal, Left**<br>*See 3 External Auditory Canal, Right* | **Ø Open**<br>**3 Percutaneous**<br>**4 Percutaneous Endoscopic**<br>**7 Via Natural or Artificial Opening**<br>**8 Via Natural or Artificial Opening Endoscopic**<br>**X External** | **Z No Device** | **X Diagnostic**<br>**Z No Qualifier** |
| **5 Middle Ear, Right**<br>Oval window<br>Tympanic cavity<br>**6 Middle Ear, Left**<br>*See 5 Middle Ear, Right*<br>**9 Auditory Ossicle, Right**<br>Incus<br>Malleus<br>Stapes | **A Auditory Ossicle, Left**<br>*See 9 Auditory Ossicle, Right*<br>**D Inner Ear, Right**<br>Bony labyrinth<br>Bony vestibule<br>Cochlea<br>Round window<br>Semicircular canal<br>**E Inner Ear, Left**<br>*See D Inner Ear, Right* | **Ø Open**<br>8 Via Natural or Artificial Opening Endoscopic | **Z No Device** | **X Diagnostic**<br>**Z No Qualifier** |
| **7 Tympanic Membrane, Right**<br>Pars flaccida<br>**8 Tympanic Membrane, Left**<br>*See 7 Tympanic Membrane, Right*<br>**F Eustachian Tube, Right**<br>Auditory tube<br>Pharyngotympanic tube<br>**G Eustachian Tube, Left**<br>*See F Eustachian Tube, Right* | **L Nasal Turbinate**<br>Inferior turbinate<br>Middle turbinate<br>Nasal concha<br>Superior turbinate<br>**N Nasopharynx**<br>Choana<br>Fossa of Rosenmuller<br>Pharyngeal recess<br>Rhinopharynx | **Ø Open**<br>**3 Percutaneous**<br>**4 Percutaneous Endoscopic**<br>**7 Via Natural or Artificial Opening**<br>**8 Via Natural or Artificial Opening Endoscopic** | **Z No Device** | **X Diagnostic**<br>**Z No Qualifier** |
| **B Mastoid Sinus, Right**<br>Mastoid air cells<br>**C Mastoid Sinus, Left**<br>*See B Mastoid Sinus, Right*<br>**M Nasal Septum**<br>Quadrangular cartilage<br>Septal cartilage<br>Vomer bone<br>**P Accessory Sinus**<br>**Q Maxillary Sinus, Right**<br>Antrum of Highmore | **R Maxillary Sinus, Left**<br>*See Q Maxillary Sinus, Right*<br>**S Frontal Sinus, Right**<br>**T Frontal Sinus, Left**<br>**U Ethmoid Sinus, Right**<br>Ethmoidal air cell<br>**V Ethmoid Sinus, Left**<br>*See U Ethmoid Sinus, Right*<br>**W Sphenoid Sinus, Right**<br>**X Sphenoid Sinus, Left** | **Ø Open**<br>**3 Percutaneous**<br>**4 Percutaneous Endoscopic**<br>8 Via Natural or Artificial Opening Endoscopic | **Z No Device** | **X Diagnostic**<br>**Z No Qualifier** |
| K **Nasal Mucosa and Soft Tissue**<br>Columella<br>External naris<br>Greater alar cartilage<br>Internal naris<br>Lateral nasal cartilage<br>Lesser alar cartilage<br>Nasal cavity<br>Nostril | | **Ø Open**<br>**3 Percutaneous**<br>**4 Percutaneous Endoscopic**<br>8 Via Natural or Artificial Opening Endoscopic<br>**X External** | **Z No Device** | **X Diagnostic**<br>**Z No Qualifier** |

**Non-OR** Ø9B[Ø,1][Ø,3,4,X]Z[X,Z]
**Non-OR** Ø9B[3,4][Ø,3,4,7,8,X]Z[X,Z]
**Non-OR** Ø9B[F,G,L,N][Ø,3,4,7,8]Z[X,Z]
**Non-OR** Ø9BM[Ø,3,4,8]ZX
**Non-OR** Ø9B[P,Q,R,S,T,U,V,W,X][3,4,8]ZX
**Non-OR** Ø9BK8Z[X,Z]

**Ø Medical and Surgical**
**9 Ear, Nose, Sinus**
**C Extirpation** Definition: Taking or cutting out solid matter from a body part

Explanation: The solid matter may be an abnormal byproduct of a biological function or a foreign body; it may be imbedded in a body part or in the lumen of a tubular body part. The solid matter may or may not have been previously broken into pieces.

| Body Part Character 4 | | Approach Character 5 | Device Character 6 | Qualifier Character 7 |
|---|---|---|---|---|
| **Ø External Ear, Right**<br>Antihelix<br>Antitragus<br>Auricle<br>Earlobe<br>Helix<br>Pinna<br>Tragus | **1 External Ear, Left**<br>*See Ø External Ear, Right* | **Ø Open**<br>**3 Percutaneous**<br>**4 Percutaneous Endoscopic**<br>**X External** | **Z No Device** | **Z No Qualifier** |
| **3 External Auditory Canal, Right**<br>External auditory meatus | **4 External Auditory Canal, Left**<br>*See 3 External Auditory Canal, Right* | **Ø Open**<br>**3 Percutaneous**<br>**4 Percutaneous Endoscopic**<br>**7 Via Natural or Artificial Opening**<br>**8 Via Natural or Artificial Opening Endoscopic**<br>**X External** | **Z No Device** | **Z No Qualifier** |
| **5 Middle Ear, Right**<br>Oval window<br>Tympanic cavity<br>**6 Middle Ear, Left**<br>*See 5 Middle Ear, Right*<br>**9 Auditory Ossicle, Right**<br>Incus<br>Malleus<br>Stapes | **A Auditory Ossicle, Left**<br>*See 9 Auditory Ossicle, Right*<br>**D Inner Ear, Right**<br>Bony labyrinth<br>Bony vestibule<br>Cochlea<br>Round window<br>Semicircular canal<br>**E Inner Ear, Left**<br>*See D Inner Ear, Right* | **Ø Open**<br>8 Via Natural or Artificial Opening Endoscopic | **Z No Device** | **Z No Qualifier** |
| **7 Tympanic Membrane, Right**<br>Pars flaccida<br>**8 Tympanic Membrane, Left**<br>*See 7 Tympanic Membrane, Right*<br>**F Eustachian Tube, Right**<br>Auditory tube<br>Pharyngotympanic tube<br>**G Eustachian Tube, Left**<br>*See F Eustachian Tube, Right* | **L Nasal Turbinate**<br>Inferior turbinate<br>Middle turbinate<br>Nasal concha<br>Superior turbinate<br>**N Nasopharynx**<br>Choana<br>Fossa of Rosenmuller<br>Pharyngeal recess<br>Rhinopharynx | **Ø Open**<br>**3 Percutaneous**<br>**4 Percutaneous Endoscopic**<br>**7 Via Natural or Artificial Opening**<br>**8 Via Natural or Artificial Opening Endoscopic** | **Z No Device** | **Z No Qualifier** |
| **B Mastoid Sinus, Right**<br>Mastoid air cells<br>**C Mastoid Sinus, Left**<br>*See B Mastoid Sinus, Right*<br>**M Nasal Septum**<br>Quadrangular cartilage<br>Septal cartilage<br>Vomer bone<br>**P Accessory Sinus**<br>**Q Maxillary Sinus, Right**<br>Antrum of Highmore | **R Maxillary Sinus, Left**<br>*See Q Maxillary Sinus, Right*<br>**S Frontal Sinus, Right**<br>**T Frontal Sinus, Left**<br>**U Ethmoid Sinus, Right**<br>Ethmoidal air cell<br>**V Ethmoid Sinus, Left**<br>*See U Ethmoid Sinus, Right*<br>**W Sphenoid Sinus, Right**<br>**X Sphenoid Sinus, Left** | **Ø Open**<br>**3 Percutaneous**<br>**4 Percutaneous Endoscopic**<br>8 Via Natural or Artificial Opening Endoscopic | **Z No Device** | **Z No Qualifier** |
| K Nasal Mucosa and Soft Tissue<br>Columella<br>External naris<br>Greater alar cartilage<br>Internal naris<br>Lateral nasal cartilage<br>Lesser alar cartilage<br>Nasal cavity<br>Nostril | | **Ø Open**<br>**3 Percutaneous**<br>**4 Percutaneous Endoscopic**<br>8 Via Natural or Artificial Opening Endoscopic<br>**X External** | **Z No Device** | **Z No Qualifier** |

**Non-OR** Ø9C[Ø,1][Ø,3,4,X]ZZ
**Non-OR** Ø9C[3,4][Ø,3,4,7,8,X]ZZ
**Non-OR** Ø9C[7,8,F,G,L][Ø,3,4,7,8]ZZ
**Non-OR** Ø9CM[Ø,3,4,8]ZZ
**Non-OR** Ø9CK8ZZ

**Ø Medical and Surgical**
**9 Ear, Nose, Sinus**
**D Extraction** Definition: Pulling or stripping out or off all or a portion of a body part by the use of force
Explanation: The qualifier DIAGNOSTIC is used to identify extraction procedures that are biopsies

| Body Part Character 4 | Approach Character 5 | Device Character 6 | Qualifier Character 7 |
|---|---|---|---|
| **7 Tympanic Membrane, Right**<br>Pars flaccida<br>**8 Tympanic Membrane, Left**<br>*See 7 Tympanic Membrane, Right*<br>**L Nasal Turbinate**<br>Inferior turbinate<br>Middle turbinate<br>Nasal concha<br>Superior turbinate | **Ø Open**<br>**3 Percutaneous**<br>**4 Percutaneous Endoscopic**<br>**7 Via Natural or Artificial Opening**<br>**8 Via Natural or Artificial Opening Endoscopic** | **Z No Device** | **Z No Qualifier** |
| **9 Auditory Ossicle, Right**<br>Incus<br>Malleus<br>Stapes<br>**A Auditory Ossicle, Left**<br>*See 9 Auditory Ossicle, Right* | **Ø Open** | **Z No Device** | **Z No Qualifier** |
| **B Mastoid Sinus, Right**<br>Mastoid air cells<br>**C Mastoid Sinus, Left**<br>*See B Mastoid Sinus, Right*<br>**M Nasal Septum**<br>Quadrangular cartilage<br>Septal cartilage<br>Vomer bone<br>**P Accessory Sinus**<br>**Q Maxillary Sinus, Right**<br>Antrum of Highmore<br>**R Maxillary Sinus, Left**<br>*See Q Maxillary Sinus, Right*<br>**S Frontal Sinus, Right**<br>**T Frontal Sinus, Left**<br>**U Ethmoid Sinus, Right**<br>Ethmoidal air cell<br>**V Ethmoid Sinus, Left**<br>*See U Ethmoid Sinus, Right*<br>**W Sphenoid Sinus, Right**<br>**X Sphenoid Sinus, Left** | **Ø Open**<br>**3 Percutaneous**<br>**4 Percutaneous Endoscopic** | **Z No Device** | **Z No Qualifier** |

**Ø Medical and Surgical**
**9 Ear, Nose, Sinus**
**H Insertion** Definition: Putting in a nonbiological appliance that monitors, assists, performs, or prevents a physiological function but does not physically take the place of a body part
Explanation: None

| Body Part Character 4 | Approach Character 5 | Device Character 6 | Qualifier Character 7 |
|---|---|---|---|
| **D Inner Ear, Right**<br>Bony labyrinth<br>Bony vestibule<br>Cochlea<br>Round window<br>Semicircular canal<br>**E Inner Ear, Left**<br>*See D Inner Ear, Right* | **Ø Open**<br>**3 Percutaneous**<br>**4 Percutaneous Endoscopic** | **4 Hearing Device, Bone Conduction**<br>**5 Hearing Device, Single Channel Cochlear Prosthesis**<br>**6 Hearing Device, Multiple Channel Cochlear Prosthesis**<br>**S Hearing Device** | **Z No Qualifier** |
| **H Ear, Right**<br>**J Ear, Left**<br>**K Nasal Mucosa and Soft Tissue**<br>Columella<br>External naris<br>Greater alar cartilage<br>Internal naris<br>Lateral nasal cartilage<br>Lesser alar cartilage<br>Nasal cavity<br>Nostril<br>**Y Sinus** | **Ø Open**<br>**3 Percutaneous**<br>**4 Percutaneous Endoscopic**<br>**7 Via Natural or Artificial Opening**<br>**8 Via Natural or Artificial Opening Endoscopic** | **Y Other Device** | **Z No Qualifier** |
| **N Nasopharynx**<br>Choana<br>Fossa of Rosenmuller<br>Pharyngeal recess<br>Rhinopharynx | **7 Via Natural or Artificial Opening**<br>**8 Via Natural or Artificial Opening Endoscopic** | **B Intraluminal Device, Airway** | **Z No Qualifier** |

**Non-OR** Ø9H[H,J][3,4,7,8]YZ
**Non-OR** Ø9H[K,Y][Ø,3,4,7,8]YZ
**Non-OR** Ø9HN[7,8]BZ

**Ø Medical and Surgical**
**9 Ear, Nose, Sinus**
**J Inspection** Definition: Visually and/or manually exploring a body part

Explanation: Visual exploration may be performed with or without optical instrumentation. Manual exploration may be performed directly or through intervening body layers.

| Body Part Character 4 | Approach Character 5 | Device Character 6 | Qualifier Character 7 |
|---|---|---|---|
| **7 Tympanic Membrane, Right**<br>Pars flaccida<br>**8 Tympanic Membrane, Left**<br>*See 7 Tympanic Membrane, Right*<br>**H Ear, Right**<br>**J Ear, Left** | **Ø Open**<br>**3 Percutaneous**<br>**4 Percutaneous Endoscopic**<br>**7 Via Natural or Artificial Opening**<br>**8 Via Natural or Artificial Opening Endoscopic**<br>**X External** | **Z No Device** | **Z No Qualifier** |
| **D Inner Ear, Right**<br>Bony labyrinth<br>Bony vestibule<br>Cochlea<br>Round window<br>Semicircular canal<br>**E Inner Ear, Left**<br>*See D Inner Ear, Right*<br>K Nasal Mucosa and Soft Tissue<br>Columella<br>External naris<br>Greater alar cartilage<br>Internal naris<br>Lateral nasal cartilage<br>Lesser alar cartilage<br>Nasal cavity<br>Nostril<br>**Y Sinus** | **Ø Open**<br>**3 Percutaneous**<br>**4 Percutaneous Endoscopic**<br>8 Via Natural or Artificial Opening Endoscopic<br>**X External** | **Z No Device** | **Z No Qualifier** |

**Non-OR** Ø9J[7,8][3,7,8,X]ZZ
**Non-OR** Ø9J[H,J][Ø,3,4,7,8,X]ZZ
**Non-OR** Ø9J[D,E][3,8,X]ZZ
**Non-OR** Ø9J[K,Y][Ø,3,4,8,X]ZZ

**Ø Medical and Surgical**
**9 Ear, Nose, Sinus**
**M Reattachment** Definition: Putting back in or on all or a portion of a separated body part to its normal location or other suitable location

Explanation: Vascular circulation and nervous pathways may or may not be reestablished

| Body Part Character 4 | Approach Character 5 | Device Character 6 | Qualifier Character 7 |
|---|---|---|---|
| **Ø External Ear, Right**<br>Antihelix<br>Antitragus<br>Auricle<br>Earlobe<br>Helix<br>Pinna<br>Tragus<br>**1 External Ear, Left**<br>*See Ø External Ear, Right*<br>K Nasal Mucosa and Soft Tissue<br>Columella<br>External naris<br>Greater alar cartilage<br>Internal naris<br>Lateral nasal cartilage<br>Lesser alar cartilage<br>Nasal cavity<br>Nostril | **X External** | **Z No Device** | **Z No Qualifier** |

**Ø Medical and Surgical**
**9 Ear, Nose, Sinus**
**N Release**　Definition: Freeing a body part from an abnormal physical constraint by cutting or by the use of force
Explanation: Some of the restraining tissue may be taken out but none of the body part is taken out

| Body Part Character 4 | | Approach Character 5 | Device Character 6 | Qualifier Character 7 |
|---|---|---|---|---|
| **Ø External Ear, Right**<br>Antihelix<br>Antitragus<br>Auricle<br>Earlobe<br>Helix<br>Pinna<br>Tragus | **1 External Ear, Left**<br>*See Ø External Ear, Right* | **Ø Open**<br>**3 Percutaneous**<br>**4 Percutaneous Endoscopic**<br>**X External** | **Z No Device** | **Z No Qualifier** |
| **3 External Auditory Canal, Right**<br>External auditory meatus | **4 External Auditory Canal, Left**<br>*See 3 External Auditory Canal, Right* | **Ø Open**<br>**3 Percutaneous**<br>**4 Percutaneous Endoscopic**<br>**7 Via Natural or Artificial Opening**<br>**8 Via Natural or Artificial Opening Endoscopic**<br>**X External** | **Z No Device** | **Z No Qualifier** |
| **5 Middle Ear, Right**<br>Oval window<br>Tympanic cavity<br>**6 Middle Ear, Left**<br>*See 5 Middle Ear, Right*<br>**9 Auditory Ossicle, Right**<br>Incus<br>Malleus<br>Stapes | **A Auditory Ossicle, Left**<br>*See 9 Auditory Ossicle, Right*<br>**D Inner Ear, Right**<br>Bony labyrinth<br>Bony vestibule<br>Cochlea<br>Round window<br>Semicircular canal<br>**E Inner Ear, Left**<br>*See D Inner Ear, Right* | **Ø Open**<br>**8 Via Natural or Artificial Opening Endoscopic** | **Z No Device** | **Z No Qualifier** |
| **7 Tympanic Membrane, Right**<br>Pars flaccida<br>**8 Tympanic Membrane, Left**<br>*See 7 Tympanic Membrane, Right*<br>**F Eustachian Tube, Right**<br>Auditory tube<br>Pharyngotympanic tube<br>**G Eustachian Tube, Left**<br>*See F Eustachian Tube, Right* | **L Nasal Turbinate**<br>Inferior turbinate<br>Middle turbinate<br>Nasal concha<br>Superior turbinate<br>**N Nasopharynx**<br>Choana<br>Fossa of Rosenmuller<br>Pharyngeal recess<br>Rhinopharynx | **Ø Open**<br>**3 Percutaneous**<br>**4 Percutaneous Endoscopic**<br>**7 Via Natural or Artificial Opening**<br>**8 Via Natural or Artificial Opening Endoscopic** | **Z No Device** | **Z No Qualifier** |
| **B Mastoid Sinus, Right**<br>Mastoid air cells<br>**C Mastoid Sinus, Left**<br>*See B Mastoid Sinus, Right*<br>**M Nasal Septum**<br>Quadrangular cartilage<br>Septal cartilage<br>Vomer bone<br>**P Accessory Sinus**<br>**Q Maxillary Sinus, Right**<br>Antrum of Highmore | **R Maxillary Sinus, Left**<br>*See Q Maxillary Sinus, Right*<br>**S Frontal Sinus, Right**<br>**T Frontal Sinus, Left**<br>**U Ethmoid Sinus, Right**<br>Ethmoidal air cell<br>**V Ethmoid Sinus, Left**<br>*See U Ethmoid Sinus, Right*<br>**W Sphenoid Sinus, Right**<br>**X Sphenoid Sinus, Left** | **Ø Open**<br>**3 Percutaneous**<br>**4 Percutaneous Endoscopic**<br>**8 Via Natural or Artificial Opening Endoscopic** | **Z No Device** | **Z No Qualifier** |
| **K Nasal Mucosa and Soft Tissue**<br>Columella<br>External naris<br>Greater alar cartilage<br>Internal naris<br>Lateral nasal cartilage<br>Lesser alar cartilage<br>Nasal cavity<br>Nostril | | **Ø Open**<br>**3 Percutaneous**<br>**4 Percutaneous Endoscopic**<br>**8 Via Natural or Artificial Opening Endoscopic**<br>**X External** | **Z No Device** | **Z No Qualifier** |

**Non-OR** Ø9N[Ø,1]XZZ
**Non-OR** Ø9N[3,4]XZZ
**Non-OR** Ø9N[F,G,L][Ø,3,4,7,8]ZZ
**Non-OR** Ø9NM[Ø,3,4,8]ZZ
**Non-OR** Ø9NK[Ø,3,4,8,X]ZZ

**Ø Medical and Surgical**
**9 Ear, Nose, Sinus**
**P Removal** Definition: Taking out or off a device from a body part

Explanation: If a device is taken out and a similar device put in without cutting or puncturing the skin or mucous membrane, the procedure is coded to the root operation CHANGE. Otherwise, the procedure for taking out a device is coded to the root operation REMOVAL.

| Body Part Character 4 | Approach Character 5 | Device Character 6 | Qualifier Character 7 |
|---|---|---|---|
| **7 Tympanic Membrane, Right**<br>Pars flaccida<br>**8 Tympanic Membrane, Left**<br>*See 7 Tympanic Membrane, Right* | **Ø Open**<br>**7 Via Natural or Artificial Opening**<br>**8 Via Natural or Artificial Opening Endoscopic**<br>**X External** | **Ø Drainage Device** | **Z No Qualifier** |
| **D Inner Ear, Right**<br>Bony labyrinth<br>Bony vestibule<br>Cochlea<br>Round window<br>Semicircular canal<br>**E Inner Ear, Left**<br>*See D Inner Ear, Right* | **Ø Open**<br>**7 Via Natural or Artificial Opening**<br>**8 Via Natural or Artificial Opening Endoscopic** | **S Hearing Device** | **Z No Qualifier** |
| **H Ear, Right**<br>**J Ear, Left**<br>**K Nasal Mucosa and Soft Tissue**<br>Columella<br>External naris<br>Greater alar cartilage<br>Internal naris<br>Lateral nasal cartilage<br>Lesser alar cartilage<br>Nasal cavity<br>Nostril | **Ø Open**<br>**3 Percutaneous**<br>**4 Percutaneous Endoscopic**<br>**7 Via Natural or Artificial Opening**<br>**8 Via Natural or Artificial Opening Endoscopic** | **Ø Drainage Device**<br>**7 Autologous Tissue Substitute**<br>**D Intraluminal Device**<br>**J Synthetic Substitute**<br>**K Nonautologous Tissue Substitute**<br>Y Other Device | **Z No Qualifier** |
| **H Ear, Right**<br>**J Ear, Left**<br>**K Nasal Mucosa and Soft Tissue**<br>Columella<br>External naris<br>Greater alar cartilage<br>Internal naris<br>Lateral nasal cartilage<br>Lesser alar cartilage<br>Nasal cavity<br>Nostril | **X External** | **Ø Drainage Device**<br>**7 Autologous Tissue Substitute**<br>**D Intraluminal Device**<br>**J Synthetic Substitute**<br>**K Nonautologous Tissue Substitute** | **Z No Qualifier** |
| **Y Sinus** | **Ø Open**<br>**3 Percutaneous**<br>**4 Percutaneous Endoscopic** | **Ø Drainage Device**<br>Y Other Device | **Z No Qualifier** |
| Y Sinus | 7 Via Natural or Artificial Opening<br>8 Via Natural or Artificial Opening Endoscopic | Y Other Device | Z No Qualifier |
| **Y Sinus** | **X External** | **Ø Drainage Device** | **Z No Qualifier** |

**Non-OR** Ø9P[7,8][Ø,7,8,X]ØZ
**Non-OR** Ø9P[H,J][3,4][Ø,J,K,Y]Z
**Non-OR** Ø9P[H,J][7,8][Ø,D,Y]Z
**Non-OR** Ø9PK[Ø,3,4,7,8][Ø,7,D,J,K,Y]Z
**Non-OR** Ø9P[H,J]X[Ø,7,D,J,K]Z
**Non-OR** Ø9PKX[Ø,7,D,J,K]Z
**Non-OR** Ø9PY[3,4]YZ
**Non-OR** Ø9PY[7,8]YZ
**Non-OR** Ø9PYXØZ

**Ø Medical and Surgical**
**9 Ear, Nose, Sinus**
**Q Repair** Definition: Restoring, to the extent possible, a body part to its normal anatomic structure and function
Explanation: Used only when the method to accomplish the repair is not one of the other root operations

| Body Part Character 4 | | Approach Character 5 | Device Character 6 | Qualifier Character 7 |
|---|---|---|---|---|
| **Ø External Ear, Right**<br>Antihelix<br>Antitragus<br>Auricle<br>Earlobe<br>Helix<br>Pinna<br>Tragus | **1 External Ear, Left**<br>*See Ø External Ear, Right*<br>**2 External Ear, Bilateral**<br>*See Ø External Ear, Right* | **Ø Open**<br>**3 Percutaneous**<br>**4 Percutaneous Endoscopic**<br>**X External** | **Z No Device** | **Z No Qualifier** |
| **3 External Auditory Canal, Right**<br>External auditory meatus<br>**4 External Auditory Canal, Left**<br>*See 3 External Auditory Canal, Right* | **F Eustachian Tube, Right**<br>Auditory tube<br>Pharyngotympanic tube<br>**G Eustachian Tube, Left**<br>*See F Eustachian Tube, Right* | **Ø Open**<br>**3 Percutaneous**<br>**4 Percutaneous Endoscopic**<br>**7 Via Natural or Artificial Opening**<br>**8 Via Natural or Artificial Opening Endoscopic**<br>**X External** | **Z No Device** | **Z No Qualifier** |
| **5 Middle Ear, Right**<br>Oval window<br>Tympanic cavity<br>**6 Middle Ear, Left**<br>*See 5 Middle Ear, Right*<br>**9 Auditory Ossicle, Right**<br>Incus<br>Malleus<br>Stapes | **A Auditory Ossicle, Left**<br>*See 9 Auditory Ossicle, Right*<br>**D Inner Ear, Right**<br>Bony labyrinth<br>Bony vestibule<br>Cochlea<br>Round window<br>Semicircular canal<br>**E Inner Ear, Left**<br>*See D Inner Ear, Right* | **Ø Open**<br>**8 Via Natural or Artificial Opening Endoscopic** | **Z No Device** | **Z No Qualifier** |
| **7 Tympanic Membrane, Right**<br>Pars flaccida<br>**8 Tympanic Membrane, Left**<br>*See 7 Tympanic Membrane, Right*<br>**L Nasal Turbinate**<br>Inferior turbinate<br>Middle turbinate<br>Nasal concha<br>Superior turbinate | **N Nasopharynx**<br>Choana<br>Fossa of Rosenmuller<br>Pharyngeal recess<br>Rhinopharynx | **Ø Open**<br>**3 Percutaneous**<br>**4 Percutaneous Endoscopic**<br>**7 Via Natural or Artificial Opening**<br>**8 Via Natural or Artificial Opening Endoscopic** | **Z No Device** | **Z No Qualifier** |
| **B Mastoid Sinus, Right**<br>Mastoid air cells<br>**C Mastoid Sinus, Left**<br>*See B Mastoid Sinus, Right*<br>**M Nasal Septum**<br>Quadrangular cartilage<br>Septal cartilage<br>Vomer bone<br>**P Accessory Sinus**<br>**Q Maxillary Sinus, Right**<br>Antrum of Highmore | **R Maxillary Sinus, Left**<br>*See Q Maxillary Sinus, Right*<br>**S Frontal Sinus, Right**<br>**T Frontal Sinus, Left**<br>**U Ethmoid Sinus, Right**<br>Ethmoidal air cell<br>**V Ethmoid Sinus, Left**<br>*See U Ethmoid Sinus, Right*<br>**W Sphenoid Sinus, Right**<br>**X Sphenoid Sinus, Left** | **Ø Open**<br>**3 Percutaneous**<br>**4 Percutaneous Endoscopic**<br>**8 Via Natural or Artificial Opening Endoscopic** | **Z No Device** | **Z No Qualifier** |
| **K Nasal Mucosa and Soft Tissue**<br>Columella<br>External naris<br>Greater alar cartilage<br>Internal naris<br>Lateral nasal cartilage<br>Lesser alar cartilage<br>Nasal cavity<br>Nostril | | **Ø Open**<br>**3 Percutaneous**<br>**4 Percutaneous Endoscopic**<br>**8 Via Natural or Artificial Opening Endoscopic**<br>**X External** | **Z No Device** | **Z No Qualifier** |

**Non-OR** Ø9Q[Ø,1,2]XZZ
**Non-OR** Ø9Q[3,4]XZZ
**Non-OR** Ø9Q[F,G][Ø,3,4,7,8,X]ZZ
**Non-OR** Ø9QKXZZ

**Ø Medical and Surgical**
**9 Ear, Nose, Sinus**
**R Replacement** Definition: Putting in or on biological or synthetic material that physically takes the place and/or function of all or a portion of a body part

Explanation: The body part may have been taken out or replaced, or may be taken out, physically eradicated, or rendered nonfunctional during the REPLACEMENT procedure. A REMOVAL procedure is coded for taking out the device used in a previous replacement procedure.

| Body Part Character 4 | Approach Character 5 | Device Character 6 | Qualifier Character 7 |
|---|---|---|---|
| **Ø External Ear, Right**<br>Antihelix<br>Antitragus<br>Auricle<br>Earlobe<br>Helix<br>Pinna<br>Tragus<br>**1 External Ear, Left**<br>*See Ø External Ear, Right*<br>**2 External Ear, Bilateral**<br>*See Ø External Ear, Right*<br>**K Nasal Mucosa and Soft Tissue**<br>Columella<br>External naris<br>Greater alar cartilage<br>Internal naris<br>Lateral nasal cartilage<br>Lesser alar cartilage<br>Nasal cavity<br>Nostril | **Ø Open**<br>**X External** | **7 Autologous Tissue Substitute**<br>**J Synthetic Substitute**<br>**K Nonautologous Tissue Substitute** | **Z No Qualifier** |
| **5 Middle Ear, Right**<br>Oval window<br>Tympanic cavity<br>**6 Middle Ear, Left**<br>*See 5 Middle Ear, Right*<br>**9 Auditory Ossicle, Right**<br>Incus<br>Malleus<br>Stapes<br>**A Auditory Ossicle, Left**<br>*See 9 Auditory Ossicle, Right*<br>**D Inner Ear, Right**<br>Bony labyrinth<br>Bony vestibule<br>Cochlea<br>Round window<br>Semicircular canal<br>**E Inner Ear, Left**<br>*See D Inner Ear, Right* | **Ø Open** | **7 Autologous Tissue Substitute**<br>**J Synthetic Substitute**<br>**K Nonautologous Tissue Substitute** | **Z No Qualifier** |
| **7 Tympanic Membrane, Right**<br>Pars flaccida<br>**8 Tympanic Membrane, Left**<br>*See 7 Tympanic Membrane, Right*<br>**N Nasopharynx**<br>Choana<br>Fossa of Rosenmuller<br>Pharyngeal recess<br>Rhinopharynx | **Ø Open**<br>**7 Via Natural or Artificial Opening**<br>**8 Via Natural or Artificial Opening Endoscopic** | **7 Autologous Tissue Substitute**<br>**J Synthetic Substitute**<br>**K Nonautologous Tissue Substitute** | **Z No Qualifier** |
| **L Nasal Turbinate**<br>Inferior turbinate<br>Middle turbinate<br>Nasal concha<br>Superior turbinate | **Ø Open**<br>**3 Percutaneous**<br>**4 Percutaneous Endoscopic**<br>**7 Via Natural or Artificial Opening**<br>**8 Via Natural or Artificial Opening Endoscopic** | **7 Autologous Tissue Substitute**<br>**J Synthetic Substitute**<br>**K Nonautologous Tissue Substitute** | **Z No Qualifier** |
| **M Nasal Septum**<br>Quadrangular cartilage<br>Septal cartilage<br>Vomer bone | **Ø Open**<br>**3 Percutaneous**<br>**4 Percutaneous Endoscopic** | **7 Autologous Tissue Substitute**<br>**J Synthetic Substitute**<br>**K Nonautologous Tissue Substitute** | **Z No Qualifier** |

**Ø Medical and Surgical**
**9 Ear, Nose, Sinus**
**S Reposition** Definition: Moving to its normal location, or other suitable location, all or a portion of a body part

Explanation: The body part is moved to a new location from an abnormal location, or from a normal location where it is not functioning correctly. The body part may or may not be cut out or off to be moved to the new location.

| Body Part Character 4 | Approach Character 5 | Device Character 6 | Qualifier Character 7 |
|---|---|---|---|
| **Ø External Ear, Right**<br>Antihelix<br>Antitragus<br>Auricle<br>Earlobe<br>Helix<br>Pinna<br>Tragus<br>**1 External Ear, Left**<br>***See*** *Ø External Ear, Right*<br>**2 External Ear, Bilateral**<br>***See*** *Ø External Ear, Right*<br>K Nasal Mucosa and Soft Tissue<br>Columella<br>External naris<br>Greater alar cartilage<br>Internal naris<br>Lateral nasal cartilage<br>Lesser alar cartilage<br>Nasal cavity<br>Nostril | **Ø Open**<br>**4 Percutaneous Endoscopic**<br>**X External** | **Z No Device** | **Z No Qualifier** |
| **7 Tympanic Membrane, Right**<br>Pars flaccida<br>**8 Tympanic Membrane, Left**<br>***See*** *7 Tympanic Membrane, Right*<br>**F Eustachian Tube, Right**<br>Auditory tube<br>Pharyngotympanic tube<br>**G Eustachian Tube, Left**<br>***See*** *F Eustachian Tube, Right*<br>**L Nasal Turbinate**<br>Inferior turbinate<br>Middle turbinate<br>Nasal concha<br>Superior turbinate | **Ø Open**<br>**4 Percutaneous Endoscopic**<br>**7 Via Natural or Artificial Opening**<br>**8 Via Natural or Artificial Opening Endoscopic** | **Z No Device** | **Z No Qualifier** |
| **9 Auditory Ossicle, Right**<br>Incus<br>Malleus<br>Stapes<br>**A Auditory Ossicle, Left**<br>***See*** *9 Auditory Ossicle, Right*<br>**M Nasal Septum**<br>Quadrangular cartilage<br>Septal cartilage<br>Vomer bone | **Ø Open**<br>**4 Percutaneous Endoscopic** | **Z No Device** | **Z No Qualifier** |

**Non-OR** Ø9S[F,G][Ø,4,7,8]ZZ

**Ø Medical and Surgical**
**9 Ear, Nose, Sinus**
**T Resection** Definition: Cutting out or off, without replacement, all of a body part
Explanation: None

| Body Part Character 4 | | Approach Character 5 | Device Character 6 | Qualifier Character 7 |
|---|---|---|---|---|
| **Ø External Ear, Right**<br>Antihelix<br>Antitragus<br>Auricle<br>Earlobe<br>Helix<br>Pinna<br>Tragus | **1 External Ear, Left**<br>*See Ø External Ear, Right* | **Ø Open**<br>**4 Percutaneous Endoscopic**<br>**X External** | **Z No Device** | **Z No Qualifier** |
| **5 Middle Ear, Right**<br>Oval window<br>Tympanic cavity<br>**6 Middle Ear, Left**<br>*See 5 Middle Ear, Right*<br>**9 Auditory Ossicle, Right**<br>Incus<br>Malleus<br>Stapes | **A Auditory Ossicle, Left**<br>*See 9 Auditory Ossicle, Right*<br>**D Inner Ear, Right**<br>Bony labyrinth<br>Bony vestibule<br>Cochlea<br>Round window<br>Semicircular canal<br>**E Inner Ear, Left**<br>*See D Inner Ear, Right* | **Ø Open**<br>8 Via Natural or Artificial Opening Endoscopic | **Z No Device** | **Z No Qualifier** |
| **7 Tympanic Membrane, Right**<br>Pars flaccida<br>**8 Tympanic Membrane, Left**<br>*See 7 Tympanic Membrane, Right*<br>**F Eustachian Tube, Right**<br>Auditory tube<br>Pharyngotympanic tube<br>**G Eustachian Tube, Left**<br>*See F Eustachian Tube, Right* | **L Nasal Turbinate**<br>Inferior turbinate<br>Middle turbinate<br>Nasal concha<br>Superior turbinate<br>**N Nasopharynx**<br>Choana<br>Fossa of Rosenmuller<br>Pharyngeal recess<br>Rhinopharynx | **Ø Open**<br>**4 Percutaneous Endoscopic**<br>**7 Via Natural or Artificial Opening**<br>**8 Via Natural or Artificial Opening Endoscopic** | **Z No Device** | **Z No Qualifier** |
| **B Mastoid Sinus, Right**<br>Mastoid air cells<br>**C Mastoid Sinus, Left**<br>*See B Mastoid Sinus, Right*<br>**M Nasal Septum**<br>Quadrangular cartilage<br>Septal cartilage<br>Vomer bone<br>**P Accessory Sinus**<br>**Q Maxillary Sinus, Right**<br>Antrum of Highmore | **R Maxillary Sinus, Left**<br>*See Q Maxillary Sinus, Right*<br>**S Frontal Sinus, Right**<br>**T Frontal Sinus, Left**<br>**U Ethmoid Sinus, Right**<br>Ethmoidal air cell<br>**V Ethmoid Sinus, Left**<br>*See U Ethmoid Sinus, Right*<br>**W Sphenoid Sinus, Right**<br>**X Sphenoid Sinus, Left** | **Ø Open**<br>**4 Percutaneous Endoscopic**<br>8 Via Natural or Artificial Opening Endoscopic | **Z No Device** | **Z No Qualifier** |
| K Nasal Mucosa and Soft Tissue<br>Columella<br>External naris<br>Greater alar cartilage<br>Internal naris<br>Lateral nasal cartilage<br>Lesser alar cartilage<br>Nasal cavity<br>Nostril | | **Ø Open**<br>**4 Percutaneous Endoscopic**<br>8 Via Natural or Artificial Opening Endoscopic<br>**X External** | **Z No Device** | **Z No Qualifier** |

**Non-OR** Ø9T[F,G][Ø,4,7,8]ZZ

Ear, Nose, Sinus

**Ø Medical and Surgical**
**9 Ear, Nose, Sinus**
**U Supplement** Definition: Putting in or on biological or synthetic material that physically reinforces and/or augments the function of a portion of a body part

Explanation: The biological material is non-living, or is living and from the same individual. The body part may have been previously replaced, and the SUPPLEMENT procedure is performed to physically reinforce and/or augment the function of the replaced body part.

| Body Part Character 4 | Approach Character 5 | Device Character 6 | Qualifier Character 7 |
|---|---|---|---|
| **Ø External Ear, Right**<br>Antihelix<br>Antitragus<br>Auricle<br>Earlobe<br>Helix<br>Pinna<br>Tragus<br>**1 External Ear, Left**<br>*See Ø External Ear, Right*<br>**2 External Ear, Bilateral**<br>*See Ø External Ear, Right* | **Ø Open**<br>**X External** | **7 Autologous Tissue Substitute**<br>**J Synthetic Substitute**<br>**K Nonautologous Tissue Substitute** | **Z No Qualifier** |
| **5 Middle Ear, Right**<br>Oval window<br>Tympanic cavity<br>**6 Middle Ear, Left**<br>*See 5 Middle Ear, Right*<br>**9 Auditory Ossicle, Right**<br>Incus<br>Malleus<br>Stapes<br>**A Auditory Ossicle, Left**<br>*See 9 Auditory Ossicle, Right*<br>**D Inner Ear, Right**<br>Bony labyrinth<br>Bony vestibule<br>Cochlea<br>Round window<br>Semicircular canal<br>**E Inner Ear, Left**<br>*See D Inner Ear, Right* | **Ø Open**<br>**8 Via Natural or Artificial Opening Endoscopic** | **7 Autologous Tissue Substitute**<br>**J Synthetic Substitute**<br>**K Nonautologous Tissue Substitute** | **Z No Qualifier** |
| **7 Tympanic Membrane, Right**<br>Pars flaccida<br>**8 Tympanic Membrane, Left**<br>*See 7 Tympanic Membrane, Right*<br>**N Nasopharynx**<br>Choana<br>Fossa of Rosenmuller<br>Pharyngeal recess<br>Rhinopharynx | **Ø Open**<br>**7 Via Natural or Artificial Opening**<br>**8 Via Natural or Artificial Opening Endoscopic** | **7 Autologous Tissue Substitute**<br>**J Synthetic Substitute**<br>**K Nonautologous Tissue Substitute** | **Z No Qualifier** |
| **K Nasal Mucosa and Soft Tissue**<br>Columella<br>External naris<br>Greater alar cartilage<br>Internal naris<br>Lateral nasal cartilage<br>Lesser alar cartilage<br>Nasal cavity<br>Nostril | **Ø Open**<br>**8 Via Natural or Artificial Opening Endoscopic**<br>**X External** | **7 Autologous Tissue Substitute**<br>**J Synthetic Substitute**<br>**K Nonautologous Tissue Substitute** | **Z No Qualifier** |
| **L Nasal Turbinate**<br>Inferior turbinate<br>Middle turbinate<br>Nasal concha<br>Superior turbinate | **Ø Open**<br>**3 Percutaneous**<br>**4 Percutaneous Endoscopic**<br>**7 Via Natural or Artificial Opening**<br>**8 Via Natural or Artificial Opening Endoscopic** | **7 Autologous Tissue Substitute**<br>**J Synthetic Substitute**<br>**K Nonautologous Tissue Substitute** | **Z No Qualifier** |
| **M Nasal Septum**<br>Quadrangular cartilage<br>Septal cartilage<br>Vomer bone | **Ø Open**<br>**3 Percutaneous**<br>**4 Percutaneous Endoscopic**<br>**8 Via Natural or Artificial Opening Endoscopic** | **7 Autologous Tissue Substitute**<br>**J Synthetic Substitute**<br>**K Nonautologous Tissue Substitute** | **Z No Qualifier** |

**Ø Medical and Surgical**
**9 Ear, Nose, Sinus**
**W Revision** Definition: Correcting, to the extent possible, a portion of a malfunctioning device or the position of a displaced device

Explanation: Revision can include correcting a malfunctioning or displaced device by taking out or putting in components of the device such as a screw or pin

| Body Part Character 4 | Approach Character 5 | Device Character 6 | Qualifier Character 7 |
|---|---|---|---|
| **7 Tympanic Membrane, Right**<br>Pars flaccida<br>**8 Tympanic Membrane, Left**<br>*See 7 Tympanic Membrane, Right*<br>**9 Auditory Ossicle, Right**<br>Incus<br>Malleus<br>Stapes<br>**A Auditory Ossicle, Left**<br>*See 9 Auditory Ossicle, Right* | **Ø Open**<br>**7 Via Natural or Artificial Opening**<br>**8 Via Natural or Artificial Opening Endoscopic** | **7 Autologous Tissue Substitute**<br>**J Synthetic Substitute**<br>**K Nonautologous Tissue Substitute** | **Z No Qualifier** |
| **D Inner Ear, Right**<br>Bony labyrinth<br>Bony vestibule<br>Cochlea<br>Round window<br>Semicircular canal<br>**E Inner Ear, Left**<br>*See D Inner Ear, Right* | **Ø Open**<br>**7 Via Natural or Artificial Opening**<br>**8 Via Natural or Artificial Opening Endoscopic** | **S Hearing Device** | **Z No Qualifier** |
| **H Ear, Right**<br>**J Ear, Left**<br>**K Nasal Mucosa and Soft Tissue**<br>Columella<br>External naris<br>Greater alar cartilage<br>Internal naris<br>Lateral nasal cartilage<br>Lesser alar cartilage<br>Nasal cavity<br>Nostril | **Ø Open**<br>**3 Percutaneous**<br>**4 Percutaneous Endoscopic**<br>**7 Via Natural or Artificial Opening**<br>**8 Via Natural or Artificial Opening Endoscopic** | **Ø Drainage Device**<br>**7 Autologous Tissue Substitute**<br>**D Intraluminal Device**<br>**J Synthetic Substitute**<br>**K Nonautologous Tissue Substitute**<br>**Y Other Device** | **Z No Qualifier** |
| **H Ear, Right**<br>**J Ear, Left**<br>**K Nasal Mucosa and Soft Tissue**<br>Columella<br>External naris<br>Greater alar cartilage<br>Internal naris<br>Lateral nasal cartilage<br>Lesser alar cartilage<br>Nasal cavity<br>Nostril | **X External** | **Ø Drainage Device**<br>**7 Autologous Tissue Substitute**<br>**D Intraluminal Device**<br>**J Synthetic Substitute**<br>**K Nonautologous Tissue Substitute** | **Z No Qualifier** |
| **Y Sinus** | **Ø Open**<br>**3 Percutaneous**<br>**4 Percutaneous Endoscopic** | **Ø Drainage Device**<br>**Y Other Device** | **Z No Qualifier** |
| **Y Sinus** | **7 Via Natural or Artificial Opening**<br>**8 Via Natural or Artificial Opening Endoscopic** | **Y Other Device** | **Z No Qualifier** |
| **Y Sinus** | **X External** | **Ø Drainage Device** | **Z No Qualifier** |

**Non-OR** Ø9W[H,J][3,4][J,K,Y]Z
**Non-OR** Ø9W[H,J][7,8][D,Y]Z
**Non-OR** Ø9WK[Ø,3,4,7,8][Ø,7,D,J,K,Y]Z
**Non-OR** Ø9W[H,J,K]X[Ø,7,D,J,K]Z
**Non-OR** Ø9WY[3,4]YZ
**Non-OR** Ø9WY[7,8]YZ
**Non-OR** Ø9WYXØZ

# Respiratory System ØB1–ØBY



## Character Meanings

This Character Meaning table is provided as a guide to assist the user in the identification of character members that may be found in this section of code tables. It **SHOULD NOT** be used to build a PCS code.

| Operation–Character 3 | Body Part–Character 4 | Approach–Character 5 | Device–Character 6 | Qualifier–Character 7 |
|---|---|---|---|---|
| 1 Bypass | Ø Tracheobronchial Tree | Ø Open | Ø Drainage Device | Ø Allogeneic |
| 2 Change | 1 Trachea | 3 Percutaneous | 1 Radioactive Element | 1 Syngeneic |
| 5 Destruction | 2 Carina | 4 Percutaneous Endoscopic | 2 Monitoring Device | 2 Zooplastic |
| 7 Dilation | 3 Main Bronchus, Right | 7 Via Natural or Artificial Opening | 3 Infusion Device | 4 Cutaneous |
| 9 Drainage | 4 Upper Lobe Bronchus, Right | 8 Via Natural or Artificial Opening Endoscopic | 7 Autologous Tissue Substitute | 6 Esophagus |
| B Excision | 5 Middle Lobe Bronchus, Right | X External | C Extraluminal Device | X Diagnostic |
| C Extirpation | 6 Lower Lobe Bronchus, Right | | D Intraluminal Device | Z No Qualifier |
| D Extraction | 7 Main Bronchus, Left | | E Intraluminal Device, Endotracheal Airway | |
| F Fragmentation | 8 Upper Lobe Bronchus, Left | | F Tracheostomy Device | |
| H Insertion | 9 Lingula Bronchus | | G Intraluminal Device, Endobronchial Valve | |
| J Inspection | B Lower Lobe Bronchus, Left | | J Synthetic Substitute | |
| L Occlusion | C Upper Lung Lobe, Right | | K Nonautologous Tissue Substitute | |
| M Reattachment | D Middle Lung Lobe, Right | | M Diaphragmatic Pacemaker Lead | |
| N Release | F Lower Lung Lobe, Right | | Y Other Device | |
| P Removal | G Upper Lung Lobe, Left | | Z No Device | |
| Q Repair | H Lung Lingula | | | |
| R Replacement | J Lower Lung Lobe, Left | | | |
| S Reposition | K Lung, Right | | | |
| T Resection | L Lung, Left | | | |
| U Supplement | M Lungs, Bilateral | | | |
| V Restriction | N Pleura, Right | | | |
| W Revision | P Pleura, Left | | | |
| Y Transplantation | Q Pleura | | | |
| | T Diaphragm | | | |

**AHA Coding Clinic for table ØB5**
**2016, 2Q, 17** Photodynamic therapy for treatment of malignant mesothelioma
**2015, 2Q, 31** Thoracoscopic talc pleurodesis

**AHA Coding Clinic for table ØB9**
**2017, 1Q, 51** Bronchoalveolar lavage
**2016, 1Q, 26** Bronchoalveolar lavage, endobronchial biopsy and transbronchial biopsy
**2016, 1Q, 27** Fiberoptic bronchoscopy with brushings and bronchoalveolar lavage

**AHA Coding Clinic for table ØBB**
**2016, 1Q, 26** Bronchoalveolar lavage, endobronchial biopsy and transbronchial biopsy
**2016, 1Q, 27** Fiberoptic bronchoscopy with brushings and bronchoalveolar lavage
**2014, 1Q, 20** Fiducial marker placement

**AHA Coding Clinic for table ØBH**
**2014, 4Q, 3-10** Mechanical ventilation

**AHA Coding Clinic for table ØBJ**
**2015, 2Q, 31** Thoracoscopic talc pleurodesis
**2014, 1Q, 20** Fiducial marker placement

**AHA Coding Clinic for table ØBN**
**2015, 3Q, 15** Vascular ring surgery with release of esophagus and trachea

**AHA Coding Clinic for table ØBQ**
**2016, 2Q, 22** Esophageal lengthening Collis gastroplasty with Nissen fundoplication and hiatal hernia
**2014, 3Q, 28** Laparoscopic Nissen fundoplication and diaphragmatic hernia repair

**AHA Coding Clinic for table ØBU**
**2015, 1Q, 28** Repair of bronchopleural fistula using omental pedicle graft

## Respiratory System

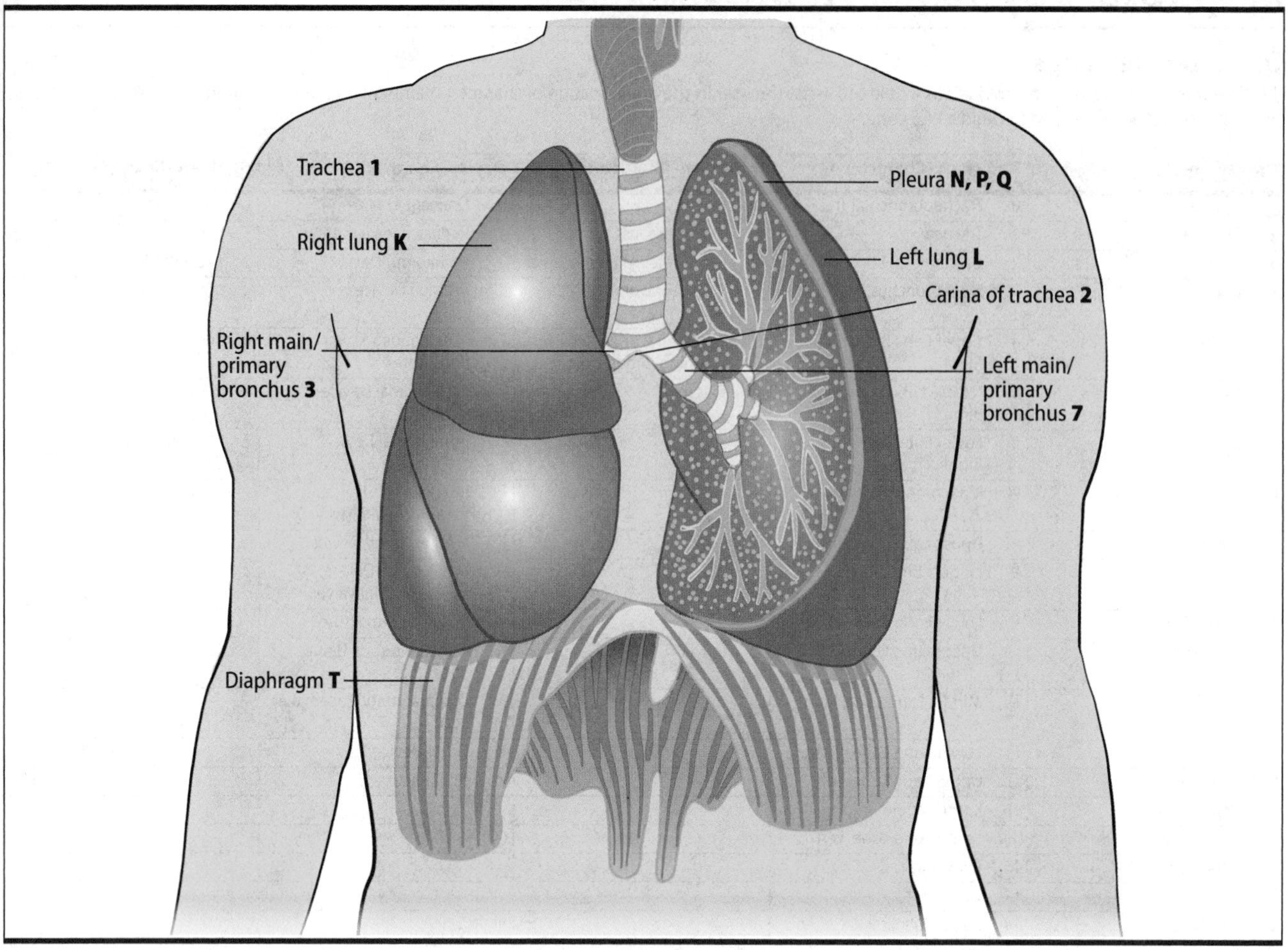

Trachea **1**
Right lung **K**
Right main/
primary
bronchus **3**
Diaphragm **T**
Pleura **N, P, Q**
Left lung **L**
Carina of trachea **2**
Left main/
primary
bronchus **7**


## Right Lung Bronchi

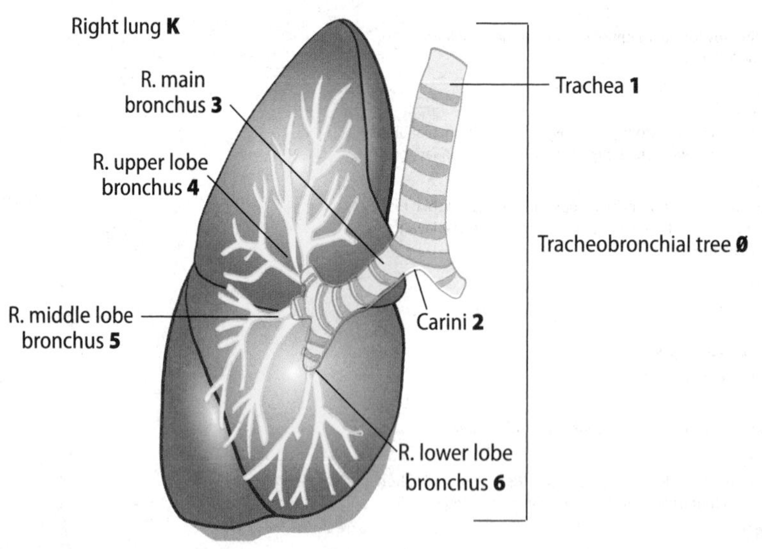

Right lung **K**
R. main
bronchus **3**
R. upper lobe
bronchus **4**
R. middle lobe
bronchus **5**
Trachea **1**
Tracheobronchial tree **Ø**
Carini **2**
R. lower lobe
bronchus **6**

**Ø Medical and Surgical**
**B Respiratory System**
**1 Bypass** Definition: Altering the route of passage of the contents of a tubular body part

Explanation: Rerouting contents of a body part to a downstream area of the normal route, to a similar route and body part, or to an abnormal route and dissimilar body part. Includes one or more anastomoses, with or without the use of a device.

| Body Part Character 4 | Approach Character 5 | Device Character 6 | Qualifier Character 7 |
|---|---|---|---|
| 1 Trachea<br>Cricoid cartilage | Ø Open | D Intraluminal Device | 6 Esophagus |
| 1 Trachea<br>Cricoid cartilage | Ø Open | F Tracheostomy Device<br>Z No Device | 4 Cutaneous |
| 1 Trachea<br>Cricoid cartilage | 3 Percutaneous<br>4 Percutaneous Endoscopic | F Tracheostomy Device<br>Z No Device | 4 Cutaneous |

DRG Non-OR ØB113[F,Z]4
Non-OR ØB11ØD6

**Ø Medical and Surgical**
**B Respiratory System**
**2 Change** Definition: Taking out or off a device from a body part and putting back an identical or similar device in or on the same body part without cutting or puncturing the skin or a mucous membrane

Explanation: All CHANGE procedures are coded using the approach EXTERNAL

| Body Part Character 4 | Approach Character 5 | Device Character 6 | Qualifier Character 7 |
|---|---|---|---|
| Ø Tracheobronchial Tree<br>K Lung, Right<br>L Lung, Left<br>Q Pleura<br>T Diaphragm | X External | Ø Drainage Device<br>Y Other Device | Z No Qualifier |
| 1 Trachea<br>Cricoid cartilage | X External | Ø Drainage Device<br>E Intraluminal Device, Endotracheal Airway<br>F Tracheostomy Device<br>Y Other Device | Z No Qualifier |

Non-OR All body part, approach, device, and qualifier values

**Ø Medical and Surgical**
**B Respiratory System**
**5 Destruction** Definition: Physical eradication of all or a portion of a body part by the direct use of energy, force, or a destructive agent

Explanation: None of the body part is physically taken out

| Body Part Character 4 | Approach Character 5 | Device Character 6 | Qualifier Character 7 |
|---|---|---|---|
| 1 Trachea<br>Cricoid cartilage<br>2 Carina<br>3 Main Bronchus, Right<br>Bronchus intermedius<br>Intermediate bronchus<br>4 Upper Lobe Bronchus, Right<br>5 Middle Lobe Bronchus, Right<br>6 Lower Lobe Bronchus, Right<br>7 Main Bronchus, Left<br>8 Upper Lobe Bronchus, Left<br>9 Lingula Bronchus<br>B Lower Lobe Bronchus, Left<br>C Upper Lung Lobe, Right<br>D Middle Lung Lobe, Right<br>F Lower Lung Lobe, Right<br>G Upper Lung Lobe, Left<br>H Lung Lingula<br>J Lower Lung Lobe, Left<br>K Lung, Right<br>L Lung, Left<br>M Lungs, Bilateral | Ø Open<br>3 Percutaneous<br>4 Percutaneous Endoscopic<br>7 Via Natural or Artificial Opening<br>8 Via Natural or Artificial Opening Endoscopic | Z No Device | Z No Qualifier |
| N Pleura, Right<br>P Pleura, Left<br>T Diaphragm | Ø Open<br>3 Percutaneous<br>4 Percutaneous Endoscopic | Z No Device | Z No Qualifier |

Non-OR ØB5[3,4,5,6,7,8,9,B][4,8]ZZ
Non-OR ØB5[C,D,F,G,H,J,K,L,M]8ZZ

**Ø Medical and Surgical**
**B Respiratory System**
**7 Dilation** Definition: Expanding an orifice or the lumen of a tubular body part

Explanation: The orifice can be a natural orifice or an artificially created orifice. Accomplished by stretching a tubular body part using intraluminal pressure or by cutting part of the orifice or wall of the tubular body part.

| Body Part Character 4 | Approach Character 5 | Device Character 6 | Qualifier Character 7 |
|---|---|---|---|
| 1 Trachea<br>Cricoid cartilage<br>2 Carina<br>3 Main Bronchus, Right<br>Bronchus intermedius<br>Intermediate bronchus<br>4 Upper Lobe Bronchus, Right<br>5 Middle Lobe Bronchus, Right<br>6 Lower Lobe Bronchus, Right<br>7 Main Bronchus, Left<br>8 Upper Lobe Bronchus, Left<br>9 Lingula Bronchus<br>B Lower Lobe Bronchus, Left | Ø Open<br>3 Percutaneous<br>4 Percutaneous Endoscopic<br>7 Via Natural or Artificial Opening<br>8 Via Natural or Artificial Opening Endoscopic | D Intraluminal Device<br>Z No Device | Z No Qualifier |

**Non-OR** ØB7[3,4,5,6,7,8,9,B][Ø,3,4,7,8][D,Z]Z

**Ø Medical and Surgical**
**B Respiratory System**
**9 Drainage** Definition: Taking or letting out fluids and/or gases from a body part

Explanation: The qualifier DIAGNOSTIC is used to identify drainage procedures that are biopsies

| Body Part Character 4 | Approach Character 5 | Device Character 6 | Qualifier Character 7 |
|---|---|---|---|
| 1 Trachea<br>Cricoid cartilage<br>2 Carina<br>3 Main Bronchus, Right<br>Bronchus intermedius<br>Intermediate bronchus<br>4 Upper Lobe Bronchus, Right<br>5 Middle Lobe Bronchus, Right<br>6 Lower Lobe Bronchus, Right<br>7 Main Bronchus, Left<br>8 Upper Lobe Bronchus, Left<br>9 Lingula Bronchus<br>B Lower Lobe Bronchus, Left<br>C Upper Lung Lobe, Right<br>D Middle Lung Lobe, Right<br>F Lower Lung Lobe, Right<br>G Upper Lung Lobe, Left<br>H Lung Lingula<br>J Lower Lung Lobe, Left<br>K Lung, Right<br>L Lung, Left<br>M Lungs, Bilateral | Ø Open<br>3 Percutaneous<br>4 Percutaneous Endoscopic<br>7 Via Natural or Artificial Opening<br>8 Via Natural or Artificial Opening Endoscopic | Ø Drainage Device | Z No Qualifier |
| 1 Trachea<br>Cricoid cartilage<br>2 Carina<br>3 Main Bronchus, Right<br>Bronchus intermedius<br>Intermediate bronchus<br>4 Upper Lobe Bronchus, Right<br>5 Middle Lobe Bronchus, Right<br>6 Lower Lobe Bronchus, Right<br>7 Main Bronchus, Left<br>8 Upper Lobe Bronchus, Left<br>9 Lingula Bronchus<br>B Lower Lobe Bronchus, Left<br>C Upper Lung Lobe, Right<br>D Middle Lung Lobe, Right<br>F Lower Lung Lobe, Right<br>G Upper Lung Lobe, Left<br>H Lung Lingula<br>J Lower Lung Lobe, Left<br>K Lung, Right<br>L Lung, Left<br>M Lungs, Bilateral | Ø Open<br>3 Percutaneous<br>4 Percutaneous Endoscopic<br>7 Via Natural or Artificial Opening<br>8 Via Natural or Artificial Opening Endoscopic | Z No Device | X Diagnostic<br>Z No Qualifier |
| N Pleura, Right<br>P Pleura, Left | Ø Open<br>3 Percutaneous<br>4 Percutaneous Endoscopic<br>8 Via Natural or Artificial Opening Endoscopic | Ø Drainage Device | Z No Qualifier |
| N Pleura, Right<br>P Pleura, Left | Ø Open<br>3 Percutaneous<br>4 Percutaneous Endoscopic<br>8 Via Natural or Artificial Opening Endoscopic | Z No Device | X Diagnostic<br>Z No Qualifier |
| T Diaphragm | Ø Open<br>3 Percutaneous<br>4 Percutaneous Endoscopic | Ø Drainage Device | Z No Qualifier |
| T Diaphragm | Ø Open<br>3 Percutaneous<br>4 Percutaneous Endoscopic | Z No Device | X Diagnostic<br>Z No Qualifier |

**Non-OR** ØB9[1,2,3,4,5,6,7,8,9,B][7,8]ØZ
**Non-OR** ØB9[1,2,3,4,5,6,7,8,9,B][3,4]ZX
**Non-OR** ØB9[1,2,3,4,5,6,7,8,9,B][7,8]Z[X,Z]
**Non-OR** ØB9[C,D,F,G,H,J,K,L,M][3,4,7]ZX
**Non-OR** ØB9[N,P][Ø,3,8]ØZ
**Non-OR** ØB9[N,P][Ø,3,8]Z[X,Z]
**Non-OR** ØB9[N,P]4ZX
**Non-OR** ØB9T[3,4]ØZ
**Non-OR** ØB9T[3,4]Z[X,Z]

**Ø Medical and Surgical**
**B Respiratory System**
**B Excision** Definition: Cutting out or off, without replacement, a portion of a body part
Explanation: The qualifier DIAGNOSTIC is used to identify excision procedures that are biopsies

| Body Part Character 4 | Approach Character 5 | Device Character 6 | Qualifier Character 7 |
|---|---|---|---|
| **1** Trachea<br>Cricoid cartilage<br>**2** Carina<br>**3** Main Bronchus, Right<br>Bronchus intermedius<br>Intermediate bronchus<br>**4** Upper Lobe Bronchus, Right<br>**5** Middle Lobe Bronchus, Right<br>**6** Lower Lobe Bronchus, Right<br>**7** Main Bronchus, Left<br>**8** Upper Lobe Bronchus, Left<br>**9** Lingula Bronchus<br>**B** Lower Lobe Bronchus, Left<br>**C** Upper Lung Lobe, Right<br>**D** Middle Lung Lobe, Right<br>**F** Lower Lung Lobe, Right<br>**G** Upper Lung Lobe, Left<br>**H** Lung Lingula<br>**J** Lower Lung Lobe, Left<br>**K** Lung, Right<br>**L** Lung, Left<br>**M** Lungs, Bilateral | **Ø** Open<br>**3** Percutaneous<br>**4** Percutaneous Endoscopic<br>**7** Via Natural or Artificial Opening<br>**8** Via Natural or Artificial Opening Endoscopic | **Z** No Device | **X** Diagnostic<br>**Z** No Qualifier |
| **N** Pleura, Right<br>**P** Pleura, Left | **Ø** Open<br>**3** Percutaneous<br>**4** Percutaneous Endoscopic<br>**8** Via Natural or Artificial Opening Endoscopic | **Z** No Device | **X** Diagnostic<br>**Z** No Qualifier |
| **T** Diaphragm | **Ø** Open<br>**3** Percutaneous<br>**4** Percutaneous Endoscopic | **Z** No Device | **X** Diagnostic<br>**Z** No Qualifier |

**Non-OR** ØBB[1,2,3,4,5,6,7,8,9,B][3,4,7,8]ZX
**Non-OR** ØBB[3,4,5,6,7,8,9,B,M][4,8]ZZ
**Non-OR** ØBB[C,D,F,G,H,J,K,L,M]3ZX
**Non-OR** ØBB[C,D,F,G,H,J,K,L]8ZZ
**Non-OR** ØBB[N,P][Ø,3]ZX

**Ø Medical and Surgical**
**B Respiratory System**
**C Extirpation** Definition: Taking or cutting out solid matter from a body part
Explanation: The solid matter may be an abnormal byproduct of a biological function or a foreign body; it may be imbedded in a body part or in the lumen of a tubular body part. The solid matter may or may not have been previously broken into pieces.

| Body Part Character 4 | Approach Character 5 | Device Character 6 | Qualifier Character 7 |
|---|---|---|---|
| **1** Trachea<br>Cricoid cartilage<br>**2** Carina<br>**3** Main Bronchus, Right<br>Bronchus intermedius<br>Intermediate bronchus<br>**4** Upper Lobe Bronchus, Right<br>**5** Middle Lobe Bronchus, Right<br>**6** Lower Lobe Bronchus, Right<br>**7** Main Bronchus, Left<br>**8** Upper Lobe Bronchus, Left<br>**9** Lingula Bronchus<br>**B** Lower Lobe Bronchus, Left<br>**C** Upper Lung Lobe, Right<br>**D** Middle Lung Lobe, Right<br>**F** Lower Lung Lobe, Right<br>**G** Upper Lung Lobe, Left<br>**H** Lung Lingula<br>**J** Lower Lung Lobe, Left<br>**K** Lung, Right<br>**L** Lung, Left<br>**M** Lungs, Bilateral | **Ø** Open<br>**3** Percutaneous<br>**4** Percutaneous Endoscopic<br>**7** Via Natural or Artificial Opening<br>**8** Via Natural or Artificial Opening Endoscopic | **Z** No Device | **Z** No Qualifier |
| **N** Pleura, Right<br>**P** Pleura, Left<br>**T** Diaphragm | **Ø** Open<br>**3** Percutaneous<br>**4** Percutaneous Endoscopic | **Z** No Device | **Z** No Qualifier |

**Non-OR** ØBC[1,2,3,4,5,6,7,8,9,B][7,8]ZZ
**Non-OR** ØBC[C,D,F,G,H,J,K,L,M]8ZZ
**Non-OR** ØBC[N,P][Ø,3,4]ZZ

**Ø Medical and Surgical**
**B Respiratory System**
**D Extraction** Definition: Pulling or stripping out or off all or a portion of a body part by the use of force

Explanation: The qualifier DIAGNOSTIC is used to identify extraction procedures that are biopsies

| Body Part Character 4 | Approach Character 5 | Device Character 6 | Qualifier Character 7 |
|---|---|---|---|
| 1 Trachea<br>Cricoid cartilage<br>2 Carina<br>3 Main Bronchus, Right<br>Bronchus intermedius<br>Intermediate bronchus<br>4 Upper Lobe Bronchus, Right<br>5 Middle Lobe Bronchus, Right<br>6 Lower Lobe Bronchus, Right<br>7 Main Bronchus, Left<br>8 Upper Lobe Bronchus, Left<br>9 Lingula Bronchus<br>B Lower Lobe Bronchus, Left<br>C Upper Lung Lobe, Right<br>D Middle Lung Lobe, Right<br>F Lower Lung Lobe, Right<br>G Upper Lung Lobe, Left<br>H Lung Lingula<br>J Lower Lung Lobe, Left<br>K Lung, Right<br>L Lung, Left<br>M Lungs, Bilateral | 4 Percutaneous Endoscopic<br>8 Via Natural or Artificial Opening Endoscopic | Z No Device | X Diagnostic |
| N Pleura, Right<br>P Pleura, Left | Ø Open<br>3 Percutaneous<br>4 Percutaneous Endoscopic | Z No Device | X Diagnostic<br>Z No Qualifier |

Non-OR ØBD[1,2,3,4,5,6,7,8,9,B,C,D,F,G,H,J,K,L,M][4,8]ZX

**Ø Medical and Surgical**
**B Respiratory System**
**F Fragmentation** Definition: Breaking solid matter in a body part into pieces

Explanation: Physical force (e.g., manual, ultrasonic) applied directly or indirectly is used to break the solid matter into pieces. The solid matter may be an abnormal byproduct of a biological function or a foreign body. The pieces of solid matter are not taken out.

| Body Part Character 4 | Approach Character 5 | Device Character 6 | Qualifier Character 7 |
|---|---|---|---|
| 1 Trachea NC<br>Cricoid cartilage<br>2 Carina NC<br>3 Main Bronchus, Right NC<br>Bronchus intermedius<br>Intermediate bronchus<br>4 Upper Lobe Bronchus, Right NC<br>5 Middle Lobe Bronchus, Right NC<br>6 Lower Lobe Bronchus, Right NC<br>7 Main Bronchus, Left NC<br>8 Upper Lobe Bronchus, Left NC<br>9 Lingula Bronchus NC<br>B Lower Lobe Bronchus, Left NC | Ø Open<br>3 Percutaneous<br>4 Percutaneous Endoscopic<br>7 Via Natural or Artificial Opening<br>8 Via Natural or Artificial Opening Endoscopic<br>X External | Z No Device | Z No Qualifier |

Non-OR ØBF[1,2,3,4,5,6,7,8,9,B]XZZ
Non-OR ØBF[3,4,5,6,7,8,9,B][7,8]ZZ
NC ØBF[1,2,3,4,5,6,7,8,9,B]XZZ

**Ø Medical and Surgical**
**B Respiratory System**
**H Insertion** Definition: Putting in a nonbiological appliance that monitors, assists, performs, or prevents a physiological function but does not physically take the place of a body part

Explanation: None

| Body Part Character 4 | Approach Character 5 | Device Character 6 | Qualifier Character 7 |
|---|---|---|---|
| **Ø Tracheobronchial Tree** | **Ø Open**<br>**3 Percutaneous**<br>**4 Percutaneous Endoscopic**<br>**7 Via Natural or Artificial Opening**<br>**8 Via Natural or Artificial Opening Endoscopic** | **1 Radioactive Element**<br>**2 Monitoring Device**<br>**3 Infusion Device**<br>**D Intraluminal Device**<br>**Y Other Device** | **Z No Qualifier** |
| **1 Trachea**<br>Cricoid cartilage | **Ø Open** | **2 Monitoring Device**<br>**D Intraluminal Device**<br>**Y Other Device** | **Z No Qualifier** |
| **1 Trachea**<br>Cricoid cartilage | **3 Percutaneous** | **D Intraluminal Device**<br>**E Intraluminal Device, Endotracheal Airway**<br>**Y Other Device** | **Z No Qualifier** |
| **1 Trachea**<br>Cricoid cartilage | **4 Percutaneous Endoscopic** | **D Intraluminal Device**<br>**Y Other Device** | **Z No Qualifier** |
| **1 Trachea**<br>Cricoid cartilage | **7 Via Natural or Artificial Opening**<br>**8 Via Natural or Artificial Opening Endoscopic** | **2 Monitoring Device**<br>**D Intraluminal Device**<br>**E Intraluminal Device, Endotracheal Airway**<br>**Y Other Device** | **Z No Qualifier** |
| **3 Main Bronchus, Right**<br>Bronchus intermedius<br>Intermediate bronchus<br>**4 Upper Lobe Bronchus, Right**<br>**5 Middle Lobe Bronchus, Right**<br>**6 Lower Lobe Bronchus, Right**<br>**7 Main Bronchus, Left**<br>**8 Upper Lobe Bronchus, Left**<br>**9 Lingula Bronchus**<br>**B Lower Lobe Bronchus, Left** | **Ø Open**<br>**3 Percutaneous**<br>**4 Percutaneous Endoscopic**<br>**7 Via Natural or Artificial Opening**<br>**8 Via Natural or Artificial Opening Endoscopic** | **G Intraluminal Device, Endobronchial Valve** | **Z No Qualifier** |
| **K Lung, Right**<br>**L Lung, Left** | **Ø Open**<br>**3 Percutaneous**<br>**4 Percutaneous Endoscopic**<br>**7 Via Natural or Artificial Opening**<br>**8 Via Natural or Artificial Opening Endoscopic** | **1 Radioactive Element**<br>**2 Monitoring Device**<br>**3 Infusion Device**<br>**Y Other Device** | **Z No Qualifier** |
| **Q Pleura** | **Ø Open**<br>**3 Percutaneous**<br>**4 Percutaneous Endoscopic**<br>**7 Via Natural or Artificial Opening**<br>**8 Via Natural or Artificial Opening Endoscopic** | **Y Other Device** | **Z No Qualifier** |
| **T Diaphragm** | **Ø Open**<br>**3 Percutaneous**<br>**4 Percutaneous Endoscopic** | **2 Monitoring Device**<br>**M Diaphragmatic Pacemaker Lead**<br>**Y Other Device** | **Z No Qualifier** |
| **T Diaphragm** | **7 Via Natural or Artificial Opening**<br>**8 Via Natural or Artificial Opening Endoscopic** | **Y Other Device** | **Z No Qualifier** |

**Non-OR** ØBHØ[3,4]YZ
**Non-OR** ØBHØ[7,8][2,3,D,Y]Z
**Non-OR** ØBH13[E,Y]Z
**Non-OR** ØBH14YZ
**Non-OR** ØBH1[7,8][2,D,E,Y]Z
**Non-OR** ØBH[3,4,5,6,7,8,9,B]8GZ
**Non-OR** ØBH[K,L][3,4]YZ
**Non-OR** ØBH[K,L][7,8][2,3,Y]Z
**Non-OR** ØBHQ[3,4,7,8]YZ
**Non-OR** ØBHT[3,4]YZ
**Non-OR** ØBHT[7,8]YZ

**Ø Medical and Surgical**
**B Respiratory System**
**J Inspection** Definition: Visually and/or manually exploring a body part

Explanation: Visual exploration may be performed with or without optical instrumentation. Manual exploration may be performed directly or through intervening body layers.

| Body Part Character 4 | Approach Character 5 | Device Character 6 | Qualifier Character 7 |
|---|---|---|---|
| Ø Tracheobronchial Tree<br>1 Trachea<br>Cricoid cartilage<br>K Lung, Right<br>L Lung, Left<br>Q Pleura<br>T Diaphragm | Ø Open<br>3 Percutaneous<br>4 Percutaneous Endoscopic<br>7 Via Natural or Artificial Opening<br>8 Via Natural or Artificial Opening Endoscopic<br>X External | Z No Device | Z No Qualifier |

Non-OR ØBJ[Ø,K,L,Q,T][3,7,8,X]ZZ
Non-OR ØBJ1[3,4,7,8,X]ZZ

**Ø Medical and Surgical**
**B Respiratory System**
**L Occlusion** Definition: Completely closing an orifice or the lumen of a tubular body part

Explanation: The orifice can be a natural orifice or an artificially created orifice

| Body Part Character 4 | Approach Character 5 | Device Character 6 | Qualifier Character 7 |
|---|---|---|---|
| 1 Trachea<br>Cricoid cartilage<br>2 Carina<br>3 Main Bronchus, Right<br>Bronchus intermedius<br>Intermediate bronchus<br>4 Upper Lobe Bronchus, Right<br>5 Middle Lobe Bronchus, Right<br>6 Lower Lobe Bronchus, Right<br>7 Main Bronchus, Left<br>8 Upper Lobe Bronchus, Left<br>9 Lingula Bronchus<br>B Lower Lobe Bronchus, Left | Ø Open<br>3 Percutaneous<br>4 Percutaneous Endoscopic | C Extraluminal Device<br>D Intraluminal Device<br>Z No Device | Z No Qualifier |
| 1 Trachea<br>Cricoid cartilage<br>2 Carina<br>3 Main Bronchus, Right<br>Bronchus intermedius<br>Intermediate bronchus<br>4 Upper Lobe Bronchus, Right<br>5 Middle Lobe Bronchus, Right<br>6 Lower Lobe Bronchus, Right<br>7 Main Bronchus, Left<br>8 Upper Lobe Bronchus, Left<br>9 Lingula Bronchus<br>B Lower Lobe Bronchus, Left | 7 Via Natural or Artificial Opening<br>8 Via Natural or Artificial Opening Endoscopic | D Intraluminal Device<br>Z No Device | Z No Qualifier |

**Ø Medical and Surgical**
**B Respiratory System**
**M Reattachment** Definition: Putting back in or on all or a portion of a separated body part to its normal location or other suitable location

Explanation: Vascular circulation and nervous pathways may or may not be reestablished

| Body Part Character 4 | Approach Character 5 | Device Character 6 | Qualifier Character 7 |
|---|---|---|---|
| **1** Trachea<br>Cricoid cartilage<br>**2** Carina<br>**3** Main Bronchus, Right<br>Bronchus intermedius<br>Intermediate bronchus<br>**4** Upper Lobe Bronchus, Right<br>**5** Middle Lobe Bronchus, Right<br>**6** Lower Lobe Bronchus, Right<br>**7** Main Bronchus, Left<br>**8** Upper Lobe Bronchus, Left<br>**9** Lingula Bronchus<br>**B** Lower Lobe Bronchus, Left<br>**C** Upper Lung Lobe, Right<br>**D** Middle Lung Lobe, Right<br>**F** Lower Lung Lobe, Right<br>**G** Upper Lung Lobe, Left<br>**H** Lung Lingula<br>**J** Lower Lung Lobe, Left<br>**K** Lung, Right<br>**L** Lung, Left<br>**T** Diaphragm | **Ø** Open | **Z** No Device | **Z** No Qualifier |

**Ø Medical and Surgical**
**B Respiratory System**
**N Release** Definition: Freeing a body part from an abnormal physical constraint by cutting or by the use of force

Explanation: Some of the restraining tissue may be taken out but none of the body part is taken out

| Body Part Character 4 | Approach Character 5 | Device Character 6 | Qualifier Character 7 |
|---|---|---|---|
| **1** Trachea<br>Cricoid cartilage<br>**2** Carina<br>**3** Main Bronchus, Right<br>Bronchus intermedius<br>Intermediate bronchus<br>**4** Upper Lobe Bronchus, Right<br>**5** Middle Lobe Bronchus, Right<br>**6** Lower Lobe Bronchus, Right<br>**7** Main Bronchus, Left<br>**8** Upper Lobe Bronchus, Left<br>**9** Lingula Bronchus<br>**B** Lower Lobe Bronchus, Left<br>**C** Upper Lung Lobe, Right<br>**D** Middle Lung Lobe, Right<br>**F** Lower Lung Lobe, Right<br>**G** Upper Lung Lobe, Left<br>**H** Lung Lingula<br>**J** Lower Lung Lobe, Left<br>**K** Lung, Right<br>**L** Lung, Left<br>**M** Lungs, Bilateral | **Ø** Open<br>**3** Percutaneous<br>**4** Percutaneous Endoscopic<br>**7** Via Natural or Artificial Opening<br>**8** Via Natural or Artificial Opening Endoscopic | **Z** No Device | **Z** No Qualifier |
| **N** Pleura, Right<br>**P** Pleura, Left<br>**T** Diaphragm | **Ø** Open<br>**3** Percutaneous<br>**4** Percutaneous Endoscopic | **Z** No Device | **Z** No Qualifier |

**Ø Medical and Surgical**
**B Respiratory System**
**P Removal** Definition: Taking out or off a device from a body part

Explanation: If a device is taken out and a similar device put in without cutting or puncturing the skin or mucous membrane, the procedure is coded to the root operation CHANGE. Otherwise, the procedure for taking out a device is coded to the root operation REMOVAL.

| Body Part Character 4 | Approach Character 5 | Device Character 6 | Qualifier Character 7 |
|---|---|---|---|
| Ø Tracheobronchial Tree | Ø Open<br>3 Percutaneous<br>4 Percutaneous Endoscopic<br>7 Via Natural or Artificial Opening<br>8 Via Natural or Artificial Opening Endoscopic | Ø Drainage Device<br>1 Radioactive Element<br>2 Monitoring Device<br>3 Infusion Device<br>7 Autologous Tissue Substitute<br>C Extraluminal Device<br>D Intraluminal Device<br>J Synthetic Substitute<br>K Nonautologous Tissue Substitute<br>Y Other Device | Z No Qualifier |
| Ø Tracheobronchial Tree | X External | Ø Drainage Device<br>1 Radioactive Element<br>2 Monitoring Device<br>3 Infusion Device<br>D Intraluminal Device | Z No Qualifier |
| 1 Trachea<br>Cricoid cartilage | Ø Open<br>3 Percutaneous<br>4 Percutaneous Endoscopic<br>7 Via Natural or Artificial Opening<br>8 Via Natural or Artificial Opening Endoscopic | Ø Drainage Device<br>2 Monitoring Device<br>7 Autologous Tissue Substitute<br>C Extraluminal Device<br>D Intraluminal Device<br>F Tracheostomy Device<br>J Synthetic Substitute<br>K Nonautologous Tissue Substitute | Z No Qualifier |
| 1 Trachea<br>Cricoid cartilage | X External | Ø Drainage Device<br>2 Monitoring Device<br>D Intraluminal Device<br>F Tracheostomy Device | Z No Qualifier |
| K Lung, Right<br>L Lung, Left | Ø Open<br>3 Percutaneous<br>4 Percutaneous Endoscopic<br>7 Via Natural or Artificial Opening<br>8 Via Natural or Artificial Opening Endoscopic | Ø Drainage Device<br>1 Radioactive Element<br>2 Monitoring Device<br>3 Infusion Device<br>Y Other Device | Z No Qualifier |
| K Lung, Right<br>L Lung, Left | X External | Ø Drainage Device<br>1 Radioactive Element<br>2 Monitoring Device<br>3 Infusion Device | Z No Qualifier |
| Q Pleura | Ø Open<br>3 Percutaneous<br>4 Percutaneous Endoscopic<br>7 Via Natural or Artificial Opening<br>8 Via Natural or Artificial Opening Endoscopic | Ø Drainage Device<br>1 Radioactive Element<br>2 Monitoring Device<br>Y Other Device | Z No Qualifier |
| Q Pleura | X External | Ø Drainage Device<br>1 Radioactive Element<br>2 Monitoring Device | Z No Qualifier |
| T Diaphragm | Ø Open<br>3 Percutaneous<br>4 Percutaneous Endoscopic<br>7 Via Natural or Artificial Opening<br>8 Via Natural or Artificial Opening Endoscopic | Ø Drainage Device<br>2 Monitoring Device<br>7 Autologous Tissue Substitute<br>J Synthetic Substitute<br>K Nonautologous Tissue Substitute<br>M Diaphragmatic Pacemaker Lead<br>Y Other Device | Z No Qualifier |
| T Diaphragm | X External | Ø Drainage Device<br>2 Monitoring Device<br>M Diaphragmatic Pacemaker Lead | Z No Qualifier |

Non-OR ØBPØ[3,4]YZ
Non-OR ØBP[7,8][Ø,2,3,D,Y]Z
Non-OR ØBPØX[Ø,1,2,3,D]Z
Non-OR ØBP1[Ø,3,4]FZ
Non-OR ØBP1[7,8][Ø,2,D,F]Z
Non-OR ØBP1X[Ø,2,D,F]Z
Non-OR ØBP[K,L][3,4]YZ
Non-OR ØBPK[7,8]1Z
Non-OR ØBP[K,L][7,8][Ø,2,3,Y]Z
Non-OR ØBP[K,L]X[Ø,1,2,3]Z
Non-OR ØBPQ[Ø,3,4,7,8][Ø,1,2,Y]Z
Non-OR ØBPQX[Ø,1,2]Z
Non-OR ØBPT[3,4]YZ
Non-OR ØBPT[7,8][Ø,2,Y]Z
Non-OR ØBPTX[Ø,2,M]Z

**Ø Medical and Surgical**
**B Respiratory System**
**Q Repair** Definition: Restoring, to the extent possible, a body part to its normal anatomic structure and function

Explanation: Used only when the method to accomplish the repair is not one of the other root operations

| Body Part Character 4 | Approach Character 5 | Device Character 6 | Qualifier Character 7 |
|---|---|---|---|
| 1 Trachea<br>Cricoid cartilage<br>2 Carina<br>3 Main Bronchus, Right<br>Bronchus intermedius<br>Intermediate bronchus<br>4 Upper Lobe Bronchus, Right<br>5 Middle Lobe Bronchus, Right<br>6 Lower Lobe Bronchus, Right<br>7 Main Bronchus, Left<br>8 Upper Lobe Bronchus, Left<br>9 Lingula Bronchus<br>B Lower Lobe Bronchus, Left<br>C Upper Lung Lobe, Right<br>D Middle Lung Lobe, Right<br>F Lower Lung Lobe, Right<br>G Upper Lung Lobe, Left<br>H Lung Lingula<br>J Lower Lung Lobe, Left<br>K Lung, Right<br>L Lung, Left<br>M Lungs, Bilateral | Ø Open<br>3 Percutaneous<br>4 Percutaneous Endoscopic<br>7 Via Natural or Artificial Opening<br>8 Via Natural or Artificial Opening Endoscopic | Z No Device | Z No Qualifier |
| N Pleura, Right<br>P Pleura, Left<br>T Diaphragm | Ø Open<br>3 Percutaneous<br>4 Percutaneous Endoscopic | Z No Device | Z No Qualifier |

**Ø Medical and Surgical**
**B Respiratory System**
**R Replacement** Definition: Putting in or on biological or synthetic material that physically takes the place and/or function of all or a portion of a body part

Explanation: The body part may have been taken out or replaced, or may be taken out, physically eradicated, or rendered nonfunctional during the REPLACEMENT procedure. A REMOVAL procedure is coded for taking out the device used in a previous replacement procedure.

| Body Part Character 4 | Approach Character 5 | Device Character 6 | Qualifier Character 7 |
|---|---|---|---|
| 1 Trachea<br>Cricoid cartilage<br>2 Carina<br>3 Main Bronchus, Right<br>Bronchus intermedius<br>Intermediate bronchus<br>4 Upper Lobe Bronchus, Right<br>5 Middle Lobe Bronchus, Right<br>6 Lower Lobe Bronchus, Right<br>7 Main Bronchus, Left<br>8 Upper Lobe Bronchus, Left<br>9 Lingula Bronchus<br>B Lower Lobe Bronchus, Left<br>T Diaphragm | Ø Open<br>4 Percutaneous Endoscopic | 7 Autologous Tissue Substitute<br>J Synthetic Substitute<br>K Nonautologous Tissue Substitute | Z No Qualifier |

**Ø Medical and Surgical**
**B Respiratory System**
**S Reposition** Definition: Moving to its normal location, or other suitable location, all or a portion of a body part

Explanation: The body part is moved to a new location from an abnormal location, or from a normal location where it is not functioning correctly. The body part may or may not be cut out or off to be moved to the new location.

| Body Part Character 4 | Approach Character 5 | Device Character 6 | Qualifier Character 7 |
|---|---|---|---|
| 1 Trachea<br>Cricoid cartilage<br>2 Carina<br>3 Main Bronchus, Right<br>Bronchus intermedius<br>Intermediate bronchus<br>4 Upper Lobe Bronchus, Right<br>5 Middle Lobe Bronchus, Right<br>6 Lower Lobe Bronchus, Right<br>7 Main Bronchus, Left<br>8 Upper Lobe Bronchus, Left<br>9 Lingula Bronchus<br>B Lower Lobe Bronchus, Left<br>C Upper Lung Lobe, Right<br>D Middle Lung Lobe, Right<br>F Lower Lung Lobe, Right<br>G Upper Lung Lobe, Left<br>H Lung Lingula<br>J Lower Lung Lobe, Left<br>K Lung, Right<br>L Lung, Left<br>T Diaphragm | Ø Open | Z No Device | Z No Qualifier |

**Ø Medical and Surgical**
**B Respiratory System**
**T Resection** Definition: Cutting out or off, without replacement, all of a body part

Explanation: None

| Body Part Character 4 | Approach Character 5 | Device Character 6 | Qualifier Character 7 |
|---|---|---|---|
| **1** Trachea<br>Cricoid cartilage<br>**2** Carina<br>**3** Main Bronchus, Right<br>Bronchus intermedius<br>Intermediate bronchus<br>**4** Upper Lobe Bronchus, Right<br>**5** Middle Lobe Bronchus, Right<br>**6** Lower Lobe Bronchus, Right<br>**7** Main Bronchus, Left<br>**8** Upper Lobe Bronchus, Left<br>**9** Lingula Bronchus<br>**B** Lower Lobe Bronchus, Left<br>**C** Upper Lung Lobe, Right<br>**D** Middle Lung Lobe, Right<br>**F** Lower Lung Lobe, Right<br>**G** Upper Lung Lobe, Left<br>**H** Lung Lingula<br>**J** Lower Lung Lobe, Left<br>**K** Lung, Right<br>**L** Lung, Left<br>**M** Lungs, Bilateral<br>**T** Diaphragm | **Ø** Open<br>**4** Percutaneous Endoscopic | **Z** No Device | **Z** No Qualifier |

**Ø Medical and Surgical**
**B Respiratory System**
**U Supplement** Definition: Putting in or on biological or synthetic material that physically reinforces and/or augments the function of a portion of a body part

Explanation: The biological material is non-living, or is living and from the same individual. The body part may have been previously replaced, and the SUPPLEMENT procedure is performed to physically reinforce and/or augment the function of the replaced body part.

| Body Part Character 4 | Approach Character 5 | Device Character 6 | Qualifier Character 7 |
|---|---|---|---|
| **1** Trachea<br>Cricoid cartilage<br>**2** Carina<br>**3** Main Bronchus, Right<br>Bronchus intermedius<br>Intermediate bronchus<br>**4** Upper Lobe Bronchus, Right<br>**5** Middle Lobe Bronchus, Right<br>**6** Lower Lobe Bronchus, Right<br>**7** Main Bronchus, Left<br>**8** Upper Lobe Bronchus, Left<br>**9** Lingula Bronchus<br>**B** Lower Lobe Bronchus, Left | **Ø** Open<br>**4** Percutaneous Endoscopic<br>**8** Via Natural or Artificial Opening Endoscopic | **7** Autologous Tissue Substitute<br>**J** Synthetic Substitute<br>**K** Nonautologous Tissue Substitute | **Z** No Qualifier |
| **T** Diaphragm | **Ø** Open<br>**4** Percutaneous Endoscopic | **7** Autologous Tissue Substitute<br>**J** Synthetic Substitute<br>**K** Nonautologous Tissue Substitute | **Z** No Qualifier |

**Ø Medical and Surgical**
**B Respiratory System**
**V Restriction** Definition: Partially closing an orifice or the lumen of a tubular body part
Explanation: The orifice can be a natural orifice or an artificially created orifice

| Body Part Character 4 | Approach Character 5 | Device Character 6 | Qualifier Character 7 |
|---|---|---|---|
| **1 Trachea**<br>Cricoid cartilage<br>**2 Carina**<br>**3 Main Bronchus, Right**<br>Bronchus intermedius<br>Intermediate bronchus<br>**4 Upper Lobe Bronchus, Right**<br>**5 Middle Lobe Bronchus, Right**<br>**6 Lower Lobe Bronchus, Right**<br>**7 Main Bronchus, Left**<br>**8 Upper Lobe Bronchus, Left**<br>**9 Lingula Bronchus**<br>**B Lower Lobe Bronchus, Left** | **Ø Open**<br>**3 Percutaneous**<br>**4 Percutaneous Endoscopic** | **C Extraluminal Device**<br>**D Intraluminal Device**<br>**Z No Device** | **Z No Qualifier** |
| **1 Trachea**<br>Cricoid cartilage<br>**2 Carina**<br>**3 Main Bronchus, Right**<br>Bronchus intermedius<br>Intermediate bronchus<br>**4 Upper Lobe Bronchus, Right**<br>**5 Middle Lobe Bronchus, Right**<br>**6 Lower Lobe Bronchus, Right**<br>**7 Main Bronchus, Left**<br>**8 Upper Lobe Bronchus, Left**<br>**9 Lingula Bronchus**<br>**B Lower Lobe Bronchus, Left** | **7 Via Natural or Artificial Opening**<br>**8 Via Natural or Artificial Opening Endoscopic** | **D Intraluminal Device**<br>**Z No Device** | **Z No Qualifier** |

**Ø Medical and Surgical**
**B Respiratory System**
**W Revision** Definition: Correcting, to the extent possible, a portion of a malfunctioning device or the position of a displaced device

Explanation: Revision can include correcting a malfunctioning or displaced device by taking out or putting in components of the device such as a screw or pin

| Body Part Character 4 | Approach Character 5 | Device Character 6 | Qualifier Character 7 |
|---|---|---|---|
| Ø Tracheobronchial Tree | Ø Open<br>3 Percutaneous<br>4 Percutaneous Endoscopic<br>7 Via Natural or Artificial Opening<br>8 Via Natural or Artificial Opening Endoscopic | Ø Drainage Device<br>2 Monitoring Device<br>3 Infusion Device<br>7 Autologous Tissue Substitute<br>C Extraluminal Device<br>D Intraluminal Device<br>J Synthetic Substitute<br>K Nonautologous Tissue Substitute<br>Y Other Device | Z No Qualifier |
| Ø Tracheobronchial Tree | X External | Ø Drainage Device<br>2 Monitoring Device<br>3 Infusion Device<br>7 Autologous Tissue Substitute<br>C Extraluminal Device<br>D Intraluminal Device<br>J Synthetic Substitute<br>K Nonautologous Tissue Substitute | Z No Qualifier |
| 1 Trachea<br>Cricoid cartilage | Ø Open<br>3 Percutaneous<br>4 Percutaneous Endoscopic<br>7 Via Natural or Artificial Opening<br>8 Via Natural or Artificial Opening Endoscopic<br>X External | Ø Drainage Device<br>2 Monitoring Device<br>7 Autologous Tissue Substitute<br>C Extraluminal Device<br>D Intraluminal Device<br>F Tracheostomy Device<br>J Synthetic Substitute<br>K Nonautologous Tissue Substitute | Z No Qualifier |
| K Lung, Right<br>L Lung, Left | Ø Open<br>3 Percutaneous<br>4 Percutaneous Endoscopic<br>7 Via Natural or Artificial Opening<br>8 Via Natural or Artificial Opening Endoscopic | Ø Drainage Device<br>2 Monitoring Device<br>3 Infusion Device<br>Y Other Device | Z No Qualifier |
| K Lung, Right<br>L Lung, Left | X External | Ø Drainage Device<br>2 Monitoring Device<br>3 Infusion Device | Z No Qualifier |
| Q Pleura | Ø Open<br>3 Percutaneous<br>4 Percutaneous Endoscopic<br>7 Via Natural or Artificial Opening<br>8 Via Natural or Artificial Opening Endoscopic | Ø Drainage Device<br>2 Monitoring Device<br>Y Other Device | Z No Qualifier |
| Q Pleura | X External | Ø Drainage Device<br>2 Monitoring Device | Z No Qualifier |
| T Diaphragm | Ø Open<br>3 Percutaneous<br>4 Percutaneous Endoscopic<br>7 Via Natural or Artificial Opening<br>8 Via Natural or Artificial Opening Endoscopic | Ø Drainage Device<br>2 Monitoring Device<br>7 Autologous Tissue Substitute<br>J Synthetic Substitute<br>K Nonautologous Tissue Substitute<br>M Diaphragmatic Pacemaker Lead<br>Y Other Device | Z No Qualifier |
| T Diaphragm | X External | Ø Drainage Device<br>2 Monitoring Device<br>7 Autologous Tissue Substitute<br>J Synthetic Substitute<br>K Nonautologous Tissue Substitute<br>M Diaphragmatic Pacemaker Lead | Z No Qualifier |

**Non-OR** ØBWØ[3,4]YZ
**Non-OR** ØBWØ[7,8][2,3,D,Y]Z
**Non-OR** ØBWØX[Ø,2,3,7,C,D,J,K]Z
**Non-OR** ØBW1X[Ø,2,7,C,D,F,J,K]Z
**Non-OR** ØBW[K,L][3,4]YZ
**Non-OR** ØBW[K,L][7,8][Ø,2,3,Y]Z
**Non-OR** ØBW[K,L]X[Ø,2,3]Z
**Non-OR** ØBWQ[Ø,3,4,7,8][Ø,2,Y]Z
**Non-OR** ØBWQX[Ø,2]Z
**Non-OR** ØBWT[3,4,7,8]YZ
**Non-OR** ØBWTX[Ø,2,7,J,K,M]Z

**Ø Medical and Surgical**
**B Respiratory System**
**Y Transplantation** Definition: Putting in or on all or a portion of a living body part taken from another individual or animal to physically take the place and/or function of all or a portion of a similar body part

Explanation: The native body part may or may not be taken out, and the transplanted body part may take over all or a portion of its function

| Body Part Character 4 | Approach Character 5 | Device Character 6 | Qualifier Character 7 |
|---|---|---|---|
| C Upper Lung Lobe, Right LC<br>D Middle Lung Lobe, Right LC<br>F Lower Lung Lobe, Right LC<br>G Upper Lung Lobe, Left LC<br>H Lung Lingula LC<br>J Lower Lung Lobe, Left LC<br>K Lung, Right LC<br>L Lung, Left LC<br>M Lungs, Bilateral LC | Ø Open | Z No Device | Ø Allogeneic<br>1 Syngeneic<br>2 Zooplastic |

LC ØBY[C,D,F,G,H,J,K,L,M]ØZ[Ø,1,2]

# Mouth and Throat ØCØ–ØCX



## Character Meanings

This Character Meaning table is provided as a guide to assist the user in the identification of character members that may be found in this section of code tables. It **SHOULD NOT** be used to build a PCS code.

| Operation–Character 3 | Body Part–Character 4 | Approach–Character 5 | Device–Character 6 | Qualifier–Character 7 |
|---|---|---|---|---|
| Ø Alteration | Ø Upper Lip | Ø Open | Ø Drainage Device | Ø Single |
| 2 Change | 1 Lower Lip | 3 Percutaneous | 1 Radioactive Element | 1 Multiple |
| 5 Destruction | 2 Hard Palate | 4 Percutaneous Endoscopic | 5 External Fixation Device | 2 All |
| 7 Dilation | 3 Soft Palate | 7 Via Natural or Artificial Opening | 7 Autologous Tissue Substitute | X Diagnostic |
| 9 Drainage | 4 Buccal Mucosa | 8 Via Natural or Artificial Opening Endoscopic | B Intraluminal Device, Airway | Z No Qualifier |
| B Excision | 5 Upper Gingiva | X External | C Extraluminal Device | |
| C Extirpation | 6 Lower Gingiva | | D Intraluminal Device | |
| D Extraction | 7 Tongue | | J Synthetic Substitute | |
| F Fragmentation | 8 Parotid Gland, Right | | K Nonautologous Tissue Substitute | |
| H Insertion | 9 Parotid Gland, Left | | Y Other Device | |
| J Inspection | A Salivary Gland | | Z No Device | |
| L Occlusion | B Parotid Duct, Right | | | |
| M Reattachment | C Parotid Duct, Left | | | |
| N Release | D Sublingual Gland, Right | | | |
| P Removal | F Sublingual Gland, Left | | | |
| Q Repair | G Submaxillary Gland, Right | | | |
| R Replacement | H Submaxillary Gland, Left | | | |
| S Reposition | J Minor Salivary Gland | | | |
| T Resection | M Pharynx | | | |
| U Supplement | N Uvula | | | |
| V Restriction | P Tonsils | | | |
| W Revision | Q Adenoids | | | |
| X Transfer | R Epiglottis | | | |
| | S Larynx | | | |
| | T Vocal Cord, Right | | | |
| | V Vocal Cord, Left | | | |
| | W Upper Tooth | | | |
| | X Lower Tooth | | | |
| | Y Mouth and Throat | | | |

**AHA Coding Clinic for table ØC9**
**2017, 2Q, 16** Incision and drainage of floor of mouth

**AHA Coding Clinic for table ØCB**
**2017, 2Q, 16** Excision of floor of mouth
**2016, 3Q, 28** Lingual tonsillectomy, tongue base excision and epiglottopexy
**2016, 2Q, 19** Biopsy of the base of tongue
**2014, 3Q, 21** Superficial parotidectomy

**AHA Coding Clinic for table ØCC**
**2016, 2Q, 20** Sialendoscopy with stone removal

**AHA Coding Clinic for table ØCQ**
**2017, 1Q, 20** Preparatory nasal adhesion repair before definitive cleft palate repair

**AHA Coding Clinic for table ØCR**
**2014, 3Q, 25** Excision of soft palate with placement of surgical obturator
**2014, 2Q, 5** Oasis acellular matrix graft
**2014, 2Q, 6** Composite grafting (synthetic versus nonautologous tissue substitute)

**AHA Coding Clinic for table ØCS**
**2016, 3Q, 28** Lingual tonsillectomy, tongue base excision and epiglottopexy

**AHA Coding Clinic for table ØCT**
**2016, 2Q, 12** Resection of malignant neoplasm of infratemporal fossa
**2014, 3Q, 21** Superficial parotidectomy
**2014, 3Q, 23** Le Fort I osteotomy

## Salivary Glands

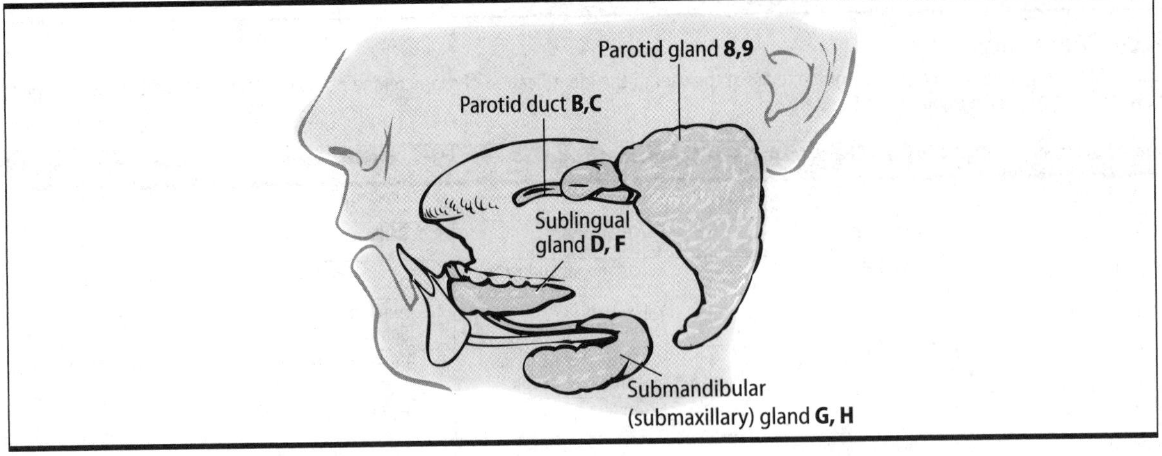
Parotid gland 8,9
Parotid duct B,C
Sublingual gland D, F
Submandibular (submaxillary) gland G, H

## Oral Anatomy

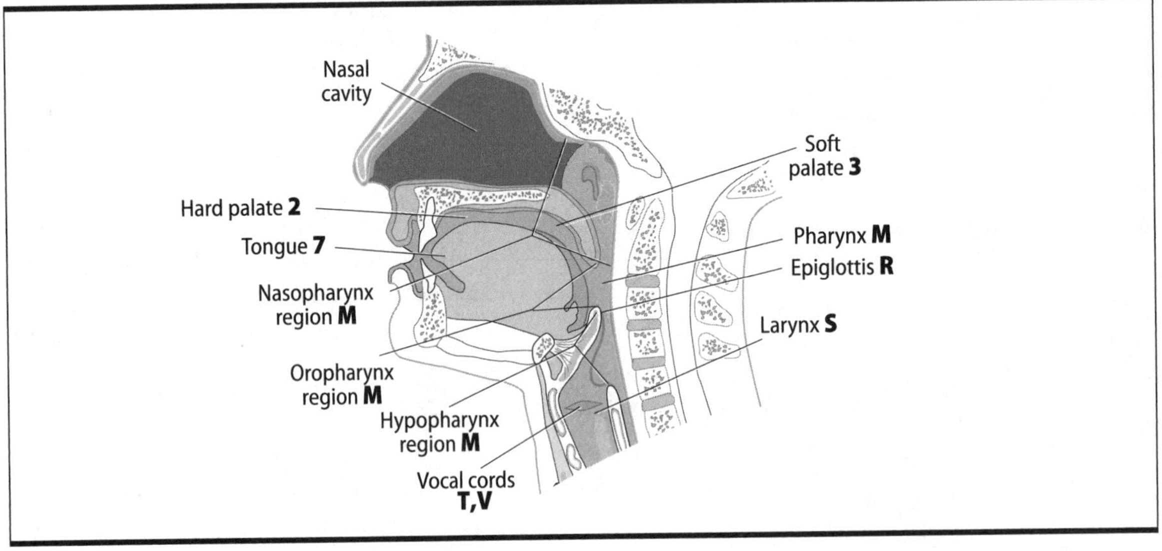
Nasal cavity
Soft palate 3
Hard palate 2
Tongue 7
Pharynx M
Epiglottis R
Nasopharynx region M
Larynx S
Oropharynx region M
Hypopharynx region M
Vocal cords T,V

## Mouth Frontal View (Upper)

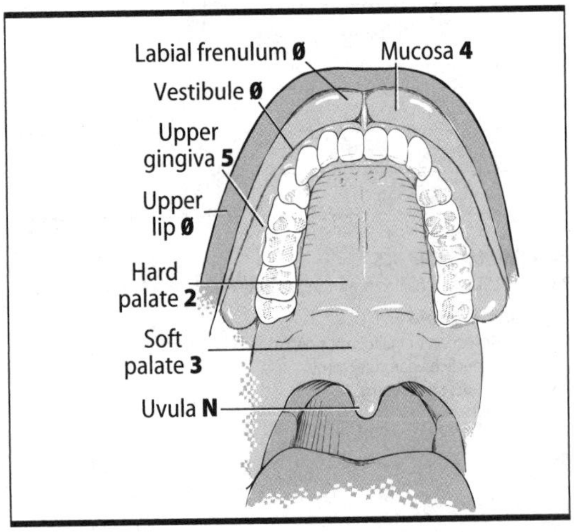
Labial frenulum Ø
Mucosa 4
Vestibule Ø
Upper gingiva 5
Upper lip Ø
Hard palate 2
Soft palate 3
Uvula N

## Mouth Frontal View (Lower)

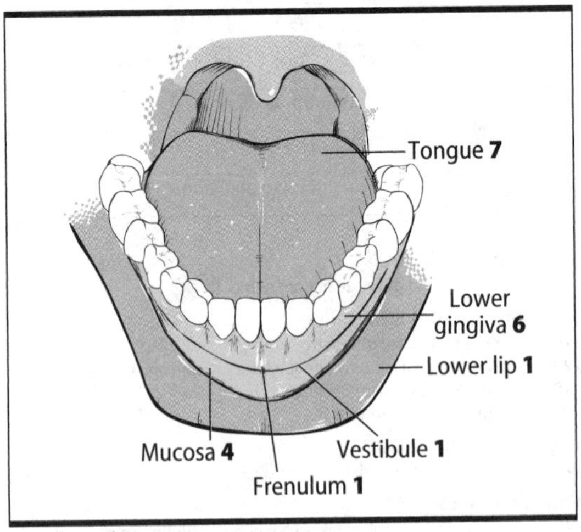
Tongue 7
Lower gingiva 6
Lower lip 1
Mucosa 4
Vestibule 1
Frenulum 1

**Ø Medical and Surgical**
**C Mouth and Throat**
**Ø Alteration** Definition: Modifying the anatomic structure of a body part without affecting the function of the body part

Explanation: Principal purpose is to improve appearance

| Body Part Character 4 | Approach Character 5 | Device Character 6 | Qualifier Character 7 |
|---|---|---|---|
| **Ø Upper Lip**<br>Frenulum labii superioris<br>Labial gland<br>Vermilion border<br>**1 Lower Lip**<br>Frenulum labii inferioris<br>Labial gland<br>Vermilion border | **X External** | **7 Autologous Tissue Substitute**<br>**J Synthetic Substitute**<br>**K Nonautologous Tissue Substitute**<br>**Z No Device** | **Z No Qualifier** |

**Ø Medical and Surgical**
**C Mouth and Throat**
**2 Change** Definition: Taking out or off a device from a body part and putting back an identical or similar device in or on the same body part without cutting or puncturing the skin or a mucous membrane

Explanation: All CHANGE procedures are coded using the approach EXTERNAL

| Body Part Character 4 | Approach Character 5 | Device Character 6 | Qualifier Character 7 |
|---|---|---|---|
| **A Salivary Gland**<br>**S Larynx**<br>Aryepiglottic fold<br>Arytenoid cartilage<br>Corniculate cartilage<br>Cuneiform cartilage<br>False vocal cord<br>Glottis<br>Rima glottidis<br>Thyroid cartilage<br>Ventricular fold<br>**Y Mouth and Throat** | **X External** | **Ø Drainage Device**<br>**Y Other Device** | **Z No Qualifier** |

Non-OR All body part, approach, device, and qualifier values

**Ø Medical and Surgical**
**C Mouth and Throat**
**5 Destruction** Definition: Physical eradication of all or a portion of a body part by the direct use of energy, force, or a destructive agent

Explanation: None of the body part is physically taken out

| Body Part Character 4 | | Approach Character 5 | Device Character 6 | Qualifier Character 7 |
|---|---|---|---|---|
| **Ø Upper Lip**<br>Frenulum labii superioris<br>Labial gland<br>Vermilion border<br>**1 Lower Lip**<br>Frenulum labii inferioris<br>Labial gland<br>Vermilion border<br>**2 Hard Palate**<br>**3 Soft Palate**<br>**4 Buccal Mucosa**<br>Buccal gland<br>Molar gland<br>Palatine gland | **5 Upper Gingiva**<br>**6 Lower Gingiva**<br>**7 Tongue**<br>Frenulum linguae<br>**N Uvula**<br>Palatine uvula<br>**P Tonsils**<br>Palatine tonsil<br>**Q Adenoids**<br>Pharyngeal tonsil | **Ø Open**<br>**3 Percutaneous**<br>**X External** | **Z No Device** | **Z No Qualifier** |
| **8 Parotid Gland, Right**<br>**9 Parotid Gland, Left**<br>**B Parotid Duct, Right**<br>Stensen's duct<br>**C Parotid Duct, Left**<br>*See B Parotid Duct, Right*<br>**D Sublingual Gland, Right** | **F Sublingual Gland, Left**<br>**G Submaxillary Gland, Right**<br>Submandibular gland<br>**H Submaxillary Gland, Left**<br>*See G Submaxillary Gland, Right*<br>**J Minor Salivary Gland**<br>Anterior lingual gland | **Ø Open**<br>**3 Percutaneous** | **Z No Device** | **Z No Qualifier** |
| **M Pharynx**<br>Base of tongue<br>Hypopharynx<br>Laryngopharynx<br>Lingual tonsil<br>Oropharynx<br>Piriform recess (sinus)<br>Tongue, base of<br>**R Epiglottis**<br>Glossoepiglottic fold | **S Larynx**<br>Aryepiglottic fold<br>Arytenoid cartilage<br>Corniculate cartilage<br>Cuneiform cartilage<br>False vocal cord<br>Glottis<br>Rima glottidis<br>Thyroid cartilage<br>Ventricular fold<br>**T Vocal Cord, Right**<br>Vocal fold<br>**V Vocal Cord, Left**<br>*See T Vocal Cord, Right* | **Ø Open**<br>**3 Percutaneous**<br>**4 Percutaneous Endoscopic**<br>**7 Via Natural or Artificial Opening**<br>**8 Via Natural or Artificial Opening Endoscopic** | **Z No Device** | **Z No Qualifier** |
| **W Upper Tooth**<br>**X Lower Tooth** | | **Ø Open**<br>**X External** | **Z No Device** | **Ø Single**<br>**1 Multiple**<br>**2 All** |

**Non-OR** ØC5[5,6][Ø,3,X]ZZ
**Non-OR** ØC5[W,X][Ø,X]Z[Ø,1,2]

**Ø Medical and Surgical**
**C Mouth and Throat**
**7 Dilation** Definition: Expanding an orifice or the lumen of a tubular body part

Explanation: The orifice can be a natural orifice or an artificially created orifice. Accomplished by stretching a tubular body part using intraluminal pressure or by cutting part of the orifice or wall of the tubular body part.

| Body Part Character 4 | Approach Character 5 | Device Character 6 | Qualifier Character 7 |
|---|---|---|---|
| **B Parotid Duct, Right**<br>Stensen's duct<br>**C Parotid Duct, Left**<br>*See B Parotid Duct, Right* | **Ø Open**<br>**3 Percutaneous**<br>**7 Via Natural or Artificial Opening** | **D Intraluminal Device**<br>**Z No Device** | **Z No Qualifier** |
| **M Pharynx**<br>Base of tongue<br>Hypopharynx<br>Laryngopharynx<br>Lingual tonsil<br>Oropharynx<br>Piriform recess (sinus)<br>Tongue, base of | **7 Via Natural or Artificial Opening**<br>**8 Via Natural or Artificial Opening Endoscopic** | **D Intraluminal Device**<br>**Z No Device** | **Z No Qualifier** |
| **S Larynx**<br>Aryepiglottic fold<br>Arytenoid cartilage<br>Corniculate cartilage<br>Cuneiform cartilage<br>False vocal cord<br>Glottis<br>Rima glottidis<br>Thyroid cartilage<br>Ventricular fold | **Ø Open**<br>**3 Percutaneous**<br>**4 Percutaneous Endoscopic**<br>**7 Via Natural or Artificial Opening**<br>**8 Via Natural or Artificial Opening Endoscopic** | **D Intraluminal Device**<br>**Z No Device** | **Z No Qualifier** |

**Non-OR** ØC7[B,C][Ø,3,7][D,Z]Z
**Non-OR** ØC7M[7,8][D,Z]Z

**Ø Medical and Surgical**
**C Mouth and Throat**
**9 Drainage** Definition: Taking or letting out fluids and/or gases from a body part

Explanation: The qualifier DIAGNOSTIC is used to identify drainage procedures that are biopsies

| Body Part Character 4 | Approach Character 5 | Device Character 6 | Qualifier Character 7 |
|---|---|---|---|
| **Ø Upper Lip**<br>Frenulum labii superioris<br>Labial gland<br>Vermilion border<br>**1 Lower Lip**<br>Frenulum labii inferioris<br>Labial gland<br>Vermilion border<br>**2 Hard Palate**<br>**3 Soft Palate**<br>**4 Buccal Mucosa**<br>Buccal gland<br>Molar gland<br>Palatine gland<br>**5 Upper Gingiva**<br>**6 Lower Gingiva**<br>**7 Tongue**<br>Frenulum linguae<br>**N Uvula**<br>Palatine uvula<br>**P Tonsils**<br>Palatine tonsil<br>**Q Adenoids**<br>Pharyngeal tonsil | **Ø Open**<br>**3 Percutaneous**<br>**X External** | **Ø Drainage Device** | **Z No Qualifier** |
| **Ø Upper Lip**<br>Frenulum labii superioris<br>Labial gland<br>Vermilion border<br>**1 Lower Lip**<br>Frenulum labii inferioris<br>Labial gland<br>Vermilion border<br>**2 Hard Palate**<br>**3 Soft Palate**<br>**4 Buccal Mucosa**<br>Buccal gland<br>Molar gland<br>Palatine gland<br>**5 Upper Gingiva**<br>**6 Lower Gingiva**<br>**7 Tongue**<br>Frenulum linguae<br>**N Uvula**<br>Palatine uvula<br>**P Tonsils**<br>Palatine tonsil<br>**Q Adenoids**<br>Pharyngeal tonsil | **Ø Open**<br>**3 Percutaneous**<br>**X External** | **Z No Device** | **X Diagnostic**<br>**Z No Qualifier** |
| **8 Parotid Gland, Right**<br>**9 Parotid Gland, Left**<br>**B Parotid Duct, Right**<br>Stensen's duct<br>**C Parotid Duct, Left**<br>*See B Parotid Duct, Right*<br>**D Sublingual Gland, Right**<br>**F Sublingual Gland, Left**<br>**G Submaxillary Gland, Right**<br>Submandibular gland<br>**H Submaxillary Gland, Left**<br>*See G Submaxillary Gland, Right*<br>**J Minor Salivary Gland**<br>Anterior lingual gland | **Ø Open**<br>**3 Percutaneous** | **Ø Drainage Device** | **Z No Qualifier** |
| **8 Parotid Gland, Right**<br>**9 Parotid Gland, Left**<br>**B Parotid Duct, Right**<br>Stensen's duct<br>**C Parotid Duct, Left**<br>*See B Parotid Duct, Right*<br>**D Sublingual Gland, Right**<br>**F Sublingual Gland, Left**<br>**G Submaxillary Gland, Right**<br>Submandibular gland<br>**H Submaxillary Gland, Left**<br>*See G Submaxillary Gland, Right*<br>**J Minor Salivary Gland**<br>Anterior lingual gland | **Ø Open**<br>**3 Percutaneous** | **Z No Device** | **X Diagnostic**<br>**Z No Qualifier** |
| **M Pharynx**<br>Base of tongue<br>Hypopharynx<br>Laryngopharynx<br>Lingual tonsil<br>Oropharynx<br>Piriform recess (sinus)<br>Tongue, base of<br>**R Epiglottis**<br>Glossoepiglottic fold<br>**S Larynx**<br>Aryepiglottic fold<br>Arytenoid cartilage<br>Corniculate cartilage<br>Cuneiform cartilage<br>False vocal cord<br>Glottis<br>Rima glottidis<br>Thyroid cartilage<br>Ventricular fold<br>**T Vocal Cord, Right**<br>Vocal fold<br>**V Vocal Cord, Left**<br>*See T Vocal Cord, Right* | **Ø Open**<br>**3 Percutaneous**<br>**4 Percutaneous Endoscopic**<br>**7 Via Natural or Artificial Opening**<br>**8 Via Natural or Artificial Opening Endoscopic** | **Ø Drainage Device** | **Z No Qualifier** |

*ØC9 Continued on next page*

**Non-OR** ØC9[Ø,1,2,3,4,7,N,P,Q]3ØZ
**Non-OR** ØC9[5,6][Ø,3,X]ØZ
**Non-OR** ØC9[Ø,1,4][Ø,3,X]ZX
**Non-OR** ØC9[Ø,1,2,3,4,7,N,P,Q]3ZZ
**Non-OR** ØC9[5,6][Ø,3,X]Z[X,Z]
**Non-OR** ØC97[3,X]ZX
**Non-OR** ØC9[8,9,B,C,D,F,G,H,J][Ø,3]ØZ
**Non-OR** ØC9[8,9,B,C,D,F,G,H,J]3ZX
**Non-OR** ØC9[8,9,B,C,D,F,G,H,J][Ø,3]ZZ
**Non-OR** ØC9[M,R,S,T,V]3ØZ

ØC9 Continued

**Ø Medical and Surgical**
**C Mouth and Throat**
**9 Drainage** Definition: Taking or letting out fluids and/or gases from a body part
Explanation: The qualifier DIAGNOSTIC is used to identify drainage procedures that are biopsies

| Body Part Character 4 | | Approach Character 5 | Device Character 6 | Qualifier Character 7 |
|---|---|---|---|---|
| **M Pharynx**<br>Base of tongue<br>Hypopharynx<br>Laryngopharynx<br>Lingual tonsil<br>Oropharynx<br>Piriform recess (sinus)<br>Tongue, base of<br>**R Epiglottis**<br>Glossoepiglottic fold | **S Larynx**<br>Aryepiglottic fold<br>Arytenoid cartilage<br>Corniculate cartilage<br>Cuneiform cartilage<br>False vocal cord<br>Glottis<br>Rima glottidis<br>Thyroid cartilage<br>Ventricular fold<br>**T Vocal Cord, Right**<br>Vocal fold<br>**V Vocal Cord, Left**<br>*See T Vocal Cord, Right* | **Ø Open**<br>**3 Percutaneous**<br>**4 Percutaneous Endoscopic**<br>**7 Via Natural or Artificial Opening**<br>**8 Via Natural or Artificial Opening Endoscopic** | **Z No Device** | **X Diagnostic**<br>**Z No Qualifier** |
| **W Upper Tooth**<br>**X Lower Tooth** | | **Ø Open**<br>**X External** | **Ø Drainage Device**<br>**Z No Device** | **Ø Single**<br>**1 Multiple**<br>**2 All** |

Non-OR ØC9M[Ø,3,4,7,8]ZX
Non-OR ØC9[M,R,S,T,V]3ZZ
Non-OR ØC9[R,S,T,V][3,4,7,8]ZX
Non-OR ØC9[W,X][Ø,X][Ø,Z][Ø,1,2]

**Ø Medical and Surgical**
**C Mouth and Throat**
**B Excision** Definition: Cutting out or off, without replacement, a portion of a body part
Explanation: The qualifier DIAGNOSTIC is used to identify excision procedures that are biopsies

| Body Part Character 4 | | Approach Character 5 | Device Character 6 | Qualifier Character 7 |
|---|---|---|---|---|
| **Ø Upper Lip**<br>Frenulum labii superioris<br>Labial gland<br>Vermilion border<br>**1 Lower Lip**<br>Frenulum labii inferioris<br>Labial gland<br>Vermilion border<br>**2 Hard Palate**<br>**3 Soft Palate**<br>**4 Buccal Mucosa**<br>Buccal gland<br>Molar gland<br>Palatine gland | **5 Upper Gingiva**<br>**6 Lower Gingiva**<br>**7 Tongue**<br>Frenulum linguae<br>**N Uvula**<br>Palatine uvula<br>**P Tonsils**<br>Palatine tonsil<br>**Q Adenoids**<br>Pharyngeal tonsil | **Ø Open**<br>**3 Percutaneous**<br>**X External** | **Z No Device** | **X Diagnostic**<br>**Z No Qualifier** |
| **8 Parotid Gland, Right**<br>**9 Parotid Gland, Left**<br>**B Parotid Duct, Right**<br>Stensen's duct<br>**C Parotid Duct, Left**<br>*See B Parotid Duct, Right*<br>**D Sublingual Gland, Right** | **F Sublingual Gland, Left**<br>**G Submaxillary Gland, Right**<br>Submandibular gland<br>**H Submaxillary Gland, Left**<br>*See G Submaxillary Gland, Right*<br>**J Minor Salivary Gland**<br>Anterior lingual gland | **Ø Open**<br>**3 Percutaneous** | **Z No Device** | **X Diagnostic**<br>**Z No Qualifier** |
| **M Pharynx**<br>Base of tongue<br>Hypopharynx<br>Laryngopharynx<br>Lingual tonsil<br>Oropharynx<br>Piriform recess (sinus)<br>Tongue, base of<br>**R Epiglottis**<br>Glossoepiglottic fold | **S Larynx**<br>Aryepiglottic fold<br>Arytenoid cartilage<br>Corniculate cartilage<br>Cuneiform cartilage<br>False vocal cord<br>Glottis<br>Rima glottidis<br>Thyroid cartilage<br>Ventricular fold<br>**T Vocal Cord, Right**<br>Vocal fold<br>**V Vocal Cord, Left**<br>*See T Vocal Cord, Right* | **Ø Open**<br>**3 Percutaneous**<br>**4 Percutaneous Endoscopic**<br>**7 Via Natural or Artificial Opening**<br>**8 Via Natural or Artificial Opening Endoscopic** | **Z No Device** | **X Diagnostic**<br>**Z No Qualifier** |
| **W Upper Tooth**<br>**X Lower Tooth** | | **Ø Open**<br>**X External** | **Z No Device** | **Ø Single**<br>**1 Multiple**<br>**2 All** |

Non-OR ØCB[Ø,1,4][Ø,3,X]ZX
Non-OR ØCB[5,6][Ø,3,X]Z[X,Z]
Non-OR ØCB7[3,X]ZX
Non-OR ØCB[8,9,B,C,D,F,G,H,J]3ZX
Non-OR ØCBM[Ø,3,4,7,8]ZX
Non-OR ØCB[R,S,T,V][3,4,7,8]ZX
Non-OR ØCB[W,X][Ø,X]Z[Ø,1,2]

**Ø Medical and Surgical**
**C Mouth and Throat**
**C Extirpation** Definition: Taking or cutting out solid matter from a body part

Explanation: The solid matter may be an abnormal byproduct of a biological function or a foreign body; it may be imbedded in a body part or in the lumen of a tubular body part. The solid matter may or may not have been previously broken into pieces.

| Body Part Character 4 | | Approach Character 5 | Device Character 6 | Qualifier Character 7 |
|---|---|---|---|---|
| **Ø Upper Lip** Frenulum labii superioris, Labial gland, Vermilion border<br>**1 Lower Lip** Frenulum labii inferioris, Labial gland, Vermilion border<br>**2 Hard Palate**<br>**3 Soft Palate**<br>**4 Buccal Mucosa** Buccal gland, Molar gland, Palatine gland | **5 Upper Gingiva**<br>**6 Lower Gingiva**<br>**7 Tongue** Frenulum linguae<br>**N Uvula** Palatine uvula<br>**P Tonsils** Palatine tonsil<br>**Q Adenoids** Pharyngeal tonsil | **Ø Open**<br>**3 Percutaneous**<br>**X External** | **Z No Device** | **Z No Qualifier** |
| **8 Parotid Gland, Right**<br>**9 Parotid Gland, Left**<br>**B Parotid Duct, Right** Stensen's duct<br>**C Parotid Duct, Left** *See B Parotid Duct, Right*<br>**D Sublingual Gland, Right** | **F Sublingual Gland, Left**<br>**G Submaxillary Gland, Right** Submandibular gland<br>**H Submaxillary Gland, Left** *See G Submaxillary Gland, Right*<br>**J Minor Salivary Gland** Anterior lingual gland | **Ø Open**<br>**3 Percutaneous** | **Z No Device** | **Z No Qualifier** |
| **M Pharynx** Base of tongue, Hypopharynx, Laryngopharynx, Lingual tonsil, Oropharynx, Piriform recess (sinus), Tongue, base of<br>**R Epiglottis** Glossoepiglottic fold | **S Larynx** Aryepiglottic fold, Arytenoid cartilage, Corniculate cartilage, Cuneiform cartilage, False vocal cord, Glottis, Rima glottidis, Thyroid cartilage, Ventricular fold<br>**T Vocal Cord, Right** Vocal fold<br>**V Vocal Cord, Left** *See T Vocal Cord, Right* | **Ø Open**<br>**3 Percutaneous**<br>**4 Percutaneous Endoscopic**<br>**7 Via Natural or Artificial Opening**<br>**8 Via Natural or Artificial Opening Endoscopic** | **Z No Device** | **Z No Qualifier** |
| **W Upper Tooth**<br>**X Lower Tooth** | | **Ø Open**<br>**X External** | **Z No Device** | **Ø Single**<br>**1 Multiple**<br>**2 All** |

**Non-OR** ØCC[Ø,1,2,3,4,7,N,P,Q]XZZ
**Non-OR** ØCC[5,6][Ø,3,X]ZZ
**Non-OR** ØCC[8,9,B,C,D,F,G,H,J][Ø,3]ZZ
**Non-OR** ØCC[M,S][7,8]ZZ
**Non-OR** ØCC[W,X][Ø,X]Z[Ø,1,2]

**Ø Medical and Surgical**
**C Mouth and Throat**
**D Extraction** Definition: Pulling or stripping out or off all or a portion of a body part by the use of force

Explanation: The qualifier DIAGNOSTIC is used to identify extraction procedures that are biopsies

| Body Part Character 4 | Approach Character 5 | Device Character 6 | Qualifier Character 7 |
|---|---|---|---|
| **T Vocal Cord, Right** Vocal fold<br>**V Vocal Cord, Left** *See T Vocal Cord, Right* | **Ø Open**<br>**3 Percutaneous**<br>**4 Percutaneous Endoscopic**<br>**7 Via Natural or Artificial Opening**<br>**8 Via Natural or Artificial Opening Endoscopic** | **Z No Device** | **Z No Qualifier** |
| **W Upper Tooth**<br>**X Lower Tooth** | **X External** | **Z No Device** | **Ø Single**<br>**1 Multiple**<br>**2 All** |

**Non-OR** ØCD[W,X]XZ[Ø,1,2]

**Ø Medical and Surgical**
**C Mouth and Throat**
**F Fragmentation** Definition: Breaking solid matter in a body part into pieces

Explanation: Physical force (e.g., manual, ultrasonic) applied directly or indirectly is used to break the solid matter into pieces. The solid matter may be an abnormal byproduct of a biological function or a foreign body. The pieces of solid matter are not taken out.

| Body Part Character 4 | Approach Character 5 | Device Character 6 | Qualifier Character 7 |
|---|---|---|---|
| **B** Parotid Duct, Right NC<br>Stensen's duct<br>**C** Parotid Duct, Left NC<br>*See B Parotid Duct, Right* | **Ø** Open<br>**3** Percutaneous<br>**7** Via Natural or Artificial Opening<br>**X** External | **Z** No Device | **Z** No Qualifier |

Non-OR All body part, approach, device, and qualifier values
NC ØCF[B,C]XZZ

**Ø Medical and Surgical**
**C Mouth and Throat**
**H Insertion** Definition: Putting in a nonbiological appliance that monitors, assists, performs, or prevents a physiological function but does not physically take the place of a body part

Explanation: None

| Body Part Character 4 | Approach Character 5 | Device Character 6 | Qualifier Character 7 |
|---|---|---|---|
| **7** Tongue<br>Frenulum linguae | **Ø** Open<br>**3** Percutaneous<br>**X** External | **1** Radioactive Element | **Z** No Qualifier |
| **A** Salivary Gland<br>**S** Larynx<br>Aryepiglottic fold<br>Arytenoid cartilage<br>Corniculate cartilage<br>Cuneiform cartilage<br>False vocal cord<br>Glottis<br>Rima glottidis<br>Thyroid cartilage<br>Ventricular fold | **Ø** Open<br>**3** Percutaneous<br>**7** Via Natural or Artificial Opening<br>**8** Via Natural or Artificial Opening Endoscopic | **Y** Other Device | **Z** No Qualifier |
| **Y** Mouth and Throat | **Ø** Open<br>**3** Percutaneous | **Y** Other Device | **Z** No Qualifier |
| **Y** Mouth and Throat | **7** Via Natural or Artificial Opening<br>**8** Via Natural or Artificial Opening Endoscopic | **B** Intraluminal Device, Airway<br>**Y** Other Device | **Z** No Qualifier |

Non-OR ØCH[A,S][3,7,8]YZ
Non-OR ØCHSØYZ
Non-OR ØCHY[Ø,3]YZ
Non-OR ØCHY[7,8][B,Y]Z

**Ø Medical and Surgical**
**C Mouth and Throat**
**J Inspection** Definition: Visually and/or manually exploring a body part

Explanation: Visual exploration may be performed with or without optical instrumentation. Manual exploration may be performed directly or through intervening body layers.

| Body Part Character 4 | Approach Character 5 | Device Character 6 | Qualifier Character 7 |
|---|---|---|---|
| **A** Salivary Gland | **Ø** Open<br>**3** Percutaneous<br>**X** External | **Z** No Device | **Z** No Qualifier |
| **S** Larynx<br>Aryepiglottic fold<br>Arytenoid cartilage<br>Corniculate cartilage<br>Cuneiform cartilage<br>False vocal cord<br>Glottis<br>Rima glottidis<br>Thyroid cartilage<br>Ventricular fold<br>**Y** Mouth and Throat | **Ø** Open<br>**3** Percutaneous<br>**4** Percutaneous Endoscopic<br>**7** Via Natural or Artificial Opening<br>**8** Via Natural or Artificial Opening Endoscopic<br>**X** External | **Z** No Device | **Z** No Qualifier |

Non-OR All body part, approach, device, and qualifier values

**Ø Medical and Surgical**
**C Mouth and Throat**
**L Occlusion** Definition: Completely closing an orifice or the lumen of a tubular body part
Explanation: The orifice can be a natural orifice or an artificially created orifice

| Body Part Character 4 | Approach Character 5 | Device Character 6 | Qualifier Character 7 |
|---|---|---|---|
| **B** Parotid Duct, Right<br>Stensen's duct<br>**C** Parotid Duct, Left<br>*See B Parotid Duct, Right* | **Ø** Open<br>**3** Percutaneous<br>**4** Percutaneous Endoscopic | **C** Extraluminal Device<br>**D** Intraluminal Device<br>**Z** No Device | **Z** No Qualifier |
| **B** Parotid Duct, Right<br>Stensen's duct<br>**C** Parotid Duct, Left<br>*See B Parotid Duct, Right* | **7** Via Natural or Artificial Opening<br>**8** Via Natural or Artificial Opening Endoscopic | **D** Intraluminal Device<br>**Z** No Device | **Z** No Qualifier |

**Ø Medical and Surgical**
**C Mouth and Throat**
**M Reattachment** Definition: Putting back in or on all or a portion of a separated body part to its normal location or other suitable location
Explanation: Vascular circulation and nervous pathways may or may not be reestablished

| Body Part Character 4 | Approach Character 5 | Device Character 6 | Qualifier Character 7 |
|---|---|---|---|
| **Ø** Upper Lip<br>Frenulum labii superioris<br>Labial gland<br>Vermilion border<br>**1** Lower Lip<br>Frenulum labii inferioris<br>Labial gland<br>Vermilion border<br>**3** Soft Palate<br>**7** Tongue<br>Frenulum linguae<br>**N** Uvula<br>Palatine uvula | **Ø** Open | **Z** No Device | **Z** No Qualifier |
| **W** Upper Tooth<br>**X** Lower Tooth | **Ø** Open<br>**X** External | **Z** No Device | **Ø** Single<br>**1** Multiple<br>**2** All |

Non-OR ØCM[W,X][Ø,X]Z[Ø,1,2]

**Ø Medical and Surgical**
**C Mouth and Throat**
**N Release** Definition: Freeing a body part from an abnormal physical constraint by cutting or by the use of force
Explanation: Some of the restraining tissue may be taken out but none of the body part is taken out

| Body Part Character 4 | Approach Character 5 | Device Character 6 | Qualifier Character 7 |
|---|---|---|---|
| **Ø Upper Lip**<br>Frenulum labii superioris<br>Labial gland<br>Vermilion border<br>**1 Lower Lip**<br>Frenulum labii inferioris<br>Labial gland<br>Vermilion border<br>**2 Hard Palate**<br>**3 Soft Palate**<br>**4 Buccal Mucosa**<br>Buccal gland<br>Molar gland<br>Palatine gland<br>**5 Upper Gingiva**<br>**6 Lower Gingiva**<br>**7 Tongue**<br>Frenulum linguae<br>**N Uvula**<br>Palatine uvula<br>**P Tonsils**<br>Palatine tonsil<br>**Q Adenoids**<br>Pharyngeal tonsil | **Ø Open**<br>**3 Percutaneous**<br>**X External** | **Z No Device** | **Z No Qualifier** |
| **8 Parotid Gland, Right**<br>**9 Parotid Gland, Left**<br>**B Parotid Duct, Right**<br>Stensen's duct<br>**C Parotid Duct, Left**<br>*See B Parotid Duct, Right*<br>**D Sublingual Gland, Right**<br>**F Sublingual Gland, Left**<br>**G Submaxillary Gland, Right**<br>Submandibular gland<br>**H Submaxillary Gland, Left**<br>*See G Submaxillary Gland, Right*<br>**J Minor Salivary Gland**<br>Anterior lingual gland | **Ø Open**<br>**3 Percutaneous** | **Z No Device** | **Z No Qualifier** |
| **M Pharynx**<br>Base of tongue<br>Hypopharynx<br>Laryngopharynx<br>Lingual tonsil<br>Oropharynx<br>Piriform recess (sinus)<br>Tongue, base of<br>**R Epiglottis**<br>Glossoepiglottic fold<br>**S Larynx**<br>Aryepiglottic fold<br>Arytenoid cartilage<br>Corniculate cartilage<br>Cuneiform cartilage<br>False vocal cord<br>Glottis<br>Rima glottidis<br>Thyroid cartilage<br>Ventricular fold<br>**T Vocal Cord, Right**<br>Vocal fold<br>**V Vocal Cord, Left**<br>*See T Vocal Cord, Right* | **Ø Open**<br>**3 Percutaneous**<br>**4 Percutaneous Endoscopic**<br>**7 Via Natural or Artificial Opening**<br>**8 Via Natural or Artificial Opening Endoscopic** | **Z No Device** | **Z No Qualifier** |
| **W Upper Tooth**<br>**X Lower Tooth** | **Ø Open**<br>**X External** | **Z No Device** | **Ø Single**<br>**1 Multiple**<br>**2 All** |

**Non-OR** ØCN[Ø,1,5,6,7][Ø,3,X]ZZ
**Non-OR** ØCN[W,X][Ø,X]Z[Ø,1,2]

**Ø Medical and Surgical**
**C Mouth and Throat**
**P Removal** Definition: Taking out or off a device from a body part

Explanation: If a device is taken out and a similar device put in without cutting or puncturing the skin or mucous membrane, the procedure is coded to the root operation CHANGE. Otherwise, the procedure for taking out a device is coded to the root operation REMOVAL.

| Body Part Character 4 | Approach Character 5 | Device Character 6 | Qualifier Character 7 |
|---|---|---|---|
| A Salivary Gland | Ø Open<br>3 Percutaneous | Ø Drainage Device<br>C Extraluminal Device<br>Y Other Device | Z No Qualifier |
| A Salivary Gland | 7 Via Natural or Artificial Opening<br>8 Via Natural or Artificial Opening Endoscopic | Y Other Device | Z No Qualifier |
| S Larynx<br>Aryepiglottic fold<br>Arytenoid cartilage<br>Corniculate cartilage<br>Cuneiform cartilage<br>False vocal cord<br>Glottis<br>Rima glottidis<br>Thyroid cartilage<br>Ventricular fold | Ø Open<br>3 Percutaneous<br>7 Via Natural or Artificial Opening<br>8 Via Natural or Artificial Opening Endoscopic | Ø Drainage Device<br>7 Autologous Tissue Substitute<br>D Intraluminal Device<br>J Synthetic Substitute<br>K Nonautologous Tissue Substitute<br>Y Other Device | Z No Qualifier |
| S Larynx<br>Aryepiglottic fold<br>Arytenoid cartilage<br>Corniculate cartilage<br>Cuneiform cartilage<br>False vocal cord<br>Glottis<br>Rima glottidis<br>Thyroid cartilage<br>Ventricular fold | X External | Ø Drainage Device<br>7 Autologous Tissue Substitute<br>D Intraluminal Device<br>J Synthetic Substitute<br>K Nonautologous Tissue Substitute | Z No Qualifier |
| Y Mouth and Throat | Ø Open<br>3 Percutaneous<br>7 Via Natural or Artificial Opening<br>8 Via Natural or Artificial Opening Endoscopic | Ø Drainage Device<br>1 Radioactive Element<br>7 Autologous Tissue Substitute<br>D Intraluminal Device<br>J Synthetic Substitute<br>K Nonautologous Tissue Substitute<br>Y Other Device | Z No Qualifier |
| Y Mouth and Throat | X External | Ø Drainage Device<br>1 Radioactive Element<br>7 Autologous Tissue Substitute<br>D Intraluminal Device<br>J Synthetic Substitute<br>K Nonautologous Tissue Substitute | Z No Qualifier |

**Non-OR** ØCPA[Ø,3][Ø,C,Y]Z
**Non-OR** ØCPA[7,8]YZ
**Non-OR** ØCPS3YZ
**Non-OR** ØCPS[7,8][Ø,D,Y]Z
**Non-OR** ØCPSX[Ø,7,D,J,K]Z
**Non-OR** ØCPY4YZ
**Non-OR** ØCPY[7,8][Ø,D,Y]Z
**Non-OR** ØCPYX[Ø,1,7,D,J,K]Z

**0 Medical and Surgical**
**C Mouth and Throat**
**Q Repair** Definition: Restoring, to the extent possible, a body part to its normal anatomic structure and function
Explanation: Used only when the method to accomplish the repair is not one of the other root operations

| Body Part Character 4 | Approach Character 5 | Device Character 6 | Qualifier Character 7 |
|---|---|---|---|
| **0 Upper Lip**<br>Frenulum labii superioris<br>Labial gland<br>Vermilion border<br>**1 Lower Lip**<br>Frenulum labii inferioris<br>Labial gland<br>Vermilion border<br>**2 Hard Palate**<br>**3 Soft Palate**<br>**4 Buccal Mucosa**<br>Buccal gland<br>Molar gland<br>Palatine gland<br>**5 Upper Gingiva**<br>**6 Lower Gingiva**<br>**7 Tongue**<br>Frenulum linguae<br>**N Uvula**<br>Palatine uvula<br>**P Tonsils**<br>Palatine tonsil<br>**Q Adenoids**<br>Pharyngeal tonsil | **0 Open**<br>**3 Percutaneous**<br>**X External** | **Z No Device** | **Z No Qualifier** |
| **8 Parotid Gland, Right**<br>**9 Parotid Gland, Left**<br>**B Parotid Duct, Right**<br>Stensen's duct<br>**C Parotid Duct, Left**<br>*See B Parotid Duct, Right*<br>**D Sublingual Gland, Right**<br>**F Sublingual Gland, Left**<br>**G Submaxillary Gland, Right**<br>Submandibular gland<br>**H Submaxillary Gland, Left**<br>*See G Submaxillary Gland, Right*<br>**J Minor Salivary Gland**<br>Anterior lingual gland | **0 Open**<br>**3 Percutaneous** | **Z No Device** | **Z No Qualifier** |
| **M Pharynx**<br>Base of tongue<br>Hypopharynx<br>Laryngopharynx<br>Lingual tonsil<br>Oropharynx<br>Piriform recess (sinus)<br>Tongue, base of<br>**R Epiglottis**<br>Glossoepiglottic fold<br>**S Larynx**<br>Aryepiglottic fold<br>Arytenoid cartilage<br>Corniculate cartilage<br>Cuneiform cartilage<br>False vocal cord<br>Glottis<br>Rima glottidis<br>Thyroid cartilage<br>Ventricular fold<br>**T Vocal Cord, Right**<br>Vocal fold<br>**V Vocal Cord, Left**<br>*See T Vocal Cord, Right* | **0 Open**<br>**3 Percutaneous**<br>**4 Percutaneous Endoscopic**<br>**7 Via Natural or Artificial Opening**<br>**8 Via Natural or Artificial Opening Endoscopic** | **Z No Device** | **Z No Qualifier** |
| **W Upper Tooth**<br>**X Lower Tooth** | **0 Open**<br>**X External** | **Z No Device** | **0 Single**<br>**1 Multiple**<br>**2 All** |

**Non-OR** 0CQ[0,1,4,7]XZZ
**Non-OR** 0CQ[5,6][0,3,X]ZZ
**Non-OR** 0CQ[W,X][0,X]Z[0,1,2]

**Ø Medical and Surgical**
**C Mouth and Throat**
**R Replacement** Definition: Putting in or on biological or synthetic material that physically takes the place and/or function of all or a portion of a body part

Explanation: The body part may have been taken out or replaced, or may be taken out, physically eradicated, or rendered nonfunctional during the REPLACEMENT procedure. A REMOVAL procedure is coded for taking out the device used in a previous replacement procedure.

| Body Part Character 4 | Approach Character 5 | Device Character 6 | Qualifier Character 7 |
|---|---|---|---|
| **Ø Upper Lip**<br>Frenulum labii superioris<br>Labial gland<br>Vermilion border<br>**1 Lower Lip**<br>Frenulum labii inferioris<br>Labial gland<br>Vermilion border<br>**2 Hard Palate**<br>**3 Soft Palate**<br>**4 Buccal Mucosa**<br>Buccal gland<br>Molar gland<br>Palatine gland<br>**5 Upper Gingiva**<br>**6 Lower Gingiva**<br>**7 Tongue**<br>Frenulum linguae<br>**N Uvula**<br>Palatine uvula | **Ø Open**<br>**3 Percutaneous**<br>**X External** | **7 Autologous Tissue Substitute**<br>**J Synthetic Substitute**<br>**K Nonautologous Tissue Substitute** | **Z No Qualifier** |
| **B Parotid Duct, Right**<br>Stensen's duct<br>**C Parotid Duct, Left**<br>*See B Parotid Duct, Right* | **Ø Open**<br>**3 Percutaneous** | **7 Autologous Tissue Substitute**<br>**J Synthetic Substitute**<br>**K Nonautologous Tissue Substitute** | **Z No Qualifier** |
| **M Pharynx**<br>Base of tongue<br>Hypopharynx<br>Laryngopharynx<br>Lingual tonsil<br>Oropharynx<br>Piriform recess (sinus)<br>Tongue, base of<br>**R Epiglottis**<br>Glossoepiglottic fold<br>**S Larynx**<br>Aryepiglottic fold<br>Arytenoid cartilage<br>Corniculate cartilage<br>Cuneiform cartilage<br>False vocal cord<br>Glottis<br>Rima glottidis<br>Thyroid cartilage<br>Ventricular fold<br>**T Vocal Cord, Right**<br>Vocal fold<br>**V Vocal Cord, Left**<br>*See T Vocal Cord, Right* | **Ø Open**<br>**7 Via Natural or Artificial Opening**<br>**8 Via Natural or Artificial Opening Endoscopic** | **7 Autologous Tissue Substitute**<br>**J Synthetic Substitute**<br>**K Nonautologous Tissue Substitute** | **Z No Qualifier** |
| **W Upper Tooth**<br>**X Lower Tooth** | **Ø Open**<br>**X External** | **7 Autologous Tissue Substitute**<br>**J Synthetic Substitute**<br>**K Nonautologous Tissue Substitute** | **Ø Single**<br>**1 Multiple**<br>**2 All** |

**Non-OR** ØCR[W,X][Ø,X][7,J,K][Ø,1,2]

**Ø Medical and Surgical**
**C Mouth and Throat**
**S Reposition** Definition: Moving to its normal location, or other suitable location, all or a portion of a body part

Explanation: The body part is moved to a new location from an abnormal location, or from a normal location where it is not functioning correctly. The body part may or may not be cut out or off to be moved to the new location.

| Body Part Character 4 | Approach Character 5 | Device Character 6 | Qualifier Character 7 |
|---|---|---|---|
| **Ø Upper Lip**<br>Frenulum labii superioris<br>Labial gland<br>Vermilion border<br>**1 Lower Lip**<br>Frenulum labii inferioris<br>Labial gland<br>Vermilion border<br>**2 Hard Palate**<br>**3 Soft Palate**<br>**7 Tongue**<br>Frenulum linguae<br>**N Uvula**<br>Palatine uvula | **Ø Open**<br>**X External** | **Z No Device** | **Z No Qualifier** |
| **B Parotid Duct, Right**<br>Stensen's duct<br>**C Parotid Duct, Left**<br>*See B Parotid Duct, Right* | **Ø Open**<br>**3 Percutaneous** | **Z No Device** | **Z No Qualifier** |
| **R Epiglottis**<br>Glossoepiglottic fold<br>**T Vocal Cord, Right**<br>Vocal fold<br>**V Vocal Cord, Left**<br>*See T Vocal Cord, Right* | **Ø Open**<br>**7 Via Natural or Artificial Opening**<br>**8 Via Natural or Artificial Opening Endoscopic** | **Z No Device** | **Z No Qualifier** |
| **W Upper Tooth**<br>**X Lower Tooth** | **Ø Open**<br>**X External** | **5 External Fixation Device**<br>**Z No Device** | **Ø Single**<br>**1 Multiple**<br>**2 All** |

**Non-OR** ØCS[W,X][Ø,X][5,Z][Ø,1,2]

**Ø Medical and Surgical**
**C Mouth and Throat**
**T Resection** Definition: Cutting out or off, without replacement, all of a body part
Explanation: None

| Body Part Character 4 | Approach Character 5 | Device Character 6 | Qualifier Character 7 |
|---|---|---|---|
| **Ø Upper Lip**<br>Frenulum labii superioris<br>Labial gland<br>Vermilion border<br>**1 Lower Lip**<br>Frenulum labii inferioris<br>Labial gland<br>Vermilion border<br>**2 Hard Palate**<br>**3 Soft Palate**<br>**7 Tongue**<br>Frenulum linguae<br>**N Uvula**<br>Palatine uvula<br>**P Tonsils**<br>Palatine tonsil<br>**Q Adenoids**<br>Pharyngeal tonsil | **Ø Open**<br>**X External** | **Z No Device** | **Z No Qualifier** |
| **8 Parotid Gland, Right**<br>**9 Parotid Gland, Left**<br>**B Parotid Duct, Right**<br>Stensen's duct<br>**C Parotid Duct, Left**<br>*See B Parotid Duct, Right*<br>**D Sublingual Gland, Right**<br>**F Sublingual Gland, Left**<br>**G Submaxillary Gland, Right**<br>Submandibular gland<br>**H Submaxillary Gland, Left**<br>*See G Submaxillary Gland, Right*<br>**J Minor Salivary Gland**<br>Anterior lingual gland | **Ø Open** | **Z No Device** | **Z No Qualifier** |
| **M Pharynx**<br>Base of tongue<br>Hypopharynx<br>Laryngopharynx<br>Lingual tonsil<br>Oropharynx<br>Piriform recess (sinus)<br>Tongue, base of<br>**R Epiglottis**<br>Glossoepiglottic fold<br>**S Larynx**<br>Aryepiglottic fold<br>Arytenoid cartilage<br>Corniculate cartilage<br>Cuneiform cartilage<br>False vocal cord<br>Glottis<br>Rima glottidis<br>Thyroid cartilage<br>Ventricular fold<br>**T Vocal Cord, Right**<br>Vocal fold<br>**V Vocal Cord, Left**<br>*See T Vocal Cord, Right* | **Ø Open**<br>**4 Percutaneous Endoscopic**<br>**7 Via Natural or Artificial Opening**<br>**8 Via Natural or Artificial Opening Endoscopic** | **Z No Device** | **Z No Qualifier** |
| **W Upper Tooth**<br>**X Lower Tooth** | **Ø Open** | **Z No Device** | **Ø Single**<br>**1 Multiple**<br>**2 All** |

**Non-OR** ØCT[W,X]ØZ[Ø,1,2]

**Ø Medical and Surgical**
**C Mouth and Throat**
**U Supplement** Definition: Putting in or on biological or synthetic material that physically reinforces and/or augments the function of a portion of a body part

Explanation: The biological material is non-living, or is living and from the same individual. The body part may have been previously replaced, and the SUPPLEMENT procedure is performed to physically reinforce and/or augment the function of the replaced body part.

| Body Part Character 4 | Approach Character 5 | Device Character 6 | Qualifier Character 7 |
|---|---|---|---|
| **Ø Upper Lip**<br>Frenulum labii superioris<br>Labial gland<br>Vermilion border<br>**1 Lower Lip**<br>Frenulum labii inferioris<br>Labial gland<br>Vermilion border<br>**2 Hard Palate**<br>**3 Soft Palate**<br>**4 Buccal Mucosa**<br>Buccal gland<br>Molar gland<br>Palatine gland<br>**5 Upper Gingiva**<br>**6 Lower Gingiva**<br>**7 Tongue**<br>Frenulum linguae<br>**N Uvula**<br>Palatine uvula | **Ø Open**<br>**3 Percutaneous**<br>**X External** | **7 Autologous Tissue Substitute**<br>**J Synthetic Substitute**<br>**K Nonautologous Tissue Substitute** | **Z No Qualifier** |
| **M Pharynx**<br>Base of tongue<br>Hypopharynx<br>Laryngopharynx<br>Lingual tonsil<br>Oropharynx<br>Piriform recess (sinus)<br>Tongue, base of<br>**R Epiglottis**<br>Glossoepiglottic fold<br>**S Larynx**<br>Aryepiglottic fold<br>Arytenoid cartilage<br>Corniculate cartilage<br>Cuneiform cartilage<br>False vocal cord<br>Glottis<br>Rima glottidis<br>Thyroid cartilage<br>Ventricular fold<br>**T Vocal Cord, Right**<br>Vocal fold<br>**V Vocal Cord, Left**<br>*See T Vocal Cord, Right* | **Ø Open**<br>**7 Via Natural or Artificial Opening**<br>**8 Via Natural or Artificial Opening Endoscopic** | **7 Autologous Tissue Substitute**<br>**J Synthetic Substitute**<br>**K Nonautologous Tissue Substitute** | **Z No Qualifier** |

Non-OR ØCU2[Ø,3]JZ

**Ø Medical and Surgical**
**C Mouth and Throat**
**V Restriction** Definition: Partially closing an orifice or the lumen of a tubular body part

Explanation: The orifice can be a natural orifice or an artificially created orifice

| Body Part Character 4 | Approach Character 5 | Device Character 6 | Qualifier Character 7 |
|---|---|---|---|
| **B Parotid Duct, Right**<br>Stensen's duct<br>**C Parotid Duct, Left**<br>*See B Parotid Duct, Right* | **Ø Open**<br>**3 Percutaneous** | **C Extraluminal Device**<br>**D Intraluminal Device**<br>**Z No Device** | **Z No Qualifier** |
| **B Parotid Duct, Right**<br>Stensen's duct<br>**C Parotid Duct, Left**<br>*See B Parotid Duct, Right* | **7 Via Natural or Artificial Opening**<br>**8 Via Natural or Artificial Opening Endoscopic** | **D Intraluminal Device**<br>**Z No Device** | **Z No Qualifier** |

**Ø Medical and Surgical**
**C Mouth and Throat**
**W Revision**

Definition: Correcting, to the extent possible, a portion of a malfunctioning device or the position of a displaced device

Explanation: Revision can include correcting a malfunctioning or displaced device by taking out or putting in components of the device such as a screw or pin

| Body Part Character 4 | Approach Character 5 | Device Character 6 | Qualifier Character 7 |
|---|---|---|---|
| A Salivary Gland | Ø Open<br>3 Percutaneous | Ø Drainage Device<br>C Extraluminal Device<br>Y Other Device | Z No Qualifier |
| A Salivary Gland | 7 Via Natural or Artificial Opening<br>8 Via Natural or Artificial Opening Endoscopic | Y Other Device | Z No Qualifier |
| A Salivary Gland | X External | Ø Drainage Device<br>C Extraluminal Device | Z No Qualifier |
| S Larynx<br>Aryepiglottic fold<br>Arytenoid cartilage<br>Corniculate cartilage<br>Cuneiform cartilage<br>False vocal cord<br>Glottis<br>Rima glottidis<br>Thyroid cartilage<br>Ventricular fold | Ø Open<br>3 Percutaneous<br>7 Via Natural or Artificial Opening<br>8 Via Natural or Artificial Opening Endoscopic | Ø Drainage Device<br>7 Autologous Tissue Substitute<br>D Intraluminal Device<br>J Synthetic Substitute<br>K Nonautologous Tissue Substitute<br>Y Other Device | Z No Qualifier |
| S Larynx<br>Aryepiglottic fold<br>Arytenoid cartilage<br>Corniculate cartilage<br>Cuneiform cartilage<br>False vocal cord<br>Glottis<br>Rima glottidis<br>Thyroid cartilage<br>Ventricular fold | X External | Ø Drainage Device<br>7 Autologous Tissue Substitute<br>D Intraluminal Device<br>J Synthetic Substitute<br>K Nonautologous Tissue Substitute | Z No Qualifier |
| Y Mouth and Throat | Ø Open<br>3 Percutaneous<br>7 Via Natural or Artificial Opening<br>8 Via Natural or Artificial Opening Endoscopic | Ø Drainage Device<br>1 Radioactive Element<br>7 Autologous Tissue Substitute<br>D Intraluminal Device<br>J Synthetic Substitute<br>K Nonautologous Tissue Substitute<br>Y Other Device | Z No Qualifier |
| Y Mouth and Throat | X External | Ø Drainage Device<br>1 Radioactive Element<br>7 Autologous Tissue Substitute<br>D Intraluminal Device<br>J Synthetic Substitute<br>K Nonautologous Tissue Substitute | Z No Qualifier |

Non-OR ØCWA[Ø,3][Ø,C,Y]Z
Non-OR ØCWA[7,8]YZ
Non-OR ØCWAX[Ø,C]Z
Non-OR ØCWS3YZ
Non-OR ØCWS[7,8]YZ
Non-OR ØCWSX[Ø,7,D,J,K]Z
Non-OR ØCWYØ7Z
Non-OR ØCWY[3,7,8]YZ
Non-OR ØCWYX[Ø,1,7,D,J,K]Z

**Ø Medical and Surgical**
**C Mouth and Throat**
**X Transfer** Definition: Moving, without taking out, all or a portion of a body part to another location to take over the function of all or a portion of a body part

Explanation: The body part transferred remains connected to its vascular and nervous supply

| Body Part Character 4 | Approach Character 5 | Device Character 6 | Qualifier Character 7 |
|---|---|---|---|
| **Ø Upper Lip**<br>Frenulum labii superioris<br>Labial gland<br>Vermilion border<br>**1 Lower Lip**<br>Frenulum labii inferioris<br>Labial gland<br>Vermilion border<br>**3 Soft Palate**<br>**4 Buccal Mucosa**<br>Buccal gland<br>Molar gland<br>Palatine gland<br>**5 Upper Gingiva**<br>**6 Lower Gingiva**<br>**7 Tongue**<br>Frenulum linguae | **Ø Open**<br>**X External** | **Z No Device** | **Z No Qualifier** |

# Gastrointestinal System ØD1–ØDY

## Character Meanings

This Character Meaning table is provided as a guide to assist the user in the identification of character members that may be found in this section of code tables. It **SHOULD NOT** be used to build a PCS code.

| Operation–Character 3 | Body Part–Character 4 | Approach–Character 5 | Device–Character 6 | Qualifier–Character 7 |
|---|---|---|---|---|
| 1 Bypass | Ø Upper Intestinal Tract | Ø Open | Ø Drainage Device | Ø Allogeneic |
| 2 Change | 1 Esophagus, Upper | 3 Percutaneous | 1 Radioactive Element | 1 Syngeneic |
| 5 Destruction | 2 Esophagus, Middle | 4 Percutaneous Endoscopic | 2 Monitoring Device | 2 Zooplastic |
| 7 Dilation | 3 Esophagus, Lower | 7 Via Natural or Artificial Opening | 3 Infusion Device | 3 Vertical |
| 8 Division | 4 Esophagogastric Junction | 8 Via Natural or Artificial Opening Endoscopic | 7 Autologous Tissue Substitute | 4 Cutaneous |
| 9 Drainage | 5 Esophagus | F Via Natural or Artificial Opening with Percutaneous Endoscopic Assistance | B Intraluminal Device, Airway | 5 Esophagus |
| B Excision | 6 Stomach | X External | C Extraluminal Device | 6 Stomach |
| C Extirpation | 7 Stomach, Pylorus | | D Intraluminal Device | 9 Duodenum |
| D Extraction | 8 Small Intestine | | J Synthetic Substitute | A Jejunum |
| F Fragmentation | 9 Duodenum | | K Nonautologous Tissue Substitute | B Ileum |
| H Insertion | A Jejunum | | L Artificial Sphincter | H Cecum |
| J Inspection | B Ileum | | M Stimulator Lead | K Ascending Colon |
| L Occlusion | C Ileocecal Valve | | U Feeding Device | L Transverse Colon |
| M Reattachment | D Lower Intestinal Tract | | Y Other Device | M Descending Colon |
| N Release | E Large Intestine | | Z No Device | N Sigmoid Colon |
| P Removal | F Large Intestine, Right | | | P Rectum |
| Q Repair | G Large Intestine, Left | | | Q Anus |
| R Replacement | H Cecum | | | X Diagnostic |
| S Reposition | J Appendix | | | Z No Qualifier |
| T Resection | K Ascending Colon | | | |
| U Supplement | L Transverse Colon | | | |
| V Restriction | M Descending Colon | | | |
| W Revision | N Sigmoid Colon | | | |
| X Transfer | P Rectum | | | |
| Y Transplantation | Q Anus | | | |
| | R Anal Sphincter | | | |
| | U Omentum | | | |
| | V Mesentery | | | |
| | W Peritoneum | | | |

**AHA Coding Clinic for table ØD1**

| | |
|---|---|
| 2017, 2Q, 17 | Billroth II (distal gastrectomy and gastrojejunostomy) |
| 2016, 2Q, 31 | Laparoscopic biliopancreatic diversion with duodenal switch |
| 2014, 4Q, 41 | Abdominoperineal resection (APR) with flap closure of perineum and colostomy |

**AHA Coding Clinic for table ØD5**

| | |
|---|---|
| 2017, 1Q, 34 | Debulking of tumor and peritoneum ablation |

**AHA Coding Clinic for table ØD7**

| | |
|---|---|
| 2014, 4Q, 40 | Dilation of gastrojejunostomy anastomosis stricture |

**AHA Coding Clinic for table ØD9**

| | |
|---|---|
| 2015, 2Q, 29 | Insertion of nasogastric tube for drainage and feeding |

**AHA Coding Clinic for table ØDB**

| | |
|---|---|
| 2017, 2Q, 17 | Billroth II (distal gastrectomy and gastrojejunostomy) |
| 2017, 1Q, 16 | Hepatic flexure versus transverse colon |
| 2016, 3Q, 3-7 | Stoma creation & takedown procedures |
| 2016, 2Q, 31 | Laparoscopic biliopancreatic diversion with duodenal switch |
| 2016, 1Q, 22 | Perineal proctectomy |
| 2016, 1Q, 24 | Endoscopic brush biopsy of esophagus |
| 2014, 4Q, 40 | Abdominoperineal resection (APR) with flap closure of perineum and colostomy |
| 2014, 3Q, 28 | Ileostomy takedown and parastomal hernia repair |
| 2014, 3Q, 32 | Pyloric-sparing Whipple procedure |

**AHA Coding Clinic for table ØDH**

| | |
|---|---|
| 2016, 3Q, 26 | Insertion of gastrostomy tube |
| 2013, 4Q,117 | Percutaneous endoscopic placement of gastrostomy tube |

**AHA Coding Clinic for table ØDJ**

| | |
|---|---|
| 2017, 2Q, 15 | Low anterior resection with sigmoidoscopy |
| 2016, 2Q, 20 | Capsule endoscopy of small intestine |
| 2015, 3Q, 24 | Esophagogastroduodenoscopy with epinephrine injection for control of bleeding |

**AHA Coding Clinic for table ØDL**

| | |
|---|---|
| 2013, 4Q, 112 | Endoscopic banding of esophageal varices |

**AHA Coding Clinic for table ØDN**

| | |
|---|---|
| 2017, 1Q, 35 | Lysis of omental and peritoneal adhesions |
| 2015, 3Q, 15 | Vascular ring surgery with release of esophagus and trachea |
| 2015, 3Q, 16 | Vascular ring surgery and double aortic arch |

**AHA Coding Clinic for table ØDQ**

| | |
|---|---|
| 2016, 3Q, 3-7 | Stoma creation & takedown procedures |
| 2016, 3Q, 26 | Insertion of gastrostomy tube |
| 2016, 1Q, 7 | Obstetrical perineal laceration repair |
| 2016, 1Q, 8 | Obstetrical perineal laceration repair |
| 2014, 4Q, 20 | Control of bleeding duodenal ulcer |

**AHA Coding Clinic for table ØDS**

| | |
|---|---|
| 2016, 3Q, 3-5 | Stoma creation & takedown procedures |

**AHA Coding Clinic for table ØDT**

| | |
|---|---|
| 2014, 4Q, 40 | Abdominoperineal resection (APR) with flap closure of perineum and colostomy |
| 2014, 4Q, 42 | Right colectomy with side-to-side functional end-to-end anastomosis |
| 2014, 3Q, 6 | Ileocecectomy including cecum, terminal ileum and appendix |
| 2014, 3Q, 6 | Right colectomy |

**AHA Coding Clinic for table ØDV**

| | |
|---|---|
| 2016, 2Q, 22 | Esophageal lengthening Collis gastroplasty with Nissen fundoplication and hiatal hernia |
| 2014, 3Q, 28 | Laparoscopic Nissen fundoplication and diaphragmatic hernia repair |

**AHA Coding Clinic for table ØDX**

| | |
|---|---|
| 2017, 2Q, 18 | Esophagectomy and esophagogastrectomy with cervical esophagogastrostomy |
| 2016, 2Q, 22 | Esophageal lengthening Collis gastroplasty with Nissen fundoplication and hiatal hernia |
| 2015, 1Q, 28 | Repair of bronchopleural fistula using omental pedicle graft |

## Upper Intestinal Tract (Ø) and Lower Intestinal Tract (D)

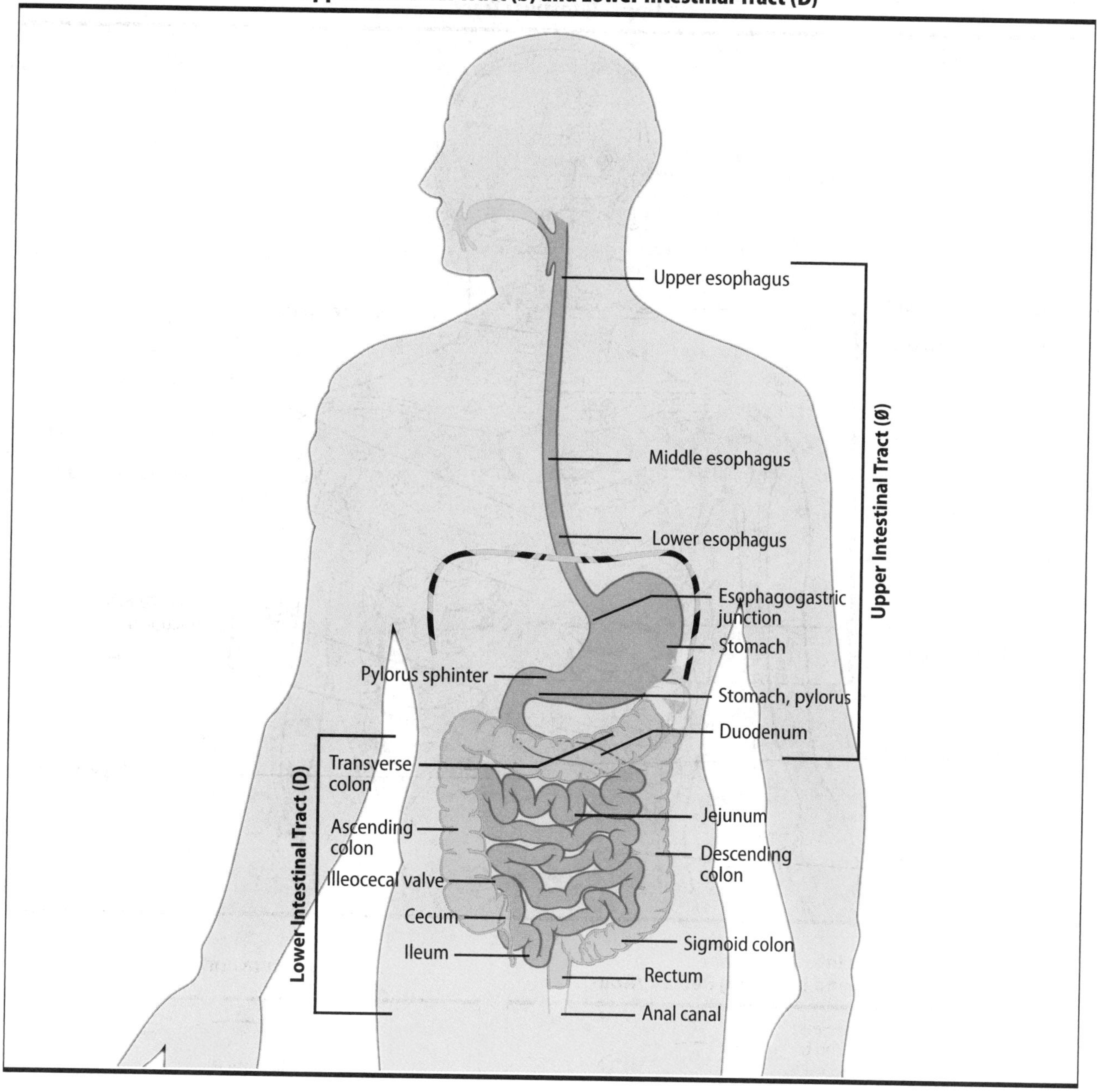
Upper esophagus
Middle esophagus
Lower esophagus
Esophagogastric junction
Stomach
Pylorus sphinter
Stomach, pylorus
Duodenum
Upper Intestinal Tract (Ø)
Transverse colon
Ascending colon
Illeocecal valve
Cecum
Ileum
Jejunum
Descending colon
Sigmoid colon
Rectum
Anal canal
Lower Intestinal Tract (D)

## Upper Intestinal Tract

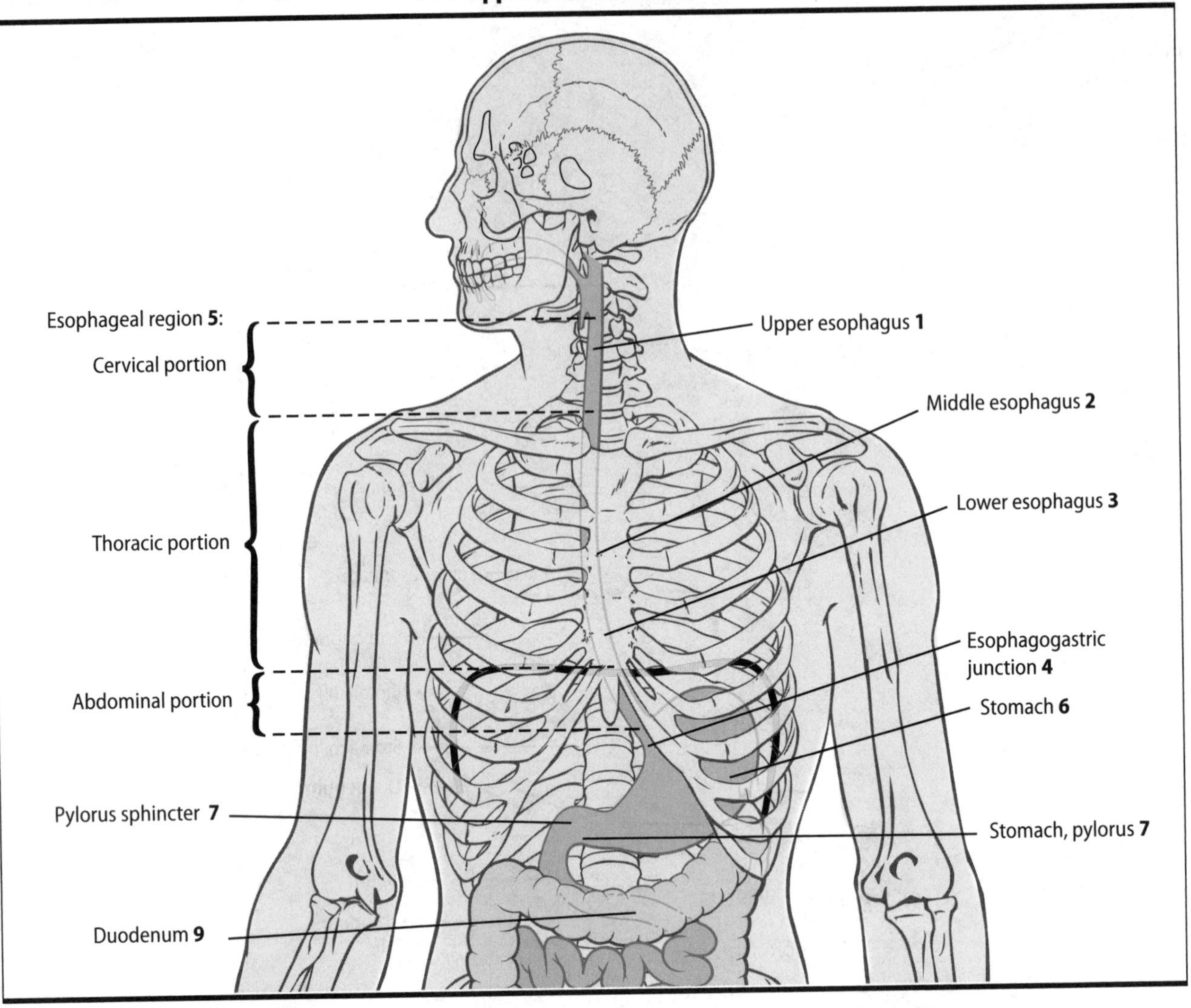
Esophageal region 5:
Cervical portion
Thoracic portion
Abdominal portion
Upper esophagus 1
Middle esophagus 2
Lower esophagus 3
Esophagogastric junction 4
Stomach 6
Pylorus sphincter 7
Stomach, pylorus 7
Duodenum 9

## Lower Intestinal Tract (Jejunum Down to and Including Rectum/Anus)

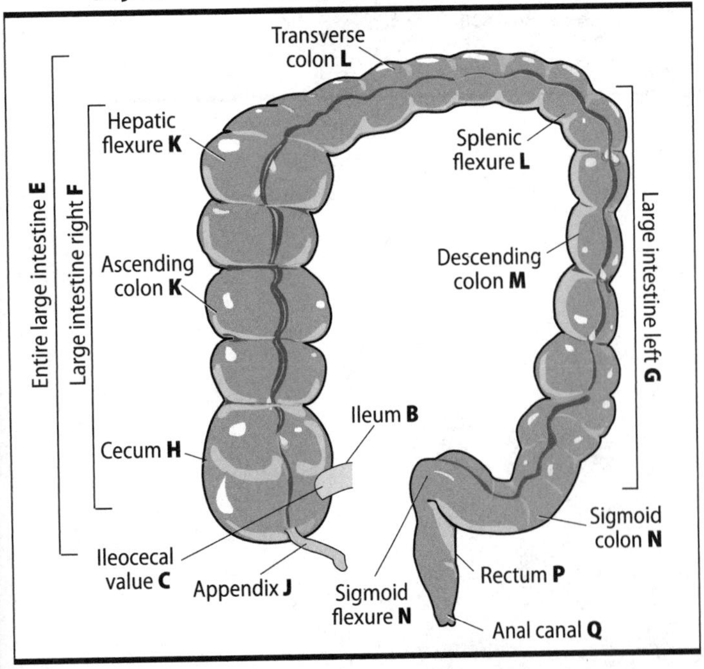
Transverse colon L
Hepatic flexure K
Splenic flexure L
Entire large intestine E
Large intestine right F
Large intestine left G
Ascending colon K
Descending colon M
Ileum B
Cecum H
Sigmoid colon N
Ileocecal value C
Appendix J
Sigmoid flexure N
Rectum P
Anal canal Q

## Rectum and Anus

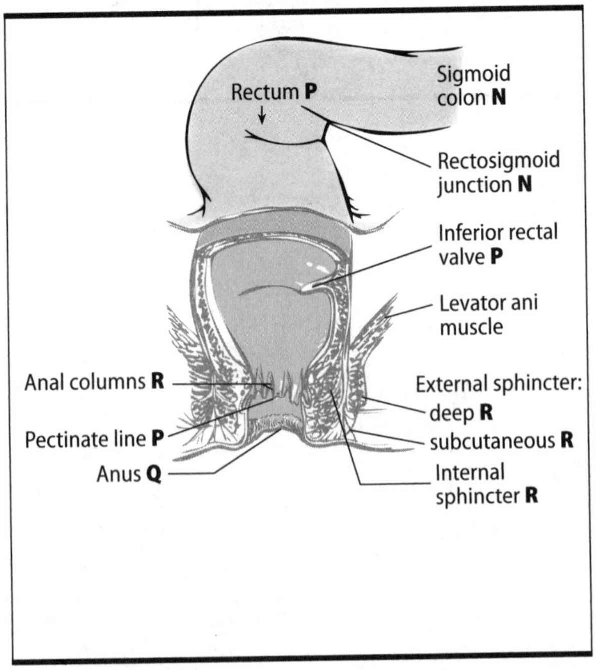
Rectum P
Sigmoid colon N
Rectosigmoid junction N
Inferior rectal valve P
Levator ani muscle
Anal columns R
External sphincter:
deep R
subcutaneous R
Pectinate line P
Anus Q
Internal sphincter R

**Ø Medical and Surgical**
**D Gastrointestinal System**
**1 Bypass** Definition: Altering the route of passage of the contents of a tubular body part

Explanation: Rerouting contents of a body part to a downstream area of the normal route, to a similar route and body part, or to an abnormal route and dissimilar body part. Includes one or more anastomoses, with or without the use of a device.

| Body Part Character 4 | Approach Character 5 | Device Character 6 | Qualifier Character 7 |
|---|---|---|---|
| **1 Esophagus, Upper** Cervical esophagus<br>**2 Esophagus, Middle** Thoracic esophagus<br>**3 Esophagus, Lower** Abdominal esophagus<br>**5 Esophagus** | **Ø Open**<br>**4 Percutaneous Endoscopic**<br>**8 Via Natural or Artificial Opening Endoscopic** | **7 Autologous Tissue Substitute**<br>**J Synthetic Substitute**<br>**K Nonautologous Tissue Substitute**<br>**Z No Device** | **4 Cutaneous**<br>**6 Stomach**<br>**9 Duodenum**<br>**A Jejunum**<br>**B Ileum** |
| **1 Esophagus, Upper** Cervical esophagus<br>**2 Esophagus, Middle** Thoracic esophagus<br>**3 Esophagus, Lower** Abdominal esophagus<br>**5 Esophagus** | **3 Percutaneous** | **J Synthetic Substitute** | **4 Cutaneous** |
| **6 Stomach**<br>**9 Duodenum** | **Ø Open**<br>**4 Percutaneous Endoscopic**<br>**8 Via Natural or Artificial Opening Endoscopic** | **7 Autologous Tissue Substitute**<br>**J Synthetic Substitute**<br>**K Nonautologous Tissue Substitute**<br>**Z No Device** | **4 Cutaneous**<br>**9 Duodenum**<br>**A Jejunum**<br>**B Ileum**<br>**L Transverse Colon** |
| **6 Stomach**<br>**9 Duodenum** | **3 Percutaneous** | **J Synthetic Substitute** | **4 Cutaneous** |
| **A Jejunum** Duodenojejunal flexure | **Ø Open**<br>**4 Percutaneous Endoscopic**<br>**8 Via Natural or Artificial Opening Endoscopic** | **7 Autologous Tissue Substitute**<br>**J Synthetic Substitute**<br>**K Nonautologous Tissue Substitute**<br>**Z No Device** | **4 Cutaneous**<br>**A Jejunum**<br>**B Ileum**<br>**H Cecum**<br>**K Ascending Colon**<br>**L Transverse Colon**<br>**M Descending Colon**<br>**N Sigmoid Colon**<br>**P Rectum**<br>**Q Anus** |
| **A Jejunum** Duodenojejunal flexure | **3 Percutaneous** | **J Synthetic Substitute** | **4 Cutaneous** |
| **B Ileum** | **Ø Open**<br>**4 Percutaneous Endoscopic**<br>**8 Via Natural or Artificial Opening Endoscopic** | **7 Autologous Tissue Substitute**<br>**J Synthetic Substitute**<br>**K Nonautologous Tissue Substitute**<br>**Z No Device** | **4 Cutaneous**<br>**B Ileum**<br>**H Cecum**<br>**K Ascending Colon**<br>**L Transverse Colon**<br>**M Descending Colon**<br>**N Sigmoid Colon**<br>**P Rectum**<br>**Q Anus** |
| **B Ileum** | **3 Percutaneous** | **J Synthetic Substitute** | **4 Cutaneous** |
| **H Cecum** | **Ø Open**<br>**4 Percutaneous Endoscopic**<br>**8 Via Natural or Artificial Opening Endoscopic** | **7 Autologous Tissue Substitute**<br>**J Synthetic Substitute**<br>**K Nonautologous Tissue Substitute**<br>**Z No Device** | **4 Cutaneous**<br>**H Cecum**<br>**K Ascending Colon**<br>**L Transverse Colon**<br>**M Descending Colon**<br>**N Sigmoid Colon**<br>**P Rectum** |
| **H Cecum** | **3 Percutaneous** | **J Synthetic Substitute** | **4 Cutaneous** |
| **K Ascending Colon** | **Ø Open**<br>**4 Percutaneous Endoscopic**<br>**8 Via Natural or Artificial Opening Endoscopic** | **7 Autologous Tissue Substitute**<br>**J Synthetic Substitute**<br>**K Nonautologous Tissue Substitute**<br>**Z No Device** | **4 Cutaneous**<br>**K Ascending Colon**<br>**L Transverse Colon**<br>**M Descending Colon**<br>**N Sigmoid Colon**<br>**P Rectum** |

***ØD1 Continued on next page***

**Non-OR** ØD16[Ø,4,8][7,J,K,Z]4
**Non-OR** ØD163J4
**HAC** ØD16[Ø,4,8][7,J,K,Z][9,A,B,L] when reported with PDx E66.Ø1 and SDx K68.11 or K95.Ø1 or K95.81 or T81.4XXA

**ØD1 Continued**

**Ø Medical and Surgical**
**D Gastrointestinal System**
**1 Bypass** Definition: Altering the route of passage of the contents of a tubular body part

Explanation: Rerouting contents of a body part to a downstream area of the normal route, to a similar route and body part, or to an abnormal route and dissimilar body part. Includes one or more anastomoses, with or without the use of a device.

| Body Part<br>Character 4 | Approach<br>Character 5 | Device<br>Character 6 | Qualifier<br>Character 7 |
|---|---|---|---|
| **K Ascending Colon** | **3 Percutaneous** | **J Synthetic Substitute** | **4 Cutaneous** |
| **L Transverse Colon**<br>Hepatic flexure<br>Splenic flexure | **Ø Open**<br>**4 Percutaneous Endoscopic**<br>**8 Via Natural or Artificial Opening Endoscopic** | **7 Autologous Tissue Substitute**<br>**J Synthetic Substitute**<br>**K Nonautologous Tissue Substitute**<br>**Z No Device** | **4 Cutaneous**<br>**L Transverse Colon**<br>**M Descending Colon**<br>**N Sigmoid Colon**<br>**P Rectum** |
| **L Transverse Colon**<br>Hepatic flexure<br>Splenic flexure | **3 Percutaneous** | **J Synthetic Substitute** | **4 Cutaneous** |
| **M Descending Colon** | **Ø Open**<br>**4 Percutaneous Endoscopic**<br>**8 Via Natural or Artificial Opening Endoscopic** | **7 Autologous Tissue Substitute**<br>**J Synthetic Substitute**<br>**K Nonautologous Tissue Substitute**<br>**Z No Device** | **4 Cutaneous**<br>**M Descending Colon**<br>**N Sigmoid Colon**<br>**P Rectum** |
| **M Descending Colon** | **3 Percutaneous** | **J Synthetic Substitute** | **4 Cutaneous** |
| **N Sigmoid Colon**<br>Rectosigmoid junction<br>Sigmoid flexure | **Ø Open**<br>**4 Percutaneous Endoscopic**<br>**8 Via Natural or Artificial Opening Endoscopic** | **7 Autologous Tissue Substitute**<br>**J Synthetic Substitute**<br>**K Nonautologous Tissue Substitute**<br>**Z No Device** | **4 Cutaneous**<br>**N Sigmoid Colon**<br>**P Rectum** |
| **N Sigmoid Colon**<br>Rectosigmoid junction<br>Sigmoid flexure | **3 Percutaneous** | **J Synthetic Substitute** | **4 Cutaneous** |

**Ø Medical and Surgical**
**D Gastrointestinal System**
**2 Change** Definition: Taking out or off a device from a body part and putting back an identical or similar device in or on the same body part without cutting or puncturing the skin or a mucous membrane

Explanation: All CHANGE procedures are coded using the approach EXTERNAL

| Body Part<br>Character 4 | Approach<br>Character 5 | Device<br>Character 6 | Qualifier<br>Character 7 |
|---|---|---|---|
| **Ø Upper Intestinal Tract**<br>**D Lower Intestinal Tract** | **X External** | **Ø Drainage Device**<br>**U Feeding Device**<br>**Y Other Device** | **Z No Qualifier** |
| **U Omentum**<br>Gastrocolic ligament<br>Gastrocolic omentum<br>Gastrohepatic omentum<br>Gastrophrenic ligament<br>Gastrosplenic ligament<br>Greater Omentum<br>Hepatogastric ligament<br>Lesser Omentum<br>**V Mesentery**<br>Mesoappendix<br>Mesocolon<br>**W Peritoneum**<br>Epiploic foramen | **X External** | **Ø Drainage Device**<br>**Y Other Device** | **Z No Qualifier** |

**Non-OR** All body part, approach, device, and qualifier values

**Ø Medical and Surgical**
**D Gastrointestinal System**
**5 Destruction** Definition: Physical eradication of all or a portion of a body part by the direct use of energy, force, or a destructive agent
Explanation: None of the body part is physically taken out

| Body Part Character 4 | Approach Character 5 | Device Character 6 | Qualifier Character 7 |
|---|---|---|---|
| 1 Esophagus, Upper<br>Cervical esophagus<br>2 Esophagus, Middle<br>Thoracic esophagus<br>3 Esophagus, Lower<br>Abdominal esophagus<br>4 Esophagogastric Junction<br>Cardia<br>Cardioesophageal junction<br>Gastroesophageal (GE) junction<br>5 Esophagus<br>6 Stomach<br>7 Stomach, Pylorus<br>Pyloric antrum<br>Pyloric canal<br>Pyloric sphincter<br>8 Small Intestine<br>9 Duodenum<br>A Jejunum<br>Duodenojejunal flexure<br>B Ileum<br>C Ileocecal Valve<br>E Large Intestine<br>F Large Intestine, Right<br>G Large Intestine, Left<br>H Cecum<br>J Appendix<br>Vermiform appendix<br>K Ascending Colon<br>L Transverse Colon<br>Hepatic flexure<br>Splenic flexure<br>M Descending Colon<br>N Sigmoid Colon<br>Rectosigmoid junction<br>Sigmoid flexure<br>P Rectum<br>Anorectal junction | Ø Open<br>3 Percutaneous<br>4 Percutaneous Endoscopic<br>7 Via Natural or Artificial Opening<br>8 Via Natural or Artificial Opening Endoscopic | Z No Device | Z No Qualifier |
| Q Anus<br>Anal orifice | Ø Open<br>3 Percutaneous<br>4 Percutaneous Endoscopic<br>7 Via Natural or Artificial Opening<br>8 Via Natural or Artificial Opening Endoscopic<br>X External | Z No Device | Z No Qualifier |
| R Anal Sphincter<br>External anal sphincter<br>Internal anal sphincter<br>U Omentum<br>Gastrocolic ligament<br>Gastrocolic omentum<br>Gastrohepatic omentum<br>Gastrophrenic ligament<br>Gastrosplenic ligament<br>Greater Omentum<br>Hepatogastric ligament<br>Lesser Omentum<br>V Mesentery<br>Mesoappendix<br>Mesocolon<br>W Peritoneum<br>Epiploic foramen | Ø Open<br>3 Percutaneous<br>4 Percutaneous Endoscopic | Z No Device | Z No Qualifier |

**Non-OR** ØD5[1,2,3,4,5,6,7,9,E,F,G,H,K,L,M,N][4,8]ZZ
**Non-OR** ØD5P[Ø,3,4,7,8]ZZ
**Non-OR** ØD5Q[4,8]ZZ
**Non-OR** ØD5R4ZZ

**Ø Medical and Surgical**
**D Gastrointestinal System**
**7 Dilation** Definition: Expanding an orifice or the lumen of a tubular body part

Explanation: The orifice can be a natural orifice or an artificially created orifice. Accomplished by stretching a tubular body part using intraluminal pressure or by cutting part of the orifice or wall of the tubular body part.

| Body Part Character 4 | Approach Character 5 | Device Character 6 | Qualifier Character 7 |
|---|---|---|---|
| **1 Esophagus, Upper**<br>Cervical esophagus<br>**2 Esophagus, Middle**<br>Thoracic esophagus<br>**3 Esophagus, Lower**<br>Abdominal esophagus<br>**4 Esophagogastric Junction**<br>Cardia<br>Cardioesophageal junction<br>Gastroesophageal (GE) junction<br>**5 Esophagus**<br>**6 Stomach**<br>**7 Stomach, Pylorus**<br>Pyloric antrum<br>Pyloric canal<br>Pyloric sphincter<br>**8 Small Intestine**<br>**9 Duodenum**<br>**A Jejunum**<br>Duodenojejunal flexure<br>**B Ileum**<br>**C Ileocecal Valve**<br>**E Large Intestine**<br>**F Large Intestine, Right**<br>**G Large Intestine, Left**<br>**H Cecum**<br>**K Ascending Colon**<br>**L Transverse Colon**<br>Hepatic flexure<br>Splenic flexure<br>**M Descending Colon**<br>**N Sigmoid Colon**<br>Rectosigmoid junction<br>Sigmoid flexure<br>**P Rectum**<br>Anorectal junction<br>**Q Anus**<br>Anal orifice | **Ø Open**<br>**3 Percutaneous**<br>**4 Percutaneous Endoscopic**<br>**7 Via Natural or Artificial Opening**<br>**8 Via Natural or Artificial Opening Endoscopic** | **D Intraluminal Device**<br>**Z No Device** | **Z No Qualifier** |

**Non-OR** ØD7[1,2,3,4,5,6,8,9,A,B,C,E,F,G,H,K,L,M,N,P,Q][7,8][D,Z]Z
**Non-OR** ØD77[4,8]DZ
**Non-OR** ØD777[D,Z]Z
**Non-OR** ØD7[8,9,A,B,C,E,F,G,H,K,L,M,N][Ø,3,4]DZ

**Ø Medical and Surgical**
**D Gastrointestinal System**
**8 Division** Definition: Cutting into a body part, without draining fluids and/or gases from the body part, in order to separate or transect a body part

Explanation: All or a portion of the body part is separated into two or more portions

| Body Part Character 4 | Approach Character 5 | Device Character 6 | Qualifier Character 7 |
|---|---|---|---|
| **4 Esophagogastric Junction**<br>Cardia<br>Cardioesophageal junction<br>Gastroesophageal (GE) junction<br>**7 Stomach, Pylorus**<br>Pyloric antrum<br>Pyloric canal<br>Pyloric sphincter | **Ø Open**<br>**3 Percutaneous**<br>**4 Percutaneous Endoscopic**<br>**7 Via Natural or Artificial Opening**<br>**8 Via Natural or Artificial Opening Endoscopic** | **Z No Device** | **Z No Qualifier** |
| **R Anal Sphincter**<br>External anal sphincter<br>Internal anal sphincter | **Ø Open**<br>**3 Percutaneous** | **Z No Device** | **Z No Qualifier** |

**Ø Medical and Surgical**
**D Gastrointestinal System**
**9 Drainage** Definition: Taking or letting out fluids and/or gases from a body part
Explanation: The qualifier DIAGNOSTIC is used to identify drainage procedures that are biopsies

| Body Part Character 4 | Approach Character 5 | Device Character 6 | Qualifier Character 7 |
|---|---|---|---|
| **1 Esophagus, Upper** Cervical esophagus **2 Esophagus, Middle** Thoracic esophagus **3 Esophagus, Lower** Abdominal esophagus **4 Esophagogastric Junction** Cardia Cardioesophageal junction Gastroesophageal (GE) junction **5 Esophagus** **6 Stomach** **7 Stomach, Pylorus** Pyloric antrum Pyloric canal Pyloric sphincter **8 Small Intestine** **9 Duodenum** **A Jejunum** Duodenojejunal flexure **B Ileum** **C Ileocecal Valve** **E Large Intestine** **F Large Intestine, Right** **G Large Intestine, Left** **H Cecum** **J Appendix** Vermiform appendix **K Ascending Colon** **L Transverse Colon** Hepatic flexure Splenic flexure **M Descending Colon** **N Sigmoid Colon** Rectosigmoid junction Sigmoid flexure **P Rectum** Anorectal junction | **Ø Open** **3 Percutaneous** **4 Percutaneous Endoscopic** **7 Via Natural or Artificial Opening** **8 Via Natural or Artificial Opening Endoscopic** | **Ø Drainage Device** | **Z No Qualifier** |
| **1 Esophagus, Upper** Cervical esophagus **2 Esophagus, Middle** Thoracic esophagus **3 Esophagus, Lower** Abdominal esophagus **4 Esophagogastric Junction** Cardia Cardioesophageal junction Gastroesophageal (GE) junction **5 Esophagus** **6 Stomach** **7 Stomach, Pylorus** Pyloric antrum Pyloric canal Pyloric sphincter **8 Small Intestine** **9 Duodenum** **A Jejunum** Duodenojejunal flexure **B Ileum** **C Ileocecal Valve** **E Large Intestine** **F Large Intestine, Right** **G Large Intestine, Left** **H Cecum** **J Appendix** Vermiform appendix **K Ascending Colon** **L Transverse Colon** Hepatic flexure Splenic flexure **M Descending Colon** **N Sigmoid Colon** Rectosigmoid junction Sigmoid flexure **P Rectum** Anorectal junction | **Ø Open** **3 Percutaneous** **4 Percutaneous Endoscopic** **7 Via Natural or Artificial Opening** **8 Via Natural or Artificial Opening Endoscopic** | **Z No Device** | **X Diagnostic** **Z No Qualifier** |
| **Q Anus** Anal orifice | **Ø Open** **3 Percutaneous** **4 Percutaneous Endoscopic** **7 Via Natural or Artificial Opening** **8 Via Natural or Artificial Opening Endoscopic** **X External** | **Ø Drainage Device** | **Z No Qualifier** |
| **Q Anus** Anal orifice | **Ø Open** **3 Percutaneous** **4 Percutaneous Endoscopic** **7 Via Natural or Artificial Opening** **8 Via Natural or Artificial Opening Endoscopic** **X External** | **Z No Device** | **X Diagnostic** **Z No Qualifier** |

***ØD9 Continued on next page***

**DRG Non-OR** ØD9[8,A,B,C]3ØZ
**DRG Non-OR** ØD9[8,A,B,C]3ZZ
**Non-OR** ØD9[1,2,3,4,5,6,7,9,E,F,G,H,J,K,L,M,N,P]3ØZ
**Non-OR** ØD9[6,7,8,9,A,B,E,F,G,H,K,L,M,N,P][7,8]ØZ
**Non-OR** ØD9[1,2,3,4,5,6,7,8,9,A,B,C,E,F,G,H,K,L,M,N,P][3,4,7,8]ZX
**Non-OR** ØD9[1,2,3,4,5,6,7,9,E,F,G,H,J,K,L,M,N,P]3ZZ
**Non-OR** ØD9Q3ØZ
**Non-OR** ØD9Q[Ø,4,7,8,X]ZX
**Non-OR** ØD9Q3Z[X,Z]

**Ø Medical and Surgical**
**D Gastrointestinal System**
**9 Drainage** Definition: Taking or letting out fluids and/or gases from a body part
Explanation: The qualifier DIAGNOSTIC is used to identify drainage procedures that are biopsies

***ØD9 Continued***

| Body Part Character 4 | Approach Character 5 | Device Character 6 | Qualifier Character 7 |
|---|---|---|---|
| **R Anal Sphincter**<br>External anal sphincter<br>Internal anal sphincter<br>**U Omentum**<br>Gastrocolic ligament<br>Gastrocolic omentum<br>Gastrohepatic omentum<br>Gastrophrenic ligament<br>Gastrosplenic ligament<br>Greater Omentum<br>Hepatogastric ligament<br>Lesser Omentum<br>**V Mesentery**<br>Mesoappendix<br>Mesocolon<br>**W Peritoneum**<br>Epiploic foramen | **Ø Open**<br>**3 Percutaneous**<br>**4 Percutaneous Endoscopic** | **Ø Drainage Device** | **Z No Qualifier** |
| **R Anal Sphincter**<br>External anal sphincter<br>Internal anal sphincter<br>**U Omentum**<br>Gastrocolic ligament<br>Gastrocolic omentum<br>Gastrohepatic omentum<br>Gastrophrenic ligament<br>Gastrosplenic ligament<br>Greater Omentum<br>Hepatogastric ligament<br>Lesser Omentum<br>**V Mesentery**<br>Mesoappendix<br>Mesocolon<br>**W Peritoneum**<br>Epiploic foramen | **Ø Open**<br>**3 Percutaneous**<br>**4 Percutaneous Endoscopic** | **Z No Device** | **X Diagnostic**<br>**Z No Qualifier** |

**Non-OR** ØD9R3ØZ
**Non-OR** ØD9U[3,4]ØZ
**Non-OR** ØD9[V,W][3,4]ØZ
**Non-OR** ØD9R[Ø,4]ZX
**Non-OR** ØD9[R,U]3Z[X,Z]
**Non-OR** ØD9U4ZZ
**Non-OR** ØD9[V,W]3Z[X,Z]
**Non-OR** ØD9[V,W]4ZZ

**Ø Medical and Surgical**
**D Gastrointestinal System**
**B Excision** Definition: Cutting out or off, without replacement, a portion of a body part
Explanation: The qualifier DIAGNOSTIC is used to identify excision procedures that are biopsies

| Body Part Character 4 | Approach Character 5 | Device Character 6 | Qualifier Character 7 |
|---|---|---|---|
| 1 Esophagus, Upper<br>Cervical esophagus<br>2 Esophagus, Middle<br>Thoracic esophagus<br>3 Esophagus, Lower<br>Abdominal esophagus<br>4 Esophagogastric Junction<br>Cardia<br>Cardioesophageal junction<br>Gastroesophageal (GE) junction<br>5 Esophagus<br>7 Stomach, Pylorus<br>Pyloric antrum<br>Pyloric canal<br>Pyloric sphincter<br>8 Small Intestine<br>9 Duodenum<br>A Jejunum<br>Duodenojejunal flexure<br>B Ileum<br>C Ileocecal Valve<br>E Large Intestine<br>F Large Intestine, Right<br>H Cecum<br>J Appendix<br>Vermiform appendix<br>K Ascending Colon<br>P Rectum<br>Anorectal junction | Ø Open<br>3 Percutaneous<br>4 Percutaneous Endoscopic<br>7 Via Natural or Artificial Opening<br>8 Via Natural or Artificial Opening Endoscopic | Z No Device | X Diagnostic<br>Z No Qualifier |
| 6 Stomach | Ø Open<br>3 Percutaneous<br>4 Percutaneous Endoscopic<br>7 Via Natural or Artificial Opening<br>8 Via Natural or Artificial Opening Endoscopic | Z No Device | 3 Vertical<br>X Diagnostic<br>Z No Qualifier |
| G Large Intestine, Left<br>L Transverse Colon<br>Hepatic flexure<br>Splenic flexure<br>M Descending Colon<br>N Sigmoid Colon<br>Rectosigmoid junction<br>Sigmoid flexure | Ø Open<br>3 Percutaneous<br>4 Percutaneous Endoscopic<br>7 Via Natural or Artificial Opening<br>8 Via Natural or Artificial Opening Endoscopic | Z No Device | X Diagnostic<br>Z No Qualifier |
| G Large Intestine, Left<br>L Transverse Colon<br>Hepatic flexure<br>Splenic flexure<br>M Descending Colon<br>N Sigmoid Colon<br>Rectosigmoid junction<br>Sigmoid flexure | F Via Natural or Artificial Opening with Percutaneous Endoscopic Assistance | Z No Device | Z No Qualifier |
| Q Anus<br>Anal orifice | Ø Open<br>3 Percutaneous<br>4 Percutaneous Endoscopic<br>7 Via Natural or Artificial Opening<br>8 Via Natural or Artificial Opening Endoscopic<br>X External | Z No Device | X Diagnostic<br>Z No Qualifier |
| R Anal Sphincter<br>External anal sphincter<br>Internal anal sphincter<br>U Omentum<br>Gastrocolic ligament<br>Gastrocolic omentum<br>Gastrohepatic omentum<br>Gastrophrenic ligament<br>Gastrosplenic ligament<br>Greater Omentum<br>Hepatogastric ligament<br>Lesser Omentum<br>V Mesentery<br>Mesoappendix<br>Mesocolon<br>W Peritoneum<br>Epiploic foramen | Ø Open<br>3 Percutaneous<br>4 Percutaneous Endoscopic | Z No Device | X Diagnostic<br>Z No Qualifier |

Non-OR ØDB[1,2,3,4,5,7,8,9,A,B,C,E,F,H,K,P][3,4,7,8]ZX
Non-OR ØDB[1,2,3,5,7,9][4,8]ZZ
Non-OR ØDB[4,E,F,H,K,P]8ZZ
Non-OR ØDB6[3,4,7,8]ZX
Non-OR ØDB6[4,8]ZZ
Non-OR ØDB[G,L,M,N][3,4,7,8]ZX
Non-OR ØDB[G,L,M,N]8ZZ
Non-OR ØDBQ[Ø,3,4,7,8,X]ZX
Non-OR ØDBQ8ZZ
Non-OR ØDBR[Ø,3,4]ZX
Non-OR ØDB[U,V,W][3,4]ZX

**Ø Medical and Surgical**
**D Gastrointestinal System**
**C Extirpation** Definition: Taking or cutting out solid matter from a body part

Explanation: The solid matter may be an abnormal byproduct of a biological function or a foreign body; it may be imbedded in a body part or in the lumen of a tubular body part. The solid matter may or may not have been previously broken into pieces.

| Body Part Character 4 | Approach Character 5 | Device Character 6 | Qualifier Character 7 |
|---|---|---|---|
| **1 Esophagus, Upper**<br>Cervical esophagus<br>**2 Esophagus, Middle**<br>Thoracic esophagus<br>**3 Esophagus, Lower**<br>Abdominal esophagus<br>**4 Esophagogastric Junction**<br>Cardia<br>Cardioesophageal junction<br>Gastroesophageal (GE) junction<br>**5 Esophagus**<br>**6 Stomach**<br>**7 Stomach, Pylorus**<br>Pyloric antrum<br>Pyloric canal<br>Pyloric sphincter<br>**8 Small Intestine**<br>**9 Duodenum**<br>**A Jejunum**<br>Duodenojejunal flexure<br>**B Ileum**<br>**C Ileocecal Valve**<br>**E Large Intestine**<br>**F Large Intestine, Right**<br>**G Large Intestine, Left**<br>**H Cecum**<br>**J Appendix**<br>Vermiform appendix<br>**K Ascending Colon**<br>**L Transverse Colon**<br>Hepatic flexure<br>Splenic flexure<br>**M Descending Colon**<br>**N Sigmoid Colon**<br>Rectosigmoid junction<br>Sigmoid flexure<br>**P Rectum**<br>Anorectal junction | **Ø Open**<br>**3 Percutaneous**<br>**4 Percutaneous Endoscopic**<br>**7 Via Natural or Artificial Opening**<br>**8 Via Natural or Artificial Opening Endoscopic** | **Z No Device** | **Z No Qualifier** |
| **Q Anus**<br>Anal orifice | **Ø Open**<br>**3 Percutaneous**<br>**4 Percutaneous Endoscopic**<br>**7 Via Natural or Artificial Opening**<br>**8 Via Natural or Artificial Opening Endoscopic**<br>**X External** | **Z No Device** | **Z No Qualifier** |
| **R Anal Sphincter**<br>External anal sphincter<br>Internal anal sphincter<br>**U Omentum**<br>Gastrocolic ligament<br>Gastrocolic omentum<br>Gastrohepatic omentum<br>Gastrophrenic ligament<br>Gastrosplenic ligament<br>Greater Omentum<br>Hepatogastric ligament<br>Lesser Omentum<br>**V Mesentery**<br>Mesoappendix<br>Mesocolon<br>**W Peritoneum**<br>Epiploic foramen | **Ø Open**<br>**3 Percutaneous**<br>**4 Percutaneous Endoscopic** | **Z No Device** | **Z No Qualifier** |

**Non-OR** ØDC[1,2,3,4,5,6,7,8,9,A,B,C,E,F,G,H,K,L,M,N,P][7,8]ZZ
**Non-OR** ØDCQ[7,8,X]ZZ

**Ø Medical and Surgical**
**D Gastrointestinal System**
**D Extraction** Definition: Pulling or stripping out or off all or a portion of a body part by the use of force

Explanation: The qualifier DIAGNOSTIC is used to identify extraction procedures that are biopsies

| Body Part Character 4 | Approach Character 5 | Device Character 6 | Qualifier Character 7 |
|---|---|---|---|
| 1 Esophagus, Upper<br>Cervical esophagus<br>2 Esophagus, Middle<br>Thoracic esophagus<br>3 Esophagus, Lower<br>Abdominal esophagus<br>4 Esophagogastric Junction<br>Cardia<br>Cardioesophageal junction<br>Gastroesophageal (GE) junction<br>5 Esophagus<br>6 Stomach<br>7 Stomach, Pylorus<br>Pyloric antrum<br>Pyloric canal<br>Pyloric sphincter<br>8 Small Intestine<br>9 Duodenum<br>A Jejunum<br>Duodenojejunal flexure<br>B Ileum<br>C Ileocecal Valve<br>E Large Intestine<br>F Large Intestine, Right<br>G Large Intestine, Left<br>H Cecum<br>J Appendix<br>Vermiform appendix<br>K Ascending Colon<br>L Transverse Colon<br>Hepatic flexure<br>Splenic flexure<br>M Descending Colon<br>N Sigmoid Colon<br>Rectosigmoid junction<br>Sigmoid flexure<br>P Rectum<br>Anorectal junction | 3 Percutaneous<br>4 Percutaneous Endoscopic<br>8 Via Natural or Artificial Opening Endoscopic | Z No Device | X Diagnostic |
| Q Anus<br>Anal orifice | 3 Percutaneous<br>4 Percutaneous Endoscopic<br>8 Via Natural or Artificial Opening Endoscopic<br>X External | Z No Device | X Diagnostic |

**Non-OR** ØDD[1,2,3,4,5,6,7,8,9,A,B,C,E,F,G,H,K,L,M,N,P][3,4,8]ZX
**Non-OR** ØDDQ[3,4,8,X]ZX

**Ø Medical and Surgical**
**D Gastrointestinal System**
**F Fragmentation** Definition: Breaking solid matter in a body part into pieces

Explanation: Physical force (e.g., manual, ultrasonic) applied directly or indirectly is used to break the solid matter into pieces. The solid matter may be an abnormal byproduct of a biological function or a foreign body. The pieces of solid matter are not taken out.

| Body Part Character 4 | Approach Character 5 | Device Character 6 | Qualifier Character 7 |
|---|---|---|---|
| 5 Esophagus NC<br>6 Stomach NC<br>8 Small Intestine NC<br>9 Duodenum NC<br>A Jejunum NC<br>Duodenojejunal flexure<br>B Ileum NC<br>E Large Intestine NC<br>F Large Intestine, Right NC<br>G Large Intestine, Left NC<br>H Cecum NC<br>J Appendix NC<br>Vermiform appendix<br>K Ascending Colon NC<br>L Transverse Colon NC<br>Hepatic flexure<br>Splenic flexure<br>M Descending Colon NC<br>N Sigmoid Colon NC<br>Rectosigmoid junction<br>Sigmoid flexure<br>P Rectum NC<br>Anorectal junction<br>Q Anus NC<br>Anal orifice | Ø Open<br>3 Percutaneous<br>4 Percutaneous Endoscopic<br>7 Via Natural or Artificial Opening<br>8 Via Natural or Artificial Opening Endoscopic<br>X External | Z No Device | Z No Qualifier |

Non-OR ØDF[5,6,8,9,A,B,E,F,G,H,J,K,L,M,N,P,Q]XZZ
NC ØDF[5,6,8,9,A,B,E,F,G,H,J,K,L,M,N,P,Q]XZZ

**Ø Medical and Surgical**
**D Gastrointestinal System**
**H Insertion** Definition: Putting in a nonbiological appliance that monitors, assists, performs, or prevents a physiological function but does not physically take the place of a body part

Explanation: None

| Body Part Character 4 | Approach Character 5 | Device Character 6 | Qualifier Character 7 |
|---|---|---|---|
| Ø Upper Intestinal Tract<br>D Lower Intestinal Tract | Ø Open<br>3 Percutaneous<br>4 Percutaneous Endoscopic<br>7 Via Natural or Artificial Opening<br>8 Via Natural or Artificial Opening Endoscopic | Y Other Device | Z No Qualifier |
| 5 Esophagus | Ø Open<br>3 Percutaneous<br>4 Percutaneous Endoscopic | 1 Radioactive Element<br>2 Monitoring Device<br>3 Infusion Device<br>D Intraluminal Device<br>U Feeding Device<br>Y Other Device | Z No Qualifier |
| 5 Esophagus | 7 Via Natural or Artificial Opening<br>8 Via Natural or Artificial Opening Endoscopic | 1 Radioactive Element<br>2 Monitoring Device<br>3 Infusion Device<br>B Intraluminal Device, Airway<br>D Intraluminal Device<br>U Feeding Device<br>Y Other Device | Z No Qualifier |
| 6 Stomach ⊞ | Ø Open<br>3 Percutaneous<br>4 Percutaneous Endoscopic | 2 Monitoring Device<br>3 Infusion Device<br>D Intraluminal Device<br>M Stimulator Lead<br>U Feeding Device<br>Y Other Device | Z No Qualifier |
| 6 Stomach | 7 Via Natural or Artificial Opening<br>8 Via Natural or Artificial Opening Endoscopic | 2 Monitoring Device<br>3 Infusion Device<br>D Intraluminal Device<br>U Feeding Device<br>Y Other Device | Z No Qualifier |
| 8 Small Intestine<br>9 Duodenum<br>A Jejunum<br>Duodenojejunal flexure<br>B Ileum | Ø Open<br>3 Percutaneous<br>4 Percutaneous Endoscopic<br>7 Via Natural or Artificial Opening<br>8 Via Natural or Artificial Opening Endoscopic | 2 Monitoring Device<br>3 Infusion Device<br>D Intraluminal Device<br>U Feeding Device | Z No Qualifier |
| E Large Intestine | Ø Open<br>3 Percutaneous<br>4 Percutaneous Endoscopic<br>7 Via Natural or Artificial Opening<br>8 Via Natural or Artificial Opening Endoscopic | D Intraluminal Device | Z No Qualifier |
| P Rectum<br>Anorectal junction | Ø Open<br>3 Percutaneous<br>4 Percutaneous Endoscopic<br>7 Via Natural or Artificial Opening<br>8 Via Natural or Artificial Opening Endoscopic | 1 Radioactive Element<br>D Intraluminal Device | Z No Qualifier |
| Q Anus<br>Anal orifice | Ø Open<br>3 Percutaneous<br>4 Percutaneous Endoscopic | D Intraluminal Device<br>L Artificial Sphincter | Z No Qualifier |
| Q Anus<br>Anal orifice | 7 Via Natural or Artificial Opening<br>8 Via Natural or Artificial Opening Endoscopic | D Intraluminal Device | Z No Qualifier |
| R Anal Sphincter<br>External anal sphincter<br>Internal anal sphincter | Ø Open<br>3 Percutaneous<br>4 Percutaneous Endoscopic | M Stimulator Lead | Z No Qualifier |

**Non-OR** ØDH[Ø,D][Ø,3,4,7,8]YZ
**Non-OR** ØDH5[Ø,3,4][D,U]Z
**Non-OR** ØDH5[3,4]YZ
**Non-OR** ØDH5[7,8][2,3,B,D,U,Y]Z
**Non-OR** ØDH6[3,4][U,Y]Z
**Non-OR** ØDH6[7,8][2,3,D,U,Y]Z
**Non-OR** ØDH[8,9,A,B][Ø,3,4][D,U]Z
**Non-OR** ØDH[8,9,A,B][7,8][2,3,D,U]Z
**Non-OR** ØDHE[Ø,3,4,7,8]DZ
**Non-OR** ØDHP[Ø,3,4,7,8]DZ

**See Appendix L for Procedure Combinations**
⊞ ØDH6[Ø,3,4]MZ

**Ø Medical and Surgical**
**D Gastrointestinal System**
**J Inspection** Definition: Visually and/or manually exploring a body part

Explanation: Visual exploration may be performed with or without optical instrumentation. Manual exploration may be performed directly or through intervening body layers.

| Body Part Character 4 | Approach Character 5 | Device Character 6 | Qualifier Character 7 |
|---|---|---|---|
| **Ø Upper Intestinal Tract**<br>**6 Stomach**<br>**D Lower Intestinal Tract** | **Ø Open**<br>**3 Percutaneous**<br>**4 Percutaneous Endoscopic**<br>**7 Via Natural or Artificial Opening**<br>**8 Via Natural or Artificial Opening Endoscopic**<br>**X External** | **Z No Device** | **Z No Qualifier** |
| **U Omentum**<br>Gastrocolic ligament<br>Gastrocolic omentum<br>Gastrohepatic omentum<br>Gastrophrenic ligament<br>Gastrosplenic ligament<br>Greater Omentum<br>Hepatogastric ligament<br>Lesser Omentum<br>**V Mesentery**<br>Mesoappendix<br>Mesocolon<br>**W Peritoneum**<br>Epiploic foramen | **Ø Open**<br>**3 Percutaneous**<br>**4 Percutaneous Endoscopic**<br>**X External** | **Z No Device** | **Z No Qualifier** |

**DRG Non-OR** ØDJ[U,V,W]3ZZ
**Non-OR** ØDJ[Ø,6,D][3,7,8,X]ZZ
**Non-OR** ØDJ[U,V,W]XZZ

**Ø Medical and Surgical**
**D Gastrointestinal System**
**L Occlusion** Definition: Completely closing an orifice or the lumen of a tubular body part
Explanation: The orifice can be a natural orifice or an artificially created orifice

| Body Part Character 4 | | Approach Character 5 | Device Character 6 | Qualifier Character 7 |
|---|---|---|---|---|
| **1 Esophagus, Upper**<br>Cervical esophagus<br>**2 Esophagus, Middle**<br>Thoracic esophagus<br>**3 Esophagus, Lower**<br>Abdominal esophagus<br>**4 Esophagogastric Junction**<br>Cardia<br>Cardioesophageal junction<br>Gastroesophageal (GE) junction<br>**5 Esophagus**<br>**6 Stomach**<br>**7 Stomach, Pylorus**<br>Pyloric antrum<br>Pyloric canal<br>Pyloric sphincter<br>**8 Small Intestine** | **9 Duodenum**<br>**A Jejunum**<br>Duodenojejunal flexure<br>**B Ileum**<br>**C Ileocecal Valve**<br>**E Large Intestine**<br>**F Large Intestine, Right**<br>**G Large Intestine, Left**<br>**H Cecum**<br>**K Ascending Colon**<br>**L Transverse Colon**<br>Hepatic flexure<br>Splenic flexure<br>**M Descending Colon**<br>**N Sigmoid Colon**<br>Rectosigmoid junction<br>Sigmoid flexure<br>**P Rectum**<br>Anorectal junction | **Ø Open**<br>**3 Percutaneous**<br>**4 Percutaneous Endoscopic** | **C Extraluminal Device**<br>**D Intraluminal Device**<br>**Z No Device** | **Z No Qualifier** |
| **1 Esophagus, Upper**<br>Cervical esophagus<br>**2 Esophagus, Middle**<br>Thoracic esophagus<br>**3 Esophagus, Lower**<br>Abdominal esophagus<br>**4 Esophagogastric Junction**<br>Cardia<br>Cardioesophageal junction<br>Gastroesophageal (GE) junction<br>**5 Esophagus**<br>**6 Stomach**<br>**7 Stomach, Pylorus**<br>Pyloric antrum<br>Pyloric canal<br>Pyloric sphincter<br>**8 Small Intestine** | **9 Duodenum**<br>**A Jejunum**<br>Duodenojejunal flexure<br>**B Ileum**<br>**C Ileocecal Valve**<br>**E Large Intestine**<br>**F Large Intestine, Right**<br>**G Large Intestine, Left**<br>**H Cecum**<br>**K Ascending Colon**<br>**L Transverse Colon**<br>Hepatic flexure<br>Splenic flexure<br>**M Descending Colon**<br>**N Sigmoid Colon**<br>Rectosigmoid junction<br>Sigmoid flexure<br>**P Rectum**<br>Anorectal junction | **7 Via Natural or Artificial Opening**<br>**8 Via Natural or Artificial Opening Endoscopic** | **D Intraluminal Device**<br>**Z No Device** | **Z No Qualifier** |
| **Q Anus**<br>Anal orifice | | **Ø Open**<br>**3 Percutaneous**<br>**4 Percutaneous Endoscopic**<br>**X External** | **C Extraluminal Device**<br>**D Intraluminal Device**<br>**Z No Device** | **Z No Qualifier** |
| **Q Anus**<br>Anal orifice | | **7 Via Natural or Artificial Opening**<br>**8 Via Natural or Artificial Opening Endoscopic** | **D Intraluminal Device**<br>**Z No Device** | **Z No Qualifier** |

**Non-OR** ØDL[1,2,3,4,5][Ø,3,4][C,D,Z]Z
**Non-OR** ØDL[1,2,3,4,5][7,8][D,Z]Z

**Ø Medical and Surgical**
**D Gastrointestinal System**
**M Reattachment** Definition: Putting back in or on all or a portion of a separated body part to its normal location or other suitable location
Explanation: Vascular circulation and nervous pathways may or may not be reestablished

| Body Part Character 4 | Approach Character 5 | Device Character 6 | Qualifier Character 7 |
|---|---|---|---|
| **5 Esophagus**<br>**6 Stomach**<br>**8 Small Intestine**<br>**9 Duodenum**<br>**A Jejunum**<br>Duodenojejunal flexure<br>**B Ileum**<br>**E Large Intestine**<br>**F Large Intestine, Right**<br>**G Large Intestine, Left**<br>**H Cecum**<br>**K Ascending Colon**<br>**L Transverse Colon**<br>Hepatic flexure<br>Splenic flexure<br>**M Descending Colon**<br>**N Sigmoid Colon**<br>Rectosigmoid junction<br>Sigmoid flexure<br>**P Rectum**<br>Anorectal junction | **Ø Open**<br>**4 Percutaneous Endoscopic** | **Z No Device** | **Z No Qualifier** |

**Ø Medical and Surgical**
**D Gastrointestinal System**
**N Release** Definition: Freeing a body part from an abnormal physical constraint by cutting or by the use of force
Explanation: Some of the restraining tissue may be taken out but none of the body part is taken out

| Body Part Character 4 | Approach Character 5 | Device Character 6 | Qualifier Character 7 |
|---|---|---|---|
| **1 Esophagus, Upper**<br>Cervical esophagus<br>**2 Esophagus, Middle**<br>Thoracic esophagus<br>**3 Esophagus, Lower**<br>Abdominal esophagus<br>**4 Esophagogastric Junction**<br>Cardia<br>Cardioesophageal junction<br>Gastroesophageal (GE) junction<br>**5 Esophagus**<br>**6 Stomach**<br>**7 Stomach, Pylorus**<br>Pyloric antrum<br>Pyloric canal<br>Pyloric sphincter<br>**8 Small Intestine**<br>**9 Duodenum**<br>**A Jejunum**<br>Duodenojejunal flexure<br>**B Ileum**<br>**C Ileocecal Valve**<br>**E Large Intestine**<br>**F Large Intestine, Right**<br>**G Large Intestine, Left**<br>**H Cecum**<br>**J Appendix**<br>Vermiform appendix<br>**K Ascending Colon**<br>**L Transverse Colon**<br>Hepatic flexure<br>Splenic flexure<br>**M Descending Colon**<br>**N Sigmoid Colon**<br>Rectosigmoid junction<br>Sigmoid flexure<br>**P Rectum**<br>Anorectal junction | **Ø Open**<br>**3 Percutaneous**<br>**4 Percutaneous Endoscopic**<br>**7 Via Natural or Artificial Opening**<br>**8 Via Natural or Artificial Opening Endoscopic** | **Z No Device** | **Z No Qualifier** |
| **Q Anus**<br>Anal orifice | **Ø Open**<br>**3 Percutaneous**<br>**4 Percutaneous Endoscopic**<br>**7 Via Natural or Artificial Opening**<br>**8 Via Natural or Artificial Opening Endoscopic**<br>**X External** | **Z No Device** | **Z No Qualifier** |
| **R Anal Sphincter**<br>External anal sphincter<br>Internal anal sphincter<br>**U Omentum**<br>Gastrocolic ligament<br>Gastrocolic omentum<br>Gastrohepatic omentum<br>Gastrophrenic ligament<br>Gastrosplenic ligament<br>Greater Omentum<br>Hepatogastric ligament<br>Lesser Omentum<br>**V Mesentery**<br>Mesoappendix<br>Mesocolon<br>**W Peritoneum**<br>Epiploic foramen | **Ø Open**<br>**3 Percutaneous**<br>**4 Percutaneous Endoscopic** | **Z No Device** | **Z No Qualifier** |

**Non-OR** ØDN[8,9,A,B,E,F,G,H,K,L,M,N][7,8]ZZ

**Ø Medical and Surgical**
**D Gastrointestinal System**
**P Removal** Definition: Taking out or off a device from a body part

Explanation: If a device is taken out and a similar device put in without cutting or puncturing the skin or mucous membrane, the procedure is coded to the root operation CHANGE. Otherwise, the procedure for taking out a device is coded to the root operation REMOVAL.

| Body Part Character 4 | Approach Character 5 | Device Character 6 | Qualifier Character 7 |
|---|---|---|---|
| Ø Upper Intestinal Tract<br>D Lower Intestinal Tract | Ø Open<br>3 Percutaneous<br>4 Percutaneous Endoscopic<br>7 Via Natural or Artificial Opening<br>8 Via Natural or Artificial Opening Endoscopic | Ø Drainage Device<br>2 Monitoring Device<br>3 Infusion Device<br>7 Autologous Tissue Substitute<br>C Extraluminal Device<br>D Intraluminal Device<br>J Synthetic Substitute<br>K Nonautologous Tissue Substitute<br>U Feeding Device<br>Y Other Device | Z No Qualifier |
| Ø Upper Intestinal Tract<br>D Lower Intestinal Tract | X External | Ø Drainage Device<br>2 Monitoring Device<br>3 Infusion Device<br>D Intraluminal Device<br>U Feeding Device | Z No Qualifier |
| 5 Esophagus | Ø Open<br>3 Percutaneous<br>4 Percutaneous Endoscopic | 1 Radioactive Element<br>2 Monitoring Device<br>3 Infusion Device<br>U Feeding Device<br>Y Other Device | Z No Qualifier |
| 5 Esophagus | 7 Via Natural or Artificial Opening<br>8 Via Natural or Artificial Opening Endoscopic | 1 Radioactive Element<br>D Intraluminal Device<br>Y Other Device | Z No Qualifier |
| 5 Esophagus | X External | 1 Radioactive Element<br>2 Monitoring Device<br>3 Infusion Device<br>D Intraluminal Device<br>U Feeding Device | Z No Qualifier |
| 6 Stomach | Ø Open<br>3 Percutaneous<br>4 Percutaneous Endoscopic | Ø Drainage Device<br>2 Monitoring Device<br>3 Infusion Device<br>7 Autologous Tissue Substitute<br>C Extraluminal Device<br>D Intraluminal Device<br>J Synthetic Substitute<br>K Nonautologous Tissue Substitute<br>M Stimulator Lead<br>U Feeding Device<br>Y Other Device | Z No Qualifier |
| 6 Stomach | 7 Via Natural or Artificial Opening<br>8 Via Natural or Artificial Opening Endoscopic | Ø Drainage Device<br>2 Monitoring Device<br>3 Infusion Device<br>7 Autologous Tissue Substitute<br>C Extraluminal Device<br>D Intraluminal Device<br>J Synthetic Substitute<br>K Nonautologous Tissue Substitute<br>U Feeding Device<br>Y Other Device | Z No Qualifier |
| 6 Stomach | X External | Ø Drainage Device<br>2 Monitoring Device<br>3 Infusion Device<br>D Intraluminal Device<br>U Feeding Device | Z No Qualifier |

***ØDP Continued on next page***

**Non-OR** ØDP[Ø,D][3,4]YZ
**Non-OR** ØDP[Ø,D][7,8][Ø,2,3,D,U,Y]Z
**Non-OR** ØDP[Ø,D]X[Ø,2,3,D,U]Z
**Non-OR** ØDP5[3,4]YZ
**Non-OR** ØDP5[7,8][1,D,Y]Z
**Non-OR** ØDP5X[1,2,3,D,U]Z
**Non-OR** ØDP6[3,4]YZ
**Non-OR** ØDP6[7,8][Ø,2,3,D,U,Y]Z
**Non-OR** ØDP6X[Ø,2,3,D,U]Z

**ØDP Continued**

**Ø Medical and Surgical**
**D Gastrointestinal System**
**P Removal** Definition: Taking out or off a device from a body part

Explanation: If a device is taken out and a similar device put in without cutting or puncturing the skin or mucous membrane, the procedure is coded to the root operation CHANGE. Otherwise, the procedure for taking out a device is coded to the root operation REMOVAL.

| Body Part Character 4 | Approach Character 5 | Device Character 6 | Qualifier Character 7 |
|---|---|---|---|
| **P Rectum**<br>Anorectal junction | **Ø Open**<br>**3 Percutaneous**<br>**4 Percutaneous Endoscopic**<br>**7 Via Natural or Artificial Opening**<br>**8 Via Natural or Artificial Opening Endoscopic**<br>**X External** | **1 Radioactive Element** | **Z No Qualifier** |
| **Q Anus**<br>Anal orifice | **Ø Open**<br>**3 Percutaneous**<br>**4 Percutaneous Endoscopic**<br>**7 Via Natural or Artificial Opening**<br>**8 Via Natural or Artificial Opening Endoscopic** | **L Artificial Sphincter** | **Z No Qualifier** |
| **R Anal Sphincter**<br>External anal sphincter<br>Internal anal sphincter | **Ø Open**<br>**3 Percutaneous**<br>**4 Percutaneous Endoscopic** | **M Stimulator Lead** | **Z No Qualifier** |
| **U Omentum**<br>Gastrocolic ligament<br>Gastrocolic omentum<br>Gastrohepatic omentum<br>Gastrophrenic ligament<br>Gastrosplenic ligament<br>Greater Omentum<br>Hepatogastric ligament<br>Lesser Omentum<br>**V Mesentery**<br>Mesoappendix<br>Mesocolon<br>**W Peritoneum**<br>Epiploic foramen | **Ø Open**<br>**3 Percutaneous**<br>**4 Percutaneous Endoscopic** | **Ø Drainage Device**<br>**1 Radioactive Element**<br>**7 Autologous Tissue Substitute**<br>**J Synthetic Substitute**<br>**K Nonautologous Tissue Substitute** | **Z No Qualifier** |

**Non-OR** ØDPP[7,8,X]1Z

**Ø Medical and Surgical**
**D Gastrointestinal System**
**Q Repair** Definition: Restoring, to the extent possible, a body part to its normal anatomic structure and function
Explanation: Used only when the method to accomplish the repair is not one of the other root operations

| Body Part Character 4 | Approach Character 5 | Device Character 6 | Qualifier Character 7 |
|---|---|---|---|
| **1 Esophagus, Upper** Cervical esophagus<br>**2 Esophagus, Middle** Thoracic esophagus<br>**3 Esophagus, Lower** Abdominal esophagus<br>**4 Esophagogastric Junction** Cardia, Cardioesophageal junction, Gastroesophageal (GE) junction<br>**5 Esophagus**<br>**6 Stomach**<br>**7 Stomach, Pylorus** Pyloric antrum, Pyloric canal, Pyloric sphincter<br>**8 Small Intestine** ⊞<br>**9 Duodenum** ⊞<br>**A Jejunum** ⊞ Duodenojejunal flexure<br>**B Ileum** ⊞<br>**C Ileocecal Valve**<br>**E Large Intestine** ⊞<br>**F Large Intestine, Right** ⊞<br>**G Large Intestine, Left** ⊞<br>**H Cecum** ⊞<br>**J Appendix** Vermiform appendix<br>**K Ascending Colon** ⊞<br>**L Transverse Colon** ⊞ Hepatic flexure, Splenic flexure<br>**M Descending Colon** ⊞<br>**N Sigmoid Colon** ⊞ Rectosigmoid junction, Sigmoid flexure<br>**P Rectum** Anorectal junction | **Ø Open**<br>**3 Percutaneous**<br>**4 Percutaneous Endoscopic**<br>**7 Via Natural or Artificial Opening**<br>**8 Via Natural or Artificial Opening Endoscopic** | **Z No Device** | **Z No Qualifier** |
| **Q Anus** Anal orifice | **Ø Open**<br>**3 Percutaneous**<br>**4 Percutaneous Endoscopic**<br>**7 Via Natural or Artificial Opening**<br>**8 Via Natural or Artificial Opening Endoscopic**<br>**X External** | **Z No Device** | **Z No Qualifier** |
| **R Anal Sphincter** External anal sphincter, Internal anal sphincter<br>**U Omentum** Gastrocolic ligament, Gastrocolic omentum, Gastrohepatic omentum, Gastrophrenic ligament, Gastrosplenic ligament, Greater Omentum, Hepatogastric ligament, Lesser Omentum<br>**V Mesentery** Mesoappendix, Mesocolon<br>**W Peritoneum** Epiploic foramen | **Ø Open**<br>**3 Percutaneous**<br>**4 Percutaneous Endoscopic** | **Z No Device** | **Z No Qualifier** |

**See Appendix L for Procedure Combinations**
⊞ ØDQ[8,9,A,B,E,F,G,H,K,L,M,N]ØZZ

**Ø Medical and Surgical**
**D Gastrointestinal System**
**R Replacement** Definition: Putting in or on biological or synthetic material that physically takes the place and/or function of all or a portion of a body part

Explanation: The body part may have been taken out or replaced, or may be taken out, physically eradicated, or rendered nonfunctional during the REPLACEMENT procedure. A REMOVAL procedure is coded for taking out the device used in a previous replacement procedure.

| Body Part Character 4 | Approach Character 5 | Device Character 6 | Qualifier Character 7 |
|---|---|---|---|
| 5 Esophagus | Ø Open<br>4 Percutaneous Endoscopic<br>7 Via Natural or Artificial Opening<br>8 Via Natural or Artificial Opening Endoscopic | 7 Autologous Tissue Substitute<br>J Synthetic Substitute<br>K Nonautologous Tissue Substitute | Z No Qualifier |
| R Anal Sphincter<br>External anal sphincter<br>Internal anal sphincter<br>U Omentum<br>Gastrocolic ligament<br>Gastrocolic omentum<br>Gastrohepatic omentum<br>Gastrophrenic ligament<br>Gastrosplenic ligament<br>Greater Omentum<br>Hepatogastric ligament<br>Lesser Omentum<br>V Mesentery<br>Mesoappendix<br>Mesocolon<br>W Peritoneum<br>Epiploic foramen | Ø Open<br>4 Percutaneous Endoscopic | 7 Autologous Tissue Substitute<br>J Synthetic Substitute<br>K Nonautologous Tissue Substitute | Z No Qualifier |

**Ø Medical and Surgical**
**D Gastrointestinal System**
**S Reposition** Definition: Moving to its normal location, or other suitable location, all or a portion of a body part

Explanation: The body part is moved to a new location from an abnormal location, or from a normal location where it is not functioning correctly. The body part may or may not be cut out or off to be moved to the new location.

| Body Part Character 4 | Approach Character 5 | Device Character 6 | Qualifier Character 7 |
|---|---|---|---|
| 5 Esophagus<br>6 Stomach<br>9 Duodenum<br>A Jejunum<br>Duodenojejunal flexure<br>B Ileum<br>H Cecum<br>K Ascending Colon<br>L Transverse Colon<br>Hepatic flexure<br>Splenic flexure<br>M Descending Colon<br>N Sigmoid Colon<br>Rectosigmoid junction<br>Sigmoid flexure<br>P Rectum<br>Anorectal junction<br>Q Anus<br>Anal orifice | Ø Open<br>4 Percutaneous Endoscopic<br>7 Via Natural or Artificial Opening<br>8 Via Natural or Artificial Opening Endoscopic<br>X External | Z No Device | Z No Qualifier |
| 8 Small Intestine<br>E Large Intestine | Ø Open<br>4 Percutaneous Endoscopic<br>7 Via Natural or Artificial Opening<br>8 Via Natural or Artificial Opening Endoscopic | Z No Device | Z No Qualifier |

**Non-OR** ØDS[5,6,9,A,B,H,K,L,M,N,P,Q]XZZ

**Ø Medical and Surgical**
**D Gastrointestinal System**
**T Resection** Definition: Cutting out or off, without replacement, all of a body part

Explanation: None

| Body Part<br>Character 4 | Approach<br>Character 5 | Device<br>Character 6 | Qualifier<br>Character 7 |
|---|---|---|---|
| **1 Esophagus, Upper**<br>Cervical esophagus<br>**2 Esophagus, Middle**<br>Thoracic esophagus<br>**3 Esophagus, Lower**<br>Abdominal esophagus<br>**4 Esophagogastric Junction**<br>Cardia<br>Cardioesophageal junction<br>Gastroesophageal (GE) junction<br>**5 Esophagus**<br>**6 Stomach**<br>**7 Stomach, Pylorus**<br>Pyloric antrum<br>Pyloric canal<br>Pyloric sphincter<br>**8 Small Intestine**<br>**9 Duodenum** ⊞<br>**A Jejunum**<br>Duodenojejunal flexure<br>**B Ileum**<br>**C Ileocecal Valve**<br>**E Large Intestine**<br>**F Large Intestine, Right**<br>**H Cecum**<br>**J Appendix**<br>Vermiform appendix<br>**K Ascending Colon**<br>**P Rectum**<br>Anorectal junction<br>**Q Anus**<br>Anal orifice | **Ø Open**<br>**4 Percutaneous Endoscopic**<br>**7 Via Natural or Artificial Opening**<br>**8 Via Natural or Artificial Opening Endoscopic** | **Z No Device** | **Z No Qualifier** |
| **G Large Intestine, Left**<br>**L Transverse Colon**<br>Hepatic flexure<br>Splenic flexure<br>**M Descending Colon**<br>**N Sigmoid Colon**<br>Rectosigmoid junction<br>Sigmoid flexure | **Ø Open**<br>**4 Percutaneous Endoscopic**<br>**7 Via Natural or Artificial Opening**<br>**8 Via Natural or Artificial Opening Endoscopic**<br>**F Via Natural or Artificial Opening with Percutaneous Endoscopic Assistance** | **Z No Device** | **Z No Qualifier** |
| **R Anal Sphincter**<br>External anal sphincter<br>Internal anal sphincter<br>**U Omentum**<br>Gastrocolic ligament<br>Gastrocolic omentum<br>Gastrohepatic omentum<br>Gastrophrenic ligament<br>Gastrosplenic ligament<br>Greater Omentum<br>Hepatogastric ligament<br>Lesser Omentum | **Ø Open**<br>**4 Percutaneous Endoscopic** | **Z No Device** | **Z No Qualifier** |

**See Appendix L for Procedure Combinations**

⊞ ØDT9ØZZ

**Ø Medical and Surgical**
**D Gastrointestinal System**
**U Supplement** Definition: Putting in or on biological or synthetic material that physically reinforces and/or augments the function of a portion of a body part

Explanation: The biological material is non-living, or is living and from the same individual. The body part may have been previously replaced, and the SUPPLEMENT procedure is performed to physically reinforce and/or augment the function of the replaced body part.

| Body Part Character 4 | Approach Character 5 | Device Character 6 | Qualifier Character 7 |
|---|---|---|---|
| **1 Esophagus, Upper**<br>Cervical esophagus<br>**2 Esophagus, Middle**<br>Thoracic esophagus<br>**3 Esophagus, Lower**<br>Abdominal esophagus<br>**4 Esophagogastric Junction**<br>Cardia<br>Cardioesophageal junction<br>Gastroesophageal (GE) junction<br>**5 Esophagus**<br>**6 Stomach**<br>**7 Stomach, Pylorus**<br>Pyloric antrum<br>Pyloric canal<br>Pyloric sphincter<br>**8 Small Intestine**<br>**9 Duodenum**<br>**A Jejunum**<br>Duodenojejunal flexure<br>**B Ileum**<br>**C Ileocecal Valve**<br>**E Large Intestine**<br>**F Large Intestine, Right**<br>**G Large Intestine, Left**<br>**H Cecum**<br>**K Ascending Colon**<br>**L Transverse Colon**<br>Hepatic flexure<br>Splenic flexure<br>**M Descending Colon**<br>**N Sigmoid Colon**<br>Rectosigmoid junction<br>Sigmoid flexure<br>**P Rectum**<br>Anorectal junction | **Ø Open**<br>**4 Percutaneous Endoscopic**<br>**7 Via Natural or Artificial Opening**<br>**8 Via Natural or Artificial Opening Endoscopic** | **7 Autologous Tissue Substitute**<br>**J Synthetic Substitute**<br>**K Nonautologous Tissue Substitute** | **Z No Qualifier** |
| **Q Anus**<br>Anal orifice | **Ø Open**<br>**4 Percutaneous Endoscopic**<br>**7 Via Natural or Artificial Opening**<br>**8 Via Natural or Artificial Opening Endoscopic**<br>**X External** | **7 Autologous Tissue Substitute**<br>**J Synthetic Substitute**<br>**K Nonautologous Tissue Substitute** | **Z No Qualifier** |
| **R Anal Sphincter**<br>External anal sphincter<br>Internal anal sphincter<br>**U Omentum**<br>Gastrocolic ligament<br>Gastrocolic omentum<br>Gastrohepatic omentum<br>Gastrophrenic ligament<br>Gastrosplenic ligament<br>Greater Omentum<br>Hepatogastric ligament<br>Lesser Omentum<br>**V Mesentery**<br>Mesoappendix<br>Mesocolon<br>**W Peritoneum**<br>Epiploic foramen | **Ø Open**<br>**4 Percutaneous Endoscopic** | **7 Autologous Tissue Substitute**<br>**J Synthetic Substitute**<br>**K Nonautologous Tissue Substitute** | **Z No Qualifier** |

**Ø Medical and Surgical**
**D Gastrointestinal System**
**V Restriction** Definition: Partially closing an orifice or the lumen of a tubular body part
Explanation: The orifice can be a natural orifice or an artificially created orifice

| Body Part Character 4 | | Approach Character 5 | Device Character 6 | Qualifier Character 7 |
|---|---|---|---|---|
| **1 Esophagus, Upper** Cervical esophagus **2 Esophagus, Middle** Thoracic esophagus **3 Esophagus, Lower** Abdominal esophagus **4 Esophagogastric Junction** Cardia Cardioesophageal junction Gastroesophageal (GE) junction **5 Esophagus** **6 Stomach** **7 Stomach, Pylorus** Pyloric antrum Pyloric canal Pyloric sphincter **8 Small Intestine** | **9 Duodenum** **A Jejunum** Duodenojejunal flexure **B Ileum** **C Ileocecal Valve** **E Large Intestine** **F Large Intestine, Right** **G Large Intestine, Left** **H Cecum** **K Ascending Colon** **L Transverse Colon** Hepatic flexure Splenic flexure **M Descending Colon** **N Sigmoid Colon** Rectosigmoid junction Sigmoid flexure **P Rectum** Anorectal junction | **Ø Open** **3 Percutaneous** **4 Percutaneous Endoscopic** | **C Extraluminal Device** **D Intraluminal Device** **Z No Device** | **Z No Qualifier** |
| **1 Esophagus, Upper** Cervical esophagus **2 Esophagus, Middle** Thoracic esophagus **3 Esophagus, Lower** Abdominal esophagus **4 Esophagogastric Junction** Cardia Cardioesophageal junction Gastroesophageal (GE) junction **5 Esophagus** **6 Stomach** NC **7 Stomach, Pylorus** Pyloric antrum Pyloric canal Pyloric sphincter **8 Small Intestine** | **9 Duodenum** **A Jejunum** Duodenojejunal flexure **B Ileum** **C Ileocecal Valve** **E Large Intestine** **F Large Intestine, Right** **G Large Intestine, Left** **H Cecum** **K Ascending Colon** **L Transverse Colon** Hepatic flexure Splenic flexure **M Descending Colon** **N Sigmoid Colon** Rectosigmoid junction Sigmoid flexure **P Rectum** Anorectal junction | **7 Via Natural or Artificial Opening** **8 Via Natural or Artificial Opening Endoscopic** | **D Intraluminal Device** **Z No Device** | **Z No Qualifier** |
| **Q Anus** Anal orifice | | **Ø Open** **3 Percutaneous** **4 Percutaneous Endoscopic** **X External** | **C Extraluminal Device** **D Intraluminal Device** **Z No Device** | **Z No Qualifier** |
| **Q Anus** Anal orifice | | **7 Via Natural or Artificial Opening** **8 Via Natural or Artificial Opening Endoscopic** | **D Intraluminal Device** **Z No Device** | **Z No Qualifier** |

**Non-OR** ØDV6[7,8]DZ
**HAC** ØDV64CZ when reported with PDx E66.Ø1 and SDx K68.11 or K95.Ø1 or K95.81 or T81.4XXA
NC ØDV6[7,8]DZ

**Ø Medical and Surgical**
**D Gastrointestinal System**
**W Revision** Definition: Correcting, to the extent possible, a portion of a malfunctioning device or the position of a displaced device

Explanation: Revision can include correcting a malfunctioning or displaced device by taking out or putting in components of the device such as a screw or pin

| Body Part Character 4 | Approach Character 5 | Device Character 6 | Qualifier Character 7 |
|---|---|---|---|
| Ø Upper Intestinal Tract<br>D Lower Intestinal Tract | Ø Open<br>3 Percutaneous<br>4 Percutaneous Endoscopic<br>7 Via Natural or Artificial Opening<br>8 Via Natural or Artificial Opening Endoscopic | Ø Drainage Device<br>2 Monitoring Device<br>3 Infusion Device<br>7 Autologous Tissue Substitute<br>C Extraluminal Device<br>D Intraluminal Device<br>J Synthetic Substitute<br>K Nonautologous Tissue Substitute<br>U Feeding Device<br>Y Other Device | Z No Qualifier |
| Ø Upper Intestinal Tract<br>D Lower Intestinal Tract | X External | Ø Drainage Device<br>2 Monitoring Device<br>3 Infusion Device<br>7 Autologous Tissue Substitute<br>C Extraluminal Device<br>D Intraluminal Device<br>J Synthetic Substitute<br>K Nonautologous Tissue Substitute<br>U Feeding Device | Z No Qualifier |
| 5 Esophagus | Ø Open<br>3 Percutaneous<br>4 Percutaneous Endoscopic | Y Other Device | Z No Qualifier |
| 5 Esophagus | 7 Via Natural or Artificial Opening<br>8 Via Natural or Artificial Opening Endoscopic | D Intraluminal Device<br>Y Other Device | Z No Qualifier |
| 5 Esophagus | X External | D Intraluminal Device | Z No Qualifier |
| 6 Stomach | Ø Open<br>3 Percutaneous<br>4 Percutaneous Endoscopic | Ø Drainage Device<br>2 Monitoring Device<br>3 Infusion Device<br>7 Autologous Tissue Substitute<br>C Extraluminal Device<br>D Intraluminal Device<br>J Synthetic Substitute<br>K Nonautologous Tissue Substitute<br>M Stimulator Lead<br>U Feeding Device<br>Y Other Device | Z No Qualifier |
| 6 Stomach | 7 Via Natural or Artificial Opening<br>8 Via Natural or Artificial Opening Endoscopic | Ø Drainage Device<br>2 Monitoring Device<br>3 Infusion Device<br>7 Autologous Tissue Substitute<br>C Extraluminal Device<br>D Intraluminal Device<br>J Synthetic Substitute<br>K Nonautologous Tissue Substitute<br>U Feeding Device<br>Y Other Device | Z No Qualifier |
| 6 Stomach | X External | Ø Drainage Device<br>2 Monitoring Device<br>3 Infusion Device<br>7 Autologous Tissue Substitute<br>C Extraluminal Device<br>D Intraluminal Device<br>J Synthetic Substitute<br>K Nonautologous Tissue Substitute<br>U Feeding Device | Z No Qualifier |

*ØDW Continued on next page*

**Non-OR** ØDW[Ø,D][3,4,7,8]YZ
**Non-OR** ØDW[Ø,D]X[Ø,2,3,7,C,D,J,K,U]Z
**Non-OR** ØDW5[Ø,3,4]YZ
**Non-OR** ØDW5[7,8]YZ
**Non-OR** ØDW5XDZ
**Non-OR** ØDW6[3,4]YZ
**Non-OR** ØDW6[7,8]YZ
**Non-OR** ØDW6X[Ø,2,3,7,C,D,J,K,U]Z

**Ø Medical and Surgical**
**D Gastrointestinal System**
**W Revision** Definition: Correcting, to the extent possible, a portion of a malfunctioning device or the position of a displaced device

Explanation: Revision can include correcting a malfunctioning or displaced device by taking out or putting in components of the device such as a screw or pin

***ØDW Continued***

| Body Part Character 4 | Approach Character 5 | Device Character 6 | Qualifier Character 7 |
|---|---|---|---|
| **8** Small Intestine<br>**E** Large Intestine | **Ø** Open<br>**4** Percutaneous Endoscopic<br>**7** Via Natural or Artificial Opening<br>**8** Via Natural or Artificial Opening Endoscopic | **7** Autologous Tissue Substitute<br>**J** Synthetic Substitute<br>**K** Nonautologous Tissue Substitute | **Z** No Qualifier |
| **Q** Anus<br>Anal orifice | **Ø** Open<br>**3** Percutaneous<br>**4** Percutaneous Endoscopic<br>**7** Via Natural or Artificial Opening<br>**8** Via Natural or Artificial Opening Endoscopic | **L** Artificial Sphincter | **Z** No Qualifier |
| **R** Anal Sphincter<br>External anal sphincter<br>Internal anal sphincter | **Ø** Open<br>**3** Percutaneous<br>**4** Percutaneous Endoscopic | **M** Stimulator Lead | **Z** No Qualifier |
| **U** Omentum<br>Gastrocolic ligament<br>Gastrocolic omentum<br>Gastrohepatic omentum<br>Gastrophrenic ligament<br>Gastrosplenic ligament<br>Greater Omentum<br>Hepatogastric ligament<br>Lesser Omentum<br>**V** Mesentery<br>Mesoappendix<br>Mesocolon<br>**W** Peritoneum<br>Epiploic foramen | **Ø** Open<br>**3** Percutaneous<br>**4** Percutaneous Endoscopic | **Ø** Drainage Device<br>**7** Autologous Tissue Substitute<br>**J** Synthetic Substitute<br>**K** Nonautologous Tissue Substitute | **Z** No Qualifier |

**Non-OR** ØDW[U,V,W][Ø,3,4]ØZ

**Ø Medical and Surgical**
**D Gastrointestinal System**
**X Transfer** Definition: Moving, without taking out, all or a portion of a body part to another location to take over the function of all or a portion of a body part

Explanation: The body part transferred remains connected to its vascular and nervous supply

| Body Part Character 4 | Approach Character 5 | Device Character 6 | Qualifier Character 7 |
|---|---|---|---|
| **6** Stomach<br>**8** Small Intestine<br>**E** Large Intestine | **Ø** Open<br>**4** Percutaneous Endoscopic | **Z** No Device | **5** Esophagus |

**Ø Medical and Surgical**
**D Gastrointestinal System**
**Y Transplantation** Definition: Putting in or on all or a portion of a living body part taken from another individual or animal to physically take the place and/or function of all or a portion of a similar body part

Explanation: The native body part may or may not be taken out, and the transplanted body part may take over all or a portion of its function

| Body Part Character 4 | Approach Character 5 | Device Character 6 | Qualifier Character 7 |
|---|---|---|---|
| **5** Esophagus<br>**6** Stomach<br>**8** Small Intestine LC<br>**E** Large Intestine LC | **Ø** Open | **Z** No Device | **Ø** Allogeneic<br>**1** Syngeneic<br>**2** Zooplastic |

**Non-OR** ØDY5ØZ[Ø,1,2]
LC ØDY[8,E]ØZ[Ø,1,2]

# Hepatobiliary System and Pancreas ØF1–ØFY

## Character Meanings

This Character Meaning table is provided as a guide to assist the user in the identification of character members that may be found in this section of code tables. It **SHOULD NOT** be used to build a PCS code.

| Operation–Character 3 | Body Part–Character 4 | Approach–Character 5 | Device–Character 6 | Qualifier–Character 7 |
|---|---|---|---|---|
| 1 Bypass | Ø Liver | Ø Open | Ø Drainage Device | Ø Allogeneic |
| 2 Change | 1 Liver, Right Lobe | 3 Percutaneous | 1 Radioactive Element | 1 Syngeneic |
| 5 Destruction | 2 Liver, Left Lobe | 4 Percutaneous Endoscopic | 2 Monitoring Device | 2 Zooplastic |
| 7 Dilation | 4 Gallbladder | 7 Via Natural or Artificial Opening | 3 Infusion Device | 3 Duodenum |
| 8 Division | 5 Hepatic Duct, Right | 8 Via Natural or Artificial Opening Endoscopic | 7 Autologous Tissue Substitute | 4 Stomach |
| 9 Drainage | 6 Hepatic Duct, Left | X External | C Extraluminal Device | 5 Hepatic Duct, Right |
| B Excision | 7 Hepatic Duct, Common | | D Intraluminal Device | 6 Hepatic Duct, Left |
| C Extirpation | 8 Cystic Duct | | J Synthetic Substitute | 7 Hepatic Duct, Caudate |
| F Fragmentation | 9 Common Bile Duct | | K Nonautologous Tissue Substitute | 8 Cystic Duct |
| H Insertion | B Hepatobiliary Duct | | Y Other Device | 9 Common Bile Duct |
| J Inspection | C Ampulla of Vater | | Z No Device | B Small Intestine |
| L Occlusion | D Pancreatic Duct | | | C Large Intestine |
| M Reattachment | F Pancreatic Duct, Accessory | | | X Diagnostic |
| N Release | G Pancreas | | | Z No Qualifier |
| P Removal | | | | |
| Q Repair | | | | |
| R Replacement | | | | |
| S Reposition | | | | |
| T Resection | | | | |
| U Supplement | | | | |
| V Restriction | | | | |
| W Revision | | | | |
| Y Transplantation | | | | |

**AHA Coding Clinic for table ØF7**
**2016, 3Q, 27** Endoscopic retrograde cholangiopancreatography with sphincterotomy and insertion of pancreatic stent
**2016, 1Q, 25** Endoscopic retrograde cholangiopancreatography with brush biopsy of pancreatic and common bile ducts
**2015, 1Q, 32** Percutaneous transhepatic biliary drainage catheter placement
**2014, 3Q, 15** Drainage of pancreatic pseudocyst

**AHA Coding Clinic for table ØF9**
**2015, 1Q, 32** Percutaneous transhepatic biliary drainage catheter placement
**2014, 3Q, 15** Drainage of pancreatic pseudocyst

**AHA Coding Clinic for table ØFB**
**2016, 3Q, 41** Open cholecystectomy with needle biopsy of liver
**2016, 1Q, 23** Endoscopic ultrasound with aspiration biopsy of common hepatic duct
**2016, 1Q, 25** Endoscopic retrograde cholangiopancreatography with brush biopsy of pancreatic and common bile ducts
**2014, 3Q, 32** Pyloric-sparing Whipple procedure

**AHA Coding Clinic for table ØFC**
**2016, 3Q, 27** Endoscopic retrograde cholangiopancreatography with sphincterotomy and insertion of pancreatic stent

**AHA Coding Clinic for table ØFQ**
**2016, 3Q, 27** Revision of common bile duct anastomosis
**2013, 4Q, 109** Separating conjoined twins

**AHA Coding Clinic for table ØFT**
**2012, 4Q, 99** Domino liver transplant

**AHA Coding Clinic for table ØFY**
**2014, 3Q, 13** Orthotopic liver transplant with end to side cavoplasty
**2012, 4Q, 99** Domino liver transplant

Hepatobiliary System and Pancreas

## Liver

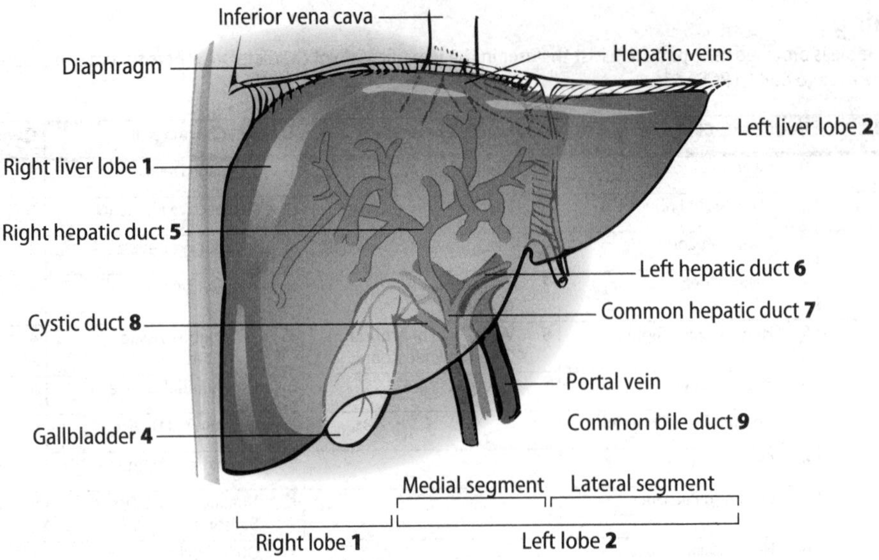


## Pancreas

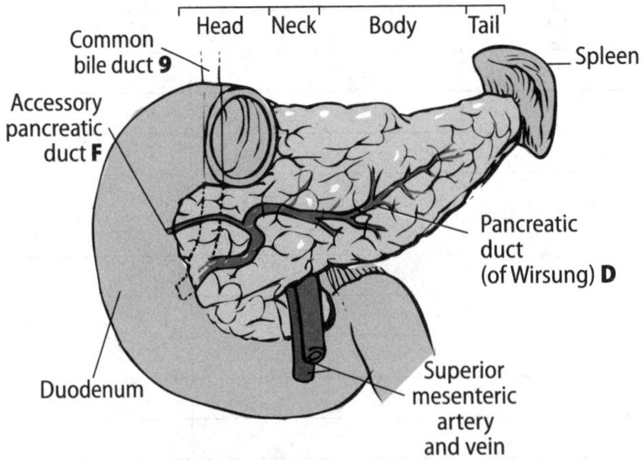


## Gallbladder and Ducts

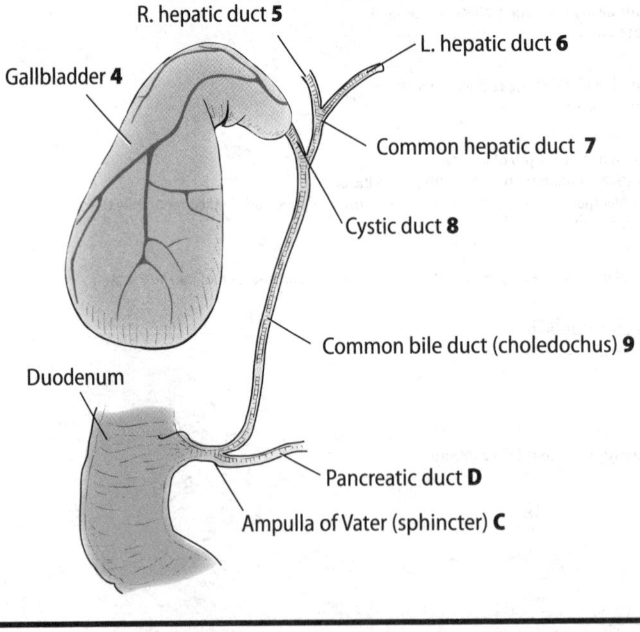

**Ø Medical and Surgical**
**F Hepatobiliary System and Pancreas**
**1 Bypass** Definition: Altering the route of passage of the contents of a tubular body part

Explanation: Rerouting contents of a body part to a downstream area of the normal route, to a similar route and body part, or to an abnormal route and dissimilar body part. Includes one or more anastomoses, with or without the use of a device.

| Body Part Character 4 | Approach Character 5 | Device Character 6 | Qualifier Character 7 |
|---|---|---|---|
| 4 Gallbladder<br>5 Hepatic Duct, Right<br>6 Hepatic Duct, Left<br>7 Hepatic Duct, Common<br>8 Cystic Duct<br>9 Common Bile Duct | Ø Open<br>4 Percutaneous Endoscopic | D Intraluminal Device<br>Z No Device | 3 Duodenum<br>4 Stomach<br>5 Hepatic Duct, Right<br>6 Hepatic Duct, Left<br>7 Hepatic Duct, Caudate<br>8 Cystic Duct<br>9 Common Bile Duct<br>B Small Intestine |
| D Pancreatic Duct<br>Duct of Wirsung<br>F Pancreatic Duct, Accessory<br>Duct of Santorini<br>G Pancreas | Ø Open<br>4 Percutaneous Endoscopic | D Intraluminal Device<br>Z No Device | 3 Duodenum<br>B Small Intestine<br>C Large Intestine |

**Ø Medical and Surgical**
**F Hepatobiliary System and Pancreas**
**2 Change** Definition: Taking out or off a device from a body part and putting back an identical or similar device in or on the same body part without cutting or puncturing the skin or a mucous membrane

Explanation: All CHANGE procedures are coded using the approach EXTERNAL

| Body Part Character 4 | Approach Character 5 | Device Character 6 | Qualifier Character 7 |
|---|---|---|---|
| Ø Liver<br>Quadrate lobe<br>4 Gallbladder<br>B Hepatobiliary Duct<br>D Pancreatic Duct<br>Duct of Wirsung<br>G Pancreas | X External | Ø Drainage Device<br>Y Other Device | Z No Qualifier |

**Non-OR** All body part, approach, device, and qualifier values

**Ø Medical and Surgical**
**F Hepatobiliary System and Pancreas**
**5 Destruction** Definition: Physical eradication of all or a portion of a body part by the direct use of energy, force, or a destructive agent

Explanation: None of the body part is physically taken out

| Body Part Character 4 | Approach Character 5 | Device Character 6 | Qualifier Character 7 |
|---|---|---|---|
| Ø Liver<br>Quadrate lobe<br>1 Liver, Right Lobe<br>2 Liver, Left Lobe | Ø Open<br>3 Percutaneous<br>4 Percutaneous Endoscopic | Z No Device | Z No Qualifier |
| 4 Gallbladder<br>G Pancreas | Ø Open<br>3 Percutaneous<br>4 Percutaneous Endoscopic<br>8 Via Natural or Artificial Opening Endoscopic | Z No Device | Z No Qualifier |
| 5 Hepatic Duct, Right<br>6 Hepatic Duct, Left<br>7 Hepatic Duct, Common<br>8 Cystic Duct<br>9 Common Bile Duct<br>C Ampulla of Vater<br>Duodenal ampulla<br>Hepatopancreatic ampulla<br>D Pancreatic Duct<br>Duct of Wirsung<br>F Pancreatic Duct, Accessory<br>Duct of Santorini | Ø Open<br>3 Percutaneous<br>4 Percutaneous Endoscopic<br>7 Via Natural or Artificial Opening<br>8 Via Natural or Artificial Opening Endoscopic | Z No Device | Z No Qualifier |

**Non-OR** ØF5G[4,8]ZZ
**Non-OR** ØF5[5,6,7,8,9,C,D,F][4,8]ZZ

Hepatobiliary System and Pancreas
ØF1–ØF5

**Ø Medical and Surgical**
**F Hepatobiliary System and Pancreas**
**7 Dilation** Definition: Expanding an orifice or the lumen of a tubular body part

Explanation: The orifice can be a natural orifice or an artificially created orifice. Accomplished by stretching a tubular body part using intraluminal pressure or by cutting part of the orifice or wall of the tubular body part.

| Body Part Character 4 | Approach Character 5 | Device Character 6 | Qualifier Character 7 |
|---|---|---|---|
| 5 Hepatic Duct, Right<br>6 Hepatic Duct, Left<br>7 Hepatic Duct, Common<br>8 Cystic Duct<br>9 Common Bile Duct<br>C Ampulla of Vater<br>Duodenal ampulla<br>Hepatopancreatic ampulla<br>D Pancreatic Duct<br>Duct of Wirsung<br>F Pancreatic Duct, Accessory<br>Duct of Santorini | Ø Open<br>3 Percutaneous<br>4 Percutaneous Endoscopic<br>7 Via Natural or Artificial Opening<br>8 Via Natural or Artificial Opening Endoscopic | D Intraluminal Device<br>Z No Device | Z No Qualifier |

**Non-OR** ØF7[5,6,7,8,9][3,4][D,Z]Z
**Non-OR** ØF7[5,6,7,8,9,D][7,8]DZ
**Non-OR** ØF7[5,6,7,8,9,C,D,F]8ZZ
**Non-OR** ØF7[D,F]4[D,Z]Z
**Non-OR** ØF7[C,F]8DZ

**See Appendix L for Procedure Combinations**
**Combo-only** ØF7[5,6,8,9,D][7,8]DZ

**Ø Medical and Surgical**
**F Hepatobiliary System and Pancreas**
**8 Division** Definition: Cutting into a body part, without draining fluids and/or gases from the body part, in order to separate or transect a body part

Explanation: All or a portion of the body part is separated into two or more portions

| Body Part Character 4 | Approach Character 5 | Device Character 6 | Qualifier Character 7 |
|---|---|---|---|
| G Pancreas | Ø Open<br>3 Percutaneous<br>4 Percutaneous Endoscopic | Z No Device | Z No Qualifier |

**Ø Medical and Surgical**
**F Hepatobiliary System and Pancreas**
**9 Drainage** Definition: Taking or letting out fluids and/or gases from a body part
Explanation: The qualifier DIAGNOSTIC is used to identify drainage procedures that are biopsies

| Body Part Character 4 | Approach Character 5 | Device Character 6 | Qualifier Character 7 |
|---|---|---|---|
| Ø Liver<br>Quadrate lobe<br>1 Liver, Right Lobe<br>2 Liver, Left Lobe | Ø Open<br>3 Percutaneous<br>4 Percutaneous Endoscopic | Ø Drainage Device | Z No Qualifier |
| Ø Liver<br>Quadrate lobe<br>1 Liver, Right Lobe<br>2 Liver, Left Lobe | Ø Open<br>3 Percutaneous<br>4 Percutaneous Endoscopic | Z No Device | X Diagnostic<br>Z No Qualifier |
| 4 Gallbladder<br>G Pancreas | Ø Open<br>3 Percutaneous<br>4 Percutaneous Endoscopic<br>8 Via Natural or Artificial Opening Endoscopic | Ø Drainage Device | Z No Qualifier |
| 4 Gallbladder<br>G Pancreas | Ø Open<br>3 Percutaneous<br>4 Percutaneous Endoscopic<br>8 Via Natural or Artificial Opening Endoscopic | Z No Device | X Diagnostic<br>Z No Qualifier |
| 5 Hepatic Duct, Right<br>6 Hepatic Duct, Left<br>7 Hepatic Duct, Common<br>8 Cystic Duct<br>9 Common Bile Duct<br>C Ampulla of Vater<br>Duodenal ampulla<br>Hepatopancreatic ampulla<br>D Pancreatic Duct<br>Duct of Wirsung<br>F Pancreatic Duct, Accessory<br>Duct of Santorini | Ø Open<br>3 Percutaneous<br>4 Percutaneous Endoscopic<br>7 Via Natural or Artificial Opening<br>8 Via Natural or Artificial Opening Endoscopic | Ø Drainage Device | Z No Qualifier |
| 5 Hepatic Duct, Right<br>6 Hepatic Duct, Left<br>7 Hepatic Duct, Common<br>8 Cystic Duct<br>9 Common Bile Duct<br>C Ampulla of Vater<br>Duodenal ampulla<br>Hepatopancreatic ampulla<br>D Pancreatic Duct<br>Duct of Wirsung<br>F Pancreatic Duct, Accessory<br>Duct of Santorini | Ø Open<br>3 Percutaneous<br>4 Percutaneous Endoscopic<br>7 Via Natural or Artificial Opening<br>8 Via Natural or Artificial Opening Endoscopic | Z No Device | X Diagnostic<br>Z No Qualifier |

Non-OR ØF9[Ø,1,2][3,4]ØZ
Non-OR ØF9[Ø,1,2][3,4]Z[X,Z]
Non-OR ØF9[4,G]8ØZ
Non-OR ØF9G3ØZ
Non-OR ØF9[4,G]8Z[X,Z]
Non-OR ØF9G3Z[XZ]
Non-OR ØF9G4ZX
Non-OR ØF9[5,6,8][3,8]ØZ
Non-OR ØF97[3,4,7,8]ØZ
Non-OR ØF99[3,8]ØZ
Non-OR ØF9C[3,4,8]ØZ
Non-OR ØF9[D,F][3,8]ØZ
Non-OR ØF9[5,6,8,9,C,D,F]3Z[X,Z]
Non-OR ØF9[5,6,8,9,C,D,F][4,7,8]ZX
Non-OR ØF9[5,6,8,D,F]8ZZ
Non-OR ØF97[3,4,7,8]Z[X,Z]
Non-OR ØF99[4,7,8]ZZ
Non-OR ØF9C[4,8]ZZ

**Ø Medical and Surgical**
**F Hepatobiliary System and Pancreas**
**B Excision** Definition: Cutting out or off, without replacement, a portion of a body part
Explanation: The qualifier DIAGNOSTIC is used to identify excision procedures that are biopsies

| Body Part Character 4 | Approach Character 5 | Device Character 6 | Qualifier Character 7 |
|---|---|---|---|
| **Ø Liver**<br>Quadrate lobe<br>**1 Liver, Right Lobe**<br>**2 Liver, Left Lobe** | **Ø Open**<br>**3 Percutaneous**<br>**4 Percutaneous Endoscopic** | **Z No Device** | **X Diagnostic**<br>**Z No Qualifier** |
| **4 Gallbladder**<br>**G Pancreas** | **Ø Open**<br>**3 Percutaneous**<br>**4 Percutaneous Endoscopic**<br>**8 Via Natural or Artificial Opening Endoscopic** | **Z No Device** | **X Diagnostic**<br>**Z No Qualifier** |
| **5 Hepatic Duct, Right**<br>**6 Hepatic Duct, Left**<br>**7 Hepatic Duct, Common**<br>**8 Cystic Duct**<br>**9 Common Bile Duct**<br>**C Ampulla of Vater**<br>Duodenal ampulla<br>Hepatopancreatic ampulla<br>**D Pancreatic Duct**<br>Duct of Wirsung<br>**F Pancreatic Duct, Accessory**<br>Duct of Santorini | **Ø Open**<br>**3 Percutaneous**<br>**4 Percutaneous Endoscopic**<br>**7 Via Natural or Artificial Opening**<br>**8 Via Natural or Artificial Opening Endoscopic** | **Z No Device** | **X Diagnostic**<br>**Z No Qualifier** |

**Non-OR** ØFB[Ø,1,2]3ZX
**Non-OR** ØFB[4,G][3,4,8]ZX
**Non-OR** ØFB[5,6,7,8,9,C,D,F][3,4,7,8]ZX
**Non-OR** ØFB[5,6,7,8,9,C,D,F][4,8]ZZ

**Ø Medical and Surgical**
**F Hepatobiliary System and Pancreas**
**C Extirpation** Definition: Taking or cutting out solid matter from a body part
Explanation: The solid matter may be an abnormal byproduct of a biological function or a foreign body; it may be imbedded in a body part or in the lumen of a tubular body part. The solid matter may or may not have been previously broken into pieces.

| Body Part Character 4 | Approach Character 5 | Device Character 6 | Qualifier Character 7 |
|---|---|---|---|
| **Ø Liver**<br>Quadrate lobe<br>**1 Liver, Right Lobe**<br>**2 Liver, Left Lobe** | **Ø Open**<br>**3 Percutaneous**<br>**4 Percutaneous Endoscopic** | **Z No Device** | **Z No Qualifier** |
| **4 Gallbladder**<br>**G Pancreas** | **Ø Open**<br>**3 Percutaneous**<br>**4 Percutaneous Endoscopic**<br>**8 Via Natural or Artificial Opening Endoscopic** | **Z No Device** | **Z No Qualifier** |
| **5 Hepatic Duct, Right**<br>**6 Hepatic Duct, Left**<br>**7 Hepatic Duct, Common**<br>**8 Cystic Duct**<br>**9 Common Bile Duct**<br>**C Ampulla of Vater**<br>Duodenal ampulla<br>Hepatopancreatic ampulla<br>**D Pancreatic Duct**<br>Duct of Wirsung<br>**F Pancreatic Duct, Accessory**<br>Duct of Santorini | **Ø Open**<br>**3 Percutaneous**<br>**4 Percutaneous Endoscopic**<br>**7 Via Natural or Artificial Opening**<br>**8 Via Natural or Artificial Opening Endoscopic** | **Z No Device** | **Z No Qualifier** |

**Non-OR** ØFC[5,6,7,8,9][3,4,7,8]ZZ
**Non-OR** ØFCC[4,8]ZZ
**Non-OR** ØFC[D,F][3,4,8]ZZ

**Ø Medical and Surgical**
**F Hepatobiliary System and Pancreas**
**F Fragmentation** Definition: Breaking solid matter in a body part into pieces

Explanation: Physical force (e.g., manual, ultrasonic) applied directly or indirectly is used to break the solid matter into pieces. The solid matter may be an abnormal byproduct of a biological function or a foreign body. The pieces of solid matter are not taken out.

| Body Part Character 4 | Approach Character 5 | Device Character 6 | Qualifier Character 7 |
|---|---|---|---|
| **4** Gallbladder NC<br>**5** Hepatic Duct, Right NC<br>**6** Hepatic Duct, Left NC<br>**7** Hepatic Duct, Common<br>**8** Cystic Duct NC<br>**9** Common Bile Duct NC<br>**C** Ampulla of Vater NC<br>Duodenal ampulla<br>Hepatopancreatic ampulla<br>**D** Pancreatic Duct NC<br>Duct of Wirsung<br>**F** Pancreatic Duct, Accessory NC<br>Duct of Santorini | **Ø** Open<br>**3** Percutaneous<br>**4** Percutaneous Endoscopic<br>**7** Via Natural or Artificial Opening<br>**8** Via Natural or Artificial Opening Endoscopic<br>**X** External | **Z** No Device | **Z** No Qualifier |

**Non-OR** ØFF[4,5,6,7,8,9,C,][8,X]ZZ
**Non-OR** ØFF[D,F][8,X]ZZ

NC ØFF[4,5,6,8,9,C,D,F]XZZ

**Ø Medical and Surgical**
**F Hepatobiliary System and Pancreas**
**H Insertion** Definition: Putting in a nonbiological appliance that monitors, assists, performs, or prevents a physiological function but does not physically take the place of a body part

Explanation: None

| Body Part Character 4 | Approach Character 5 | Device Character 6 | Qualifier Character 7 |
|---|---|---|---|
| **Ø** Liver<br>Quadrate lobe<br>**4** Gallbladder<br>**G** Pancreas | **Ø** Open<br>**3** Percutaneous<br>**4** Percutaneous Endoscopic | **2** Monitoring Device<br>**3** Infusion Device<br>**Y** Other Device | **Z** No Qualifier |
| **1** Liver, Right Lobe<br>**2** Liver, Left Lobe | **Ø** Open<br>**3** Percutaneous<br>**4** Percutaneous Endoscopic | **2** Monitoring Device<br>**3** Infusion Device | **Z** No Qualifier |
| **B** Hepatobiliary Duct<br>**D** Pancreatic Duct<br>Duct of Wirsung | **Ø** Open<br>**3** Percutaneous<br>**4** Percutaneous Endoscopic<br>**7** Via Natural or Artificial Opening<br>**8** Via Natural or Artificial Opening Endoscopic | **1** Radioactive Element<br>**2** Monitoring Device<br>**3** Infusion Device<br>**D** Intraluminal Device<br>**Y** Other Device | **Z** No Qualifier |

**Non-OR** ØFH[Ø,4,G][Ø,3,4]3Z
**Non-OR** ØFH[Ø,4,G][3,4]YZ
**Non-OR** ØFH[1,2][Ø,3,4]3Z
**Non-OR** ØFH[B,D][Ø,3,4]3Z
**Non-OR** ØFH[B,D]4DZ
**Non-OR** ØFH[B,D][7,8][2,3]Z
**Non-OR** ØFH[B,D]8DZ
**Non-OR** ØFH[B,D][3,4,7,8]YZ

**See Appendix L for Procedure Combinations**
**Combo-only** ØFHB8DZ

**Ø Medical and Surgical**
**F Hepatobiliary System and Pancreas**
**J Inspection** Definition: Visually and/or manually exploring a body part
Explanation: Visual exploration may be performed with or without optical instrumentation. Manual exploration may be performed directly or through intervening body layers.

| Body Part Character 4 | Approach Character 5 | Device Character 6 | Qualifier Character 7 |
|---|---|---|---|
| Ø Liver<br>Quadrate lobe | Ø Open<br>3 Percutaneous<br>4 Percutaneous Endoscopic<br>X External | Z No Device | Z No Qualifier |
| 4 Gallbladder<br>G Pancreas | Ø Open<br>3 Percutaneous<br>4 Percutaneous Endoscopic<br>8 Via Natural or Artificial Opening Endoscopic<br>X External | Z No Device | Z No Qualifier |
| B Hepatobiliary Duct<br>D Pancreatic Duct<br>Duct of Wirsung | Ø Open<br>3 Percutaneous<br>4 Percutaneous Endoscopic<br>7 Via Natural or Artificial Opening<br>8 Via Natural or Artificial Opening Endoscopic | Z No Device | Z No Qualifier |

DRG Non-OR ØFJ[Ø,G]3ZZ
DRG Non-OR ØFJD[3,7,8]ZZ
Non-OR ØFJØXZZ
Non-OR ØFJ43ZZ
Non-OR ØFJ[4,G][8,X]ZZ
Non-OR ØFJB[3,7,8]ZZ

**Ø Medical and Surgical**
**F Hepatobiliary System and Pancreas**
**L Occlusion** Definition: Completely closing an orifice or the lumen of a tubular body part
Explanation: The orifice can be a natural orifice or an artificially created orifice

| Body Part Character 4 | Approach Character 5 | Device Character 6 | Qualifier Character 7 |
|---|---|---|---|
| 5 Hepatic Duct, Right<br>6 Hepatic Duct, Left<br>7 Hepatic Duct, Common<br>8 Cystic Duct<br>9 Common Bile Duct<br>C Ampulla of Vater<br>Duodenal ampulla<br>Hepatopancreatic ampulla<br>D Pancreatic Duct<br>Duct of Wirsung<br>F Pancreatic Duct, Accessory<br>Duct of Santorini | Ø Open<br>3 Percutaneous<br>4 Percutaneous Endoscopic | C Extraluminal Device<br>D Intraluminal Device<br>Z No Device | Z No Qualifier |
| 5 Hepatic Duct, Right<br>6 Hepatic Duct, Left<br>7 Hepatic Duct, Common<br>8 Cystic Duct<br>9 Common Bile Duct<br>C Ampulla of Vater<br>Duodenal ampulla<br>Hepatopancreatic ampulla<br>D Pancreatic Duct<br>Duct of Wirsung<br>F Pancreatic Duct, Accessory<br>Duct of Santorini | 7 Via Natural or Artificial Opening<br>8 Via Natural or Artificial Opening Endoscopic | D Intraluminal Device<br>Z No Device | Z No Qualifier |

Non-OR ØFL[5,6,7,8,9][3,4][C,D,Z]Z
Non-OR ØFL[5,6,7,8,9][7,8][D,Z]Z

**Ø Medical and Surgical**
**F Hepatobiliary System and Pancreas**
**M Reattachment** Definition: Putting back in or on all or a portion of a separated body part to its normal location or other suitable location
Explanation: Vascular circulation and nervous pathways may or may not be reestablished

| Body Part Character 4 | Approach Character 5 | Device Character 6 | Qualifier Character 7 |
|---|---|---|---|
| **Ø** Liver<br>Quadrate lobe<br>**1** Liver, Right Lobe<br>**2** Liver, Left Lobe<br>**4** Gallbladder<br>**5** Hepatic Duct, Right<br>**6** Hepatic Duct, Left<br>**7** Hepatic Duct, Common<br>**8** Cystic Duct<br>**9** Common Bile Duct<br>**C** Ampulla of Vater<br>Duodenal ampulla<br>Hepatopancreatic ampulla<br>**D** Pancreatic Duct<br>Duct of Wirsung<br>**F** Pancreatic Duct, Accessory<br>Duct of Santorini<br>**G** Pancreas | **Ø** Open<br>**4** Percutaneous Endoscopic | **Z** No Device | **Z** No Qualifier |

Non-OR ØFM[4,5,6,7,8,9]4ZZ

**Ø Medical and Surgical**
**F Hepatobiliary System and Pancreas**
**N Release** Definition: Freeing a body part from an abnormal physical constraint by cutting or by the use of force
Explanation: Some of the restraining tissue may be taken out but none of the body part is taken out

| Body Part Character 4 | Approach Character 5 | Device Character 6 | Qualifier Character 7 |
|---|---|---|---|
| **Ø** Liver<br>Quadrate lobe<br>**1** Liver, Right Lobe<br>**2** Liver, Left Lobe | **Ø** Open<br>**3** Percutaneous<br>**4** Percutaneous Endoscopic | **Z** No Device | **Z** No Qualifier |
| **4** Gallbladder<br>**G** Pancreas | **Ø** Open<br>**3** Percutaneous<br>**4** Percutaneous Endoscopic<br>**8** Via Natural or Artificial Opening Endoscopic | **Z** No Device | **Z** No Qualifier |
| **5** Hepatic Duct, Right<br>**6** Hepatic Duct, Left<br>**7** Hepatic Duct, Common<br>**8** Cystic Duct<br>**9** Common Bile Duct<br>**C** Ampulla of Vater<br>Duodenal ampulla<br>Hepatopancreatic ampulla<br>**D** Pancreatic Duct<br>Duct of Wirsung<br>**F** Pancreatic Duct, Accessory<br>Duct of Santorini | **Ø** Open<br>**3** Percutaneous<br>**4** Percutaneous Endoscopic<br>**7** Via Natural or Artificial Opening<br>**8** Via Natural or Artificial Opening Endoscopic | **Z** No Device | **Z** No Qualifier |

**Ø Medical and Surgical**
**F Hepatobiliary System and Pancreas**
**P Removal** Definition: Taking out or off a device from a body part

Explanation: If a device is taken out and a similar device put in without cutting or puncturing the skin or mucous membrane, the procedure is coded to the root operation CHANGE. Otherwise, the procedure for taking out a device is coded to the root operation REMOVAL.

| Body Part Character 4 | Approach Character 5 | Device Character 6 | Qualifier Character 7 |
|---|---|---|---|
| **Ø Liver**<br>Quadrate lobe | **Ø Open**<br>**3 Percutaneous**<br>**4 Percutaneous Endoscopic** | **Ø Drainage Device**<br>**2 Monitoring Device**<br>**3 Infusion Device**<br>Y Other Device | **Z No Qualifier** |
| **Ø Liver**<br>Quadrate lobe | **X External** | **Ø Drainage Device**<br>**2 Monitoring Device**<br>**3 Infusion Device** | **Z No Qualifier** |
| **4 Gallbladder**<br>**G Pancreas** | **Ø Open**<br>**3 Percutaneous**<br>**4 Percutaneous Endoscopic** | **Ø Drainage Device**<br>**2 Monitoring Device**<br>**3 Infusion Device**<br>**D Intraluminal Device**<br>Y Other Device | **Z No Qualifier** |
| **4 Gallbladder**<br>**G Pancreas** | **X External** | **Ø Drainage Device**<br>**2 Monitoring Device**<br>**3 Infusion Device**<br>**D Intraluminal Device** | **Z No Qualifier** |
| **B Hepatobiliary Duct**<br>**D Pancreatic Duct**<br>Duct of Wirsung | **Ø Open**<br>**3 Percutaneous**<br>**4 Percutaneous Endoscopic**<br>**7 Via Natural or Artificial Opening**<br>**8 Via Natural or Artificial Opening Endoscopic** | **Ø Drainage Device**<br>**1 Radioactive Element**<br>**2 Monitoring Device**<br>**3 Infusion Device**<br>**7 Autologous Tissue Substitute**<br>**C Extraluminal Device**<br>**D Intraluminal Device**<br>**J Synthetic Substitute**<br>**K Nonautologous Tissue Substitute**<br>Y Other Device | **Z No Qualifier** |
| **B Hepatobiliary Duct**<br>**D Pancreatic Duct**<br>Duct of Wirsung | **X External** | **Ø Drainage Device**<br>**1 Radioactive Element**<br>**2 Monitoring Device**<br>**3 Infusion Device**<br>**D Intraluminal Device** | **Z No Qualifier** |

Non-OR ØFPØ[3,4]YZ
Non-OR ØFPØX[Ø,2,3]Z
Non-OR ØFP[4,G][3,4]YZ
Non-OR ØFP4X[Ø,2,3,D]Z
Non-OR ØFPGX[Ø,2,3]Z
Non-OR ØFP[B,D][3,4]YZ
Non-OR ØFP[B,D][7,8][Ø,2,3,D,Y]Z
Non-OR ØFP[B,D]X[Ø,1,2,3,D]Z

**See Appendix L for Procedure Combinations**
Combo-only ØFP[B,D]XDZ

**Ø Medical and Surgical**
**F Hepatobiliary System and Pancreas**
**Q Repair** Definition: Restoring, to the extent possible, a body part to its normal anatomic structure and function

Explanation: Used only when the method to accomplish the repair is not one of the other root operations

| Body Part Character 4 | Approach Character 5 | Device Character 6 | Qualifier Character 7 |
|---|---|---|---|
| **Ø Liver**<br>Quadrate lobe<br>**1 Liver, Right Lobe**<br>**2 Liver, Left Lobe** | **Ø Open**<br>**3 Percutaneous**<br>**4 Percutaneous Endoscopic** | **Z No Device** | **Z No Qualifier** |
| **4 Gallbladder**<br>**G Pancreas** | **Ø Open**<br>**3 Percutaneous**<br>**4 Percutaneous Endoscopic**<br>8 Via Natural or Artificial Opening Endoscopic | **Z No Device** | **Z No Qualifier** |
| **5 Hepatic Duct, Right**<br>**6 Hepatic Duct, Left**<br>7 Hepatic Duct, Common<br>**8 Cystic Duct**<br>**9 Common Bile Duct**<br>**C Ampulla of Vater**<br>Duodenal ampulla<br>Hepatopancreatic ampulla<br>**D Pancreatic Duct**<br>Duct of Wirsung<br>**F Pancreatic Duct, Accessory**<br>Duct of Santorini | **Ø Open**<br>**3 Percutaneous**<br>**4 Percutaneous Endoscopic**<br>**7 Via Natural or Artificial Opening**<br>**8 Via Natural or Artificial Opening Endoscopic** | **Z No Device** | **Z No Qualifier** |

**Ø Medical and Surgical**
**F Hepatobiliary System and Pancreas**
**R Replacement** Definition: Putting in or on biological or synthetic material that physically takes the place and/or function of all or a portion of a body part

Explanation: The body part may have been taken out or replaced, or may be taken out, physically eradicated, or rendered nonfunctional during the REPLACEMENT procedure. A REMOVAL procedure is coded for taking out the device used in a previous replacement procedure.

| Body Part Character 4 | Approach Character 5 | Device Character 6 | Qualifier Character 7 |
|---|---|---|---|
| 5 Hepatic Duct, Right<br>6 Hepatic Duct, Left<br>7 Hepatic Duct, Common<br>8 Cystic Duct<br>9 Common Bile Duct<br>C Ampulla of Vater<br>Duodenal ampulla<br>Hepatopancreatic ampulla<br>D Pancreatic Duct<br>Duct of Wirsung<br>F Pancreatic Duct, Accessory<br>Duct of Santorini | Ø Open<br>4 Percutaneous Endoscopic<br>8 Via Natural or Artificial Opening Endoscopic | 7 Autologous Tissue Substitute<br>J Synthetic Substitute<br>K Nonautologous Tissue Substitute | Z No Qualifier |

**Ø Medical and Surgical**
**F Hepatobiliary System and Pancreas**
**S Reposition** Definition: Moving to its normal location, or other suitable location, all or a portion of a body part

Explanation: The body part is moved to a new location from an abnormal location, or from a normal location where it is not functioning correctly. The body part may or may not be cut out or off to be moved to the new location.

| Body Part Character 4 | Approach Character 5 | Device Character 6 | Qualifier Character 7 |
|---|---|---|---|
| Ø Liver<br>Quadrate lobe<br>4 Gallbladder<br>5 Hepatic Duct, Right<br>6 Hepatic Duct, Left<br>7 Hepatic Duct, Common<br>8 Cystic Duct<br>9 Common Bile Duct<br>C Ampulla of Vater<br>Duodenal ampulla<br>Hepatopancreatic ampulla<br>D Pancreatic Duct<br>Duct of Wirsung<br>F Pancreatic Duct, Accessory<br>Duct of Santorini<br>G Pancreas | Ø Open<br>4 Percutaneous Endoscopic | Z No Device | Z No Qualifier |

**Ø Medical and Surgical**
**F Hepatobiliary System and Pancreas**
**T Resection** Definition: Cutting out or off, without replacement, all of a body part

Explanation: None

| Body Part Character 4 | Approach Character 5 | Device Character 6 | Qualifier Character 7 |
|---|---|---|---|
| Ø Liver<br>Quadrate lobe<br>1 Liver, Right Lobe<br>2 Liver, Left Lobe<br>4 Gallbladder<br>G Pancreas ⊞ | Ø Open<br>4 Percutaneous Endoscopic | Z No Device | Z No Qualifier |
| 5 Hepatic Duct, Right<br>6 Hepatic Duct, Left<br>7 Hepatic Duct, Common<br>8 Cystic Duct<br>9 Common Bile Duct<br>C Ampulla of Vater<br>Duodenal ampulla<br>Hepatopancreatic ampulla<br>D Pancreatic Duct<br>Duct of Wirsung<br>F Pancreatic Duct, Accessory<br>Duct of Santorini | Ø Open<br>4 Percutaneous Endoscopic<br>7 Via Natural or Artificial Opening<br>8 Via Natural or Artificial Opening Endoscopic | Z No Device | Z No Qualifier |

Non-OR ØFT[D,F][4,8]ZZ

See Appendix L for Procedure Combinations
⊞ ØFTGØZZ

**Ø Medical and Surgical**
**F Hepatobiliary System and Pancreas**
**U Supplement** Definition: Putting in or on biological or synthetic material that physically reinforces and/or augments the function of a portion of a body part

Explanation: The biological material is non-living, or is living and from the same individual. The body part may have been previously replaced, and the SUPPLEMENT procedure is performed to physically reinforce and/or augment the function of the replaced body part.

| Body Part Character 4 | Approach Character 5 | Device Character 6 | Qualifier Character 7 |
|---|---|---|---|
| 5 Hepatic Duct, Right<br>6 Hepatic Duct, Left<br>7 Hepatic Duct, Common<br>8 Cystic Duct<br>9 Common Bile Duct<br>C Ampulla of Vater<br>Duodenal ampulla<br>Hepatopancreatic ampulla<br>D Pancreatic Duct<br>Duct of Wirsung<br>F Pancreatic Duct, Accessory<br>Duct of Santorini | Ø Open<br>3 Percutaneous<br>4 Percutaneous Endoscopic<br>8 Via Natural or Artificial Opening Endoscopic | 7 Autologous Tissue Substitute<br>J Synthetic Substitute<br>K Nonautologous Tissue Substitute | Z No Qualifier |

**Ø Medical and Surgical**
**F Hepatobiliary System and Pancreas**
**V Restriction** Definition: Partially closing an orifice or the lumen of a tubular body part

Explanation: The orifice can be a natural orifice or an artificially created orifice

| Body Part Character 4 | Approach Character 5 | Device Character 6 | Qualifier Character 7 |
|---|---|---|---|
| 5 Hepatic Duct, Right<br>6 Hepatic Duct, Left<br>7 Hepatic Duct, Common<br>8 Cystic Duct<br>9 Common Bile Duct<br>C Ampulla of Vater<br>Duodenal ampulla<br>Hepatopancreatic ampulla<br>D Pancreatic Duct<br>Duct of Wirsung<br>F Pancreatic Duct, Accessory<br>Duct of Santorini | Ø Open<br>3 Percutaneous<br>4 Percutaneous Endoscopic | C Extraluminal Device<br>D Intraluminal Device<br>Z No Device | Z No Qualifier |
| 5 Hepatic Duct, Right<br>6 Hepatic Duct, Left<br>7 Hepatic Duct, Common<br>8 Cystic Duct<br>9 Common Bile Duct<br>C Ampulla of Vater<br>Duodenal ampulla<br>Hepatopancreatic ampulla<br>D Pancreatic Duct<br>Duct of Wirsung<br>F Pancreatic Duct, Accessory<br>Duct of Santorini | 7 Via Natural or Artificial Opening<br>8 Via Natural or Artificial Opening Endoscopic | D Intraluminal Device<br>Z No Device | Z No Qualifier |

Non-OR ØFV[5,6,7,8,9][3,4][C,D,Z]Z
Non-OR ØFV[5,6,7,8,9][7,8][D,Z]Z

**Ø Medical and Surgical**
**F Hepatobiliary System and Pancreas**
**W Revision** Definition: Correcting, to the extent possible, a portion of a malfunctioning device or the position of a displaced device

Explanation: Revision can include correcting a malfunctioning or displaced device by taking out or putting in components of the device such as a screw or pin

| Body Part Character 4 | Approach Character 5 | Device Character 6 | Qualifier Character 7 |
|---|---|---|---|
| Ø Liver<br>Quadrate lobe | Ø Open<br>3 Percutaneous<br>4 Percutaneous Endoscopic | Ø Drainage Device<br>2 Monitoring Device<br>3 Infusion Device<br>Y Other Device | Z No Qualifier |
| Ø Liver<br>Quadrate lobe | X External | Ø Drainage Device<br>2 Monitoring Device<br>3 Infusion Device | Z No Qualifier |
| 4 Gallbladder<br>G Pancreas | Ø Open<br>3 Percutaneous<br>4 Percutaneous Endoscopic | Ø Drainage Device<br>2 Monitoring Device<br>3 Infusion Device<br>D Intraluminal Device<br>Y Other Device | Z No Qualifier |
| 4 Gallbladder<br>G Pancreas | X External | Ø Drainage Device<br>2 Monitoring Device<br>3 Infusion Device<br>D Intraluminal Device | Z No Qualifier |
| B Hepatobiliary Duct<br>D Pancreatic Duct<br>Duct of Wirsung | Ø Open<br>3 Percutaneous<br>4 Percutaneous Endoscopic<br>7 Via Natural or Artificial Opening<br>8 Via Natural or Artificial Opening Endoscopic | Ø Drainage Device<br>2 Monitoring Device<br>3 Infusion Device<br>7 Autologous Tissue Substitute<br>C Extraluminal Device<br>D Intraluminal Device<br>J Synthetic Substitute<br>K Nonautologous Tissue Substitute<br>Y Other Device | Z No Qualifier |
| B Hepatobiliary Duct<br>D Pancreatic Duct<br>Duct of Wirsung | X External | Ø Drainage Device<br>2 Monitoring Device<br>3 Infusion Device<br>7 Autologous Tissue Substitute<br>C Extraluminal Device<br>D Intraluminal Device<br>J Synthetic Substitute<br>K Nonautologous Tissue Substitute | Z No Qualifier |

Non-OR ØFWØ[3,4]YZ
Non-OR ØFWØX[Ø,2,3]Z
Non-OR ØFW[4,G][3,4]YZ
Non-OR ØFW[4,G]X[Ø,2,3,D]Z
Non-OR ØFW[B,D][3,4,7,8]YZ
Non-OR ØFW[B,D]X[Ø,2,3,7,C,D,J,K]Z

**Ø Medical and Surgical**
**F Hepatobiliary System and Pancreas**
**Y Transplantation** Definition: Putting in or on all or a portion of a living body part taken from another individual or animal to physically take the place and/or function of all or a portion of a similar body part

Explanation: The native body part may or may not be taken out, and the transplanted body part may take over all or a portion of its function

| Body Part Character 4 | Approach Character 5 | Device Character 6 | Qualifier Character 7 |
|---|---|---|---|
| Ø Liver LC<br>Quadrate lobe<br>G Pancreas ⊞ LC NC | Ø Open | Z No Device | Ø Allogeneic<br>1 Syngeneic<br>2 Zooplastic |

LC ØFYØØZ[Ø,1,2]
LC ØFYGØZ[Ø,1]
NC ØFYGØZ2
NC ØFYGØZ[Ø,1] If reported alone without one of the following procedures ØTYØØZ[Ø,1,2], ØTY1ØZ[Ø,1,2] and without one of the following diagnoses E1Ø.1Ø-E1Ø.9, E89.1

See Appendix L for Procedure Combinations
⊞ ØFYGØZ[Ø,1,2]

# Endocrine System ØG2–ØGW



## Character Meanings

This Character Meaning table is provided as a guide to assist the user in the identification of character members that may be found in this section of code tables. It **SHOULD NOT** be used to build a PCS code.

| Operation–Character 3 | | Body Part–Character 4 | | Approach–Character 5 | | Device–Character 6 | | Qualifier–Character 7 | |
|---|---|---|---|---|---|---|---|---|---|
| 2 | Change | Ø | Pituitary Gland | Ø | Open | Ø | Drainage Device | X | Diagnostic |
| 5 | Destruction | 1 | Pineal Body | 3 | Percutaneous | 2 | Monitoring Device | Z | No Qualifier |
| 8 | Division | 2 | Adrenal Gland, Left | 4 | Percutaneous Endoscopic | 3 | Infusion Device | | |
| 9 | Drainage | 3 | Adrenal Gland, Right | X | External | Y | Other Device | | |
| B | Excision | 4 | Adrenal Glands, Bilateral | | | Z | No Device | | |
| C | Extirpation | 5 | Adrenal Gland | | | | | | |
| H | Insertion | 6 | Carotid Body, Left | | | | | | |
| J | Inspection | 7 | Carotid Body, Right | | | | | | |
| M | Reattachment | 8 | Carotid Bodies, Bilateral | | | | | | |
| N | Release | 9 | Para-aortic Body | | | | | | |
| P | Removal | B | Coccygeal Glomus | | | | | | |
| Q | Repair | C | Glomus Jugulare | | | | | | |
| S | Reposition | D | Aortic Body | | | | | | |
| T | Resection | F | Paraganglion Extremity | | | | | | |
| W | Revision | G | Thyroid Gland Lobe, Left | | | | | | |
| | | H | Thyroid Gland Lobe, Right | | | | | | |
| | | J | Thyroid Gland Isthmus | | | | | | |
| | | K | Thyroid Gland | | | | | | |
| | | L | Superior Parathyroid Gland, Right | | | | | | |
| | | M | Superior Parathyroid Gland, Left | | | | | | |
| | | N | Inferior Parathyroid Gland, Right | | | | | | |
| | | P | Inferior Parathyroid Gland, Left | | | | | | |
| | | Q | Parathyroid Glands, Multiple | | | | | | |
| | | R | Parathyroid Gland | | | | | | |
| | | S | Endocrine Gland | | | | | | |

**AHA Coding Clinic for table ØGB**

**2017, 2Q, 20** Near total thyroidectomy

**2014, 3Q, 22** Transsphenoidal removal of pituitary tumor and fat graft placement

**AHA Coding Clinic for table ØGT**

**2017, 2Q, 20** Near total thyroidectomy

## Endocrine System

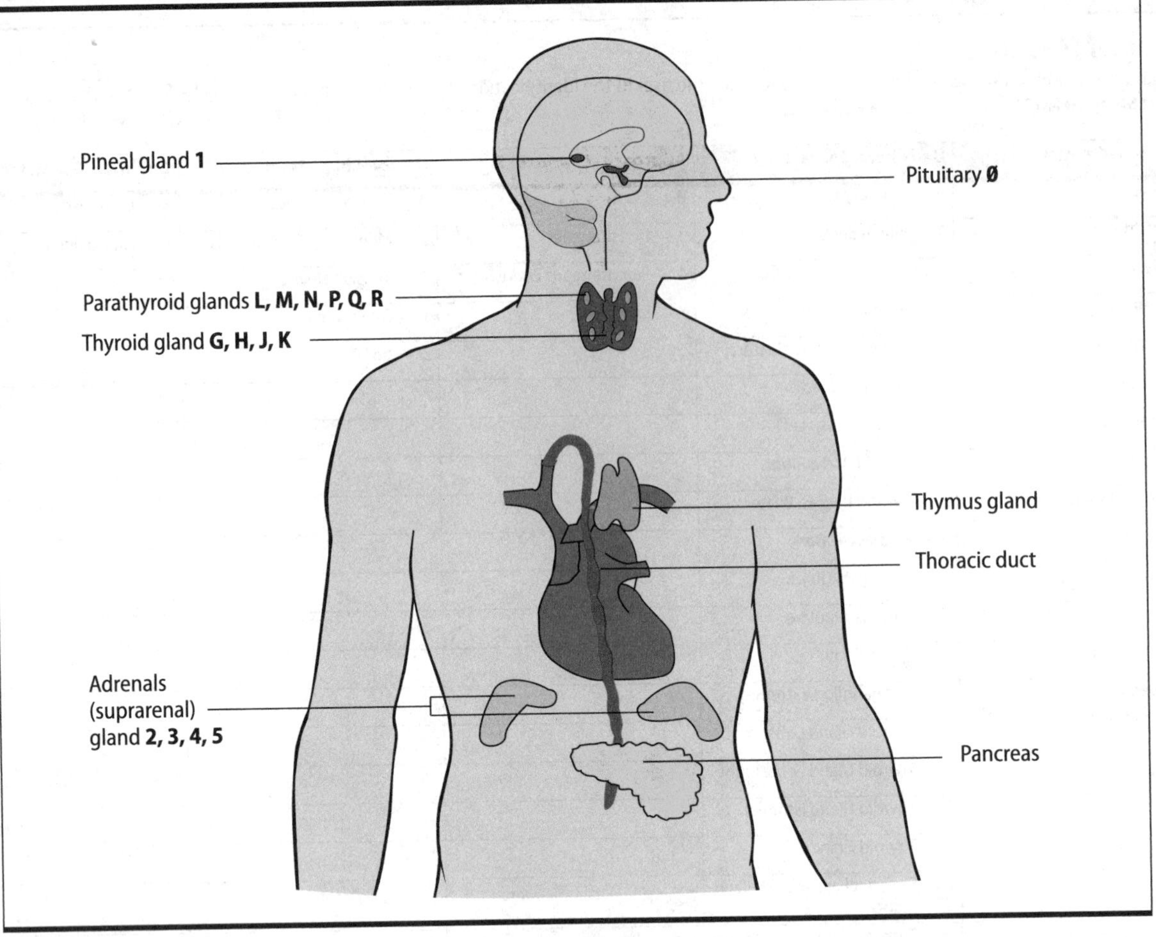
Pineal gland **1**
Pituitary **Ø**
Parathyroid glands **L, M, N, P, Q, R**
Thyroid gland **G, H, J, K**
Thymus gland
Thoracic duct
Adrenals (suprarenal) gland **2, 3, 4, 5**
Pancreas

## Left Adrenal Gland

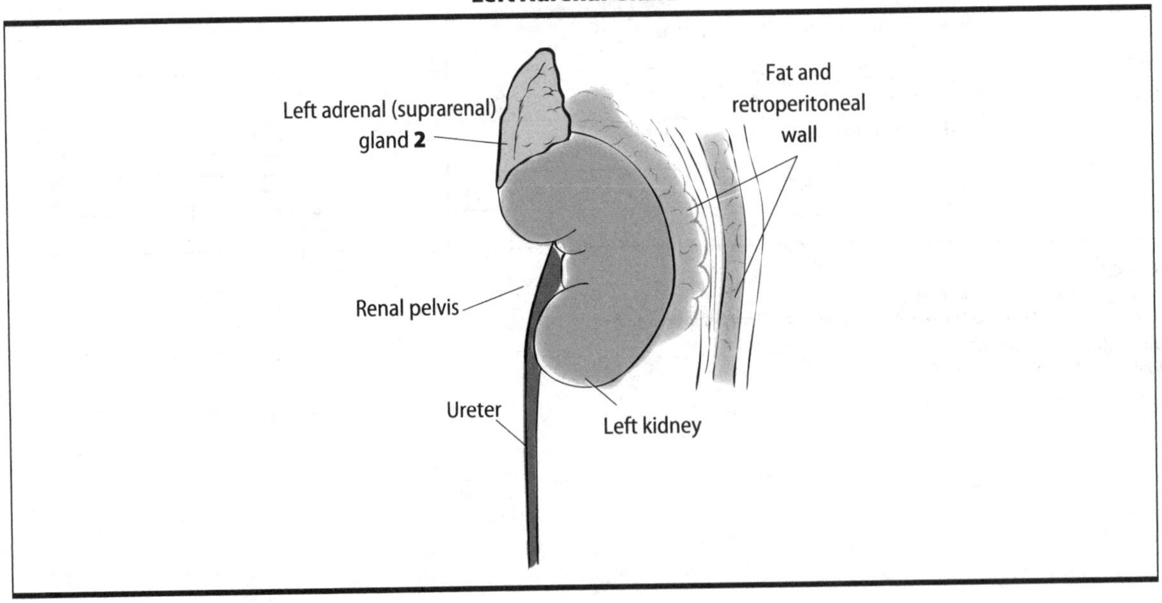
Left adrenal (suprarenal) gland **2**
Fat and retroperitoneal wall
Renal pelvis
Ureter
Left kidney

## Thyroid

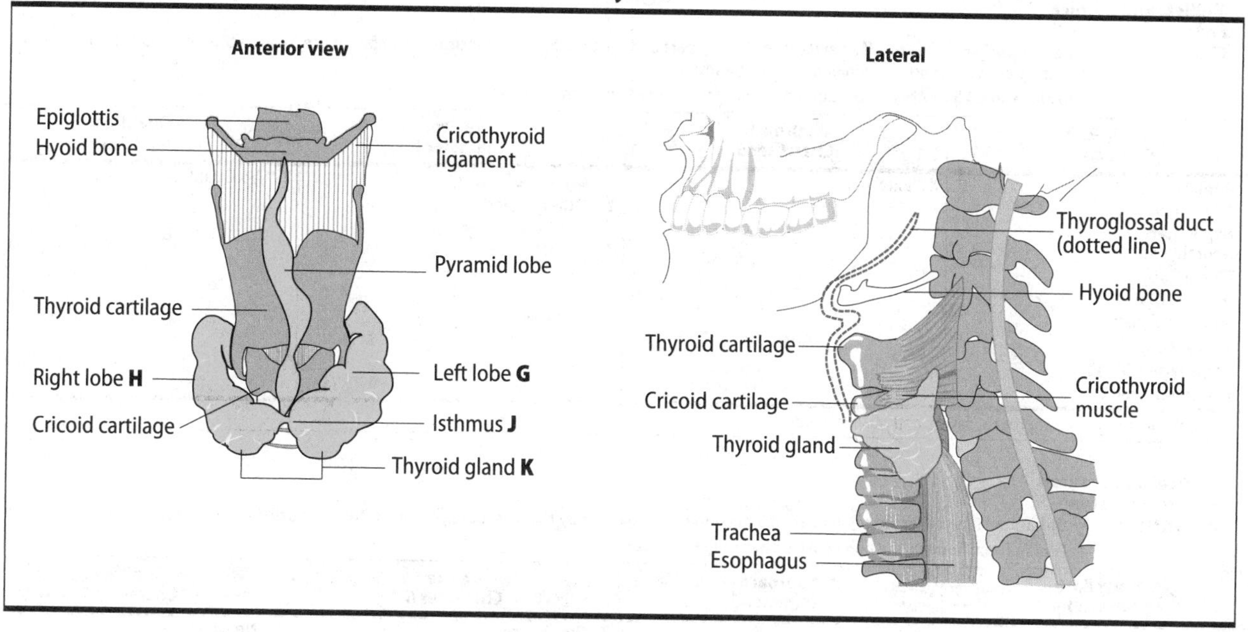
Anterior view
Epiglottis
Hyoid bone
Cricothyroid ligament
Pyramid lobe
Thyroid cartilage
Right lobe **H**
Left lobe **G**
Cricoid cartilage
Isthmus **J**
Thyroid gland **K**
Lateral
Thyroglossal duct (dotted line)
Hyoid bone
Thyroid cartilage
Cricoid cartilage
Cricothyroid muscle
Thyroid gland
Trachea
Esophagus

## Thyroid and Parathyroid Glands

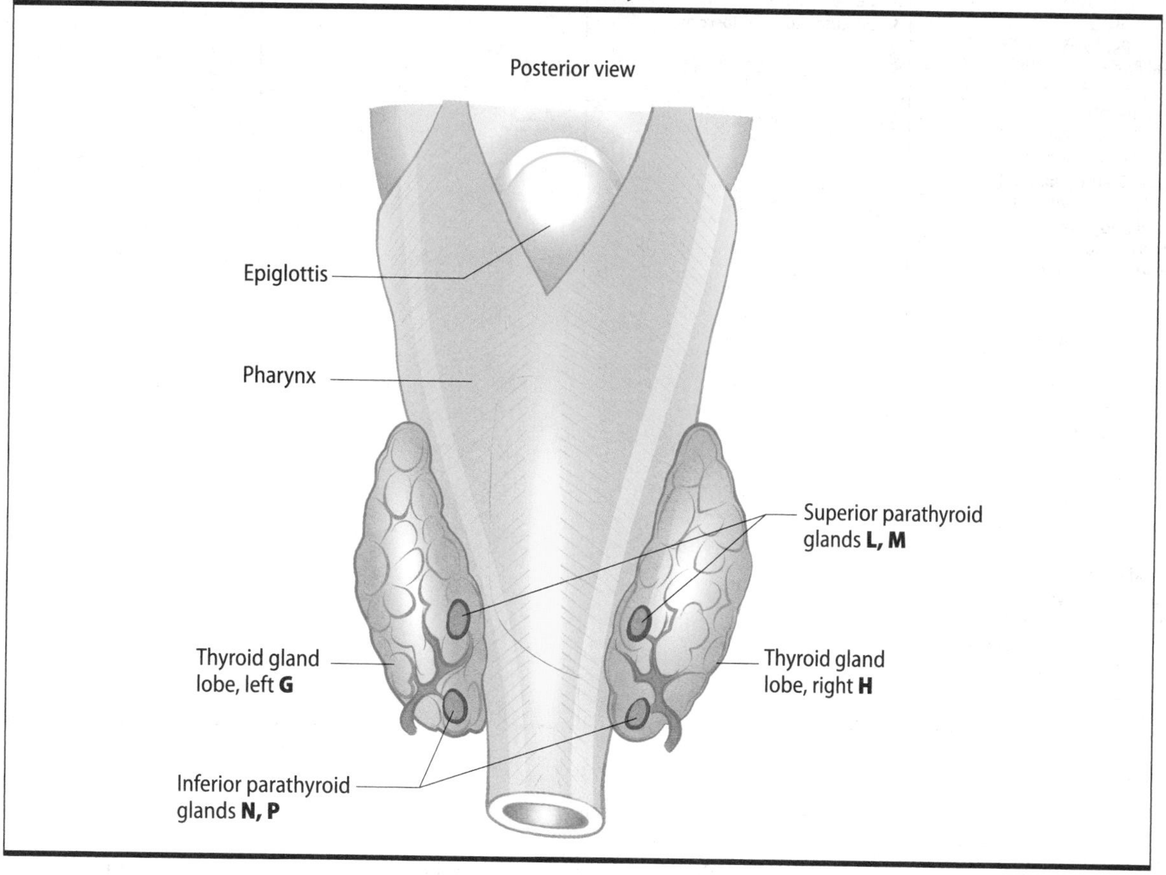
Posterior view
Epiglottis
Pharynx
Superior parathyroid glands **L, M**
Thyroid gland lobe, left **G**
Thyroid gland lobe, right **H**
Inferior parathyroid glands **N, P**

**Ø Medical and Surgical**
**G Endocrine System**
**2 Change** Definition: Taking out or off a device from a body part and putting back an identical or similar device in or on the same body part without cutting or puncturing the skin or a mucous membrane

Explanation: All CHANGE procedures are coded using the approach EXTERNAL

| Body Part Character 4 | Approach Character 5 | Device Character 6 | Qualifier Character 7 |
|---|---|---|---|
| **Ø Pituitary Gland**<br>Adenohypophysis<br>Hypophysis<br>Neurohypophysis<br>**1 Pineal Body**<br>**5 Adrenal Gland**<br>Suprarenal gland<br>**K Thyroid Gland**<br>**R Parathyroid Gland**<br>**S Endocrine Gland** | **X External** | **Ø Drainage Device**<br>**Y Other Device** | **Z No Qualifier** |

Non-OR All body part, approach, device, and qualifier values

**Ø Medical and Surgical**
**G Endocrine System**
**5 Destruction** Definition: Physical eradication of all or a portion of a body part by the direct use of energy, force, or a destructive agent

Explanation: None of the body part is physically taken out

| Body Part Character 4 | Approach Character 5 | Device Character 6 | Qualifier Character 7 |
|---|---|---|---|
| **Ø Pituitary Gland**<br>Adenohypophysis<br>Hypophysis<br>Neurohypophysis<br>**1 Pineal Body**<br>**2 Adrenal Gland, Left**<br>Suprarenal gland<br>**3 Adrenal Gland, Right**<br>*See 2 Adrenal Gland, Left*<br>**4 Adrenal Glands, Bilateral**<br>*See 2 Adrenal Gland, Left*<br>**6 Carotid Body, Left**<br>Carotid glomus<br>**7 Carotid Body, Right**<br>*See 6 Carotid Body, Left*<br>**8 Carotid Bodies, Bilateral**<br>*See 6 Carotid Body, Left*<br>**9 Para-aortic Body**<br>**B Coccygeal Glomus**<br>Coccygeal body<br>**C Glomus Jugulare**<br>Jugular body<br>**D Aortic Body**<br>**F Paraganglion Extremity**<br>**G Thyroid Gland Lobe, Left**<br>**H Thyroid Gland Lobe, Right**<br>**K Thyroid Gland**<br>**L Superior Parathyroid Gland, Right**<br>**M Superior Parathyroid Gland, Left**<br>**N Inferior Parathyroid Gland, Right**<br>**P Inferior Parathyroid Gland, Left**<br>**Q Parathyroid Glands, Multiple**<br>**R Parathyroid Gland** | **Ø Open**<br>**3 Percutaneous**<br>**4 Percutaneous Endoscopic** | **Z No Device** | **Z No Qualifier** |

**Ø Medical and Surgical**
**G Endocrine System**
**8 Division** Definition: Cutting into a body part, without draining fluids and/or gases from the body part, in order to separate or transect a body part

Explanation: All or a portion of the body part is separated into two or more portions

| Body Part Character 4 | Approach Character 5 | Device Character 6 | Qualifier Character 7 |
|---|---|---|---|
| **Ø Pituitary Gland**<br>Adenohypophysis<br>Hypophysis<br>Neurohypophysis<br>**J Thyroid Gland Isthmus** | **Ø Open**<br>**3 Percutaneous**<br>**4 Percutaneous Endoscopic** | **Z No Device** | **Z No Qualifier** |

**Ø Medical and Surgical**
**G Endocrine System**
**9 Drainage** Definition: Taking or letting out fluids and/or gases from a body part
Explanation: The qualifier DIAGNOSTIC is used to identify drainage procedures that are biopsies

| Body Part Character 4 | Approach Character 5 | Device Character 6 | Qualifier Character 7 |
|---|---|---|---|
| **Ø Pituitary Gland**<br>Adenohypophysis<br>Hypophysis<br>Neurohypophysis<br>**1 Pineal Body**<br>**2 Adrenal Gland, Left**<br>Suprarenal gland<br>**3 Adrenal Gland, Right**<br>*See 2 Adrenal Gland, Left*<br>**4 Adrenal Glands, Bilateral**<br>*See 2 Adrenal Gland, Left*<br>**6 Carotid Body, Left**<br>Carotid glomus<br>**7 Carotid Body, Right**<br>*See 6 Carotid Body, Left*<br>**8 Carotid Bodies, Bilateral**<br>*See 6 Carotid Body, Left*<br>**9 Para-aortic Body**<br>**B Coccygeal Glomus**<br>Coccygeal body<br>**C Glomus Jugulare**<br>Jugular body<br>**D Aortic Body**<br>**F Paraganglion Extremity**<br>**G Thyroid Gland Lobe, Left**<br>**H Thyroid Gland Lobe, Right**<br>**K Thyroid Gland**<br>**L Superior Parathyroid Gland, Right**<br>**M Superior Parathyroid Gland, Left**<br>**N Inferior Parathyroid Gland, Right**<br>**P Inferior Parathyroid Gland, Left**<br>**Q Parathyroid Glands, Multiple**<br>**R Parathyroid Gland** | **Ø Open**<br>**3 Percutaneous**<br>**4 Percutaneous Endoscopic** | **Ø Drainage Device** | **Z No Qualifier** |
| **Ø Pituitary Gland**<br>Adenohypophysis<br>Hypophysis<br>Neurohypophysis<br>**1 Pineal Body**<br>**2 Adrenal Gland, Left**<br>Suprarenal gland<br>**3 Adrenal Gland, Right**<br>*See 2 Adrenal Gland, Left*<br>**4 Adrenal Glands, Bilateral**<br>*See 2 Adrenal Gland, Left*<br>**6 Carotid Body, Left**<br>Carotid glomus<br>**7 Carotid Body, Right**<br>*See 6 Carotid Body, Left*<br>**8 Carotid Bodies, Bilateral**<br>*See 6 Carotid Body, Left*<br>**9 Para-aortic Body**<br>**B Coccygeal Glomus**<br>Coccygeal body<br>**C Glomus Jugulare**<br>Jugular body<br>**D Aortic Body**<br>**F Paraganglion Extremity**<br>**G Thyroid Gland Lobe, Left**<br>**H Thyroid Gland Lobe, Right**<br>**K Thyroid Gland**<br>**L Superior Parathyroid Gland, Right**<br>**M Superior Parathyroid Gland, Left**<br>**N Inferior Parathyroid Gland, Right**<br>**P Inferior Parathyroid Gland, Left**<br>**Q Parathyroid Glands, Multiple**<br>**R Parathyroid Gland** | **Ø Open**<br>**3 Percutaneous**<br>**4 Percutaneous Endoscopic** | **Z No Device** | **X Diagnostic**<br>**Z No Qualifier** |

**Non-OR** ØG9[Ø,1,2,3,4,6,7,8,9,B,C,D,F,G,H,K,L,M,N,P,Q,R]3ØZ
**Non-OR** ØG9[G,H,K,L,M,N,P,Q,R]4ØZ
**Non-OR** ØG9[2,3,4,G,H,K][3,4]ZX
**Non-OR** ØG9[Ø,1,2,3,4,6,7,8,9,B,C,D,F,G,H,K,L,M,N,P,Q,R]3ZZ
**Non-OR** ØG9[G,H,K,L,M,N,P,Q,R]4ZZ

**Ø Medical and Surgical**
**G Endocrine System**
**B Excision** Definition: Cutting out or off, without replacement, a portion of a body part
Explanation: The qualifier DIAGNOSTIC is used to identify excision procedures that are biopsies

| Body Part Character 4 | Approach Character 5 | Device Character 6 | Qualifier Character 7 |
|---|---|---|---|
| **Ø Pituitary Gland**<br>Adenohypophysis<br>Hypophysis<br>Neurohypophysis<br>**1 Pineal Body**<br>**2 Adrenal Gland, Left**<br>Suprarenal gland<br>**3 Adrenal Gland, Right**<br>*See 2 Adrenal Gland, Left*<br>**4 Adrenal Glands, Bilateral**<br>*See 2 Adrenal Gland, Left*<br>**6 Carotid Body, Left**<br>Carotid glomus<br>**7 Carotid Body, Right**<br>*See 6 Carotid Body, Left*<br>**8 Carotid Bodies, Bilateral**<br>*See 6 Carotid Body, Left*<br>**9 Para-aortic Body**<br>**B Coccygeal Glomus**<br>Coccygeal body<br>**C Glomus Jugulare**<br>Jugular body<br>**D Aortic Body**<br>**F Paraganglion Extremity**<br>**G Thyroid Gland Lobe, Left**<br>**H Thyroid Gland Lobe, Right**<br>**J Thyroid Gland Isthmus**<br>**L Superior Parathyroid Gland, Right**<br>**M Superior Parathyroid Gland, Left**<br>**N Inferior Parathyroid Gland, Right**<br>**P Inferior Parathyroid Gland, Left**<br>**Q Parathyroid Glands, Multiple**<br>**R Parathyroid Gland** | **Ø Open**<br>**3 Percutaneous**<br>**4 Percutaneous Endoscopic** | **Z No Device** | **X Diagnostic**<br>**Z No Qualifier** |

**Non-OR** ØGB[2,3,4,G,H][3,4]ZX

**Ø Medical and Surgical**
**G Endocrine System**
**C Extirpation** Definition: Taking or cutting out solid matter from a body part
Explanation: The solid matter may be an abnormal byproduct of a biological function or a foreign body; it may be imbedded in a body part or in the lumen of a tubular body part. The solid matter may or may not have been previously broken into pieces.

| Body Part Character 4 | Approach Character 5 | Device Character 6 | Qualifier Character 7 |
|---|---|---|---|
| **Ø Pituitary Gland**<br>Adenohypophysis<br>Hypophysis<br>Neurohypophysis<br>**1 Pineal Body**<br>**2 Adrenal Gland, Left**<br>Suprarenal gland<br>**3 Adrenal Gland, Right**<br>*See 2 Adrenal Gland, Left*<br>**4 Adrenal Glands, Bilateral**<br>*See 2 Adrenal Gland, Left*<br>**6 Carotid Body, Left**<br>Carotid glomus<br>**7 Carotid Body, Right**<br>*See 6 Carotid Body, Left*<br>**8 Carotid Bodies, Bilateral**<br>*See 6 Carotid Body, Left*<br>**9 Para-aortic Body**<br>**B Coccygeal Glomus**<br>Coccygeal body<br>**C Glomus Jugulare**<br>Jugular body<br>**D Aortic Body**<br>**F Paraganglion Extremity**<br>**G Thyroid Gland Lobe, Left**<br>**H Thyroid Gland Lobe, Right**<br>**K Thyroid Gland**<br>**L Superior Parathyroid Gland, Right**<br>**M Superior Parathyroid Gland, Left**<br>**N Inferior Parathyroid Gland, Right**<br>**P Inferior Parathyroid Gland, Left**<br>**Q Parathyroid Glands, Multiple**<br>**R Parathyroid Gland** | **Ø Open**<br>**3 Percutaneous**<br>**4 Percutaneous Endoscopic** | **Z No Device** | **Z No Qualifier** |

**Ø Medical and Surgical**
**G Endocrine System**
**H Insertion** Definition: Putting in a nonbiological appliance that monitors, assists, performs, or prevents a physiological function but does not physically take the place of a body part

Explanation: None

| Body Part Character 4 | Approach Character 5 | Device Character 6 | Qualifier Character 7 |
|---|---|---|---|
| S Endocrine Gland | Ø Open<br>3 Percutaneous<br>4 Percutaneous Endoscopic | 2 Monitoring Device<br>3 Infusion Device<br>Y Other Device | Z No Qualifier |

Non-OR ØGHS[3,4]YZ

**Ø Medical and Surgical**
**G Endocrine System**
**J Inspection** Definition: Visually and/or manually exploring a body part

Explanation: Visual exploration may be performed with or without optical instrumentation. Manual exploration may be performed directly or through intervening body layers.

| Body Part Character 4 | Approach Character 5 | Device Character 6 | Qualifier Character 7 |
|---|---|---|---|
| Ø Pituitary Gland<br>Adenohypophysis<br>Hypophysis<br>Neurohypophysis<br>1 Pineal Body<br>5 Adrenal Gland<br>Suprarenal gland<br>K Thyroid Gland<br>R Parathyroid Gland<br>S Endocrine Gland | Ø Open<br>3 Percutaneous<br>4 Percutaneous Endoscopic | Z No Device | Z No Qualifier |

Non-OR ØGJ[Ø,1,5,K,R,S]3ZZ

**Ø Medical and Surgical**
**G Endocrine System**
**M Reattachment** Definition: Putting back in or on all or a portion of a separated body part to its normal location or other suitable location

Explanation: Vascular circulation and nervous pathways may or may not be reestablished

| Body Part Character 4 | Approach Character 5 | Device Character 6 | Qualifier Character 7 |
|---|---|---|---|
| 2 Adrenal Gland, Left<br>Suprarenal gland<br>3 Adrenal Gland, Right<br>*See 2 Adrenal Gland, Left*<br>G Thyroid Gland Lobe, Left<br>H Thyroid Gland Lobe, Right<br>L Superior Parathyroid Gland, Right<br>M Superior Parathyroid Gland, Left<br>N Inferior Parathyroid Gland, Right<br>P Inferior Parathyroid Gland, Left<br>Q Parathyroid Glands, Multiple<br>R Parathyroid Gland | Ø Open<br>4 Percutaneous Endoscopic | Z No Device | Z No Qualifier |

**Ø Medical and Surgical**
**G Endocrine System**
**N Release** Definition: Freeing a body part from an abnormal physical constraint by cutting or by the use of force
Explanation: Some of the restraining tissue may be taken out but none of the body part is taken out

| Body Part Character 4 | Approach Character 5 | Device Character 6 | Qualifier Character 7 |
|---|---|---|---|
| **Ø Pituitary Gland**<br>Adenohypophysis<br>Hypophysis<br>Neurohypophysis<br>**1 Pineal Body**<br>**2 Adrenal Gland, Left**<br>Suprarenal gland<br>**3 Adrenal Gland, Right**<br>*See 2 Adrenal Gland, Left*<br>**4 Adrenal Glands, Bilateral**<br>*See 2 Adrenal Gland, Left*<br>**6 Carotid Body, Left**<br>Carotid glomus<br>**7 Carotid Body, Right**<br>*See 6 Carotid Body, Left*<br>**8 Carotid Bodies, Bilateral**<br>*See 6 Carotid Body, Left*<br>**9 Para-aortic Body**<br>**B Coccygeal Glomus**<br>Coccygeal body<br>**C Glomus Jugulare**<br>Jugular body<br>**D Aortic Body**<br>**F Paraganglion Extremity**<br>**G Thyroid Gland Lobe, Left**<br>**H Thyroid Gland Lobe, Right**<br>**K Thyroid Gland**<br>**L Superior Parathyroid Gland, Right**<br>**M Superior Parathyroid Gland, Left**<br>**N Inferior Parathyroid Gland, Right**<br>**P Inferior Parathyroid Gland, Left**<br>**Q Parathyroid Glands, Multiple**<br>**R Parathyroid Gland** | **Ø Open**<br>**3 Percutaneous**<br>**4 Percutaneous Endoscopic** | **Z No Device** | **Z No Qualifier** |

**Non-OR** ØGN[6,7,8,9,B,C,D,F][Ø,3,4]ZZ

**Ø Medical and Surgical**
**G Endocrine System**
**P Removal** Definition: Taking out or off a device from a body part
Explanation: If a device is taken out and a similar device put in without cutting or puncturing the skin or mucous membrane, the procedure is coded to the root operation CHANGE. Otherwise, the procedure for taking out a device is coded to the root operation REMOVAL.

| Body Part Character 4 | Approach Character 5 | Device Character 6 | Qualifier Character 7 |
|---|---|---|---|
| **Ø Pituitary Gland**<br>Adenohypophysis<br>Hypophysis<br>Neurohypophysis<br>**1 Pineal Body**<br>**5 Adrenal Gland**<br>Suprarenal gland<br>**K Thyroid Gland**<br>**R Parathyroid Gland** | **Ø Open**<br>**3 Percutaneous**<br>**4 Percutaneous Endoscopic**<br>**X External** | **Ø Drainage Device** | **Z No Qualifier** |
| **S Endocrine Gland** | **Ø Open**<br>**3 Percutaneous**<br>**4 Percutaneous Endoscopic** | **Ø Drainage Device**<br>**2 Monitoring Device**<br>**3 Infusion Device**<br>**Y Other Device** | **Z No Qualifier** |
| **S Endocrine Gland** | **X External** | **Ø Drainage Device**<br>**2 Monitoring Device**<br>**3 Infusion Device** | **Z No Qualifier** |

**Non-OR** ØGP[Ø,1,5,K,R]XØZ
**Non-OR** ØGPS[3,4]YZ
**Non-OR** ØGPSX[Ø,2,3]Z

**Ø Medical and Surgical**
**G Endocrine System**
**Q Repair** Definition: Restoring, to the extent possible, a body part to its normal anatomic structure and function

Explanation: Used only when the method to accomplish the repair is not one of the other root operations

| Body Part Character 4 | Approach Character 5 | Device Character 6 | Qualifier Character 7 |
|---|---|---|---|
| **Ø Pituitary Gland**<br>Adenohypophysis<br>Hypophysis<br>Neurohypophysis<br>**1 Pineal Body**<br>**2 Adrenal Gland, Left**<br>Suprarenal gland<br>**3 Adrenal Gland, Right**<br>*See 2 Adrenal Gland, Left*<br>**4 Adrenal Glands, Bilateral**<br>*See 2 Adrenal Gland, Left*<br>**6 Carotid Body, Left**<br>Carotid glomus<br>**7 Carotid Body, Right**<br>*See 6 Carotid Body, Left*<br>**8 Carotid Bodies, Bilateral**<br>*See 6 Carotid Body, Left*<br>**9 Para-aortic Body**<br>**B Coccygeal Glomus**<br>Coccygeal body<br>**C Glomus Jugulare**<br>Jugular body<br>**D Aortic Body**<br>**F Paraganglion Extremity**<br>**G Thyroid Gland Lobe, Left**<br>**H Thyroid Gland Lobe, Right**<br>**J Thyroid Gland Isthmus**<br>**K Thyroid Gland**<br>**L Superior Parathyroid Gland, Right**<br>**M Superior Parathyroid Gland, Left**<br>**N Inferior Parathyroid Gland, Right**<br>**P Inferior Parathyroid Gland, Left**<br>**Q Parathyroid Glands, Multiple**<br>**R Parathyroid Gland** | **Ø Open**<br>**3 Percutaneous**<br>**4 Percutaneous Endoscopic** | **Z No Device** | **Z No Qualifier** |

**Ø Medical and Surgical**
**G Endocrine System**
**S Reposition** Definition: Moving to its normal location, or other suitable location, all or a portion of a body part

Explanation: The body part is moved to a new location from an abnormal location, or from a normal location where it is not functioning correctly. The body part may or may not be cut out or off to be moved to the new location.

| Body Part Character 4 | Approach Character 5 | Device Character 6 | Qualifier Character 7 |
|---|---|---|---|
| **2 Adrenal Gland, Left**<br>Suprarenal gland<br>**3 Adrenal Gland, Right**<br>*See 2 Adrenal Gland, Left*<br>**G Thyroid Gland Lobe, Left**<br>**H Thyroid Gland Lobe, Right**<br>**L Superior Parathyroid Gland, Right**<br>**M Superior Parathyroid Gland, Left**<br>**N Inferior Parathyroid Gland, Right**<br>**P Inferior Parathyroid Gland, Left**<br>**Q Parathyroid Glands, Multiple**<br>**R Parathyroid Gland** | Ø Open<br>4 Percutaneous Endoscopic | Z No Device | Z No Qualifier |

**Ø Medical and Surgical**
**G Endocrine System**
**T Resection** Definition: Cutting out or off, without replacement, all of a body part

Explanation: None

| Body Part Character 4 | Approach Character 5 | Device Character 6 | Qualifier Character 7 |
|---|---|---|---|
| **Ø Pituitary Gland**<br>Adenohypophysis<br>Hypophysis<br>Neurohypophysis<br>**1 Pineal Body**<br>**2 Adrenal Gland, Left**<br>Suprarenal gland<br>**3 Adrenal Gland, Right**<br>*See 2 Adrenal Gland, Left*<br>**4 Adrenal Glands, Bilateral**<br>*See 2 Adrenal Gland, Left*<br>**6 Carotid Body, Left**<br>Carotid glomus<br>**7 Carotid Body, Right**<br>*See 6 Carotid Body, Left*<br>**8 Carotid Bodies, Bilateral**<br>*See 6 Carotid Body, Left*<br>**9 Para-aortic Body**<br>**B Coccygeal Glomus**<br>Coccygeal body<br>**C Glomus Jugulare**<br>Jugular body<br>**D Aortic Body**<br>**F Paraganglion Extremity**<br>**G Thyroid Gland Lobe, Left**<br>**H Thyroid Gland Lobe, Right**<br>**J Thyroid Gland Isthmus**<br>**K Thyroid Gland**<br>**L Superior Parathyroid Gland, Right**<br>**M Superior Parathyroid Gland, Left**<br>**N Inferior Parathyroid Gland, Right**<br>**P Inferior Parathyroid Gland, Left**<br>**Q Parathyroid Glands, Multiple**<br>**R Parathyroid Gland** | **Ø Open**<br>**4 Percutaneous Endoscopic** | **Z No Device** | **Z No Qualifier** |

**Non-OR** ØGT[6,7,8,9,B,C,D,F][Ø,4]ZZ

**Ø Medical and Surgical**
**G Endocrine System**
**W Revision** Definition: Correcting, to the extent possible, a portion of a malfunctioning device or the position of a displaced device

Explanation: Revision can include correcting a malfunctioning or displaced device by taking out or putting in components of the device such as a screw or pin

| Body Part Character 4 | Approach Character 5 | Device Character 6 | Qualifier Character 7 |
|---|---|---|---|
| **Ø Pituitary Gland**<br>Adenohypophysis<br>Hypophysis<br>Neurohypophysis<br>**1 Pineal Body**<br>**5 Adrenal Gland**<br>Suprarenal gland<br>**K Thyroid Gland**<br>**R Parathyroid Gland** | **Ø Open**<br>**3 Percutaneous**<br>**4 Percutaneous Endoscopic**<br>**X External** | **Ø Drainage Device** | **Z No Qualifier** |
| **S Endocrine Gland** | **Ø Open**<br>**3 Percutaneous**<br>**4 Percutaneous Endoscopic** | **Ø Drainage Device**<br>**2 Monitoring Device**<br>**3 Infusion Device**<br>**Y Other Device** | **Z No Qualifier** |
| **S Endocrine Gland** | **X External** | **Ø Drainage Device**<br>**2 Monitoring Device**<br>**3 Infusion Device** | **Z No Qualifier** |

**Non-OR** ØGW[Ø,1,5,K,R]XØZ
**Non-OR** ØGWS[3,4]YZ
**Non-OR** ØGWSX[Ø,2,3]Z

# Skin and Breast ØHØ–ØHX

## Character Meanings*

This Character Meaning table is provided as a guide to assist the user in the identification of character members that may be found in this section of code tables. It **SHOULD NOT** be used to build a PCS code.

| Operation–Character 3 | Body Part–Character 4 | Approach–Character 5 | Device–Character 6 | Qualifier–Character 7 |
|---|---|---|---|---|
| Ø Alteration | Ø Skin, Scalp | Ø Open | Ø Drainage Device | 3 Full Thickness |
| 2 Change | 1 Skin, Face | 3 Percutaneous | 1 Radioactive Element | 4 Partial Thickness |
| 5 Destruction | 2 Skin, Right Ear | 7 Via Natural or Artificial Opening | 7 Autologous Tissue Substitute | 5 Latissimus Dorsi Myocutaneous Flap |
| 8 Division | 3 Skin, Left Ear | 8 Via Natural or Artificial Opening Endoscopic | J Synthetic Substitute | 6 Transverse Rectus Abdominis Myocutaneous Flap |
| 9 Drainage | 4 Skin, Neck | X External | K Nonautologous Tissue Substitute | 7 Deep Inferior Epigastric Artery Perforator Flap |
| B Excision | 5 Skin, Chest | | N Tissue Expander | 8 Superficial Inferior Epigastric Artery Flap |
| C Extirpation | 6 Skin, Back | | Y Other Device | 9 Gluteal Artery Perforator Flap |
| D Extraction | 7 Skin, Abdomen | | Z No Device | D Multiple |
| H Insertion | 8 Skin, Buttock | | | X Diagnostic |
| J Inspection | 9 Skin, Perineum | | | Z No Qualifier |
| M Reattachment | A Skin, Inguinal | | | |
| N Release | B Skin, Right Upper Arm | | | |
| P Removal | C Skin, Left Upper Arm | | | |
| Q Repair | D Skin, Right Lower Arm | | | |
| R Replacement | E Skin, Left Lower Arm | | | |
| S Reposition | F Skin, Right Hand | | | |
| T Resection | G Skin, Left Hand | | | |
| U Supplement | H Skin, Right Upper Leg | | | |
| W Revision | J Skin, Left Upper Leg | | | |
| X Transfer | K Skin, Right Lower Leg | | | |
| | L Skin, Left Lower Leg | | | |
| | M Skin, Right Foot | | | |
| | N Skin, Left Foot | | | |
| | P Skin | | | |
| | Q Finger Nail | | | |
| | R Toe Nail | | | |
| | S Hair | | | |
| | T Breast, Right | | | |
| | U Breast, Left | | | |
| | V Breast, Bilateral | | | |
| | W Nipple, Right | | | |
| | X Nipple, Left | | | |
| | Y Supernumerary Breast | | | |

* Includes skin and breast glands and ducts.

**AHA Coding Clinic for table ØHB**
**2016, 3Q, 29** Closure of bilateral alveolar clefts
**2015, 3Q, 3-8** Excisional and nonexcisional debridement

**AHA Coding Clinic for table ØHD**
**2016, 1Q, 40** Nonexcisional debridement of skin and subcutaneous tissue
**2015, 3Q, 3-8** Excisional and nonexcisional debridement

**AHA Coding Clinic for table ØHH**
**2014, 2Q, 12** Pedicle latissimus myocutaneous flap with placement of breast tissue expanders
**2013, 4Q, 107** Breast tissue expander placement using acellular dermal matrix

**AHA Coding Clinic for table ØHP**
**2016, 2Q, 27** Removal of nonviable transverse rectus abdominis myocutaneous (TRAM) flaps

**AHA Coding Clinic for table ØHQ**
**2016, 1Q, 7** Obstetrical perineal laceration repair
**2014, 4Q, 31** Delayed wound closure following fracture treatment

**AHA Coding Clinic for table ØHR**
**2017, 1Q, 35** Epifix® allograft
**2014, 3Q, 14** Application of TheraSkin® and excisional debridement

**AHA Coding Clinic for table ØHT**
**2014, 4Q, 34** Skin-sparing mastectomy

## Integumentary Anatomy

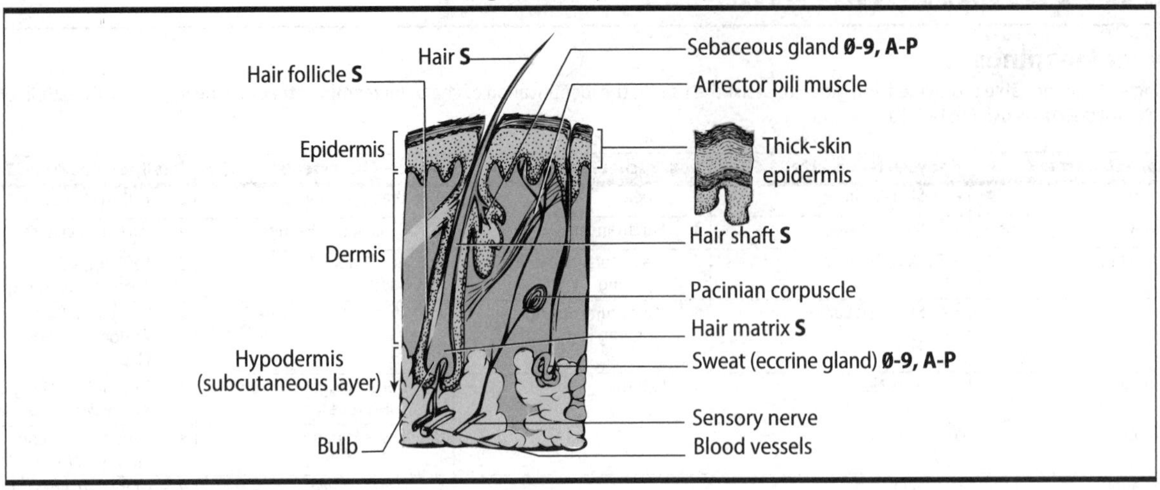
Hair S
Hair follicle S
Sebaceous gland Ø-9, A-P
Arrector pili muscle
Epidermis
Thick-skin epidermis
Dermis
Hair shaft S
Pacinian corpuscle
Hair matrix S
Hypodermis (subcutaneous layer)
Sweat (eccrine gland) Ø-9, A-P
Sensory nerve
Bulb
Blood vessels

## Nail Anatomy

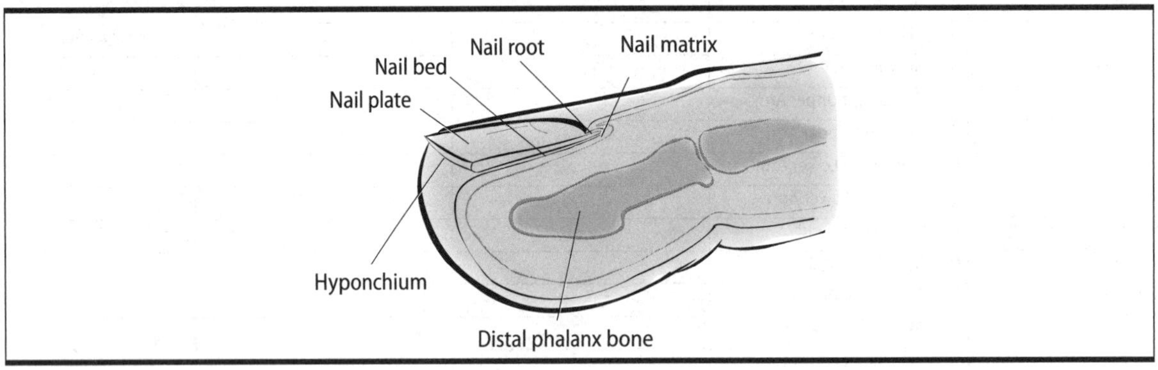
Nail root
Nail matrix
Nail bed
Nail plate
Hyponchium
Distal phalanx bone

## Breast

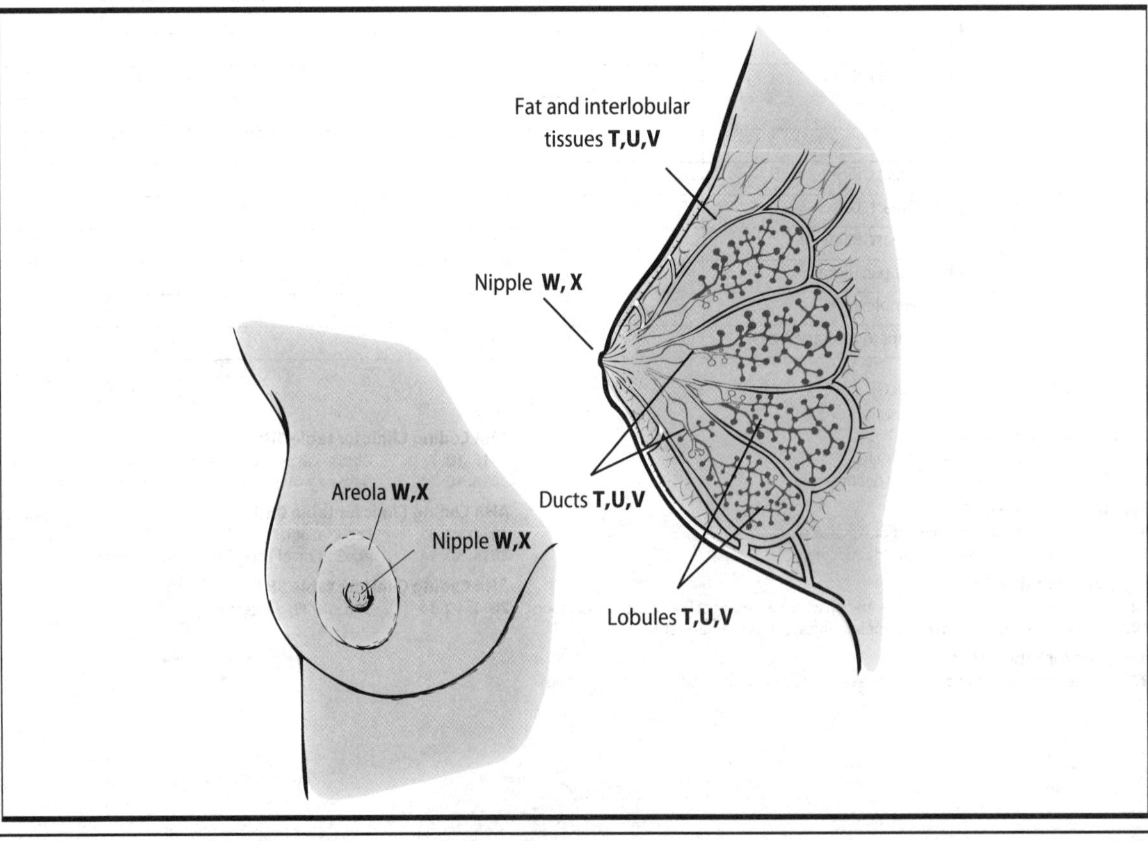
Fat and interlobular tissues T,U,V
Nipple W, X
Ducts T,U,V
Areola W,X
Nipple W,X
Lobules T,U,V

**Ø Medical and Surgical**
**H Skin and Breast**
**Ø Alteration** Definition: Modifying the anatomic structure of a body part without affecting the function of the body part
Explanation: Principal purpose is to improve appearance

| Body Part Character 4 | Approach Character 5 | Device Character 6 | Qualifier Character 7 |
|---|---|---|---|
| **T** Breast, Right<br>Mammary duct<br>Mammary gland<br>**U** Breast, Left<br>*See T Breast, Right*<br>**V** Breast, Bilateral<br>*See T Breast, Right* | **Ø** Open<br>**3** Percutaneous<br>**X** External | **7** Autologous Tissue Substitute<br>**J** Synthetic Substitute<br>**K** Nonautologous Tissue Substitute<br>**Z** No Device | **Z** No Qualifier |

Non-OR ØHØ[T,U,V]3JZ

**Ø Medical and Surgical**
**H Skin and Breast**
**2 Change** Definition: Taking out or off a device from a body part and putting back an identical or similar device in or on the same body part without cutting or puncturing the skin or a mucous membrane
Explanation: All CHANGE procedures are coded using the approach EXTERNAL

| Body Part Character 4 | Approach Character 5 | Device Character 6 | Qualifier Character 7 |
|---|---|---|---|
| **P** Skin<br>Dermis<br>Epidermis<br>Sebaceous gland<br>Sweat gland<br>**T** Breast, Right<br>Mammary duct<br>Mammary gland<br>**U** Breast, Left<br>*See T Breast, Right* | **X** External | **Ø** Drainage Device<br>**Y** Other Device | **Z** No Qualifier |

Non-OR All body part, approach, device, and qualifier values

**Ø Medical and Surgical**
**H Skin and Breast**
**5 Destruction** Definition: Physical eradication of all or a portion of a body part by the direct use of energy, force, or a destructive agent
Explanation: None of the body part is physically taken out

| Body Part Character 4 | | Approach Character 5 | Device Character 6 | Qualifier Character 7 |
|---|---|---|---|---|
| **Ø** Skin, Scalp<br>**1** Skin, Face<br>**2** Skin, Right Ear<br>**3** Skin, Left Ear<br>**4** Skin, Neck<br>**5** Skin, Chest<br>**6** Skin, Back<br>**7** Skin, Abdomen<br>**8** Skin, Buttock<br>**9** Skin, Perineum<br>**A** Skin, Inguinal<br>**B** Skin, Right Upper Arm | **C** Skin, Left Upper Arm<br>**D** Skin, Right Lower Arm<br>**E** Skin, Left Lower Arm<br>**F** Skin, Right Hand<br>**G** Skin, Left Hand<br>**H** Skin, Right Upper Leg<br>**J** Skin, Left Upper Leg<br>**K** Skin, Right Lower Leg<br>**L** Skin, Left Lower Leg<br>**M** Skin, Right Foot<br>**N** Skin, Left Foot | **X** External | **Z** No Device | **D** Multiple<br>**Z** No Qualifier |
| **Q** Finger Nail<br>Nail bed<br>Nail plate | **R** Toe Nail<br>*See Q Finger Nail* | **X** External | **Z** No Device | **Z** No Qualifier |
| **T** Breast, Right<br>Mammary duct<br>Mammary gland<br>**U** Breast, Left<br>*See T Breast, Right*<br>**V** Breast, Bilateral<br>*See T Breast, Right* | **W** Nipple, Right<br>Areola<br>**X** Nipple, Left<br>*See W Nipple, Right* | **Ø** Open<br>**3** Percutaneous<br>**7** Via Natural or Artificial Opening<br>**8** Via Natural or Artificial Opening Endoscopic<br>**X** External | **Z** No Device | **Z** No Qualifier |

DRG Non-OR ØH5[Ø,1,4,5,6,7,8,9,A,B,C,D,E,F,G,H,J,K,L,M,N]XZ[D,Z]
DRG Non-OR ØH5[Q,R]XZZ
Non-OR ØH5[2,3]XZ[D,Z]

**Ø Medical and Surgical**
**H Skin and Breast**
**8 Division** Definition: Cutting into a body part, without draining fluids and/or gases from the body part, in order to separate or transect a body part
Explanation: All or a portion of the body part is separated into two or more portions

| Body Part Character 4 | | Approach Character 5 | Device Character 6 | Qualifier Character 7 |
|---|---|---|---|---|
| **Ø** Skin, Scalp<br>**1** Skin, Face<br>**2** Skin, Right Ear<br>**3** Skin, Left Ear<br>**4** Skin, Neck<br>**5** Skin, Chest<br>**6** Skin, Back<br>**7** Skin, Abdomen<br>**8** Skin, Buttock<br>**9** Skin, Perineum<br>**A** Skin, Inguinal<br>**B** Skin, Right Upper Arm | **C** Skin, Left Upper Arm<br>**D** Skin, Right Lower Arm<br>**E** Skin, Left Lower Arm<br>**F** Skin, Right Hand<br>**G** Skin, Left Hand<br>**H** Skin, Right Upper Leg<br>**J** Skin, Left Upper Leg<br>**K** Skin, Right Lower Leg<br>**L** Skin, Left Lower Leg<br>**M** Skin, Right Foot<br>**N** Skin, Left Foot | **X** External | **Z** No Device | **Z** No Qualifier |

**Non-OR** All body part, approach, device, and qualifier values

**Ø Medical and Surgical**
**H Skin and Breast**
**9 Drainage** Definition: Taking or letting out fluids and/or gases from a body part
Explanation: The qualifier DIAGNOSTIC is used to identify drainage procedures that are biopsies

| Body Part Character 4 | | Approach Character 5 | Device Character 6 | Qualifier Character 7 |
|---|---|---|---|---|
| **Ø** Skin, Scalp<br>**1** Skin, Face<br>**2** Skin, Right Ear<br>**3** Skin, Left Ear<br>**4** Skin, Neck<br>**5** Skin, Chest<br>**6** Skin, Back<br>**7** Skin, Abdomen<br>**8** Skin, Buttock<br>**9** Skin, Perineum<br>**A** Skin, Inguinal<br>**B** Skin, Right Upper Arm<br>**C** Skin, Left Upper Arm<br>**D** Skin, Right Lower Arm | **E** Skin, Left Lower Arm<br>**F** Skin, Right Hand<br>**G** Skin, Left Hand<br>**H** Skin, Right Upper Leg<br>**J** Skin, Left Upper Leg<br>**K** Skin, Right Lower Leg<br>**L** Skin, Left Lower Leg<br>**M** Skin, Right Foot<br>**N** Skin, Left Foot<br>**Q** Finger Nail<br>Nail bed<br>Nail plate<br>**R** Toe Nail<br>*See Q Finger Nail* | **X** External | **Ø** Drainage Device | **Z** No Qualifier |
| **Ø** Skin, Scalp<br>**1** Skin, Face<br>**2** Skin, Right Ear<br>**3** Skin, Left Ear<br>**4** Skin, Neck<br>**5** Skin, Chest<br>**6** Skin, Back<br>**7** Skin, Abdomen<br>**8** Skin, Buttock<br>**9** Skin, Perineum<br>**A** Skin, Inguinal<br>**B** Skin, Right Upper Arm<br>**C** Skin, Left Upper Arm<br>**D** Skin, Right Lower Arm | **E** Skin, Left Lower Arm<br>**F** Skin, Right Hand<br>**G** Skin, Left Hand<br>**H** Skin, Right Upper Leg<br>**J** Skin, Left Upper Leg<br>**K** Skin, Right Lower Leg<br>**L** Skin, Left Lower Leg<br>**M** Skin, Right Foot<br>**N** Skin, Left Foot<br>**Q** Finger Nail<br>Nail bed<br>Nail plate<br>**R** Toe Nail<br>*See Q Finger Nail* | **X** External | **Z** No Device | **X** Diagnostic<br>**Z** No Qualifier |
| **T** Breast, Right<br>Mammary duct<br>Mammary gland<br>**U** Breast, Left<br>*See T Breast, Right*<br>**V** Breast, Bilateral<br>*See T Breast, Right* | **W** Nipple, Right<br>Areola<br>**X** Nipple, Left<br>*See W Nipple, Right* | **Ø** Open<br>**3** Percutaneous<br>**7** Via Natural or Artificial Opening<br>**8** Via Natural or Artificial Opening Endoscopic<br>**X** External | **Ø** Drainage Device | **Z** No Qualifier |
| **T** Breast, Right<br>Mammary duct<br>Mammary gland<br>**U** Breast, Left<br>*See T Breast, Right*<br>**V** Breast, Bilateral<br>*See T Breast, Right* | **W** Nipple, Right<br>Areola<br>**X** Nipple, Left<br>*See W Nipple, Right* | **Ø** Open<br>**3** Percutaneous<br>**7** Via Natural or Artificial Opening<br>**8** Via Natural or Artificial Opening Endoscopic<br>**X** External | **Z** No Device | **X** Diagnostic<br>**Z** No Qualifier |

**Non-OR** ØH9[Ø,1,2,3,4,5,6,7,8,A,B,C,D,E,F,G,H,J,K,L,M,N,Q,R]XØZ
**Non-OR** ØH9[Ø,1,2,3,4,5,6,7,8,A,B,C,D,E,F,G,H,J,K,L,M,N,Q,R]XZ[X,Z]
**Non-OR** ØH99XZX
**Non-OR** ØH9[T,U,V,W,X][Ø,3,7,8,X]ØZ
**Non-OR** ØH9[T,U,V,W,X][3,7,8,X]Z[X,Z]
**Non-OR** ØH9[T,U,V,W,X]ØZZ

**Ø Medical and Surgical**
**H Skin and Breast**
**B Excision** Definition: Cutting out or off, without replacement, a portion of a body part
Explanation: The qualifier DIAGNOSTIC is used to identify excision procedures that are biopsies

| Body Part Character 4 | Approach Character 5 | Device Character 6 | Qualifier Character 7 |
|---|---|---|---|
| **Ø Skin, Scalp**<br>**1 Skin, Face**<br>**2 Skin, Right Ear**<br>**3 Skin, Left Ear**<br>**4 Skin, Neck**<br>**5 Skin, Chest**<br>**6 Skin, Back**<br>**7 Skin, Abdomen**<br>**8 Skin, Buttock**<br>**9 Skin, Perineum**<br>**A Skin, Inguinal**<br>**B Skin, Right Upper Arm**<br>**C Skin, Left Upper Arm**<br>**D Skin, Right Lower Arm**<br>**E Skin, Left Lower Arm**<br>**F Skin, Right Hand**<br>**G Skin, Left Hand**<br>**H Skin, Right Upper Leg**<br>**J Skin, Left Upper Leg**<br>**K Skin, Right Lower Leg**<br>**L Skin, Left Lower Leg**<br>**M Skin, Right Foot**<br>**N Skin, Left Foot**<br>**Q Finger Nail**<br>Nail bed<br>Nail plate<br>**R Toe Nail**<br>*See Q Finger Nail* | **X External** | **Z No Device** | **X Diagnostic**<br>**Z No Qualifier** |
| **T Breast, Right**<br>Mammary duct<br>Mammary gland<br>**U Breast, Left**<br>*See T Breast, Right*<br>**V Breast, Bilateral**<br>*See T Breast, Right*<br>**W Nipple, Right**<br>Areola<br>**X Nipple, Left**<br>*See W Nipple, Right*<br>**Y Supernumerary Breast** | **Ø Open**<br>**3 Percutaneous**<br>**7 Via Natural or Artificial Opening**<br>**8 Via Natural or Artificial Opening Endoscopic**<br>**X External** | **Z No Device** | **X Diagnostic**<br>**Z No Qualifier** |

**DRG Non-OR** ØHB9XZZ
**Non-OR** ØHB[Ø,1,2,3,4,5,6,7,8,A,B,C,D,E,F,G,H,J,K,L,M,N,Q,R]XZ[X,Z]
**Non-OR** ØHB9XZX
**Non-OR** ØHB[T,U,V,W,X,Y][3,7,8,X]ZX

**Ø Medical and Surgical**
**H Skin and Breast**
**C Extirpation** Definition: Taking or cutting out solid matter from a body part

Explanation: The solid matter may be an abnormal byproduct of a biological function or a foreign body; it may be imbedded in a body part or in the lumen of a tubular body part. The solid matter may or may not have been previously broken into pieces.

| Body Part Character 4 | Approach Character 5 | Device Character 6 | Qualifier Character 7 |
|---|---|---|---|
| **Ø** Skin, Scalp<br>**1** Skin, Face<br>**2** Skin, Right Ear<br>**3** Skin, Left Ear<br>**4** Skin, Neck<br>**5** Skin, Chest<br>**6** Skin, Back<br>**7** Skin, Abdomen<br>**8** Skin, Buttock<br>**9** Skin, Perineum<br>**A** Skin, Inguinal<br>**B** Skin, Right Upper Arm<br>**C** Skin, Left Upper Arm<br>**D** Skin, Right Lower Arm<br>**E** Skin, Left Lower Arm<br>**F** Skin, Right Hand<br>**G** Skin, Left Hand<br>**H** Skin, Right Upper Leg<br>**J** Skin, Left Upper Leg<br>**K** Skin, Right Lower Leg<br>**L** Skin, Left Lower Leg<br>**M** Skin, Right Foot<br>**N** Skin, Left Foot<br>**Q** Finger Nail<br>Nail bed<br>Nail plate<br>**R** Toe Nail<br>*See Q Finger Nail* | **X** External | **Z** No Device | **Z** No Qualifier |
| **T** Breast, Right<br>Mammary duct<br>Mammary gland<br>**U** Breast, Left<br>*See T Breast, Right*<br>**V** Breast, Bilateral<br>*See T Breast, Right*<br>**W** Nipple, Right<br>Areola<br>**X** Nipple, Left<br>*See W Nipple, Right* | **Ø** Open<br>**3** Percutaneous<br>**7** Via Natural or Artificial Opening<br>**8** Via Natural or Artificial Opening Endoscopic<br>**X** External | **Z** No Device | **Z** No Qualifier |

**Non-OR** All body part, approach, device and qualifier values

**Ø Medical and Surgical**
**H Skin and Breast**
**D Extraction** Definition: Pulling or stripping out or off all or a portion of a body part by the use of force
Explanation: The qualifier DIAGNOSTIC is used to identify extraction procedures that are biopsies

| Body Part Character 4 | Approach Character 5 | Device Character 6 | Qualifier Character 7 |
|---|---|---|---|
| Ø Skin, Scalp<br>1 Skin, Face<br>2 Skin, Right Ear<br>3 Skin, Left Ear<br>4 Skin, Neck<br>5 Skin, Chest<br>6 Skin, Back<br>7 Skin, Abdomen<br>8 Skin, Buttock<br>9 Skin, Perineum<br>A Skin, Inguinal<br>B Skin, Right Upper Arm<br>C Skin, Left Upper Arm<br>D Skin, Right Lower Arm<br>E Skin, Left Lower Arm<br>F Skin, Right Hand<br>G Skin, Left Hand<br>H Skin, Right Upper Leg<br>J Skin, Left Upper Leg<br>K Skin, Right Lower Leg<br>L Skin, Left Lower Leg<br>M Skin, Right Foot<br>N Skin, Left Foot<br>Q Finger Nail<br>Nail bed<br>Nail plate<br>R Toe Nail<br>*See Q Finger Nail*<br>S Hair | X External | Z No Device | Z No Qualifier |

**Non-OR** All body part, approach, device, and qualifier values

**Ø Medical and Surgical**
**H Skin and Breast**
**H Insertion** Definition: Putting in a nonbiological appliance that monitors, assists, performs, or prevents a physiological function but does not physically take the place of a body part
Explanation: None

| Body Part Character 4 | Approach Character 5 | Device Character 6 | Qualifier Character 7 |
|---|---|---|---|
| P Skin | X External | Y Other Device | Z No Qualifier |
| T Breast, Right<br>Mammary duct<br>Mammary gland<br>U Breast, Left<br>*See T Breast, Right* | Ø Open<br>3 Percutaneous<br>7 Via Natural or Artificial Opening<br>8 Via Natural or Artificial Opening Endoscopic | 1 Radioactive Element<br>N Tissue Expander<br>Y Other Device | Z No Qualifier |
| T Breast, Right<br>Mammary duct<br>Mammary gland<br>U Breast, Left<br>*See T Breast, Right* | X External | 1 Radioactive Element | Z No Qualifier |
| V Breast, Bilateral<br>*See T Breast, Right*<br>W Nipple, Right<br>Areola<br>X Nipple, Left<br>*See W Nipple, Right* | Ø Open<br>3 Percutaneous<br>7 Via Natural or Artificial Opening<br>8 Via Natural or Artificial Opening Endoscopic | 1 Radioactive Element<br>N Tissue Expander | Z No Qualifier |
| V Breast, Bilateral<br>*See T Breast, Right*<br>W Nipple, Right<br>Areola<br>X Nipple, Left<br>*See W Nipple, Right* | X External | 1 Radioactive Element | Z No Qualifier |

**Non-OR** ØHHPXYZ
**Non-OR** ØHH[T,U][3,7,8]YZ

**Ø Medical and Surgical**
**H Skin and Breast**
**J Inspection** Definition: Visually and/or manually exploring a body part

Explanation: Visual exploration may be performed with or without optical instrumentation. Manual exploration may be performed directly or through intervening body layers.

| Body Part Character 4 | Approach Character 5 | Device Character 6 | Qualifier Character 7 |
|---|---|---|---|
| **P Skin**<br>Dermis<br>Epidermis<br>Sebaceous gland<br>Sweat gland<br>**Q Finger Nail**<br>Nail bed<br>Nail plate<br>**R Toe Nail**<br>*See Q Finger Nail* | **X External** | **Z No Device** | **Z No Qualifier** |
| **T Breast, Right**<br>Mammary duct<br>Mammary gland<br>**U Breast, Left**<br>*See T Breast, Right* | **Ø Open**<br>**3 Percutaneous**<br>**7 Via Natural or Artificial Opening**<br>**8 Via Natural or Artificial Opening Endoscopic**<br>**X External** | **Z No Device** | **Z No Qualifier** |

**Non-OR** All body part, approach, device and qualifier values

**Ø Medical and Surgical**
**H Skin and Breast**
**M Reattachment** Definition: Putting back in or on all or a portion of a separated body part to its normal location or other suitable location

Explanation: Vascular circulation and nervous pathways may or may not be reestablished

| Body Part Character 4 | Approach Character 5 | Device Character 6 | Qualifier Character 7 |
|---|---|---|---|
| **Ø Skin, Scalp**<br>**1 Skin, Face**<br>**2 Skin, Right Ear**<br>**3 Skin, Left Ear**<br>**4 Skin, Neck**<br>**5 Skin, Chest**<br>**6 Skin, Back**<br>**7 Skin, Abdomen**<br>**8 Skin, Buttock**<br>**9 Skin, Perineum**<br>**A Skin, Inguinal**<br>**B Skin, Right Upper Arm**<br>**C Skin, Left Upper Arm**<br>**D Skin, Right Lower Arm**<br>**E Skin, Left Lower Arm**<br>**F Skin, Right Hand**<br>**G Skin, Left Hand**<br>**H Skin, Right Upper Leg**<br>**J Skin, Left Upper Leg**<br>**K Skin, Right Lower Leg**<br>**L Skin, Left Lower Leg**<br>**M Skin, Right Foot**<br>**N Skin, Left Foot**<br>**T Breast, Right**<br>Mammary duct<br>Mammary gland<br>**U Breast, Left**<br>*See T Breast, Right*<br>**V Breast, Bilateral**<br>*See T Breast, Right*<br>**W Nipple, Right**<br>Areola<br>**X Nipple, Left**<br>*See W Nipple, Right* | **X External** | **Z No Device** | **Z No Qualifier** |

**Non-OR** ØHMØXZZ

**Ø Medical and Surgical**
**H Skin and Breast**
**N Release** Definition: Freeing a body part from an abnormal physical constraint by cutting or by the use of force
Explanation: Some of the restraining tissue may be taken out but none of the body part is taken out

| Body Part Character 4 | Approach Character 5 | Device Character 6 | Qualifier Character 7 |
|---|---|---|---|
| **Ø** Skin, Scalp<br>**1** Skin, Face<br>**2** Skin, Right Ear<br>**3** Skin, Left Ear<br>**4** Skin, Neck<br>**5** Skin, Chest<br>**6** Skin, Back<br>**7** Skin, Abdomen<br>**8** Skin, Buttock<br>**9** Skin, Perineum<br>**A** Skin, Inguinal<br>**B** Skin, Right Upper Arm<br>**C** Skin, Left Upper Arm<br>**D** Skin, Right Lower Arm<br>**E** Skin, Left Lower Arm<br>**F** Skin, Right Hand<br>**G** Skin, Left Hand<br>**H** Skin, Right Upper Leg<br>**J** Skin, Left Upper Leg<br>**K** Skin, Right Lower Leg<br>**L** Skin, Left Lower Leg<br>**M** Skin, Right Foot<br>**N** Skin, Left Foot<br>**Q** Finger Nail<br>Nail bed<br>Nail plate<br>**R** Toe Nail<br>*See Q Finger Nail* | **X** External | **Z** No Device | **Z** No Qualifier |
| **T** Breast, Right<br>Mammary duct<br>Mammary gland<br>**U** Breast, Left<br>*See T Breast, Right*<br>**V** Breast, Bilateral<br>*See T Breast, Right*<br>**W** Nipple, Right<br>Areola<br>**X** Nipple, Left<br>*See W Nipple, Right* | **Ø** Open<br>**3** Percutaneous<br>**7** Via Natural or Artificial Opening<br>**8** Via Natural or Artificial Opening Endoscopic<br>**X** External | **Z** No Device | **Z** No Qualifier |

**Ø Medical and Surgical**
**H Skin and Breast**
**P Removal** Definition: Taking out or off a device from a body part

Explanation: If a device is taken out and a similar device put in without cutting or puncturing the skin or mucous membrane, the procedure is coded to the root operation CHANGE. Otherwise, the procedure for taking out a device is coded to the root operation REMOVAL.

| Body Part Character 4 | Approach Character 5 | Device Character 6 | Qualifier Character 7 |
|---|---|---|---|
| **P Skin**<br>Dermis<br>Epidermis<br>Sebaceous gland<br>Sweat gland | **X External** | **Ø Drainage Device**<br>**7 Autologous Tissue Substitute**<br>**J Synthetic Substitute**<br>**K Nonautologous Tissue Substitute**<br>Y Other Device | **Z No Qualifier** |
| **Q Finger Nail**<br>Nail bed<br>Nail plate<br>**R Toe Nail**<br>*See Q Finger Nail* | **X External** | **Ø Drainage Device**<br>**7 Autologous Tissue Substitute**<br>**J Synthetic Substitute**<br>**K Nonautologous Tissue Substitute** | **Z No Qualifier** |
| **S Hair** | **X External** | **7 Autologous Tissue Substitute**<br>**J Synthetic Substitute**<br>**K Nonautologous Tissue Substitute** | **Z No Qualifier** |
| **T Breast, Right**<br>Mammary duct<br>Mammary gland<br>**U Breast, Left**<br>*See T Breast, Right* | **Ø Open**<br>**3 Percutaneous**<br>**7 Via Natural or Artificial Opening**<br>**8 Via Natural or Artificial Opening Endoscopic** | **Ø Drainage Device**<br>**1 Radioactive Element**<br>**7 Autologous Tissue Substitute**<br>**J Synthetic Substitute**<br>**K Nonautologous Tissue Substitute**<br>**N Tissue Expander**<br>Y Other Device | **Z No Qualifier** |
| **T Breast, Right**<br>Mammary duct<br>Mammary gland<br>**U Breast, Left**<br>*See T Breast, Right* | **X External** | **Ø Drainage Device**<br>**1 Radioactive Element**<br>**7 Autologous Tissue Substitute**<br>**J Synthetic Substitute**<br>**K Nonautologous Tissue Substitute** | **Z No Qualifier** |

**Non-OR** ØHPPX[Ø,7,J,K,Y]Z
**Non-OR** ØHP[Q,R]X[Ø,7,J,K]Z
**Non-OR** ØHPSX[7,J,K]Z
**Non-OR** ØHP[T,U][Ø,3][Ø,1,7,K,Y]Z
**Non-OR** ØHP[T,U][7,8][Ø,1,7,J,K,N,Y]Z
**Non-OR** ØHP[T,U]X[Ø,1,7,J,K]Z

**Ø Medical and Surgical**
**H Skin and Breast**
**Q Repair** Definition: Restoring, to the extent possible, a body part to its normal anatomic structure and function
Explanation: Used only when the method to accomplish the repair is not one of the other root operations

| Body Part Character 4 | Approach Character 5 | Device Character 6 | Qualifier Character 7 |
|---|---|---|---|
| **Ø** Skin, Scalp<br>**1** Skin, Face<br>**2** Skin, Right Ear<br>**3** Skin, Left Ear<br>**4** Skin, Neck<br>**5** Skin, Chest<br>**6** Skin, Back<br>**7** Skin, Abdomen<br>**8** Skin, Buttock<br>**9** Skin, Perineum<br>**A** Skin, Inguinal<br>**B** Skin, Right Upper Arm<br>**C** Skin, Left Upper Arm<br>**D** Skin, Right Lower Arm<br>**E** Skin, Left Lower Arm<br>**F** Skin, Right Hand<br>**G** Skin, Left Hand<br>**H** Skin, Right Upper Leg<br>**J** Skin, Left Upper Leg<br>**K** Skin, Right Lower Leg<br>**L** Skin, Left Lower Leg<br>**M** Skin, Right Foot<br>**N** Skin, Left Foot<br>**Q** Finger Nail<br>Nail bed<br>Nail plate<br>**R** Toe Nail<br>*See Q Finger Nail* | **X** External | **Z** No Device | **Z** No Qualifier |
| **T** Breast, Right<br>Mammary duct<br>Mammary gland<br>**U** Breast, Left<br>*See T Breast, Right*<br>**V** Breast, Bilateral<br>*See T Breast, Right*<br>**W** Nipple, Right<br>Areola<br>**X** Nipple, Left<br>*See W Nipple, Right*<br>**Y** Supernumerary Breast | **Ø** Open<br>**3** Percutaneous<br>**7** Via Natural or Artificial Opening<br>**8** Via Natural or Artificial Opening Endoscopic<br>**X** External | **Z** No Device | **Z** No Qualifier |

**DRG Non-OR** ØHQ9XZZ
**Non-OR** ØHQ[Ø,1,2,3,4,5,6,7,8,A,B,C,D,E,F,G,H,J,K,L,M,N]XZZ
**Non-OR** ØHQ[T,U,V,Y]XZZ

**Ø Medical and Surgical**
**H Skin and Breast**
**R Replacement** Definition: Putting in or on biological or synthetic material that physically takes the place and/or function of all or a portion of a body part

Explanation: The body part may have been taken out or replaced, or may be taken out, physically eradicated, or rendered nonfunctional during the REPLACEMENT procedure. A REMOVAL procedure is coded for taking out the device used in a previous replacement procedure.

| Body Part Character 4 | Approach Character 5 | Device Character 6 | Qualifier Character 7 |
|---|---|---|---|
| **Ø** Skin, Scalp<br>**1** Skin, Face<br>**2** Skin, Right Ear<br>**3** Skin, Left Ear<br>**4** Skin, Neck<br>**5** Skin, Chest<br>**6** Skin, Back<br>**7** Skin, Abdomen<br>**8** Skin, Buttock<br>**9** Skin, Perineum<br>**A** Skin, Inguinal<br>**B** Skin, Right Upper Arm<br>**C** Skin, Left Upper Arm<br>**D** Skin, Right Lower Arm<br>**E** Skin, Left Lower Arm<br>**F** Skin, Right Hand<br>**G** Skin, Left Hand<br>**H** Skin, Right Upper Leg<br>**J** Skin, Left Upper Leg<br>**K** Skin, Right Lower Leg<br>**L** Skin, Left Lower Leg<br>**M** Skin, Right Foot<br>**N** Skin, Left Foot | **X** External | **7** Autologous Tissue Substitute<br>**K** Nonautologous Tissue Substitute | **3** Full Thickness<br>**4** Partial Thickness |
| **Ø** Skin, Scalp<br>**1** Skin, Face<br>**2** Skin, Right Ear<br>**3** Skin, Left Ear<br>**4** Skin, Neck<br>**5** Skin, Chest<br>**6** Skin, Back<br>**7** Skin, Abdomen<br>**8** Skin, Buttock<br>**9** Skin, Perineum<br>**A** Skin, Inguinal<br>**B** Skin, Right Upper Arm<br>**C** Skin, Left Upper Arm<br>**D** Skin, Right Lower Arm<br>**E** Skin, Left Lower Arm<br>**F** Skin, Right Hand<br>**G** Skin, Left Hand<br>**H** Skin, Right Upper Leg<br>**J** Skin, Left Upper Leg<br>**K** Skin, Right Lower Leg<br>**L** Skin, Left Lower Leg<br>**M** Skin, Right Foot<br>**N** Skin, Left Foot | **X** External | **J** Synthetic Substitute | **3** Full Thickness<br>**4** Partial Thickness<br>**Z** No Qualifier |
| **Q** Finger Nail<br>Nail bed<br>Nail plate<br>**R** Toe Nail<br>*See Q Finger Nail*<br>**S** Hair | **X** External | **7** Autologous Tissue Substitute<br>**J** Synthetic Substitute<br>**K** Nonautologous Tissue Substitute | **Z** No Qualifier |
| **T** Breast, Right<br>Mammary duct<br>Mammary gland<br>**U** Breast, Left<br>*See T Breast, Right*<br>**V** Breast, Bilateral<br>*See T Breast, Right* | **Ø** Open | **7** Autologous Tissue Substitute | **5** Latissimus Dorsi Myocutaneous Flap<br>**6** Transverse Rectus Abdominis Myocutaneous Flap<br>**7** Deep Inferior Epigastric Artery Perforator Flap<br>**8** Superficial Inferior Epigastric Artery Flap<br>**9** Gluteal Artery Perforator Flap<br>**Z** No Qualifier |
| **T** Breast, Right<br>Mammary duct<br>Mammary gland<br>**U** Breast, Left<br>*See T Breast, Right*<br>**V** Breast, Bilateral<br>*See T Breast, Right* | **Ø** Open | **J** Synthetic Substitute<br>**K** Nonautologous Tissue Substitute | **Z** No Qualifier |
| **T** Breast, Right ⊞<br>Mammary duct<br>Mammary gland<br>**U** Breast, Left ⊞<br>*See T Breast, Right*<br>**V** Breast, Bilateral ⊞<br>*See T Breast, Right* | **3** Percutaneous<br>**X** External | **7** Autologous Tissue Substitute<br>**J** Synthetic Substitute<br>**K** Nonautologous Tissue Substitute | **Z** No Qualifier |
| **W** Nipple, Right<br>Areola<br>**X** Nipple, Left<br>*See W Nipple, Right* | **Ø** Open<br>**3** Percutaneous<br>**X** External | **7** Autologous Tissue Substitute<br>**J** Synthetic Substitute<br>**K** Nonautologous Tissue Substitute | **Z** No Qualifier |

Non-OR ØHRSX7Z

**See Appendix L for Procedure Combinations**
⊞ ØHR[T,U,V]37Z

**Ø Medical and Surgical**
**H Skin and Breast**
**S Reposition** Definition: Moving to its normal location, or other suitable location, all or a portion of a body part

Explanation: The body part is moved to a new location from an abnormal location, or from a normal location where it is not functioning correctly. The body part may or may not be cut out or off to be moved to the new location.

| Body Part Character 4 | Approach Character 5 | Device Character 6 | Qualifier Character 7 |
|---|---|---|---|
| **S** Hair<br>**W** Nipple, Right<br>Areola<br>**X** Nipple, Left<br>*See W Nipple, Right* | **X** External | **Z** No Device | **Z** No Qualifier |
| **T** Breast, Right<br>Mammary duct<br>Mammary gland<br>**U** Breast, Left<br>*See T Breast, Right*<br>**V** Breast, Bilateral<br>*See T Breast, Right* | **Ø** Open | **Z** No Device | **Z** No Qualifier |

Non-OR ØHSSXZZ

**Ø Medical and Surgical**
**H Skin and Breast**
**T Resection** Definition: Cutting out or off, without replacement, all of a body part

Explanation: None

| Body Part Character 4 | Approach Character 5 | Device Character 6 | Qualifier Character 7 |
|---|---|---|---|
| **Q** Finger Nail<br>Nail bed<br>Nail plate<br>**R** Toe Nail<br>*See Q Finger Nail*<br>**W** Nipple, Right<br>Areola<br>**X** Nipple, Left<br>*See W Nipple, Right* | **X** External | **Z** No Device | **Z** No Qualifier |
| **T** Breast, Right ⊞<br>Mammary duct<br>Mammary gland<br>**U** Breast, Left ⊞<br>*See T Breast, Right*<br>**V** Breast, Bilateral ⊞<br>*See T Breast, Right*<br>**Y** Supernumerary Breast | **Ø** Open | **Z** No Device | **Z** No Qualifier |

Non-OR ØHT[Q,R]XZZ

**See Appendix L for Procedure Combinations**
⊞ ØHT[T,U,V]ØZZ

**Ø Medical and Surgical**
**H Skin and Breast**
**U Supplement** Definition: Putting in or on biological or synthetic material that physically reinforces and/or augments the function of a portion of a body part

Explanation: The biological material is non-living, or is living and from the same individual. The body part may have been previously replaced, and the SUPPLEMENT procedure is performed to physically reinforce and/or augment the function of the replaced body part.

| Body Part Character 4 | Approach Character 5 | Device Character 6 | Qualifier Character 7 |
|---|---|---|---|
| **T** Breast, Right<br>Mammary duct<br>Mammary gland<br>**U** Breast, Left<br>*See T Breast, Right*<br>**V** Breast, Bilateral<br>*See T Breast, Right*<br>**W** Nipple, Right<br>Areola<br>**X** Nipple, Left<br>*See W Nipple, Right* | **Ø** Open<br>**3** Percutaneous<br>**7** Via Natural or Artificial Opening<br>**8** Via Natural or Artificial Opening Endoscopic<br>**X** External | **7** Autologous Tissue Substitute<br>**J** Synthetic Substitute<br>**K** Nonautologous Tissue Substitute | **Z** No Qualifier |

Non-OR ØHU[T,U,V]3JZ

**Ø Medical and Surgical**
**H Skin and Breast**
**W Revision**

Definition: Correcting, to the extent possible, a portion of a malfunctioning device or the position of a displaced device

Explanation: Revision can include correcting a malfunctioning or displaced device by taking out or putting in components of the device such as a screw or pin

| Body Part Character 4 | Approach Character 5 | Device Character 6 | Qualifier Character 7 |
|---|---|---|---|
| **P Skin**<br>Dermis<br>Epidermis<br>Sebaceous gland<br>Sweat gland | **X External** | **Ø Drainage Device**<br>**7 Autologous Tissue Substitute**<br>**J Synthetic Substitute**<br>**K Nonautologous Tissue Substitute**<br>Y Other Device | **Z No Qualifier** |
| **Q Finger Nail**<br>Nail bed<br>Nail plate<br>**R Toe Nail**<br>*See Q Finger Nail* | **X External** | **Ø Drainage Device**<br>**7 Autologous Tissue Substitute**<br>**J Synthetic Substitute**<br>**K Nonautologous Tissue Substitute** | **Z No Qualifier** |
| **S Hair** | **X External** | **7 Autologous Tissue Substitute**<br>**J Synthetic Substitute**<br>**K Nonautologous Tissue Substitute** | **Z No Qualifier** |
| **T Breast, Right**<br>Mammary duct<br>Mammary gland<br>**U Breast, Left**<br>*See T Breast, Right* | **Ø Open**<br>**3 Percutaneous**<br>**7 Via Natural or Artificial Opening**<br>**8 Via Natural or Artificial Opening Endoscopic** | **Ø Drainage Device**<br>**7 Autologous Tissue Substitute**<br>**J Synthetic Substitute**<br>**K Nonautologous Tissue Substitute**<br>**N Tissue Expander**<br>Y Other Device | **Z No Qualifier** |
| **T Breast, Right**<br>Mammary duct<br>Mammary gland<br>**U Breast, Left**<br>*See T Breast, Right* | **X External** | **Ø Drainage Device**<br>**7 Autologous Tissue Substitute**<br>**J Synthetic Substitute**<br>**K Nonautologous Tissue Substitute** | **Z No Qualifier** |

**Non-OR** ØHWPX[Ø,7,J,K,Y]Z
**Non-OR** ØHW[Q,R]X[Ø,7,J,K]Z
**Non-OR** ØHWSX[7,J,K]Z
**Non-OR** ØHW[T,U][Ø,3][Ø,7,K,N,Y]Z
**Non-OR** ØHW[T,U][7,8][Ø,7,J,K,N,Y]Z
**Non-OR** ØHW[T,U]X[Ø,7,J,K]Z

**Ø Medical and Surgical**
**H Skin and Breast**
**X Transfer**

Definition: Moving, without taking out, all or a portion of a body part to another location to take over the function of all or a portion of a body part

Explanation: The body part transferred remains connected to its vascular and nervous supply

| Body Part Character 4 | Approach Character 5 | Device Character 6 | Qualifier Character 7 |
|---|---|---|---|
| **Ø Skin, Scalp**<br>**1 Skin, Face**<br>**2 Skin, Right Ear**<br>**3 Skin, Left Ear**<br>**4 Skin, Neck**<br>**5 Skin, Chest**<br>**6 Skin, Back**<br>**7 Skin, Abdomen**<br>**8 Skin, Buttock**<br>**9 Skin, Perineum**<br>A Skin, Inguinal<br>**B Skin, Right Upper Arm**<br>**C Skin, Left Upper Arm**<br>**D Skin, Right Lower Arm**<br>**E Skin, Left Lower Arm**<br>**F Skin, Right Hand**<br>**G Skin, Left Hand**<br>**H Skin, Right Upper Leg**<br>**J Skin, Left Upper Leg**<br>**K Skin, Right Lower Leg**<br>**L Skin, Left Lower Leg**<br>**M Skin, Right Foot**<br>**N Skin, Left Foot** | **X External** | **Z No Device** | **Z No Qualifier** |

# Subcutaneous Tissue and Fascia ØJØ–ØJX

## Character Meanings

This Character Meaning table is provided as a guide to assist the user in the identification of character members that may be found in this section of code tables. It **SHOULD NOT** be used to build a PCS code.

| Operation–Character 3 | | Body Part–Character 4 | | Approach–Character 5 | | Device–Character 6 | | Qualifier–Character 7 | |
|---|---|---|---|---|---|---|---|---|---|
| Ø | Alteration | Ø | Subcutaneous Tissue and Fascia, Scalp | Ø | Open | Ø | Drainage Device OR Monitoring Device, Hemodynamic | B | Skin and Subcutaneous Tissue |
| 2 | Change | 1 | Subcutaneous Tissue and Fascia, Face | 3 | Percutaneous | 1 | Radioactive Element | C | Skin, Subcutaneous Tissue and Fascia |
| 5 | Destruction | 4 | Subcutaneous Tissue and Fascia, Right Neck | X | External | 2 | Monitoring Device | X | Diagnostic |
| 8 | Division | 5 | Subcutaneous Tissue and Fascia, Left Neck | | | 3 | Infusion Device | Z | No Qualifier |
| 9 | Drainage | 6 | Subcutaneous Tissue and Fascia, Chest | | | 4 | Pacemaker, Single Chamber | | |
| B | Excision | 7 | Subcutaneous Tissue and Fascia, Back | | | 5 | Pacemaker, Single Chamber Rate Responsive | | |
| C | Extirpation | 8 | Subcutaneous Tissue and Fascia, Abdomen | | | 6 | Pacemaker, Dual Chamber | | |
| D | Extraction | 9 | Subcutaneous Tissue and Fascia, Buttock | | | 7 | Autologous Tissue Substitute OR Cardiac Resynchronization Pacemaker Pulse Generator | | |
| H | Insertion | B | Subcutaneous Tissue and Fascia, Perineum | | | 8 | Defibrillator Generator | | |
| J | Inspection | C | Subcutaneous Tissue and Fascia, Pelvic Region | | | 9 | Cardiac Resynchronization Defibrillator Pulse Generator | | |
| N | Release | D | Subcutaneous Tissue and Fascia, Right Upper Arm | | | A | Contractility Modulation Device | | |
| P | Removal | F | Subcutaneous Tissue and Fascia, Left Upper Arm | | | B | Stimulator Generator, Single Array | | |
| Q | Repair | G | Subcutaneous Tissue and Fascia, Right Lower Arm | | | C | Stimulator Generator, Single Array Rechargeable | | |
| R | Replacement | H | Subcutaneous Tissue and Fascia, Left Lower Arm | | | D | Stimulator Generator, Multiple Array | | |
| U | Supplement | J | Subcutaneous Tissue and Fascia, Right Hand | | | E | Stimulator Generator, Multiple Array Rechargeable | | |
| W | Revision | K | Subcutaneous Tissue and Fascia, Left Hand | | | H | Contraceptive Device | | |
| X | Transfer | L | Subcutaneous Tissue and Fascia, Right Upper Leg | | | J | Synthetic Substitute | | |
| | | M | Subcutaneous Tissue and Fascia, Left Upper Leg | | | K | Nonautologous Tissue Substitute | | |
| | | N | Subcutaneous Tissue and Fascia, Right Lower Leg | | | M | Stimulator Generator | | |
| | | P | Subcutaneous Tissue and Fascia, Left Lower Leg | | | N | Tissue Expander | | |
| | | Q | Subcutaneous Tissue and Fascia, Right Foot | | | P | Cardiac Rhythm Related Device | | |
| | | R | Subcutaneous Tissue and Fascia, Left Foot | | | V | Infusion Device, Pump | | |
| | | S | Subcutaneous Tissue and Fascia, Head and Neck | | | W | Vascular Access Device, Totally Implantable | | |
| | | T | Subcutaneous Tissue and Fascia, Trunk | | | X | Vascular Access Device, Tunneled | | |
| | | V | Subcutaneous Tissue and Fascia, Upper Extremity | | | Y | Other Device | | |
| | | W | Subcutaneous Tissue and Fascia, Lower Extremity | | | Z | No Device | | |

**AHA Coding Clinic for table ØJ2**

| | |
|---|---|
| **2017, 2Q, 26** | Exchange of tunneled catheter |

**AHA Coding Clinic for table ØJ9**

| | |
|---|---|
| **2015, 3Q, 23** | Incision and drainage of multiple abscess cavities using vessel loop |

**AHA Coding Clinic for table ØJB**

| | |
|---|---|
| **2015, 3Q, 3-8** | Excisional and nonexcisional debridement |
| **2015, 2Q, 13** | Transfer of free flap to reconstruct orbital defect |
| **2015, 1Q, 29** | Fistulectomy with placement of seton |
| **2014, 4Q, 38** | Abdominoplasty and abdominal wall plication for hernia repair |
| **2014, 3Q, 22** | Transsphenoidal removal of pituitary tumor and fat graft placement |

**AHA Coding Clinic for table ØJD**

| | |
|---|---|
| **2016, 3Q, 20** | VersaJet™ nonexcisional debridement of leg muscle |
| **2016, 3Q, 21** | Nonexcisional debridement of infected lumbar wound |
| **2016, 3Q, 21** | Nonexcisional pulsed lavage debridement |
| **2016, 3Q, 22** | Debridement of bone and tendon using Tenex ultrasound device |
| **2016, 1Q, 40** | Nonexcisional debridement of skin and subcutaneous tissue |
| **2015, 3Q, 3-8** | Excisional and nonexcisional debridement |
| **2015, 1Q, 23** | Non-Excisional debridement with lavage of wound |

**AHA Coding Clinic for table ØJH**

| | |
|---|---|
| **2017, 2Q, 24** | Tunneled catheter versus totally implantable catheter |
| **2017, 2Q, 26** | Exchange of tunneled catheter |
| **2016, 4Q, 97-98** | Phrenic neurostimulator |
| **2016, 2Q, 14** | Insertion of peritoneal totally implantable venous access device |
| **2016, 2Q, 15** | Removal and replacement of tunneled internal jugular catheter |
| **2015, 4Q, 14** | New Section X codes—New Technology procedures |
| **2015, 4Q, 30-31** | Vascular access devices |
| **2015, 2Q, 33** | Totally implantable central venous access device (Port-a-Cath) |
| **2014, 3Q, 19** | End of life replacement of Baclofen pump |
| **2013, 4Q, 116** | Device character for Port-A-Cath placement |
| **2012, 4Q, 104** | Placement of subcutaneous implantable cardioverter defibrillator |

**AHA Coding Clinic for table ØJP**

| | |
|---|---|
| **2016, 2Q, 15** | Removal and replacement of tunneled internal jugular catheter |
| **2015, 4Q, 31** | Vascular access devices |
| **2014, 3Q, 19** | End of life replacement of Baclofen pump |
| **2013, 4Q, 109** | Separating conjoined twins |
| **2012, 4Q, 104** | Placement of subcutaneous implantable cardioverter defibrillator |

**AHA Coding Clinic for table ØJQ**

| | |
|---|---|
| **2014, 4Q, 44** | Posterior colporrhaphy/rectocele repair |

**AHA Coding Clinic for table ØJR**

| | |
|---|---|
| **2015, 2Q, 13** | Transfer of free flap to reconstruct orbital defect |

**AHA Coding Clinic for table ØJW**

| | |
|---|---|
| **2015, 4Q, 33** | Externalization of peritoneal dialysis catheter |
| **2015, 2Q, 9** | Revision of ventriculoperitoneal (VP) shunt |
| **2012, 4Q, 104** | Placement of subcutaneous implantable cardioverter defibrillator |

**AHA Coding Clinic for table ØJX**

| | |
|---|---|
| **2014, 3Q, 18** | Placement of reverse sural fasciocutaneous pedicle flap |
| **2013, 4Q, 109** | Separating conjoined twins |

**Ø Medical and Surgical**
**J Subcutaneous Tissue and Fascia**
**Ø Alteration** Definition: Modifying the anatomic structure of a body part without affecting the function of the body part
Explanation: Principal purpose is to improve appearance

| Body Part Character 4 | | Approach Character 5 | Device Character 6 | Qualifier Character 7 |
|---|---|---|---|---|
| **1 Subcutaneous Tissue and Fascia, Face**<br>Masseteric fascia<br>Orbital fascia<br>**4 Subcutaneous Tissue and Fascia, Right Neck**<br>Deep cervical fascia<br>Pretracheal fascia<br>Prevertebral fascia<br>**5 Subcutaneous Tissue and Fascia, Left Neck**<br>*See 4 Subcutaneous Tissue and Fascia, Right Neck*<br>**6 Subcutaneous Tissue and Fascia, Chest**<br>Pectoral fascia<br>**7 Subcutaneous Tissue and Fascia, Back**<br>**8 Subcutaneous Tissue and Fascia, Abdomen**<br>**9 Subcutaneous Tissue and Fascia, Buttock**<br>**D Subcutaneous Tissue and Fascia, Right Upper Arm**<br>Axillary fascia<br>Deltoid fascia<br>Infraspinatus fascia<br>Subscapular aponeurosis<br>Supraspinatus fascia | **F Subcutaneous Tissue and Fascia, Left Upper Arm**<br>*See D Subcutaneous Tissue and Fascia, Right Upper Arm*<br>**G Subcutaneous Tissue and Fascia, Right Lower Arm**<br>Antebrachial fascia<br>Bicipital aponeurosis<br>**H Subcutaneous Tissue and Fascia, Left Lower Arm**<br>*See G Subcutaneous Tissue and Fascia, Right Lower Arm*<br>**L Subcutaneous Tissue and Fascia, Right Upper Leg**<br>Crural fascia<br>Fascia lata<br>Iliac fascia<br>Iliotibial tract (band)<br>**M Subcutaneous Tissue and Fascia, Left Upper Leg**<br>*See L Subcutaneous Tissue and Fascia, Right Upper Leg*<br>**N Subcutaneous Tissue and Fascia, Right Lower Leg**<br>**P Subcutaneous Tissue and Fascia, Left Lower Leg** | **Ø Open**<br>**3 Percutaneous** | **Z No Device** | **Z No Qualifier** |

**Ø Medical and Surgical**
**J Subcutaneous Tissue and Fascia**
**2 Change** Definition: Taking out or off a device from a body part and putting back an identical or similar device in or on the same body part without cutting or puncturing the skin or a mucous membrane
Explanation: All CHANGE procedures are coded using the approach EXTERNAL

| Body Part Character 4 | Approach Character 5 | Device Character 6 | Qualifier Character 7 |
|---|---|---|---|
| **S Subcutaneous Tissue and Fascia, Head and Neck**<br>**T Subcutaneous Tissue and Fascia, Trunk**<br>External oblique aponeurosis<br>Transversalis fascia<br>**V Subcutaneous Tissue and Fascia, Upper Extremity**<br>**W Subcutaneous Tissue and Fascia, Lower Extremity** | **X External** | **Ø Drainage Device**<br>**Y Other Device** | **Z No Qualifier** |

**Non-OR** All body part, approach, device, and qualifier values

**Ø Medical and Surgical**
**J Subcutaneous Tissue and Fascia**
**5 Destruction** Definition: Physical eradication of all or a portion of a body part by the direct use of energy, force, or a destructive agent
Explanation: None of the body part is physically taken out

| Body Part Character 4 | Approach Character 5 | Device Character 6 | Qualifier Character 7 |
|---|---|---|---|
| **Ø** Subcutaneous Tissue and Fascia, Scalp<br>Galea aponeurotica<br>**1** Subcutaneous Tissue and Fascia, Face<br>Masseteric fascia<br>Orbital fascia<br>**4** Subcutaneous Tissue and Fascia, Right Neck<br>Deep cervical fascia<br>Pretracheal fascia<br>Prevertebral fascia<br>**5** Subcutaneous Tissue and Fascia, Left Neck<br>*See 4 Subcutaneous Tissue and Fascia, Right Neck*<br>**6** Subcutaneous Tissue and Fascia, Chest<br>Pectoral fascia<br>**7** Subcutaneous Tissue and Fascia, Back<br>**8** Subcutaneous Tissue and Fascia, Abdomen<br>**9** Subcutaneous Tissue and Fascia, Buttock<br>**B** Subcutaneous Tissue and Fascia, Perineum<br>**C** Subcutaneous Tissue and Fascia, Pelvic Region<br>**D** Subcutaneous Tissue and Fascia, Right Upper Arm<br>Axillary fascia<br>Deltoid fascia<br>Infraspinatus fascia<br>Subscapular aponeurosis<br>Supraspinatus fascia<br>**F** Subcutaneous Tissue and Fascia, Left Upper Arm<br>*See D Subcutaneous Tissue and Fascia, Right Upper Arm*<br>**G** Subcutaneous Tissue and Fascia, Right Lower Arm<br>Antebrachial fascia<br>Bicipital aponeurosis<br>**H** Subcutaneous Tissue and Fascia, Left Lower Arm<br>*See G Subcutaneous Tissue and Fascia, Right Lower Arm*<br>**J** Subcutaneous Tissue and Fascia, Right Hand<br>Palmar fascia (aponeurosis)<br>**K** Subcutaneous Tissue and Fascia, Left Hand<br>*See J Subcutaneous Tissue and Fascia, Right Hand*<br>**L** Subcutaneous Tissue and Fascia, Right Upper Leg<br>Crural fascia<br>Fascia lata<br>Iliac fascia<br>Iliotibial tract (band)<br>**M** Subcutaneous Tissue and Fascia, Left Upper Leg<br>*See L Subcutaneous Tissue and Fascia, Right Upper Leg*<br>**N** Subcutaneous Tissue and Fascia, Right Lower Leg<br>**P** Subcutaneous Tissue and Fascia, Left Lower Leg<br>**Q** Subcutaneous Tissue and Fascia, Right Foot<br>Plantar fascia (aponeurosis)<br>**R** Subcutaneous Tissue and Fascia, Left Foot<br>*See Q Subcutaneous Tissue and Fascia, Right Foot* | **Ø** Open<br>**3** Percutaneous | **Z** No Device | **Z** No Qualifier |

DRG Non-OR All body part, approach, device, and qualifier values

**Ø Medical and Surgical**
**J Subcutaneous Tissue and Fascia**
**8 Division** Definition: Cutting into a body part, without draining fluids and/or gases from the body part, in order to separate or transect a body part
Explanation: All or a portion of the body part is separated into two or more portions

| Body Part Character 4 | Approach Character 5 | Device Character 6 | Qualifier Character 7 |
|---|---|---|---|
| **Ø Subcutaneous Tissue and Fascia, Scalp** Galea aponeurotica<br>**1 Subcutaneous Tissue and Fascia, Face** Masseteric fascia, Orbital fascia<br>**4 Subcutaneous Tissue and Fascia, Right Neck** Deep cervical fascia, Pretracheal fascia, Prevertebral fascia<br>**5 Subcutaneous Tissue and Fascia, Left Neck** *See 4 Subcutaneous Tissue and Fascia, Right Neck*<br>**6 Subcutaneous Tissue and Fascia, Chest** Pectoral fascia<br>**7 Subcutaneous Tissue and Fascia, Back**<br>**8 Subcutaneous Tissue and Fascia, Abdomen**<br>**9 Subcutaneous Tissue and Fascia, Buttock**<br>**B Subcutaneous Tissue and Fascia, Perineum**<br>**C Subcutaneous Tissue and Fascia, Pelvic Region**<br>**D Subcutaneous Tissue and Fascia, Right Upper Arm** Axillary fascia, Deltoid fascia, Infraspinatus fascia, Subscapular aponeurosis, Supraspinatus fascia<br>**F Subcutaneous Tissue and Fascia, Left Upper Arm** *See D Subcutaneous Tissue and Fascia, Right Upper Arm*<br>**G Subcutaneous Tissue and Fascia, Right Lower Arm** Antebrachial fascia, Bicipital aponeurosis<br>**H Subcutaneous Tissue and Fascia, Left Lower Arm** *See G Subcutaneous Tissue and Fascia, Right Lower Arm*<br>**J Subcutaneous Tissue and Fascia, Right Hand** Palmar fascia (aponeurosis)<br>**K Subcutaneous Tissue and Fascia, Left Hand** *See J Subcutaneous Tissue and Fascia, Right Hand*<br>**L Subcutaneous Tissue and Fascia, Right Upper Leg** Crural fascia, Fascia lata, Iliac fascia, Iliotibial tract (band)<br>**M Subcutaneous Tissue and Fascia, Left Upper Leg** *See L Subcutaneous Tissue and Fascia, Right Upper Leg*<br>**N Subcutaneous Tissue and Fascia, Right Lower Leg**<br>**P Subcutaneous Tissue and Fascia, Left Lower Leg**<br>**Q Subcutaneous Tissue and Fascia, Right Foot** Plantar fascia (aponeurosis)<br>**R Subcutaneous Tissue and Fascia, Left Foot** *See Q Subcutaneous Tissue and Fascia, Right Foot*<br>**S Subcutaneous Tissue and Fascia, Head and Neck**<br>**T Subcutaneous Tissue and Fascia, Trunk** External oblique aponeurosis, Transversalis fascia<br>**V Subcutaneous Tissue and Fascia, Upper Extremity**<br>**W Subcutaneous Tissue and Fascia, Lower Extremity** | Ø Open<br>3 Percutaneous | Z No Device | Z No Qualifier |

**Ø Medical and Surgical**
**J Subcutaneous Tissue and Fascia**
**9 Drainage** Definition: Taking or letting out fluids and/or gases from a body part
Explanation: The qualifier DIAGNOSTIC is used to identify drainage procedures that are biopsies

| Body Part Character 4 | Approach Character 5 | Device Character 6 | Qualifier Character 7 |
|---|---|---|---|
| **Ø Subcutaneous Tissue and Fascia, Scalp** Galea aponeurotica<br>**1 Subcutaneous Tissue and Fascia, Face** Masseteric fascia; Orbital fascia<br>**4 Subcutaneous Tissue and Fascia, Right Neck** Deep cervical fascia; Pretracheal fascia; Prevertebral fascia<br>**5 Subcutaneous Tissue and Fascia, Left Neck** *See 4 Subcutaneous Tissue and Fascia, Right Neck*<br>**6 Subcutaneous Tissue and Fascia, Chest** Pectoral fascia<br>**7 Subcutaneous Tissue and Fascia, Back**<br>**8 Subcutaneous Tissue and Fascia, Abdomen**<br>**9 Subcutaneous Tissue and Fascia, Buttock**<br>**B Subcutaneous Tissue and Fascia, Perineum**<br>**C Subcutaneous Tissue and Fascia, Pelvic Region**<br>**D Subcutaneous Tissue and Fascia, Right Upper Arm** Axillary fascia; Deltoid fascia; Infraspinatus fascia; Subscapular aponeurosis; Supraspinatus fascia<br>**F Subcutaneous Tissue and Fascia, Left Upper Arm** *See D Subcutaneous Tissue and Fascia, Right Upper Arm*<br>**G Subcutaneous Tissue and Fascia, Right Lower Arm** Antebrachial fascia; Bicipital aponeurosis<br>**H Subcutaneous Tissue and Fascia, Left Lower Arm** *See G Subcutaneous Tissue and Fascia, Right Lower Arm*<br>**J Subcutaneous Tissue and Fascia, Right Hand** Palmar fascia (aponeurosis)<br>**K Subcutaneous Tissue and Fascia, Left Hand** *See J Subcutaneous Tissue and Fascia, Right Hand*<br>**L Subcutaneous Tissue and Fascia, Right Upper Leg** Crural fascia; Fascia lata; Iliac fascia; Iliotibial tract (band)<br>**M Subcutaneous Tissue and Fascia, Left Upper Leg** *See L Subcutaneous Tissue and Fascia, Right Upper Leg*<br>**N Subcutaneous Tissue and Fascia, Right Lower Leg**<br>**P Subcutaneous Tissue and Fascia, Left Lower Leg**<br>**Q Subcutaneous Tissue and Fascia, Right Foot** Plantar fascia (aponeurosis)<br>**R Subcutaneous Tissue and Fascia, Left Foot** *See Q Subcutaneous Tissue and Fascia, Right Foot* | **Ø Open**<br>**3 Percutaneous** | **Ø Drainage Device** | **Z No Qualifier** |

***ØJ9 Continued on next page***

**Non-OR** ØJ9[Ø,1,4,5,6,7,8,9,B,C,D,F,G,H,J,K,L,M,N,P,Q,R][Ø,3]ØZ

**Ø Medical and Surgical**
**J Subcutaneous Tissue and Fascia**
**9 Drainage** Definition: Taking or letting out fluids and/or gases from a body part
Explanation: The qualifier DIAGNOSTIC is used to identify drainage procedures that are biopsies

***ØJ9 Continued***

| Body Part Character 4 | Approach Character 5 | Device Character 6 | Qualifier Character 7 |
|---|---|---|---|
| **Ø Subcutaneous Tissue and Fascia, Scalp**<br>Galea aponeurotica<br>**1 Subcutaneous Tissue and Fascia, Face**<br>Masseteric fascia<br>Orbital fascia<br>**4 Subcutaneous Tissue and Fascia, Right Neck**<br>Deep cervical fascia<br>Pretracheal fascia<br>Prevertebral fascia<br>**5 Subcutaneous Tissue and Fascia, Left Neck**<br>***See*** *4 Subcutaneous Tissue and Fascia, Right Neck*<br>**6 Subcutaneous Tissue and Fascia, Chest**<br>Pectoral fascia<br>**7 Subcutaneous Tissue and Fascia, Back**<br>**8 Subcutaneous Tissue and Fascia, Abdomen**<br>**9 Subcutaneous Tissue and Fascia, Buttock**<br>**B Subcutaneous Tissue and Fascia, Perineum**<br>**C Subcutaneous Tissue and Fascia, Pelvic Region**<br>**D Subcutaneous Tissue and Fascia, Right Upper Arm**<br>Axillary fascia<br>Deltoid fascia<br>Infraspinatus fascia<br>Subscapular aponeurosis<br>Supraspinatus fascia<br>**F Subcutaneous Tissue and Fascia, Left Upper Arm**<br>***See*** *D Subcutaneous Tissue and Fascia, Right Upper Arm*<br>**G Subcutaneous Tissue and Fascia, Right Lower Arm**<br>Antebrachial fascia<br>Bicipital aponeurosis<br>**H Subcutaneous Tissue and Fascia, Left Lower Arm**<br>***See*** *G Subcutaneous Tissue and Fascia, Right Lower Arm*<br>**J Subcutaneous Tissue and Fascia, Right Hand**<br>Palmar fascia (aponeurosis)<br>**K Subcutaenous Tissue and Fascia, Left Hand**<br>***See*** *J Subcutaneous Tissue and Fascia, Right Hand*<br>**L Subcutaneous Tissue and Fascia, Right Upper Leg**<br>Crural fascia<br>Fascia lata<br>Iliac fascia<br>Iliotibial tract (band)<br>**M Subcutaneous Tissue and Fascia, Left Upper Leg**<br>***See*** *L Subcutaneous Tissue and Fascia, Right Upper Leg*<br>**N Subcutaneous Tissue and Fascia, Right Lower Leg**<br>**P Subcutaneous Tissue and Fascia, Left Lower Leg**<br>**Q Subcutaneous Tissue and Fascia, Right Foot**<br>Plantar fascia (aponeurosis)<br>**R Subcutaneous Tissue and Fascia, Left Foot**<br>***See*** *Q Subcutaneous Tissue and Fascia, Right Foot* | **Ø** Open<br>**3** Percutaneous | **Z** No Device | **X** Diagnostic<br>**Z** No Qualifier |

**Non-OR** ØJ9[Ø,1,4,5,6,7,8,9,B,C,D,F,G,H,J,K,L,M,N,P,Q,R][Ø,3]ZX
**Non-OR** ØJ9[Ø,1,4,5,6,7,8,9,B,C,D,F,G,H,L,M,N,P,Q,R][Ø,3]ZZ
**Non-OR** ØJ9[J,K][Ø,3]ZZ

**Ø Medical and Surgical**
**J Subcutaneous Tissue and Fascia**
**B Excision** Definition: Cutting out or off, without replacement, a portion of a body part
Explanation: The qualifier DIAGNOSTIC is used to identify excision procedures that are biopsies

| Body Part Character 4 | | Approach Character 5 | Device Character 6 | Qualifier Character 7 |
|---|---|---|---|---|
| **Ø Subcutaneous Tissue and Fascia, Scalp**<br>Galea aponeurotica<br>**1 Subcutaneous Tissue and Fascia, Face**<br>Masseteric fascia<br>Orbital fascia<br>**4 Subcutaneous Tissue and Fascia, Right Neck**<br>Deep cervical fascia<br>Pretracheal fascia<br>Prevertebral fascia<br>**5 Subcutaneous Tissue and Fascia, Left Neck**<br>*See 4 Subcutaneous Tissue and Fascia, Right Neck*<br>**6 Subcutaneous Tissue and Fascia, Chest**<br>Pectoral fascia<br>**7 Subcutaneous Tissue and Fascia, Back**<br>**8 Subcutaneous Tissue and Fascia, Abdomen**<br>**9 Subcutaneous Tissue and Fascia, Buttock**<br>**B Subcutaneous Tissue and Fascia, Perineum**<br>**C Subcutaneous Tissue and Fascia, Pelvic Region**<br>**D Subcutaneous Tissue and Fascia, Right Upper Arm**<br>Axillary fascia<br>Deltoid fascia<br>Infraspinatus fascia<br>Subscapular aponeurosis<br>Supraspinatus fascia<br>**F Subcutaneous Tissue and Fascia, Left Upper Arm**<br>*See D Subcutaneous Tissue and Fascia, Right Upper Arm* | **G Subcutaneous Tissue and Fascia, Right Lower Arm**<br>Antebrachial fascia<br>Bicipital aponeurosis<br>**H Subcutaneous Tissue and Fascia, Left Lower Arm**<br>*See G Subcutaneous Tissue and Fascia, Right Lower Arm*<br>**J Subcutaneous Tissue and Fascia, Right Hand**<br>Palmar fascia (aponeurosis)<br>**K Subcutaneous Tissue and Fascia, Left Hand**<br>*See J Subcutaneous Tissue and Fascia, Right Hand*<br>**L Subcutaneous Tissue and Fascia, Right Upper Leg**<br>Crural fascia<br>Fascia lata<br>Iliac fascia<br>Iliotibial tract (band)<br>**M Subcutaneous Tissue and Fascia, Left Upper Leg**<br>*See L Subcutaneous Tissue and Fascia, Right Upper Leg*<br>**N Subcutaneous Tissue and Fascia, Right Lower Leg**<br>**P Subcutaneous Tissue and Fascia, Left Lower Leg**<br>**Q Subcutaneous Tissue and Fascia, Right Foot**<br>Plantar fascia (aponeurosis)<br>**R Subcutaneous Tissue and Fascia, Left Foot**<br>*See Q Subcutaneous Tissue and Fascia, Right Foot* | **Ø Open**<br>**3 Percutaneous** | **Z No Device** | **X Diagnostic**<br>**Z No Qualifier** |

**DRG Non-OR** ØJB[Ø,4,5,6,7,8,9,B,C,D,F,G,H,L,M,N,P,Q,R]3ZZ
**Non-OR** ØJB[Ø,1,4,5,6,7,8,9,B,C,D,F,G,H,J,K,L,M,N,P,Q,R][Ø,3]ZX

**Ø Medical and Surgical**
**J Subcutaneous Tissue and Fascia**
**C Extirpation** Definition: Taking or cutting out solid matter from a body part

Explanation: The solid matter may be an abnormal byproduct of a biological function or a foreign body; it may be imbedded in a body part or in the lumen of a tubular body part. The solid matter may or may not have been previously broken into pieces.

| Body Part Character 4 | | Approach Character 5 | Device Character 6 | Qualifier Character 7 |
|---|---|---|---|---|
| **Ø Subcutaneous Tissue and Fascia, Scalp**<br>Galea aponeurotica<br>**1 Subcutaneous Tissue and Fascia, Face**<br>Masseteric fascia<br>Orbital fascia<br>**4 Subcutaneous Tissue and Fascia, Right Neck**<br>Deep cervical fascia<br>Pretracheal fascia<br>Prevertebral fascia<br>**5 Subcutaneous Tissue and Fascia, Left Neck**<br>***See*** *4 Subcutaneous Tissue and Fascia, Right Neck*<br>**6 Subcutaneous Tissue and Fascia, Chest**<br>Pectoral fascia<br>**7 Subcutaneous Tissue and Fascia, Back**<br>**8 Subcutaneous Tissue and Fascia, Abdomen**<br>**9 Subcutaneous Tissue and Fascia, Buttock**<br>**B Subcutaneous Tissue and Fascia, Perineum**<br>**C Subcutaneous Tissue and Fascia, Pelvic Region**<br>**D Subcutaneous Tissue and Fascia, Right Upper Arm**<br>Axillary fascia<br>Deltoid fascia<br>Infraspinatus fascia<br>Subscapular aponeurosis<br>Supraspinatus fascia<br>**F Subcutaneous Tissue and Fascia, Left Upper Arm**<br>***See*** *D Subcutaneous Tissue and Fascia, Right Upper Arm* | **G Subcutaneous Tissue and Fascia, Right Lower Arm**<br>Antebrachial fascia<br>Bicipital aponeurosis<br>**H Subcutaneous Tissue and Fascia, Left Lower Arm**<br>***See*** *G Subcutaneous Tissue and Fascia, Right Lower Arm*<br>**J Subcutaneous Tissue and Fascia, Right Hand**<br>Palmar fascia (aponeurosis)<br>**K Subcutaneous Tissue and Fascia, Left Hand**<br>***See*** *J Subcutaneous Tissue and Fascia, Right Hand*<br>**L Subcutaneous Tissue and Fascia, Right Upper Leg**<br>Crural fascia<br>Fascia lata<br>Iliac fascia<br>Iliotibial tract (band)<br>**M Subcutaneous Tissue and Fascia, Left Upper Leg**<br>***See*** *L Subcutaneous Tissue and Fascia, Right Upper Leg*<br>**N Subcutaneous Tissue and Fascia, Right Lower Leg**<br>**P Subcutaneous Tissue and Fascia, Left Lower Leg**<br>**Q Subcutaneous Tissue and Fascia, Right Foot**<br>Plantar fascia (aponeurosis)<br>**R Subcutaneous Tissue and Fascia, Left Foot**<br>***See*** *Q Subcutaneous Tissue and Fascia, Right Foot* | **Ø Open**<br>**3 Percutaneous** | **Z No Device** | **Z No Qualifier** |

**Non-OR** All body part, approach, device, and qualifier values

**Ø Medical and Surgical**
**J Subcutaneous Tissue and Fascia**
**D Extraction** Definition: Pulling or stripping out or off all or a portion of a body part by the use of force
Explanation: The qualifier DIAGNOSTIC is used to identify extraction procedures that are biopsies

| Body Part Character 4 | Approach Character 5 | Device Character 6 | Qualifier Character 7 |
|---|---|---|---|
| **Ø Subcutaneous Tissue and Fascia, Scalp**<br>Galea aponeurotica<br>**1 Subcutaneous Tissue and Fascia, Face**<br>Masseteric fascia<br>Orbital fascia<br>**4 Subcutaneous Tissue and Fascia, Right Neck**<br>Deep cervical fascia<br>Pretracheal fascia<br>Prevertebral fascia<br>**5 Subcutaneous Tissue and Fascia, Left Neck**<br>*See 4 Subcutaneous Tissue and Fascia, Right Neck*<br>**6 Subcutaneous Tissue and Fascia, Chest** ⊞<br>Pectoral fascia<br>**7 Subcutaneous Tissue and Fascia, Back** ⊞<br>**8 Subcutaneous Tissue and Fascia, Abdomen** ⊞<br>**9 Subcutaneous Tissue and Fascia, Buttock** ⊞<br>**B Subcutaneous Tissue and Fascia, Perineum**<br>**C Subcutaneous Tissue and Fascia, Pelvic Region**<br>**D Subcutaneous Tissue and Fascia, Right Upper Arm**<br>Axillary fascia<br>Deltoid fascia<br>Infraspinatus fascia<br>Subscapular aponeurosis<br>Supraspinatus fascia<br>**F Subcutaneous Tissue and Fascia, Left Upper Arm**<br>*See D Subcutaneous Tissue and Fascia, Right Upper Arm*<br>**G Subcutaneous Tissue and Fascia, Right Lower Arm**<br>Antebrachial fascia<br>Bicipital aponeurosis<br>**H Subcutaneous Tissue and Fascia, Left Lower Arm**<br>*See G Subcutaneous Tissue and Fascia, Right Lower Arm*<br>**J Subcutaneous Tissue and Fascia, Right Hand**<br>Palmar fascia (aponeurosis)<br>**K Subcutaneous Tissue and Fascia, Left Hand**<br>*See J Subcutaneous Tissue and Fascia, Right Hand*<br>**L Subcutaneous Tissue and Fascia, Right Upper Leg**<br>Crural fascia<br>Fascia lata<br>Iliac fascia<br>Iliotibial tract (band)<br>**M Subcutaneous Tissue and Fascia, Left Upper Leg**<br>*See L Subcutaneous Tissue and Fascia, Right Upper Leg*<br>**N Subcutaneous Tissue and Fascia, Right Lower Leg**<br>**P Subcutaneous Tissue and Fascia, Left Lower Leg**<br>**Q Subcutaneous Tissue and Fascia, Right Foot**<br>Plantar fascia (aponeurosis)<br>**R Subcutaneous Tissue and Fascia, Left Foot**<br>*See Q Subcutaneous Tissue and Fascia, Right Foot* | **Ø** Open<br>**3** Percutaneous | **Z** No Device | **Z** No Qualifier |

**Non-OR** All body part, approach, device, and qualifier values

**See Appendix L for Procedure Combinations**
⊞ ØJD[6,7,8,9,L,M]3ZZ

**Ø Medical and Surgical**
**J Subcutaneous Tissue and Fascia**
**H Insertion** Definition: Putting in a nonbiological appliance that monitors, assists, performs, or prevents a physiological function but does not physically take the place of a body part
Explanation: None

| Body Part Character 4 | Approach Character 5 | Device Character 6 | Qualifier Character 7 |
|---|---|---|---|
| **Ø Subcutaneous Tissue and Fascia, Scalp**<br>Galea aponeurotica<br>**1 Subcutaneous Tissue and Fascia, Face**<br>Masseteric fascia<br>Orbital fascia<br>**4 Subcutaneous Tissue and Fascia, Right Neck**<br>Deep cervical fascia<br>Pretracheal fascia<br>Prevertebral fascia<br>**5 Subcutaneous Tissue and Fascia, Left Neck**<br>*See 4 Subcutaneous Tissue and Fascia, Right Neck*<br>**9 Subcutaneous Tissue and Fascia, Buttock**<br>**B Subcutaneous Tissue and Fascia, Perineum**<br>**C Subcutaneous Tissue and Fascia, Pelvic Region**<br>**J Subcutaneous Tissue and Fascia, Right Hand**<br>Palmar fascia (aponeurosis)<br>**K Subcutaneous Tissue and Fascia, Left Hand**<br>*See J Subcutaneous Tissue and Fascia, Right Hand*<br>**Q Subcutaneous Tissue and Fascia, Right Foot**<br>Plantar fascia (aponeurosis)<br>**R Subcutaneous Tissue and Fascia, Left Foot**<br>*See Q Subcutaneous Tissue and Fascia, Right Foot* | **Ø** Open<br>**3** Percutaneous | **N** Tissue Expander | **Z** No Qualifier |

***ØJH Continued on next page***

**Ø Medical and Surgical**
**J Subcutaneous Tissue and Fascia**
**H Insertion** Definition: Putting in a nonbiological appliance that monitors, assists, performs, or prevents a physiological function but does not physically take the place of a body part
Explanation: None

*ØJH Continued*

| Body Part Character 4 | Approach Character 5 | Device Character 6 | Qualifier Character 7 |
|---|---|---|---|
| **6** Subcutaneous Tissue and Fascia, Chest ⊞<br>Pectoral fascia<br>**8** Subcutaneous Tissue and Fascia, Abdomen ⊞ NC | **Ø** Open<br>**3** Percutaneous | **Ø** Monitoring Device, Hemodynamic<br>**2** Monitoring Device<br>**4** Pacemaker, Single Chamber<br>**5** Pacemaker, Single Chamber Rate Responsive<br>**6** Pacemaker, Dual Chamber<br>**7** Cardiac Resynchronization Pacemaker Pulse Generator<br>**8** Defibrillator Generator<br>**9** Cardiac Resynchronization Defibrillator Pulse Generator<br>**A** Contractility Modulation Device<br>**B** Stimulator Generator, Single Array<br>**C** Stimulator Generator, Single Array Rechargeable<br>**D** Stimulator Generator, Multiple Array<br>**E** Stimulator Generator, Multiple Array Rechargeable<br>**H** Contraceptive Device<br>**M** Stimulator Generator<br>**N** Tissue Expander<br>**P** Cardiac Rhythm Related Device<br>**V** Infusion Device, Pump<br>**W** Vascular Access Device, Totally Implantable<br>**X** Vascular Access Device, Tunneled | **Z** No Qualifier |
| **7** Subcutaneous Tissue and Fascia, Back ⊞ NC | **Ø** Open<br>**3** Percutaneous | **B** Stimulator Generator, Single Array<br>**C** Stimulator Generator, Single Array Rechargeable<br>**D** Stimulator Generator, Multiple Array<br>**E** Stimulator Generator, Multiple Array Rechargeable<br>**M** Stimulator Generator<br>**N** Tissue Expander<br>**V** Infusion Device, Pump | **Z** No Qualifier |
| **D** Subcutaneous Tissue and Fascia, Right Upper Arm<br>Axillary fascia<br>Deltoid fascia<br>Infraspinatus fascia<br>Subscapular aponeurosis<br>Supraspinatus fascia<br>**F** Subcutaneous Tissue and Fascia, Left Upper Arm<br>*See D Subcutaneous Tissue and Fascia, Right Upper Arm*<br>**G** Subcutaneous Tissue and Fascia, Right Lower Arm<br>Antebrachial fascia<br>Bicipital aponeurosis<br>**H** Subcutaneous Tissue and Fascia, Left Lower Arm<br>*See G Subcutaneous Tissue and Fascia, Right Lower Arm*<br>**L** Subcutaneous Tissue and Fascia, Right Upper Leg<br>Crural fascia<br>Fascia lata<br>Iliac fascia<br>Iliotibial tract (band)<br>**M** Subcutaneous Tissue and Fascia, Left Upper Leg<br>*See L Subcutaneous Tissue and Fascia, Right Upper Leg*<br>**N** Subcutaneous Tissue and Fascia, Right Lower Leg<br>**P** Subcutaneous Tissue and Fascia, Left Lower Leg | **Ø** Open<br>**3** Percutaneous | **H** Contraceptive Device<br>**N** Tissue Expander<br>**V** Infusion Device, Pump<br>**W** Vascular Access Device, Totally Implantable<br>**X** Vascular Access Device, Tunneled | **Z** No Qualifier |
| **S** Subcutaneous Tissue and Fascia, Head and Neck<br>**V** Subcutaneous Tissue and Fascia, Upper Extremity<br>**W** Subcutaneous Tissue and Fascia, Lower Extremity | **Ø** Open<br>**3** Percutaneous | **1** Radioactive Element<br>**3** Infusion Device<br>**Y** Other Device | **Z** No Qualifier |
| **T** Subcutaneous Tissue and Fascia, Trunk<br>External oblique aponeurosis<br>Transversalis fascia | **Ø** Open<br>**3** Percutaneous | **1** Radioactive Element<br>**3** Infusion Device<br>**V** Infusion Device, Pump<br>**Y** Other Device | **Z** No Qualifier |

DRG Non-OR ØJH6[Ø,3][4,5,6,H,W,X]Z
DRG Non-OR ØJH8[Ø,3][2,4,5,6,H,W,X]Z
DRG Non-OR ØJH[D,F,G,H,L,M][Ø,3][W,X]Z
DRG Non-OR ØJHNØ[W,X]Z
DRG Non-OR ØJHN3[H,W,X]Z
DRG Non-OR ØJHP[Ø,3][H,W,X]Z
Non-OR ØJH[D,F,G,H,L,M][Ø,3]HZ
Non-OR ØJHNØHZ
Non-OR ØJH[S,V,W][Ø,3][3,Y]Z
Non-OR ØJHT[Ø,3][3,Y]Z

HAC ØJH[6,8][Ø,3][4,5,6,7,8,9,P]Z when reported with SDx K68.11 or T81.4XXA or T82.6XXA or T82.7XXA
HAC ØJH63XZ when reported with SDx J95.811
NC ØJH8[Ø,3]MZ
NC ØJH7[Ø,3]MZ

**See Appendix L for Procedure Combinations**
⊞ ØJH[6,8][Ø,3][8,9,A,B,C,D,E]Z
⊞ ØJH7[Ø,3][B,C,D,E]Z

**Ø Medical and Surgical**
**J Subcutaneous Tissue and Fascia**
**J Inspection** Definition: Visually and/or manually exploring a body part

Explanation: Visual exploration may be performed with or without optical instrumentation. Manual exploration may be performed directly or through intervening body layers.

| Body Part Character 4 | Approach Character 5 | Device Character 6 | Qualifier Character 7 |
|---|---|---|---|
| **S Subcutaneous Tissue and Fascia, Head and Neck**<br>**T Subcutaneous Tissue and Fascia, Trunk**<br>External oblique aponeurosis<br>Transversalis fascia<br>**V Subcutaneous Tissue and Fascia, Upper Extremity**<br>**W Subcutaneous Tissue and Fascia, Lower Extremity** | **Ø** Open<br>**3** Percutaneous<br>**X** External | **Z** No Device | **Z** No Qualifier |

**Non-OR** All body part, approach, device, and qualifier values

**Ø Medical and Surgical**
**J Subcutaneous Tissue and Fascia**
**N Release** Definition: Freeing a body part from an abnormal physical constraint by cutting or by the use of force

Explanation: Some of the restraining tissue may be taken out but none of the body part is taken out

| Body Part Character 4 | Approach Character 5 | Device Character 6 | Qualifier Character 7 |
|---|---|---|---|
| **Ø Subcutaneous Tissue and Fascia, Scalp**<br>Galea aponeurotica<br>**1 Subcutaneous Tissue and Fascia, Face**<br>Masseteric fascia<br>Orbital fascia<br>**4 Subcutaneous Tissue and Fascia, Right Neck**<br>Deep cervical fascia<br>Pretracheal fascia<br>Prevertebral fascia<br>**5 Subcutaneous Tissue and Fascia, Left Neck**<br>***See*** *4 Subcutaneous Tissue and Fascia, Right Neck*<br>**6 Subcutaneous Tissue and Fascia, Chest**<br>Pectoral fascia<br>**7 Subcutaneous Tissue and Fascia, Back**<br>**8 Subcutaneous Tissue and Fascia, Abdomen**<br>**9 Subcutaneous Tissue and Fascia, Buttock**<br>**B Subcutaneous Tissue and Fascia, Perineum**<br>**C Subcutaneous Tissue and Fascia, Pelvic Region**<br>**D Subcutaneous Tissue and Fascia, Right Upper Arm**<br>Axillary fascia<br>Deltoid fascia<br>Infraspinatus fascia<br>Subscapular aponeurosis<br>Supraspinatus fascia<br>**F Subcutaneous Tissue and Fascia, Left Upper Arm**<br>***See*** *D Subcutaneous Tissue and Fascia, Right Upper Arm*<br>**G Subcutaneous Tissue and Fascia, Right Lower Arm**<br>Antebrachial fascia<br>Bicipital aponeurosis<br>**H Subcutaneous Tissue and Fascia, Left Lower Arm**<br>***See*** *G Subcutaneous Tissue and Fascia, Right Lower Arm*<br>**J Subcutaneous Tissue and Fascia, Right Hand**<br>Palmar fascia (aponeurosis)<br>**K Subcutaneous Tissue and Fascia, Left Hand**<br>***See*** *J Subcutaneous Tissue and Fascia, Right Hand*<br>**L Subcutaneous Tissue and Fascia, Right Upper Leg**<br>Crural fascia<br>Fascia lata<br>Iliac fascia<br>Iliotibial tract (band)<br>**M Subcutaneous Tissue and Fascia, Left Upper Leg**<br>***See*** *L Subcutaneous Tissue and Fascia, Right Upper Leg*<br>**N Subcutaneous Tissue and Fascia, Right Lower Leg**<br>**P Subcutaneous Tissue and Fascia, Left Lower Leg**<br>**Q Subcutaneous Tissue and Fascia, Right Foot**<br>Plantar fascia (aponeurosis)<br>**R Subcutaneous Tissue and Fascia, Left Foot**<br>***See*** *Q Subcutaneous Tissue and Fascia, Right Foot* | **Ø** Open<br>**3** Percutaneous<br>**X** External | **Z** No Device | **Z** No Qualifier |

**Non-OR** ØJN[Ø,1,4,5,6,7,8,9,B,C,D,F,G,H,J,K,L,M,N,P,Q,R]XZZ

**Ø Medical and Surgical**
**J Subcutaneous Tissue and Fascia**
**P Removal** Definition: Taking out or off a device from a body part

Explanation: If a device is taken out and a similar device put in without cutting or puncturing the skin or mucous membrane, the procedure is coded to the root operation CHANGE. Otherwise, the procedure for taking out a device is coded to the root operation REMOVAL.

| Body Part Character 4 | Approach Character 5 | Device Character 6 | Qualifier Character 7 |
|---|---|---|---|
| S Subcutaneous Tissue and Fascia, Head and Neck | Ø Open<br>3 Percutaneous | Ø Drainage Device<br>1 Radioactive Element<br>3 Infusion Device<br>7 Autologous Tissue Substitute<br>J Synthetic Substitute<br>K Nonautologous Tissue Substitute<br>N Tissue Expander<br>Y Other Device | Z No Qualifier |
| S Subcutaneous Tissue and Fascia, Head and Neck | X External | Ø Drainage Device<br>1 Radioactive Element<br>3 Infusion Device | Z No Qualifier |
| T Subcutaneous Tissue and Fascia, Trunk<br>External oblique aponeurosis<br>Transversalis fascia | Ø Open<br>3 Percutaneous | Ø Drainage Device<br>1 Radioactive Element<br>2 Monitoring Device<br>3 Infusion Device<br>7 Autologous Tissue Substitute<br>H Contraceptive Device<br>J Synthetic Substitute<br>K Nonautologous Tissue Substitute<br>M Stimulator Generator<br>N Tissue Expander<br>P Cardiac Rhythm Related Device<br>V Infusion Device, Pump<br>W Vascular Access Device, Totally Implantable<br>X Vascular Access Device, Tunneled<br>Y Other Device | Z No Qualifier |
| T Subcutaneous Tissue and Fascia, Trunk<br>External oblique aponeurosis<br>Transversalis fascia | X External | Ø Drainage Device<br>1 Radioactive Element<br>2 Monitoring Device<br>3 Infusion Device<br>H Contraceptive Device<br>V Infusion Device, Pump<br>X Vascular Access Device, Tunneled | Z No Qualifier |
| V Subcutaneous Tissue and Fascia, Upper Extremity<br>W Subcutaneous Tissue and Fascia, Lower Extremity | Ø Open<br>3 Percutaneous | Ø Drainage Device<br>1 Radioactive Element<br>3 Infusion Device<br>7 Autologous Tissue Substitute<br>H Contraceptive Device<br>J Synthetic Substitute<br>K Nonautologous Tissue Substitute<br>N Tissue Expander<br>V Infusion Device, Pump<br>W Vascular Access Device, Totally Implantable<br>X Vascular Access Device, Tunneled<br>Y Other Device | Z No Qualifier |
| V Subcutaneous Tissue and Fascia, Upper Extremity<br>W Subcutaneous Tissue and Fascia, Lower Extremity | X External | Ø Drainage Device<br>1 Radioactive Element<br>3 Infusion Device<br>H Contraceptive Device<br>V Infusion Device, Pump<br>X Vascular Access Device, Tunneled | Z No Qualifier |

**Non-OR** ØJPS[Ø,3][Ø,1,3,7,J,K,N,Y]Z
**Non-OR** ØJPSX[Ø,1,3]Z
**Non-OR** ØJPT[Ø,3][Ø,1,2,3,7,H,J,K,M,N,V,W,X,Y]Z
**Non-OR** ØJPTX[Ø,1,2,3,H,V,X]Z
**Non-OR** ØJP[V,W][Ø,3][Ø,1,3,7,H,J,K,N,V,W,X,Y]Z
**Non-OR** ØJP[V,W]X[Ø,1,3,H,V,X]Z
**HAC** ØJPT[Ø,3]PZ when reported with SDx K68.11 or T81.4XXA or T82.6XXA or T82.7XXA

**Ø Medical and Surgical**
**J Subcutaneous Tissue and Fascia**
**Q Repair** Definition: Restoring, to the extent possible, a body part to its normal anatomic structure and function
Explanation: Used only when the method to accomplish the repair is not one of the other root operations

| Body Part Character 4 | | Approach Character 5 | Device Character 6 | Qualifier Character 7 |
|---|---|---|---|---|
| **Ø Subcutaneous Tissue and Fascia, Scalp**<br>Galea aponeurotica<br>**1 Subcutaneous Tissue and Fascia, Face**<br>Masseteric fascia<br>Orbital fascia<br>**4 Subcutaneous Tissue and Fascia, Right Neck**<br>Deep cervical fascia<br>Pretracheal fascia<br>Prevertebral fascia<br>**5 Subcutaneous Tissue and Fascia, Left Neck**<br>*See 4 Subcutaneous Tissue and Fascia, Right Neck*<br>**6 Subcutaneous Tissue and Fascia, Chest**<br>Pectoral fascia<br>**7 Subcutaneous Tissue and Fascia, Back**<br>**8 Subcutaneous Tissue and Fascia, Abdomen**<br>**9 Subcutaneous Tissue and Fascia, Buttock**<br>**B Subcutaneous Tissue and Fascia, Perineum**<br>**C Subcutaneous Tissue and Fascia, Pelvic Region**<br>**D Subcutaneous Tissue and Fascia, Right Upper Arm**<br>Axillary fascia<br>Deltoid fascia<br>Infraspinatus fascia<br>Subscapular aponeurosis<br>Supraspinatus fascia<br>**F Subcutaneous Tissue and Fascia, Left Upper Arm**<br>*See D Subcutaneous Tissue and Fascia, Right Upper Arm* | **G Subcutaneous Tissue and Fascia, Right Lower Arm**<br>Antebrachial fascia<br>Bicipital aponeurosis<br>**H Subcutaneous Tissue and Fascia, Left Lower Arm**<br>*See G Subcutaneous Tissue and Fascia, Right Lower Arm*<br>**J Subcutaneous Tissue and Fascia, Right Hand**<br>Palmar fascia (aponeurosis)<br>**K Subcutaneous Tissue and Fascia, Left Hand**<br>*See J Subcutaneous Tissue and Fascia, Right Hand*<br>**L Subcutaneous Tissue and Fascia, Right Upper Leg**<br>Crural fascia<br>Fascia lata<br>Iliac fascia<br>Iliotibial tract (band)<br>**M Subcutaneous Tissue and Fascia, Left Upper Leg**<br>*See L Subcutaneous Tissue and Fascia, Right Upper Leg*<br>**N Subcutaneous Tissue and Fascia, Right Lower Leg**<br>**P Subcutaneous Tissue and Fascia, Left Lower Leg**<br>**Q Subcutaneous Tissue and Fascia, Right Foot**<br>Plantar fascia (aponeurosis)<br>**R Subcutaneous Tissue and Fascia, Left Foot**<br>*See Q Subcutaneous Tissue and Fascia, Right Foot* | **Ø Open**<br>**3 Percutaneous** | **Z No Device** | **Z No Qualifier** |

**Non-OR** All body part, approach, device, and qualifier values

**Ø Medical and Surgical**
**J Subcutaneous Tissue and Fascia**
**R Replacement** Definition: Putting in or on biological or synthetic material that physically takes the place and/or function of all or a portion of a body part

Explanation: The body part may have been taken out or replaced, or may be taken out, physically eradicated, or rendered nonfunctional during the REPLACEMENT procedure. A REMOVAL procedure is coded for taking out the device used in a previous replacement procedure.

| Body Part Character 4 | Approach Character 5 | Device Character 6 | Qualifier Character 7 |
|---|---|---|---|
| **Ø Subcutaneous Tissue and Fascia, Scalp** Galea aponeurotica<br>**1 Subcutaneous Tissue and Fascia, Face** Masseteric fascia; Orbital fascia<br>**4 Subcutaneous Tissue and Fascia, Right Neck** Deep cervical fascia; Pretracheal fascia; Prevertebral fascia<br>**5 Subcutaneous Tissue and Fascia, Left Neck** *See 4 Subcutaneous Tissue and Fascia, Right Neck*<br>**6 Subcutaneous Tissue and Fascia, Chest** Pectoral fascia<br>**7 Subcutaneous Tissue and Fascia, Back**<br>**8 Subcutaneous Tissue and Fascia, Abdomen**<br>**9 Subcutaneous Tissue and Fascia, Buttock**<br>**B Subcutaneous Tissue and Fascia, Perineum**<br>**C Subcutaneous Tissue and Fascia, Pelvic Region**<br>**D Subcutaneous Tissue and Fascia, Right Upper Arm** Axillary fascia; Deltoid fascia; Infraspinatus fascia; Subscapular aponeurosis; Supraspinatus fascia<br>**F Subcutaneous Tissue and Fascia, Left Upper Arm** *See D Subcutaneous Tissue and Fascia, Right Upper Arm*<br>**G Subcutaneous Tissue and Fascia, Right Lower Arm** Antebrachial fascia; Bicipital aponeurosis<br>**H Subcutaneous Tissue and Fascia, Left Lower Arm** *See G Subcutaneous Tissue and Fascia, Right Lower Arm*<br>**J Subcutaneous Tissue and Fascia, Right Hand** Palmar fascia (aponeurosis)<br>**K Subcutaneous Tissue and Fascia, Left Hand** *See J Subcutaneous Tissue and Fascia, Right Hand*<br>**L Subcutaneous Tissue and Fascia, Right Upper Leg** Crural fascia; Fascia lata; Iliac fascia; Iliotibial tract (band)<br>**M Subcutaneous Tissue and Fascia, Left Upper Leg** *See L Subcutaneous Tissue and Fascia, Right Upper Leg*<br>**N Subcutaneous Tissue and Fascia, Right Lower Leg**<br>**P Subcutaneous Tissue and Fascia, Left Lower Leg**<br>**Q Subcutaneous Tissue and Fascia, Right Foot** Plantar fascia (aponeurosis)<br>**R Subcutaneous Tissue and Fascia, Left Foot** *See Q Subcutaneous Tissue and Fascia, Right Foot* | **Ø Open**<br>**3 Percutaneous** | **7 Autologous Tissue Substitute**<br>**J Synthetic Substitute**<br>**K Nonautologous Tissue Substitute** | **Z No Qualifier** |

**Ø Medical and Surgical**
**J Subcutaneous Tissue and Fascia**
**U Supplement:** Definition: Putting in or on biological or synthetic material that physically reinforces and/or augments the function of a portion of a body part

Explanation: The biological material is non-living, or is living and from the same individual. The body part may have been previously replaced, and the SUPPLEMENT procedure is performed to physically reinforce and/or augment the function of the replaced body part.

| Body Part Character 4 | Approach Character 5 | Device Character 6 | Qualifier Character 7 |
|---|---|---|---|
| **Ø Subcutaneous Tissue and Fascia, Scalp** Galea aponeurotica<br>**1 Subcutaneous Tissue and Fascia, Face** Masseteric fascia; Orbital fascia<br>**4 Subcutaneous Tissue and Fascia, Right Neck** Deep cervical fascia; Pretracheal fascia; Prevertebral fascia<br>**5 Subcutaneous Tissue and Fascia, Left Neck** ***See*** *4 Subcutaneous Tissue and Fascia, Right Neck*<br>**6 Subcutaneous Tissue and Fascia, Chest** Pectoral fascia<br>**7 Subcutaneous Tissue and Fascia, Back**<br>**8 Subcutaneous Tissue and Fascia, Abdomen**<br>**9 Subcutaneous Tissue and Fascia, Buttock**<br>**B Subcutaneous Tissue and Fascia, Perineum**<br>**C Subcutaneous Tissue and Fascia, Pelvic Region**<br>**D Subcutaneous Tissue and Fascia, Right Upper Arm** Axillary fascia; Deltoid fascia; Infraspinatus fascia; Subscapular aponeurosis; Supraspinatus fascia<br>**F Subcutaneous Tissue and Fascia, Left Upper Arm** ***See*** *D Subcutaneous Tissue and Fascia, Right Upper Arm*<br>**G Subcutaneous Tissue and Fascia, Right Lower Arm** Antebrachial fascia; Bicipital aponeurosis<br>**H Subcutaneous Tissue and Fascia, Left Lower Arm** ***See*** *G Subcutaneous Tissue and Fascia, Right Lower Arm*<br>**J Subcutaneous Tissue and Fascia, Right Hand** Palmar fascia (aponeurosis)<br>**K Subcutaneous Tissue and Fascia, Left Hand** ***See*** *J Subcutaneous Tissue and Fascia, Right Hand*<br>**L Subcutaneous Tissue and Fascia, Right Upper Leg** Crural fascia; Fascia lata; Iliac fascia; Iliotibial tract (band)<br>**M Subcutaneous Tissue and Fascia, Left Upper Leg** ***See*** *L Subcutaneous Tissue and Fascia, Right Upper Leg*<br>**N Subcutaneous Tissue and Fascia, Right Lower Leg**<br>**P Subcutaneous Tissue and Fascia, Left Lower Leg**<br>**Q Subcutaneous Tissue and Fascia, Right Foot** Plantar fascia (aponeurosis)<br>**R Subcutaneous Tissue and Fascia, Left Foot** ***See*** *Q Subcutaneous Tissue and Fascia, Right Foot* | **Ø Open**<br>**3 Percutaneous** | **7 Autologous Tissue Substitute**<br>**J Synthetic Substitute**<br>**K Nonautologous Tissue Substitute** | **Z No Qualifier** |

**Ø Medical and Surgical**
**J Subcutaneous Tissue and Fascia**
**W Revision**

Definition: Correcting, to the extent possible, a portion of a malfunctioning device or the position of a displaced device

Explanation: Revision can include correcting a malfunctioning or displaced device by taking out or putting in components of the device such as a screw or pin

| Body Part Character 4 | Approach Character 5 | Device Character 6 | Qualifier Character 7 |
|---|---|---|---|
| S Subcutaneous Tissue and Fascia, Head and Neck | Ø Open<br>3 Percutaneous | Ø Drainage Device<br>3 Infusion Device<br>7 Autologous Tissue Substitute<br>J Synthetic Substitute<br>K Nonautologous Tissue Substitute<br>N Tissue Expander<br>Y Other Device | Z No Qualifier |
| S Subcutaneous Tissue and Fascia, Head and Neck | X External | Ø Drainage Device<br>3 Infusion Device<br>7 Autologous Tissue Substitute<br>J Synthetic Substitute<br>K Nonautologous Tissue Substitute<br>N Tissue Expander | Z No Qualifier |
| T Subcutaneous Tissue and Fascia, Trunk<br>External oblique aponeurosis<br>Transversalis fascia | Ø Open<br>3 Percutaneous | Ø Drainage Device<br>2 Monitoring Device<br>3 Infusion Device<br>7 Autologous Tissue Substitute<br>H Contraceptive Device<br>J Synthetic Substitute<br>K Nonautologous Tissue Substitute<br>M Stimulator Generator<br>N Tissue Expander<br>P Cardiac Rhythm Related Device<br>V Infusion Device, Pump<br>W Vascular Access Device, Totally Implantable<br>X Vascular Access Device, Tunneled<br>Y Other Device | Z No Qualifier |
| T Subcutaneous Tissue and Fascia, Trunk<br>External oblique aponeurosis<br>Transversalis fascia | X External | Ø Drainage Device<br>2 Monitoring Device<br>3 Infusion Device<br>7 Autologous Tissue Substitute<br>H Contraceptive Device<br>J Synthetic Substitute<br>K Nonautologous Tissue Substitute<br>M Stimulator Generator<br>N Tissue Expander<br>P Cardiac Rhythm Related Device<br>V Infusion Device, Pump<br>W Vascular Access Device, Totally Implantable<br>X Vascular Access Device, Tunneled | Z No Qualifier |
| V Subcutaneous Tissue and Fascia, Upper Extremity<br>W Subcutaneous Tissue and Fascia, Lower Extremity | Ø Open<br>3 Percutaneous | Ø Drainage Device<br>3 Infusion Device<br>7 Autologous Tissue Substitute<br>H Contraceptive Device<br>J Synthetic Substitute<br>K Nonautologous Tissue Substitute<br>N Tissue Expander<br>V Infusion Device, Pump<br>W Vascular Access Device, Totally Implantable<br>X Vascular Access Device, Tunneled<br>Y Other Device | Z No Qualifier |
| V Subcutaneous Tissue and Fascia, Upper Extremity<br>W Subcutaneous Tissue and Fascia, Lower Extremity | X External | Ø Drainage Device<br>3 Infusion Device<br>7 Autologous Tissue Substitute<br>H Contraceptive Device<br>J Synthetic Substitute<br>K Nonautologous Tissue Substitute<br>N Tissue Expander<br>V Infusion Device, Pump<br>W Vascular Access Device, Totally Implantable<br>X Vascular Access Device, Tunneled | Z No Qualifier |

DRG Non-OR ØJWS[Ø,3][Ø,3,7,J,K,N,Y]Z
DRG Non-OR ØJWT[Ø,3][Ø,3,7,H,J,K,N,V,W,X]Z
DRG Non-OR ØJW[V,W][Ø,3][Ø,3,7,H,J,K,N,V,W,X,Y]Z
Non-OR ØJWSX[Ø,3,7,J,K,N]Z
Non-OR ØJWT3YZ
Non-OR ØJWTX[Ø,2,3,7,H,J,K,N,P,V,W,X]Z
Non-OR ØJW[V,W]X[Ø,3,7,H,J,K,N,V,W,X]Z

HAC ØJWT[Ø,3]PZ when reported with SDx K68.11 or T81.4XXA or T82.6XXA or T82.7XXA

**Ø Medical and Surgical**
**J Subcutaneous Tissue and Fascia**
**X Transfer** Definition: Moving, without taking out, all or a portion of a body part to another location to take over the function of all or a portion of a body part
Explanation: The body part transferred remains connected to its vascular and nervous supply

| Body Part Character 4 | Approach Character 5 | Device Character 6 | Qualifier Character 7 |
|---|---|---|---|
| **Ø Subcutaneous Tissue and Fascia, Scalp** Galea aponeurotica<br>**1 Subcutaneous Tissue and Fascia, Face** Masseteric fascia; Orbital fascia<br>**4 Subcutaneous Tissue and Fascia, Right Neck** Deep cervical fascia; Pretracheal fascia; Prevertebral fascia<br>**5 Subcutaneous Tissue and Fascia, Left Neck** *See 4 Subcutaneous Tissue and Fascia, Right Neck*<br>**6 Subcutaneous Tissue and Fascia, Chest** Pectoral fascia<br>**7 Subcutaneous Tissue and Fascia, Back**<br>**8 Subcutaneous Tissue and Fascia, Abdomen**<br>**9 Subcutaneous Tissue and Fascia, Buttock**<br>**B Subcutaneous Tissue and Fascia, Perineum**<br>**C Subcutaneous Tissue and Fascia, Pelvic Region**<br>**D Subcutaneous Tissue and Fascia, Right Upper Arm** Axillary fascia; Deltoid fascia; Infraspinatus fascia; Subscapular aponeurosis; Supraspinatus fascia<br>**F Subcutaneous Tissue and Fascia, Left Upper Arm** *See D Subcutaneous Tissue and Fascia, Right Upper Arm*<br>**G Subcutaneous Tissue and Fascia, Right Lower Arm** Antebrachial fascia; Bicipital aponeurosis<br>**H Subcutaneous Tissue and Fascia, Left Lower Arm** *See G Subcutaneous Tissue and Fascia, Right Lower Arm*<br>**J Subcutaneous Tissue and Fascia, Right Hand** Palmar fascia (aponeurosis)<br>**K Subcutaneous Tissue and Fascia, Left Hand** *See J Subcutaneous Tissue and Fascia, Right Hand*<br>**L Subcutaneous Tissue and Fascia, Right Upper Leg** Crural fascia; Fascia lata; Iliac fascia; Iliotibial tract (band)<br>**M Subcutaneous Tissue and Fascia, Left Upper Leg** *See L Subcutaneous Tissue and Fascia, Right Upper Leg*<br>**N Subcutaneous Tissue and Fascia, Right Lower Leg**<br>**P Subcutaneous Tissue and Fascia, Left Lower Leg**<br>**Q Subcutaneous Tissue and Fascia, Right Foot** Plantar fascia (aponeurosis)<br>**R Subcutaneous Tissue and Fascia, Left Foot** *See Q Subcutaneous Tissue and Fascia, Right Foot* | **Ø Open**<br>**3 Percutaneous** | **Z No Device** | **B Skin and Subcutaneous Tissue**<br>**C Skin, Subcutaneous Tissue and Fascia**<br>**Z No Qualifier** |

# Muscles ØK2–ØKX

## Character Meanings

This Character Meaning table is provided as a guide to assist the user in the identification of character members that may be found in this section of code tables. It **SHOULD NOT** be used to build a PCS code.

| Operation–Character 3 | | Body Part–Character 4 | | Approach–Character 5 | | Device–Character 6 | | Qualifier–Character 7 | |
|---|---|---|---|---|---|---|---|---|---|
| 2 | Change | Ø | Head Muscle | Ø | Open | Ø | Drainage Device | Ø | Skin |
| 5 | Destruction | 1 | Facial Muscle | 3 | Percutaneous | 7 | Autologous Tissue Substitute | 1 | Subcutaneous Tissue |
| 8 | Division | 2 | Neck Muscle, Right | 4 | Percutaneous Endoscopic | J | Synthetic Substitute | 2 | Skin and Subcutaneous Tissue |
| 9 | Drainage | 3 | Neck Muscle, Left | X | External | K | Nonautologous Tissue Substitute | 5 | Latissimus Dorsi Myocutaneous Flap |
| B | Excision | 4 | Tongue, Palate, Pharynx Muscle | | | M | Stimulator Lead | 6 | Transverse Rectus Abdominis Myocutaneous Flap |
| C | Extirpation | 5 | Shoulder Muscle, Right | | | Y | Other Device | 7 | Deep Inferior Epigastric Artery Perforator Flap |
| D | Extraction | 6 | Shoulder Muscle, Left | | | Z | No Device | 8 | Superficial Inferior Epigastric Artery Flap |
| H | Insertion | 7 | Upper Arm Muscle, Right | | | | | 9 | Gluteal Artery Perforator Flap |
| J | Inspection | 8 | Upper Arm Muscle, Left | | | | | X | Diagnostic |
| M | Reattachment | 9 | Lower Arm and Wrist Muscle, Right | | | | | Z | No Qualifier |
| N | Release | B | Lower Arm and Wrist Muscle, Left | | | | | | |
| P | Removal | C | Hand Muscle, Right | | | | | | |
| Q | Repair | D | Hand Muscle, Left | | | | | | |
| R | Replacement | F | Trunk Muscle, Right | | | | | | |
| S | Reposition | G | Trunk Muscle, Left | | | | | | |
| T | Resection | H | Thorax Muscle, Right | | | | | | |
| U | Supplement | J | Thorax Muscle, Left | | | | | | |
| W | Revision | K | Abdomen Muscle, Right | | | | | | |
| X | Transfer | L | Abdomen Muscle, Left | | | | | | |
| | | M | Perineum Muscle | | | | | | |
| | | N | Hip Muscle, Right | | | | | | |
| | | P | Hip Muscle, Left | | | | | | |
| | | Q | Upper Leg Muscle, Right | | | | | | |
| | | R | Upper Leg Muscle, Left | | | | | | |
| | | S | Lower Leg Muscle, Right | | | | | | |
| | | T | Lower Leg Muscle, Left | | | | | | |
| | | V | Foot Muscle, Right | | | | | | |
| | | W | Foot Muscle, Left | | | | | | |
| | | X | Upper Muscle | | | | | | |
| | | Y | Lower Muscle | | | | | | |

**AHA Coding Clinic for table ØKB**

**2016, 3Q, 20** Excisional debridement of sacrum
**2015, 3Q, 3-8** Excisional and nonexcisional debridement

**AHA Coding Clinic for table ØKN**

**2017, 2Q, 12** Compartment syndrome and fasciotomy of foot
**2017, 2Q, 13** Compartment syndrome and fasciotomy of leg
**2015, 2Q, 22** Arthroscopic subacromial decompression
**2014, 4Q, 39** Abdominal component release with placement of mesh for hernia repair

**AHA Coding Clinic for table ØKQ**

**2016, 2Q, 34** Assisted vaginal delivery
**2016, 1Q, 7** Obstetrical perineal laceration repair
**2014, 4Q, 43** Second degree obstetric perineal laceration
**2013, 4Q, 120** Repair of second degree perineum obstetric laceration

**AHA Coding Clinic for table ØKS**

**2017, 1Q, 41** Manual reduction of hernia

**AHA Coding Clinic for table ØKT**

**2016, 2Q, 12** Resection of malignant neoplasm of infratemporal fossa
**2015, 1Q, 38** Abdominoperineal resection with flap closure of the perineum and colostomy

**AHA Coding Clinic for table ØKX**

**2016, 3Q, 30** Resection of femur with interposition arthroplasty
**2015, 3Q, 33** Cleft lip repair using Millard rotation advancement
**2015, 2Q, 26** Pharyngeal flap to soft palate
**2014, 4Q, 41** Abdominoperineal resection (APR) with flap closure of perineum and colostomy
**2014, 2Q, 10** Transverse abdominomyocutaneous (TRAM) breast reconstruction
**2014, 2Q, 12** Pedicle latissimus myocutaneous flap with placement of breast tissue expanders

# Muscles

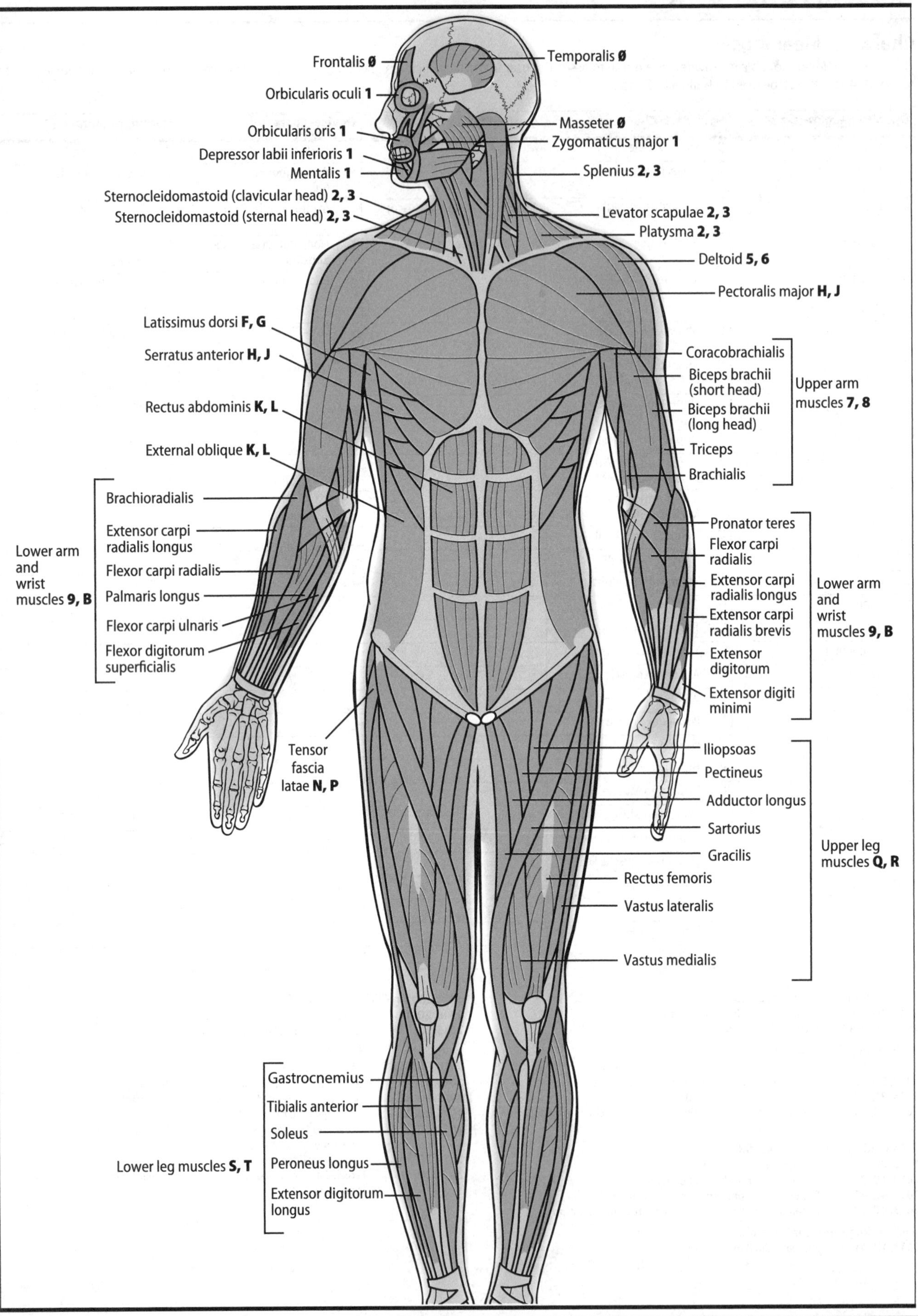
Frontalis Ø
Temporalis Ø
Orbicularis oculi 1
Masseter Ø
Orbicularis oris 1
Zygomaticus major 1
Depressor labii inferioris 1
Mentalis 1
Splenius 2, 3
Sternocleidomastoid (clavicular head) 2, 3
Sternocleidomastoid (sternal head) 2, 3
Levator scapulae 2, 3
Platysma 2, 3
Deltoid 5, 6
Pectoralis major H, J
Latissimus dorsi F, G
Serratus anterior H, J
Coracobrachialis
Biceps brachii (short head)
Biceps brachii (long head)
Triceps
Brachialis
Upper arm muscles 7, 8
Rectus abdominis K, L
External oblique K, L
Brachioradialis
Extensor carpi radialis longus
Flexor carpi radialis
Palmaris longus
Flexor carpi ulnaris
Flexor digitorum superficialis
Lower arm and wrist muscles 9, B
Pronator teres
Flexor carpi radialis
Extensor carpi radialis longus
Extensor carpi radialis brevis
Extensor digitorum
Extensor digiti minimi
Lower arm and wrist muscles 9, B
Tensor fascia latae N, P
Iliopsoas
Pectineus
Adductor longus
Sartorius
Gracilis
Rectus femoris
Vastus lateralis
Vastus medialis
Upper leg muscles Q, R
Gastrocnemius
Tibialis anterior
Soleus
Peroneus longus
Extensor digitorum longus
Lower leg muscles S, T

**Ø Medical and Surgical**
**K Muscles**
**2 Change** Definition: Taking out or off a device from a body part and putting back an identical or similar device in or on the same body part without cutting or puncturing the skin or a mucous membrane

Explanation: All CHANGE procedures are coded using the approach EXTERNAL

| Body Part Character 4 | Approach Character 5 | Device Character 6 | Qualifier Character 7 |
|---|---|---|---|
| X Upper Muscle<br>Y Lower Muscle | X External | Ø Drainage Device<br>Y Other Device | Z No Qualifier |

Non-OR All body part, approach, device, and qualifier values

**Ø Medical and Surgical**
**K Muscles**
**5 Destruction** Definition: Physical eradication of all or a portion of a body part by the direct use of energy, force, or a destructive agent

Explanation: None of the body part is physically taken out

| Body Part Character 4 | Approach Character 5 | Device Character 6 | Qualifier Character 7 |
|---|---|---|---|
| **Ø Head Muscle**<br>Auricularis muscle<br>Masseter muscle<br>Pterygoid muscle<br>Splenius capitis muscle<br>Temporalis muscle<br>Temporoparietalis muscle<br>**1 Facial Muscle**<br>Buccinator muscle<br>Corrugator supercilii muscle<br>Depressor anguli oris muscle<br>Depressor labii inferioris muscle<br>Depressor septi nasi muscle<br>Depressor supercilii muscle<br>Levator anguli oris muscle<br>Levator labii superioris alaeque nasi muscle<br>Levator labii superioris muscle<br>Mentalis muscle<br>Nasalis muscle<br>Occipitofrontalis muscle<br>Orbicularis oris muscle<br>Procerus muscle<br>Risorius muscle<br>Zygomaticus muscle<br>**2 Neck Muscle, Right**<br>Anterior vertebral muscle<br>Arytenoid muscle<br>Cricothyroid muscle<br>Infrahyoid muscle<br>Levator scapulae muscle<br>Platysma muscle<br>Scalene muscle<br>Splenius cervicis muscle<br>Sternocleidomastoid muscle<br>Suprahyoid muscle<br>Thyroarytenoid muscle<br>**3 Neck Muscle, Left**<br>*See 2 Neck Muscle, Right*<br>**4 Tongue, Palate, Pharynx Muscle**<br>Chondroglossus muscle<br>Genioglossus muscle<br>Hyoglossus muscle<br>Inferior longitudinal muscle<br>Levator veli palatini muscle<br>Palatoglossal muscle<br>Palatopharyngeal muscle<br>Pharyngeal constrictor muscle<br>Salpingopharyngeus muscle<br>Styloglossus muscle<br>Stylopharyngeus muscle<br>Superior longitudinal muscle<br>Tensor veli palatini muscle<br>**5 Shoulder Muscle, Right**<br>Deltoid muscle<br>Infraspinatus muscle<br>Subscapularis muscle<br>Supraspinatus muscle<br>Teres major muscle<br>Teres minor muscle<br>**6 Shoulder Muscle, Left**<br>*See 5 Shoulder Muscle, Right*<br>**7 Upper Arm Muscle, Right**<br>Biceps brachii muscle<br>Brachialis muscle<br>Coracobrachialis muscle<br>Triceps brachii muscle<br>**8 Upper Arm Muscle, Left**<br>*See 7 Upper Arm Muscle, Right*<br>**9 Lower Arm and Wrist Muscle, Right**<br>Anatomical snuffbox<br>Brachioradialis muscle<br>Extensor carpi radialis muscle<br>Extensor carpi ulnaris muscle<br>Flexor carpi radialis muscle<br>Flexor carpi ulnaris muscle<br>Flexor pollicis longus muscle<br>Palmaris longus muscle<br>Pronator quadratus muscle<br>Pronator teres muscle<br>**B Lower Arm and Wrist Muscle, Left**<br>*See 9 Lower Arm and Wrist Muscle, Right*<br>**C Hand Muscle, Right**<br>Hypothenar muscle<br>Palmar interosseous muscle<br>Thenar muscle<br>**D Hand Muscle, Left**<br>*See C Hand Muscle, Right*<br>**F Trunk Muscle, Right**<br>Coccygeus muscle<br>Erector spinae muscle<br>Interspinalis muscle<br>Intertransversarius muscle<br>Latissimus dorsi muscle<br>Quadratus lumborum muscle<br>Rhomboid major muscle<br>Rhomboid minor muscle<br>Serratus posterior muscle<br>Transversospinalis muscle<br>Trapezius muscle<br>**G Trunk Muscle, Left**<br>*See F Trunk Muscle, Right*<br>**H Thorax Muscle, Right**<br>Intercostal muscle<br>Levatores costarum muscle<br>Pectoralis major muscle<br>Pectoralis minor muscle<br>Serratus anterior muscle<br>Subclavius muscle<br>Subcostal muscle<br>Transverse thoracis muscle<br>**J Thorax Muscle, Left**<br>*See H Thorax Muscle, Right*<br>**K Abdomen Muscle, Right**<br>External oblique muscle<br>Internal oblique muscle<br>Pyramidalis muscle<br>Rectus abdominis muscle<br>Transversus abdominis muscle<br>**L Abdomen Muscle, Left**<br>*See K Abdomen Muscle, Right*<br>**M Perineum Muscle**<br>Bulbospongiosus muscle<br>Cremaster muscle<br>Deep transverse perineal muscle<br>Ischiocavernosus muscle<br>Levator ani muscle<br>Superficial transverse perineal muscle<br>**N Hip Muscle, Right**<br>Gemellus muscle<br>Gluteus maximus muscle<br>Gluteus medius muscle<br>Gluteus minimus muscle<br>Iliacus muscle<br>Obturator muscle<br>Piriformis muscle<br>Psoas muscle<br>Quadratus femoris muscle<br>Tensor fasciae latae muscle<br>**P Hip Muscle, Left**<br>*See N Hip Muscle, Right*<br>**Q Upper Leg Muscle, Right**<br>Adductor brevis muscle<br>Adductor longus muscle<br>Adductor magnus muscle<br>Biceps femoris muscle<br>Gracilis muscle<br>Pectineus muscle<br>Quadriceps (femoris)<br>Rectus femoris muscle<br>Sartorius muscle<br>Semimembranosus muscle<br>Semitendinosus muscle<br>Vastus intermedius muscle<br>Vastus lateralis muscle<br>Vastus medialis muscle<br>**R Upper Leg Muscle, Left**<br>*See Q Upper Leg Muscle, Right*<br>**S Lower Leg Muscle, Right**<br>Extensor digitorum longus muscle<br>Extensor hallucis longus muscle<br>Fibularis brevis muscle<br>Fibularis longus muscle<br>Flexor digitorum longus muscle<br>Flexor hallucis longus muscle<br>Gastrocnemius muscle<br>Peroneus brevis muscle<br>Peroneus longus muscle<br>Popliteus muscle<br>Soleus muscle<br>Tibialis anterior muscle<br>Tibialis posterior muscle<br>**T Lower Leg Muscle, Left**<br>*See S Lower Leg Muscle, Right*<br>**V Foot Muscle, Right**<br>Abductor hallucis muscle<br>Adductor hallucis muscle<br>Extensor digitorum brevis muscle<br>Extensor hallucis brevis muscle<br>Flexor digitorum brevis muscle<br>Flexor hallucis brevis muscle<br>Quadratus plantae muscle<br>**W Foot Muscle, Left**<br>*See V Foot Muscle, Right* | Ø Open<br>3 Percutaneous<br>4 Percutaneous Endoscopic | Z No Device | Z No Qualifier |

**Ø Medical and Surgical**
**K Muscles**
**8 Division** Definition: Cutting into a body part, without draining fluids and/or gases from the body part, in order to separate or transect a body part
Explanation: All or a portion of the body part is separated into two or more portions

| Body Part Character 4 | Approach Character 5 | Device Character 6 | Qualifier Character 7 |
|---|---|---|---|
| **Ø Head Muscle**<br>Auricularis muscle<br>Masseter muscle<br>Pterygoid muscle<br>Splenius capitis muscle<br>Temporalis muscle<br>Temporoparietalis muscle | **Ø Open** | **Z No Device** | **Z No Qualifier** |
| **1 Facial Muscle**<br>Buccinator muscle<br>Corrugator supercilii muscle<br>Depressor anguli oris muscle<br>Depressor labii inferioris muscle<br>Depressor septi nasi muscle<br>Depressor supercilii muscle<br>Levator anguli oris muscle<br>Levator labii superioris alaeque nasi muscle<br>Levator labii superioris muscle<br>Mentalis muscle<br>Nasalis muscle<br>Occipitofrontalis muscle<br>Orbicularis oris muscle<br>Procerus muscle<br>Risorius muscle<br>Zygomaticus muscle | **3 Percutaneous** | | |
| **2 Neck Muscle, Right**<br>Anterior vertebral muscle<br>Arytenoid muscle<br>Cricothyroid muscle<br>Infrahyoid muscle<br>Levator scapulae muscle<br>Platysma muscle<br>Scalene muscle<br>Splenius cervicis muscle<br>Sternocleidomastoid muscle<br>Suprahyoid muscle<br>Thyroarytenoid muscle | **4 Percutaneous Endoscopic** | | |
| **3 Neck Muscle, Left**<br>*See 2 Neck Muscle, Right* | | | |
| **4 Tongue, Palate, Pharynx Muscle**<br>Chondroglossus muscle<br>Genioglossus muscle<br>Hyoglossus muscle<br>Inferior longitudinal muscle<br>Levator veli palatini muscle<br>Palatoglossal muscle<br>Palatopharyngeal muscle<br>Pharyngeal constrictor muscle<br>Salpingopharyngeus muscle<br>Styloglossus muscle<br>Stylopharyngeus muscle<br>Superior longitudinal muscle<br>Tensor veli palatini muscle | | | |
| **5 Shoulder Muscle, Right**<br>Deltoid muscle<br>Infraspinatus muscle<br>Subscapularis muscle<br>Supraspinatus muscle<br>Teres major muscle<br>Teres minor muscle | | | |
| **6 Shoulder Muscle, Left**<br>*See 5 Shoulder Muscle, Right* | | | |
| **7 Upper Arm Muscle, Right**<br>Biceps brachii muscle<br>Brachialis muscle<br>Coracobrachialis muscle<br>Triceps brachii muscle | | | |
| **8 Upper Arm Muscle, Left**<br>*See 7 Upper Arm Muscle, Right* | | | |
| **9 Lower Arm and Wrist Muscle, Right**<br>Anatomical snuffbox<br>Brachioradialis muscle<br>Extensor carpi radialis muscle<br>Extensor carpi ulnaris muscle<br>Flexor carpi radialis muscle<br>Flexor carpi ulnaris muscle<br>Flexor pollicis longus muscle<br>Palmaris longus muscle<br>Pronator quadratus muscle<br>Pronator teres muscle | | | |
| **B Lower Arm and Wrist Muscle, Left**<br>*See 9 Lower Arm and Wrist Muscle, Right* | | | |
| **C Hand Muscle, Right**<br>Hypothenar muscle<br>Palmar interosseous muscle<br>Thenar muscle | | | |
| **D Hand Muscle, Left**<br>*See C Hand Muscle, Right* | | | |
| **F Trunk Muscle, Right**<br>Coccygeus muscle<br>Erector spinae muscle<br>Interspinalis muscle<br>Intertransversarius muscle<br>Latissimus dorsi muscle<br>Quadratus lumborum muscle<br>Rhomboid major muscle<br>Rhomboid minor muscle<br>Serratus posterior muscle<br>Transversospinalis muscle<br>Trapezius muscle | | | |
| **G Trunk Muscle, Left**<br>*See F Trunk Muscle, Right* | | | |
| **H Thorax Muscle, Right**<br>Intercostal muscle<br>Levatores costarum muscle<br>Pectoralis major muscle<br>Pectoralis minor muscle<br>Serratus anterior muscle<br>Subclavius muscle<br>Subcostal muscle<br>Transverse thoracis muscle | | | |
| **J Thorax Muscle, Left**<br>*See H Thorax Muscle, Right* | | | |
| **K Abdomen Muscle, Right**<br>External oblique muscle<br>Internal oblique muscle<br>Pyramidalis muscle<br>Rectus abdominis muscle<br>Transversus abdominis muscle | | | |
| **L Abdomen Muscle, Left**<br>*See K Abdomen Muscle, Right* | | | |
| **M Perineum Muscle**<br>Bulbospongiosus muscle<br>Cremaster muscle<br>Deep transverse perineal muscle<br>Ischiocavernosus muscle<br>Levator ani muscle<br>Superficial transverse perineal muscle | | | |
| **N Hip Muscle, Right**<br>Gemellus muscle<br>Gluteus maximus muscle<br>Gluteus medius muscle<br>Gluteus minimus muscle<br>Iliacus muscle<br>Obturator muscle<br>Piriformis muscle<br>Psoas muscle<br>Quadratus femoris muscle<br>Tensor fasciae latae muscle | | | |
| **P Hip Muscle, Left**<br>*See N Hip Muscle, Right* | | | |
| **Q Upper Leg Muscle, Right**<br>Adductor brevis muscle<br>Adductor longus muscle<br>Adductor magnus muscle<br>Biceps femoris muscle<br>Gracilis muscle<br>Pectineus muscle<br>Quadriceps (femoris)<br>Rectus femoris muscle<br>Sartorius muscle<br>Semimembranosus muscle<br>Semitendinosus muscle<br>Vastus intermedius muscle<br>Vastus lateralis muscle<br>Vastus medialis muscle | | | |
| **R Upper Leg Muscle, Left**<br>*See Q Upper Leg Muscle, Right* | | | |
| **S Lower Leg Muscle, Right**<br>Extensor digitorum longus muscle<br>Extensor hallucis longus muscle<br>Fibularis brevis muscle<br>Fibularis longus muscle<br>Flexor digitorum longus muscle<br>Flexor hallucis longus muscle<br>Gastrocnemius muscle<br>Peroneus brevis muscle<br>Peroneus longus muscle<br>Popliteus muscle<br>Soleus muscle<br>Tibialis anterior muscle<br>Tibialis posterior muscle | | | |
| **T Lower Leg Muscle, Left**<br>*See S Lower Leg Muscle, Right* | | | |
| **V Foot Muscle, Right**<br>Abductor hallucis muscle<br>Adductor hallucis muscle<br>Extensor digitorum brevis muscle<br>Extensor hallucis brevis muscle<br>Flexor digitorum brevis muscle<br>Flexor hallucis brevis muscle<br>Quadratus plantae muscle | | | |
| **W Foot Muscle, Left**<br>*See V Foot Muscle, Right* | | | |

**Ø Medical and Surgical**
**K Muscles**
**9 Drainage** Definition: Taking or letting out fluids and/or gases from a body part
Explanation: The qualifier DIAGNOSTIC is used to identify drainage procedures that are biopsies

| Body Part Character 4 | Approach Character 5 | Device Character 6 | Qualifier Character 7 |
|---|---|---|---|
| **Ø Head Muscle**<br>Auricularis muscle<br>Masseter muscle<br>Pterygoid muscle<br>Splenius capitis muscle<br>Temporalis muscle<br>Temporoparietalis muscle<br>**1 Facial Muscle**<br>Buccinator muscle<br>Corrugator supercilii muscle<br>Depressor anguli oris muscle<br>Depressor labii inferioris muscle<br>Depressor septi nasi muscle<br>Depressor supercilii muscle<br>Levator anguli oris muscle<br>Levator labii superioris alaeque nasi muscle<br>Levator labii superioris muscle<br>Mentalis muscle<br>Nasalis muscle<br>Occipitofrontalis muscle<br>Orbicularis oris muscle<br>Procerus muscle<br>Risorius muscle<br>Zygomaticus muscle<br>**2 Neck Muscle, Right**<br>Anterior vertebral muscle<br>Arytenoid muscle<br>Cricothyroid muscle<br>Infrahyoid muscle<br>Levator scapulae muscle<br>Platysma muscle<br>Scalene muscle<br>Splenius cervicis muscle<br>Sternocleidomastoid muscle<br>Suprahyoid muscle<br>Thyroarytenoid muscle<br>**3 Neck Muscle, Left**<br>*See 2 Neck Muscle, Right*<br>**4 Tongue, Palate, Pharynx Muscle**<br>Chondroglossus muscle<br>Genioglossus muscle<br>Hyoglossus muscle<br>Inferior longitudinal muscle<br>Levator veli palatini muscle<br>Palatoglossal muscle<br>Palatopharyngeal muscle<br>Pharyngeal constrictor muscle<br>Salpingopharyngeus muscle<br>Styloglossus muscle<br>Stylopharyngeus muscle<br>Superior longitudinal muscle<br>Tensor veli palatini muscle<br>**5 Shoulder Muscle, Right**<br>Deltoid muscle<br>Infraspinatus muscle<br>Subscapularis muscle<br>Supraspinatus muscle<br>Teres major muscle<br>Teres minor muscle<br>**6 Shoulder Muscle, Left**<br>*See 5 Shoulder Muscle, Right*<br>**7 Upper Arm Muscle, Right**<br>Biceps brachii muscle<br>Brachialis muscle<br>Coracobrachialis muscle<br>Triceps brachii muscle<br>**8 Upper Arm Muscle, Left**<br>*See 7 Upper Arm Muscle, Right*<br>**9 Lower Arm and Wrist Muscle, Right**<br>Anatomical snuffbox<br>Brachioradialis muscle<br>Extensor carpi radialis muscle<br>Extensor carpi ulnaris muscle<br>Flexor carpi radialis muscle<br>Flexor carpi ulnaris muscle<br>Flexor pollicis longus muscle<br>Palmaris longus muscle<br>Pronator quadratus muscle<br>Pronator teres muscle<br>**B Lower Arm and Wrist Muscle, Left**<br>*See 9 Lower Arm and Wrist Muscle, Right*<br>**C Hand Muscle, Right**<br>Hypothenar muscle<br>Palmar interosseous muscle<br>Thenar muscle<br>**D Hand Muscle, Left**<br>*See C Hand Muscle, Right*<br>**F Trunk Muscle, Right**<br>Coccygeus muscle<br>Erector spinae muscle<br>Interspinalis muscle<br>Intertransversarius muscle<br>Latissimus dorsi muscle<br>Quadratus lumborum muscle<br>Rhomboid major muscle<br>Rhomboid minor muscle<br>Serratus posterior muscle<br>Transversospinalis muscle<br>Trapezius muscle<br>**G Trunk Muscle, Left**<br>*See F Trunk Muscle, Right*<br>**H Thorax Muscle, Right**<br>Intercostal muscle<br>Levatores costarum muscle<br>Pectoralis major muscle<br>Pectoralis minor muscle<br>Serratus anterior muscle<br>Subclavius muscle<br>Subcostal muscle<br>Transverse thoracis muscle<br>**J Thorax Muscle, Left**<br>*See H Thorax Muscle, Right*<br>**K Abdomen Muscle, Right**<br>External oblique muscle<br>Internal oblique muscle<br>Pyramidalis muscle<br>Rectus abdominis muscle<br>Transversus abdominis muscle<br>**L Abdomen Muscle, Left**<br>*See K Abdomen Muscle, Right*<br>**M Perineum Muscle**<br>Bulbospongiosus muscle<br>Cremaster muscle<br>Deep transverse perineal muscle<br>Ischiocavernosus muscle<br>Levator ani muscle<br>Superficial transverse perineal muscle<br>**N Hip Muscle, Right**<br>Gemellus muscle<br>Gluteus maximus muscle<br>Gluteus medius muscle<br>Gluteus minimus muscle<br>Iliacus muscle<br>Obturator muscle<br>Piriformis muscle<br>Psoas muscle<br>Quadratus femoris muscle<br>Tensor fasciae latae muscle<br>**P Hip Muscle, Left**<br>*See N Hip Muscle, Right*<br>**Q Upper Leg Muscle, Right**<br>Adductor brevis muscle<br>Adductor longus muscle<br>Adductor magnus muscle<br>Biceps femoris muscle<br>Gracilis muscle<br>Pectineus muscle<br>Quadriceps (femoris)<br>Rectus femoris muscle<br>Sartorius muscle<br>Semimembranosus muscle<br>Semitendinosus muscle<br>Vastus intermedius muscle<br>Vastus lateralis muscle<br>Vastus medialis muscle<br>**R Upper Leg Muscle, Left**<br>*See Q Upper Leg Muscle, Right*<br>**S Lower Leg Muscle, Right**<br>Extensor digitorum longus muscle<br>Extensor hallucis longus muscle<br>Fibularis brevis muscle<br>Fibularis longus muscle<br>Flexor digitorum longus muscle<br>Flexor hallucis longus muscle<br>Gastrocnemius muscle<br>Peroneus brevis muscle<br>Peroneus longus muscle<br>Popliteus muscle<br>Soleus muscle<br>Tibialis anterior muscle<br>Tibialis posterior muscle<br>**T Lower Leg Muscle, Left**<br>*See S Lower Leg Muscle, Right*<br>**V Foot Muscle, Right**<br>Abductor hallucis muscle<br>Adductor hallucis muscle<br>Extensor digitorum brevis muscle<br>Extensor hallucis brevis muscle<br>Flexor digitorum brevis muscle<br>Flexor hallucis brevis muscle<br>Quadratus plantae muscle<br>**W Foot Muscle, Left**<br>*See V Foot Muscle, Right* | **Ø Open**<br>**3 Percutaneous**<br>**4 Percutaneous Endoscopic** | **Ø Drainage Device** | **Z No Qualifier** |

**Non-OR** ØK9[Ø,1,2,3,4,5,6,7,8,9,B,C,D,F,G,H,J,K,L,M,N,P,Q,R,S,T,V,W]3ØZ

ØK9 Continued on next page

**ØK9 Continued**

**Ø Medical and Surgical**
**K Muscles**
**9 Drainage** Definition: Taking or letting out fluids and/or gases from a body part

Explanation: The qualifier DIAGNOSTIC is used to identify drainage procedures that are biopsies

| Body Part Character 4 | Approach Character 5 | Device Character 6 | Qualifier Character 7 |
|---|---|---|---|
| **Ø Head Muscle**<br>Auricularis muscle<br>Masseter muscle<br>Pterygoid muscle<br>Splenius capitis muscle<br>Temporalis muscle<br>Temporoparietalis muscle<br>**1 Facial Muscle**<br>Buccinator muscle<br>Corrugator supercilii muscle<br>Depressor anguli oris muscle<br>Depressor labii inferioris muscle<br>Depressor septi nasi muscle<br>Depressor supercilii muscle<br>Levator anguli oris muscle<br>Levator labii superioris alaeque nasi muscle<br>Levator labii superioris muscle<br>Mentalis muscle<br>Nasalis muscle<br>Occipitofrontalis muscle<br>Orbicularis oris muscle<br>Procerus muscle<br>Risorius muscle<br>Zygomaticus muscle<br>**2 Neck Muscle, Right**<br>Anterior vertebral muscle<br>Arytenoid muscle<br>Cricothyroid muscle<br>Infrahyoid muscle<br>Levator scapulae muscle<br>Platysma muscle<br>Scalene muscle<br>Splenius cervicis muscle<br>Sternocleidomastoid muscle<br>Suprahyoid muscle<br>Thyroarytenoid muscle<br>**3 Neck Muscle, Left**<br>*See 2 Neck Muscle, Right*<br>**4 Tongue, Palate, Pharynx Muscle**<br>Chondroglossus muscle<br>Genioglossus muscle<br>Hyoglossus muscle<br>Inferior longitudinal muscle<br>Levator veli palatini muscle<br>Palatoglossal muscle<br>Palatopharyngeal muscle<br>Pharyngeal constrictor muscle<br>Salpingopharyngeus muscle<br>Styloglossus muscle<br>Stylopharyngeus muscle<br>Superior longitudinal muscle<br>Tensor veli palatini muscle<br>**5 Shoulder Muscle, Right**<br>Deltoid muscle<br>Infraspinatus muscle<br>Subscapularis muscle<br>Supraspinatus muscle<br>Teres major muscle<br>Teres minor muscle<br>**6 Shoulder Muscle, Left**<br>*See 5 Shoulder Muscle, Right*<br>**7 Upper Arm Muscle, Right**<br>Biceps brachii muscle<br>Brachialis muscle<br>Coracobrachialis muscle<br>Triceps brachii muscle<br>**8 Upper Arm Muscle, Left**<br>*See 7 Upper Arm Muscle, Right*<br>**9 Lower Arm and Wrist Muscle, Right**<br>Anatomical snuffbox<br>Brachioradialis muscle<br>Extensor carpi radialis muscle<br>Extensor carpi ulnaris muscle<br>Flexor carpi radialis muscle<br>Flexor carpi ulnaris muscle<br>Flexor pollicis longus muscle<br>Palmaris longus muscle<br>Pronator quadratus muscle<br>Pronator teres muscle<br>**B Lower Arm and Wrist Muscle, Left**<br>*See 9 Lower Arm and Wrist Muscle, Right*<br>**C Hand Muscle, Right**<br>Hypothenar muscle<br>Palmar interosseous muscle<br>Thenar muscle<br>**D Hand Muscle, Left**<br>*See C Hand Muscle, Right*<br>**F Trunk Muscle, Right**<br>Coccygeus muscle<br>Erector spinae muscle<br>Interspinalis muscle<br>Intertransversarius muscle<br>Latissimus dorsi muscle<br>Quadratus lumborum muscle<br>Rhomboid major muscle<br>Rhomboid minor muscle<br>Serratus posterior muscle<br>Transversospinalis muscle<br>Trapezius muscle<br>**G Trunk Muscle, Left**<br>*See F Trunk Muscle, Right*<br>**H Thorax Muscle, Right**<br>Intercostal muscle<br>Levatores costarum muscle<br>Pectoralis major muscle<br>Pectoralis minor muscle<br>Serratus anterior muscle<br>Subclavius muscle<br>Subcostal muscle<br>Transverse thoracis muscle<br>**J Thorax Muscle, Left**<br>*See H Thorax Muscle, Right*<br>**K Abdomen Muscle, Right**<br>External oblique muscle<br>Internal oblique muscle<br>Pyramidalis muscle<br>Rectus abdominis muscle<br>Transversus abdominis muscle<br>**L Abdomen Muscle, Left**<br>*See K Abdomen Muscle, Right*<br>**M Perineum Muscle**<br>Bulbospongiosus muscle<br>Cremaster muscle<br>Deep transverse perineal muscle<br>Ischiocavernosus muscle<br>Levator ani muscle<br>Superficial transverse perineal muscle<br>**N Hip Muscle, Right**<br>Gemellus muscle<br>Gluteus maximus muscle<br>Gluteus medius muscle<br>Gluteus minimus muscle<br>Iliacus muscle<br>Obturator muscle<br>Piriformis muscle<br>Psoas muscle<br>Quadratus femoris muscle<br>Tensor fasciae latae muscle<br>**P Hip Muscle, Left**<br>*See N Hip Muscle, Right*<br>**Q Upper Leg Muscle, Right**<br>Adductor brevis muscle<br>Adductor longus muscle<br>Adductor magnus muscle<br>Biceps femoris muscle<br>Gracilis muscle<br>Pectineus muscle<br>Quadriceps (femoris)<br>Rectus femoris muscle<br>Sartorius muscle<br>Semimembranosus muscle<br>Semitendinosus muscle<br>Vastus intermedius muscle<br>Vastus lateralis muscle<br>Vastus medialis muscle<br>**R Upper Leg Muscle, Left**<br>*See Q Upper Leg Muscle, Right*<br>**S Lower Leg Muscle, Right**<br>Extensor digitorum longus muscle<br>Extensor hallucis longus muscle<br>Fibularis brevis muscle<br>Fibularis longus muscle<br>Flexor digitorum longus muscle<br>Flexor hallucis longus muscle<br>Gastrocnemius muscle<br>Peroneus brevis muscle<br>Peroneus longus muscle<br>Popliteus muscle<br>Soleus muscle<br>Tibialis anterior muscle<br>Tibialis posterior muscle<br>**T Lower Leg Muscle, Left**<br>*See S Lower Leg Muscle, Right*<br>**V Foot Muscle, Right**<br>Abductor hallucis muscle<br>Adductor hallucis muscle<br>Extensor digitorum brevis muscle<br>Extensor hallucis brevis muscle<br>Flexor digitorum brevis muscle<br>Flexor hallucis brevis muscle<br>Quadratus plantae muscle<br>**W Foot Muscle, Left**<br>*See V Foot Muscle, Right* | **Ø Open**<br>**3 Percutaneous**<br>**4 Percutaneous Endoscopic** | **Z No Device** | **X Diagnostic**<br>**Z No Qualifier** |

**Non-OR** ØK9[Ø,1,2,3,4,5,6,7,8,9,B,C,D,F,G,H,J,K,L,M,N,P,Q,R,S,T,V,W]3ZZ
**Non-OR** ØK9[C,D][3,4]ZZ

**Ø Medical and Surgical**
**K Muscles**
**B Excision**

Definition: Cutting out or off, without replacement, a portion of a body part

Explanation: The qualifier DIAGNOSTIC is used to identify excision procedures that are biopsies

| Body Part Character 4 | Approach Character 5 | Device Character 6 | Qualifier Character 7 |
|---|---|---|---|
| **Ø Head Muscle**<br>Auricularis muscle<br>Masseter muscle<br>Pterygoid muscle<br>Splenius capitis muscle<br>Temporalis muscle<br>Temporoparietalis muscle<br>**1 Facial Muscle**<br>Buccinator muscle<br>Corrugator supercilii muscle<br>Depressor anguli oris muscle<br>Depressor labii inferioris muscle<br>Depressor septi nasi muscle<br>Depressor supercilii muscle<br>Levator anguli oris muscle<br>Levator labii superioris alaeque nasi muscle<br>Levator labii superioris muscle<br>Mentalis muscle<br>Nasalis muscle<br>Occipitofrontalis muscle<br>Orbicularis oris muscle<br>Procerus muscle<br>Risorius muscle<br>Zygomaticus muscle<br>**2 Neck Muscle, Right**<br>Anterior vertebral muscle<br>Arytenoid muscle<br>Cricothyroid muscle<br>Infrahyoid muscle<br>Levator scapulae muscle<br>Platysma muscle<br>Scalene muscle<br>Splenius cervicis muscle<br>Sternocleidomastoid muscle<br>Suprahyoid muscle<br>Thyroarytenoid muscle<br>**3 Neck Muscle, Left**<br>*See 2 Neck Muscle, Right*<br>**4 Tongue, Palate, Pharynx Muscle**<br>Chondroglossus muscle<br>Genioglossus muscle<br>Hyoglossus muscle<br>Inferior longitudinal muscle<br>Levator veli palatini muscle<br>Palatoglossal muscle<br>Palatopharyngeal muscle<br>Pharyngeal constrictor muscle<br>Salpingopharyngeus muscle<br>Styloglossus muscle<br>Stylopharyngeus muscle<br>Superior longitudinal muscle<br>Tensor veli palatini muscle<br>**5 Shoulder Muscle, Right**<br>Deltoid muscle<br>Infraspinatus muscle<br>Subscapularis muscle<br>Supraspinatus muscle<br>Teres major muscle<br>Teres minor muscle<br>**6 Shoulder Muscle, Left**<br>*See 5 Shoulder Muscle, Right*<br>**7 Upper Arm Muscle, Right**<br>Biceps brachii muscle<br>Brachialis muscle<br>Coracobrachialis muscle<br>Triceps brachii muscle<br>**8 Upper Arm Muscle, Left**<br>*See 7 Upper Arm Muscle, Right*<br>**9 Lower Arm and Wrist Muscle, Right**<br>Anatomical snuffbox<br>Brachioradialis muscle<br>Extensor carpi radialis muscle<br>Extensor carpi ulnaris muscle<br>Flexor carpi radialis muscle<br>Flexor carpi ulnaris muscle<br>Flexor pollicis longus muscle<br>Palmaris longus muscle<br>Pronator quadratus muscle<br>Pronator teres muscle<br>**B Lower Arm and Wrist Muscle, Left**<br>*See 9 Lower Arm and Wrist Muscle, Right*<br>**C Hand Muscle, Right**<br>Hypothenar muscle<br>Palmar interosseous muscle<br>Thenar muscle<br>**D Hand Muscle, Left**<br>*See C Hand Muscle, Right*<br>**F Trunk Muscle, Right**<br>Coccygeus muscle<br>Erector spinae muscle<br>Interspinalis muscle<br>Intertransversarius muscle<br>Latissimus dorsi muscle<br>Quadratus lumborum muscle<br>Rhomboid major muscle<br>Rhomboid minor muscle<br>Serratus posterior muscle<br>Transversospinalis muscle<br>Trapezius muscle<br>**G Trunk Muscle, Left**<br>*See F Trunk Muscle, Right*<br>**H Thorax Muscle, Right**<br>Intercostal muscle<br>Levatores costarum muscle<br>Pectoralis major muscle<br>Pectoralis minor muscle<br>Serratus anterior muscle<br>Subclavius muscle<br>Subcostal muscle<br>Transverse thoracis muscle<br>**J Thorax Muscle, Left**<br>*See H Thorax Muscle, Right*<br>**K Abdomen Muscle, Right**<br>External oblique muscle<br>Internal oblique muscle<br>Pyramidalis muscle<br>Rectus abdominis muscle<br>Transversus abdominis muscle<br>**L Abdomen Muscle, Left**<br>*See K Abdomen Muscle, Right*<br>**M Perineum Muscle**<br>Bulbospongiosus muscle<br>Cremaster muscle<br>Deep transverse perineal muscle<br>Ischiocavernosus muscle<br>Levator ani muscle<br>Superficial transverse perineal muscle<br>**N Hip Muscle, Right**<br>Gemellus muscle<br>Gluteus maximus muscle<br>Gluteus medius muscle<br>Gluteus minimus muscle<br>Iliacus muscle<br>Obturator muscle<br>Piriformis muscle<br>Psoas muscle<br>Quadratus femoris muscle<br>Tensor fasciae latae muscle<br>**P Hip Muscle, Left**<br>*See N Hip Muscle, Right*<br>**Q Upper Leg Muscle, Right**<br>Adductor brevis muscle<br>Adductor longus muscle<br>Adductor magnus muscle<br>Biceps femoris muscle<br>Gracilis muscle<br>Pectineus muscle<br>Quadriceps (femoris)<br>Rectus femoris muscle<br>Sartorius muscle<br>Semimembranosus muscle<br>Semitendinosus muscle<br>Vastus intermedius muscle<br>Vastus lateralis muscle<br>Vastus medialis muscle<br>**R Upper Leg Muscle, Left**<br>*See Q Upper Leg Muscle, Right*<br>**S Lower Leg Muscle, Right**<br>Extensor digitorum longus muscle<br>Extensor hallucis longus muscle<br>Fibularis brevis muscle<br>Fibularis longus muscle<br>Flexor digitorum longus muscle<br>Flexor hallucis longus muscle<br>Gastrocnemius muscle<br>Peroneus brevis muscle<br>Peroneus longus muscle<br>Popliteus muscle<br>Soleus muscle<br>Tibialis anterior muscle<br>Tibialis posterior muscle<br>**T Lower Leg Muscle, Left**<br>*See S Lower Leg Muscle, Right*<br>**V Foot Muscle, Right**<br>Abductor hallucis muscle<br>Adductor hallucis muscle<br>Extensor digitorum brevis muscle<br>Extensor hallucis brevis muscle<br>Flexor digitorum brevis muscle<br>Flexor hallucis brevis muscle<br>Quadratus plantae muscle<br>**W Foot Muscle, Left**<br>*See V Foot Muscle, Right* | **Ø Open**<br>**3 Percutaneous**<br>**4 Percutaneous Endoscopic** | **Z No Device** | **X Diagnostic**<br>**Z No Qualifier** |

**Ø Medical and Surgical**
**K Muscles**
**C Extirpation** Definition: Taking or cutting out solid matter from a body part

Explanation: The solid matter may be an abnormal byproduct of a biological function or a foreign body; it may be imbedded in a body part or in the lumen of a tubular body part. The solid matter may or may not have been previously broken into pieces.

| Body Part Character 4 | Approach Character 5 | Device Character 6 | Qualifier Character 7 |
|---|---|---|---|
| **Ø Head Muscle** Auricularis muscle; Masseter muscle; Pterygoid muscle; Splenius capitis muscle; Temporalis muscle; Temporoparietalis muscle<br>**1 Facial Muscle** Buccinator muscle; Corrugator supercilii muscle; Depressor anguli oris muscle; Depressor labii inferioris muscle; Depressor septi nasi muscle; Depressor supercilii muscle; Levator anguli oris muscle; Levator labii superioris alaeque nasi muscle; Levator labii superioris muscle; Mentalis muscle; Nasalis muscle; Occipitofrontalis muscle; Orbicularis oris muscle; Procerus muscle; Risorius muscle; Zygomaticus muscle<br>**2 Neck Muscle, Right** Anterior vertebral muscle; Arytenoid muscle; Cricothyroid muscle; Infrahyoid muscle; Levator scapulae muscle; Platysma muscle; Scalene muscle; Splenius cervicis muscle; Sternocleidomastoid muscle; Suprahyoid muscle; Thyroarytenoid muscle<br>**3 Neck Muscle, Left** *See 2 Neck Muscle, Right*<br>**4 Tongue, Palate, Pharynx Muscle** Chondroglossus muscle; Genioglossus muscle; Hyoglossus muscle; Inferior longitudinal muscle; Levator veli palatini muscle; Palatoglossal muscle; Palatopharyngeal muscle; Pharyngeal constrictor muscle; Salpingopharyngeus muscle; Styloglossus muscle; Stylopharyngeus muscle; Superior longitudinal muscle; Tensor veli palatini muscle<br>**5 Shoulder Muscle, Right** Deltoid muscle; Infraspinatus muscle; Subscapularis muscle; Supraspinatus muscle; Teres major muscle; Teres minor muscle<br>**6 Shoulder Muscle, Left** *See 5 Shoulder Muscle, Right*<br>**7 Upper Arm Muscle, Right** Biceps brachii muscle; Brachialis muscle; Coracobrachialis muscle; Triceps brachii muscle<br>**8 Upper Arm Muscle, Left** *See 7 Upper Arm Muscle, Right*<br>**9 Lower Arm and Wrist Muscle, Right** Anatomical snuffbox; Brachioradialis muscle; Extensor carpi radialis muscle; Extensor carpi ulnaris muscle; Flexor carpi radialis muscle; Flexor carpi ulnaris muscle; Flexor pollicis longus muscle; Palmaris longus muscle; Pronator quadratus muscle; Pronator teres muscle<br>**B Lower Arm and Wrist Muscle, Left** *See 9 Lower Arm and Wrist Muscle, Right*<br>**C Hand Muscle, Right** Hypothenar muscle; Palmar interosseous muscle; Thenar muscle<br>**D Hand Muscle, Left** *See C Hand Muscle, Right*<br>**F Trunk Muscle, Right** Coccygeus muscle; Erector spinae muscle; Interspinalis muscle; Intertransversarius muscle; Latissimus dorsi muscle; Quadratus lumborum muscle; Rhomboid major muscle; Rhomboid minor muscle; Serratus posterior muscle; Transversospinalis muscle; Trapezius muscle<br>**G Trunk Muscle, Left** *See F Trunk Muscle, Right*<br>**H Thorax Muscle, Right** Intercostal muscle; Levatores costarum muscle; Pectoralis major muscle; Pectoralis minor muscle; Serratus anterior muscle; Subclavius muscle; Subcostal muscle; Transverse thoracis muscle<br>**J Thorax Muscle, Left** *See H Thorax Muscle, Right*<br>**K Abdomen Muscle, Right** External oblique muscle; Internal oblique muscle; Pyramidalis muscle; Rectus abdominis muscle; Transversus abdominis muscle<br>**L Abdomen Muscle, Left** *See K Abdomen Muscle, Right*<br>**M Perineum Muscle** Bulbospongiosus muscle; Cremaster muscle; Deep transverse perineal muscle; Ischiocavernosus muscle; Levator ani muscle; Superficial transverse perineal muscle<br>**N Hip Muscle, Right** Gemellus muscle; Gluteus maximus muscle; Gluteus medius muscle; Gluteus minimus muscle; Iliacus muscle; Obturator muscle; Piriformis muscle; Psoas muscle; Quadratus femoris muscle; Tensor fasciae latae muscle<br>**P Hip Muscle, Left** *See N Hip Muscle, Right*<br>**Q Upper Leg Muscle, Right** Adductor brevis muscle; Adductor longus muscle; Adductor magnus muscle; Biceps femoris muscle; Gracilis muscle; Pectineus muscle; Quadriceps (femoris); Rectus femoris muscle; Sartorius muscle; Semimembranosus muscle; Semitendinosus muscle; Vastus intermedius muscle; Vastus lateralis muscle; Vastus medialis muscle<br>**R Upper Leg Muscle, Left** *See Q Upper Leg Muscle, Right*<br>**S Lower Leg Muscle, Right** Extensor digitorum longus muscle; Extensor hallucis longus muscle; Fibularis brevis muscle; Fibularis longus muscle; Flexor digitorum longus muscle; Flexor hallucis longus muscle; Gastrocnemius muscle; Peroneus brevis muscle; Peroneus longus muscle; Popliteus muscle; Soleus muscle; Tibialis anterior muscle; Tibialis posterior muscle<br>**T Lower Leg Muscle, Left** *See S Lower Leg Muscle, Right*<br>**V Foot Muscle, Right** Abductor hallucis muscle; Adductor hallucis muscle; Extensor digitorum brevis muscle; Extensor hallucis brevis muscle; Flexor digitorum brevis muscle; Flexor hallucis brevis muscle; Quadratus plantae muscle<br>**W Foot Muscle, Left** *See V Foot Muscle, Right* | **Ø Open**<br>**3 Percutaneous**<br>**4 Percutaneous Endoscopic** | **Z No Device** | **Z No Qualifier** |

**Ø Medical and Surgical**
**K Muscles**
**D Extraction** Definition: Pulling or stripping out or off all or a portion of a body part by the use of force
Explanation: The qualifier DIAGNOSTIC is used to identify extraction procedures that are biopsies

| Body Part Character 4 | Approach Character 5 | Device Character 6 | Qualifier Character 7 |
|---|---|---|---|
| Ø Head Muscle<br>Auricularis muscle<br>Masseter muscle<br>Pterygoid muscle<br>Splenius capitis muscle<br>Temporalis muscle<br>Temporoparietalis muscle<br>1 Facial Muscle<br>Buccinator muscle<br>Corrugator supercilii muscle<br>Depressor anguli oris muscle<br>Depressor labii inferioris muscle<br>Depressor septi nasi muscle<br>Depressor supercilii muscle<br>Levator anguli oris muscle<br>Levator labii superioris alaeque nasi muscle<br>Levator labii superioris muscle<br>Mentalis muscle<br>Nasalis muscle<br>Occipitofrontalis muscle<br>Orbicularis oris muscle<br>Procerus muscle<br>Risorius muscle<br>Zygomaticus muscle<br>2 Neck Muscle, Right<br>Anterior vertebral muscle<br>Arytenoid muscle<br>Cricothyroid muscle<br>Infrahyoid muscle<br>Levator scapulae muscle<br>Platysma muscle<br>Scalene muscle<br>Splenius cervicis muscle<br>Sternocleidomastoid muscle<br>Suprahyoid muscle<br>Thyroarytenoid muscle<br>3 Neck Muscle, Left<br>***See** 2 Neck Muscle, Right*<br>4 Tongue, Palate, Pharynx Muscle<br>Chondroglossus muscle<br>Genioglossus muscle<br>Hyoglossus muscle<br>Inferior longitudinal muscle<br>Levator veli palatini muscle<br>Palatoglossal muscle<br>Palatopharyngeal muscle<br>Pharyngeal constrictor muscle<br>Salpingopharyngeus muscle<br>Styloglossus muscle<br>Stylopharyngeus muscle<br>Superior longitudinal muscle<br>Tensor veli palatini muscle<br>5 Shoulder Muscle, Right<br>Deltoid muscle<br>Infraspinatus muscle<br>Subscapularis muscle<br>Supraspinatus muscle<br>Teres major muscle<br>Teres minor muscle<br>6 Shoulder Muscle, Left<br>***See** 5 Shoulder Muscle, Right*<br>7 Upper Arm Muscle, Right<br>Biceps brachii muscle<br>Brachialis muscle<br>Coracobrachialis muscle<br>Triceps brachii muscle<br>8 Upper Arm Muscle, Left<br>***See** 7 Upper Arm Muscle, Right*<br>9 Lower Arm and Wrist Muscle, Right<br>Anatomical snuffbox<br>Brachioradialis muscle<br>Extensor carpi radialis muscle<br>Extensor carpi ulnaris muscle<br>Flexor carpi radialis muscle<br>Flexor carpi ulnaris muscle<br>Flexor pollicis longus muscle<br>Palmaris longus muscle<br>Pronator quadratus muscle<br>Pronator teres muscle<br>B Lower Arm and Wrist Muscle, Left<br>***See** 9 Lower Arm and Wrist Muscle, Right*<br>C Hand Muscle, Right<br>Hypothenar muscle<br>Palmar interosseous muscle<br>Thenar muscle<br>D Hand Muscle, Left<br>***See** C Hand Muscle, Right*<br>F Trunk Muscle, Right<br>Coccygeus muscle<br>Erector spinae muscle<br>Interspinalis muscle<br>Intertransversarius muscle<br>Latissimus dorsi muscle<br>Quadratus lumborum muscle<br>Rhomboid major muscle<br>Rhomboid minor muscle<br>Serratus posterior muscle<br>Transversospinalis muscle<br>Trapezius muscle<br>G Trunk Muscle, Left<br>***See** F Trunk Muscle, Right*<br>H Thorax Muscle, Right<br>Intercostal muscle<br>Levatores costarum muscle<br>Pectoralis major muscle<br>Pectoralis minor muscle<br>Serratus anterior muscle<br>Subclavius muscle<br>Subcostal muscle<br>Transverse thoracis muscle<br>J Thorax Muscle, Left<br>***See** H Thorax Muscle, Right*<br>K Abdomen Muscle, Right<br>External oblique muscle<br>Internal oblique muscle<br>Pyramidalis muscle<br>Rectus abdominis muscle<br>Transversus abdominis muscle<br>L Abdomen Muscle, Left<br>***See** K Abdomen Muscle, Right*<br>M Perineum Muscle<br>Bulbospongiosus muscle<br>Cremaster muscle<br>Deep transverse perineal muscle<br>Ischiocavernosus muscle<br>Levator ani muscle<br>Superficial transverse perineal muscle<br>N Hip Muscle, Right<br>Gemellus muscle<br>Gluteus maximus muscle<br>Gluteus medius muscle<br>Gluteus minimus muscle<br>Iliacus muscle<br>Obturator muscle<br>Piriformis muscle<br>Psoas muscle<br>Quadratus femoris muscle<br>Tensor fasciae latae muscle<br>P Hip Muscle, Left<br>***See** N Hip Muscle, Right*<br>Q Upper Leg Muscle, Right<br>Adductor brevis muscle<br>Adductor longus muscle<br>Adductor magnus muscle<br>Biceps femoris muscle<br>Gracilis muscle<br>Pectineus muscle<br>Quadriceps (femoris)<br>Rectus femoris muscle<br>Sartorius muscle<br>Semimembranosus muscle<br>Semitendinosus muscle<br>Vastus intermedius muscle<br>Vastus lateralis muscle<br>Vastus medialis muscle<br>R Upper Leg Muscle, Left<br>***See** Q Upper Leg Muscle, Right*<br>S Lower Leg Muscle, Right<br>Extensor digitorum longus muscle<br>Extensor hallucis longus muscle<br>Fibularis brevis muscle<br>Fibularis longus muscle<br>Flexor digitorum longus muscle<br>Flexor hallucis longus muscle<br>Gastrocnemius muscle<br>Peroneus brevis muscle<br>Peroneus longus muscle<br>Popliteus muscle<br>Soleus muscle<br>Tibialis anterior muscle<br>Tibialis posterior muscle<br>T Lower Leg Muscle, Left<br>***See** S Lower Leg Muscle, Right*<br>V Foot Muscle, Right<br>Abductor hallucis muscle<br>Adductor hallucis muscle<br>Extensor digitorum brevis muscle<br>Extensor hallucis brevis muscle<br>Flexor digitorum brevis muscle<br>Flexor hallucis brevis muscle<br>Quadratus plantae muscle<br>W Foot Muscle, Left<br>***See** V Foot Muscle, Right* | Ø Open | Z No Device | Z No Qualifier |

**Ø Medical and Surgical**
**K Muscles**
**H Insertion** Definition: Putting in a nonbiological appliance that monitors, assists, performs, or prevents a physiological function but does not physically take the place of a body part

Explanation: None

| Body Part Character 4 | Approach Character 5 | Device Character 6 | Qualifier Character 7 |
|---|---|---|---|
| **X** Upper Muscle<br>**Y** Lower Muscle | **Ø** Open<br>**3** Percutaneous<br>**4** Percutaneous Endoscopic | **M** Stimulator Lead<br>**Y** Other Device | **Z** No Qualifier |

Non-OR ØKH[X,Y][3,4]YZ

**Ø Medical and Surgical**
**K Muscles**
**J Inspection** Definition: Visually and/or manually exploring a body part

Explanation: Visual exploration may be performed with or without optical instrumentation. Manual exploration may be performed directly or through intervening body layers.

| Body Part Character 4 | Approach Character 5 | Device Character 6 | Qualifier Character 7 |
|---|---|---|---|
| **X** Upper Muscle<br>**Y** Lower Muscle | **Ø** Open<br>**3** Percutaneous<br>**4** Percutaneous Endoscopic<br>**X** External | **Z** No Device | **Z** No Qualifier |

Non-OR ØKJ[X,Y][3,X]ZZ

**Ø Medical and Surgical**
**K Muscles**
**M Reattachment** Definition: Putting back in or on all or a portion of a separated body part to its normal location or other suitable location
Explanation: Vascular circulation and nervous pathways may or may not be reestablished

| Body Part Character 4 | Approach Character 5 | Device Character 6 | Qualifier Character 7 |
|---|---|---|---|
| **Ø Head Muscle**<br>Auricularis muscle<br>Masseter muscle<br>Pterygoid muscle<br>Splenius capitis muscle<br>Temporalis muscle<br>Temporoparietalis muscle | **Ø Open**<br>**4 Percutaneous Endoscopic** | **Z No Device** | **Z No Qualifier** |
| **1 Facial Muscle**<br>Buccinator muscle<br>Corrugator supercilii muscle<br>Depressor anguli oris muscle<br>Depressor labii inferioris muscle<br>Depressor septi nasi muscle<br>Depressor supercilii muscle<br>Levator anguli oris muscle<br>Levator labii superioris alaeque nasi muscle<br>Levator labii superioris muscle<br>Mentalis muscle<br>Nasalis muscle<br>Occipitofrontalis muscle<br>Orbicularis oris muscle<br>Procerus muscle<br>Risorius muscle<br>Zygomaticus muscle | | | |
| **2 Neck Muscle, Right**<br>Anterior vertebral muscle<br>Arytenoid muscle<br>Cricothyroid muscle<br>Infrahyoid muscle<br>Levator scapulae muscle<br>Platysma muscle<br>Scalene muscle<br>Splenius cervicis muscle<br>Sternocleidomastoid muscle<br>Suprahyoid muscle<br>Thyroarytenoid muscle | | | |
| **3 Neck Muscle, Left**<br>*See 2 Neck Muscle, Right* | | | |
| **4 Tongue, Palate, Pharynx Muscle**<br>Chondroglossus muscle<br>Genioglossus muscle<br>Hyoglossus muscle<br>Inferior longitudinal muscle<br>Levator veli palatini muscle<br>Palatoglossal muscle<br>Palatopharyngeal muscle<br>Pharyngeal constrictor muscle<br>Salpingopharyngeus muscle<br>Styloglossus muscle<br>Stylopharyngeus muscle<br>Superior longitudinal muscle<br>Tensor veli palatini muscle | | | |
| **5 Shoulder Muscle, Right**<br>Deltoid muscle<br>Infraspinatus muscle<br>Subscapularis muscle<br>Supraspinatus muscle<br>Teres major muscle<br>Teres minor muscle | | | |
| **6 Shoulder Muscle, Left**<br>*See 5 Shoulder Muscle, Right* | | | |
| **7 Upper Arm Muscle, Right**<br>Biceps brachii muscle<br>Brachialis muscle<br>Coracobrachialis muscle<br>Triceps brachii muscle | | | |
| **8 Upper Arm Muscle, Left**<br>*See 7 Upper Arm Muscle, Right* | | | |
| **9 Lower Arm and Wrist Muscle, Right**<br>Anatomical snuffbox<br>Brachioradialis muscle<br>Extensor carpi radialis muscle<br>Extensor carpi ulnaris muscle<br>Flexor carpi radialis muscle<br>Flexor carpi ulnaris muscle<br>Flexor pollicis longus muscle<br>Palmaris longus muscle<br>Pronator quadratus muscle<br>Pronator teres muscle | | | |
| **B Lower Arm and Wrist Muscle, Left**<br>*See 9 Lower Arm and Wrist Muscle, Right* | | | |
| **C Hand Muscle, Right**<br>Hypothenar muscle<br>Palmar interosseous muscle<br>Thenar muscle | | | |
| **D Hand Muscle, Left**<br>*See C Hand Muscle, Right* | | | |
| **F Trunk Muscle, Right**<br>Coccygeus muscle<br>Erector spinae muscle<br>Interspinalis muscle<br>Intertransversarius muscle<br>Latissimus dorsi muscle<br>Quadratus lumborum muscle<br>Rhomboid major muscle<br>Rhomboid minor muscle<br>Serratus posterior muscle<br>Transversospinalis muscle<br>Trapezius muscle | | | |
| **G Trunk Muscle, Left**<br>*See F Trunk Muscle, Right* | | | |
| **H Thorax Muscle, Right**<br>Intercostal muscle<br>Levatores costarum muscle<br>Pectoralis major muscle<br>Pectoralis minor muscle<br>Serratus anterior muscle<br>Subclavius muscle<br>Subcostal muscle<br>Transverse thoracis muscle | | | |
| **J Thorax Muscle, Left**<br>*See H Thorax Muscle, Right* | | | |
| **K Abdomen Muscle, Right**<br>External oblique muscle<br>Internal oblique muscle<br>Pyramidalis muscle<br>Rectus abdominis muscle<br>Transversus abdominis muscle | | | |
| **L Abdomen Muscle, Left**<br>*See K Abdomen Muscle, Right* | | | |
| **M Perineum Muscle**<br>Bulbospongiosus muscle<br>Cremaster muscle<br>Deep transverse perineal muscle<br>Ischiocavernosus muscle<br>Levator ani muscle<br>Superficial transverse perineal muscle | | | |
| **N Hip Muscle, Right**<br>Gemellus muscle<br>Gluteus maximus muscle<br>Gluteus medius muscle<br>Gluteus minimus muscle<br>Iliacus muscle<br>Obturator muscle<br>Piriformis muscle<br>Psoas muscle<br>Quadratus femoris muscle<br>Tensor fasciae latae muscle | | | |
| **P Hip Muscle, Left**<br>*See N Hip Muscle, Right* | | | |
| **Q Upper Leg Muscle, Right**<br>Adductor brevis muscle<br>Adductor longus muscle<br>Adductor magnus muscle<br>Biceps femoris muscle<br>Gracilis muscle<br>Pectineus muscle<br>Quadriceps (femoris)<br>Rectus femoris muscle<br>Sartorius muscle<br>Semimembranosus muscle<br>Semitendinosus muscle<br>Vastus intermedius muscle<br>Vastus lateralis muscle<br>Vastus medialis muscle | | | |
| **R Upper Leg Muscle, Left**<br>*See Q Upper Leg Muscle, Right* | | | |
| **S Lower Leg Muscle, Right**<br>Extensor digitorum longus muscle<br>Extensor hallucis longus muscle<br>Fibularis brevis muscle<br>Fibularis longus muscle<br>Flexor digitorum longus muscle<br>Flexor hallucis longus muscle<br>Gastrocnemius muscle<br>Peroneus brevis muscle<br>Peroneus longus muscle<br>Popliteus muscle<br>Soleus muscle<br>Tibialis anterior muscle<br>Tibialis posterior muscle | | | |
| **T Lower Leg Muscle, Left**<br>*See S Lower Leg Muscle, Right* | | | |
| **V Foot Muscle, Right**<br>Abductor hallucis muscle<br>Adductor hallucis muscle<br>Extensor digitorum brevis muscle<br>Extensor hallucis brevis muscle<br>Flexor digitorum brevis muscle<br>Flexor hallucis brevis muscle<br>Quadratus plantae muscle | | | |
| **W Foot Muscle, Left**<br>*See V Foot Muscle, Right* | | | |

**Ø Medical and Surgical**
**K Muscles**
**N Release**

Definition: Freeing a body part from an abnormal physical constraint by cutting or by the use of force
Explanation: Some of the restraining tissue may be taken out but none of the body part is taken out

| Body Part Character 4 | Approach Character 5 | Device Character 6 | Qualifier Character 7 |
|---|---|---|---|
| **Ø Head Muscle**<br>Auricularis muscle<br>Masseter muscle<br>Pterygoid muscle<br>Splenius capitis muscle<br>Temporalis muscle<br>Temporoparietalis muscle<br>**1 Facial Muscle**<br>Buccinator muscle<br>Corrugator supercilii muscle<br>Depressor anguli oris muscle<br>Depressor labii inferioris muscle<br>Depressor septi nasi muscle<br>Depressor supercilii muscle<br>Levator anguli oris muscle<br>Levator labii superioris alaeque nasi muscle<br>Levator labii superioris muscle<br>Mentalis muscle<br>Nasalis muscle<br>Occipitofrontalis muscle<br>Orbicularis oris muscle<br>Procerus muscle<br>Risorius muscle<br>Zygomaticus muscle<br>**2 Neck Muscle, Right**<br>Anterior vertebral muscle<br>Arytenoid muscle<br>Cricothyroid muscle<br>Infrahyoid muscle<br>Levator scapulae muscle<br>Platysma muscle<br>Scalene muscle<br>Splenius cervicis muscle<br>Sternocleidomastoid muscle<br>Suprahyoid muscle<br>Thyroarytenoid muscle<br>**3 Neck Muscle, Left**<br>*See 2 Neck Muscle, Right*<br>**4 Tongue, Palate, Pharynx Muscle**<br>Chondroglossus muscle<br>Genioglossus muscle<br>Hyoglossus muscle<br>Inferior longitudinal muscle<br>Levator veli palatini muscle<br>Palatoglossal muscle<br>Palatopharyngeal muscle<br>Pharyngeal constrictor muscle<br>Salpingopharyngeus muscle<br>Styloglossus muscle<br>Stylopharyngeus muscle<br>Superior longitudinal muscle<br>Tensor veli palatini muscle<br>**5 Shoulder Muscle, Right**<br>Deltoid muscle<br>Infraspinatus muscle<br>Subscapularis muscle<br>Supraspinatus muscle<br>Teres major muscle<br>Teres minor muscle<br>**6 Shoulder Muscle, Left**<br>*See 5 Shoulder Muscle, Right*<br>**7 Upper Arm Muscle, Right**<br>Biceps brachii muscle<br>Brachialis muscle<br>Coracobrachialis muscle<br>Triceps brachii muscle<br>**8 Upper Arm Muscle, Left**<br>*See 7 Upper Arm Muscle, Right*<br>**9 Lower Arm and Wrist Muscle, Right**<br>Anatomical snuffbox<br>Brachioradialis muscle<br>Extensor carpi radialis muscle<br>Extensor carpi ulnaris muscle<br>Flexor carpi radialis muscle<br>Flexor carpi ulnaris muscle<br>Flexor pollicis longus muscle<br>Palmaris longus muscle<br>Pronator quadratus muscle<br>Pronator teres muscle<br>**B Lower Arm and Wrist Muscle, Left**<br>*See 9 Lower Arm and Wrist Muscle, Right*<br>**C Hand Muscle, Right**<br>Hypothenar muscle<br>Palmar interosseous muscle<br>Thenar muscle<br>**D Hand Muscle, Left**<br>*See C Hand Muscle, Right*<br>**F Trunk Muscle, Right**<br>Coccygeus muscle<br>Erector spinae muscle<br>Interspinalis muscle<br>Intertransversarius muscle<br>Latissimus dorsi muscle<br>Quadratus lumborum muscle<br>Rhomboid major muscle<br>Rhomboid minor muscle<br>Serratus posterior muscle<br>Transversospinalis muscle<br>Trapezius muscle<br>**G Trunk Muscle, Left**<br>*See F Trunk Muscle, Right*<br>**H Thorax Muscle, Right**<br>Intercostal muscle<br>Levatores costarum muscle<br>Pectoralis major muscle<br>Pectoralis minor muscle<br>Serratus anterior muscle<br>Subclavius muscle<br>Subcostal muscle<br>Transverse thoracis muscle<br>**J Thorax Muscle, Left**<br>*See H Thorax Muscle, Right*<br>**K Abdomen Muscle, Right**<br>External oblique muscle<br>Internal oblique muscle<br>Pyramidalis muscle<br>Rectus abdominis muscle<br>Transversus abdominis muscle<br>**L Abdomen Muscle, Left**<br>*See K Abdomen Muscle, Right*<br>**M Perineum Muscle**<br>Bulbospongiosus muscle<br>Cremaster muscle<br>Deep transverse perineal muscle<br>Ischiocavernosus muscle<br>Levator ani muscle<br>Superficial transverse perineal muscle<br>**N Hip Muscle, Right**<br>Gemellus muscle<br>Gluteus maximus muscle<br>Gluteus medius muscle<br>Gluteus minimus muscle<br>Iliacus muscle<br>Obturator muscle<br>Piriformis muscle<br>Psoas muscle<br>Quadratus femoris muscle<br>Tensor fasciae latae muscle<br>**P Hip Muscle, Left**<br>*See N Hip Muscle, Right*<br>**Q Upper Leg Muscle, Right**<br>Adductor brevis muscle<br>Adductor longus muscle<br>Adductor magnus muscle<br>Biceps femoris muscle<br>Gracilis muscle<br>Pectineus muscle<br>Quadriceps (femoris)<br>Rectus femoris muscle<br>Sartorius muscle<br>Semimembranosus muscle<br>Semitendinosus muscle<br>Vastus intermedius muscle<br>Vastus lateralis muscle<br>Vastus medialis muscle<br>**R Upper Leg Muscle, Left**<br>*See Q Upper Leg Muscle, Right*<br>**S Lower Leg Muscle, Right**<br>Extensor digitorum longus muscle<br>Extensor hallucis longus muscle<br>Fibularis brevis muscle<br>Fibularis longus muscle<br>Flexor digitorum longus muscle<br>Flexor hallucis longus muscle<br>Gastrocnemius muscle<br>Peroneus brevis muscle<br>Peroneus longus muscle<br>Popliteus muscle<br>Soleus muscle<br>Tibialis anterior muscle<br>Tibialis posterior muscle<br>**T Lower Leg Muscle, Left**<br>*See S Lower Leg Muscle, Right*<br>**V Foot Muscle, Right**<br>Abductor hallucis muscle<br>Adductor hallucis muscle<br>Extensor digitorum brevis muscle<br>Extensor hallucis brevis muscle<br>Flexor digitorum brevis muscle<br>Flexor hallucis brevis muscle<br>Quadratus plantae muscle<br>**W Foot Muscle, Left**<br>*See V Foot Muscle, Right* | **Ø Open**<br>**3 Percutaneous**<br>**4 Percutaneous Endoscopic**<br>**X External** | **Z No Device** | **Z No Qualifier** |

**Non-OR** ØKN[Ø,1,2,3,4,5,6,7,8,9,B,C,D,F,G,H,J,K,L,M,N,P,Q,R,S,T,V,W]XZZ

**Ø Medical and Surgical**
**K Muscles**
**P Removal**

Definition: Taking out or off a device from a body part

Explanation: If a device is taken out and a similar device put in without cutting or puncturing the skin or mucous membrane, the procedure is coded to the root operation CHANGE. Otherwise, the procedure for taking out a device is coded to the root operation REMOVAL.

| Body Part Character 4 | Approach Character 5 | Device Character 6 | Qualifier Character 7 |
|---|---|---|---|
| X Upper Muscle<br>Y Lower Muscle | Ø Open<br>3 Percutaneous<br>4 Percutaneous Endoscopic | Ø Drainage Device<br>7 Autologous Tissue Substitute<br>J Synthetic Substitute<br>K Nonautologous Tissue Substitute<br>M Stimulator Lead<br>Y Other Device | Z No Qualifier |
| X Upper Muscle<br>Y Lower Muscle | X External | Ø Drainage Device<br>M Stimulator Lead | Z No Qualifier |

Non-OR ØKP[X,Y][3,4]YZ
Non-OR ØKP[X,Y]X[Ø,M]Z

**Ø Medical and Surgical**
**K Muscles**
**Q Repair** Definition: Restoring, to the extent possible, a body part to its normal anatomic structure and function

Explanation: Used only when the method to accomplish the repair is not one of the other root operations

| Body Part Character 4 | Approach Character 5 | Device Character 6 | Qualifier Character 7 |
|---|---|---|---|
| **Ø Head Muscle**<br>Auricularis muscle<br>Masseter muscle<br>Pterygoid muscle<br>Splenius capitis muscle<br>Temporalis muscle<br>Temporoparietalis muscle<br>**1 Facial Muscle**<br>Buccinator muscle<br>Corrugator supercilii muscle<br>Depressor anguli oris muscle<br>Depressor labii inferioris muscle<br>Depressor septi nasi muscle<br>Depressor supercilii muscle<br>Levator anguli oris muscle<br>Levator labii superioris alaeque nasi muscle<br>Levator labii superioris muscle<br>Mentalis muscle<br>Nasalis muscle<br>Occipitofrontalis muscle<br>Orbicularis oris muscle<br>Procerus muscle<br>Risorius muscle<br>Zygomaticus muscle<br>**2 Neck Muscle, Right**<br>Anterior vertebral muscle<br>Arytenoid muscle<br>Cricothyroid muscle<br>Infrahyoid muscle<br>Levator scapulae muscle<br>Platysma muscle<br>Scalene muscle<br>Splenius cervicis muscle<br>Sternocleidomastoid muscle<br>Suprahyoid muscle<br>Thyroarytenoid muscle<br>**3 Neck Muscle, Left**<br>*See 2 Neck Muscle, Right*<br>**4 Tongue, Palate, Pharynx Muscle**<br>Chondroglossus muscle<br>Genioglossus muscle<br>Hyoglossus muscle<br>Inferior longitudinal muscle<br>Levator veli palatini muscle<br>Palatoglossal muscle<br>Palatopharyngeal muscle<br>Pharyngeal constrictor muscle<br>Salpingopharyngeus muscle<br>Styloglossus muscle<br>Stylopharyngeus muscle<br>Superior longitudinal muscle<br>Tensor veli palatini muscle<br>**5 Shoulder Muscle, Right**<br>Deltoid muscle<br>Infraspinatus muscle<br>Subscapularis muscle<br>Supraspinatus muscle<br>Teres major muscle<br>Teres minor muscle<br>**6 Shoulder Muscle, Left**<br>*See 5 Shoulder Muscle, Right*<br>**7 Upper Arm Muscle, Right**<br>Biceps brachii muscle<br>Brachialis muscle<br>Coracobrachialis muscle<br>Triceps brachii muscle<br>**8 Upper Arm Muscle, Left**<br>*See 7 Upper Arm Muscle, Right*<br>**9 Lower Arm and Wrist Muscle, Right**<br>Anatomical snuffbox<br>Brachioradialis muscle<br>Extensor carpi radialis muscle<br>Extensor carpi ulnaris muscle<br>Flexor carpi radialis muscle<br>Flexor carpi ulnaris muscle<br>Flexor pollicis longus muscle<br>Palmaris longus muscle<br>Pronator quadratus muscle<br>Pronator teres muscle<br>**B Lower Arm and Wrist Muscle, Left**<br>*See 9 Lower Arm and Wrist Muscle, Right*<br>**C Hand Muscle, Right**<br>Hypothenar muscle<br>Palmar interosseous muscle<br>Thenar muscle<br>**D Hand Muscle, Left**<br>*See C Hand Muscle, Right*<br>**F Trunk Muscle, Right**<br>Coccygeus muscle<br>Erector spinae muscle<br>Interspinalis muscle<br>Intertransversarius muscle<br>Latissimus dorsi muscle<br>Quadratus lumborum muscle<br>Rhomboid major muscle<br>Rhomboid minor muscle<br>Serratus posterior muscle<br>Transversospinalis muscle<br>Trapezius muscle<br>**G Trunk Muscle, Left**<br>*See F Trunk Muscle, Right*<br>**H Thorax Muscle, Right**<br>Intercostal muscle<br>Levatores costarum muscle<br>Pectoralis major muscle<br>Pectoralis minor muscle<br>Serratus anterior muscle<br>Subclavius muscle<br>Subcostal muscle<br>Transverse thoracis muscle<br>**J Thorax Muscle, Left**<br>*See H Thorax Muscle, Right*<br>**K Abdomen Muscle, Right**<br>External oblique muscle<br>Internal oblique muscle<br>Pyramidalis muscle<br>Rectus abdominis muscle<br>Transversus abdominis muscle<br>**L Abdomen Muscle, Left**<br>*See K Abdomen Muscle, Right*<br>**M Perineum Muscle**<br>Bulbospongiosus muscle<br>Cremaster muscle<br>Deep transverse perineal muscle<br>Ischiocavernosus muscle<br>Levator ani muscle<br>Superficial transverse perineal muscle<br>**N Hip Muscle, Right**<br>Gemellus muscle<br>Gluteus maximus muscle<br>Gluteus medius muscle<br>Gluteus minimus muscle<br>Iliacus muscle<br>Obturator muscle<br>Piriformis muscle<br>Psoas muscle<br>Quadratus femoris muscle<br>Tensor fasciae latae muscle<br>**P Hip Muscle, Left**<br>*See N Hip Muscle, Right*<br>**Q Upper Leg Muscle, Right**<br>Adductor brevis muscle<br>Adductor longus muscle<br>Adductor magnus muscle<br>Biceps femoris muscle<br>Gracilis muscle<br>Pectineus muscle<br>Quadriceps (femoris)<br>Rectus femoris muscle<br>Sartorius muscle<br>Semimembranosus muscle<br>Semitendinosus muscle<br>Vastus intermedius muscle<br>Vastus lateralis muscle<br>Vastus medialis muscle<br>**R Upper Leg Muscle, Left**<br>*See Q Upper Leg Muscle, Right*<br>**S Lower Leg Muscle, Right**<br>Extensor digitorum longus muscle<br>Extensor hallucis longus muscle<br>Fibularis brevis muscle<br>Fibularis longus muscle<br>Flexor digitorum longus muscle<br>Flexor hallucis longus muscle<br>Gastrocnemius muscle<br>Peroneus brevis muscle<br>Peroneus longus muscle<br>Popliteus muscle<br>Soleus muscle<br>Tibialis anterior muscle<br>Tibialis posterior muscle<br>**T Lower Leg Muscle, Left**<br>*See S Lower Leg Muscle, Right*<br>**V Foot Muscle, Right**<br>Abductor hallucis muscle<br>Adductor hallucis muscle<br>Extensor digitorum brevis muscle<br>Extensor hallucis brevis muscle<br>Flexor digitorum brevis muscle<br>Flexor hallucis brevis muscle<br>Quadratus plantae muscle<br>**W Foot Muscle, Left**<br>*See V Foot Muscle, Right* | **Ø Open**<br>**3 Percutaneous**<br>**4 Percutaneous Endoscopic** | **Z No Device** | **Z No Qualifier** |

**Ø Medical and Surgical**
**K Muscles**
**R Replacement** Definition: Putting in or on biological or synthetic material that physically takes the place and/or function of all or a portion of a body part

Explanation: The body part may have been taken out or replaced, or may be taken out, physically eradicated, or rendered nonfunctional during the REPLACEMENT procedure. A REMOVAL procedure is coded for taking out the device used in a previous replacement procedure.

| Body Part Character 4 | Approach Character 5 | Device Character 6 | Qualifier Character 7 |
|---|---|---|---|
| **Ø Head Muscle**<br>Auricularis muscle<br>Masseter muscle<br>Pterygoid muscle<br>Splenius capitis muscle<br>Temporalis muscle<br>Temporoparietalis muscle<br>**1 Facial Muscle**<br>Buccinator muscle<br>Corrugator supercilii muscle<br>Depressor anguli oris muscle<br>Depressor labii inferioris muscle<br>Depressor septi nasi muscle<br>Depressor supercilii muscle<br>Levator anguli oris muscle<br>Levator labii superioris alaeque nasi muscle<br>Levator labii superioris muscle<br>Mentalis muscle<br>Nasalis muscle<br>Occipitofrontalis muscle<br>Orbicularis oris muscle<br>Procerus muscle<br>Risorius muscle<br>Zygomaticus muscle<br>**2 Neck Muscle, Right**<br>Anterior vertebral muscle<br>Arytenoid muscle<br>Cricothyroid muscle<br>Infrahyoid muscle<br>Levator scapulae muscle<br>Platysma muscle<br>Scalene muscle<br>Splenius cervicis muscle<br>Sternocleidomastoid muscle<br>Suprahyoid muscle<br>Thyroarytenoid muscle<br>**3 Neck Muscle, Left**<br>**See** *2 Neck Muscle, Right*<br>**4 Tongue, Palate, Pharynx Muscle**<br>Chondroglossus muscle<br>Genioglossus muscle<br>Hyoglossus muscle<br>Inferior longitudinal muscle<br>Levator veli palatini muscle<br>Palatoglossal muscle<br>Palatopharyngeal muscle<br>Pharyngeal constrictor muscle<br>Salpingopharyngeus muscle<br>Styloglossus muscle<br>Stylopharyngeus muscle<br>Superior longitudinal muscle<br>Tensor veli palatini muscle<br>**5 Shoulder Muscle, Right**<br>Deltoid muscle<br>Infraspinatus muscle<br>Subscapularis muscle<br>Supraspinatus muscle<br>Teres major muscle<br>Teres minor muscle<br>**6 Shoulder Muscle, Left**<br>**See** *5 Shoulder Muscle, Right*<br>**7 Upper Arm Muscle, Right**<br>Biceps brachii muscle<br>Brachialis muscle<br>Coracobrachialis muscle<br>Triceps brachii muscle<br>**8 Upper Arm Muscle, Left**<br>**See** *7 Upper Arm Muscle, Right*<br>**9 Lower Arm and Wrist Muscle, Right**<br>Anatomical snuffbox<br>Brachioradialis muscle<br>Extensor carpi radialis muscle<br>Extensor carpi ulnaris muscle<br>Flexor carpi radialis muscle<br>Flexor carpi ulnaris muscle<br>Flexor pollicis longus muscle<br>Palmaris longus muscle<br>Pronator quadratus muscle<br>Pronator teres muscle<br>**B Lower Arm and Wrist Muscle, Left**<br>**See** *9 Lower Arm and Wrist Muscle, Right*<br>**C Hand Muscle, Right**<br>Hypothenar muscle<br>Palmar interosseous muscle<br>Thenar muscle<br>**D Hand Muscle, Left**<br>**See** *C Hand Muscle, Right*<br>**F Trunk Muscle, Right**<br>Coccygeus muscle<br>Erector spinae muscle<br>Interspinalis muscle<br>Intertransversarius muscle<br>Latissimus dorsi muscle<br>Quadratus lumborum muscle<br>Rhomboid major muscle<br>Rhomboid minor muscle<br>Serratus posterior muscle<br>Transversospinalis muscle<br>Trapezius muscle<br>**G Trunk Muscle, Left**<br>**See** *F Trunk Muscle, Right*<br>**H Thorax Muscle, Right**<br>Intercostal muscle<br>Levatores costarum muscle<br>Pectoralis major muscle<br>Pectoralis minor muscle<br>Serratus anterior muscle<br>Subclavius muscle<br>Subcostal muscle<br>Transverse thoracis muscle<br>**J Thorax Muscle, Left**<br>**See** *H Thorax Muscle, Right*<br>**K Abdomen Muscle, Right**<br>External oblique muscle<br>Internal oblique muscle<br>Pyramidalis muscle<br>Rectus abdominis muscle<br>Transversus abdominis muscle<br>**L Abdomen Muscle, Left**<br>**See** *K Abdomen Muscle, Right*<br>**M Perineum Muscle**<br>Bulbospongiosus muscle<br>Cremaster muscle<br>Deep transverse perineal muscle<br>Ischiocavernosus muscle<br>Levator ani muscle<br>Superficial transverse perineal muscle<br>**N Hip Muscle, Right**<br>Gemellus muscle<br>Gluteus maximus muscle<br>Gluteus medius muscle<br>Gluteus minimus muscle<br>Iliacus muscle<br>Obturator muscle<br>Piriformis muscle<br>Psoas muscle<br>Quadratus femoris muscle<br>Tensor fasciae latae muscle<br>**P Hip Muscle, Left**<br>**See** *N Hip Muscle, Right*<br>**Q Upper Leg Muscle, Right**<br>Adductor brevis muscle<br>Adductor longus muscle<br>Adductor magnus muscle<br>Biceps femoris muscle<br>Gracilis muscle<br>Pectineus muscle<br>Quadriceps (femoris)<br>Rectus femoris muscle<br>Sartorius muscle<br>Semimembranosus muscle<br>Semitendinosus muscle<br>Vastus intermedius muscle<br>Vastus lateralis muscle<br>Vastus medialis muscle<br>**R Upper Leg Muscle, Left**<br>**See** *Q Upper Leg Muscle, Right*<br>**S Lower Leg Muscle, Right**<br>Extensor digitorum longus muscle<br>Extensor hallucis longus muscle<br>Fibularis brevis muscle<br>Fibularis longus muscle<br>Flexor digitorum longus muscle<br>Flexor hallucis longus muscle<br>Gastrocnemius muscle<br>Peroneus brevis muscle<br>Peroneus longus muscle<br>Popliteus muscle<br>Soleus muscle<br>Tibialis anterior muscle<br>Tibialis posterior muscle<br>**T Lower Leg Muscle, Left**<br>**See** *S Lower Leg Muscle, Right*<br>**V Foot Muscle, Right**<br>Abductor hallucis muscle<br>Adductor hallucis muscle<br>Extensor digitorum brevis muscle<br>Extensor hallucis brevis muscle<br>Flexor digitorum brevis muscle<br>Flexor hallucis brevis muscle<br>Quadratus plantae muscle<br>**W Foot Muscle, Left**<br>**See** *V Foot Muscle, Right* | **Ø** Open<br>**4** Percutaneous Endoscopic | **7** Autologous Tissue Substitute<br>**J** Synthetic Substitute<br>**K** Nonautologous Tissue Substitute | **Z** No Qualifier |

**Ø Medical and Surgical**
**K Muscles**
**S Reposition** Definition: Moving to its normal location, or other suitable location, all or a portion of a body part

Explanation: The body part is moved to a new location from an abnormal location, or from a normal location where it is not functioning correctly. The body part may or may not be cut out or off to be moved to the new location.

| Body Part Character 4 | | | Approach Character 5 | Device Character 6 | Qualifier Character 7 |
|---|---|---|---|---|---|
| **Ø Head Muscle**<br>Auricularis muscle<br>Masseter muscle<br>Pterygoid muscle<br>Splenius capitis muscle<br>Temporalis muscle<br>Temporoparietalis muscle<br>**1 Facial Muscle**<br>Buccinator muscle<br>Corrugator supercilii muscle<br>Depressor anguli oris muscle<br>Depressor labii inferioris muscle<br>Depressor septi nasi muscle<br>Depressor supercilii muscle<br>Levator anguli oris muscle<br>Levator labii superioris alaeque nasi muscle<br>Levator labii superioris muscle<br>Mentalis muscle<br>Nasalis muscle<br>Occipitofrontalis muscle<br>Orbicularis oris muscle<br>Procerus muscle<br>Risorius muscle<br>Zygomaticus muscle<br>**2 Neck Muscle, Right**<br>Anterior vertebral muscle<br>Arytenoid muscle<br>Cricothyroid muscle<br>Infrahyoid muscle<br>Levator scapulae muscle<br>Platysma muscle<br>Scalene muscle<br>Splenius cervicis muscle<br>Sternocleidomastoid muscle<br>Suprahyoid muscle<br>Thyroarytenoid muscle<br>**3 Neck Muscle, Left**<br>*See 2 Neck Muscle, Right*<br>**4 Tongue, Palate, Pharynx Muscle**<br>Chondroglossus muscle<br>Genioglossus muscle<br>Hyoglossus muscle<br>Inferior longitudinal muscle<br>Levator veli palatini muscle<br>Palatoglossal muscle<br>Palatopharyngeal muscle<br>Pharyngeal constrictor muscle<br>Salpingopharyngeus muscle<br>Styloglossus muscle<br>Stylopharyngeus muscle<br>Superior longitudinal muscle<br>Tensor veli palatini muscle<br>**5 Shoulder Muscle, Right**<br>Deltoid muscle<br>Infraspinatus muscle<br>Subscapularis muscle<br>Supraspinatus muscle<br>Teres major muscle<br>Teres minor muscle<br>**6 Shoulder Muscle, Left**<br>*See 5 Shoulder Muscle, Right* | **7 Upper Arm Muscle, Right**<br>Biceps brachii muscle<br>Brachialis muscle<br>Coracobrachialis muscle<br>Triceps brachii muscle<br>**8 Upper Arm Muscle, Left**<br>*See 7 Upper Arm Muscle, Right*<br>**9 Lower Arm and Wrist Muscle, Right**<br>Anatomical snuffbox<br>Brachioradialis muscle<br>Extensor carpi radialis muscle<br>Extensor carpi ulnaris muscle<br>Flexor carpi radialis muscle<br>Flexor carpi ulnaris muscle<br>Flexor pollicis longus muscle<br>Palmaris longus muscle<br>Pronator quadratus muscle<br>Pronator teres muscle<br>**B Lower Arm and Wrist Muscle, Left**<br>*See 9 Lower Arm and Wrist Muscle, Right*<br>**C Hand Muscle, Right**<br>Hypothenar muscle<br>Palmar interosseous muscle<br>Thenar muscle<br>**D Hand Muscle, Left**<br>*See C Hand Muscle, Right*<br>**F Trunk Muscle, Right**<br>Coccygeus muscle<br>Erector spinae muscle<br>Interspinalis muscle<br>Intertransversarius muscle<br>Latissimus dorsi muscle<br>Quadratus lumborum muscle<br>Rhomboid major muscle<br>Rhomboid minor muscle<br>Serratus posterior muscle<br>Transversospinalis muscle<br>Trapezius muscle<br>**G Trunk Muscle, Left**<br>*See F Trunk Muscle, Right*<br>**H Thorax Muscle, Right**<br>Intercostal muscle<br>Levatores costarum muscle<br>Pectoralis major muscle<br>Pectoralis minor muscle<br>Serratus anterior muscle<br>Subclavius muscle<br>Subcostal muscle<br>Transverse thoracis muscle<br>**J Thorax Muscle, Left**<br>*See H Thorax Muscle, Right*<br>**K Abdomen Muscle, Right**<br>External oblique muscle<br>Internal oblique muscle<br>Pyramidalis muscle<br>Rectus abdominis muscle<br>Transversus abdominis muscle<br>**L Abdomen Muscle, Left**<br>*See K Abdomen Muscle, Right* | **M Perineum Muscle**<br>Bulbospongiosus muscle<br>Cremaster muscle<br>Deep transverse perineal muscle<br>Ischiocavernosus muscle<br>Levator ani muscle<br>Superficial transverse perineal muscle<br>**N Hip Muscle, Right**<br>Gemellus muscle<br>Gluteus maximus muscle<br>Gluteus medius muscle<br>Gluteus minimus muscle<br>Iliacus muscle<br>Obturator muscle<br>Piriformis muscle<br>Psoas muscle<br>Quadratus femoris muscle<br>Tensor fasciae latae muscle<br>**P Hip Muscle, Left**<br>*See N Hip Muscle, Right*<br>**Q Upper Leg Muscle, Right**<br>Adductor brevis muscle<br>Adductor longus muscle<br>Adductor magnus muscle<br>Biceps femoris muscle<br>Gracilis muscle<br>Pectineus muscle<br>Quadriceps (femoris)<br>Rectus femoris muscle<br>Sartorius muscle<br>Semimembranosus muscle<br>Semitendinosus muscle<br>Vastus intermedius muscle<br>Vastus lateralis muscle<br>Vastus medialis muscle<br>**R Upper Leg Muscle, Left**<br>*See Q Upper Leg Muscle, Right*<br>**S Lower Leg Muscle, Right**<br>Extensor digitorum longus muscle<br>Extensor hallucis longus muscle<br>Fibularis brevis muscle<br>Fibularis longus muscle<br>Flexor digitorum longus muscle<br>Flexor hallucis longus muscle<br>Gastrocnemius muscle<br>Peroneus brevis muscle<br>Peroneus longus muscle<br>Popliteus muscle<br>Soleus muscle<br>Tibialis anterior muscle<br>Tibialis posterior muscle<br>**T Lower Leg Muscle, Left**<br>*See S Lower Leg Muscle, Right*<br>**V Foot Muscle, Right**<br>Abductor hallucis muscle<br>Adductor hallucis muscle<br>Extensor digitorum brevis muscle<br>Extensor hallucis brevis muscle<br>Flexor digitorum brevis muscle<br>Flexor hallucis brevis muscle<br>Quadratus plantae muscle<br>**W Foot Muscle, Left**<br>*See V Foot Muscle, Right* | **Ø Open**<br>**4 Percutaneous Endoscopic** | **Z No Device** | **Z No Qualifier** |

**Ø Medical and Surgical**
**K Muscles**
**T Resection** Definition: Cutting out or off, without replacement, all of a body part

Explanation: None

| Body Part Character 4 | Approach Character 5 | Device Character 6 | Qualifier Character 7 |
|---|---|---|---|
| **Ø Head Muscle**<br>Auricularis muscle<br>Masseter muscle<br>Pterygoid muscle<br>Splenius capitis muscle<br>Temporalis muscle<br>Temporoparietalis muscle<br>**1 Facial Muscle**<br>Buccinator muscle<br>Corrugator supercilii muscle<br>Depressor anguli oris muscle<br>Depressor labii inferioris muscle<br>Depressor septi nasi muscle<br>Depressor supercilii muscle<br>Levator anguli oris muscle<br>Levator labii superioris alaeque nasi muscle<br>Levator labii superioris muscle<br>Mentalis muscle<br>Nasalis muscle<br>Occipitofrontalis muscle<br>Orbicularis oris muscle<br>Procerus muscle<br>Risorius muscle<br>Zygomaticus muscle<br>**2 Neck Muscle, Right**<br>Anterior vertebral muscle<br>Arytenoid muscle<br>Cricothyroid muscle<br>Infrahyoid muscle<br>Levator scapulae muscle<br>Platysma muscle<br>Scalene muscle<br>Splenius cervicis muscle<br>Sternocleidomastoid muscle<br>Suprahyoid muscle<br>Thyroarytenoid muscle<br>**3 Neck Muscle, Left**<br>*See 2 Neck Muscle, Right*<br>**4 Tongue, Palate, Pharynx Muscle**<br>Chondroglossus muscle<br>Genioglossus muscle<br>Hyoglossus muscle<br>Inferior longitudinal muscle<br>Levator veli palatini muscle<br>Palatoglossal muscle<br>Palatopharyngeal muscle<br>Pharyngeal constrictor muscle<br>Salpingopharyngeus muscle<br>Styloglossus muscle<br>Stylopharyngeus muscle<br>Superior longitudinal muscle<br>Tensor veli palatini muscle<br>**5 Shoulder Muscle, Right**<br>Deltoid muscle<br>Infraspinatus muscle<br>Subscapularis muscle<br>Supraspinatus muscle<br>Teres major muscle<br>Teres minor muscle<br>**6 Shoulder Muscle, Left**<br>*See 5 Shoulder Muscle, Right*<br>**7 Upper Arm Muscle, Right**<br>Biceps brachii muscle<br>Brachialis muscle<br>Coracobrachialis muscle<br>Triceps brachii muscle<br>**8 Upper Arm Muscle, Left**<br>*See 7 Upper Arm Muscle, Right*<br>**9 Lower Arm and Wrist Muscle, Right**<br>Anatomical snuffbox<br>Brachioradialis muscle<br>Extensor carpi radialis muscle<br>Extensor carpi ulnaris muscle<br>Flexor carpi radialis muscle<br>Flexor carpi ulnaris muscle<br>Flexor pollicis longus muscle<br>Palmaris longus muscle<br>Pronator quadratus muscle<br>Pronator teres muscle<br>**B Lower Arm and Wrist Muscle, Left**<br>*See 9 Lower Arm and Wrist Muscle, Right*<br>**C Hand Muscle, Right**<br>Hypothenar muscle<br>Palmar interosseous muscle<br>Thenar muscle<br>**D Hand Muscle, Left**<br>*See C Hand Muscle, Right*<br>**F Trunk Muscle, Right**<br>Coccygeus muscle<br>Erector spinae muscle<br>Interspinalis muscle<br>Intertransversarius muscle<br>Latissimus dorsi muscle<br>Quadratus lumborum muscle<br>Rhomboid major muscle<br>Rhomboid minor muscle<br>Serratus posterior muscle<br>Transversospinalis muscle<br>Trapezius muscle<br>**G Trunk Muscle, Left**<br>*See F Trunk Muscle, Right*<br>**H Thorax Muscle, Right** ⊞<br>Intercostal muscle<br>Levatores costarum muscle<br>Pectoralis major muscle<br>Pectoralis minor muscle<br>Serratus anterior muscle<br>Subclavius muscle<br>Subcostal muscle<br>Transverse thoracis muscle<br>**J Thorax Muscle, Left** ⊞<br>*See H Thorax Muscle, Right*<br>**K Abdomen Muscle, Right**<br>External oblique muscle<br>Internal oblique muscle<br>Pyramidalis muscle<br>Rectus abdominis muscle<br>Transversus abdominis muscle<br>**L Abdomen Muscle, Left**<br>*See K Abdomen Muscle, Right*<br>**M Perineum Muscle**<br>Bulbospongiosus muscle<br>Cremaster muscle<br>Deep transverse perineal muscle<br>Ischiocavernosus muscle<br>Levator ani muscle<br>Superficial transverse perineal muscle<br>**N Hip Muscle, Right**<br>Gemellus muscle<br>Gluteus maximus muscle<br>Gluteus medius muscle<br>Gluteus minimus muscle<br>Iliacus muscle<br>Obturator muscle<br>Piriformis muscle<br>Psoas muscle<br>Quadratus femoris muscle<br>Tensor fasciae latae muscle<br>**P Hip Muscle, Left**<br>*See N Hip Muscle, Right*<br>**Q Upper Leg Muscle, Right**<br>Adductor brevis muscle<br>Adductor longus muscle<br>Adductor magnus muscle<br>Biceps femoris muscle<br>Gracilis muscle<br>Pectineus muscle<br>Quadriceps (femoris)<br>Rectus femoris muscle<br>Sartorius muscle<br>Semimembranosus muscle<br>Semitendinosus muscle<br>Vastus intermedius muscle<br>Vastus lateralis muscle<br>Vastus medialis muscle<br>**R Upper Leg Muscle, Left**<br>*See Q Upper Leg Muscle, Right*<br>**S Lower Leg Muscle, Right**<br>Extensor digitorum longus muscle<br>Extensor hallucis longus muscle<br>Fibularis brevis muscle<br>Fibularis longus muscle<br>Flexor digitorum longus muscle<br>Flexor hallucis longus muscle<br>Gastrocnemius muscle<br>Peroneus brevis muscle<br>Peroneus longus muscle<br>Popliteus muscle<br>Soleus muscle<br>Tibialis anterior muscle<br>Tibialis posterior muscle<br>**T Lower Leg Muscle, Left**<br>*See S Lower Leg Muscle, Right*<br>**V Foot Muscle, Right**<br>Abductor hallucis muscle<br>Adductor hallucis muscle<br>Extensor digitorum brevis muscle<br>Extensor hallucis brevis muscle<br>Flexor digitorum brevis muscle<br>Flexor hallucis brevis muscle<br>Quadratus plantae muscle<br>**W Foot Muscle, Left**<br>*See V Foot Muscle, Right* | **Ø Open**<br>**4 Percutaneous Endoscopic** | **Z No Device** | **Z No Qualifier** |

**See Appendix L for Procedure Combinations**

⊞ ØKT[H,J]ØZZ

**Ø Medical and Surgical**
**K Muscles**
**U Supplement**

Definition: Putting in or on biological or synthetic material that physically reinforces and/or augments the function of a portion of a body part

Explanation: The biological material is non-living, or is living and from the same individual. The body part may have been previously replaced, and the SUPPLEMENT procedure is performed to physically reinforce and/or augment the function of the replaced body part.

| Body Part Character 4 | Approach Character 5 | Device Character 6 | Qualifier Character 7 |
|---|---|---|---|
| **Ø Head Muscle**<br>Auriculakris muscle<br>Masseter muscle<br>Pterygoid muscle<br>Splenius capitis muscle<br>Temporalis muscle<br>Temporoparietalis muscle<br>**1 Facial Muscle**<br>Buccinator muscle<br>Corrugator supercilii muscle<br>Depressor anguli oris muscle<br>Depressor labii inferioris muscle<br>Depressor septi nasi muscle<br>Depressor supercilii muscle<br>Levator anguli oris muscle<br>Levator labii superioris alaeque nasi muscle<br>Levator labii superioris muscle<br>Mentalis muscle<br>Nasalis muscle<br>Occipitofrontalis muscle<br>Orbicularis oris muscle<br>Procerus muscle<br>Risorius muscle<br>Zygomaticus muscle<br>**2 Neck Muscle, Right**<br>Anterior vertebral muscle<br>Arytenoid muscle<br>Cricothyroid muscle<br>Infrahyoid muscle<br>Levator scapulae muscle<br>Platysma muscle<br>Scalene muscle<br>Splenius cervicis muscle<br>Sternocleidomastoid muscle<br>Suprahyoid muscle<br>Thyroarytenoid muscle<br>**3 Neck Muscle, Left**<br>*See 2 Neck Muscle, Right*<br>**4 Tongue, Palate, Pharynx Muscle**<br>Chondroglossus muscle<br>Genioglossus muscle<br>Hyoglossus muscle<br>Inferior longitudinal muscle<br>Levator veli palatini muscle<br>Palatoglossal muscle<br>Palatopharyngeal muscle<br>Pharyngeal constrictor muscle<br>Salpingopharyngeus muscle<br>Styloglossus muscle<br>Stylopharyngeus muscle<br>Superior longitudinal muscle<br>Tensor veli palatini muscle<br>**5 Shoulder Muscle, Right**<br>Deltoid muscle<br>Infraspinatus muscle<br>Subscapularis muscle<br>Supraspinatus muscle<br>Teres major muscle<br>Teres minor muscle<br>**6 Shoulder Muscle, Left**<br>*See 5 Shoulder Muscle, Right*<br>**7 Upper Arm Muscle, Right**<br>Biceps brachii muscle<br>Brachialis muscle<br>Coracobrachialis muscle<br>Triceps brachii muscle<br>**8 Upper Arm Muscle, Left**<br>*See 7 Upper Arm Muscle, Right*<br>**9 Lower Arm and Wrist Muscle, Right**<br>Anatomical snuffbox<br>Brachioradialis muscle<br>Extensor carpi radialis muscle<br>Extensor carpi ulnaris muscle<br>Flexor carpi radialis muscle<br>Flexor carpi ulnaris muscle<br>Flexor pollicis longus muscle<br>Palmaris longus muscle<br>Pronator quadratus muscle<br>Pronator teres muscle<br>**B Lower Arm and Wrist Muscle, Left**<br>*See 9 Lower Arm and Wrist Muscle, Right*<br>**C Hand Muscle, Right**<br>Hypothenar muscle<br>Palmar interosseous muscle<br>Thenar muscle<br>**D Hand Muscle, Left**<br>*See C Hand Muscle, Right*<br>**F Trunk Muscle, Right**<br>Coccygeus muscle<br>Erector spinae muscle<br>Interspinalis muscle<br>Intertransversarius muscle<br>Latissimus dorsi muscle<br>Quadratus lumborum muscle<br>Rhomboid major muscle<br>Rhomboid minor muscle<br>Serratus posterior muscle<br>Transversospinalis muscle<br>Trapezius muscle<br>**G Trunk Muscle, Left**<br>*See F Trunk Muscle, Right*<br>**H Thorax Muscle, Right**<br>Intercostal muscle<br>Levatores costarum muscle<br>Pectoralis major muscle<br>Pectoralis minor muscle<br>Serratus anterior muscle<br>Subclavius muscle<br>Subcostal muscle<br>Transverse thoracis muscle<br>**J Thorax Muscle, Left**<br>*See H Thorax Muscle, Right*<br>**M Perineum Muscle**<br>Bulbospongiosus muscle<br>Cremaster muscle<br>Deep transverse perineal muscle<br>Ischiocavernosus muscle<br>Levator ani muscle<br>Superficial transverse perineal muscle<br>**N Hip Muscle, Right**<br>Gemellus muscle<br>Gluteus maximus muscle<br>Gluteus medius muscle<br>Gluteus minimus muscle<br>Iliacus muscle<br>Obturator muscle<br>Piriformis muscle<br>Psoas muscle<br>Quadratus femoris muscle<br>Tensor fasciae latae muscle<br>**P Hip Muscle, Left**<br>*See N Hip Muscle, Right*<br>**Q Upper Leg Muscle, Right**<br>Adductor brevis muscle<br>Adductor longus muscle<br>Adductor magnus muscle<br>Biceps femoris muscle<br>Gracilis muscle<br>Pectineus muscle<br>Quadriceps (femoris)<br>Rectus femoris muscle<br>Sartorius muscle<br>Semimembranosus muscle<br>Semitendinosus muscle<br>Vastus intermedius muscle<br>Vastus lateralis muscle<br>Vastus medialis muscle<br>**R Upper Leg Muscle, Left**<br>*See Q Upper Leg Muscle, Right*<br>**S Lower Leg Muscle, Right**<br>Extensor digitorum longus muscle<br>Extensor hallucis longus muscle<br>Fibularis brevis muscle<br>Fibularis longus muscle<br>Flexor digitorum longus muscle<br>Flexor hallucis longus muscle<br>Gastrocnemius muscle<br>Peroneus brevis muscle<br>Peroneus longus muscle<br>Popliteus muscle<br>Soleus muscle<br>Tibialis anterior muscle<br>Tibialis posterior muscle<br>**T Lower Leg Muscle, Left**<br>*See S Lower Leg Muscle, Right*<br>**V Foot Muscle, Right**<br>Abductor hallucis muscle<br>Adductor hallucis muscle<br>Extensor digitorum brevis muscle<br>Extensor hallucis brevis muscle<br>Flexor digitorum brevis muscle<br>Flexor hallucis brevis muscle<br>Quadratus plantae muscle<br>**W Foot Muscle, Left**<br>*See V Foot Muscle, Right* | **Ø Open**<br>**4 Percutaneous Endoscopic** | **7 Autologous Tissue Substitute**<br>**J Synthetic Substitute**<br>**K Nonautologous Tissue Substitute** | **Z No Qualifier** |

**Ø Medical and Surgical**
**K Muscles**
**W Revision**

Definition: Correcting, to the extent possible, a portion of a malfunctioning device or the position of a displaced device

Explanation: Revision can include correcting a malfunctioning or displaced device by taking out or putting in components of the device such as a screw or pin

| Body Part Character 4 | Approach Character 5 | Device Character 6 | Qualifier Character 7 |
|---|---|---|---|
| **X** Upper Muscle<br>**Y** Lower Muscle | **Ø** Open<br>**3** Percutaneous<br>**4** Percutaneous Endoscopic | **Ø** Drainage Device<br>**7** Autologous Tissue Substitute<br>**J** Synthetic Substitute<br>**K** Nonautologous Tissue Substitute<br>**M** Stimulator Lead<br>**Y** Other Device | **Z** No Qualifier |
| **X** Upper Muscle<br>**Y** Lower Muscle | **X** External | **Ø** Drainage Device<br>**7** Autologous Tissue Substitute<br>**J** Synthetic Substitute<br>**K** Nonautologous Tissue Substitute<br>**M** Stimulator Lead | **Z** No Qualifier |

**Non-OR** ØKW[X,Y][3,4]YZ
**Non-OR** ØKW[X,Y]X[Ø,7,J,K,M]Z

**Ø Medical and Surgical**
**K Muscles**
**X Transfer**

Definition: Moving, without taking out, all or a portion of a body part to another location to take over the function of all or a portion of a body part
Explanation: The body part transferred remains connected to its vascular and nervous supply

| Body Part Character 4 | Approach Character 5 | Device Character 6 | Qualifier Character 7 |
|---|---|---|---|
| **Ø Head Muscle**<br>Auricularis muscle<br>Masseter muscle<br>Pterygoid muscle<br>Splenius capitis muscle<br>Temporalis muscle<br>Temporoparietalis muscle<br>**1 Facial Muscle**<br>Buccinator muscle<br>Corrugator supercilii muscle<br>Depressor anguli oris muscle<br>Depressor labii inferioris muscle<br>Depressor septi nasi muscle<br>Depressor supercilii muscle<br>Levator anguli oris muscle<br>Levator labii superioris alaeque nasi muscle<br>Levator labii superioris muscle<br>Mentalis muscle<br>Nasalis muscle<br>Occipitofrontalis muscle<br>Orbicularis oris muscle<br>Procerus muscle<br>Risorius muscle<br>Zygomaticus muscle<br>**2 Neck Muscle, Right**<br>Anterior vertebral muscle<br>Arytenoid muscle<br>Cricothyroid muscle<br>Infrahyoid muscle<br>Levator scapulae muscle<br>Platysma muscle<br>Scalene muscle<br>Splenius cervicis muscle<br>Sternocleidomastoid muscle<br>Suprahyoid muscle<br>Thyroarytenoid muscle<br>**3 Neck Muscle, Left**<br>**See** *2 Neck Muscle, Right*<br>**4 Tongue, Palate, Pharynx Muscle**<br>Chondroglossus muscle<br>Genioglossus muscle<br>Hyoglossus muscle<br>Inferior longitudinal muscle<br>Levator veli palatini muscle<br>Palatoglossal muscle<br>Palatopharyngeal muscle<br>Pharyngeal constrictor muscle<br>Salpingopharyngeus muscle<br>Styloglossus muscle<br>Stylopharyngeus muscle<br>Superior longitudinal muscle<br>Tensor veli palatini muscle<br>**5 Shoulder Muscle, Right**<br>Deltoid muscle<br>Infraspinatus muscle<br>Subscapularis muscle<br>Supraspinatus muscle<br>Teres major muscle<br>Teres minor muscle<br>**6 Shoulder Muscle, Left**<br>**See** *5 Shoulder Muscle, Right*<br>**7 Upper Arm Muscle, Right**<br>Biceps brachii muscle<br>Brachialis muscle<br>Coracobrachialis muscle<br>Triceps brachii muscle<br>**8 Upper Arm Muscle, Left**<br>**See** *7 Upper Arm Muscle, Right*<br>**9 Lower Arm and Wrist Muscle, Right**<br>Anatomical snuffbox<br>Brachioradialis muscle<br>Extensor carpi radialis muscle<br>Extensor carpi ulnaris muscle<br>Flexor carpi radialis muscle<br>Flexor carpi ulnaris muscle<br>Flexor pollicis longus muscle<br>Palmaris longus muscle<br>Pronator quadratus muscle<br>Pronator teres muscle<br>**B Lower Arm and Wrist Muscle, Left**<br>**See** *9 Lower Arm and Wrist Muscle, Right*<br>**C Hand Muscle, Right**<br>Hypothenar muscle<br>Palmar interosseous muscle<br>Thenar muscle<br>**D Hand Muscle, Left**<br>**See** *C Hand Muscle, Right*<br>**H Thorax Muscle, Right**<br>Intercostal muscle<br>Levatores costarum muscle<br>Pectoralis major muscle<br>Pectoralis minor muscle<br>Serratus anterior muscle<br>Subclavius muscle<br>Subcostal muscle<br>Transverse thoracis muscle<br>**J Thorax Muscle, Left**<br>**See** *H Thorax Muscle, Right*<br>**M Perineum Muscle**<br>Bulbospongiosus muscle<br>Cremaster muscle<br>Deep transverse perineal muscle<br>Ischiocavernosus muscle<br>Levator ani muscle<br>Superficial transverse perineal muscle<br>**N Hip Muscle, Right**<br>Gemellus muscle<br>Gluteus maximus muscle<br>Gluteus medius muscle<br>Gluteus minimus muscle<br>Iliacus muscle<br>Obturator muscle<br>Piriformis muscle<br>Psoas muscle<br>Quadratus femoris muscle<br>Tensor fasciae latae muscle<br>**P Hip Muscle, Left**<br>**See** *N Hip Muscle, Right*<br>**Q Upper Leg Muscle, Right**<br>Adductor brevis muscle<br>Adductor longus muscle<br>Adductor magnus muscle<br>Biceps femoris muscle<br>Gracilis muscle<br>Pectineus muscle<br>Quadriceps (femoris)<br>Rectus femoris muscle<br>Sartorius muscle<br>Semimembranosus muscle<br>Semitendinosus muscle<br>Vastus intermedius muscle<br>Vastus lateralis muscle<br>Vastus medialis muscle<br>**R Upper Leg Muscle, Left**<br>**See** *Q Upper Leg Muscle, Right*<br>**S Lower Leg Muscle, Right**<br>Extensor digitorum longus muscle<br>Extensor hallucis longus muscle<br>Fibularis brevis muscle<br>Fibularis longus muscle<br>Flexor digitorum longus muscle<br>Flexor hallucis longus muscle<br>Gastrocnemius muscle<br>Peroneus brevis muscle<br>Peroneus longus muscle<br>Popliteus muscle<br>Soleus muscle<br>Tibialis anterior muscle<br>Tibialis posterior muscle<br>**T Lower Leg Muscle, Left**<br>**See** *S Lower Leg Muscle, Right*<br>**V Foot Muscle, Right**<br>Abductor hallucis muscle<br>Adductor hallucis muscle<br>Extensor digitorum brevis muscle<br>Extensor hallucis brevis muscle<br>Flexor digitorum brevis muscle<br>Flexor hallucis brevis muscle<br>Quadratus plantae muscle<br>**W Foot Muscle, Left**<br>**See** *V Foot Muscle, Right* | **Ø Open**<br>**4 Percutaneous Endoscopic** | **Z No Device** | **Ø Skin**<br>**1 Subcutaneous Tissue**<br>**2 Skin and Subcutaneous Tissue**<br>**Z No Qualifier** |

***ØKX Continued on next page***

**Ø Medical and Surgical**
**K Muscles**
**X Transfer**

**ØKX Continued**

Definition: Moving, without taking out, all or a portion of a body part to another location to take over the function of all or a portion of a body part
Explanation: The body part transferred remains connected to its vascular and nervous supply

| Body Part Character 4 | Approach Character 5 | Device Character 6 | Qualifier Character 7 |
|---|---|---|---|
| **F Trunk Muscle, Right**<br>Coccygeus muscle<br>Erector spinae muscle<br>Interspinalis muscle<br>Intertransversarius muscle<br>Latissimus dorsi muscle<br>Quadratus lumborum muscle<br>Rhomboid major muscle<br>Rhomboid minor muscle<br>Serratus posterior muscle<br>Transversospinalis muscle<br>Trapezius muscle<br>**G Trunk Muscle, Left**<br>*See F Trunk Muscle, Right* | Ø Open<br>4 Percutaneous Endoscopic | Z No Device | Ø Skin<br>1 Subcutaneous Tissue<br>2 Skin and Subcutaneous Tissue<br>5 Latissimus Dorsi Myocutaneous Flap<br>7 Deep Inferior Epigastric Artery Perforator Flap<br>8 Superficial Inferior Epigastric Artery Flap<br>9 Gluteal Artery Perforator Flap<br>Z No Qualifier |
| **K Abdomen Muscle, Right**<br>External oblique muscle<br>Internal oblique muscle<br>Pyramidalis muscle<br>Rectus abdominis muscle<br>Transversus abdominis muscle<br>**L Abdomen Muscle, Left**<br>*See K Abdomen Muscle, Right* | Ø Open<br>4 Percutaneous Endoscopic | Z No Device | Ø Skin<br>1 Subcutaneous Tissue<br>2 Skin and Subcutaneous Tissue<br>6 Transverse Rectus Abdominis Myocutaneous Flap<br>Z No Qualifier |

# Tendons ØL2–ØLX

## Character Meanings*

This Character Meaning table is provided as a guide to assist the user in the identification of character members that may be found in this section of code tables. It **SHOULD NOT** be used to build a PCS code.

| Operation–Character 3 | Body Part–Character 4 | Approach–Character 5 | Device–Character 6 | Qualifier–Character 7 |
|---|---|---|---|---|
| 2 Change | Ø Head and Neck Tendon | Ø Open | Ø Drainage Device | X Diagnostic |
| 5 Destruction | 1 Shoulder Tendon, Right | 3 Percutaneous | 7 Autologous Tissue Substitute | Z No Qualifier |
| 8 Division | 2 Shoulder Tendon, Left | 4 Percutaneous Endoscopic | J Synthetic Substitute | |
| 9 Drainage | 3 Upper Arm Tendon, Right | X External | K Nonautologous Tissue Substitute | |
| B Excision | 4 Upper Arm Tendon, Left | | Y Other Device | |
| C Extirpation | 5 Lower Arm and Wrist Tendon, Right | | Z No Device | |
| D Extraction | 6 Lower Arm and Wrist Tendon, Left | | | |
| H Insertion | 7 Hand Tendon, Right | | | |
| J Inspection | 8 Hand Tendon, Left | | | |
| M Reattachment | 9 Trunk Tendon, Right | | | |
| N Release | B Trunk Tendon, Left | | | |
| P Removal | C Thorax Tendon, Right | | | |
| Q Repair | D Thorax Tendon, Left | | | |
| R Replacement | F Abdomen Tendon, Right | | | |
| S Reposition | G Abdomen Tendon, Left | | | |
| T Resection | H Perineum Tendon | | | |
| U Supplement | J Hip Tendon, Right | | | |
| W Revision | K Hip Tendon, Left | | | |
| X Transfer | L Upper Leg Tendon, Right | | | |
| | M Upper Leg Tendon, Left | | | |
| | N Lower Leg Tendon, Right | | | |
| | P Lower Leg Tendon, Left | | | |
| | Q Knee Tendon, Right | | | |
| | R Knee Tendon, Left | | | |
| | S Ankle Tendon, Right | | | |
| | T Ankle Tendon, Left | | | |
| | V Foot Tendon, Right | | | |
| | W Foot Tendon, Left | | | |
| | X Upper Tendon | | | |
| | Y Lower Tendon | | | |

* Includes synovial membrane.

**AHA Coding Clinic for table ØL8**
**2016, 3Q, 30** Resection of femur with interposition arthroplasty

**AHA Coding Clinic for table ØLB**
**2017, 2Q, 21** Arthroscopic anterior cruciate ligament revision using autograft with anterolateral ligament reconstruction
**2015, 3Q, 26** Thumb arthroplasty with resection of trapezium
**2014, 3Q, 14** Application of TheraSkin® and excisional debridement
**2014, 3Q, 18** Placement of reverse sural fasciocutaneous pedicle flap

**AHA Coding Clinic for table ØLQ**
**2016, 3Q, 32** Rotator cuff repair, tenodesis, decompression, acromioplasty and coracoplasty
**2015, 2Q, 11** Repair of patellar and quadriceps tendons with allograft
**2013, 3Q, 20** Superior labrum anterior posterior (SLAP) repair and subacromial decompression

**AHA Coding Clinic for table ØLS**
**2016, 3Q, 32** Rotator cuff repair, tenodesis, decompression, acromioplasty and coracoplasty
**2015, 3Q, 14** Endoprosthetic replacement of humerus and tendon reattachment

**AHA Coding Clinic for table ØLU**
**2015, 2Q, 11** Repair of patellar and quadriceps tendons with allograft

## Foot Tendons

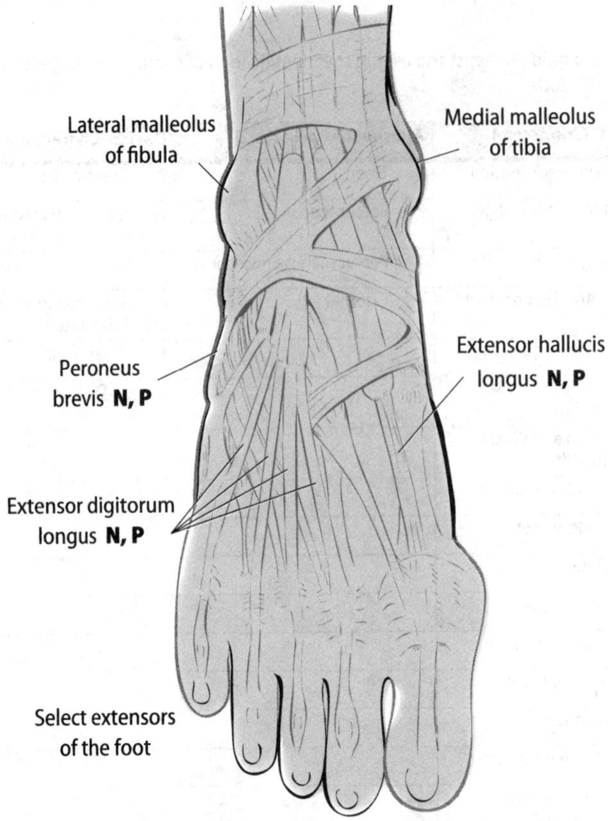
Lateral malleolus of fibula
Medial malleolus of tibia
Peroneus brevis **N, P**
Extensor hallucis longus **N, P**
Extensor digitorum longus **N, P**
Select extensors of the foot

## Shoulder Tendons

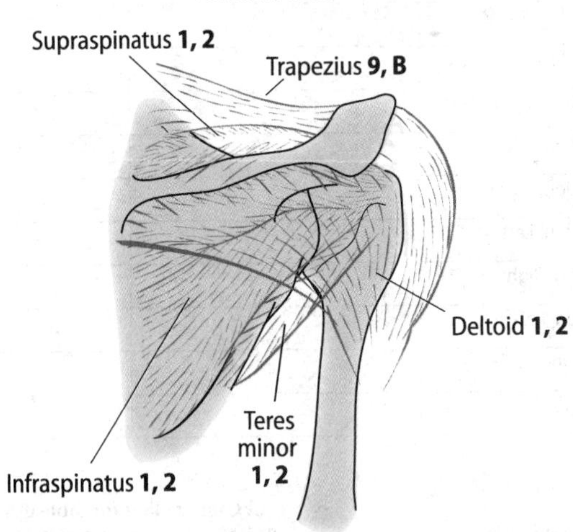
Posterior view
Supraspinatus **1, 2**
Trapezius **9, B**
Deltoid **1, 2**
Teres minor **1, 2**
Infraspinatus **1, 2**

## Tendons of Wrist and Hand

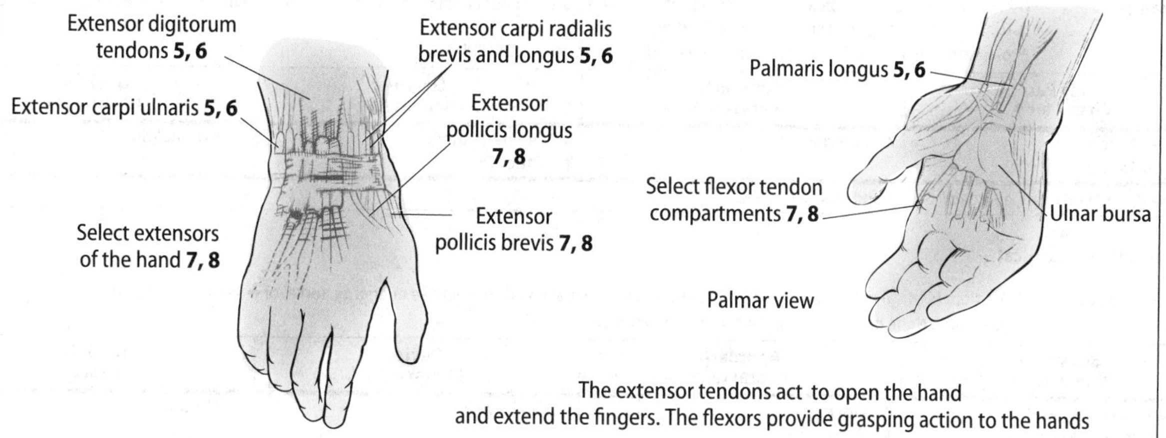

Extensor digitorum tendons **5, 6**
Extensor carpi ulnaris **5, 6**
Select extensors of the hand **7, 8**
Extensor carpi radialis brevis and longus **5, 6**
Extensor pollicis longus **7, 8**
Extensor pollicis brevis **7, 8**
Palmaris longus **5, 6**
Select flexor tendon compartments **7, 8**
Ulnar bursa
Palmar view


The extensor tendons act to open the hand and extend the fingers. The flexors provide grasping action to the hands

## Leg Muscles and Tendons

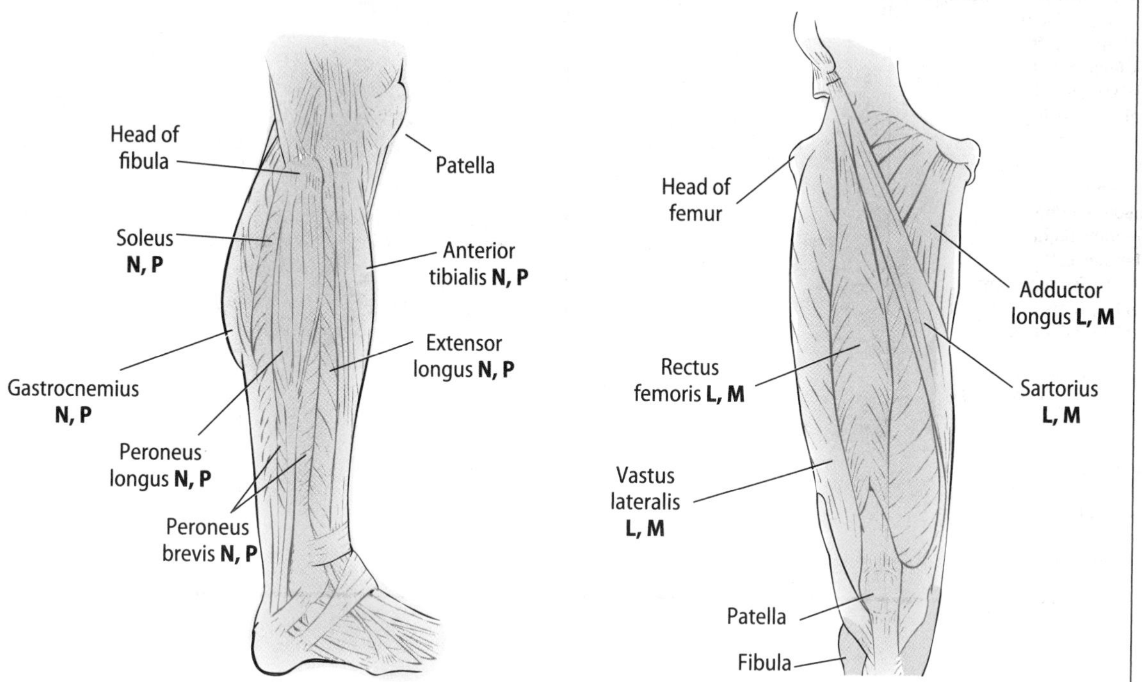

Head of fibula
Patella
Soleus **N, P**
Anterior tibialis **N, P**
Gastrocnemius **N, P**
Extensor longus **N, P**
Peroneus longus **N, P**
Peroneus brevis **N, P**
Head of femur
Adductor longus **L, M**
Rectus femoris **L, M**
Sartorius **L, M**
Vastus lateralis **L, M**
Patella
Fibula

**Ø Medical and Surgical**
**L Tendons**
**2 Change**

Definition: Taking out or off a device from a body part and putting back an identical or similar device in or on the same body part without cutting or puncturing the skin or a mucous membrane

Explanation: All CHANGE procedures are coded using the approach EXTERNAL

| Body Part Character 4 | Approach Character 5 | Device Character 6 | Qualifier Character 7 |
|---|---|---|---|
| X Upper Tendon<br>Y Lower Tendon | X External | Ø Drainage Device<br>Y Other Device | Z No Qualifier |

Non-OR All body part, approach, device, and qualifier values

**Ø Medical and Surgical**
**L Tendons**
**5 Destruction**

Definition: Physical eradication of all or a portion of a body part by the direct use of energy, force, or a destructive agent

Explanation: None of the body part is physically taken out

| Body Part Character 4 | Approach Character 5 | Device Character 6 | Qualifier Character 7 |
|---|---|---|---|
| Ø Head and Neck Tendon<br>1 Shoulder Tendon, Right<br>2 Shoulder Tendon, Left<br>3 Upper Arm Tendon, Right<br>4 Upper Arm Tendon, Left<br>5 Lower Arm and Wrist Tendon, Right<br>6 Lower Arm and Wrist Tendon, Left<br>7 Hand Tendon, Right<br>8 Hand Tendon, Left<br>9 Trunk Tendon, Right<br>B Trunk Tendon, Left<br>C Thorax Tendon, Right<br>D Thorax Tendon, Left<br>F Abdomen Tendon, Right<br>G Abdomen Tendon, Left<br>H Perineum Tendon<br>J Hip Tendon, Right<br>K Hip Tendon, Left<br>L Upper Leg Tendon, Right<br>M Upper Leg Tendon, Left<br>N Lower Leg Tendon, Right<br>Achilles tendon<br>P Lower Leg Tendon, Left<br>*See N Lower Leg Tendon, Right*<br>Q Knee Tendon, Right<br>Patellar tendon<br>R Knee Tendon, Left<br>*See Q Knee Tendon, Right*<br>S Ankle Tendon, Right<br>T Ankle Tendon, Left<br>V Foot Tendon, Right<br>W Foot Tendon, Left | Ø Open<br>3 Percutaneous<br>4 Percutaneous Endoscopic | Z No Device | Z No Qualifier |

**Ø Medical and Surgical**
**L Tendons**
**8 Division**

Definition: Cutting into a body part, without draining fluids and/or gases from the body part, in order to separate or transect a body part
Explanation: All or a portion of the body part is separated into two or more portions

| Body Part Character 4 | Approach Character 5 | Device Character 6 | Qualifier Character 7 |
|---|---|---|---|
| **Ø** Head and Neck Tendon<br>**1** Shoulder Tendon, Right<br>**2** Shoulder Tendon, Left<br>**3** Upper Arm Tendon, Right<br>**4** Upper Arm Tendon, Left<br>**5** Lower Arm and Wrist Tendon, Right<br>**6** Lower Arm and Wrist Tendon, Left<br>**7** Hand Tendon, Right<br>**8** Hand Tendon, Left<br>**9** Trunk Tendon, Right<br>**B** Trunk Tendon, Left<br>**C** Thorax Tendon, Right<br>**D** Thorax Tendon, Left<br>**F** Abdomen Tendon, Right<br>**G** Abdomen Tendon, Left<br>**H** Perineum Tendon<br>**J** Hip Tendon, Right<br>**K** Hip Tendon, Left<br>**L** Upper Leg Tendon, Right<br>**M** Upper Leg Tendon, Left<br>**N** Lower Leg Tendon, Right<br>Achilles tendon<br>**P** Lower Leg Tendon, Left<br>*See N Lower Leg Tendon, Right*<br>**Q** Knee Tendon, Right<br>Patellar tendon<br>**R** Knee Tendon, Left<br>*See Q Knee Tendon, Right*<br>**S** Ankle Tendon, Right<br>**T** Ankle Tendon, Left<br>**V** Foot Tendon, Right<br>**W** Foot Tendon, Left | **Ø** Open<br>**3** Percutaneous<br>**4** Percutaneous Endoscopic | **Z** No Device | **Z** No Qualifier |

**Ø Medical and Surgical**
**L Tendons**
**9 Drainage** Definition: Taking or letting out fluids and/or gases from a body part
Explanation: The qualifier DIAGNOSTIC is used to identify drainage procedures that are biopsies

| Body Part Character 4 | Approach Character 5 | Device Character 6 | Qualifier Character 7 |
|---|---|---|---|
| Ø Head and Neck Tendon<br>1 Shoulder Tendon, Right<br>2 Shoulder Tendon, Left<br>3 Upper Arm Tendon, Right<br>4 Upper Arm Tendon, Left<br>5 Lower Arm and Wrist Tendon, Right<br>6 Lower Arm and Wrist Tendon, Left<br>7 Hand Tendon, Right<br>8 Hand Tendon, Left<br>9 Trunk Tendon, Right<br>B Trunk Tendon, Left<br>C Thorax Tendon, Right<br>D Thorax Tendon, Left<br>F Abdomen Tendon, Right<br>G Abdomen Tendon, Left<br>H Perineum Tendon<br>J Hip Tendon, Right<br>K Hip Tendon, Left<br>L Upper Leg Tendon, Right<br>M Upper Leg Tendon, Left<br>N Lower Leg Tendon, Right<br>Achilles tendon<br>P Lower Leg Tendon, Left<br>*See N Lower Leg Tendon, Right*<br>Q Knee Tendon, Right<br>Patellar tendon<br>R Knee Tendon, Left<br>*See Q Knee Tendon, Right*<br>S Ankle Tendon, Right<br>T Ankle Tendon, Left<br>V Foot Tendon, Right<br>W Foot Tendon, Left | Ø Open<br>3 Percutaneous<br>4 Percutaneous Endoscopic | Ø Drainage Device | Z No Qualifier |
| Ø Head and Neck Tendon<br>1 Shoulder Tendon, Right<br>2 Shoulder Tendon, Left<br>3 Upper Arm Tendon, Right<br>4 Upper Arm Tendon, Left<br>5 Lower Arm and Wrist Tendon, Right<br>6 Lower Arm and Wrist Tendon, Left<br>7 Hand Tendon, Right<br>8 Hand Tendon, Left<br>9 Trunk Tendon, Right<br>B Trunk Tendon, Left<br>C Thorax Tendon, Right<br>D Thorax Tendon, Left<br>F Abdomen Tendon, Right<br>G Abdomen Tendon, Left<br>H Perineum Tendon<br>J Hip Tendon, Right<br>K Hip Tendon, Left<br>L Upper Leg Tendon, Right<br>M Upper Leg Tendon, Left<br>N Lower Leg Tendon, Right<br>Achilles tendon<br>P Lower Leg Tendon, Left<br>*See N Lower Leg Tendon, Right*<br>Q Knee Tendon, Right<br>Patellar tendon<br>R Knee Tendon, Left<br>*See Q Knee Tendon, Right*<br>S Ankle Tendon, Right<br>T Ankle Tendon, Left<br>V Foot Tendon, Right<br>W Foot Tendon, Left | Ø Open<br>3 Percutaneous<br>4 Percutaneous Endoscopic | Z No Device | X Diagnostic<br>Z No Qualifier |

**Non-OR** ØL9[Ø,1,2,3,4,5,6,7,8,9,B,C,D,F,G,H,J,K,L,M,N,P,Q,R,S,T,V,W]3ØZ
**Non-OR** ØL9[Ø,1,2,3,4,5,6,7,8,9,B,C,D,F,G,H,J,K,L,M,N,P,Q,R,S,T,V,W]3ZZ
**Non-OR** ØL9[7,8]4ZZ

**Ø Medical and Surgical**
**L Tendons**
**B Excision** Definition: Cutting out or off, without replacement, a portion of a body part
Explanation: The qualifier DIAGNOSTIC is used to identify excision procedures that are biopsies

| Body Part Character 4 | Approach Character 5 | Device Character 6 | Qualifier Character 7 |
|---|---|---|---|
| **Ø** Head and Neck Tendon<br>**1** Shoulder Tendon, Right<br>**2** Shoulder Tendon, Left<br>**3** Upper Arm Tendon, Right<br>**4** Upper Arm Tendon, Left<br>**5** Lower Arm and Wrist Tendon, Right<br>**6** Lower Arm and Wrist Tendon, Left<br>**7** Hand Tendon, Right<br>**8** Hand Tendon, Left<br>**9** Trunk Tendon, Right<br>**B** Trunk Tendon, Left<br>**C** Thorax Tendon, Right<br>**D** Thorax Tendon, Left<br>**F** Abdomen Tendon, Right<br>**G** Abdomen Tendon, Left<br>**H** Perineum Tendon<br>**J** Hip Tendon, Right<br>**K** Hip Tendon, Left<br>**L** Upper Leg Tendon, Right<br>**M** Upper Leg Tendon, Left<br>**N** Lower Leg Tendon, Right<br>Achilles tendon<br>**P** Lower Leg Tendon, Left<br>*See N Lower Leg Tendon, Right*<br>**Q** Knee Tendon, Right<br>Patellar tendon<br>**R** Knee Tendon, Left<br>*See Q Knee Tendon, Right*<br>**S** Ankle Tendon, Right<br>**T** Ankle Tendon, Left<br>**V** Foot Tendon, Right<br>**W** Foot Tendon, Left | **Ø** Open<br>**3** Percutaneous<br>**4** Percutaneous Endoscopic | **Z** No Device | **X** Diagnostic<br>**Z** No Qualifier |

**Ø Medical and Surgical**
**L Tendons**
**C Extirpation** Definition: Taking or cutting out solid matter from a body part

Explanation: The solid matter may be an abnormal byproduct of a biological function or a foreign body; it may be imbedded in a body part or in the lumen of a tubular body part. The solid matter may or may not have been previously broken into pieces.

| Body Part Character 4 | Approach Character 5 | Device Character 6 | Qualifier Character 7 |
|---|---|---|---|
| **Ø** Head and Neck Tendon<br>**1** Shoulder Tendon, Right<br>**2** Shoulder Tendon, Left<br>**3** Upper Arm Tendon, Right<br>**4** Upper Arm Tendon, Left<br>**5** Lower Arm and Wrist Tendon, Right<br>**6** Lower Arm and Wrist Tendon, Left<br>**7** Hand Tendon, Right<br>**8** Hand Tendon, Left<br>**9** Trunk Tendon, Right<br>**B** Trunk Tendon, Left<br>**C** Thorax Tendon, Right<br>**D** Thorax Tendon, Left<br>**F** Abdomen Tendon, Right<br>**G** Abdomen Tendon, Left<br>**H** Perineum Tendon<br>**J** Hip Tendon, Right<br>**K** Hip Tendon, Left<br>**L** Upper Leg Tendon, Right<br>**M** Upper Leg Tendon, Left<br>**N** Lower Leg Tendon, Right<br>Achilles tendon<br>**P** Lower Leg Tendon, Left<br>*See N Lower Leg Tendon, Right*<br>**Q** Knee Tendon, Right<br>Patellar tendon<br>**R** Knee Tendon, Left<br>*See Q Knee Tendon, Right*<br>**S** Ankle Tendon, Right<br>**T** Ankle Tendon, Left<br>**V** Foot Tendon, Right<br>**W** Foot Tendon, Left | **Ø** Open<br>**3** Percutaneous<br>**4** Percutaneous Endoscopic | **Z** No Device | **Z** No Qualifier |

**Ø Medical and Surgical**
**L Tendons**
**D Extraction** Definition: Pulling or stripping out or off all or a portion of a body part by the use of force
Explanation: The qualifier DIAGNOSTIC is used to identify extraction procedures that are biopsies

| Body Part Character 4 | Approach Character 5 | Device Character 6 | Qualifier Character 7 |
|---|---|---|---|
| Ø Head and Neck Tendon<br>1 Shoulder Tendon, Right<br>2 Shoulder Tendon, Left<br>3 Upper Arm Tendon, Right<br>4 Upper Arm Tendon, Left<br>5 Lower Arm and Wrist Tendon, Right<br>6 Lower Arm and Wrist Tendon, Left<br>7 Hand Tendon, Right<br>8 Hand Tendon, Left<br>9 Trunk Tendon, Right<br>B Trunk Tendon, Left<br>C Thorax Tendon, Right<br>D Thorax Tendon, Left<br>F Abdomen Tendon, Right<br>G Abdomen Tendon, Left<br>H Perineum Tendon<br>J Hip Tendon, Right<br>K Hip Tendon, Left<br>L Upper Leg Tendon, Right<br>M Upper Leg Tendon, Left<br>N Lower Leg Tendon, Right<br>Achilles tendon<br>P Lower Leg Tendon, Left<br>*See N Lower Leg Tendon, Right*<br>Q Knee Tendon, Right<br>Patellar tendon<br>R Knee Tendon, Left<br>*See Q Knee Tendon, Right*<br>S Ankle Tendon, Right<br>T Ankle Tendon, Left<br>V Foot Tendon, Right<br>W Foot Tendon, Left | Ø Open | Z No Device | Z No Qualifier |

**Ø Medical and Surgical**
**L Tendons**
**H Insertion** Definition: Putting in a nonbiological appliance that monitors, assists, performs, or prevents a physiological function but does not physically take the place of a body part
Explanation: None

| Body Part Character 4 | Approach Character 5 | Device Character 6 | Qualifier Character 7 |
|---|---|---|---|
| X Upper Tendon<br>Y Lower Tendon | Ø Open<br>3 Percutaneous<br>4 Percutaneous Endoscopic | Y Other Device | Z No Qualifier |

**Non-OR** ØLH[X,Y][3,4]YZ

**Ø Medical and Surgical**
**L Tendons**
**J Inspection** Definition: Visually and/or manually exploring a body part
Explanation: Visual exploration may be performed with or without optical instrumentation. Manual exploration may be performed directly or through intervening body layers.

| Body Part Character 4 | Approach Character 5 | Device Character 6 | Qualifier Character 7 |
|---|---|---|---|
| X Upper Tendon<br>Y Lower Tendon | Ø Open<br>3 Percutaneous<br>4 Percutaneous Endoscopic<br>X External | Z No Device | Z No Qualifier |

**Non-OR** ØLJ[X,Y][3,X]ZZ

**Ø Medical and Surgical**
**L Tendons**
**M Reattachment** Definition: Putting back in or on all or a portion of a separated body part to its normal location or other suitable location
Explanation: Vascular circulation and nervous pathways may or may not be reestablished

| Body Part Character 4 | Approach Character 5 | Device Character 6 | Qualifier Character 7 |
|---|---|---|---|
| **Ø** Head and Neck Tendon<br>**1** Shoulder Tendon, Right<br>**2** Shoulder Tendon, Left<br>**3** Upper Arm Tendon, Right<br>**4** Upper Arm Tendon, Left<br>**5** Lower Arm and Wrist Tendon, Right<br>**6** Lower Arm and Wrist Tendon, Left<br>**7** Hand Tendon, Right<br>**8** Hand Tendon, Left<br>**9** Trunk Tendon, Right<br>**B** Trunk Tendon, Left<br>**C** Thorax Tendon, Right<br>**D** Thorax Tendon, Left<br>**F** Abdomen Tendon, Right<br>**G** Abdomen Tendon, Left<br>**H** Perineum Tendon<br>**J** Hip Tendon, Right<br>**K** Hip Tendon, Left<br>**L** Upper Leg Tendon, Right<br>**M** Upper Leg Tendon, Left<br>**N** Lower Leg Tendon, Right<br>Achilles tendon<br>**P** Lower Leg Tendon, Left<br>*See N Lower Leg Tendon, Right*<br>**Q** Knee Tendon, Right<br>Patellar tendon<br>**R** Knee Tendon, Left<br>*See Q Knee Tendon, Right*<br>**S** Ankle Tendon, Right<br>**T** Ankle Tendon, Left<br>**V** Foot Tendon, Right<br>**W** Foot Tendon, Left | **Ø** Open<br>**4** Percutaneous Endoscopic | **Z** No Device | **Z** No Qualifier |

**Ø Medical and Surgical**
**L Tendons**
**N Release** Definition: Freeing a body part from an abnormal physical constraint by cutting or by the use of force
Explanation: Some of the restraining tissue may be taken out but none of the body part is taken out

| Body Part Character 4 | Approach Character 5 | Device Character 6 | Qualifier Character 7 |
|---|---|---|---|
| **Ø** Head and Neck Tendon<br>**1** Shoulder Tendon, Right<br>**2** Shoulder Tendon, Left<br>**3** Upper Arm Tendon, Right<br>**4** Upper Arm Tendon, Left<br>**5** Lower Arm and Wrist Tendon, Right<br>**6** Lower Arm and Wrist Tendon, Left<br>**7** Hand Tendon, Right<br>**8** Hand Tendon, Left<br>**9** Trunk Tendon, Right<br>**B** Trunk Tendon, Left<br>**C** Thorax Tendon, Right<br>**D** Thorax Tendon, Left<br>**F** Abdomen Tendon, Right<br>**G** Abdomen Tendon, Left<br>**H** Perineum Tendon<br>**J** Hip Tendon, Right<br>**K** Hip Tendon, Left<br>**L** Upper Leg Tendon, Right<br>**M** Upper Leg Tendon, Left<br>**N** Lower Leg Tendon, Right<br>Achilles tendon<br>**P** Lower Leg Tendon, Left<br>*See N Lower Leg Tendon, Right*<br>**Q** Knee Tendon, Right<br>Patellar tendon<br>**R** Knee Tendon, Left<br>*See Q Knee Tendon, Right*<br>**S** Ankle Tendon, Right<br>**T** Ankle Tendon, Left<br>**V** Foot Tendon, Right<br>**W** Foot Tendon, Left | **Ø** Open<br>**3** Percutaneous<br>**4** Percutaneous Endoscopic<br>**X** External | **Z** No Device | **Z** No Qualifier |

**Non-OR** ØLN[Ø,1,2,3,4,5,6,7,8,9,B,C,D,F,G,H,J,K,L,M,N,P,Q,R,S,T,V,W]XZZ

**Ø Medical and Surgical**
**L Tendons**
**P Removal**

Definition: Taking out or off a device from a body part

Explanation: If a device is taken out and a similar device put in without cutting or puncturing the skin or mucous membrane, the procedure is coded to the root operation CHANGE. Otherwise, the procedure for taking out a device is coded to the root operation REMOVAL.

| Body Part Character 4 | Approach Character 5 | Device Character 6 | Qualifier Character 7 |
|---|---|---|---|
| X Upper Tendon<br>Y Lower Tendon | Ø Open<br>3 Percutaneous<br>4 Percutaneous Endoscopic | Ø Drainage Device<br>7 Autologous Tissue Substitute<br>J Synthetic Substitute<br>K Nonautologous Tissue Substitute<br>Y Other Device | Z No Qualifier |
| X Upper Tendon<br>Y Lower Tendon | X External | Ø Drainage Device | Z No Qualifier |

Non-OR ØLP[X,Y]3ØZ
Non-OR ØLP[X,Y][3,4]YZ
Non-OR ØLP[X,Y]XØZ

**Ø Medical and Surgical**
**L Tendons**
**Q Repair**

Definition: Restoring, to the extent possible, a body part to its normal anatomic structure and function

Explanation: Used only when the method to accomplish the repair is not one of the other root operations

| Body Part Character 4 | Approach Character 5 | Device Character 6 | Qualifier Character 7 |
|---|---|---|---|
| Ø Head and Neck Tendon<br>1 Shoulder Tendon, Right<br>2 Shoulder Tendon, Left<br>3 Upper Arm Tendon, Right<br>4 Upper Arm Tendon, Left<br>5 Lower Arm and Wrist Tendon, Right<br>6 Lower Arm and Wrist Tendon, Left<br>7 Hand Tendon, Right<br>8 Hand Tendon, Left<br>9 Trunk Tendon, Right<br>B Trunk Tendon, Left<br>C Thorax Tendon, Right<br>D Thorax Tendon, Left<br>F Abdomen Tendon, Right<br>G Abdomen Tendon, Left<br>H Perineum Tendon<br>J Hip Tendon, Right<br>K Hip Tendon, Left<br>L Upper Leg Tendon, Right<br>M Upper Leg Tendon, Left<br>N Lower Leg Tendon, Right<br>Achilles tendon<br>P Lower Leg Tendon, Left<br>*See N Lower Leg Tendon, Right*<br>Q Knee Tendon, Right<br>Patellar tendon<br>R Knee Tendon, Left<br>*See Q Knee Tendon, Right*<br>S Ankle Tendon, Right<br>T Ankle Tendon, Left<br>V Foot Tendon, Right<br>W Foot Tendon, Left | Ø Open<br>3 Percutaneous<br>4 Percutaneous Endoscopic | Z No Device | Z No Qualifier |

**Ø Medical and Surgical**
**L Tendons**
**R Replacement** Definition: Putting in or on biological or synthetic material that physically takes the place and/or function of all or a portion of a body part

Explanation: The body part may have been taken out or replaced, or may be taken out, physically eradicated, or rendered nonfunctional during the REPLACEMENT procedure. A REMOVAL procedure is coded for taking out the device used in a previous replacement procedure.

| Body Part Character 4 | Approach Character 5 | Device Character 6 | Qualifier Character 7 |
|---|---|---|---|
| **Ø** Head and Neck Tendon<br>**1** Shoulder Tendon, Right<br>**2** Shoulder Tendon, Left<br>**3** Upper Arm Tendon, Right<br>**4** Upper Arm Tendon, Left<br>**5** Lower Arm and Wrist Tendon, Right<br>**6** Lower Arm and Wrist Tendon, Left<br>**7** Hand Tendon, Right<br>**8** Hand Tendon, Left<br>**9** Trunk Tendon, Right<br>**B** Trunk Tendon, Left<br>**C** Thorax Tendon, Right<br>**D** Thorax Tendon, Left<br>**F** Abdomen Tendon, Right<br>**G** Abdomen Tendon, Left<br>**H** Perineum Tendon<br>**J** Hip Tendon, Right<br>**K** Hip Tendon, Left<br>**L** Upper Leg Tendon, Right<br>**M** Upper Leg Tendon, Left<br>**N** Lower Leg Tendon, Right<br>Achilles tendon<br>**P** Lower Leg Tendon, Left<br>*See N Lower Leg Tendon, Right*<br>**Q** Knee Tendon, Right<br>Patellar tendon<br>**R** Knee Tendon, Left<br>*See Q Knee Tendon, Right*<br>**S** Ankle Tendon, Right<br>**T** Ankle Tendon, Left<br>**V** Foot Tendon, Right<br>**W** Foot Tendon, Left | **Ø** Open<br>**4** Percutaneous Endoscopic | **7** Autologous Tissue Substitute<br>**J** Synthetic Substitute<br>**K** Nonautologous Tissue Substitute | **Z** No Qualifier |

**Ø Medical and Surgical**
**L Tendons**
**S Reposition** Definition: Moving to its normal location, or other suitable location, all or a portion of a body part

Explanation: The body part is moved to a new location from an abnormal location, or from a normal location where it is not functioning correctly. The body part may or may not be cut out or off to be moved to the new location.

| Body Part Character 4 | Approach Character 5 | Device Character 6 | Qualifier Character 7 |
|---|---|---|---|
| **Ø** Head and Neck Tendon<br>**1** Shoulder Tendon, Right<br>**2** Shoulder Tendon, Left<br>**3** Upper Arm Tendon, Right<br>**4** Upper Arm Tendon, Left<br>**5** Lower Arm and Wrist Tendon, Right<br>**6** Lower Arm and Wrist Tendon, Left<br>**7** Hand Tendon, Right<br>**8** Hand Tendon, Left<br>**9** Trunk Tendon, Right<br>**B** Trunk Tendon, Left<br>**C** Thorax Tendon, Right<br>**D** Thorax Tendon, Left<br>**F** Abdomen Tendon, Right<br>**G** Abdomen Tendon, Left<br>**H** Perineum Tendon<br>**J** Hip Tendon, Right<br>**K** Hip Tendon, Left<br>**L** Upper Leg Tendon, Right<br>**M** Upper Leg Tendon, Left<br>**N** Lower Leg Tendon, Right<br>Achilles tendon<br>**P** Lower Leg Tendon, Left<br>*See N Lower Leg Tendon, Right*<br>**Q** Knee Tendon, Right<br>Patellar tendon<br>**R** Knee Tendon, Left<br>*See Q Knee Tendon, Right*<br>**S** Ankle Tendon, Right<br>**T** Ankle Tendon, Left<br>**V** Foot Tendon, Right<br>**W** Foot Tendon, Left | **Ø** Open<br>**4** Percutaneous Endoscopic | **Z** No Device | **Z** No Qualifier |

**Ø Medical and Surgical**
**L Tendons**
**T Resection** Definition: Cutting out or off, without replacement, all of a body part

Explanation: None

| Body Part Character 4 | Approach Character 5 | Device Character 6 | Qualifier Character 7 |
|---|---|---|---|
| **Ø** Head and Neck Tendon<br>**1** Shoulder Tendon, Right<br>**2** Shoulder Tendon, Left<br>**3** Upper Arm Tendon, Right<br>**4** Upper Arm Tendon, Left<br>**5** Lower Arm and Wrist Tendon, Right<br>**6** Lower Arm and Wrist Tendon, Left<br>**7** Hand Tendon, Right<br>**8** Hand Tendon, Left<br>**9** Trunk Tendon, Right<br>**B** Trunk Tendon, Left<br>**C** Thorax Tendon, Right<br>**D** Thorax Tendon, Left<br>**F** Abdomen Tendon, Right<br>**G** Abdomen Tendon, Left<br>**H** Perineum Tendon<br>**J** Hip Tendon, Right<br>**K** Hip Tendon, Left<br>**L** Upper Leg Tendon, Right<br>**M** Upper Leg Tendon, Left<br>**N** Lower Leg Tendon, Right<br>Achilles tendon<br>**P** Lower Leg Tendon, Left<br>*See N Lower Leg Tendon, Right*<br>**Q** Knee Tendon, Right<br>Patellar tendon<br>**R** Knee Tendon, Left<br>*See Q Knee Tendon, Right*<br>**S** Ankle Tendon, Right<br>**T** Ankle Tendon, Left<br>**V** Foot Tendon, Right<br>**W** Foot Tendon, Left | **Ø** Open<br>**4** Percutaneous Endoscopic | **Z** No Device | **Z** No Qualifier |

**Ø Medical and Surgical**
**L Tendons**
**U Supplement** Definition: Putting in or on biological or synthetic material that physically reinforces and/or augments the function of a portion of a body part

Explanation: The biological material is non-living, or is living and from the same individual. The body part may have been previously replaced, and the SUPPLEMENT procedure is performed to physically reinforce and/or augment the function of the replaced body part.

| Body Part Character 4 | Approach Character 5 | Device Character 6 | Qualifier Character 7 |
|---|---|---|---|
| **Ø** Head and Neck Tendon<br>**1** Shoulder Tendon, Right<br>**2** Shoulder Tendon, Left<br>**3** Upper Arm Tendon, Right<br>**4** Upper Arm Tendon, Left<br>**5** Lower Arm and Wrist Tendon, Right<br>**6** Lower Arm and Wrist Tendon, Left<br>**7** Hand Tendon, Right<br>**8** Hand Tendon, Left<br>**9** Trunk Tendon, Right<br>**B** Trunk Tendon, Left<br>**C** Thorax Tendon, Right<br>**D** Thorax Tendon, Left<br>**F** Abdomen Tendon, Right<br>**G** Abdomen Tendon, Left<br>**H** Perineum Tendon<br>**J** Hip Tendon, Right<br>**K** Hip Tendon, Left<br>**L** Upper Leg Tendon, Right<br>**M** Upper Leg Tendon, Left<br>**N** Lower Leg Tendon, Right<br>Achilles tendon<br>**P** Lower Leg Tendon, Left<br>*See N Lower Leg Tendon, Right*<br>**Q** Knee Tendon, Right<br>Patellar tendon<br>**R** Knee Tendon, Left<br>*See Q Knee Tendon, Right*<br>**S** Ankle Tendon, Right<br>**T** Ankle Tendon, Left<br>**V** Foot Tendon, Right<br>**W** Foot Tendon, Left | **Ø** Open<br>**4** Percutaneous Endoscopic | **7** Autologous Tissue Substitute<br>**J** Synthetic Substitute<br>**K** Nonautologous Tissue Substitute | **Z** No Qualifier |

**Ø Medical and Surgical**
**L Tendons**
**W Revision**

Definition: Correcting, to the extent possible, a portion of a malfunctioning device or the position of a displaced device

Explanation: Revision can include correcting a malfunctioning or displaced device by taking out or putting in components of the device such as a screw or pin

| Body Part Character 4 | Approach Character 5 | Device Character 6 | Qualifier Character 7 |
|---|---|---|---|
| X Upper Tendon<br>Y Lower Tendon | Ø Open<br>3 Percutaneous<br>4 Percutaneous Endoscopic | Ø Drainage Device<br>7 Autologous Tissue Substitute<br>J Synthetic Substitute<br>K Nonautologous Tissue Substitute<br>Y Other Device | Z No Qualifier |
| X Upper Tendon<br>Y Lower Tendon | X External | Ø Drainage Device<br>7 Autologous Tissue Substitute<br>J Synthetic Substitute<br>K Nonautologous Tissue Substitute | Z No Qualifier |

Non-OR ØLW[X,Y][3,4]YZ
Non-OR ØLW[X,Y]X[Ø,7,J,K]Z

**Ø Medical and Surgical**
**L Tendons**
**X Transfer**

Definition: Moving, without taking out, all or a portion of a body part to another location to take over the function of all or a portion of a body part

Explanation: The body part transferred remains connected to its vascular and nervous supply

| Body Part Character 4 | Approach Character 5 | Device Character 6 | Qualifier Character 7 |
|---|---|---|---|
| Ø Head and Neck Tendon<br>1 Shoulder Tendon, Right<br>2 Shoulder Tendon, Left<br>3 Upper Arm Tendon, Right<br>4 Upper Arm Tendon, Left<br>5 Lower Arm and Wrist Tendon, Right<br>6 Lower Arm and Wrist Tendon, Left<br>7 Hand Tendon, Right<br>8 Hand Tendon, Left<br>9 Trunk Tendon, Right<br>B Trunk Tendon, Left<br>C Thorax Tendon, Right<br>D Thorax Tendon, Left<br>F Abdomen Tendon, Right<br>G Abdomen Tendon, Left<br>H Perineum Tendon<br>J Hip Tendon, Right<br>K Hip Tendon, Left<br>L Upper Leg Tendon, Right<br>M Upper Leg Tendon, Left<br>N Lower Leg Tendon, Right<br>Achilles tendon<br>P Lower Leg Tendon, Left<br>*See N Lower Leg Tendon, Right*<br>Q Knee Tendon, Right<br>Patellar tendon<br>R Knee Tendon, Left<br>*See Q Knee Tendon, Right*<br>S Ankle Tendon, Right<br>T Ankle Tendon, Left<br>V Foot Tendon, Right<br>W Foot Tendon, Left | Ø Open<br>4 Percutaneous Endoscopic | Z No Device | Z No Qualifier |

# Bursae and Ligaments ØM2–ØMX



## Character Meanings*

This Character Meaning table is provided as a guide to assist the user in the identification of character members that may be found in this section of code tables. It **SHOULD NOT** be used to build a PCS code.

| Operation–Character 3 | | Body Part–Character 4 | | Approach–Character 5 | | Device–Character 6 | | Qualifier–Character 7 | |
|---|---|---|---|---|---|---|---|---|---|
| 2 | Change | Ø | Head and Neck Bursa and Ligament | Ø | Open | Ø | Drainage Device | X | Diagnostic |
| 5 | Destruction | 1 | Shoulder Bursa and Ligament, Right | 3 | Percutaneous | 7 | Autologous Tissue Substitute | Z | No Qualifier |
| 8 | Division | 2 | Shoulder Bursa and Ligament, Left | 4 | Percutaneous Endoscopic | J | Synthetic Substitute | | |
| 9 | Drainage | 3 | Elbow Bursa and Ligament, Right | X | External | K | Nonautologous Tissue Substitute | | |
| B | Excision | 4 | Elbow Bursa and Ligament, Left | | | Y | Other Device | | |
| C | Extirpation | 5 | Wrist Bursa and Ligament, Right | | | Z | No Device | | |
| D | Extraction | 6 | Wrist Bursa and Ligament, Left | | | | | | |
| H | Insertion | 7 | Hand Bursa and Ligament, Right | | | | | | |
| J | Inspection | 8 | Hand Bursa and Ligament, Left | | | | | | |
| M | Reattachment | 9 | Upper Extremity Bursa and Ligament, Right | | | | | | |
| N | Release | B | Upper Extremity Bursa and Ligament, Left | | | | | | |
| P | Removal | C | Upper Spine Bursa and Ligament | | | | | | |
| Q | Repair | D | Lower Spine Bursa and Ligament | | | | | | |
| R | Replacement | F | Sternum Bursa and Ligament | | | | | | |
| S | Reposition | G | Rib(s) Bursa and Ligament | | | | | | |
| T | Resection | H | Abdomen Bursa and Ligament, Right | | | | | | |
| U | Supplement | J | Abdomen Bursa and Ligament, Left | | | | | | |
| W | Revision | K | Perineum Bursa and Ligament | | | | | | |
| X | Transfer | L | Hip Bursa and Ligament, Right | | | | | | |
| | | M | Hip Bursa and Ligament, Left | | | | | | |
| | | N | Knee Bursa and Ligament, Right | | | | | | |
| | | P | Knee Bursa and Ligament, Left | | | | | | |
| | | Q | Ankle Bursa and Ligament, Right | | | | | | |
| | | R | Ankle Bursa and Ligament, Left | | | | | | |
| | | S | Foot Bursa and Ligament, Right | | | | | | |
| | | T | Foot Bursa and Ligament, Left | | | | | | |
| | | V | Lower Extremity Bursa and Ligament, Right | | | | | | |
| | | W | Lower Extremity Bursa and Ligament, Left | | | | | | |
| | | X | Upper Bursa and Ligament | | | | | | |
| | | Y | Lower Bursa and Ligament | | | | | | |

* Includes synovial membrane.

**AHA Coding Clinic for table ØMM**
**2013, 3Q, 20** Superior labrum anterior posterior (SLAP) repair and subacromial decompression

**AHA Coding Clinic for table ØMQ**
**2014, 3Q, 9** Interspinous ligamentoplasty

**AHA Coding Clinic for table ØMT**
**2017, 2Q, 21** Arthroscopic anterior cruciate ligament revision using autograft with anterolateral ligament reconstruction

**AHA Coding Clinic for table ØMU**
**2017, 2Q, 21** Arthroscopic anterior cruciate ligament revision using autograft with anterolateral ligament reconstruction

## Shoulder Anatomy

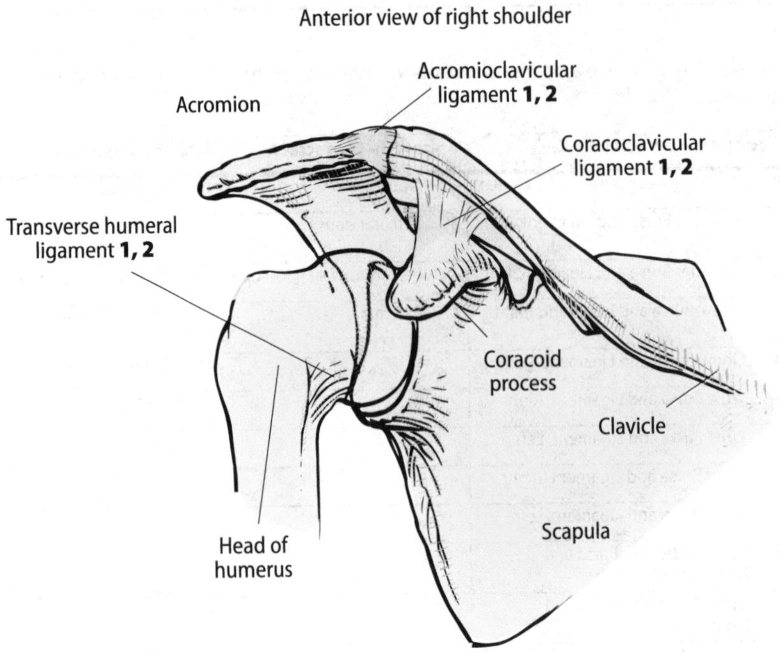
Anterior view of right shoulder
Acromion
Acromioclavicular ligament **1, 2**
Coracoclavicular ligament **1, 2**
Transverse humeral ligament **1, 2**
Coracoid process
Clavicle
Head of humerus
Scapula

## Knee Bursae

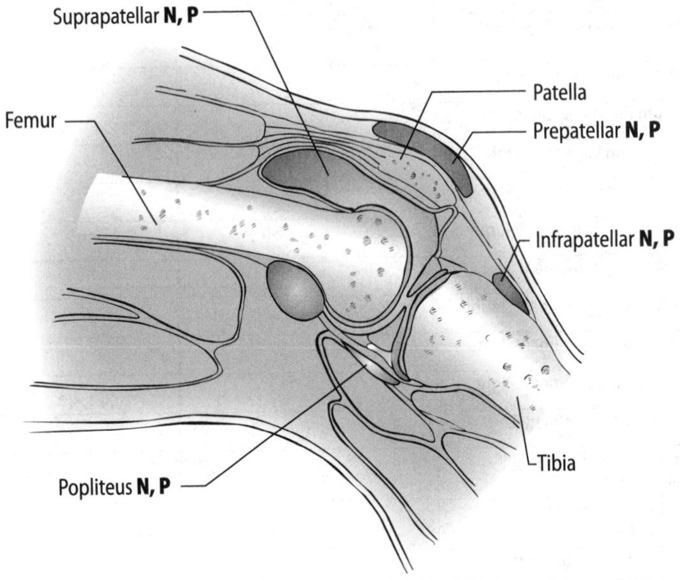
Suprapatellar **N, P**
Patella
Femur
Prepatellar **N, P**
Infrapatellar **N, P**
Tibia
Popliteus **N, P**

## Knee Ligaments

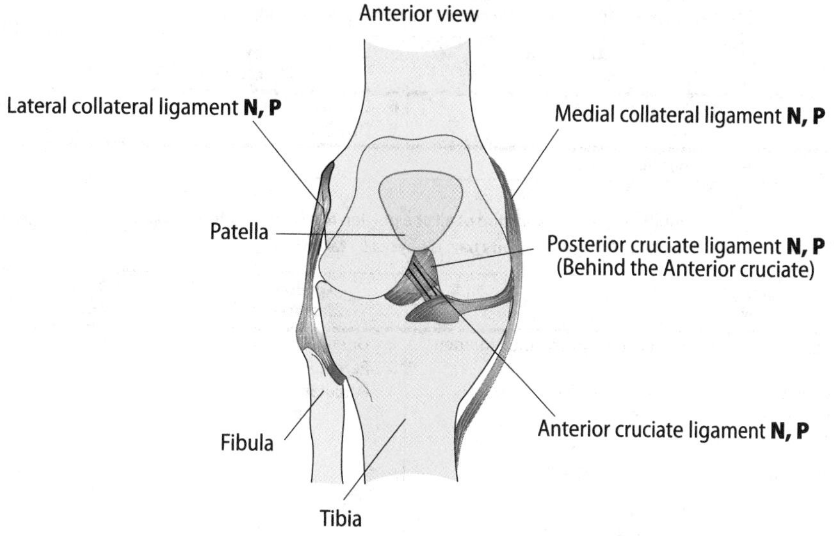
Anterior view
Lateral collateral ligament **N, P**
Medial collateral ligament **N, P**
Patella
Posterior cruciate ligament **N, P**
(Behind the Anterior cruciate)
Fibula
Anterior cruciate ligament **N, P**
Tibia

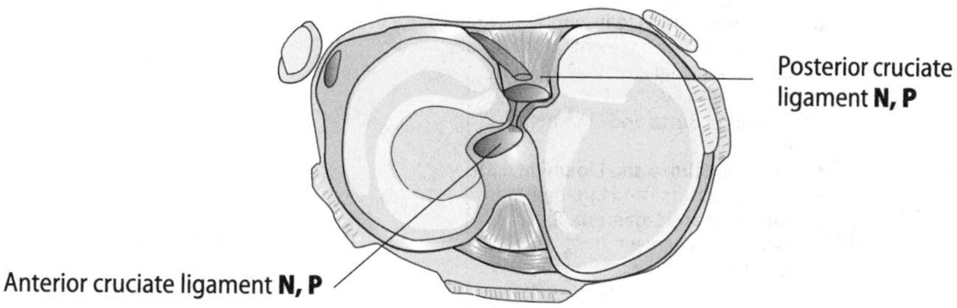
Posterior cruciate ligament **N, P**
Anterior cruciate ligament **N, P**

## Wrist Ligaments

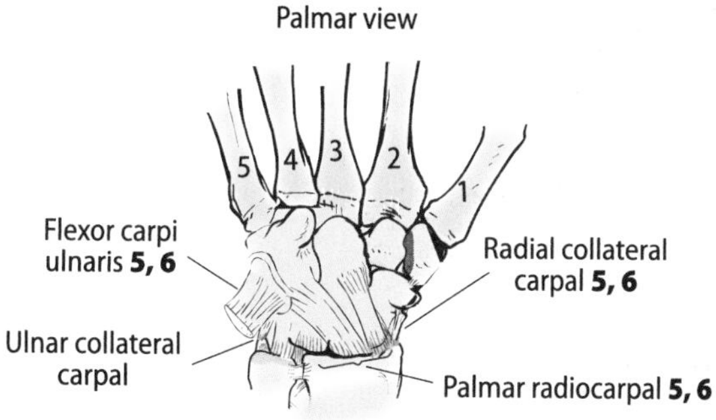
Palmar view
5
4
3
2
1
Flexor carpi ulnaris **5, 6**
Radial collateral carpal **5, 6**
Ulnar collateral carpal
Palmar radiocarpal **5, 6**

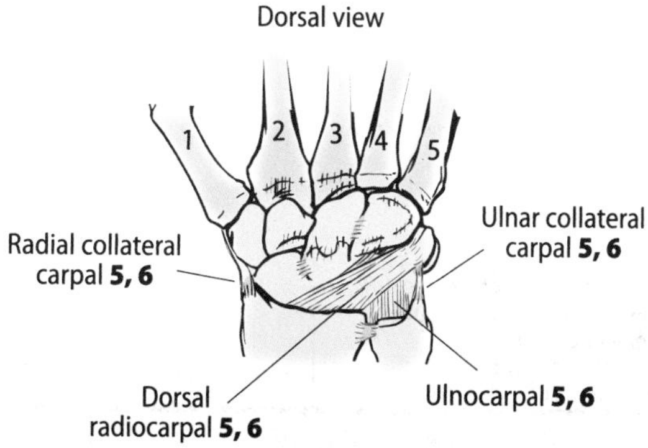
Dorsal view
1
2
3
4
5
Radial collateral carpal **5, 6**
Ulnar collateral carpal **5, 6**
Dorsal radiocarpal **5, 6**
Ulnocarpal **5, 6**

**Ø Medical and Surgical**
**M Bursae and Ligaments**
**2 Change**

Definition: Taking out or off a device from a body part and putting back an identical or similar device in or on the same body part without cutting or puncturing the skin or a mucous membrane

Explanation: All CHANGE procedures are coded using the approach EXTERNAL

| Body Part Character 4 | Approach Character 5 | Device Character 6 | Qualifier Character 7 |
|---|---|---|---|
| **X** Upper Bursa and Ligament<br>**Y** Lower Bursa and Ligament | **X** External | **Ø** Drainage Device<br>**Y** Other Device | **Z** No Qualifier |

Non-OR All body part, approach, device, and qualifier values

**Ø Medical and Surgical**
**M Bursae and Ligaments**
**5 Destruction**

Definition: Physical eradication of all or a portion of a body part by the direct use of energy, force, or a destructive agent

Explanation: None of the body part is physically taken out

| Body Part Character 4 | Approach Character 5 | Device Character 6 | Qualifier Character 7 |
|---|---|---|---|
| **Ø Head and Neck Bursa and Ligament**<br>Alar ligament of axis<br>Cervical interspinous ligament<br>Cervical intertransverse ligament<br>Cervical ligamentum flavum<br>Interspinous ligament<br>Lateral temporomandibular ligament<br>Sphenomandibular ligament<br>Stylomandibular ligament<br>Transverse ligament of atlas<br>**1 Shoulder Bursa and Ligament, Right**<br>Acromioclavicular ligament<br>Coracoacromial ligament<br>Coracoclavicular ligament<br>Coracohumeral ligament<br>Costoclavicular ligament<br>Glenohumeral ligament<br>Interclavicular ligament<br>Sternoclavicular ligament<br>Subacromial bursa<br>Transverse humeral ligament<br>Transverse scapular ligament<br>**2 Shoulder Bursa and Ligament, Left**<br>*See 1 Shoulder Bursa and Ligament, Right*<br>**3 Elbow Bursa and Ligament, Right**<br>Annular ligament<br>Olecranon bursa<br>Radial collateral ligament<br>Ulnar collateral ligament<br>**4 Elbow Bursa and Ligament, Left**<br>*See 3 Elbow Bursa and Ligament, Right*<br>**5 Wrist Bursa and Ligament, Right**<br>Palmar ulnocarpal ligament<br>Radial collateral carpal ligament<br>Radiocarpal ligament<br>Radioulnar ligament<br>Ulnar collateral carpal ligament<br>**6 Wrist Bursa and Ligament, Left**<br>*See 5 Wrist Bursa and Ligament, Right*<br>**7 Hand Bursa and Ligament, Right**<br>Carpometacarpal ligament<br>Intercarpal ligament<br>Interphalangeal ligament<br>Lunotriquetral ligament<br>Metacarpal ligament<br>Metacarpophalangeal ligament<br>Pisohamate ligament<br>Pisometacarpal ligament<br>Scapholunate ligament<br>Scaphotrapezium ligament<br>**8 Hand Bursa and Ligament, Left**<br>*See 7 Hand Bursa and Ligament, Right*<br>**9 Upper Extremity Bursa and Ligament, Right**<br>**B Upper Extremity Bursa and Ligament, Left**<br>**C Upper Spine Bursa and Ligament**<br>Interspinous ligament<br>Intertransverse ligament<br>Ligamentum flavum<br>Supraspinous ligament<br>**D Lower Spine Bursa and Ligament**<br>Iliolumbar ligament<br>Interspinous ligament<br>Intertransverse ligament<br>Ligamentum flavum<br>Sacrococcygeal ligament<br>Sacroiliac ligament<br>Sacrospinous ligament<br>Sacrotuberous ligament<br>Supraspinous ligament<br>**F Sternum Bursa and Ligament**<br>Costotransverse ligament<br>Costoxiphoid ligament<br>Sternocostal ligament<br>**G Rib(s) Bursa and Ligament**<br>Costotransverse ligament<br>Costoxiphoid ligament<br>Sternocostal ligament<br>**H Abdomen Bursa and Ligament, Right**<br>**J Abdomen Bursa and Ligament, Left**<br>**K Perineum Bursa and Ligament**<br>**L Hip Bursa and Ligament, Right**<br>Iliofemoral ligament<br>Ischiofemoral ligament<br>Pubofemoral ligament<br>Transverse acetabular ligament<br>Trochanteric bursa<br>**M Hip Bursa and Ligament, Left**<br>*See L Hip Bursa and Ligament, Right*<br>**N Knee Bursa and Ligament, Right**<br>Anterior cruciate ligament (ACL)<br>Lateral collateral ligament (LCL)<br>Ligament of head of fibula<br>Medial collateral ligament (MCL)<br>Patellar ligament<br>Popliteal ligament<br>Posterior cruciate ligament (PCL)<br>Prepatellar bursa<br>**P Knee Bursa and Ligament, Left**<br>*See N Knee Bursa and Ligament, Right*<br>**Q Ankle Bursa and Ligament, Right**<br>Calcaneofibular ligament<br>Deltoid ligament<br>Ligament of the lateral malleolus<br>Talofibular ligament<br>**R Ankle Bursa and Ligament, Left**<br>*See Q Ankle Bursa and Ligament, Right*<br>**S Foot Bursa and Ligament, Right**<br>Calcaneocuboid ligament<br>Cuneonavicular ligament<br>Intercuneiform ligament<br>Interphalangeal ligament<br>Metatarsal ligament<br>Metatarsophalangeal ligament<br>Subtalar ligament<br>Talocalcaneal ligament<br>Talocalcaneonavicular ligament<br>Tarsometatarsal ligament<br>**T Foot Bursa and Ligament, Left**<br>*See S Foot Bursa and Ligament, Right*<br>**V Lower Extremity Bursa and Ligament, Right**<br>**W Lower Extremity Bursa and Ligament, Left** | **Ø** Open<br>**3** Percutaneous<br>**4** Percutaneous Endoscopic | **Z** No Device | **Z** No Qualifier |

**Ø Medical and Surgical**
**M Bursae and Ligaments**
**8 Division** Definition: Cutting into a body part, without draining fluids and/or gases from the body part, in order to separate or transect a body part
Explanation: All or a portion of the body part is separated into two or more portions

| Body Part Character 4 | Approach Character 5 | Device Character 6 | Qualifier Character 7 |
|---|---|---|---|
| **Ø Head and Neck Bursa and Ligament**<br>Alar ligament of axis<br>Cervical interspinous ligament<br>Cervical intertransverse ligament<br>Cervical ligamentum flavum<br>Interspinous ligament<br>Lateral temporomandibular ligament<br>Sphenomandibular ligament<br>Stylomandibular ligament<br>Transverse ligament of atlas<br>**1 Shoulder Bursa and Ligament, Right**<br>Acromioclavicular ligament<br>Coracoacromial ligament<br>Coracoclavicular ligament<br>Coracohumeral ligament<br>Costoclavicular ligament<br>Glenohumeral ligament<br>Interclavicular ligament<br>Sternoclavicular ligament<br>Subacromial bursa<br>Transverse humeral ligament<br>Transverse scapular ligament<br>**2 Shoulder Bursa and Ligament, Left**<br>*See 1 Shoulder Bursa and Ligament, Right*<br>**3 Elbow Bursa and Ligament, Right**<br>Annular ligament<br>Olecranon bursa<br>Radial collateral ligament<br>Ulnar collateral ligament<br>**4 Elbow Bursa and Ligament, Left**<br>*See 3 Elbow Bursa and Ligament, Right*<br>**5 Wrist Bursa and Ligament, Right**<br>Palmar ulnocarpal ligament<br>Radial collateral carpal ligament<br>Radiocarpal ligament<br>Radioulnar ligament<br>Ulnar collateral carpal ligament<br>**6 Wrist Bursa and Ligament, Left**<br>*See 5 Wrist Bursa and Ligament, Right*<br>**7 Hand Bursa and Ligament, Right**<br>Carpometacarpal ligament<br>Intercarpal ligament<br>Interphalangeal ligament<br>Lunotriquetral ligament<br>Metacarpal ligament<br>Metacarpophalangeal ligament<br>Pisohamate ligament<br>Pisometacarpal ligament<br>Scapholunate ligament<br>Scaphotrapezium ligament<br>**8 Hand Bursa and Ligament, Left**<br>*See 7 Hand Bursa and Ligament, Right*<br>**9 Upper Extremity Bursa and Ligament, Right**<br>**B Upper Extremity Bursa and Ligament, Left**<br>**C Upper Spine Bursa and Ligament**<br>Interspinous ligament<br>Intertransverse ligament<br>Ligamentum flavum<br>Supraspinous ligament<br>**D Lower Spine Bursa and Ligament**<br>Iliolumbar ligament<br>Interspinous ligament<br>Intertransverse ligament<br>Ligamentum flavum<br>Sacrococcygeal ligament<br>Sacroiliac ligament<br>Sacrospinous ligament<br>Sacrotuberous ligament<br>Supraspinous ligament<br>**F Sternum Bursa and Ligament**<br>Costotransverse ligament<br>Costoxiphoid ligament<br>Sternocostal ligament<br>**G Rib(s) Bursa and Ligament**<br>Costotransverse ligament<br>Costoxiphoid ligament<br>Sternocostal ligament<br>**H Abdomen Bursa and Ligament, Right**<br>**J Abdomen Bursa and Ligament, Left**<br>**K Perineum Bursa and Ligament**<br>**L Hip Bursa and Ligament, Right**<br>Iliofemoral ligament<br>Ischiofemoral ligament<br>Pubofemoral ligament<br>Transverse acetabular ligament<br>Trochanteric bursa<br>**M Hip Bursa and Ligament, Left**<br>*See L Hip Bursa and Ligament, Right*<br>**N Knee Bursa and Ligament, Right**<br>Anterior cruciate ligament (ACL)<br>Lateral collateral ligament (LCL)<br>Ligament of head of fibula<br>Medial collateral ligament (MCL)<br>Patellar ligament<br>Popliteal ligament<br>Posterior cruciate ligament (PCL)<br>Prepatellar bursa<br>**P Knee Bursa and Ligament, Left**<br>*See N Knee Bursa and Ligament, Right*<br>**Q Ankle Bursa and Ligament, Right**<br>Calcaneofibular ligament<br>Deltoid ligament<br>Ligament of the lateral malleolus<br>Talofibular ligament<br>**R Ankle Bursa and Ligament, Left**<br>*See Q Ankle Bursa and Ligament, Right*<br>**S Foot Bursa and Ligament, Right**<br>Calcaneocuboid ligament<br>Cuneonavicular ligament<br>Intercuneiform ligament<br>Interphalangeal ligament<br>Metatarsal ligament<br>Metatarsophalangeal ligament<br>Subtalar ligament<br>Talocalcaneal ligament<br>Talocalcaneonavicular ligament<br>Tarsometatarsal ligament<br>**T Foot Bursa and Ligament, Left**<br>*See S Foot Bursa and Ligament, Right*<br>**V Lower Extremity Bursa and Ligament, Right**<br>**W Lower Extremity Bursa and Ligament, Left** | **Ø** Open<br>**3** Percutaneous<br>**4** Percutaneous Endoscopic | **Z** No Device | **Z** No Qualifier |

**Ø Medical and Surgical**
**M Bursae and Ligaments**
**9 Drainage** Definition: Taking or letting out fluids and/or gases from a body part

Explanation: The qualifier DIAGNOSTIC is used to identify drainage procedures that are biopsies

| Body Part Character 4 | Approach Character 5 | Device Character 6 | Qualifier Character 7 |
|---|---|---|---|
| **Ø Head and Neck Bursa and Ligament**<br>Alar ligament of axis<br>Cervical interspinous ligament<br>Cervical intertransverse ligament<br>Cervical ligamentum flavum<br>Interspinous ligament<br>Lateral temporomandibular ligament<br>Sphenomandibular ligament<br>Stylomandibular ligament<br>Transverse ligament of atlas<br>**1 Shoulder Bursa and Ligament, Right**<br>Acromioclavicular ligament<br>Coracoacromial ligament<br>Coracoclavicular ligament<br>Coracohumeral ligament<br>Costoclavicular ligament<br>Glenohumeral ligament<br>Interclavicular ligament<br>Sternoclavicular ligament<br>Subacromial bursa<br>Transverse humeral ligament<br>Transverse scapular ligament<br>**2 Shoulder Bursa and Ligament, Left**<br>**See** *1 Shoulder Bursa and Ligament, Right*<br>**3 Elbow Bursa and Ligament, Right**<br>Annular ligament<br>Olecranon bursa<br>Radial collateral ligament<br>Ulnar collateral ligament<br>**4 Elbow Bursa and Ligament, Left**<br>**See** *3 Elbow Bursa and Ligament, Right*<br>**5 Wrist Bursa and Ligament, Right**<br>Palmar ulnocarpal ligament<br>Radial collateral carpal ligament<br>Radiocarpal ligament<br>Radioulnar ligament<br>Ulnar collateral carpal ligament<br>**6 Wrist Bursa and Ligament, Left**<br>**See** *5 Wrist Bursa and Ligament, Right*<br>**7 Hand Bursa and Ligament, Right**<br>Carpometacarpal ligament<br>Intercarpal ligament<br>Interphalangeal ligament<br>Lunotriquetral ligament<br>Metacarpal ligament<br>Metacarpophalangeal ligament<br>Pisohamate ligament<br>Pisometacarpal ligament<br>Scapholunate ligament<br>Scaphotrapezium ligament<br>**8 Hand Bursa and Ligament, Left**<br>**See** *7 Hand Bursa and Ligament, Right*<br>**9 Upper Extremity Bursa and Ligament, Right**<br>**B Upper Extremity Bursa and Ligament, Left**<br>**C Upper Spine Bursa and Ligament**<br>Interspinous ligament<br>Intertransverse ligament<br>Ligamentum flavum<br>Supraspinous ligament<br>**D Lower Spine Bursa and Ligament**<br>Iliolumbar ligament<br>Interspinous ligament<br>Intertransverse ligament<br>Ligamentum flavum<br>Sacrococcygeal ligament<br>Sacroiliac ligament<br>Sacrospinous ligament<br>Sacrotuberous ligament<br>Supraspinous ligament<br>**F Sternum Bursa and Ligament**<br>Costotransverse ligament<br>Costoxiphoid ligament<br>Sternocostal ligament<br>**G Rib(s) Bursa and Ligament**<br>Costotransverse ligament<br>Costoxiphoid ligament<br>Sternocostal ligament<br>**H Abdomen Bursa and Ligament, Right**<br>**J Abdomen Bursa and Ligament, Left**<br>**K Perineum Bursa and Ligament**<br>**L Hip Bursa and Ligament, Right**<br>Iliofemoral ligament<br>Ischiofemoral ligament<br>Pubofemoral ligament<br>Transverse acetabular ligament<br>Trochanteric bursa<br>**M Hip Bursa and Ligament, Left**<br>**See** *L Hip Bursa and Ligament, Right*<br>**N Knee Bursa and Ligament, Right**<br>Anterior cruciate ligament (ACL)<br>Lateral collateral ligament (LCL)<br>Ligament of head of fibula<br>Medial collateral ligament (MCL)<br>Patellar ligament<br>Popliteal ligament<br>Posterior cruciate ligament (PCL)<br>Prepatellar bursa<br>**P Knee Bursa and Ligament, Left**<br>**See** *N Knee Bursa and Ligament, Right*<br>**Q Ankle Bursa and Ligament, Right**<br>Calcaneofibular ligament<br>Deltoid ligament<br>Ligament of the lateral malleolus<br>Talofibular ligament<br>**R Ankle Bursa and Ligament, Left**<br>**See** *Q Ankle Bursa and Ligament, Right*<br>**S Foot Bursa and Ligament, Right**<br>Calcaneocuboid ligament<br>Cuneonavicular ligament<br>Intercuneiform ligament<br>Interphalangeal ligament<br>Metatarsal ligament<br>Metatarsophalangeal ligament<br>Subtalar ligament<br>Talocalcaneal ligament<br>Talocalcaneonavicular ligament<br>Tarsometatarsal ligament<br>**T Foot Bursa and Ligament, Left**<br>**See** *S Foot Bursa and Ligament, Right*<br>**V Lower Extremity Bursa and Ligament, Right**<br>**W Lower Extremity Bursa and Ligament, Left** | **Ø Open**<br>**3 Percutaneous**<br>**4 Percutaneous Endoscopic** | **Ø Drainage Device** | **Z No Qualifier** |

***ØM9 Continued on next page***

**Non-OR** ØM9[Ø,1,2,3,4,5,6,7,8,9,B,C,D,F,G,H,J,K,L,M,N,,P,Q,R,S,T,V,W]3ØZ
**Non-OR** ØM9[1,2,3,4,7,8,9,B,C,D,F,G,H,J,K,L,M,V,W]4ØZ

ØM9 Continued

**Ø Medical and Surgical**
**M Bursae and Ligaments**
**9 Drainage** Definition: Taking or letting out fluids and/or gases from a body part
Explanation: The qualifier DIAGNOSTIC is used to identify drainage procedures that are biopsies

| Body Part Character 4 | Approach Character 5 | Device Character 6 | Qualifier Character 7 |
|---|---|---|---|
| **Ø Head and Neck Bursa and Ligament**<br>Alar ligament of axis<br>Cervical interspinous ligament<br>Cervical intertransverse ligament<br>Cervical ligamentum flavum<br>Interspinous ligament<br>Lateral temporomandibular ligament<br>Sphenomandibular ligament<br>Stylomandibular ligament<br>Transverse ligament of atlas<br>**1 Shoulder Bursa and Ligament, Right**<br>Acromioclavicular ligament<br>Coracoacromial ligament<br>Coracoclavicular ligament<br>Coracohumeral ligament<br>Costoclavicular ligament<br>Glenohumeral ligament<br>Interclavicular ligament<br>Sternoclavicular ligament<br>Subacromial bursa<br>Transverse humeral ligament<br>Transverse scapular ligament<br>**2 Shoulder Bursa and Ligament, Left**<br>*See 1 Shoulder Bursa and Ligament, Right*<br>**3 Elbow Bursa and Ligament, Right**<br>Annular ligament<br>Olecranon bursa<br>Radial collateral ligament<br>Ulnar collateral ligament<br>**4 Elbow Bursa and Ligament, Left**<br>*See 3 Elbow Bursa and Ligament, Right*<br>**5 Wrist Bursa and Ligament, Right**<br>Palmar ulnocarpal ligament<br>Radial collateral carpal ligament<br>Radiocarpal ligament<br>Radioulnar ligament<br>Ulnar collateral carpal ligament<br>**6 Wrist Bursa and Ligament, Left**<br>*See 5 Wrist Bursa and Ligament, Right*<br>**7 Hand Bursa and Ligament, Right**<br>Carpometacarpal ligament<br>Intercarpal ligament<br>Interphalangeal ligament<br>Lunotriquetral ligament<br>Metacarpal ligament<br>Metacarpophalangeal ligament<br>Pisohamate ligament<br>Pisometacarpal ligament<br>Scapholunate ligament<br>Scaphotrapezium ligament<br>**8 Hand Bursa and Ligament, Left**<br>*See 7 Hand Bursa and Ligament, Right*<br>**9 Upper Extremity Bursa and Ligament, Right**<br>**B Upper Extremity Bursa and Ligament, Left**<br>**C Upper Spine Bursa and Ligament**<br>Interspinous ligament<br>Intertransverse ligament<br>Ligamentum flavum<br>Supraspinous ligament<br>**D Lower Spine Bursa and Ligament**<br>Iliolumbar ligament<br>Interspinous ligament<br>Intertransverse ligament<br>Ligamentum flavum<br>Sacrococcygeal ligament<br>Sacroiliac ligament<br>Sacrospinous ligament<br>Sacrotuberous ligament<br>Supraspinous ligament<br>**F Sternum Bursa and Ligament**<br>Costotransverse ligament<br>Costoxiphoid ligament<br>Sternocostal ligament<br>**G Rib(s) Bursa and Ligament**<br>Costotransverse ligament<br>Costoxiphoid ligament<br>Sternocostal ligament<br>**H Abdomen Bursa and Ligament, Right**<br>**J Abdomen Bursa and Ligament, Left**<br>**K Perineum Bursa and Ligament**<br>**L Hip Bursa and Ligament, Right**<br>Iliofemoral ligament<br>Ischiofemoral ligament<br>Pubofemoral ligament<br>Transverse acetabular ligament<br>Trochanteric bursa<br>**M Hip Bursa and Ligament, Left**<br>*See L Hip Bursa and Ligament, Right*<br>**N Knee Bursa and Ligament, Right**<br>Anterior cruciate ligament (ACL)<br>Lateral collateral ligament (LCL)<br>Ligament of head of fibula<br>Medial collateral ligament (MCL)<br>Patellar ligament<br>Popliteal ligament<br>Posterior cruciate ligament (PCL)<br>Prepatellar bursa<br>**P Knee Bursa and Ligament, Left**<br>*See N Knee Bursa and Ligament, Right*<br>**Q Ankle Bursa and Ligament, Right**<br>Calcaneofibular ligament<br>Deltoid ligament<br>Ligament of the lateral malleolus<br>Talofibular ligament<br>**R Ankle Bursa and Ligament, Left**<br>*See Q Ankle Bursa and Ligament, Right*<br>**S Foot Bursa and Ligament, Right**<br>Calcaneocuboid ligament<br>Cuneonavicular ligament<br>Intercuneiform ligament<br>Interphalangeal ligament<br>Metatarsal ligament<br>Metatarsophalangeal ligament<br>Subtalar ligament<br>Talocalcaneal ligament<br>Talocalcaneonavicular ligament<br>Tarsometatarsal ligament<br>**T Foot Bursa and Ligament, Left**<br>*See S Foot Bursa and Ligament, Right*<br>**V Lower Extremity Bursa and Ligament, Right**<br>**W Lower Extremity Bursa and Ligament, Left** | **Ø Open**<br>**3 Percutaneous**<br>**4 Percutaneous Endoscopic** | **Z No Device** | **X Diagnostic**<br>**Z No Qualifier** |

**Non-OR** ØM9[Ø,1,2,3,4,5,6,7,8,C,D,F,G,L,M,N,P,Q,R,S,T][Ø,3,4]ZX
**Non-OR** ØM9[Ø,1,2,3,4,5,6,7,8,9,B,C,D,F,G,H,J,K,L,M,N,,P,Q,R,S,T,V,W]3ZZ
**Non-OR** ØM9[Ø,5,6,7,8,9,B,C,D,F,G,H,J,K,N,P,Q,R,S,T,V,W]4ZZ

**Ø Medical and Surgical**
**M Bursae and Ligaments**
**B Excision** Definition: Cutting out or off, without replacement, a portion of a body part

Explanation: The qualifier DIAGNOSTIC is used to identify excision procedures that are biopsies

| Body Part Character 4 | | Approach Character 5 | Device Character 6 | Qualifier Character 7 |
|---|---|---|---|---|
| **Ø Head and Neck Bursa and Ligament**<br>Alar ligament of axis<br>Cervical interspinous ligament<br>Cervical intertransverse ligament<br>Cervical ligamentum flavum<br>Interspinous ligament<br>Lateral temporomandibular ligament<br>Sphenomandibular ligament<br>Stylomandibular ligament<br>Transverse ligament of atlas<br>**1 Shoulder Bursa and Ligament, Right**<br>Acromioclavicular ligament<br>Coracoacromial ligament<br>Coracoclavicular ligament<br>Coracohumeral ligament<br>Costoclavicular ligament<br>Glenohumeral ligament<br>Interclavicular ligament<br>Sternoclavicular ligament<br>Subacromial bursa<br>Transverse humeral ligament<br>Transverse scapular ligament<br>**2 Shoulder Bursa and Ligament, Left**<br>*See 1 Shoulder Bursa and Ligament, Right*<br>**3 Elbow Bursa and Ligament, Right**<br>Annular ligament<br>Olecranon bursa<br>Radial collateral ligament<br>Ulnar collateral ligament<br>**4 Elbow Bursa and Ligament, Left**<br>*See 3 Elbow Bursa and Ligament, Right*<br>**5 Wrist Bursa and Ligament, Right**<br>Palmar ulnocarpal ligament<br>Radial collateral carpal ligament<br>Radiocarpal ligament<br>Radioulnar ligament<br>Ulnar collateral carpal ligament<br>**6 Wrist Bursa and Ligament, Left**<br>*See 5 Wrist Bursa and Ligament, Right*<br>**7 Hand Bursa and Ligament, Right**<br>Carpometacarpal ligament<br>Intercarpal ligament<br>Interphalangeal ligament<br>Lunotriquetral ligament<br>Metacarpal ligament<br>Metacarpophalangeal ligament<br>Pisohamate ligament<br>Pisometacarpal ligament<br>Scapholunate ligament<br>Scaphotrapezium ligament<br>**8 Hand Bursa and Ligament, Left**<br>*See 7 Hand Bursa and Ligament, Right*<br>**9 Upper Extremity Bursa and Ligament, Right**<br>**B Upper Extremity Bursa and Ligament, Left**<br>**C Upper Spine Bursa and Ligament**<br>Interspinous ligament<br>Intertransverse ligament<br>Ligamentum flavum<br>Supraspinous ligament | **D Lower Spine Bursa and Ligament**<br>Iliolumbar ligament<br>Interspinous ligament<br>Intertransverse ligament<br>Ligamentum flavum<br>Sacrococcygeal ligament<br>Sacroiliac ligament<br>Sacrospinous ligament<br>Sacrotuberous ligament<br>Supraspinous ligament<br>**F Sternum Bursa and Ligament**<br>Costotransverse ligament<br>Costoxiphoid ligament<br>Sternocostal ligament<br>**G Rib(s) Bursa and Ligament**<br>Costotransverse ligament<br>Costoxiphoid ligament<br>Sternocostal ligament<br>**H Abdomen Bursa and Ligament, Right**<br>**J Abdomen Bursa and Ligament, Left**<br>**K Perineum Bursa and Ligament**<br>**L Hip Bursa and Ligament, Right**<br>Iliofemoral ligament<br>Ischiofemoral ligament<br>Pubofemoral ligament<br>Transverse acetabular ligament<br>Trochanteric bursa<br>**M Hip Bursa and Ligament, Left**<br>*See L Hip Bursa and Ligament, Right*<br>**N Knee Bursa and Ligament, Right**<br>Anterior cruciate ligament (ACL)<br>Lateral collateral ligament (LCL)<br>Ligament of head of fibula<br>Medial collateral ligament (MCL)<br>Patellar ligament<br>Popliteal ligament<br>Posterior cruciate ligament (PCL)<br>Prepatellar bursa<br>**P Knee Bursa and Ligament, Left**<br>*See N Knee Bursa and Ligament, Right*<br>**Q Ankle Bursa and Ligament, Right**<br>Calcaneofibular ligament<br>Deltoid ligament<br>Ligament of the lateral malleolus<br>Talofibular ligament<br>**R Ankle Bursa and Ligament, Left**<br>*See Q Ankle Bursa and Ligament, Right*<br>**S Foot Bursa and Ligament, Right**<br>Calcaneocuboid ligament<br>Cuneonavicular ligament<br>Intercuneiform ligament<br>Interphalangeal ligament<br>Metatarsal ligament<br>Metatarsophalangeal ligament<br>Subtalar ligament<br>Talocalcaneal ligament<br>Talocalcaneonavicular ligament<br>Tarsometatarsal ligament<br>**T Foot Bursa and Ligament, Left**<br>*See S Foot Bursa and Ligament, Right*<br>**V Lower Extremity Bursa and Ligament, Right**<br>**W Lower Extremity Bursa and Ligament, Left** | **Ø Open**<br>**3 Percutaneous**<br>**4 Percutaneous Endoscopic** | **Z No Device** | **X Diagnostic**<br>**Z No Qualifier** |

Non-OR ØMB[Ø,1,2,3,4,5,6,7,8,B,C,D,F,G,L,M,N,P,Q,R,S,T][Ø,3,4]ZX
Non-OR ØMB94ZX

**Ø Medical and Surgical**
**M Bursae and Ligaments**
**C Extirpation** Definition: Taking or cutting out solid matter from a body part

Explanation: The solid matter may be an abnormal byproduct of a biological function or a foreign body; it may be imbedded in a body part or in the lumen of a tubular body part. The solid matter may or may not have been previously broken into pieces.

| Body Part Character 4 | | Approach Character 5 | Device Character 6 | Qualifier Character 7 |
|---|---|---|---|---|
| **Ø Head and Neck Bursa and Ligament**<br>Alar ligament of axis<br>Cervical interspinous ligament<br>Cervical intertransverse ligament<br>Cervical ligamentum flavum<br>Interspinous ligament<br>Lateral temporomandibular ligament<br>Sphenomandibular ligament<br>Stylomandibular ligament<br>Transverse ligament of atlas<br>**1 Shoulder Bursa and Ligament, Right**<br>Acromioclavicular ligament<br>Coracoacromial ligament<br>Coracoclavicular ligament<br>Coracohumeral ligament<br>Costoclavicular ligament<br>Glenohumeral ligament<br>Interclavicular ligament<br>Sternoclavicular ligament<br>Subacromial bursa<br>Transverse humeral ligament<br>Transverse scapular ligament<br>**2 Shoulder Bursa and Ligament, Left**<br>*See 1 Shoulder Bursa and Ligament, Right*<br>**3 Elbow Bursa and Ligament, Right**<br>Annular ligament<br>Olecranon bursa<br>Radial collateral ligament<br>Ulnar collateral ligament<br>**4 Elbow Bursa and Ligament, Left**<br>*See 3 Elbow Bursa and Ligament, Right*<br>**5 Wrist Bursa and Ligament, Right**<br>Palmar ulnocarpal ligament<br>Radial collateral carpal ligament<br>Radiocarpal ligament<br>Radioulnar ligament<br>Ulnar collateral carpal ligament<br>**6 Wrist Bursa and Ligament, Left**<br>*See 5 Wrist Bursa and Ligament, Right*<br>**7 Hand Bursa and Ligament, Right**<br>Carpometacarpal ligament<br>Intercarpal ligament<br>Interphalangeal ligament<br>Lunotriquetral ligament<br>Metacarpal ligament<br>Metacarpophalangeal ligament<br>Pisohamate ligament<br>Pisometacarpal ligament<br>Scapholunate ligament<br>Scaphotrapezium ligament<br>**8 Hand Bursa and Ligament, Left**<br>*See 7 Hand Bursa and Ligament, Right*<br>**9 Upper Extremity Bursa and Ligament, Right**<br>**B Upper Extremity Bursa and Ligament, Left**<br>C Upper Spine Bursa and Ligament<br>Interspinous ligament<br>Intertransverse ligament<br>Ligamentum flavum<br>Supraspinous ligament | D Lower Spine Bursa and Ligament<br>Iliolumbar ligament<br>Interspinous ligament<br>Intertransverse ligament<br>Ligamentum flavum<br>Sacrococcygeal ligament<br>Sacroiliac ligament<br>Sacrospinous ligament<br>Sacrotuberous ligament<br>Supraspinous ligament<br>F Sternum Bursa and Ligament<br>Costotransverse ligament<br>Costoxiphoid ligament<br>Sternocostal ligament<br>G Rib(s) Bursa and Ligament<br>Costotransverse ligament<br>Costoxiphoid ligament<br>Sternocostal ligament<br>**H Abdomen Bursa and Ligament, Right**<br>**J Abdomen Bursa and Ligament, Left**<br>**K Perineum Bursa and Ligament**<br>**L Hip Bursa and Ligament, Right**<br>Iliofemoral ligament<br>Ischiofemoral ligament<br>Pubofemoral ligament<br>Transverse acetabular ligament<br>Trochanteric bursa<br>**M Hip Bursa and Ligament, Left**<br>*See L Hip Bursa and Ligament, Right*<br>**N Knee Bursa and Ligament, Right**<br>Anterior cruciate ligament (ACL)<br>Lateral collateral ligament (LCL)<br>Ligament of head of fibula<br>Medial collateral ligament (MCL)<br>Patellar ligament<br>Popliteal ligament<br>Posterior cruciate ligament (PCL)<br>Prepatellar bursa<br>**P Knee Bursa and Ligament, Left**<br>*See N Knee Bursa and Ligament, Right*<br>**Q Ankle Bursa and Ligament, Right**<br>Calcaneofibular ligament<br>Deltoid ligament<br>Ligament of the lateral malleolus<br>Talofibular ligament<br>**R Ankle Bursa and Ligament, Left**<br>*See Q Ankle Bursa and Ligament, Right*<br>**S Foot Bursa and Ligament, Right**<br>Calcaneocuboid ligament<br>Cuneonavicular ligament<br>Intercuneiform ligament<br>Interphalangeal ligament<br>Metatarsal ligament<br>Metatarsophalangeal ligament<br>Subtalar ligament<br>Talocalcaneal ligament<br>Talocalcaneonavicular ligament<br>Tarsometatarsal ligament<br>**T Foot Bursa and Ligament, Left**<br>*See S Foot Bursa and Ligament, Right*<br>**V Lower Extremity Bursa and Ligament, Right**<br>**W Lower Extremity Bursa and Ligament, Left** | **Ø Open**<br>**3 Percutaneous**<br>**4 Percutaneous Endoscopic** | **Z No Device** | **Z No Qualifier** |

**Ø Medical and Surgical**
**M Bursae and Ligaments**
**D Extraction** Definition: Pulling or stripping out or off all or a portion of a body part by the use of force

Explanation: The qualifier DIAGNOSTIC is used to identify extraction procedures that are biopsies

| Body Part Character 4 | | Approach Character 5 | Device Character 6 | Qualifier Character 7 |
|---|---|---|---|---|
| **Ø Head and Neck Bursa and Ligament**<br>Alar ligament of axis<br>Cervical interspinous ligament<br>Cervical intertransverse ligament<br>Cervical ligamentum flavum<br>Interspinous ligament<br>Lateral temporomandibular ligament<br>Sphenomandibular ligament<br>Stylomandibular ligament<br>Transverse ligament of atlas<br>**1 Shoulder Bursa and Ligament, Right**<br>Acromioclavicular ligament<br>Coracoacromial ligament<br>Coracoclavicular ligament<br>Coracohumeral ligament<br>Costoclavicular ligament<br>Glenohumeral ligament<br>Interclavicular ligament<br>Sternoclavicular ligament<br>Subacromial bursa<br>Transverse humeral ligament<br>Transverse scapular ligament<br>**2 Shoulder Bursa and Ligament, Left**<br>***See** 1 Shoulder Bursa and Ligament, Right*<br>**3 Elbow Bursa and Ligament, Right**<br>Annular ligament<br>Olecranon bursa<br>Radial collateral ligament<br>Ulnar collateral ligament<br>**4 Elbow Bursa and Ligament, Left**<br>***See** 3 Elbow Bursa and Ligament, Right*<br>**5 Wrist Bursa and Ligament, Right**<br>Palmar ulnocarpal ligament<br>Radial collateral carpal ligament<br>Radiocarpal ligament<br>Radioulnar ligament<br>Ulnar collateral carpal ligament<br>**6 Wrist Bursa and Ligament, Left**<br>***See** 5 Wrist Bursa and Ligament, Right*<br>**7 Hand Bursa and Ligament, Right**<br>Carpometacarpal ligament<br>Intercarpal ligament<br>Interphalangeal ligament<br>Lunotriquetral ligament<br>Metacarpal ligament<br>Metacarpophalangeal ligament<br>Pisohamate ligament<br>Pisometacarpal ligament<br>Scapholunate ligament<br>Scaphotrapezium ligament<br>**8 Hand Bursa and Ligament, Left**<br>***See** 7 Hand Bursa and Ligament, Right*<br>**9 Upper Extremity Bursa and Ligament, Right**<br>**B Upper Extremity Bursa and Ligament, Left**<br>**C Upper Spine Bursa and Ligament**<br>Interspinous ligament<br>Intertransverse ligament<br>Ligamentum flavum<br>Supraspinous ligament | **D Lower Spine Bursa and Ligament**<br>Iliolumbar ligament<br>Interspinous ligament<br>Intertransverse ligament<br>Ligamentum flavum<br>Sacrococcygeal ligament<br>Sacroiliac ligament<br>Sacrospinous ligament<br>Sacrotuberous ligament<br>Supraspinous ligament<br>**F Sternum Bursa and Ligament**<br>Costotransverse ligament<br>Costoxiphoid ligament<br>Sternocostal ligament<br>**G Rib(s) Bursa and Ligament**<br>Costotransverse ligament<br>Costoxiphoid ligament<br>Sternocostal ligament<br>**H Abdomen Bursa and Ligament, Right**<br>**J Abdomen Bursa and Ligament, Left**<br>**K Perineum Bursa and Ligament**<br>**L Hip Bursa and Ligament, Right**<br>Iliofemoral ligament<br>Ischiofemoral ligament<br>Pubofemoral ligament<br>Transverse acetabular ligament<br>Trochanteric bursa<br>**M Hip Bursa and Ligament, Left**<br>***See** L Hip Bursa and Ligament, Right*<br>**N Knee Bursa and Ligament, Right**<br>Anterior cruciate ligament (ACL)<br>Lateral collateral ligament (LCL)<br>Ligament of head of fibula<br>Medial collateral ligament (MCL)<br>Patellar ligament<br>Popliteal ligament<br>Posterior cruciate ligament (PCL)<br>Prepatellar bursa<br>**P Knee Bursa and Ligament, Left**<br>***See** N Knee Bursa and Ligament, Right*<br>**Q Ankle Bursa and Ligament, Right**<br>Calcaneofibular ligament<br>Deltoid ligament<br>Ligament of the lateral malleolus<br>Talofibular ligament<br>**R Ankle Bursa and Ligament, Left**<br>***See** Q Ankle Bursa and Ligament, Right*<br>**S Foot Bursa and Ligament, Right**<br>Calcaneocuboid ligament<br>Cuneonavicular ligament<br>Intercuneiform ligament<br>Interphalangeal ligament<br>Metatarsal ligament<br>Metatarsophalangeal ligament<br>Subtalar ligament<br>Talocalcaneal ligament<br>Talocalcaneonavicular ligament<br>Tarsometatarsal ligament<br>**T Foot Bursa and Ligament, Left**<br>***See** S Foot Bursa and Ligament, Right*<br>**V Lower Extremity Bursa and Ligament, Right**<br>**W Lower Extremity Bursa and Ligament, Left** | **Ø Open**<br>**3 Percutaneous**<br>**4 Percutaneous Endoscopic** | **Z No Device** | **Z No Qualifier** |

**Ø Medical and Surgical**
**M Bursae and Ligaments**
**H Insertion** Definition: Putting in a nonbiological appliance that monitors, assists, performs, or prevents a physiological function but does not physically take the place of a body part

Explanation: None

| Body Part Character 4 | Approach Character 5 | Device Character 6 | Qualifier Character 7 |
|---|---|---|---|
| X Upper Bursa and Ligament<br>Y Lower Bursa and Ligament | Ø Open<br>3 Percutaneous<br>4 Percutaneous Endoscopic | Y Other Device | Z No Qualifier |

**Non-OR** ØMH[X,Y][3,4]YZ

**Ø Medical and Surgical**
**M Bursae and Ligaments**
**J Inspection** Definition: Visually and/or manually exploring a body part

Explanation: Visual exploration may be performed with or without optical instrumentation. Manual exploration may be performed directly or through intervening body layers.

| Body Part Character 4 | Approach Character 5 | Device Character 6 | Qualifier Character 7 |
|---|---|---|---|
| X Upper Bursa and Ligament<br>Y Lower Bursa and Ligament | Ø Open<br>3 Percutaneous<br>4 Percutaneous Endoscopic<br>X External | Z No Device | Z No Qualifier |

**Non-OR** ØMJ[X,Y][3,X]ZZ

**Ø Medical and Surgical**
**M Bursae and Ligaments**
**M Reattachment** Definition: Putting back in or on all or a portion of a separated body part to its normal location or other suitable location
Explanation: Vascular circulation and nervous pathways may or may not be reestablished

| Body Part Character 4 | Approach Character 5 | Device Character 6 | Qualifier Character 7 |
|---|---|---|---|
| **Ø Head and Neck Bursa and Ligament**<br>Alar ligament of axis<br>Cervical interspinous ligament<br>Cervical intertransverse ligament<br>Cervical ligamentum flavum<br>Interspinous ligament<br>Lateral temporomandibular ligament<br>Sphenomandibular ligament<br>Stylomandibular ligament<br>Transverse ligament of atlas<br>**1 Shoulder Bursa and Ligament, Right**<br>Acromioclavicular ligament<br>Coracoacromial ligament<br>Coracoclavicular ligament<br>Coracohumeral ligament<br>Costoclavicular ligament<br>Glenohumeral ligament<br>Interclavicular ligament<br>Sternoclavicular ligament<br>Subacromial bursa<br>Transverse humeral ligament<br>Transverse scapular ligament<br>**2 Shoulder Bursa and Ligament, Left**<br>*See 1 Shoulder Bursa and Ligament, Right*<br>**3 Elbow Bursa and Ligament, Right**<br>Annular ligament<br>Olecranon bursa<br>Radial collateral ligament<br>Ulnar collateral ligament<br>**4 Elbow Bursa and Ligament, Left**<br>*See 3 Elbow Bursa and Ligament, Right*<br>**5 Wrist Bursa and Ligament, Right**<br>Palmar ulnocarpal ligament<br>Radial collateral carpal ligament<br>Radiocarpal ligament<br>Radioulnar ligament<br>Ulnar collateral carpal ligament<br>**6 Wrist Bursa and Ligament, Left**<br>*See 5 Wrist Bursa and Ligament, Right*<br>**7 Hand Bursa and Ligament, Right**<br>Carpometacarpal ligament<br>Intercarpal ligament<br>Interphalangeal ligament<br>Lunotriquetral ligament<br>Metacarpal ligament<br>Metacarpophalangeal ligament<br>Pisohamate ligament<br>Pisometacarpal ligament<br>Scapholunate ligament<br>Scaphotrapezium ligament<br>**8 Hand Bursa and Ligament, Left**<br>*See 7 Hand Bursa and Ligament, Right*<br>**9 Upper Extremity Bursa and Ligament, Right**<br>**B Upper Extremity Bursa and Ligament, Left**<br>**C Upper Spine Bursa and Ligament**<br>Interspinous ligament<br>Intertransverse ligament<br>Ligamentum flavum<br>Supraspinous ligament<br>**D Lower Spine Bursa and Ligament**<br>Iliolumbar ligament<br>Interspinous ligament<br>Intertransverse ligament<br>Ligamentum flavum<br>Sacrococcygeal ligament<br>Sacroiliac ligament<br>Sacrospinous ligament<br>Sacrotuberous ligament<br>Supraspinous ligament<br>**F Sternum Bursa and Ligament**<br>Costotransverse ligament<br>Costoxiphoid ligament<br>Sternocostal ligament<br>**G Rib(s) Bursa and Ligament**<br>Costotransverse ligament<br>Costoxiphoid ligament<br>Sternocostal ligament<br>**H Abdomen Bursa and Ligament, Right**<br>**J Abdomen Bursa and Ligament, Left**<br>**K Perineum Bursa and Ligament**<br>**L Hip Bursa and Ligament, Right**<br>Iliofemoral ligament<br>Ischiofemoral ligament<br>Pubofemoral ligament<br>Transverse acetabular ligament<br>Trochanteric bursa<br>**M Hip Bursa and Ligament, Left**<br>*See L Hip Bursa and Ligament, Right*<br>**N Knee Bursa and Ligament, Right**<br>Anterior cruciate ligament (ACL)<br>Lateral collateral ligament (LCL)<br>Ligament of head of fibula<br>Medial collateral ligament (MCL)<br>Patellar ligament<br>Popliteal ligament<br>Posterior cruciate ligament (PCL)<br>Prepatellar bursa<br>**P Knee Bursa and Ligament, Left**<br>*See N Knee Bursa and Ligament, Right*<br>**Q Ankle Bursa and Ligament, Right**<br>Calcaneofibular ligament<br>Deltoid ligament<br>Ligament of the lateral malleolus<br>Talofibular ligament<br>**R Ankle Bursa and Ligament, Left**<br>*See Q Ankle Bursa and Ligament, Right*<br>**S Foot Bursa and Ligament, Right**<br>Calcaneocuboid ligament<br>Cuneonavicular ligament<br>Intercuneiform ligament<br>Interphalangeal ligament<br>Metatarsal ligament<br>Metatarsophalangeal ligament<br>Subtalar ligament<br>Talocalcaneal ligament<br>Talocalcaneonavicular ligament<br>Tarsometatarsal ligament<br>**T Foot Bursa and Ligament, Left**<br>*See S Foot Bursa and Ligament, Right*<br>**V Lower Extremity Bursa and Ligament, Right**<br>**W Lower Extremity Bursa and Ligament, Left** | **Ø Open**<br>**4 Percutaneous Endoscopic** | **Z No Device** | **Z No Qualifier** |

**Ø Medical and Surgical**
**M Bursae and Ligaments**
**N Release** Definition: Freeing a body part from an abnormal physical constraint by cutting or by the use of force
Explanation: Some of the restraining tissue may be taken out but none of the body part is taken out

| Body Part Character 4 | Approach Character 5 | Device Character 6 | Qualifier Character 7 |
|---|---|---|---|
| **Ø Head and Neck Bursa and Ligament**<br>Alar ligament of axis<br>Cervical interspinous ligament<br>Cervical intertransverse ligament<br>Cervical ligamentum flavum<br>Interspinous ligament<br>Lateral temporomandibular ligament<br>Sphenomandibular ligament<br>Stylomandibular ligament<br>Transverse ligament of atlas<br>**1 Shoulder Bursa and Ligament, Right**<br>Acromioclavicular ligament<br>Coracoacromial ligament<br>Coracoclavicular ligament<br>Coracohumeral ligament<br>Costoclavicular ligament<br>Glenohumeral ligament<br>Interclavicular ligament<br>Sternoclavicular ligament<br>Subacromial bursa<br>Transverse humeral ligament<br>Transverse scapular ligament<br>**2 Shoulder Bursa and Ligament, Left**<br>*See 1 Shoulder Bursa and Ligament, Right*<br>**3 Elbow Bursa and Ligament, Right**<br>Annular ligament<br>Olecranon bursa<br>Radial collateral ligament<br>Ulnar collateral ligament<br>**4 Elbow Bursa and Ligament, Left**<br>*See 3 Elbow Bursa and Ligament, Right*<br>**5 Wrist Bursa and Ligament, Right**<br>Palmar ulnocarpal ligament<br>Radial collateral carpal ligament<br>Radiocarpal ligament<br>Radioulnar ligament<br>Ulnar collateral carpal ligament<br>**6 Wrist Bursa and Ligament, Left**<br>*See 5 Wrist Bursa and Ligament, Right*<br>**7 Hand Bursa and Ligament, Right**<br>Carpometacarpal ligament<br>Intercarpal ligament<br>Interphalangeal ligament<br>Lunotriquetral ligament<br>Metacarpal ligament<br>Metacarpophalangeal ligament<br>Pisohamate ligament<br>Pisometacarpal ligament<br>Scapholunate ligament<br>Scaphotrapezium ligament<br>**8 Hand Bursa and Ligament, Left**<br>*See 7 Hand Bursa and Ligament, Right*<br>**9 Upper Extremity Bursa and Ligament, Right**<br>**B Upper Extremity Bursa and Ligament, Left**<br>**C Upper Spine Bursa and Ligament**<br>Interspinous ligament<br>Intertransverse ligament<br>Ligamentum flavum<br>Supraspinous ligament<br>**D Lower Spine Bursa and Ligament**<br>Iliolumbar ligament<br>Interspinous ligament<br>Intertransverse ligament<br>Ligamentum flavum<br>Sacrococcygeal ligament<br>Sacroiliac ligament<br>Sacrospinous ligament<br>Sacrotuberous ligament<br>Supraspinous ligament<br>**F Sternum Bursa and Ligament**<br>Costotransverse ligament<br>Costoxiphoid ligament<br>Sternocostal ligament<br>**G Rib(s) Bursa and Ligament**<br>Costotransverse ligament<br>Costoxiphoid ligament<br>Sternocostal ligament<br>**H Abdomen Bursa and Ligament, Right**<br>**J Abdomen Bursa and Ligament, Left**<br>**K Perineum Bursa and Ligament**<br>**L Hip Bursa and Ligament, Right**<br>Iliofemoral ligament<br>Ischiofemoral ligament<br>Pubofemoral ligament<br>Transverse acetabular ligament<br>Trochanteric bursa<br>**M Hip Bursa and Ligament, Left**<br>*See L Hip Bursa and Ligament, Right*<br>**N Knee Bursa and Ligament, Right**<br>Anterior cruciate ligament (ACL)<br>Lateral collateral ligament (LCL)<br>Ligament of head of fibula<br>Medial collateral ligament (MCL)<br>Patellar ligament<br>Popliteal ligament<br>Posterior cruciate ligament (PCL)<br>Prepatellar bursa<br>**P Knee Bursa and Ligament, Left**<br>*See N Knee Bursa and Ligament, Right*<br>**Q Ankle Bursa and Ligament, Right**<br>Calcaneofibular ligament<br>Deltoid ligament<br>Ligament of the lateral malleolus<br>Talofibular ligament<br>**R Ankle Bursa and Ligament, Left**<br>*See Q Ankle Bursa and Ligament, Right*<br>**S Foot Bursa and Ligament, Right**<br>Calcaneocuboid ligament<br>Cuneonavicular ligament<br>Intercuneiform ligament<br>Interphalangeal ligament<br>Metatarsal ligament<br>Metatarsophalangeal ligament<br>Subtalar ligament<br>Talocalcaneal ligament<br>Talocalcaneonavicular ligament<br>Tarsometatarsal ligament<br>**T Foot Bursa and Ligament, Left**<br>*See S Foot Bursa and Ligament, Right*<br>**V Lower Extremity Bursa and Ligament, Right**<br>**W Lower Extremity Bursa and Ligament, Left** | **Ø Open**<br>**3 Percutaneous**<br>**4 Percutaneous Endoscopic**<br>**X External** | **Z No Device** | **Z No Qualifier** |

**Non-OR** ØMN[Ø,1,2,3,4,5,6,7,8,9,B,C,D,F,G,H,J,K,L,M,N,P,Q,R,S,T,V,W]XZZ

**Ø Medical and Surgical**
**M Bursae and Ligaments**
**P Removal** Definition: Taking out or off a device from a body part

Explanation: If a device is taken out and a similar device put in without cutting or puncturing the skin or mucous membrane, the procedure is coded to the root operation CHANGE. Otherwise, the procedure for taking out a device is coded to the root operation REMOVAL.

| Body Part Character 4 | Approach Character 5 | Device Character 6 | Qualifier Character 7 |
|---|---|---|---|
| X Upper Bursa and Ligament<br>Y Lower Bursa and Ligament | Ø Open<br>3 Percutaneous<br>4 Percutaneous Endoscopic | Ø Drainage Device<br>7 Autologous Tissue Substitute<br>J Synthetic Substitute<br>K Nonautologous Tissue Substitute<br>Y Other Device | Z No Qualifier |
| X Upper Bursa and Ligament<br>Y Lower Bursa and Ligament | X External | Ø Drainage Device | Z No Qualifier |

Non-OR ØMP[X,Y]3ØZ
Non-OR ØMP[X,Y][3,4]YZ
Non-OR ØMP[X,Y]XØZ

**Ø Medical and Surgical**
**M Bursae and Ligaments**
**Q Repair** Definition: Restoring, to the extent possible, a body part to its normal anatomic structure and function
Explanation: Used only when the method to accomplish the repair is not one of the other root operations

| Body Part Character 4 | Approach Character 5 | Device Character 6 | Qualifier Character 7 |
|---|---|---|---|
| **Ø Head and Neck Bursa and Ligament**<br>Alar ligament of axis<br>Cervical interspinous ligament<br>Cervical intertransverse ligament<br>Cervical ligamentum flavum<br>Interspinous ligament<br>Lateral temporomandibular ligament<br>Sphenomandibular ligament<br>Stylomandibular ligament<br>Transverse ligament of atlas<br>**1 Shoulder Bursa and Ligament, Right**<br>Acromioclavicular ligament<br>Coracoacromial ligament<br>Coracoclavicular ligament<br>Coracohumeral ligament<br>Costoclavicular ligament<br>Glenohumeral ligament<br>Interclavicular ligament<br>Sternoclavicular ligament<br>Subacromial bursa<br>Transverse humeral ligament<br>Transverse scapular ligament<br>**2 Shoulder Bursa and Ligament, Left**<br>**See** *1 Shoulder Bursa and Ligament, Right*<br>**3 Elbow Bursa and Ligament, Right**<br>Annular ligament<br>Olecranon bursa<br>Radial collateral ligament<br>Ulnar collateral ligament<br>**4 Elbow Bursa and Ligament, Left**<br>**See** *3 Elbow Bursa and Ligament, Right*<br>**5 Wrist Bursa and Ligament, Right**<br>Palmar ulnocarpal ligament<br>Radial collateral carpal ligament<br>Radiocarpal ligament<br>Radioulnar ligament<br>Ulnar collateral carpal ligament<br>**6 Wrist Bursa and Ligament, Left**<br>**See** *5 Wrist Bursa and Ligament, Right*<br>**7 Hand Bursa and Ligament, Right**<br>Carpometacarpal ligament<br>Intercarpal ligament<br>Interphalangeal ligament<br>Lunotriquetral ligament<br>Metacarpal ligament<br>Metacarpophalangeal ligament<br>Pisohamate ligament<br>Pisometacarpal ligament<br>Scapholunate ligament<br>Scaphotrapezium ligament<br>**8 Hand Bursa and Ligament, Left**<br>**See** *7 Hand Bursa and Ligament, Right*<br>**9 Upper Extremity Bursa and Ligament, Right**<br>**B Upper Extremity Bursa and Ligament, Left**<br>C Upper Spine Bursa and Ligament<br>Interspinous ligament<br>Intertransverse ligament<br>Ligamentum flavum<br>Supraspinous ligament<br>D Lower Spine Bursa and Ligament<br>Iliolumbar ligament<br>Interspinous ligament<br>Intertransverse ligament<br>Ligamentum flavum<br>Sacrococcygeal ligament<br>Sacroiliac ligament<br>Sacrospinous ligament<br>Sacrotuberous ligament<br>Supraspinous ligament<br>F Sternum Bursa and Ligament<br>Costotransverse ligament<br>Costoxiphoid ligament<br>Sternocostal ligament<br>G Rib(s) Bursa and Ligament<br>Costotransverse ligament<br>Costoxiphoid ligament<br>Sternocostal ligament<br>**H Abdomen Bursa and Ligament, Right**<br>**J Abdomen Bursa and Ligament, Left**<br>**K Perineum Bursa and Ligament**<br>**L Hip Bursa and Ligament, Right**<br>Iliofemoral ligament<br>Ischiofemoral ligament<br>Pubofemoral ligament<br>Transverse acetabular ligament<br>Trochanteric bursa<br>**M Hip Bursa and Ligament, Left**<br>**See** *L Hip Bursa and Ligament, Right*<br>**N Knee Bursa and Ligament, Right**<br>Anterior cruciate ligament (ACL)<br>Lateral collateral ligament (LCL)<br>Ligament of head of fibula<br>Medial collateral ligament (MCL)<br>Patellar ligament<br>Popliteal ligament<br>Posterior cruciate ligament (PCL)<br>Prepatellar bursa<br>**P Knee Bursa and Ligament, Left**<br>**See** *N Knee Bursa and Ligament, Right*<br>**Q Ankle Bursa and Ligament, Right**<br>Calcaneofibular ligament<br>Deltoid ligament<br>Ligament of the lateral malleolus<br>Talofibular ligament<br>**R Ankle Bursa and Ligament, Left**<br>**See** *Q Ankle Bursa and Ligament, Right*<br>**S Foot Bursa and Ligament, Right**<br>Calcaneocuboid ligament<br>Cuneonavicular ligament<br>Intercuneiform ligament<br>Interphalangeal ligament<br>Metatarsal ligament<br>Metatarsophalangeal ligament<br>Subtalar ligament<br>Talocalcaneal ligament<br>Talocalcaneonavicular ligament<br>Tarsometatarsal ligament<br>**T Foot Bursa and Ligament, Left**<br>**See** *S Foot Bursa and Ligament, Right*<br>**V Lower Extremity Bursa and Ligament, Right**<br>**W Lower Extremity Bursa and Ligament, Left** | **Ø Open**<br>**3 Percutaneous**<br>**4 Percutaneous Endoscopic** | **Z No Device** | **Z No Qualifier** |

**Ø Medical and Surgical**
**M Bursae and Ligaments**
**R Replacement** Definition: Putting in or on biological or synthetic material that physically takes the place and/or function of all or a portion of a body part

Explanation: The body part may have been taken out or replaced, or may be taken out, physically eradicated, or rendered nonfunctional during the REPLACEMENT procedure. A REMOVAL procedure is coded for taking out the device used in a previous replacement procedure.

| Body Part Character 4 | Approach Character 5 | Device Character 6 | Qualifier Character 7 |
|---|---|---|---|
| **Ø Head and Neck Bursa and Ligament**<br>Alar ligament of axis<br>Cervical interspinous ligament<br>Cervical intertransverse ligament<br>Cervical ligamentum flavum<br>Interspinous ligament<br>Lateral temporomandibular ligament<br>Sphenomandibular ligament<br>Stylomandibular ligament<br>Transverse ligament of atlas<br>**1 Shoulder Bursa and Ligament, Right**<br>Acromioclavicular ligament<br>Coracoacromial ligament<br>Coracoclavicular ligament<br>Coracohumeral ligament<br>Costoclavicular ligament<br>Glenohumeral ligament<br>Interclavicular ligament<br>Sternoclavicular ligament<br>Subacromial bursa<br>Transverse humeral ligament<br>Transverse scapular ligament<br>**2 Shoulder Bursa and Ligament, Left**<br>**See** *1 Shoulder Bursa and Ligament, Right*<br>**3 Elbow Bursa and Ligament, Right**<br>Annular ligament<br>Olecranon bursa<br>Radial collateral ligament<br>Ulnar collateral ligament<br>**4 Elbow Bursa and Ligament, Left**<br>**See** *3 Elbow Bursa and Ligament, Right*<br>**5 Wrist Bursa and Ligament, Right**<br>Palmar ulnocarpal ligament<br>Radial collateral carpal ligament<br>Radiocarpal ligament<br>Radioulnar ligament<br>Ulnar collateral carpal ligament<br>**6 Wrist Bursa and Ligament, Left**<br>**See** *5 Wrist Bursa and Ligament, Right*<br>**7 Hand Bursa and Ligament, Right**<br>Carpometacarpal ligament<br>Intercarpal ligament<br>Interphalangeal ligament<br>Lunotriquetral ligament<br>Metacarpal ligament<br>Metacarpophalangeal ligament<br>Pisohamate ligament<br>Pisometacarpal ligament<br>Scapholunate ligament<br>Scaphotrapezium ligament<br>**8 Hand Bursa and Ligament, Left**<br>**See** *7 Hand Bursa and Ligament, Right*<br>**9 Upper Extremity Bursa and Ligament, Right**<br>**B Upper Extremity Bursa and Ligament, Left**<br>**C Upper Spine Bursa and Ligament**<br>Interspinous ligament<br>Intertransverse ligament<br>Ligamentum flavum<br>Supraspinous ligament<br>**D Lower Spine Bursa and Ligament**<br>Iliolumbar ligament<br>Interspinous ligament<br>Intertransverse ligament<br>Ligamentum flavum<br>Sacrococcygeal ligament<br>Sacroiliac ligament<br>Sacrospinous ligament<br>Sacrotuberous ligament<br>Supraspinous ligament<br>**F Sternum Bursa and Ligament**<br>Costotransverse ligament<br>Costoxiphoid ligament<br>Sternocostal ligament<br>**G Rib(s) Bursa and Ligament**<br>Costotransverse ligament<br>Costoxiphoid ligament<br>Sternocostal ligament<br>**H Abdomen Bursa and Ligament, Right**<br>**J Abdomen Bursa and Ligament, Left**<br>**K Perineum Bursa and Ligament**<br>**L Hip Bursa and Ligament, Right**<br>Iliofemoral ligament<br>Ischiofemoral ligament<br>Pubofemoral ligament<br>Transverse acetabular ligament<br>Trochanteric bursa<br>**M Hip Bursa and Ligament, Left**<br>**See** *L Hip Bursa and Ligament, Right*<br>**N Knee Bursa and Ligament, Right**<br>Anterior cruciate ligament (ACL)<br>Lateral collateral ligament (LCL)<br>Ligament of head of fibula<br>Medial collateral ligament (MCL)<br>Patellar ligament<br>Popliteal ligament<br>Posterior cruciate ligament (PCL)<br>Prepatellar bursa<br>**P Knee Bursa and Ligament, Left**<br>**See** *N Knee Bursa and Ligament, Right*<br>**Q Ankle Bursa and Ligament, Right**<br>Calcaneofibular ligament<br>Deltoid ligament<br>Ligament of the lateral malleolus<br>Talofibular ligament<br>**R Ankle Bursa and Ligament, Left**<br>**See** *Q Ankle Bursa and Ligament, Right*<br>**S Foot Bursa and Ligament, Right**<br>Calcaneocuboid ligament<br>Cuneonavicular ligament<br>Intercuneiform ligament<br>Interphalangeal ligament<br>Metatarsal ligament<br>Metatarsophalangeal ligament<br>Subtalar ligament<br>Talocalcaneal ligament<br>Talocalcaneonavicular ligament<br>Tarsometatarsal ligament<br>**T Foot Bursa and Ligament, Left**<br>**See** *S Foot Bursa and Ligament, Right*<br>**V Lower Extremity Bursa and Ligament, Right**<br>**W Lower Extremity Bursa and Ligament, Left** | **Ø Open**<br>**4 Percutaneous Endoscopic** | **7 Autologous Tissue Substitute**<br>**J Synthetic Substitute**<br>**K Nonautologous Tissue Substitute** | **Z No Qualifier** |

**Ø Medical and Surgical**
**M Bursae and Ligaments**
**S Reposition** Definition: Moving to its normal location, or other suitable location, all or a portion of a body part

Explanation: The body part is moved to a new location from an abnormal location, or from a normal location where it is not functioning correctly. The body part may or may not be cut out or off to be moved to the new location.

| Body Part Character 4 | Approach Character 5 | Device Character 6 | Qualifier Character 7 |
|---|---|---|---|
| **Ø Head and Neck Bursa and Ligament**<br>Alar ligament of axis<br>Cervical interspinous ligament<br>Cervical intertransverse ligament<br>Cervical ligamentum flavum<br>Interspinous ligament<br>Lateral temporomandibular ligament<br>Sphenomandibular ligament<br>Stylomandibular ligament<br>Transverse ligament of atlas<br>**1 Shoulder Bursa and Ligament, Right**<br>Acromioclavicular ligament<br>Coracoacromial ligament<br>Coracoclavicular ligament<br>Coracohumeral ligament<br>Costoclavicular ligament<br>Glenohumeral ligament<br>Interclavicular ligament<br>Sternoclavicular ligament<br>Subacromial bursa<br>Transverse humeral ligament<br>Transverse scapular ligament<br>**2 Shoulder Bursa and Ligament, Left**<br>***See*** *1 Shoulder Bursa and Ligament, Right*<br>**3 Elbow Bursa and Ligament, Right**<br>Annular ligament<br>Olecranon bursa<br>Radial collateral ligament<br>Ulnar collateral ligament<br>**4 Elbow Bursa and Ligament, Left**<br>***See*** *3 Elbow Bursa and Ligament, Right*<br>**5 Wrist Bursa and Ligament, Right**<br>Palmar ulnocarpal ligament<br>Radial collateral carpal ligament<br>Radiocarpal ligament<br>Radioulnar ligament<br>Ulnar collateral carpal ligament<br>**6 Wrist Bursa and Ligament, Left**<br>***See*** *5 Wrist Bursa and Ligament, Right*<br>**7 Hand Bursa and Ligament, Right**<br>Carpometacarpal ligament<br>Intercarpal ligament<br>Interphalangeal ligament<br>Lunotriquetral ligament<br>Metacarpal ligament<br>Metacarpophalangeal ligament<br>Pisohamate ligament<br>Pisometacarpal ligament<br>Scapholunate ligament<br>Scaphotrapezium ligament<br>**8 Hand Bursa and Ligament, Left**<br>***See*** *7 Hand Bursa and Ligament, Right*<br>**9 Upper Extremity Bursa and Ligament, Right**<br>**B Upper Extremity Bursa and Ligament, Left**<br>C Upper Spine Bursa and Ligament<br>Interspinous ligament<br>Intertransverse ligament<br>Ligamentum flavum<br>Supraspinous ligament<br>D Lower Spine Bursa and Ligament<br>Iliolumbar ligament<br>Interspinous ligament<br>Intertransverse ligament<br>Ligamentum flavum<br>Sacrococcygeal ligament<br>Sacroiliac ligament<br>Sacrospinous ligament<br>Sacrotuberous ligament<br>Supraspinous ligament<br>F Sternum Bursa and Ligament<br>Costotransverse ligament<br>Costoxiphoid ligament<br>Sternocostal ligament<br>G Rib(s) Bursa and Ligament<br>Costotransverse ligament<br>Costoxiphoid ligament<br>Sternocostal ligament<br>**H Abdomen Bursa and Ligament, Right**<br>**J Abdomen Bursa and Ligament, Left**<br>**K Perineum Bursa and Ligament**<br>**L Hip Bursa and Ligament, Right**<br>Iliofemoral ligament<br>Ischiofemoral ligament<br>Pubofemoral ligament<br>Transverse acetabular ligament<br>Trochanteric bursa<br>**M Hip Bursa and Ligament, Left**<br>***See*** *L Hip Bursa and Ligament, Right*<br>**N Knee Bursa and Ligament, Right**<br>Anterior cruciate ligament (ACL)<br>Lateral collateral ligament (LCL)<br>Ligament of head of fibula<br>Medial collateral ligament (MCL)<br>Patellar ligament<br>Popliteal ligament<br>Posterior cruciate ligament (PCL)<br>Prepatellar bursa<br>**P Knee Bursa and Ligament, Left**<br>***See*** *N Knee Bursa and Ligament, Right*<br>**Q Ankle Bursa and Ligament, Right**<br>Calcaneofibular ligament<br>Deltoid ligament<br>Ligament of the lateral malleolus<br>Talofibular ligament<br>**R Ankle Bursa and Ligament, Left**<br>***See*** *Q Ankle Bursa and Ligament, Right*<br>**S Foot Bursa and Ligament, Right**<br>Calcaneocuboid ligament<br>Cuneonavicular ligament<br>Intercuneiform ligament<br>Interphalangeal ligament<br>Metatarsal ligament<br>Metatarsophalangeal ligament<br>Subtalar ligament<br>Talocalcaneal ligament<br>Talocalcaneonavicular ligament<br>Tarsometatarsal ligament<br>**T Foot Bursa and Ligament, Left**<br>***See*** *S Foot Bursa and Ligament, Right*<br>**V Lower Extremity Bursa and Ligament, Right**<br>**W Lower Extremity Bursa and Ligament, Left** | **Ø Open**<br>**4 Percutaneous Endoscopic** | **Z No Device** | **Z No Qualifier** |

**Ø Medical and Surgical**
**M Bursae and Ligaments**
**T Resection** Definition: Cutting out or off, without replacement, all of a body part

Explanation: None

| Body Part Character 4 | Approach Character 5 | Device Character 6 | Qualifier Character 7 |
|---|---|---|---|
| **Ø Head and Neck Bursa and Ligament**<br>Alar ligament of axis<br>Cervical interspinous ligament<br>Cervical intertransverse ligament<br>Cervical ligamentum flavum<br>Interspinous ligament<br>Lateral temporomandibular ligament<br>Sphenomandibular ligament<br>Stylomandibular ligament<br>Transverse ligament of atlas<br>**1 Shoulder Bursa and Ligament, Right**<br>Acromioclavicular ligament<br>Coracoacromial ligament<br>Coracoclavicular ligament<br>Coracohumeral ligament<br>Costoclavicular ligament<br>Glenohumeral ligament<br>Interclavicular ligament<br>Sternoclavicular ligament<br>Subacromial bursa<br>Transverse humeral ligament<br>Transverse scapular ligament<br>**2 Shoulder Bursa and Ligament, Left**<br>*See 1 Shoulder Bursa and Ligament, Right*<br>**3 Elbow Bursa and Ligament, Right**<br>Annular ligament<br>Olecranon bursa<br>Radial collateral ligament<br>Ulnar collateral ligament<br>**4 Elbow Bursa and Ligament, Left**<br>*See 3 Elbow Bursa and Ligament, Right*<br>**5 Wrist Bursa and Ligament, Right**<br>Palmar ulnocarpal ligament<br>Radial collateral carpal ligament<br>Radiocarpal ligament<br>Radioulnar ligament<br>Ulnar collateral carpal ligament<br>**6 Wrist Bursa and Ligament, Left**<br>*See 5 Wrist Bursa and Ligament, Right*<br>**7 Hand Bursa and Ligament, Right**<br>Carpometacarpal ligament<br>Intercarpal ligament<br>Interphalangeal ligament<br>Lunotriquetral ligament<br>Metacarpal ligament<br>Metacarpophalangeal ligament<br>Pisohamate ligament<br>Pisometacarpal ligament<br>Scapholunate ligament<br>Scaphotrapezium ligament<br>**8 Hand Bursa and Ligament, Left**<br>*See 7 Hand Bursa and Ligament, Right*<br>**9 Upper Extremity Bursa and Ligament, Right**<br>**B Upper Extremity Bursa and Ligament, Left**<br>**C Upper Spine Bursa and Ligament**<br>Interspinous ligament<br>Intertransverse ligament<br>Ligamentum flavum<br>Supraspinous ligament<br>**D Lower Spine Bursa and Ligament**<br>Iliolumbar ligament<br>Interspinous ligament<br>Intertransverse ligament<br>Ligamentum flavum<br>Sacrococcygeal ligament<br>Sacroiliac ligament<br>Sacrospinous ligament<br>Sacrotuberous ligament<br>Supraspinous ligament<br>**F Sternum Bursa and Ligament**<br>Costotransverse ligament<br>Costoxiphoid ligament<br>Sternocostal ligament<br>**G Rib(s) Bursa and Ligament**<br>Costotransverse ligament<br>Costoxiphoid ligament<br>Sternocostal ligament<br>**H Abdomen Bursa and Ligament, Right**<br>**J Abdomen Bursa and Ligament, Left**<br>**K Perineum Bursa and Ligament**<br>**L Hip Bursa and Ligament, Right**<br>Iliofemoral ligament<br>Ischiofemoral ligament<br>Pubofemoral ligament<br>Transverse acetabular ligament<br>Trochanteric bursa<br>**M Hip Bursa and Ligament, Left**<br>*See L Hip Bursa and Ligament, Right*<br>**N Knee Bursa and Ligament, Right**<br>Anterior cruciate ligament (ACL)<br>Lateral collateral ligament (LCL)<br>Ligament of head of fibula<br>Medial collateral ligament (MCL)<br>Patellar ligament<br>Popliteal ligament<br>Posterior cruciate ligament (PCL)<br>Prepatellar bursa<br>**P Knee Bursa and Ligament, Left**<br>*See N Knee Bursa and Ligament, Right*<br>**Q Ankle Bursa and Ligament, Right**<br>Calcaneofibular ligament<br>Deltoid ligament<br>Ligament of the lateral malleolus<br>Talofibular ligament<br>**R Ankle Bursa and Ligament, Left**<br>*See Q Ankle Bursa and Ligament, Right*<br>**S Foot Bursa and Ligament, Right**<br>Calcaneocuboid ligament<br>Cuneonavicular ligament<br>Intercuneiform ligament<br>Interphalangeal ligament<br>Metatarsal ligament<br>Metatarsophalangeal ligament<br>Subtalar ligament<br>Talocalcaneal ligament<br>Talocalcaneonavicular ligament<br>Tarsometatarsal ligament<br>**T Foot Bursa and Ligament, Left**<br>*See S Foot Bursa and Ligament, Right*<br>**V Lower Extremity Bursa and Ligament, Right**<br>**W Lower Extremity Bursa and Ligament, Left** | **Ø Open**<br>**4 Percutaneous Endoscopic** | **Z No Device** | **Z No Qualifier** |

**Ø Medical and Surgical**
**M Bursae and Ligaments**
**U Supplement** Definition: Putting in or on biological or synthetic material that physically reinforces and/or augments the function of a portion of a body part

Explanation: The biological material is non-living, or is living and from the same individual. The body part may have been previously replaced, and the SUPPLEMENT procedure is performed to physically reinforce and/or augment the function of the replaced body part.

| Body Part Character 4 | Approach Character 5 | Device Character 6 | Qualifier Character 7 |
|---|---|---|---|
| **Ø Head and Neck Bursa and Ligament**<br>Alar ligament of axis<br>Cervical interspinous ligament<br>Cervical intertransverse ligament<br>Cervical ligamentum flavum<br>Interspinous ligament<br>Lateral temporomandibular ligament<br>Sphenomandibular ligament<br>Stylomandibular ligament<br>Transverse ligament of atlas<br>**1 Shoulder Bursa and Ligament, Right**<br>Acromioclavicular ligament<br>Coracoacromial ligament<br>Coracoclavicular ligament<br>Coracohumeral ligament<br>Costoclavicular ligament<br>Glenohumeral ligament<br>Interclavicular ligament<br>Sternoclavicular ligament<br>Subacromial bursa<br>Transverse humeral ligament<br>Transverse scapular ligament<br>**2 Shoulder Bursa and Ligament, Left**<br>*See 1 Shoulder Bursa and Ligament, Right*<br>**3 Elbow Bursa and Ligament, Right**<br>Annular ligament<br>Olecranon bursa<br>Radial collateral ligament<br>Ulnar collateral ligament<br>**4 Elbow Bursa and Ligament, Left**<br>*See 3 Elbow Bursa and Ligament, Right*<br>**5 Wrist Bursa and Ligament, Right**<br>Palmar ulnocarpal ligament<br>Radial collateral carpal ligament<br>Radiocarpal ligament<br>Radioulnar ligament<br>Ulnar collateral carpal ligament<br>**6 Wrist Bursa and Ligament, Left**<br>*See 5 Wrist Bursa and Ligament, Right*<br>**7 Hand Bursa and Ligament, Right**<br>Carpometacarpal ligament<br>Intercarpal ligament<br>Interphalangeal ligament<br>Lunotriquetral ligament<br>Metacarpal ligament<br>Metacarpophalangeal ligament<br>Pisohamate ligament<br>Pisometacarpal ligament<br>Scapholunate ligament<br>Scaphotrapezium ligament<br>**8 Hand Bursa and Ligament, Left**<br>*See 7 Hand Bursa and Ligament, Right*<br>**9 Upper Extremity Bursa and Ligament, Right**<br>**B Upper Extremity Bursa and Ligament, Left**<br>**C Upper Spine Bursa and Ligament**<br>Interspinous ligament<br>Intertransverse ligament<br>Ligamentum flavum<br>Supraspinous ligament<br>**D Lower Spine Bursa and Ligament**<br>Iliolumbar ligament<br>Interspinous ligament<br>Intertransverse ligament<br>Ligamentum flavum<br>Sacrococcygeal ligament<br>Sacroiliac ligament<br>Sacrospinous ligament<br>Sacrotuberous ligament<br>Supraspinous ligament<br>**F Sternum Bursa and Ligament**<br>Costotransverse ligament<br>Costoxiphoid ligament<br>Sternocostal ligament<br>**G Rib(s) Bursa and Ligament**<br>Costotransverse ligament<br>Costoxiphoid ligament<br>Sternocostal ligament<br>**H Abdomen Bursa and Ligament, Right**<br>**J Abdomen Bursa and Ligament, Left**<br>**K Perineum Bursa and Ligament**<br>**L Hip Bursa and Ligament, Right**<br>Iliofemoral ligament<br>Ischiofemoral ligament<br>Pubofemoral ligament<br>Transverse acetabular ligament<br>Trochanteric bursa<br>**M Hip Bursa and Ligament, Left**<br>*See L Hip Bursa and Ligament, Right*<br>**N Knee Bursa and Ligament, Right**<br>Anterior cruciate ligament (ACL)<br>Lateral collateral ligament (LCL)<br>Ligament of head of fibula<br>Medial collateral ligament (MCL)<br>Patellar ligament<br>Popliteal ligament<br>Posterior cruciate ligament (PCL)<br>Prepatellar bursa<br>**P Knee Bursa and Ligament, Left**<br>*See N Knee Bursa and Ligament, Right*<br>**Q Ankle Bursa and Ligament, Right**<br>Calcaneofibular ligament<br>Deltoid ligament<br>Ligament of the lateral malleolus<br>Talofibular ligament<br>**R Ankle Bursa and Ligament, Left**<br>*See Q Ankle Bursa and Ligament, Right*<br>**S Foot Bursa and Ligament, Right**<br>Calcaneocuboid ligament<br>Cuneonavicular ligament<br>Intercuneiform ligament<br>Interphalangeal ligament<br>Metatarsal ligament<br>Metatarsophalangeal ligament<br>Subtalar ligament<br>Talocalcaneal ligament<br>Talocalcaneonavicular ligament<br>Tarsometatarsal ligament<br>**T Foot Bursa and Ligament, Left**<br>*See S Foot Bursa and Ligament, Right*<br>**V Lower Extremity Bursa and Ligament, Right**<br>**W Lower Extremity Bursa and Ligament, Left** | **Ø Open**<br>**4 Percutaneous Endoscopic** | **7 Autologous Tissue Substitute**<br>**J Synthetic Substitute**<br>**K Nonautologous Tissue Substitute** | **Z No Qualifier** |

**Ø Medical and Surgical**
**M Bursae and Ligaments**
**W Revision**

Definition: Correcting, to the extent possible, a portion of a malfunctioning device or the position of a displaced device

Explanation: Revision can include correcting a malfunctioning or displaced device by taking out or putting in components of the device such as a screw or pin

| Body Part Character 4 | Approach Character 5 | Device Character 6 | Qualifier Character 7 |
|---|---|---|---|
| X Upper Bursa and Ligament<br>Y Lower Bursa and Ligament | Ø Open<br>3 Percutaneous<br>4 Percutaneous Endoscopic | Ø Drainage Device<br>7 Autologous Tissue Substitute<br>J Synthetic Substitute<br>K Nonautologous Tissue Substitute<br>Y Other Device | Z No Qualifier |
| X Upper Bursa and Ligament<br>Y Lower Bursa and Ligament | X External | Ø Drainage Device<br>7 Autologous Tissue Substitute<br>J Synthetic Substitute<br>K Nonautologous Tissue Substitute | Z No Qualifier |

Non-OR ØMW[X,Y][3,4]YZ
Non-OR ØMW[X,Y]X[Ø,7,J,K]Z

**Ø Medical and Surgical**
**M Bursae and Ligaments**
**X Transfer** Definition: Moving, without taking out, all or a portion of a body part to another location to take over the function of all or a portion of a body part
Explanation: The body part transferred remains connected to its vascular and nervous supply

| Body Part Character 4 | | Approach Character 5 | Device Character 6 | Qualifier Character 7 |
|---|---|---|---|---|
| **Ø Head and Neck Bursa and Ligament**<br>Alar ligament of axis<br>Cervical interspinous ligament<br>Cervical intertransverse ligament<br>Cervical ligamentum flavum<br>Interspinous ligament<br>Lateral temporomandibular ligament<br>Sphenomandibular ligament<br>Stylomandibular ligament<br>Transverse ligament of atlas<br>**1 Shoulder Bursa and Ligament, Right**<br>Acromioclavicular ligament<br>Coracoacromial ligament<br>Coracoclavicular ligament<br>Coracohumeral ligament<br>Costoclavicular ligament<br>Glenohumeral ligament<br>Interclavicular ligament<br>Sternoclavicular ligament<br>Subacromial bursa<br>Transverse humeral ligament<br>Transverse scapular ligament<br>**2 Shoulder Bursa and Ligament, Left**<br>*See 1 Shoulder Bursa and Ligament, Right*<br>**3 Elbow Bursa and Ligament, Right**<br>Annular ligament<br>Olecranon bursa<br>Radial collateral ligament<br>Ulnar collateral ligament<br>**4 Elbow Bursa and Ligament, Left**<br>*See 3 Elbow Bursa and Ligament, Right*<br>**5 Wrist Bursa and Ligament, Right**<br>Palmar ulnocarpal ligament<br>Radial collateral carpal ligament<br>Radiocarpal ligament<br>Radioulnar ligament<br>Ulnar collateral carpal ligament<br>**6 Wrist Bursa and Ligament, Left**<br>*See 5 Wrist Bursa and Ligament, Right*<br>**7 Hand Bursa and Ligament, Right**<br>Carpometacarpal ligament<br>Intercarpal ligament<br>Interphalangeal ligament<br>Lunotriquetral ligament<br>Metacarpal ligament<br>Metacarpophalangeal ligament<br>Pisohamate ligament<br>Pisometacarpal ligament<br>Scapholunate ligament<br>Scaphotrapezium ligament<br>**8 Hand Bursa and Ligament, Left**<br>*See 7 Hand Bursa and Ligament, Right*<br>**9 Upper Extremity Bursa and Ligament, Right**<br>**B Upper Extremity Bursa and Ligament, Left**<br>**C Upper Spine Bursa and Ligament**<br>Interspinous ligament<br>Intertransverse ligament<br>Ligamentum flavum<br>Supraspinous ligament | **D Lower Spine Bursa and Ligament**<br>Iliolumbar ligament<br>Interspinous ligament<br>Intertransverse ligament<br>Ligamentum flavum<br>Sacrococcygeal ligament<br>Sacroiliac ligament<br>Sacrospinous ligament<br>Sacrotuberous ligament<br>Supraspinous ligament<br>**F Sternum Bursa and Ligament**<br>Costotransverse ligament<br>Costoxiphoid ligament<br>Sternocostal ligament<br>**G Rib(s) Bursa and Ligament**<br>Costotransverse ligament<br>Costoxiphoid ligament<br>Sternocostal ligament<br>**H Abdomen Bursa and Ligament, Right**<br>**J Abdomen Bursa and Ligament, Left**<br>**K Perineum Bursa and Ligament**<br>**L Hip Bursa and Ligament, Right**<br>Iliofemoral ligament<br>Ischiofemoral ligament<br>Pubofemoral ligament<br>Transverse acetabular ligament<br>Trochanteric bursa<br>**M Hip Bursa and Ligament, Left**<br>*See L Hip Bursa and Ligament, Right*<br>**N Knee Bursa and Ligament, Right**<br>Anterior cruciate ligament (ACL)<br>Lateral collateral ligament (LCL)<br>Ligament of head of fibula<br>Medial collateral ligament (MCL)<br>Patellar ligament<br>Popliteal ligament<br>Posterior cruciate ligament (PCL)<br>Prepatellar bursa<br>**P Knee Bursa and Ligament, Left**<br>*See N Knee Bursa and Ligament, Right*<br>**Q Ankle Bursa and Ligament, Right**<br>Calcaneofibular ligament<br>Deltoid ligament<br>Ligament of the lateral malleolus<br>Talofibular ligament<br>**R Ankle Bursa and Ligament, Left**<br>*See Q Ankle Bursa and Ligament, Right*<br>**S Foot Bursa and Ligament, Right**<br>Calcaneocuboid ligament<br>Cuneonavicular ligament<br>Intercuneiform ligament<br>Interphalangeal ligament<br>Metatarsal ligament<br>Metatarsophalangeal ligament<br>Subtalar ligament<br>Talocalcaneal ligament<br>Talocalcaneonavicular ligament<br>Tarsometatarsal ligament<br>**T Foot Bursa and Ligament, Left**<br>*See S Foot Bursa and Ligament, Right*<br>**V Lower Extremity Bursa and Ligament, Right**<br>**W Lower Extremity Bursa and Ligament, Left** | **Ø Open**<br>**4 Percutaneous Endoscopic** | **Z No Device** | **Z No Qualifier** |

# Head and Facial Bones ØN2–ØNW

## Character Meanings

This Character Meaning table is provided as a guide to assist the user in the identification of character members that may be found in this section of code tables. It **SHOULD NOT** be used to build a PCS code.

| Operation–Character 3 | Body Part–Character 4 | Approach–Character 5 | Device–Character 6 | Qualifier–Character 7 |
|---|---|---|---|---|
| 2 Change | Ø Skull | Ø Open | Ø Drainage Device | X Diagnostic |
| 5 Destruction | 1 Frontal Bone | 3 Percutaneous | 4 Internal Fixation Device | Z No Qualifier |
| 8 Division | 3 Parietal Bone, Right | 4 Percutaneous Endoscopic | 5 External Fixation Device | |
| 9 Drainage | 4 Parietal Bone, Left | X External | 7 Autologous Tissue Substitute | |
| B Excision | 5 Temporal Bone, Right | | J Synthetic Substitute | |
| C Extirpation | 6 Temporal Bone, Left | | K Nonautologous Tissue Substitute | |
| D Extraction | 7 Occipital Bone | | M Bone Growth Stimulator | |
| H Insertion | B Nasal Bone | | N Neurostimulator Generator | |
| J Inspection | C Sphenoid Bone | | S Hearing Device | |
| N Release | F Ethmoid Bone, Right | | Y Other Device | |
| P Removal | G Ethmoid Bone, Left | | Z No Device | |
| Q Repair | H Lacrimal Bone, Right | | | |
| R Replacement | J Lacrimal Bone, Left | | | |
| S Reposition | K Palatine Bone, Right | | | |
| T Resection | L Palatine Bone, Left | | | |
| U Supplement | M Zygomatic Bone, Right | | | |
| W Revision | N Zygomatic Bone, Left | | | |
| | P Orbit, Right | | | |
| | Q Orbit, Left | | | |
| | R Maxilla | | | |
| | T Mandible, Right | | | |
| | V Mandible, Left | | | |
| | W Facial Bone | | | |
| | X Hyoid Bone | | | |

**AHA Coding Clinic for table ØNB**
**2017, 1Q, 20** Preparatory nasal adhesion repair before definitive cleft palate repair
**2015, 3Q, 3-8** Excisional and nonexcisional debridement
**2015, 2Q, 12** Orbital exenteration

**AHA Coding Clinic for table ØNH**
**2015, 3Q, 13** Nonexcisional debridement of cranial wound with removal and replacement of hardware

**AHA Coding Clinic for table ØNP**
**2015, 3Q, 13** Nonexcisional debridement of cranial wound with removal and replacement of hardware

**AHA Coding Clinic for table ØNR**
**2017, 1Q, 23** Reconstruction of mandible using titanium and bone
**2014, 3Q, 7** Hemi-cranioplasty for repair of cranial defect

**AHA Coding Clinic for table ØNQ**
**2016, 3Q, 29** Closure of bilateral alveolar clefts

**AHA Coding Clinic for table ØNS**
**2017, 1Q, 20** Preparatory nasal adhesion repair before definitive cleft palate repair
**2016, 2Q, 30** Clipping (occlusion) of cerebral artery, decompressive craniectomy and storage of bone flap in abdominal wall
**2015, 3Q, 17** Craniosynostosis with cranial vault reconstruction
**2015, 3Q, 27** Moyamoya disease and hemispheric pial synagiosis with craniotomy
**2014, 3Q, 23** Le Fort I osteotomy
**2013, 3Q, 24** Distraction osteogenesis
**2013, 3Q, 25** Fracture of frontal bone with repair and coagulation for hemostasis

**AHA Coding Clinic for table ØNU**
**2016, 3Q, 29** Closure of bilateral alveolar clefts
**2013, 3Q, 24** Distraction osteogenesis

## Head and Facial Bones

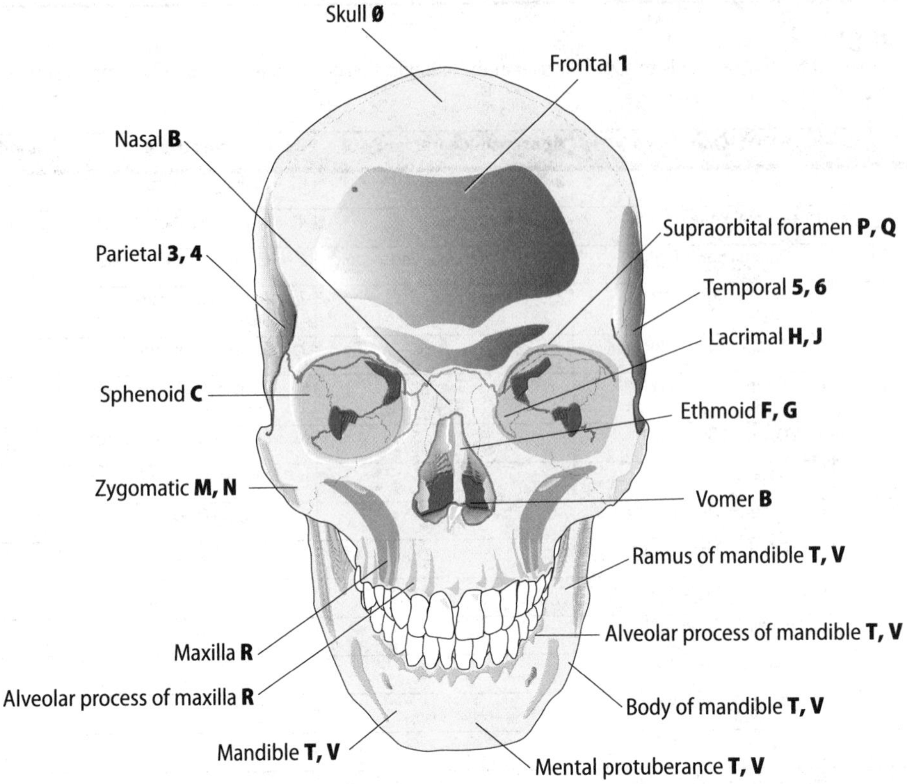
Skull Ø
Frontal 1
Nasal B
Supraorbital foramen P, Q
Parietal 3, 4
Temporal 5, 6
Lacrimal H, J
Sphenoid C
Ethmoid F, G
Zygomatic M, N
Vomer B
Ramus of mandible T, V
Alveolar process of mandible T, V
Maxilla R
Alveolar process of maxilla R
Body of mandible T, V
Mandible T, V
Mental protuberance T, V

## Skull Bones

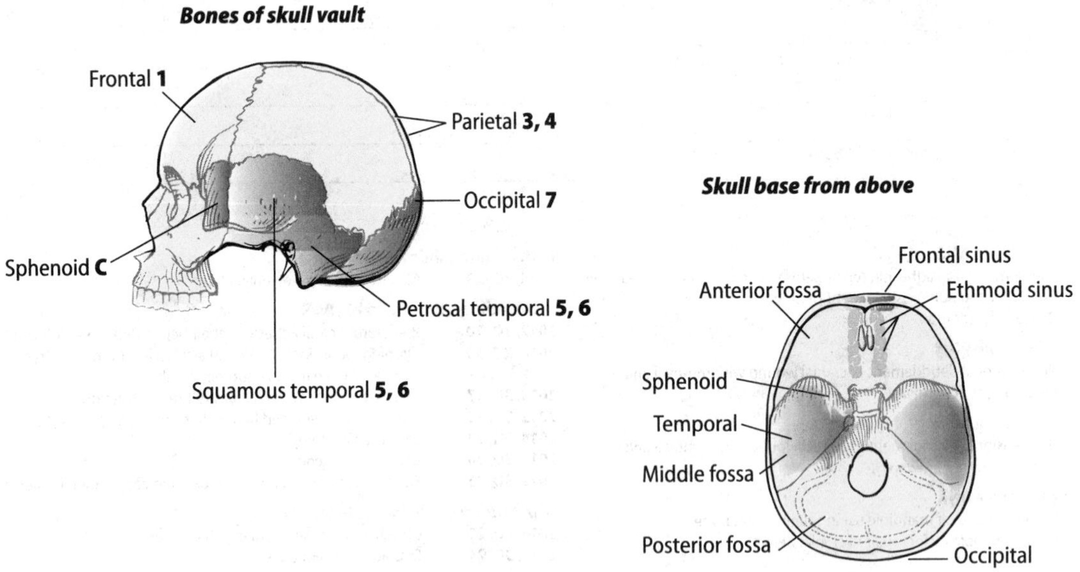
Bones of skull vault
Frontal 1
Parietal 3, 4
Occipital 7
Sphenoid C
Petrosal temporal 5, 6
Squamous temporal 5, 6
Skull base from above
Frontal sinus
Anterior fossa
Ethmoid sinus
Sphenoid
Temporal
Middle fossa
Posterior fossa
Occipital

**Ø Medical and Surgical**
**N Head and Facial Bones**
**2 Change** Definition: Taking out or off a device from a body part and putting back an identical or similar device in or on the same body part without cutting or puncturing the skin or a mucous membrane
Explanation: All CHANGE procedures are coded using the approach EXTERNAL

| Body Part Character 4 | Approach Character 5 | Device Character 6 | Qualifier Character 7 |
|---|---|---|---|
| **Ø Skull**<br>**B Nasal Bone**<br>Vomer of nasal septum<br>**W Facial Bone** | **X External** | **Ø Drainage Device**<br>**Y Other Device** | **Z No Qualifier** |

Non-OR All body part, approach, device, and qualifier values

**Ø Medical and Surgical**
**N Head and Facial Bones**
**5 Destruction** Definition: Physical eradication of all or a portion of a body part by the direct use of energy, force, or a destructive agent
Explanation: None of the body part is physically taken out

| Body Part Character 4 | Approach Character 5 | Device Character 6 | Qualifier Character 7 |
|---|---|---|---|
| **Ø Skull**<br>**1 Frontal Bone**<br>Zygomatic process of frontal bone<br>**3 Parietal Bone, Right**<br>**4 Parietal Bone, Left**<br>**5 Temporal Bone, Right**<br>Mastoid process<br>Petrous part of temporal bone<br>Tympanic part of temporal bone<br>Zygomatic process of temporal bone<br>**6 Temporal Bone, Left**<br>*See 5 Temporal Bone, Right*<br>**7 Occipital Bone**<br>Foramen magnum<br>**B Nasal Bone**<br>Vomer of nasal septum<br>**C Sphenoid Bone**<br>Greater wing<br>Lesser wing<br>Optic foramen<br>Pterygoid process<br>Sella turcica<br>**F Ethmoid Bone, Right**<br>Cribriform plate<br>**G Ethmoid Bone, Left**<br>*See F Ethmoid Bone, Right*<br>**H Lacrimal Bone, Right**<br>**J Lacrimal Bone, Left**<br>**K Palatine Bone, Right**<br>**L Palatine Bone, Left**<br>**M Zygomatic Bone, Right**<br>**N Zygomatic Bone, Left**<br>**P Orbit, Right**<br>Bony orbit<br>Orbital portion of ethmoid bone<br>Orbital portion of frontal bone<br>Orbital portion of lacrimal bone<br>Orbital portion of maxilla<br>Orbital portion of palatine bone<br>Orbital portion of sphenoid bone<br>Orbital portion of zygomatic bone<br>**Q Orbit, Left**<br>*See P Orbit, Right*<br>**R Maxilla**<br>Alveolar process of maxilla<br>**T Mandible, Right**<br>Alveolar process of mandible<br>Condyloid process<br>Mandibular notch<br>Mental foramen<br>**V Mandible, Left**<br>*See T Mandible, Right*<br>**X Hyoid Bone** | **Ø Open**<br>**3 Percutaneous**<br>**4 Percutaneous Endoscopic** | **Z No Device** | **Z No Qualifier** |

**Ø Medical and Surgical**
**N Head and Facial Bones**
**8 Division** Definition: Cutting into a body part, without draining fluids and/or gases from the body part, in order to separate or transect a body part
Explanation: All or a portion of the body part is separated into two or more portions

| Body Part Character 4 | Approach Character 5 | Device Character 6 | Qualifier Character 7 |
|---|---|---|---|
| **Ø Skull**<br>**1 Frontal Bone**<br>Zygomatic process of frontal bone<br>**3 Parietal Bone, Right**<br>**4 Parietal Bone, Left**<br>**5 Temporal Bone, Right**<br>Mastoid process<br>Petrous part of temporal bone<br>Tympanic part of temporal bone<br>Zygomatic process of temporal bone<br>**6 Temporal Bone, Left**<br>*See 5 Temporal Bone, Right*<br>**7 Occipital Bone**<br>Foramen magnum<br>**B Nasal Bone**<br>Vomer of nasal septum<br>**C Sphenoid Bone**<br>Greater wing<br>Lesser wing<br>Optic foramen<br>Pterygoid process<br>Sella turcica<br>**F Ethmoid Bone, Right**<br>Cribriform plate<br>**G Ethmoid Bone, Left**<br>*See F Ethmoid Bone, Right*<br>**H Lacrimal Bone, Right**<br>**J Lacrimal Bone, Left**<br>**K Palatine Bone, Right**<br>**L Palatine Bone, Left**<br>**M Zygomatic Bone, Right**<br>**N Zygomatic Bone, Left**<br>**P Orbit, Right**<br>Bony orbit<br>Orbital portion of ethmoid bone<br>Orbital portion of frontal bone<br>Orbital portion of lacrimal bone<br>Orbital portion of maxilla<br>Orbital portion of palatine bone<br>Orbital portion of sphenoid bone<br>Orbital portion of zygomatic bone<br>**Q Orbit, Left**<br>*See P Orbit, Right*<br>**R Maxilla**<br>Alveolar process of maxilla<br>**T Mandible, Right**<br>Alveolar process of mandible<br>Condyloid process<br>Mandibular notch<br>Mental foramen<br>**V Mandible, Left**<br>*See T Mandible, Right*<br>**X Hyoid Bone** | **Ø Open**<br>**3 Percutaneous**<br>**4 Percutaneous Endoscopic** | **Z No Device** | **Z No Qualifier** |

**Non-OR** ØN8B[Ø,3,4]ZZ

**Ø Medical and Surgical**
**N Head and Facial Bones**
**9 Drainage** Definition: Taking or letting out fluids and/or gases from a body part
Explanation: The qualifier DIAGNOSTIC is used to identify drainage procedures that are biopsies

| Body Part Character 4 | Approach Character 5 | Device Character 6 | Qualifier Character 7 |
|---|---|---|---|
| **Ø Skull**<br>**1 Frontal Bone**<br>Zygomatic process of frontal bone<br>**3 Parietal Bone, Right**<br>**4 Parietal Bone, Left**<br>**5 Temporal Bone, Right**<br>Mastoid process<br>Petrous part of temporal bone<br>Tympanic part of temporal bone<br>Zygomatic process of temporal bone<br>**6 Temporal Bone, Left**<br>*See 5 Temporal Bone, Right*<br>**7 Occipital Bone**<br>Foramen magnum<br>**B Nasal Bone**<br>Vomer of nasal septum<br>**C Sphenoid Bone**<br>Greater wing<br>Lesser wing<br>Optic foramen<br>Pterygoid process<br>Sella turcica<br>**F Ethmoid Bone, Right**<br>Cribriform plate<br>**G Ethmoid Bone, Left**<br>*See F Ethmoid Bone, Right*<br>**H Lacrimal Bone, Right**<br>**J Lacrimal Bone, Left**<br>**K Palatine Bone, Right**<br>**L Palatine Bone, Left**<br>**M Zygomatic Bone, Right**<br>**N Zygomatic Bone, Left**<br>**P Orbit, Right**<br>Bony orbit<br>Orbital portion of ethmoid bone<br>Orbital portion of frontal bone<br>Orbital portion of lacrimal bone<br>Orbital portion of maxilla<br>Orbital portion of palatine bone<br>Orbital portion of sphenoid bone<br>Orbital portion of zygomatic bone<br>**Q Orbit, Left**<br>*See P Orbit, Right*<br>**R Maxilla**<br>Alveolar process of maxilla<br>**T Mandible, Right**<br>Alveolar process of mandible<br>Condyloid process<br>Mandibular notch<br>Mental foramen<br>**V Mandible, Left**<br>*See T Mandible, Right*<br>**X Hyoid Bone** | **Ø Open**<br>**3 Percutaneous**<br>**4 Percutaneous Endoscopic** | **Ø Drainage Device** | **Z No Qualifier** |

***ØN9 Continued on next page***

**Non-OR** ØN9[Ø,1,3,4,5,6,7,C,F,G,H,J,K,L,M,N,P,Q,X]3ØZ
**Non-OR** ØN9[B,R,T,V][Ø,3,4]ØZ

ØN9 Continued

**Ø Medical and Surgical**
**N Head and Facial Bones**
**9 Drainage** Definition: Taking or letting out fluids and/or gases from a body part
Explanation: The qualifier DIAGNOSTIC is used to identify drainage procedures that are biopsies

| Body Part Character 4 | Approach Character 5 | Device Character 6 | Qualifier Character 7 |
|---|---|---|---|
| **Ø Skull**<br>**1 Frontal Bone**<br>Zygomatic process of frontal bone<br>**3 Parietal Bone, Right**<br>**4 Parietal Bone, Left**<br>**5 Temporal Bone, Right**<br>Mastoid process<br>Petrous part of temporal bone<br>Tympanic part of temporal bone<br>Zygomatic process of temporal bone<br>**6 Temporal Bone, Left**<br>*See 5 Temporal Bone, Right*<br>**7 Occipital Bone**<br>Foramen magnum<br>**B Nasal Bone**<br>Vomer of nasal septum<br>**C Sphenoid Bone**<br>Greater wing<br>Lesser wing<br>Optic foramen<br>Pterygoid process<br>Sella turcica<br>**F Ethmoid Bone, Right**<br>Cribriform plate<br>**G Ethmoid Bone, Left**<br>*See F Ethmoid Bone, Right*<br>**H Lacrimal Bone, Right**<br>**J Lacrimal Bone, Left**<br>**K Palatine Bone, Right**<br>**L Palatine Bone, Left**<br>**M Zygomatic Bone, Right**<br>**N Zygomatic Bone, Left**<br>**P Orbit, Right**<br>Bony orbit<br>Orbital portion of ethmoid bone<br>Orbital portion of frontal bone<br>Orbital portion of lacrimal bone<br>Orbital portion of maxilla<br>Orbital portion of palatine bone<br>Orbital portion of sphenoid bone<br>Orbital portion of zygomatic bone<br>**Q Orbit, Left**<br>*See P Orbit, Right*<br>**R Maxilla**<br>Alveolar process of maxilla<br>**T Mandible, Right**<br>Alveolar process of mandible<br>Condyloid process<br>Mandibular notch<br>Mental foramen<br>**V Mandible, Left**<br>*See T Mandible, Right*<br>**X Hyoid Bone** | **Ø Open**<br>**3 Percutaneous**<br>**4 Percutaneous Endoscopic** | **Z No Device** | **X Diagnostic**<br>**Z No Qualifier** |

**Non-OR** ØN9[Ø,1,3,4,5,6,7,C,F,G,H,J,K,L,M,N,P,Q,X]3ZZ
**Non-OR** ØN9B[Ø,3,4]Z[X,Z]
**Non-OR** ØN9[R,T,V][Ø,3,4]ZZ

**Ø Medical and Surgical**
**N Head and Facial Bones**
**B Excision** Definition: Cutting out or off, without replacement, a portion of a body part
Explanation: The qualifier DIAGNOSTIC is used to identify excision procedures that are biopsies

| Body Part Character 4 | Approach Character 5 | Device Character 6 | Qualifier Character 7 |
|---|---|---|---|
| Ø Skull<br>1 Frontal Bone<br>Zygomatic process of frontal bone<br>3 Parietal Bone, Right<br>4 Parietal Bone, Left<br>5 Temporal Bone, Right<br>Mastoid process<br>Petrous part of temporal bone<br>Tympanic part of temporal bone<br>Zygomatic process of temporal bone<br>6 Temporal Bone, Left<br>*See 5 Temporal Bone, Right*<br>7 Occipital Bone<br>Foramen magnum<br>B Nasal Bone<br>Vomer of nasal septum<br>C Sphenoid Bone<br>Greater wing<br>Lesser wing<br>Optic foramen<br>Pterygoid process<br>Sella turcica<br>F Ethmoid Bone, Right<br>Cribriform plate<br>G Ethmoid Bone, Left<br>*See F Ethmoid Bone, Right*<br>H Lacrimal Bone, Right<br>J Lacrimal Bone, Left<br>K Palatine Bone, Right<br>L Palatine Bone, Left<br>M Zygomatic Bone, Right<br>N Zygomatic Bone, Left<br>P Orbit, Right<br>Bony orbit<br>Orbital portion of ethmoid bone<br>Orbital portion of frontal bone<br>Orbital portion of lacrimal bone<br>Orbital portion of maxilla<br>Orbital portion of palatine bone<br>Orbital portion of sphenoid bone<br>Orbital portion of zygomatic bone<br>Q Orbit, Left<br>*See P Orbit, Right*<br>R Maxilla<br>Alveolar process of maxilla<br>T Mandible, Right<br>Alveolar process of mandible<br>Condyloid process<br>Mandibular notch<br>Mental foramen<br>V Mandible, Left<br>*See T Mandible, Right*<br>X Hyoid Bone | Ø Open<br>3 Percutaneous<br>4 Percutaneous Endoscopic | Z No Device | X Diagnostic<br>Z No Qualifier |

Non-OR ØNB[B,R,T,V][Ø,3,4]ZX

**Ø Medical and Surgical**
**N Head and Facial Bones**
**C Extirpation** Definition: Taking or cutting out solid matter from a body part

Explanation: The solid matter may be an abnormal byproduct of a biological function or a foreign body; it may be imbedded in a body part or in the lumen of a tubular body part. The solid matter may or may not have been previously broken into pieces.

| Body Part Character 4 | Approach Character 5 | Device Character 6 | Qualifier Character 7 |
|---|---|---|---|
| 1 Frontal Bone<br>Zygomatic process of frontal bone<br>**3 Parietal Bone, Right**<br>**4 Parietal Bone, Left**<br>**5 Temporal Bone, Right**<br>Mastoid process<br>Petrous part of temporal bone<br>Tympanic part of temporal bone<br>Zygomatic process of temporal bone<br>**6 Temporal Bone, Left**<br>*See 5 Temporal Bone, Right*<br>7 Occipital Bone<br>Foramen magnum<br>**B Nasal Bone**<br>Vomer of nasal septum<br>C Sphenoid Bone<br>Greater wing<br>Lesser wing<br>Optic foramen<br>Pterygoid process<br>Sella turcica<br>**F Ethmoid Bone, Right**<br>Cribriform plate<br>**G Ethmoid Bone, Left**<br>*See F Ethmoid Bone, Right*<br>**H Lacrimal Bone, Right**<br>**J Lacrimal Bone, Left**<br>**K Palatine Bone, Right**<br>**L Palatine Bone, Left**<br>**M Zygomatic Bone, Right**<br>**N Zygomatic Bone, Left**<br>**P Orbit, Right**<br>Bony orbit<br>Orbital portion of ethmoid bone<br>Orbital portion of frontal bone<br>Orbital portion of lacrimal bone<br>Orbital portion of maxilla<br>Orbital portion of palatine bone<br>Orbital portion of sphenoid bone<br>Orbital portion of zygomatic bone<br>**Q Orbit, Left**<br>*See P Orbit, Right*<br>R Maxilla<br>Alveolar process of maxilla<br>**T Mandible, Right**<br>Alveolar process of mandible<br>Condyloid process<br>Mandibular notch<br>Mental foramen<br>**V Mandible, Left**<br>*See T Mandible, Right*<br>**X Hyoid Bone** | **Ø Open**<br>**3 Percutaneous**<br>**4 Percutaneous Endoscopic** | **Z No Device** | **Z No Qualifier** |

**Non-OR** ØNC[B,R,T,V][Ø,3,4]ZZ

**Ø Medical and Surgical**
**N Head and Facial Bones**
**D Extraction** Definition: Pulling or stripping out or off all or a portion of a body part by the use of force
Explanation: The qualifier DIAGNOSTIC is used to identify extraction procedures that are biopsies

| Body Part Character 4 | Approach Character 5 | Device Character 6 | Qualifier Character 7 |
|---|---|---|---|
| Ø Skull<br>1 Frontal Bone<br>Zygomatic process of frontal bone<br>3 Parietal Bone, Right<br>4 Parietal Bone, Left<br>5 Temporal Bone, Right<br>Mastoid process<br>Petrous part of temporal bone<br>Tympanic part of temporal bone<br>Zygomatic process of temporal bone<br>6 Temporal Bone, Left<br>*See 5 Temporal Bone, Right*<br>7 Occipital Bone<br>Foramen magnum<br>B Nasal Bone<br>Vomer of nasal septum<br>C Sphenoid Bone<br>Greater wing<br>Lesser wing<br>Optic foramen<br>Pterygoid process<br>Sella turcica<br>F Ethmoid Bone, Right<br>Cribriform plate<br>G Ethmoid Bone, Left<br>*See F Ethmoid Bone, Right*<br>H Lacrimal Bone, Right<br>J Lacrimal Bone, Left<br>K Palatine Bone, Right<br>L Palatine Bone, Left<br>M Zygomatic Bone, Right<br>N Zygomatic Bone, Left<br>P Orbit, Right<br>Bony orbit<br>Orbital portion of ethmoid bone<br>Orbital portion of frontal bone<br>Orbital portion of lacrimal bone<br>Orbital portion of maxilla<br>Orbital portion of palatine bone<br>Orbital portion of sphenoid bone<br>Orbital portion of zygomatic bone<br>Q Orbit, Left<br>*See P Orbit, Right*<br>R Maxilla<br>Alveolar process of maxilla<br>T Mandible, Right<br>Alveolar process of mandible<br>Condyloid process<br>Mandibular notch<br>Mental foramen<br>V Mandible, Left<br>*See T Mandible, Right*<br>X Hyoid Bone | Ø Open | Z No Device | Z No Qualifier |

**Ø Medical and Surgical**
**N Head and Facial Bones**
**H Insertion** Definition: Putting in a nonbiological appliance that monitors, assists, performs, or prevents a physiological function but does not physically take the place of a body part

Explanation: None

| Body Part Character 4 | Approach Character 5 | Device Character 6 | Qualifier Character 7 |
|---|---|---|---|
| **Ø Skull** ⊞ | **Ø Open** | **4 Internal Fixation Device**<br>**5 External Fixation Device**<br>**M Bone Growth Stimulator**<br>**N Neurostimulator Generator** | **Z No Qualifier** |
| **Ø Skull** | **3 Percutaneous**<br>**4 Percutaneous Endoscopic** | **4 Internal Fixation Device**<br>**5 External Fixation Device**<br>**M Bone Growth Stimulator** | **Z No Qualifier** |
| **1 Frontal Bone**<br>Zygomatic process of frontal bone<br>**3 Parietal Bone, Right**<br>**4 Parietal Bone, Left**<br>**7 Occipital Bone**<br>Foramen magnum<br>**C Sphenoid Bone**<br>Greater wing<br>Lesser wing<br>Optic foramen<br>Pterygoid process<br>Sella turcica<br>**F Ethmoid Bone, Right**<br>Cribriform plate<br>**G Ethmoid Bone, Left**<br>*See F Ethmoid Bone, Right*<br>**H Lacrimal Bone, Right**<br>**J Lacrimal Bone, Left**<br>**K Palatine Bone, Right**<br>**L Palatine Bone, Left**<br>**M Zygomatic Bone, Right**<br>**N Zygomatic Bone, Left**<br>**P Orbit, Right**<br>Bony orbit<br>Orbital portion of ethmoid bone<br>Orbital portion of frontal bone<br>Orbital portion of lacrimal bone<br>Orbital portion of maxilla<br>Orbital portion of palatine bone<br>Orbital portion of sphenoid bone<br>Orbital portion of zygomatic bone<br>**Q Orbit, Left**<br>*See P Orbit, Right*<br>**X Hyoid Bone** | **Ø Open**<br>**3 Percutaneous**<br>**4 Percutaneous Endoscopic** | **4 Internal Fixation Device** | **Z No Qualifier** |
| **5 Temporal Bone, Right**<br>Mastoid process<br>Petrous part of temporal bone<br>Tympanic part of temporal bone<br>Zygomatic process of temporal bone<br>**6 Temporal Bone, Left**<br>*See 5 Temporal Bone, Right* | **Ø Open**<br>**3 Percutaneous**<br>**4 Percutaneous Endoscopic** | **4 Internal Fixation Device**<br>**S Hearing Device** | **Z No Qualifier** |
| **B Nasal Bone**<br>Vomer of nasal septum | **Ø Open**<br>**3 Percutaneous**<br>**4 Percutaneous Endoscopic** | **4 Internal Fixation Device**<br>**M Bone Growth Stimulator** | **Z No Qualifier** |
| **R Maxilla**<br>Alveolar process of maxilla<br>**T Mandible, Right**<br>Alveolar process of mandible<br>Condyloid process<br>Mandibular notch<br>Mental foramen<br>**V Mandible, Left**<br>*See T Mandible, Right* | **Ø Open**<br>**3 Percutaneous**<br>**4 Percutaneous Endoscopic** | **4 Internal Fixation Device**<br>**5 External Fixation Device** | **Z No Qualifier** |
| **W Facial Bone** | **Ø Open**<br>**3 Percutaneous**<br>**4 Percutaneous Endoscopic** | **M Bone Growth Stimulator** | **Z No Qualifier** |

**Non-OR** ØNHØØ5Z
**Non-OR** ØNHØ[3,4]5Z
**Non-OR** ØNHB[Ø,3,4][4,M]Z

**See Appendix L for Procedure Combinations**
⊞ ØNHØØNZ

**Ø Medical and Surgical**
**N Head and Facial Bones**
**J Inspection** Definition: Visually and/or manually exploring a body part

Explanation: Visual exploration may be performed with or without optical instrumentation. Manual exploration may be performed directly or through intervening body layers.

| Body Part Character 4 | Approach Character 5 | Device Character 6 | Qualifier Character 7 |
|---|---|---|---|
| **Ø Skull**<br>**B Nasal Bone**<br>Vomer of nasal septum<br>**W Facial Bone** | **Ø Open**<br>**3 Percutaneous**<br>**4 Percutaneous Endoscopic**<br>**X External** | **Z No Device** | **Z No Qualifier** |

Non-OR ØNJ[Ø,B,W][3,X]ZZ

**Ø Medical and Surgical**
**N Head and Facial Bones**
**N Release** Definition: Freeing a body part from an abnormal physical constraint by cutting or by the use of force

Explanation: Some of the restraining tissue may be taken out but none of the body part is taken out

| Body Part Character 4 | Approach Character 5 | Device Character 6 | Qualifier Character 7 |
|---|---|---|---|
| **1 Frontal Bone**<br>Zygomatic process of frontal bone<br>**3 Parietal Bone, Right**<br>**4 Parietal Bone, Left**<br>**5 Temporal Bone, Right**<br>Mastoid process<br>Petrous part of temporal bone<br>Tympanic part of temporal bone<br>Zygomatic process of temporal bone<br>**6 Temporal Bone, Left**<br>*See 5 Temporal Bone, Right*<br>**7 Occipital Bone**<br>Foramen magnum<br>**B Nasal Bone**<br>Vomer of nasal septum<br>**C Sphenoid Bone**<br>Greater wing<br>Lesser wing<br>Optic foramen<br>Pterygoid process<br>Sella turcica<br>**F Ethmoid Bone, Right**<br>Cribriform plate<br>**G Ethmoid Bone, Left**<br>*See F Ethmoid Bone, Right*<br>**H Lacrimal Bone, Right**<br>**J Lacrimal Bone, Left**<br>**K Palatine Bone, Right**<br>**L Palatine Bone, Left**<br>**M Zygomatic Bone, Right**<br>**N Zygomatic Bone, Left**<br>**P Orbit, Right**<br>Bony orbit<br>Orbital portion of ethmoid bone<br>Orbital portion of frontal bone<br>Orbital portion of lacrimal bone<br>Orbital portion of maxilla<br>Orbital portion of palatine bone<br>Orbital portion of sphenoid bone<br>Orbital portion of zygomatic bone<br>**Q Orbit, Left**<br>*See P Orbit, Right*<br>**R Maxilla**<br>Alveolar process of maxilla<br>**T Mandible, Right**<br>Alveolar process of mandible<br>Condyloid process<br>Mandibular notch<br>Mental foramen<br>**V Mandible, Left**<br>*See T Mandible, Right*<br>**X Hyoid Bone** | **Ø Open**<br>**3 Percutaneous**<br>**4 Percutaneous Endoscopic** | **Z No Device** | **Z No Qualifier** |

Non-OR ØNNB[Ø,3,4]ZZ

**Ø Medical and Surgical**
**N Head and Facial Bones**
**P Removal** Definition: Taking out or off a device from a body part

Explanation: If a device is taken out and a similar device put in without cutting or puncturing the skin or mucous membrane, the procedure is coded to the root operation CHANGE. Otherwise, the procedure for taking out a device is coded to the root operation REMOVAL.

| Body Part Character 4 | Approach Character 5 | Device Character 6 | Qualifier Character 7 |
|---|---|---|---|
| **Ø** Skull | **Ø** Open | **Ø** Drainage Device<br>**4** Internal Fixation Device<br>**5** External Fixation Device<br>**7** Autologous Tissue Substitute<br>**J** Synthetic Substitute<br>**K** Nonautologous Tissue Substitute<br>**M** Bone Growth Stimulator<br>**N** Neurostimulator Generator<br>**S** Hearing Device | **Z** No Qualifier |
| **Ø** Skull | **3** Percutaneous<br>**4** Percutaneous Endoscopic | **Ø** Drainage Device<br>**4** Internal Fixation Device<br>**5** External Fixation Device<br>**7** Autologous Tissue Substitute<br>**J** Synthetic Substitute<br>**K** Nonautologous Tissue Substitute<br>**M** Bone Growth Stimulator<br>**S** Hearing Device | **Z** No Qualifier |
| **Ø** Skull | **X** External | **Ø** Drainage Device<br>**4** Internal Fixation Device<br>**5** External Fixation Device<br>**M** Bone Growth Stimulator<br>**S** Hearing Device | **Z** No Qualifier |
| **B** Nasal Bone<br>Vomer of nasal septum<br>**W** Facial Bone | **Ø** Open<br>**3** Percutaneous<br>**4** Percutaneous Endoscopic | **Ø** Drainage Device<br>**4** Internal Fixation Device<br>**7** Autologous Tissue Substitute<br>**J** Synthetic Substitute<br>**K** Nonautologous Tissue Substitute<br>**M** Bone Growth Stimulator | **Z** No Qualifier |
| **B** Nasal Bone<br>Vomer of nasal septum<br>**W** Facial Bone | **X** External | **Ø** Drainage Device<br>**4** Internal Fixation Device<br>**M** Bone Growth Stimulator | **Z** No Qualifier |

**Non-OR** ØNPØ[3,4]5Z
**Non-OR** ØNPØX[Ø,5]Z
**Non-OR** ØNPB[Ø,3,4][Ø,4,7,J,K,M]Z
**Non-OR** ØNPBX[Ø,4,M]Z
**Non-OR** ØNPWX[Ø,M]Z

**Ø Medical and Surgical**
**N Head and Facial Bones**
**Q Repair** Definition: Restoring, to the extent possible, a body part to its normal anatomic structure and function
Explanation: Used only when the method to accomplish the repair is not one of the other root operations

| Body Part Character 4 | Approach Character 5 | Device Character 6 | Qualifier Character 7 |
|---|---|---|---|
| **Ø Skull**<br>**1 Frontal Bone**<br>Zygomatic process of frontal bone<br>**3 Parietal Bone, Right**<br>**4 Parietal Bone, Left**<br>**5 Temporal Bone, Right**<br>Mastoid process<br>Petrous part of temporal bone<br>Tympanic part of temporal bone<br>Zygomatic process of temporal bone<br>**6 Temporal Bone, Left**<br>*See 5 Temporal Bone, Right*<br>**7 Occipital Bone**<br>Foramen magnum<br>**B Nasal Bone**<br>Vomer of nasal septum<br>**C Sphenoid Bone**<br>Greater wing<br>Lesser wing<br>Optic foramen<br>Pterygoid process<br>Sella turcica<br>**F Ethmoid Bone, Right**<br>Cribriform plate<br>**G Ethmoid Bone, Left**<br>*See F Ethmoid Bone, Right*<br>**H Lacrimal Bone, Right**<br>**J Lacrimal Bone, Left**<br>**K Palatine Bone, Right**<br>**L Palatine Bone, Left**<br>**M Zygomatic Bone, Right**<br>**N Zygomatic Bone, Left**<br>**P Orbit, Right**<br>Bony orbit<br>Orbital portion of ethmoid bone<br>Orbital portion of frontal bone<br>Orbital portion of lacrimal bone<br>Orbital portion of maxilla<br>Orbital portion of palatine bone<br>Orbital portion of sphenoid bone<br>Orbital portion of zygomatic bone<br>**Q Orbit, Left**<br>*See P Orbit, Right*<br>**R Maxilla**<br>Alveolar process of maxilla<br>**T Mandible, Right**<br>Alveolar process of mandible<br>Condyloid process<br>Mandibular notch<br>Mental foramen<br>**V Mandible, Left**<br>*See T Mandible, Right*<br>**X Hyoid Bone** | **Ø Open**<br>**3 Percutaneous**<br>**4 Percutaneous Endoscopic**<br>**X External** | **Z No Device** | **Z No Qualifier** |

**Non-OR** ØNQ[Ø,1,3,4,5,6,7,B,C,F,G,H,J,K,L,M,N,P,Q,R,T,V,X]XZZ

**Ø Medical and Surgical**
**N Head and Facial Bones**
**R Replacement** Definition: Putting in or on biological or synthetic material that physically takes the place and/or function of all or a portion of a body part

Explanation: The body part may have been taken out or replaced, or may be taken out, physically eradicated, or rendered nonfunctional during the REPLACEMENT procedure. A REMOVAL procedure is coded for taking out the device used in a previous replacement procedure.

| Body Part Character 4 | Approach Character 5 | Device Character 6 | Qualifier Character 7 |
|---|---|---|---|
| Ø Skull<br>1 Frontal Bone<br>Zygomatic process of frontal bone<br>3 Parietal Bone, Right<br>4 Parietal Bone, Left<br>5 Temporal Bone, Right<br>Mastoid process<br>Petrous part of temporal bone<br>Tympanic part of temporal bone<br>Zygomatic process of temporal bone<br>6 Temporal Bone, Left<br>*See 5 Temporal Bone, Right*<br>7 Occipital Bone<br>Foramen magnum<br>B Nasal Bone<br>Vomer of nasal septum<br>C Sphenoid Bone<br>Greater wing<br>Lesser wing<br>Optic foramen<br>Pterygoid process<br>Sella turcica<br>F Ethmoid Bone, Right<br>Cribriform plate<br>G Ethmoid Bone, Left<br>*See F Ethmoid Bone, Right*<br>H Lacrimal Bone, Right<br>J Lacrimal Bone, Left<br>K Palatine Bone, Right<br>L Palatine Bone, Left<br>M Zygomatic Bone, Right<br>N Zygomatic Bone, Left<br>P Orbit, Right<br>Bony orbit<br>Orbital portion of ethmoid bone<br>Orbital portion of frontal bone<br>Orbital portion of lacrimal bone<br>Orbital portion of maxilla<br>Orbital portion of palatine bone<br>Orbital portion of sphenoid bone<br>Orbital portion of zygomatic bone<br>Q Orbit, Left<br>*See P Orbit, Right*<br>R Maxilla<br>Alveolar process of maxilla<br>T Mandible, Right<br>Alveolar process of mandible<br>Condyloid process<br>Mandibular notch<br>Mental foramen<br>V Mandible, Left<br>*See T Mandible, Right*<br>X Hyoid Bone | Ø Open<br>3 Percutaneous<br>4 Percutaneous Endoscopic | 7 Autologous Tissue Substitute<br>J Synthetic Substitute<br>K Nonautologous Tissue Substitute | Z No Qualifier |

**Ø Medical and Surgical**
**N Head and Facial Bones**
**S Reposition** Definition: Moving to its normal location, or other suitable location, all or a portion of a body part

Explanation: The body part is moved to a new location from an abnormal location, or from a normal location where it is not functioning correctly. The body part may or may not be cut out or off to be moved to the new location.

| Body Part Character 4 | Approach Character 5 | Device Character 6 | Qualifier Character 7 |
|---|---|---|---|
| **Ø Skull**<br>**R Maxilla**<br>Alveolar process of maxilla<br>**T Mandible, Right**<br>Alveolar process of mandible<br>Condyloid process<br>Mandibular notch<br>Mental foramen<br>**V Mandible, Left**<br>*See T Mandible, Right* | **Ø Open**<br>**3 Percutaneous**<br>**4 Percutaneous Endoscopic** | **4 Internal Fixation Device**<br>**5 External Fixation Device**<br>**Z No Device** | **Z No Qualifier** |
| **Ø Skull**<br>**R Maxilla**<br>Alveolar process of maxilla<br>**T Mandible, Right**<br>Alveolar process of mandible<br>Condyloid process<br>Mandibular notch<br>Mental foramen<br>**V Mandible, Left**<br>*See T Mandible, Right* | **X External** | **Z No Device** | **Z No Qualifier** |
| **1 Frontal Bone**<br>Zygomatic process of frontal bone<br>**3 Parietal Bone, Right**<br>**4 Parietal Bone, Left**<br>**5 Temporal Bone, Right**<br>Mastoid process<br>Petrous part of temporal bone<br>Tympanic part of temporal bone<br>Zygomatic process of temporal bone<br>**6 Temporal Bone, Left**<br>*See 5 Temporal Bone, Right*<br>**7 Occipital Bone**<br>Foramen magnum<br>**B Nasal Bone**<br>Vomer of nasal septum<br>**C Sphenoid Bone**<br>Greater wing<br>Lesser wing<br>Optic foramen<br>Pterygoid process<br>Sella turcica<br>**F Ethmoid Bone, Right**<br>Cribriform plate<br>**G Ethmoid Bone, Left**<br>*See F Ethmoid Bone, Right*<br>**H Lacrimal Bone, Right**<br>**J Lacrimal Bone, Left**<br>**K Palatine Bone, Right**<br>**L Palatine Bone, Left**<br>**M Zygomatic Bone, Right**<br>**N Zygomatic Bone, Left**<br>**P Orbit, Right**<br>Bony orbit<br>Orbital portion of ethmoid bone<br>Orbital portion of frontal bone<br>Orbital portion of lacrimal bone<br>Orbital portion of maxilla<br>Orbital portion of palatine bone<br>Orbital portion of sphenoid bone<br>Orbital portion of zygomatic bone<br>**Q Orbit, Left**<br>*See P Orbit, Right*<br>**X Hyoid Bone** | **Ø Open**<br>**3 Percutaneous**<br>**4 Percutaneous Endoscopic** | **4 Internal Fixation Device**<br>**Z No Device** | **Z No Qualifier** |

***ØNS Continued on next page***

**Non-OR** ØNS[R,T,V][3,4][4,5,Z]Z
**Non-OR** ØNS[Ø,R,T,V]XZZ
**Non-OR** ØNS[B,C,F,G,H,J,K,L,M,N,P,Q,X][3,4][4,Z]Z

**ØNS Continued**

**Ø Medical and Surgical**
**N Head and Facial Bones**
**S Reposition** Definition: Moving to its normal location, or other suitable location, all or a portion of a body part

Explanation: The body part is moved to a new location from an abnormal location, or from a normal location where it is not functioning correctly. The body part may or may not be cut out or off to be moved to the new location.

| Body Part Character 4 | Approach Character 5 | Device Character 6 | Qualifier Character 7 |
|---|---|---|---|
| 1 Frontal Bone<br>Zygomatic process of frontal bone<br>3 Parietal Bone, Right<br>4 Parietal Bone, Left<br>5 Temporal Bone, Right<br>Mastoid process<br>Petrous part of temporal bone<br>Tympanic part of temporal bone<br>Zygomatic process of temporal bone<br>6 Temporal Bone, Left<br>*See 5 Temporal Bone, Right*<br>7 Occipital Bone<br>Foramen magnum<br>B Nasal Bone<br>Vomer of nasal septum<br>C Sphenoid Bone<br>Greater wing<br>Lesser wing<br>Optic foramen<br>Pterygoid process<br>Sella turcica<br>F Ethmoid Bone, Right<br>Cribriform plate<br>G Ethmoid Bone, Left<br>*See F Ethmoid Bone, Right*<br>H Lacrimal Bone, Right<br>J Lacrimal Bone, Left<br>K Palatine Bone, Right<br>L Palatine Bone, Left<br>M Zygomatic Bone, Right<br>N Zygomatic Bone, Left<br>P Orbit, Right<br>Bony orbit<br>Orbital portion of ethmoid bone<br>Orbital portion of frontal bone<br>Orbital portion of lacrimal bone<br>Orbital portion of maxilla<br>Orbital portion of palatine bone<br>Orbital portion of sphenoid bone<br>Orbital portion of zygomatic bone<br>Q Orbit, Left<br>*See P Orbit, Right*<br>X Hyoid Bone | X External | Z No Device | Z No Qualifier |

**Non-OR** ØNS[1,3,4,5,6,7,B,C,F,G,H,J,K,L,M,N,P,Q,X]XZZ

**Ø Medical and Surgical**
**N Head and Facial Bones**
**T Resection** Definition: Cutting out or off, without replacement, all of a body part
Explanation: None

| Body Part Character 4 | Approach Character 5 | Device Character 6 | Qualifier Character 7 |
|---|---|---|---|
| 1 Frontal Bone<br>Zygomatic process of frontal bone<br>**3 Parietal Bone, Right**<br>**4 Parietal Bone, Left**<br>**5 Temporal Bone, Right**<br>Mastoid process<br>Petrous part of temporal bone<br>Tympanic part of temporal bone<br>Zygomatic process of temporal bone<br>**6 Temporal Bone, Left**<br>*See 5 Temporal Bone, Right*<br>7 Occipital Bone<br>Foramen magnum<br>**B Nasal Bone**<br>Vomer of nasal septum<br>C Sphenoid Bone<br>Greater wing<br>Lesser wing<br>Optic foramen<br>Pterygoid process<br>Sella turcica<br>**F Ethmoid Bone, Right**<br>Cribriform plate<br>**G Ethmoid Bone, Left**<br>*See F Ethmoid Bone, Right*<br>**H Lacrimal Bone, Right**<br>**J Lacrimal Bone, Left**<br>**K Palatine Bone, Right**<br>**L Palatine Bone, Left**<br>**M Zygomatic Bone, Right**<br>**N Zygomatic Bone, Left**<br>**P Orbit, Right**<br>Bony orbit<br>Orbital portion of ethmoid bone<br>Orbital portion of frontal bone<br>Orbital portion of lacrimal bone<br>Orbital portion of maxilla<br>Orbital portion of palatine bone<br>Orbital portion of sphenoid bone<br>Orbital portion of zygomatic bone<br>**Q Orbit, Left**<br>*See P Orbit, Right*<br>R Maxilla<br>Alveolar process of maxilla<br>**T Mandible, Right**<br>Alveolar process of mandible<br>Condyloid process<br>Mandibular notch<br>Mental foramen<br>**V Mandible, Left**<br>*See T Mandible, Right*<br>**X Hyoid Bone** | Ø Open | Z No Device | Z No Qualifier |

**Ø Medical and Surgical**
**N Head and Facial Bones**
**U Supplement** Definition: Putting in or on biological or synthetic material that physically reinforces and/or augments the function of a portion of a body part

Explanation: The biological material is non-living, or is living and from the same individual. The body part may have been previously replaced, and the SUPPLEMENT procedure is performed to physically reinforce and/or augment the function of the replaced body part.

| Body Part Character 4 | Approach Character 5 | Device Character 6 | Qualifier Character 7 |
|---|---|---|---|
| **Ø Skull**<br>**1 Frontal Bone**<br>Zygomatic process of frontal bone<br>**3 Parietal Bone, Right**<br>**4 Parietal Bone, Left**<br>**5 Temporal Bone, Right**<br>Mastoid process<br>Petrous part of temporal bone<br>Tympanic part of temporal bone<br>Zygomatic process of temporal bone<br>**6 Temporal Bone, Left**<br>*See 5 Temporal Bone, Right*<br>**7 Occipital Bone**<br>Foramen magnum<br>**B Nasal Bone**<br>Vomer of nasal septum<br>**C Sphenoid Bone**<br>Greater wing<br>Lesser wing<br>Optic foramen<br>Pterygoid process<br>Sella turcica<br>**F Ethmoid Bone, Right**<br>Cribriform plate<br>**G Ethmoid Bone, Left**<br>*See F Ethmoid Bone, Right*<br>**H Lacrimal Bone, Right**<br>**J Lacrimal Bone, Left**<br>**K Palatine Bone, Right**<br>**L Palatine Bone, Left**<br>**M Zygomatic Bone, Right**<br>**N Zygomatic Bone, Left**<br>**P Orbit, Right**<br>Bony orbit<br>Orbital portion of ethmoid bone<br>Orbital portion of frontal bone<br>Orbital portion of lacrimal bone<br>Orbital portion of maxilla<br>Orbital portion of palatine bone<br>Orbital portion of sphenoid bone<br>Orbital portion of zygomatic bone<br>**Q Orbit, Left**<br>*See P Orbit, Right*<br>**R Maxilla**<br>Alveolar process of maxilla<br>**T Mandible, Right**<br>Alveolar process of mandible<br>Condyloid process<br>Mandibular notch<br>Mental foramen<br>**V Mandible, Left**<br>*See T Mandible, Right*<br>**X Hyoid Bone** | **Ø Open**<br>**3 Percutaneous**<br>**4 Percutaneous Endoscopic** | **7 Autologous Tissue Substitute**<br>**J Synthetic Substitute**<br>**K Nonautologous Tissue Substitute** | **Z No Qualifier** |

**Ø Medical and Surgical**
**N Head and Facial Bones**
**W Revision**

Definition: Correcting, to the extent possible, a portion of a malfunctioning device or the position of a displaced device

Explanation: Revision can include correcting a malfunctioning or displaced device by taking out or putting in components of the device such as a screw or pin

| Body Part Character 4 | Approach Character 5 | Device Character 6 | Qualifier Character 7 |
|---|---|---|---|
| Ø Skull | Ø Open | Ø Drainage Device<br>4 Internal Fixation Device<br>5 External Fixation Device<br>7 Autologous Tissue Substitute<br>J Synthetic Substitute<br>K Nonautologous Tissue Substitute<br>M Bone Growth Stimulator<br>N Neurostimulator Generator<br>S Hearing Device | Z No Qualifier |
| Ø Skull | 3 Percutaneous<br>4 Percutaneous Endoscopic<br>X External | Ø Drainage Device<br>4 Internal Fixation Device<br>5 External Fixation Device<br>7 Autologous Tissue Substitute<br>J Synthetic Substitute<br>K Nonautologous Tissue Substitute<br>M Bone Growth Stimulator<br>S Hearing Device | Z No Qualifier |
| B Nasal Bone<br>Vomer of nasal septum<br>W Facial Bone | Ø Open<br>3 Percutaneous<br>4 Percutaneous Endoscopic<br>X External | Ø Drainage Device<br>4 Internal Fixation Device<br>7 Autologous Tissue Substitute<br>J Synthetic Substitute<br>K Nonautologous Tissue Substitute<br>M Bone Growth Stimulator | Z No Qualifier |

**Non-OR** ØNWØX[Ø,4,5,7,J,K,M,S]Z
**Non-OR** ØNWB[Ø,3,4,X][Ø,4,7,J,K,M]Z
**Non-OR** ØNWWX[Ø,4,7,J,K,M]Z

# Upper Bones ØP2–ØPW



## Character Meanings

This Character Meaning table is provided as a guide to assist the user in the identification of character members that may be found in this section of code tables. It **SHOULD NOT** be used to build a PCS code.

| Operation–Character 3 | Body Part–Character 4 | Approach–Character 5 | Device–Character 6 | Qualifier–Character 7 |
|---|---|---|---|---|
| 2 Change | Ø Sternum | Ø Open | Ø Drainage Device OR Internal Fixation Device, Rigid Plate | X Diagnostic |
| 5 Destruction | 1 Ribs, 1 to 2 | 3 Percutaneous | 4 Internal Fixation Device | Z No Qualifier |
| 8 Division | 2 Ribs, 3 or more | 4 Percutaneous Endoscopic | 5 External Fixation Device | |
| 9 Drainage | 3 Cervical Vertebra | X External | 6 Internal Fixation Device, Intramedullary | |
| B Excision | 4 Thoracic Vertebra | | 7 Autologous Tissue Substitute | |
| C Extirpation | 5 Scapula, Right | | 8 External Fixation Device, Limb Lengthening | |
| D Extraction | 6 Scapula, Left | | B External Fixation Device, Monoplanar | |
| H Insertion | 7 Glenoid Cavity, Right | | C External Fixation Device, Ring | |
| J Inspection | 8 Glenoid Cavity, Left | | D External Fixation Device, Hybrid | |
| N Release | 9 Clavicle, Right | | J Synthetic Substitute | |
| P Removal | B Clavicle, Left | | K Nonautologous Tissue Substitute | |
| Q Repair | C Humeral Head, Right | | M Bone Growth Stimulator | |
| R Replacement | D Humeral Head, Left | | Y Other Device | |
| S Reposition | F Humeral Shaft, Right | | Z No Device | |
| T Resection | G Humeral Shaft, Left | | | |
| U Supplement | H Radius, Right | | | |
| W Revision | J Radius, Left | | | |
| | K Ulna, Right | | | |
| | L Ulna, Left | | | |
| | M Carpal, Right | | | |
| | N Carpal, Left | | | |
| | P Metacarpal, Right | | | |
| | Q Metacarpal, Left | | | |
| | R Thumb Phalanx, Right | | | |
| | S Thumb Phalanx, Left | | | |
| | T Finger Phalanx, Right | | | |
| | V Finger Phalanx, Left | | | |
| | Y Upper Bone | | | |

**AHA Coding Clinic for table ØPB**

**2015, 3Q, 3-8** Excisional and nonexcisional debridement
**2015, 2Q, 34** Decompressive laminectomy
**2013, 4Q, 109** Separating conjoined twins
**2013, 4Q, 116** Spinal decompression
**2013, 3Q, 20** Superior labrum anterior posterior (SLAP) repair and subacromialdecompression
**2012, 4Q, 101** Rib resection with reconstruction of anterior chest wall
**2012, 2Q, 19** Multiple decompressive cervical laminectomies

**AHA Coding Clinic for table ØPH**

**2017, 2Q, 20** Exchange of intramedullary antibiotic impregnated spacer
**2016, 4Q, 117** Placement of magnetic growth rods
**2014, 4Q, 28** Removal and replacement of displaced growing rods

**AHA Coding Clinic for table ØPP**

**2017, 2Q, 20** Exchange of intramedullary antibiotic impregnated spacer
**2016, 4Q, 117** Placement of magnetic growth rods
**2014, 4Q, 28** Removal and replacement of displaced growing rods

**AHA Coding Clinic for table ØPS**

**2016, 1Q, 21** Elongation derotation flexion casting
**2015, 4Q, 33** Ravitch operation
**2015, 2Q, 35** Application of tongs to reduce and stabilize cervical fracture
**2014, 4Q, 26** Placement of vertical expandable prosthetic titanium rib (VEPTR)
**2014, 4Q, 32** Open reduction internal fixation of fracture with debridement
**2014, 3Q, 33** Radial fracture treatment with open reduction internal fixation, and release of carpal ligament

**AHA Coding Clinic for table ØPT**

**2015, 3Q, 26** Thumb arthroplasty with resection of trapezium

**AHA Coding Clinic for table ØPU**

**2015, 2Q, 20** Cervical laminoplasty
**2013, 4Q, 109** Separating conjoined twins

**AHA Coding Clinic for table ØPW**

**2014, 4Q, 26** Adjustment of VEPTR lengthening mechanism
**2014, 4Q, 27** Bilateral lengthening of growing rods

## Upper Bones

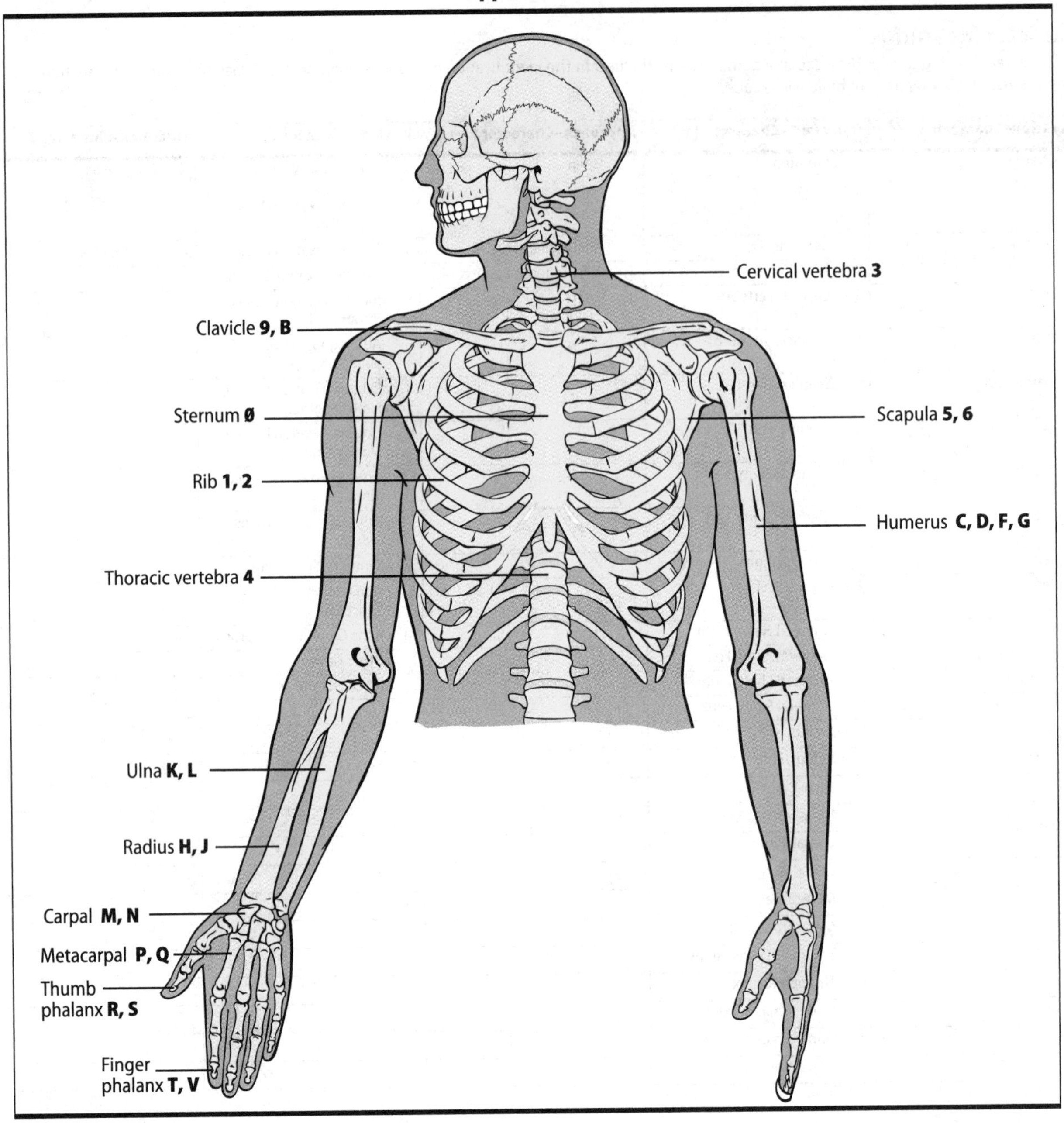
Cervical vertebra 3
Clavicle 9, B
Sternum Ø
Scapula 5, 6
Rib 1, 2
Humerus C, D, F, G
Thoracic vertebra 4
Ulna K, L
Radius H, J
Carpal M, N
Metacarpal P, Q
Thumb phalanx R, S
Finger phalanx T, V

## Humerus and Scapula

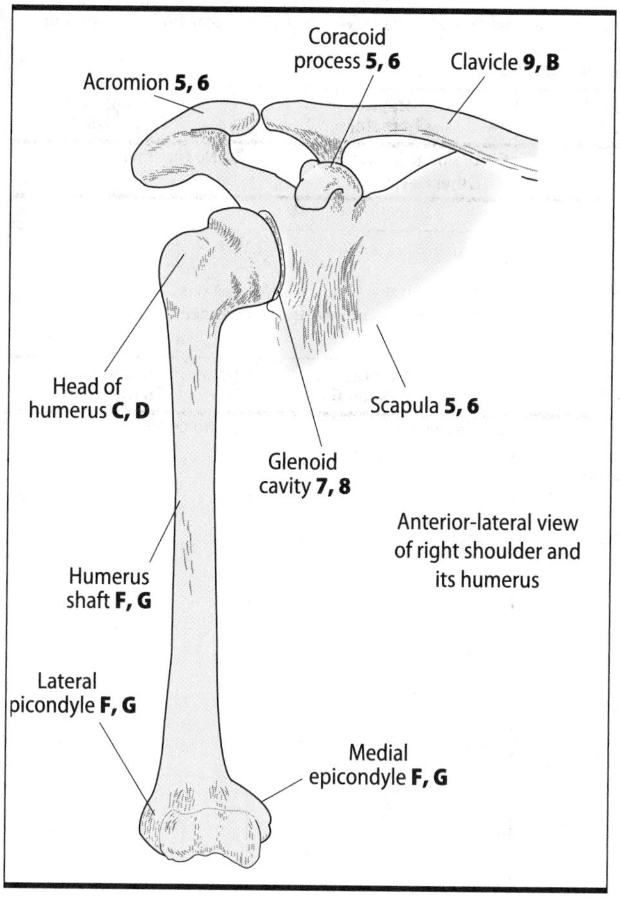
Coracoid process 5, 6
Clavicle 9, B
Acromion 5, 6
Head of humerus C, D
Scapula 5, 6
Glenoid cavity 7, 8
Anterior-lateral view of right shoulder and its humerus
Humerus shaft F, G
Lateral picondyle F, G
Medial epicondyle F, G

## Radius and Ulna

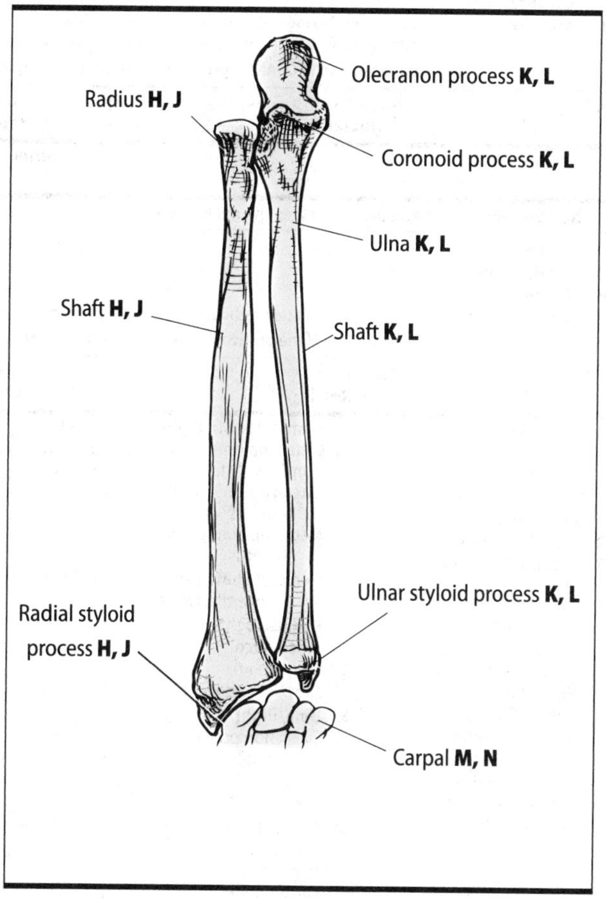
Olecranon process K, L
Radius H, J
Coronoid process K, L
Ulna K, L
Shaft H, J
Shaft K, L
Ulnar styloid process K, L
Radial styloid process H, J
Carpal M, N

## Hand

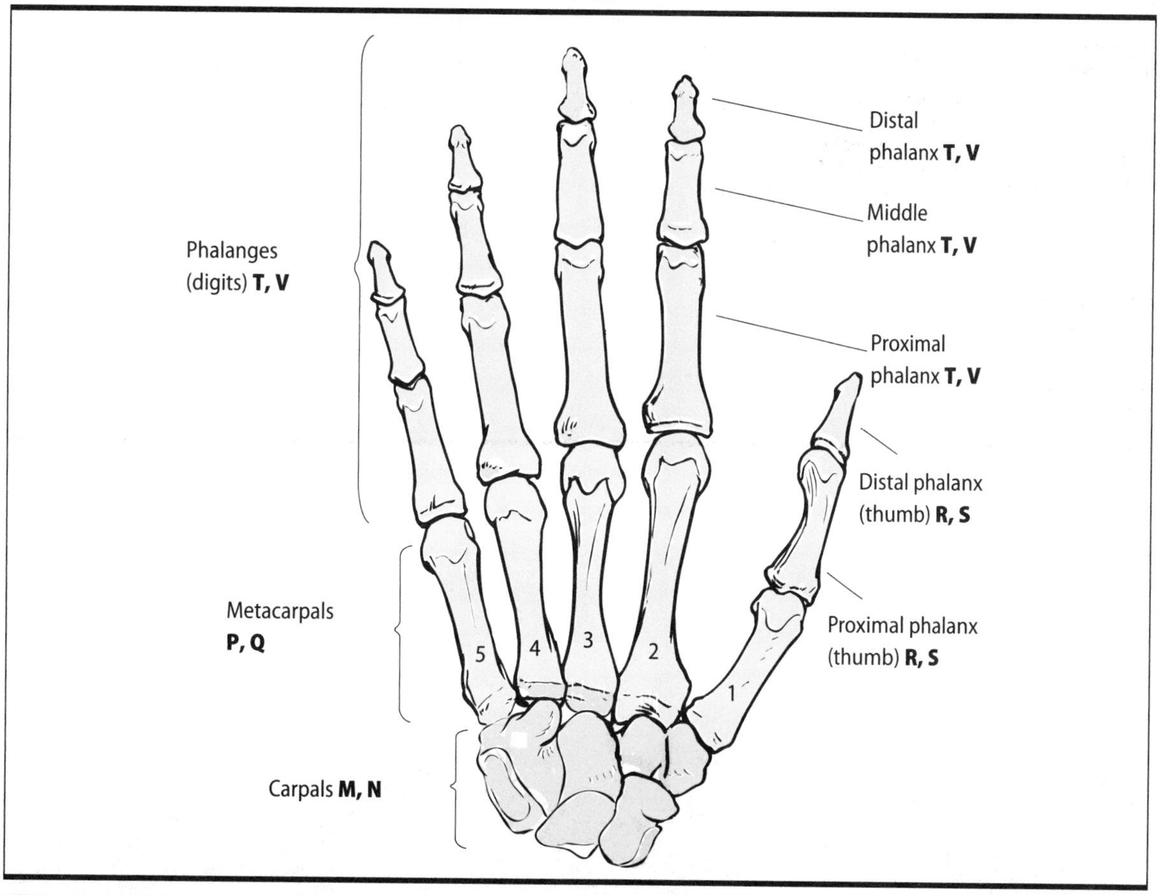
Distal phalanx T, V
Middle phalanx T, V
Phalanges (digits) T, V
Proximal phalanx T, V
Distal phalanx (thumb) R, S
Metacarpals P, Q
Proximal phalanx (thumb) R, S
5
4
3
2
1
Carpals M, N

**Ø Medical and Surgical**
**P Upper Bones**
**2 Change**

Definition: Taking out or off a device from a body part and putting back an identical or similar device in or on the same body part without cutting or puncturing the skin or a mucous membrane

Explanation: All CHANGE procedures are coded using the approach EXTERNAL

| Body Part Character 4 | Approach Character 5 | Device Character 6 | Qualifier Character 7 |
|---|---|---|---|
| **Y** Upper Bone | **X** External | **Ø** Drainage Device<br>**Y** Other Device | **Z** No Qualifier |

**Non-OR** All body part, approach, device, and qualifier values

**Ø Medical and Surgical**
**P Upper Bones**
**5 Destruction**

Definition: Physical eradication of all or a portion of a body part by the direct use of energy, force, or a destructive agent

Explanation: None of the body part is physically taken out

| Body Part Character 4 | Approach Character 5 | Device Character 6 | Qualifier Character 7 |
|---|---|---|---|
| **Ø Sternum**<br>Manubrium<br>Suprasternal notch<br>Xiphoid process<br>**1** Ribs, 1 to 2<br>**2** Ribs, 3 or More<br>**3 Cervical Vertebra**<br>Dens<br>Odontoid process<br>Spinous process<br>Transverse foramen<br>Transverse process<br>Vertebral arch<br>Vertebral body<br>Vertebral foramen<br>Vertebral lamina<br>Vertebral pedicle<br>**4 Thoracic Vertebra**<br>Spinous process<br>Transverse process<br>Vertebral arch<br>Vertebral body<br>Vertebral foramen<br>Vertebral lamina<br>Vertebral pedicle<br>**5 Scapula, Right**<br>Acromion (process)<br>Coracoid process<br>**6 Scapula, Left**<br>*See 5 Scapula, Right*<br>**7 Glenoid Cavity, Right**<br>Glenoid fossa (of scapula)<br>**8 Glenoid Cavity, Left**<br>*See 7 Glenoid Cavity, Right*<br>**9 Clavicle, Right**<br>**B Clavicle, Left**<br>**C Humeral Head, Right**<br>Greater tuberosity<br>Lesser tuberosity<br>Neck of humerus (anatomical)(surgical)<br>**D Humeral Head, Left**<br>*See C Humeral Head, Right*<br>**F Humeral Shaft, Right**<br>Distal humerus<br>Humerus, distal<br>Lateral epicondyle of humerus<br>Medial epicondyle of humerus<br>**G Humeral Shaft, Left**<br>*See F Humeral Shaft, Right*<br>**H Radius, Right**<br>Ulnar notch<br>**J Radius, Left**<br>*See H Radius, Right*<br>**K Ulna, Right**<br>Olecranon process<br>Radial notch<br>**L Ulna, Left**<br>*See K Ulna, Right*<br>**M Carpal, Right**<br>Capitate bone<br>Hamate bone<br>Lunate bone<br>Pisiform bone<br>Scaphoid bone<br>Trapezium bone<br>Trapezoid bone<br>Triquetral bone<br>**N Carpal, Left**<br>*See M Carpal, Right*<br>**P Metacarpal, Right**<br>**Q Metacarpal, Left**<br>**R Thumb Phalanx, Right**<br>**S Thumb Phalanx, Left**<br>**T Finger Phalanx, Right**<br>**V Finger Phalanx, Left** | **Ø** Open<br>**3** Percutaneous<br>**4** Percutaneous Endoscopic | **Z** No Device | **Z** No Qualifier |

**Ø Medical and Surgical**
**P Upper Bones**
**8 Division**

Definition: Cutting into a body part, without draining fluids and/or gases from the body part, in order to separate or transect a body part
Explanation: All or a portion of the body part is separated into two or more portions

| Body Part Character 4 | Approach Character 5 | Device Character 6 | Qualifier Character 7 |
|---|---|---|---|
| **Ø Sternum**<br>Manubrium<br>Suprasternal notch<br>Xiphoid process<br>**1 Ribs, 1 to 2**<br>**2 Ribs, 3 or More**<br>**3 Cervical Vertebra**<br>Dens<br>Odontoid process<br>Spinous process<br>Transverse foramen<br>Transverse process<br>Vertebral arch<br>Vertebral body<br>Vertebral foramen<br>Vertebral lamina<br>Vertebral pedicle<br>**4 Thoracic Vertebra**<br>Spinous process<br>Transverse process<br>Vertebral arch<br>Vertebral body<br>Vertebral foramen<br>Vertebral lamina<br>Vertebral pedicle<br>**5 Scapula, Right**<br>Acromion (process)<br>Coracoid process<br>**6 Scapula, Left**<br>*See 5 Scapula, Right*<br>**7 Glenoid Cavity, Right**<br>Glenoid fossa (of scapula)<br>**8 Glenoid Cavity, Left**<br>*See 7 Glenoid Cavity, Right*<br>**9 Clavicle, Right**<br>**B Clavicle, Left**<br>**C Humeral Head, Right**<br>Greater tuberosity<br>Lesser tuberosity<br>Neck of humerus (anatomical)(surgical)<br>**D Humeral Head, Left**<br>*See C Humeral Head, Right*<br>**F Humeral Shaft, Right**<br>Distal humerus<br>Humerus, distal<br>Lateral epicondyle of humerus<br>Medial epicondyle of humerus<br>**G Humeral Shaft, Left**<br>*See F Humeral Shaft, Right*<br>**H Radius, Right**<br>Ulnar notch<br>**J Radius, Left**<br>*See H Radius, Right*<br>**K Ulna, Right**<br>Olecranon process<br>Radial notch<br>**L Ulna, Left**<br>*See K Ulna, Right*<br>**M Carpal, Right**<br>Capitate bone<br>Hamate bone<br>Lunate bone<br>Pisiform bone<br>Scaphoid bone<br>Trapezium bone<br>Trapezoid bone<br>Triquetral bone<br>**N Carpal, Left**<br>*See M Carpal, Right*<br>**P Metacarpal, Right**<br>**Q Metacarpal, Left**<br>**R Thumb Phalanx, Right**<br>**S Thumb Phalanx, Left**<br>**T Finger Phalanx, Right**<br>**V Finger Phalanx, Left** | **Ø Open**<br>**3 Percutaneous**<br>**4 Percutaneous Endoscopic** | **Z No Device** | **Z No Qualifier** |

**Ø Medical and Surgical**
**P Upper Bones**
**9 Drainage** Definition: Taking or letting out fluids and/or gases from a body part

Explanation: The qualifier DIAGNOSTIC is used to identify drainage procedures that are biopsies

| Body Part Character 4 | Approach Character 5 | Device Character 6 | Qualifier Character 7 |
|---|---|---|---|
| **Ø Sternum**<br>Manubrium<br>Suprasternal notch<br>Xiphoid process<br>**1 Ribs, 1 to 2**<br>**2 Ribs, 3 or More**<br>**3 Cervical Vertebra**<br>Dens<br>Odontoid process<br>Spinous process<br>Transverse foramen<br>Transverse process<br>Vertebral arch<br>Vertebral body<br>Vertebral foramen<br>Vertebral lamina<br>Vertebral pedicle<br>**4 Thoracic Vertebra**<br>Spinous process<br>Transverse process<br>Vertebral arch<br>Vertebral body<br>Vertebral foramen<br>Vertebral lamina<br>Vertebral pedicle<br>**5 Scapula, Right**<br>Acromion (process)<br>Coracoid process<br>**6 Scapula, Left**<br>***See** 5 Scapula, Right*<br>**7 Glenoid Cavity, Right**<br>Glenoid fossa (of scapula)<br>**8 Glenoid Cavity, Left**<br>***See** 7 Glenoid Cavity, Right*<br>**9 Clavicle, Right**<br>**B Clavicle, Left**<br>**C Humeral Head, Right**<br>Greater tuberosity<br>Lesser tuberosity<br>Neck of humerus (anatomical)(surgical)<br>**D Humeral Head, Left**<br>***See** C Humeral Head, Right*<br>**F Humeral Shaft, Right**<br>Distal humerus<br>Humerus, distal<br>Lateral epicondyle of humerus<br>Medial epicondyle of humerus<br>**G Humeral Shaft, Left**<br>***See** F Humeral Shaft, Right*<br>**H Radius, Right**<br>Ulnar notch<br>**J Radius, Left**<br>***See** H Radius, Right*<br>**K Ulna, Right**<br>Olecranon process<br>Radial notch<br>**L Ulna, Left**<br>***See** K Ulna, Right*<br>**M Carpal, Right**<br>Capitate bone<br>Hamate bone<br>Lunate bone<br>Pisiform bone<br>Scaphoid bone<br>Trapezium bone<br>Trapezoid bone<br>Triquetral bone<br>**N Carpal, Left**<br>***See** M Carpal, Right*<br>**P Metacarpal, Right**<br>**Q Metacarpal, Left**<br>**R Thumb Phalanx, Right**<br>**S Thumb Phalanx, Left**<br>**T Finger Phalanx, Right**<br>**V Finger Phalanx, Left** | **Ø Open**<br>**3 Percutaneous**<br>**4 Percutaneous Endoscopic** | **Ø Drainage Device** | **Z No Qualifier** |

***ØP9 Continued on next page***

**Non-OR** ØP9[Ø,1,2,3,4,5,6,7,8,9,B,C,D,F,G,H,J,K,L,M,N,P,Q,R,S,T,V]3ØZ

**Ø Medical and Surgical**
**P Upper Bones**
**9 Drainage**

*ØP9 Continued*

Definition: Taking or letting out fluids and/or gases from a body part
Explanation: The qualifier DIAGNOSTIC is used to identify drainage procedures that are biopsies

| Body Part Character 4 | Approach Character 5 | Device Character 6 | Qualifier Character 7 |
|---|---|---|---|
| **Ø Sternum**<br>Manubrium<br>Suprasternal notch<br>Xiphoid process<br>**1 Ribs, 1 to 2**<br>**2 Ribs, 3 or More**<br>**3 Cervical Vertebra**<br>Dens<br>Odontoid process<br>Spinous process<br>Transverse foramen<br>Transverse process<br>Vertebral arch<br>Vertebral body<br>Vertebral foramen<br>Vertebral lamina<br>Vertebral pedicle<br>**4 Thoracic Vertebra**<br>Spinous process<br>Transverse process<br>Vertebral arch<br>Vertebral body<br>Vertebral foramen<br>Vertebral lamina<br>Vertebral pedicle<br>**5 Scapula, Right**<br>Acromion (process)<br>Coracoid process<br>**6 Scapula, Left**<br>*See 5 Scapula, Right*<br>**7 Glenoid Cavity, Right**<br>Glenoid fossa (of scapula)<br>**8 Glenoid Cavity, Left**<br>*See 7 Glenoid Cavity, Right*<br>**9 Clavicle, Right**<br>**B Clavicle, Left**<br>**C Humeral Head, Right**<br>Greater tuberosity<br>Lesser tuberosity<br>Neck of humerus (anatomical)(surgical)<br>**D Humeral Head, Left**<br>*See C Humeral Head, Right*<br>**F Humeral Shaft, Right**<br>Distal humerus<br>Humerus, distal<br>Lateral epicondyle of humerus<br>Medial epicondyle of humerus<br>**G Humeral Shaft, Left**<br>*See F Humeral Shaft, Right*<br>**H Radius, Right**<br>Ulnar notch<br>**J Radius, Left**<br>*See H Radius, Right*<br>**K Ulna, Right**<br>Olecranon process<br>Radial notch<br>**L Ulna, Left**<br>*See K Ulna, Right*<br>**M Carpal, Right**<br>Capitate bone<br>Hamate bone<br>Lunate bone<br>Pisiform bone<br>Scaphoid bone<br>Trapezium bone<br>Trapezoid bone<br>Triquetral bone<br>**N Carpal, Left**<br>*See M Carpal, Right*<br>**P Metacarpal, Right**<br>**Q Metacarpal, Left**<br>**R Thumb Phalanx, Right**<br>**S Thumb Phalanx, Left**<br>**T Finger Phalanx, Right**<br>**V Finger Phalanx, Left** | **Ø Open**<br>**3 Percutaneous**<br>**4 Percutaneous Endoscopic** | **Z No Device** | **X Diagnostic**<br>**Z No Qualifier** |

**Non-OR** ØP9[Ø,1,2,3,4,5,6,7,8,9,B,C,D,F,G,H,J,K,L,M,N,P,Q,R,S,T,V]3ZZ

**Ø Medical and Surgical**
**P Upper Bones**
**B Excision** Definition: Cutting out or off, without replacement, a portion of a body part
Explanation: The qualifier DIAGNOSTIC is used to identify excision procedures that are biopsies

| Body Part Character 4 | | Approach Character 5 | Device Character 6 | Qualifier Character 7 |
|---|---|---|---|---|
| **Ø Sternum**<br>Manubrium<br>Suprasternal notch<br>Xiphoid process<br>**1 Ribs, 1 to 2**<br>**2 Ribs, 3 or More**<br>**3 Cervical Vertebra**<br>Dens<br>Odontoid process<br>Spinous process<br>Transverse foramen<br>Transverse process<br>Vertebral arch<br>Vertebral body<br>Vertebral foramen<br>Vertebral lamina<br>Vertebral pedicle<br>**4 Thoracic Vertebra**<br>Spinous process<br>Transverse process<br>Vertebral arch<br>Vertebral body<br>Vertebral foramen<br>Vertebral lamina<br>Vertebral pedicle<br>**5 Scapula, Right**<br>Acromion (process)<br>Coracoid process<br>**6 Scapula, Left**<br>*See 5 Scapula, Right*<br>**7 Glenoid Cavity, Right**<br>Glenoid fossa (of scapula)<br>**8 Glenoid Cavity, Left**<br>*See 7 Glenoid Cavity, Right*<br>**9 Clavicle, Right**<br>**B Clavicle, Left**<br>**C Humeral Head, Right**<br>Greater tuberosity<br>Lesser tuberosity<br>Neck of humerus (anatomical)(surgical)<br>**D Humeral Head, Left**<br>*See C Humeral Head, Right* | **F Humeral Shaft, Right**<br>Distal humerus<br>Humerus, distal<br>Lateral epicondyle of humerus<br>Medial epicondyle of humerus<br>**G Humeral Shaft, Left**<br>*See F Humeral Shaft, Right*<br>**H Radius, Right**<br>Ulnar notch<br>**J Radius, Left**<br>*See H Radius, Right*<br>**K Ulna, Right**<br>Olecranon process<br>Radial notch<br>**L Ulna, Left**<br>*See K Ulna, Right*<br>**M Carpal, Right**<br>Capitate bone<br>Hamate bone<br>Lunate bone<br>Pisiform bone<br>Scaphoid bone<br>Trapezium bone<br>Trapezoid bone<br>Triquetral bone<br>**N Carpal, Left**<br>*See M Carpal, Right*<br>**P Metacarpal, Right**<br>**Q Metacarpal, Left**<br>**R Thumb Phalanx, Right**<br>**S Thumb Phalanx, Left**<br>**T Finger Phalanx, Right**<br>**V Finger Phalanx, Left** | **Ø Open**<br>**3 Percutaneous**<br>**4 Percutaneous Endoscopic** | **Z No Device** | **X Diagnostic**<br>**Z No Qualifier** |

**Ø Medical and Surgical**
**P Upper Bones**
**C Extirpation** Definition: Taking or cutting out solid matter from a body part

Explanation: The solid matter may be an abnormal byproduct of a biological function or a foreign body; it may be imbedded in a body part or in the lumen of a tubular body part. The solid matter may or may not have been previously broken into pieces.

| Body Part Character 4 | | Approach Character 5 | Device Character 6 | Qualifier Character 7 |
|---|---|---|---|---|
| **Ø Sternum**<br>Manubrium<br>Suprasternal notch<br>Xiphoid process<br>**1 Ribs, 1 to 2**<br>**2 Ribs, 3 or More**<br>**3 Cervical Vertebra**<br>Dens<br>Odontoid process<br>Spinous process<br>Transverse foramen<br>Transverse process<br>Vertebral arch<br>Vertebral body<br>Vertebral foramen<br>Vertebral lamina<br>Vertebral pedicle<br>**4 Thoracic Vertebra**<br>Spinous process<br>Transverse process<br>Vertebral arch<br>Vertebral body<br>Vertebral foramen<br>Vertebral lamina<br>Vertebral pedicle<br>**5 Scapula, Right**<br>Acromion (process)<br>Coracoid process<br>**6 Scapula, Left**<br>*See 5 Scapula, Right*<br>**7 Glenoid Cavity, Right**<br>Glenoid fossa (of scapula)<br>**8 Glenoid Cavity, Left**<br>*See 7 Glenoid Cavity, Right*<br>**9 Clavicle, Right**<br>**B Clavicle, Left**<br>**C Humeral Head, Right**<br>Greater tuberosity<br>Lesser tuberosity<br>Neck of humerus (anatomical)(surgical)<br>**D Humeral Head, Left**<br>*See C Humeral Head, Right* | **F Humeral Shaft, Right**<br>Distal humerus<br>Humerus, distal<br>Lateral epicondyle of humerus<br>Medial epicondyle of humerus<br>**G Humeral Shaft, Left**<br>*See F Humeral Shaft, Right*<br>**H Radius, Right**<br>Ulnar notch<br>**J Radius, Left**<br>*See H Radius, Right*<br>**K Ulna, Right**<br>Olecranon process<br>Radial notch<br>**L Ulna, Left**<br>*See K Ulna, Right*<br>**M Carpal, Right**<br>Capitate bone<br>Hamate bone<br>Lunate bone<br>Pisiform bone<br>Scaphoid bone<br>Trapezium bone<br>Trapezoid bone<br>Triquetral bone<br>**N Carpal, Left**<br>*See M Carpal, Right*<br>**P Metacarpal, Right**<br>**Q Metacarpal, Left**<br>**R Thumb Phalanx, Right**<br>**S Thumb Phalanx, Left**<br>**T Finger Phalanx, Right**<br>**V Finger Phalanx, Left** | **Ø Open**<br>**3 Percutaneous**<br>**4 Percutaneous Endoscopic** | **Z No Device** | **Z No Qualifier** |

**Ø Medical and Surgical**
**P Upper Bones**
**D Extraction** Definition: Pulling or stripping out or off all or a portion of a body part by the use of force
Explanation: The qualifier DIAGNOSTIC is used to identify extraction procedures that are biopsies

| Body Part Character 4 | | Approach Character 5 | Device Character 6 | Qualifier Character 7 |
|---|---|---|---|---|
| **Ø** Sternum<br>Manubrium<br>Suprasternal notch<br>Xiphoid process<br>**1** Ribs, 1 to 2<br>**2** Ribs, 3 or More<br>**3** Cervical Vertebra<br>Dens<br>Odontoid process<br>Spinous process<br>Transverse foramen<br>Transverse process<br>Vertebral arch<br>Vertebral body<br>Vertebral foramen<br>Vertebral lamina<br>Vertebral pedicle<br>**4** Thoracic Vertebra<br>Spinous process<br>Transverse process<br>Vertebral arch<br>Vertebral body<br>Vertebral foramen<br>Vertebral lamina<br>Vertebral pedicle<br>**5** Scapula, Right<br>Acromion (process)<br>Coracoid process<br>**6** Scapula, Left<br>***See*** *5 Scapula, Right*<br>**7** Glenoid Cavity, Right<br>Glenoid fossa (of scapula)<br>**8** Glenoid Cavity, Left<br>***See*** *7 Glenoid Cavity, Right*<br>**9** Clavicle, Right<br>**B** Clavicle, Left<br>**C** Humeral Head, Right<br>Greater tuberosity<br>Lesser tuberosity<br>Neck of humerus (anatomical)(surgical)<br>**D** Humeral Head, Left<br>***See*** *C Humeral Head, Right* | **F** Humeral Shaft, Right<br>Distal humerus<br>Humerus, distal<br>Lateral epicondyle of humerus<br>Medial epicondyle of humerus<br>**G** Humeral Shaft, Left<br>***See*** *F Humeral Shaft, Right*<br>**H** Radius, Right<br>Ulnar notch<br>**J** Radius, Left<br>***See*** *H Radius, Right*<br>**K** Ulna, Right<br>Olecranon process<br>Radial notch<br>**L** Ulna, Left<br>***See*** *K Ulna, Right*<br>**M** Carpal, Right<br>Capitate bone<br>Hamate bone<br>Lunate bone<br>Pisiform bone<br>Scaphoid bone<br>Trapezium bone<br>Trapezoid bone<br>Triquetral bone<br>**N** Carpal, Left<br>***See*** *M Carpal, Right*<br>**P** Metacarpal, Right<br>**Q** Metacarpal, Left<br>**R** Thumb Phalanx, Right<br>**S** Thumb Phalanx, Left<br>**T** Finger Phalanx, Right<br>**V** Finger Phalanx, Left | **Ø** Open | **Z** No Device | **Z** No Qualifier |

**Ø Medical and Surgical**
**P Upper Bones**
**H Insertion**

Definition: Putting in a nonbiological appliance that monitors, assists, performs, or prevents a physiological function but does not physically take the place of a body part

Explanation: None

| Body Part Character 4 | | Approach Character 5 | Device Character 6 | Qualifier Character 7 |
|---|---|---|---|---|
| **Ø Sternum**<br>Manubrium<br>Suprasternal notch<br>Xiphoid process | | **Ø Open**<br>**3 Percutaneous**<br>**4 Percutaneous Endoscopic** | **Ø Internal Fixation Device, Rigid Plate**<br>**4 Internal Fixation Device** | **Z No Qualifier** |
| **1 Ribs, 1 to 2**<br>**2 Ribs, 3 or More**<br>**3 Cervical Vertebra**<br>Dens<br>Odontoid process<br>Spinous process<br>Transverse foramen<br>Transverse process<br>Vertebral arch<br>Vertebral body<br>Vertebral foramen<br>Vertebral lamina<br>Vertebral pedicle<br>**4 Thoracic Vertebra**<br>Spinous process<br>Transverse process<br>Vertebral arch<br>Vertebral body<br>Vertebral foramen<br>Vertebral lamina<br>Vertebral pedicle | **5 Scapula, Right**<br>Acromion (process)<br>Coracoid process<br>**6 Scapula, Left**<br>*See 5 Scapula, Right*<br>**7 Glenoid Cavity, Right**<br>Glenoid fossa (of scapula)<br>**8 Glenoid Cavity, Left**<br>*See 7 Glenoid Cavity, Right*<br>**9 Clavicle, Right**<br>**B Clavicle, Left** | **Ø Open**<br>**3 Percutaneous**<br>**4 Percutaneous Endoscopic** | **4 Internal Fixation Device** | **Z No Qualifier** |
| **C Humeral Head, Right**<br>Greater tuberosity<br>Lesser tuberosity<br>Neck of humerus (anatomical)(surgical)<br>**D Humeral Head, Left**<br>*See C Humeral Head, Right*<br>**F Humeral Shaft, Right**<br>Distal humerus<br>Humerus, distal<br>Lateral epicondyle of humerus<br>Medial epicondyle of humerus | **G Humeral Shaft, Left**<br>*See F Humeral Shaft, Right*<br>**H Radius, Right**<br>Ulnar notch<br>**J Radius, Left**<br>*See H Radius, Right*<br>**K Ulna, Right**<br>Olecranon process<br>Radial notch<br>**L Ulna, Left**<br>*See K Ulna, Right* | **Ø Open**<br>**3 Percutaneous**<br>**4 Percutaneous Endoscopic** | **4 Internal Fixation Device**<br>**5 External Fixation Device**<br>**6 Internal Fixation Device, Intramedullary**<br>**8 External Fixation Device, Limb Lengthening**<br>**B External Fixation Device, Monoplanar**<br>**C External Fixation Device, Ring**<br>**D External Fixation Device, Hybrid** | **Z No Qualifier** |
| **M Carpal, Right**<br>Capitate bone<br>Hamate bone<br>Lunate bone<br>Pisiform bone<br>Scaphoid bone<br>Trapezium bone<br>Trapezoid bone<br>Triquetral bone<br>**N Carpal, Left**<br>*See M Carpal, Right* | **P Metacarpal, Right**<br>**Q Metacarpal, Left**<br>**R Thumb Phalanx, Right**<br>**S Thumb Phalanx, Left**<br>**T Finger Phalanx, Right**<br>**V Finger Phalanx, Left** | **Ø Open**<br>**3 Percutaneous**<br>**4 Percutaneous Endoscopic** | **4 Internal Fixation Device**<br>**5 External Fixation Device** | **Z No Qualifier** |
| **Y Upper Bone** | | **Ø Open**<br>**3 Percutaneous**<br>**4 Percutaneous Endoscopic** | **M Bone Growth Stimulator** | **Z No Qualifier** |

**Non-OR** ØPH[C,D,F,G,H,J,K,L][Ø,3,4]8Z

**Ø Medical and Surgical**
**P Upper Bones**
**J Inspection**

Definition: Visually and/or manually exploring a body part

Explanation: Visual exploration may be performed with or without optical instrumentation. Manual exploration may be performed directly or through intervening body layers.

| Body Part Character 4 | Approach Character 5 | Device Character 6 | Qualifier Character 7 |
|---|---|---|---|
| Y Upper Bone | Ø Open<br>3 Percutaneous<br>4 Percutaneous Endoscopic<br>X External | Z No Device | Z No Qualifier |

Non-OR ØPJY[3,X]ZZ

**Ø Medical and Surgical**
**P Upper Bones**
**N Release**

Definition: Freeing a body part from an abnormal physical constraint by cutting or by the use of force

Explanation: Some of the restraining tissue may be taken out but none of the body part is taken out

| Body Part Character 4 | | Approach Character 5 | Device Character 6 | Qualifier Character 7 |
|---|---|---|---|---|
| **Ø Sternum**<br>Manubrium<br>Suprasternal notch<br>Xiphoid process<br>**1 Ribs, 1 to 2**<br>**2 Ribs, 3 or More**<br>**3 Cervical Vertebra**<br>Dens<br>Odontoid process<br>Spinous process<br>Transverse foramen<br>Transverse process<br>Vertebral arch<br>Vertebral body<br>Vertebral foramen<br>Vertebral lamina<br>Vertebral pedicle<br>**4 Thoracic Vertebra**<br>Spinous process<br>Transverse process<br>Vertebral arch<br>Vertebral body<br>Vertebral foramen<br>Vertebral lamina<br>Vertebral pedicle<br>**5 Scapula, Right**<br>Acromion (process)<br>Coracoid process<br>**6 Scapula, Left**<br>*See 5 Scapula, Right*<br>**7 Glenoid Cavity, Right**<br>Glenoid fossa (of scapula)<br>**8 Glenoid Cavity, Left**<br>*See 7 Glenoid Cavity, Right*<br>**9 Clavicle, Right**<br>**B Clavicle, Left**<br>**C Humeral Head, Right**<br>Greater tuberosity<br>Lesser tuberosity<br>Neck of humerus (anatomical) (surgical)<br>**D Humeral Head, Left**<br>*See C Humeral Head, Right* | **F Humeral Shaft, Right**<br>Distal humerus<br>Humerus, distal<br>Lateral epicondyle of humerus<br>Medial epicondyle of humerus<br>**G Humeral Shaft, Left**<br>*See F Humeral Shaft, Right*<br>**H Radius, Right**<br>Ulnar notch<br>**J Radius, Left**<br>*See H Radius, Right*<br>**K Ulna, Right**<br>Olecranon process<br>Radial notch<br>**L Ulna, Left**<br>*See K Ulna, Right*<br>**M Carpal, Right**<br>Capitate bone<br>Hamate bone<br>Lunate bone<br>Pisiform bone<br>Scaphoid bone<br>Trapezium bone<br>Trapezoid bone<br>Triquetral bone<br>**N Carpal, Left**<br>*See M Carpal, Right*<br>**P Metacarpal, Right**<br>**Q Metacarpal, Left**<br>**R Thumb Phalanx, Right**<br>**S Thumb Phalanx, Left**<br>**T Finger Phalanx, Right**<br>**V Finger Phalanx, Left** | Ø Open<br>3 Percutaneous<br>4 Percutaneous Endoscopic | Z No Device | Z No Qualifier |

**Ø Medical and Surgical**
**P Upper Bones**
**P Removal** Definition: Taking out or off a device from a body part

Explanation: If a device is taken out and a similar device put in without cutting or puncturing the skin or mucous membrane, the procedure is coded to the root operation CHANGE. Otherwise, the procedure for taking out a device is coded to the root operation REMOVAL.

| Body Part Character 4 | Approach Character 5 | Device Character 6 | Qualifier Character 7 |
|---|---|---|---|
| **Ø Sternum**<br>Manubrium<br>Suprasternal notch<br>Xiphoid process<br>**1 Ribs, 1 to 2**<br>**2 Ribs, 3 or More**<br>**3 Cervical Vertebra**<br>Dens<br>Odontoid process<br>Spinous process<br>Transverse foramen<br>Transverse process<br>Vertebral arch<br>Vertebral body<br>Vertebral foramen<br>Vertebral lamina<br>Vertebral pedicle<br>**4 Thoracic Vertebra**<br>Spinous process<br>Transverse process<br>Vertebral arch<br>Vertebral body<br>Vertebral foramen<br>Vertebral lamina<br>Vertebral pedicle<br>**5 Scapula, Right**<br>Acromion (process)<br>Coracoid process<br>**6 Scapula, Left**<br>*See 5 Scapula, Right*<br>**7 Glenoid Cavity, Right**<br>Glenoid fossa (of scapula)<br>**8 Glenoid Cavity, Left**<br>*See 7 Glenoid Cavity, Right*<br>**9 Clavicle, Right**<br>**B Clavicle, Left** | **Ø Open**<br>**3 Percutaneous**<br>**4 Percutaneous Endoscopic** | **4 Internal Fixation Device**<br>**7 Autologous Tissue Substitute**<br>**J Synthetic Substitute**<br>**K Nonautologous Tissue Substitute** | **Z No Qualifier** |
| **Ø Sternum**<br>Manubrium<br>Suprasternal notch<br>Xiphoid process<br>**1 Ribs, 1 to 2**<br>**2 Ribs, 3 or More**<br>**3 Cervical Vertebra**<br>Dens<br>Odontoid process<br>Spinous process<br>Transverse foramen<br>Transverse process<br>Vertebral arch<br>Vertebral body<br>Vertebral foramen<br>Vertebral lamina<br>Vertebral pedicle<br>**4 Thoracic Vertebra**<br>Spinous process<br>Transverse process<br>Vertebral arch<br>Vertebral body<br>Vertebral foramen<br>Vertebral lamina<br>Vertebral pedicle<br>**5 Scapula, Right**<br>Acromion (process)<br>Coracoid process<br>**6 Scapula, Left**<br>*See 5 Scapula, Right*<br>**7 Glenoid Cavity, Right**<br>Glenoid fossa (of scapula)<br>**8 Glenoid Cavity, Left**<br>*See 7 Glenoid Cavity, Right*<br>**9 Clavicle, Right**<br>**B Clavicle, Left** | **X External** | **4 Internal Fixation Device** | **Z No Qualifier** |
| **C Humeral Head, Right**<br>Greater tuberosity<br>Lesser tuberosity<br>Neck of humerus (anatomical) (surgical)<br>**D Humeral Head, Left**<br>*See C Humeral Head, Right*<br>**F Humeral Shaft, Right**<br>Distal humerus<br>Humerus, distal<br>Lateral epicondyle of humerus<br>Medial epicondyle of humerus<br>**G Humeral Shaft, Left**<br>*See F Humeral Shaft, Right*<br>**H Radius, Right**<br>Ulnar notch<br>**J Radius, Left**<br>*See H Radius, Right*<br>**K Ulna, Right**<br>Olecranon process<br>Radial notch<br>**L Ulna, Left**<br>*See K Ulna, Right*<br>**M Carpal, Right**<br>Capitate bone<br>Hamate bone<br>Lunate bone<br>Pisiform bone<br>Scaphoid bone<br>Trapezium bone<br>Trapezoid bone<br>Triquetral bone<br>**N Carpal, Left**<br>*See M Carpal, Right*<br>**P Metacarpal, Right**<br>**Q Metacarpal, Left**<br>**R Thumb Phalanx, Right**<br>**S Thumb Phalanx, Left**<br>**T Finger Phalanx, Right**<br>**V Finger Phalanx, Left** | **Ø Open**<br>**3 Percutaneous**<br>**4 Percutaneous Endoscopic** | **4 Internal Fixation Device**<br>**5 External Fixation Device**<br>**7 Autologous Tissue Substitute**<br>**J Synthetic Substitute**<br>**K Nonautologous Tissue Substitute** | **Z No Qualifier** |

***ØPP Continued on next page***

**Non-OR** ØPP[Ø,1,2,3,4,5,6,7,8,9,B]X4Z

**ØPP Continued**

**Ø Medical and Surgical**
**P Upper Bones**
**P Removal**

Definition: Taking out or off a device from a body part

Explanation: If a device is taken out and a similar device put in without cutting or puncturing the skin or mucous membrane, the procedure is coded to the root operation CHANGE. Otherwise, the procedure for taking out a device is coded to the root operation REMOVAL.

| Body Part Character 4 | Approach Character 5 | Device Character 6 | Qualifier Character 7 |
|---|---|---|---|
| **C Humeral Head, Right**<br>Greater tuberosity<br>Lesser tuberosity<br>Neck of humerus (anatomical) (surgical)<br>**D Humeral Head, Left**<br>*See C Humeral Head, Right*<br>**F Humeral Shaft, Right**<br>Distal humerus<br>Humerus, distal<br>Lateral epicondyle of humerus<br>Medial epicondyle of humerus<br>**G Humeral Shaft, Left**<br>*See F Humeral Shaft, Right*<br>**H Radius, Right**<br>Ulnar notch<br>**J Radius, Left**<br>*See H Radius, Right*<br>**K Ulna, Right**<br>Olecranon process<br>Radial notch<br>**L Ulna, Left**<br>*See K Ulna, Right*<br>**M Carpal, Right**<br>Capitate bone<br>Hamate bone<br>Lunate bone<br>Pisiform bone<br>Scaphoid bone<br>Trapezium bone<br>Trapezoid bone<br>Triquetral bone<br>**N Carpal, Left**<br>*See M Carpal, Right*<br>**P Metacarpal, Right**<br>**Q Metacarpal, Left**<br>**R Thumb Phalanx, Right**<br>**S Thumb Phalanx, Left**<br>**T Finger Phalanx, Right**<br>**V Finger Phalanx, Left** | **X External** | **4 Internal Fixation Device**<br>**5 External Fixation Device** | **Z No Qualifier** |
| **Y Upper Bone** | **Ø Open**<br>**3 Percutaneous**<br>**4 Percutaneous Endoscopic**<br>**X External** | **Ø Drainage Device**<br>**M Bone Growth Stimulator** | **Z No Qualifier** |

Non-OR ØPP[C,D,F,G,H,J,K,L,M,N,P,Q,R,S,T,V]X[4,5]Z
Non-OR ØPPY3ØZ
Non-OR ØPPYX[Ø,M]Z

**Ø Medical and Surgical**
**P Upper Bones**
**Q Repair**

Definition: Restoring, to the extent possible, a body part to its normal anatomic structure and function
Explanation: Used only when the method to accomplish the repair is not one of the other root operations

| Body Part Character 4 | Approach Character 5 | Device Character 6 | Qualifier Character 7 |
|---|---|---|---|
| **Ø Sternum**<br>Manubrium<br>Suprasternal notch<br>Xiphoid process<br>**1 Ribs, 1 to 2**<br>**2 Ribs, 3 or More**<br>**3 Cervical Vertebra**<br>Dens<br>Odontoid process<br>Spinous process<br>Transverse foramen<br>Transverse process<br>Vertebral arch<br>Vertebral body<br>Vertebral foramen<br>Vertebral lamina<br>Vertebral pedicle<br>**4 Thoracic Vertebra**<br>Spinous process<br>Transverse process<br>Vertebral arch<br>Vertebral body<br>Vertebral foramen<br>Vertebral lamina<br>Vertebral pedicle<br>**5 Scapula, Right**<br>Acromion (process)<br>Coracoid process<br>**6 Scapula, Left**<br>*See 5 Scapula, Right*<br>**7 Glenoid Cavity, Right**<br>Glenoid fossa (of scapula)<br>**8 Glenoid Cavity, Left**<br>*See 7 Glenoid Cavity, Right*<br>**9 Clavicle, Right**<br>**B Clavicle, Left**<br>**C Humeral Head, Right**<br>Greater tuberosity<br>Lesser tuberosity<br>Neck of humerus (anatomical)(surgical)<br>**D Humeral Head, Left**<br>*See C Humeral Head, Right*<br>**F Humeral Shaft, Right**<br>Distal humerus<br>Humerus, distal<br>Lateral epicondyle of humerus<br>Medial epicondyle of humerus<br>**G Humeral Shaft, Left**<br>*See F Humeral Shaft, Right*<br>**H Radius, Right**<br>Ulnar notch<br>**J Radius, Left**<br>*See H Radius, Right*<br>**K Ulna, Right**<br>Olecranon process<br>Radial notch<br>**L Ulna, Left**<br>*See K Ulna, Right*<br>**M Carpal, Right**<br>Capitate bone<br>Hamate bone<br>Lunate bone<br>Pisiform bone<br>Scaphoid bone<br>Trapezium bone<br>Trapezoid bone<br>Triquetral bone<br>**N Carpal, Left**<br>*See M Carpal, Right*<br>**P Metacarpal, Right**<br>**Q Metacarpal, Left**<br>**R Thumb Phalanx, Right**<br>**S Thumb Phalanx, Left**<br>**T Finger Phalanx, Right**<br>**V Finger Phalanx, Left** | **Ø Open**<br>**3 Percutaneous**<br>**4 Percutaneous Endoscopic**<br>**X External** | **Z** No Device | **Z** No Qualifier |

**Non-OR** ØPQ[Ø,1,2,3,4,5,6,7,8,9,B,C,D,F,G,H,J,K,L,M,N,P,Q,R,S,T,V]XZZ

**Ø Medical and Surgical**
**P Upper Bones**
**R Replacement**

Definition: Putting in or on biological or synthetic material that physically takes the place and/or function of all or a portion of a body part

Explanation: The body part may have been taken out or replaced, or may be taken out, physically eradicated, or rendered nonfunctional during the REPLACEMENT procedure. A REMOVAL procedure is coded for taking out the device used in a previous replacement procedure.

| Body Part Character 4 | Approach Character 5 | Device Character 6 | Qualifier Character 7 |
|---|---|---|---|
| **Ø Sternum**<br>Manubrium<br>Suprasternal notch<br>Xiphoid process<br>**1 Ribs, 1 to 2**<br>**2 Ribs, 3 or More**<br>**3 Cervical Vertebra**<br>Dens<br>Odontoid process<br>Spinous process<br>Transverse foramen<br>Transverse process<br>Vertebral arch<br>Vertebral body<br>Vertebral foramen<br>Vertebral lamina<br>Vertebral pedicle<br>**4 Thoracic Vertebra**<br>Spinous process<br>Transverse process<br>Vertebral arch<br>Vertebral body<br>Vertebral foramen<br>Vertebral lamina<br>Vertebral pedicle<br>**5 Scapula, Right**<br>Acromion (process)<br>Coracoid process<br>**6 Scapula, Left**<br>*See 5 Scapula, Right*<br>**7 Glenoid Cavity, Right**<br>Glenoid fossa (of scapula)<br>**8 Glenoid Cavity, Left**<br>*See 7 Glenoid Cavity, Right*<br>**9 Clavicle, Right**<br>**B Clavicle, Left**<br>**C Humeral Head, Right**<br>Greater tuberosity<br>Lesser tuberosity<br>Neck of humerus (anatomical)(surgical)<br>**D Humeral Head, Left**<br>*See C Humeral Head, Right*<br>**F Humeral Shaft, Right**<br>Distal humerus<br>Humerus, distal<br>Lateral epicondyle of humerus<br>Medial epicondyle of humerus<br>**G Humeral Shaft, Left**<br>*See F Humeral Shaft, Right*<br>**H Radius, Right**<br>Ulnar notch<br>**J Radius, Left**<br>*See H Radius, Right*<br>**K Ulna, Right**<br>Olecranon process<br>Radial notch<br>**L Ulna, Left**<br>*See K Ulna, Right*<br>**M Carpal, Right**<br>Capitate bone<br>Hamate bone<br>Lunate bone<br>Pisiform bone<br>Scaphoid bone<br>Trapezium bone<br>Trapezoid bone<br>Triquetral bone<br>**N Carpal, Left**<br>*See M Carpal, Right*<br>**P Metacarpal, Right**<br>**Q Metacarpal, Left**<br>**R Thumb Phalanx, Right**<br>**S Thumb Phalanx, Left**<br>**T Finger Phalanx, Right**<br>**V Finger Phalanx, Left** | **Ø Open**<br>**3 Percutaneous**<br>**4 Percutaneous Endoscopic** | **7 Autologous Tissue Substitute**<br>**J Synthetic Substitute**<br>**K Nonautologous Tissue Substitute** | **Z No Qualifier** |

**Ø Medical and Surgical**
**P Upper Bones**
**S Reposition**

Definition: Moving to its normal location, or other suitable location, all or a portion of a body part

Explanation: The body part is moved to a new location from an abnormal location, or from a normal location where it is not functioning correctly. The body part may or may not be cut out or off to be moved to the new location.

| Body Part Character 4 | | Approach Character 5 | Device Character 6 | Qualifier Character 7 |
|---|---|---|---|---|
| **Ø Sternum**<br>Manubrium<br>Suprasternal notch<br>Xiphoid process | | **Ø Open**<br>**3 Percutaneous**<br>**4 Percutaneous Endoscopic** | **Ø Internal Fixation Device, Rigid Plate**<br>**4 Internal Fixation Device**<br>**Z No Device** | **Z No Qualifier** |
| **Ø Sternum**<br>Manubrium<br>Suprasternal notch<br>Xiphoid process | | **X External** | **Z No Device** | **Z No Qualifier** |
| **1 Ribs, 1 to 2**<br>**2 Ribs, 3 or More**<br>**3 Cervical Vertebra** ⊞<br>Dens<br>Odontoid process<br>Spinous process<br>Transverse foramen<br>Transverse process<br>Vertebral arch<br>Vertebral body<br>Vertebral foramen<br>Vertebral lamina<br>Vertebral pedicle<br>**4 Thoracic Vertebra** ⊞<br>Spinous process<br>Transverse process<br>Vertebral arch<br>Vertebral body<br>Vertebral foramen<br>Vertebral lamina<br>Vertebral pedicle | **5 Scapula, Right**<br>Acromion (process)<br>Coracoid process<br>**6 Scapula, Left**<br>*See 5 Scapula, Right*<br>**7 Glenoid Cavity, Right**<br>Glenoid fossa (of scapula)<br>**8 Glenoid Cavity, Left**<br>*See 7 Glenoid Cavity, Right*<br>**9 Clavicle, Right**<br>**B Clavicle, Left** | **Ø Open**<br>**3 Percutaneous**<br>**4 Percutaneous Endoscopic** | **4 Internal Fixation Device**<br>**Z No Device** | **Z No Qualifier** |
| **1 Ribs, 1 to 2**<br>**2 Ribs, 3 or More**<br>**3 Cervical Vertebra**<br>Dens<br>Odontoid process<br>Spinous process<br>Transverse foramen<br>Transverse process<br>Vertebral arch<br>Vertebral body<br>Vertebral foramen<br>Vertebral lamina<br>Vertebral pedicle<br>**4 Thoracic Vertebra**<br>Spinous process<br>Transverse process<br>Vertebral arch<br>Vertebral body<br>Vertebral foramen<br>Vertebral lamina<br>Vertebral pedicle | **5 Scapula, Right**<br>Acromion (process)<br>Coracoid process<br>**6 Scapula, Left**<br>*See 5 Scapula, Right*<br>**7 Glenoid Cavity, Right**<br>Glenoid fossa (of scapula)<br>**8 Glenoid Cavity, Left**<br>*See 7 Glenoid Cavity, Right*<br>**9 Clavicle, Right**<br>**B Clavicle, Left** | **X External** | **Z No Device** | **Z No Qualifier** |
| **C Humeral Head, Right**<br>Greater tuberosity<br>Lesser tuberosity<br>Neck of humerus (anatomical)(surgical)<br>**D Humeral Head, Left**<br>*See C Humeral Head, Right*<br>**F Humeral Shaft, Right**<br>Distal humerus<br>Humerus, distal<br>Lateral epicondyle of humerus<br>Medial epicondyle of humerus | **G Humeral Shaft, Left**<br>*See F Humeral Shaft, Right*<br>**H Radius, Right**<br>Ulnar notch<br>**J Radius, Left**<br>*See H Radius, Right*<br>**K Ulna, Right**<br>Olecranon process<br>Radial notch<br>**L Ulna, Left**<br>*See K Ulna, Right* | **Ø Open**<br>**3 Percutaneous**<br>**4 Percutaneous Endoscopic** | **4 Internal Fixation Device**<br>**5 External Fixation Device**<br>**6 Internal Fixation Device, Intramedullary**<br>**B External Fixation Device, Monoplanar**<br>**C External Fixation Device, Ring**<br>**D External Fixation Device, Hybrid**<br>**Z No Device** | **Z No Qualifier** |

*ØPS Continued on next page*

**Non-OR** ØPSØ[3,4]ZZ
**Non-OR** ØPSØXZZ
**Non-OR** ØPS[1,2,5,6,7,8,9,B][3,4]ZZ
**Non-OR** ØPS[1,2,3,4,5,6,7,8,9,B]XZZ
**Non-OR** ØPS[C,D,F,G,H,J,K,L][3,4]ZZ

**See Appendix L for Procedure Combinations**
⊞ ØPS[3,4]3ZZ

## ØPS Continued

**Ø Medical and Surgical**
**P Upper Bones**
**S Reposition**

Definition: Moving to its normal location, or other suitable location, all or a portion of a body part

Explanation: The body part is moved to a new location from an abnormal location, or from a normal location where it is not functioning correctly. The body part may or may not be cut out or off to be moved to the new location.

| Body Part Character 4 | | Approach Character 5 | Device Character 6 | Qualifier Character 7 |
|---|---|---|---|---|
| **C Humeral Head, Right**<br>Greater tuberosity<br>Lesser tuberosity<br>Neck of humerus (anatomical)(surgical)<br>**D Humeral Head, Left**<br>*See C Humeral Head, Right*<br>**F Humeral Shaft, Right**<br>Distal humerus<br>Humerus, distal<br>Lateral epicondyle of humerus<br>Medial epicondyle of humerus | **G Humeral Shaft, Left**<br>*See F Humeral Shaft, Right*<br>**H Radius, Right**<br>Ulnar notch<br>**J Radius, Left**<br>*See H Radius, Right*<br>**K Ulna, Right**<br>Olecranon process<br>Radial notch<br>**L Ulna, Left**<br>*See K Ulna, Right* | **X External** | **Z No Device** | **Z No Qualifier** |
| **M Carpal, Right**<br>Capitate bone<br>Hamate bone<br>Lunate bone<br>Pisiform bone<br>Scaphoid bone<br>Trapezium bone<br>Trapezoid bone<br>Triquetral bone | **N Carpal, Left**<br>*See M Carpal, Right*<br>**P Metacarpal, Right**<br>**Q Metacarpal, Left**<br>**R Thumb Phalanx, Right**<br>**S Thumb Phalanx, Left**<br>**T Finger Phalanx, Right**<br>**V Finger Phalanx, Left** | **Ø Open**<br>**3 Percutaneous**<br>**4 Percutaneous Endoscopic** | **4 Internal Fixation Device**<br>**5 External Fixation Device**<br>**Z No Device** | **Z No Qualifier** |
| **M Carpal, Right**<br>Capitate bone<br>Hamate bone<br>Lunate bone<br>Pisiform bone<br>Scaphoid bone<br>Trapezium bone<br>Trapezoid bone<br>Triquetral bone | **N Carpal, Left**<br>*See M Carpal, Right*<br>**P Metacarpal, Right**<br>**Q Metacarpal, Left**<br>**R Thumb Phalanx, Right**<br>**S Thumb Phalanx, Left**<br>**T Finger Phalanx, Right**<br>**V Finger Phalanx, Left** | **X External** | **Z No Device** | **Z No Qualifier** |

Non-OR ØPS[C,D,F,G,H,J,K,L]XZZ
Non-OR ØPS[M,N,P,Q,R,S,T,V][3,4]ZZ
Non-OR ØPS[M,N,P,Q,R,S,T,V]XZZ

**Ø Medical and Surgical**
**P Upper Bones**
**T Resection**

Definition: Cutting out or off, without replacement, all of a body part

Explanation: None

| Body Part Character 4 | | Approach Character 5 | Device Character 6 | Qualifier Character 7 |
|---|---|---|---|---|
| **Ø Sternum**<br>Manubrium<br>Suprasternal notch<br>Xiphoid process<br>**1 Ribs, 1 to 2**<br>**2 Ribs, 3 or More**<br>**5 Scapula, Right**<br>Acromion (process)<br>Coracoid process<br>**6 Scapula, Left**<br>*See 5 Scapula, Right*<br>**7 Glenoid Cavity, Right**<br>Glenoid fossa (of scapula)<br>**8 Glenoid Cavity, Left**<br>*See 7 Glenoid Cavity, Right*<br>**9 Clavicle, Right**<br>**B Clavicle, Left**<br>**C Humeral Head, Right**<br>Greater tuberosity<br>Lesser tuberosity<br>Neck of humerus (anatomical) (surgical)<br>**D Humeral Head, Left**<br>*See C Humeral Head, Right*<br>**F Humeral Shaft, Right**<br>Distal humerus<br>Humerus, distal<br>Lateral epicondyle of humerus<br>Medial epicondyle of humerus | **G Humeral Shaft, Left**<br>*See F Humeral Shaft, Right*<br>**H Radius, Right**<br>Ulnar notch<br>**J Radius, Left**<br>*See H Radius, Right*<br>**K Ulna, Right**<br>Olecranon process<br>Radial notch<br>**L Ulna, Left**<br>*See K Ulna, Right*<br>**M Carpal, Right**<br>Capitate bone<br>Hamate bone<br>Lunate bone<br>Pisiform bone<br>Scaphoid bone<br>Trapezium bone<br>Trapezoid bone<br>Triquetral bone<br>**N Carpal, Left**<br>*See M Carpal, Right*<br>**P Metacarpal, Right**<br>**Q Metacarpal, Left**<br>**R Thumb Phalanx, Right**<br>**S Thumb Phalanx, Left**<br>**T Finger Phalanx, Right**<br>**V Finger Phalanx, Left** | **Ø Open** | **Z No Device** | **Z No Qualifier** |

**Ø Medical and Surgical**
**P Upper Bones**
**U Supplement**

Definition: Putting in or on biological or synthetic material that physically reinforces and/or augments the function of a portion of a body part

Explanation: The biological material is non-living, or is living and from the same individual. The body part may have been previously replaced, and the SUPPLEMENT procedure is performed to physically reinforce and/or augment the function of the replaced body part.

| Body Part Character 4 | Approach Character 5 | Device Character 6 | Qualifier Character 7 |
|---|---|---|---|
| **Ø Sternum**<br>Manubrium<br>Suprasternal notch<br>Xiphoid process<br>1 Ribs, 1 to 2<br>2 Ribs, 3 or More<br>**3 Cervical Vertebra** ⊞<br>Dens<br>Odontoid process<br>Spinous process<br>Transverse foramen<br>Transverse process<br>Vertebral arch<br>Vertebral body<br>Vertebral foramen<br>Vertebral lamina<br>Vertebral pedicle<br>**4 Thoracic Vertebra** ⊞<br>Spinous process<br>Transverse process<br>Vertebral arch<br>Vertebral body<br>Vertebral foramen<br>Vertebral lamina<br>Vertebral pedicle<br>**5 Scapula, Right**<br>Acromion (process)<br>Coracoid process<br>**6 Scapula, Left**<br>*See 5 Scapula, Right*<br>**7 Glenoid Cavity, Right**<br>Glenoid fossa (of scapula)<br>**8 Glenoid Cavity, Left**<br>*See 7 Glenoid Cavity, Right*<br>**9 Clavicle, Right**<br>**B Clavicle, Left**<br>**C Humeral Head, Right**<br>Greater tuberosity<br>Lesser tuberosity<br>Neck of humerus (anatomical) (surgical)<br>**D Humeral Head, Left**<br>*See C Humeral Head, Right*<br>**F Humeral Shaft, Right**<br>Distal humerus<br>Humerus, distal<br>Lateral epicondyle of humerus<br>Medial epicondyle of humerus<br>**G Humeral Shaft, Left**<br>*See F Humeral Shaft, Right*<br>**H Radius, Right**<br>Ulnar notch<br>**J Radius, Left**<br>*See H Radius, Right*<br>**K Ulna, Right**<br>Olecranon process<br>Radial notch<br>**L Ulna, Left**<br>*See K Ulna, Right*<br>**M Carpal, Right**<br>Capitate bone<br>Hamate bone<br>Lunate bone<br>Pisiform bone<br>Scaphoid bone<br>Trapezium bone<br>Trapezoid bone<br>Triquetral bone<br>**N Carpal, Left**<br>*See M Carpal, Right*<br>**P Metacarpal, Right**<br>**Q Metacarpal, Left**<br>**R Thumb Phalanx, Right**<br>**S Thumb Phalanx, Left**<br>**T Finger Phalanx, Right**<br>**V Finger Phalanx, Left** | **Ø Open**<br>**3 Percutaneous**<br>**4 Percutaneous Endoscopic** | **7 Autologous Tissue Substitute**<br>**J Synthetic Substitute**<br>**K Nonautologous Tissue Substitute** | **Z No Qualifier** |

**See Appendix L for Procedure Combinations**
⊞ ØPU[3,4]3JZ

**Ø Medical and Surgical**
**P Upper Bones**
**W Revision**

Definition: Correcting, to the extent possible, a portion of a malfunctioning device or the position of a displaced device

Explanation: Revision can include correcting a malfunctioning or displaced device by taking out or putting in components of the device such as a screw or pin

| Body Part Character 4 | Approach Character 5 | Device Character 6 | Qualifier Character 7 |
|---|---|---|---|
| **Ø Sternum**<br>Manubrium<br>Suprasternal notch<br>Xiphoid process<br>**1 Ribs, 1 to 2**<br>**2 Ribs, 3 or More**<br>**3 Cervical Vertebra**<br>Dens<br>Odontoid process<br>Spinous process<br>Transverse foramen<br>Transverse process<br>Vertebral arch<br>Vertebral body<br>Vertebral foramen<br>Vertebral lamina<br>Vertebral pedicle<br>**4 Thoracic Vertebra**<br>Spinous process<br>Transverse process<br>Vertebral arch<br>Vertebral body<br>Vertebral foramen<br>Vertebral lamina<br>Vertebral pedicle<br>**5 Scapula, Right**<br>Acromion (process)<br>Coracoid process<br>**6 Scapula, Left**<br>*See 5 Scapula, Right*<br>**7 Glenoid Cavity, Right**<br>Glenoid fossa (of scapula)<br>**8 Glenoid Cavity, Left**<br>*See 7 Glenoid Cavity, Right*<br>**9 Clavicle, Right**<br>**B Clavicle, Left** | **Ø Open**<br>**3 Percutaneous**<br>**4 Percutaneous Endoscopic**<br>**X External** | **4 Internal Fixation Device**<br>**7 Autologous Tissue Substitute**<br>**J Synthetic Substitute**<br>**K Nonautologous Tissue Substitute** | **Z No Qualifier** |
| **C Humeral Head, Right**<br>Greater tuberosity<br>Lesser tuberosity<br>Neck of humerus (anatomical)(surgical)<br>**D Humeral Head, Left**<br>*See C Humeral Head, Right*<br>**F Humeral Shaft, Right**<br>Distal humerus<br>Humerus, distal<br>Lateral epicondyle of humerus<br>Medial epicondyle of humerus<br>**G Humeral Shaft, Left**<br>*See F Humeral Shaft, Right*<br>**H Radius, Right**<br>Ulnar notch<br>**J Radius, Left**<br>*See H Radius, Right*<br>**K Ulna, Right**<br>Olecranon process<br>Radial notch<br>**L Ulna, Left**<br>*See K Ulna, Right*<br>**M Carpal, Right**<br>Capitate bone<br>Hamate bone<br>Lunate bone<br>Pisiform bone<br>Scaphoid bone<br>Trapezium bone<br>Trapezoid bone<br>Triquetral bone<br>**N Carpal, Left**<br>*See M Carpal, Right*<br>**P Metacarpal, Right**<br>**Q Metacarpal, Left**<br>**R Thumb Phalanx, Right**<br>**S Thumb Phalanx, Left**<br>**T Finger Phalanx, Right**<br>**V Finger Phalanx, Left** | **Ø Open**<br>**3 Percutaneous**<br>**4 Percutaneous Endoscopic**<br>**X External** | **4 Internal Fixation Device**<br>**5 External Fixation Device**<br>**7 Autologous Tissue Substitute**<br>**J Synthetic Substitute**<br>**K Nonautologous Tissue Substitute** | **Z No Qualifier** |
| **Y Upper Bone** | **Ø Open**<br>**3 Percutaneous**<br>**4 Percutaneous Endoscopic**<br>**X External** | **Ø Drainage Device**<br>**M Bone Growth Stimulator** | **Z No Qualifier** |

Non-OR ØPW[Ø,1,2,3,4,5,6,7,8,9,B]X[4,7,J,K]Z
Non-OR ØPW[C,D,F,G,H,J,K,L,M,N,P,Q,R,S,T,V]X[4,5,7,J,K]Z
Non-OR ØPWYX[Ø,M]Z

# Lower Bones ØQ2–ØQW

## Character Meanings

This Character Meaning table is provided as a guide to assist the user in the identification of character members that may be found in this section of code tables. It **SHOULD NOT** be used to build a PCS code.

| Operation–Character 3 | Body Part–Character 4 | Approach–Character 5 | Device–Character 6 | Qualifier–Character 7 |
|---|---|---|---|---|
| 2 Change | Ø Lumbar Vertebra | Ø Open | Ø Drainage Device | 2 Sesamoid Bone(s) 1st Toe |
| 5 Destruction | 1 Sacrum | 3 Percutaneous | 4 Internal Fixation Device | X Diagnostic |
| 8 Division | 2 Pelvic Bone, Right | 4 Percutaneous Endoscopic | 5 External Fixation Device | Z No Qualifier |
| 9 Drainage | 3 Pelvic Bone, Left | X External | 6 Internal Fixation Device, Intramedullary | |
| B Excision | 4 Acetabulum, Right | | 7 Autologous Tissue Substitute | |
| C Extirpation | 5 Acetabulum, Left | | 8 External Fixation Device, Limb Lengthening | |
| D Extraction | 6 Upper Femur, Right | | B External Fixation Device, Monoplanar | |
| H Insertion | 7 Upper Femur, Left | | C External Fixation Device, Ring | |
| J Inspection | 8 Femoral Shaft, Right | | D External Fixation Device, Hybrid | |
| N Release | 9 Femoral Shaft, Left | | J Synthetic Substitute | |
| P Removal | B Lower Femur, Right | | K Nonautologous Tissue Substitute | |
| Q Repair | C Lower Femur, Left | | M Bone Growth Stimulator | |
| R Replacement | D Patella, Right | | Y Other Device | |
| S Reposition | F Patella, Left | | Z No Device | |
| T Resection | G Tibia, Right | | | |
| U Supplement | H Tibia, Left | | | |
| W Revision | J Fibula, Right | | | |
| | K Fibula, Left | | | |
| | L Tarsal, Right | | | |
| | M Tarsal, Left | | | |
| | N Metatarsal, Right | | | |
| | P Metatarsal, Left | | | |
| | Q Toe Phalanx, Right | | | |
| | R Toe Phalanx, Left | | | |
| | S Coccyx | | | |
| | Y Lower Bone | | | |

**AHA Coding Clinic for table ØQ8**
**2016, 2Q, 31** Periacetabular ostectomy for repair of congenital hip dysplasia

**AHA Coding Clinic for table ØQB**
**2017, 1Q, 23** Reconstruction of mandible using titanium and bone
**2016, 3Q, 30** Resection of femur with interposition arthroplasty
**2015, 3Q, 3-8** Excisional and nonexcisional debridement
**2015, 3Q, 26** Femoral head resection
**2015, 2Q, 34** Decompressive laminectomy
**2014, 4Q, 25** Femoroacetabular impingement and labral tear with repair
**2014, 2Q, 6** Posterior lumbar fusion with discectomy
**2013, 4Q, 116** Spinal decompression
**2013, 2Q, 39** Ankle fusion, osteotomy, and removal of hardware
**2012, 2Q, 19** Multiple decompressive cervical laminectomies

**AHA Coding Clinic for table ØQH**
**2017, 1Q, 21** Staged scoliosis surgery with iliac fixation and spinal fusion
**2016, 3Q, 34** Tibial/fibula epiphysiodesis

**AHA Coding Clinic for table ØQP**
**2015, 2Q, 6** Planned implant break

**AHA Coding Clinic for table ØQQ**
**2014, 3Q, 24** Repair of lipomyelomeningocele and tethered cord

**AHA Coding Clinic for table ØQR**
**2017, 1Q, 22** Total knee replacement and patellar component
**2016, 3Q, 30** Resection of femur with interposition arthroplasty

**AHA Coding Clinic for table ØQS**
**2016, 3Q, 34** Tibial/fibula epiphysiodesis
**2014, 4Q, 29** Rotational osteosynthesis
**2014, 4Q, 31** Reposition of femur for correction of valgus and recurvatum deformities

**AHA Coding Clinic for table ØQT**
**2017, 1Q, 22** Chopart amputation of foot
**2016, 3Q, 30** Resection of femur with interposition arthroplasty
**2015, 3Q, 26** Femoral head resection
**2014, 4Q, 29** Rotational osteosynthesis

**AHA Coding Clinic for table ØQU**
**2015, 3Q, 18** Total hip replacement with acetabular reconstruction
**2014, 4Q, 31** Reposition of femur for correction of valgus and recurvatum deformities
**2014, 2Q, 12** Percutaneous vertebroplasty using cement
**2013, 2Q, 35** Use of bone void filler in grafting

## Lower Bones

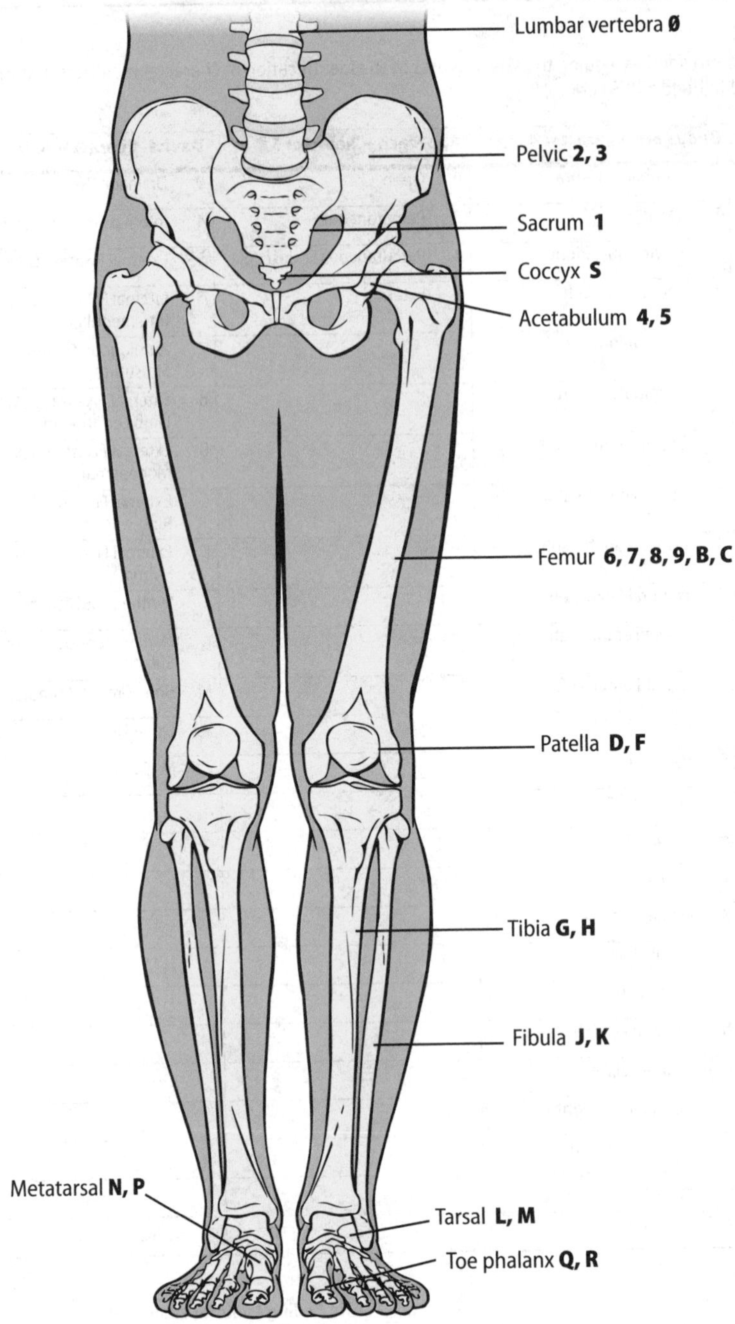
Lumbar vertebra Ø
Pelvic 2, 3
Sacrum 1
Coccyx S
Acetabulum 4, 5
Femur 6, 7, 8, 9, B, C
Patella D, F
Tibia G, H
Fibula J, K
Metatarsal N, P
Tarsal L, M
Toe phalanx Q, R

## Hip Bone Anatomy

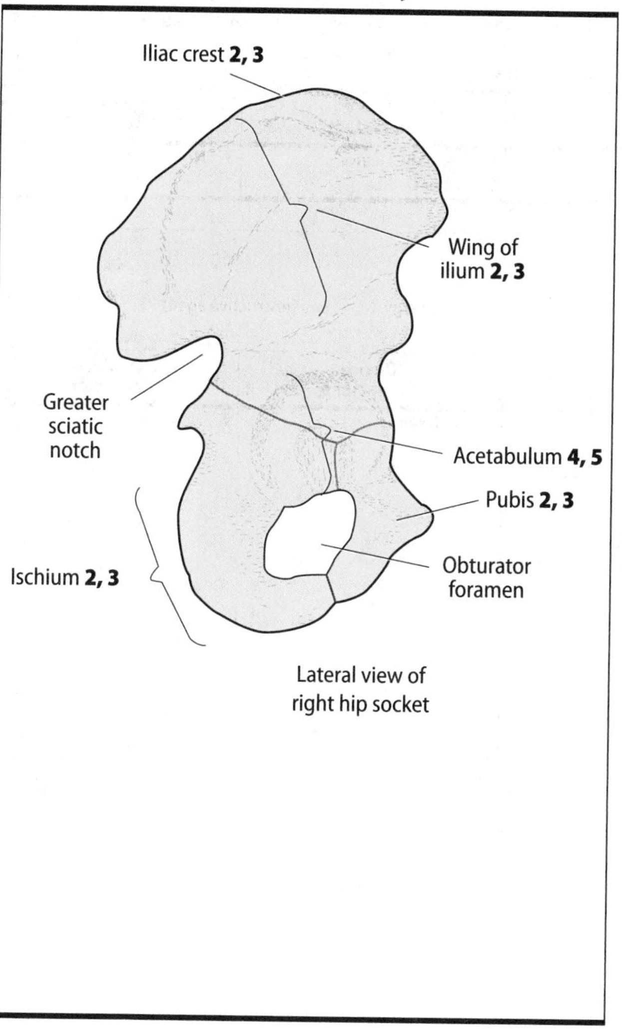
Iliac crest 2, 3
Wing of ilium 2, 3
Greater sciatic notch
Acetabulum 4, 5
Pubis 2, 3
Ischium 2, 3
Obturator foramen

Lateral view of right hip socket

## Pelvic and Lower Extremity Bones

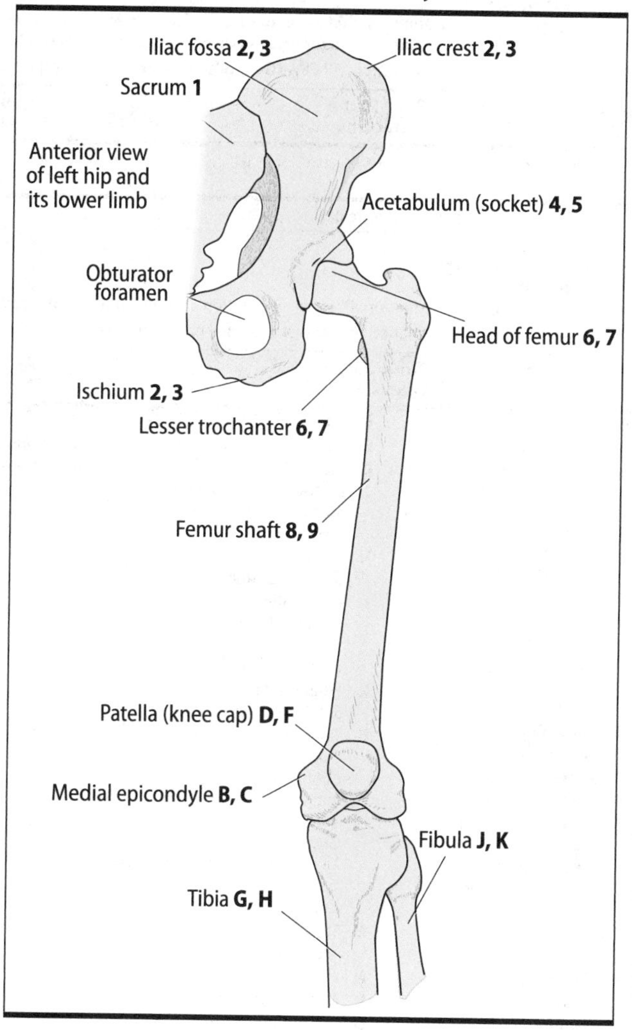
Iliac fossa 2, 3
Iliac crest 2, 3
Sacrum 1
Anterior view of left hip and its lower limb
Acetabulum (socket) 4, 5
Obturator foramen
Head of femur 6, 7
Ischium 2, 3
Lesser trochanter 6, 7
Femur shaft 8, 9
Patella (knee cap) D, F
Medial epicondyle B, C
Fibula J, K
Tibia G, H

## Foot Bones

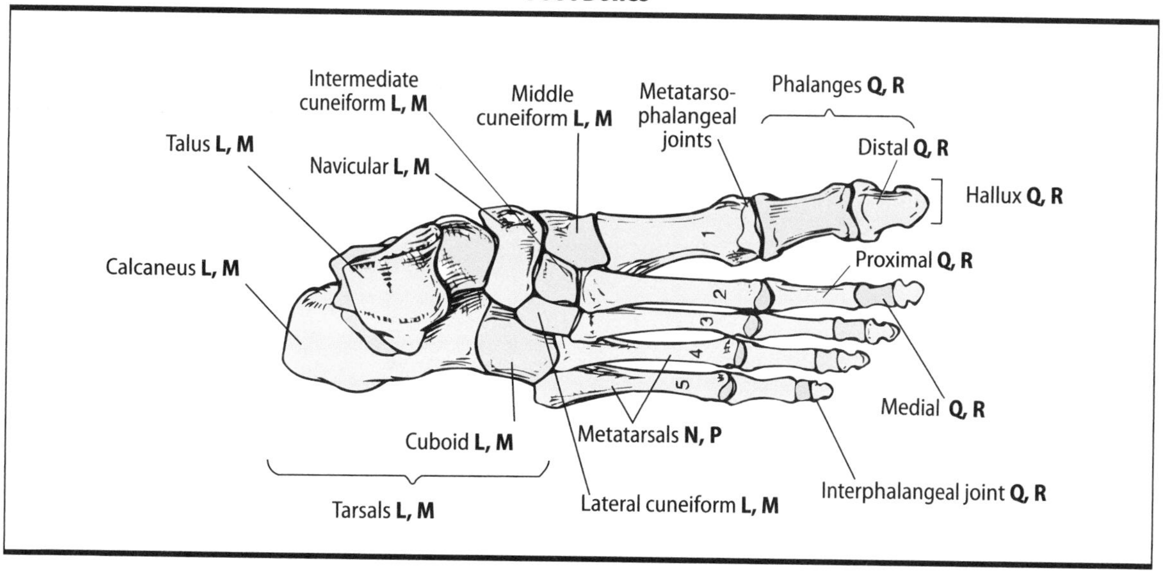
Intermediate cuneiform L, M
Middle cuneiform L, M
Metatarso-phalangeal joints
Phalanges Q, R
Talus L, M
Navicular L, M
Distal Q, R
Hallux Q, R
Calcaneus L, M
Proximal Q, R
1
2
3
4
5
Medial Q, R
Cuboid L, M
Metatarsals N, P
Tarsals L, M
Lateral cuneiform L, M
Interphalangeal joint Q, R

**Ø Medical and Surgical**
**Q Lower Bones**
**2 Change** Definition: Taking out or off a device from a body part and putting back an identical or similar device in or on the same body part without cutting or puncturing the skin or a mucous membrane

Explanation: All CHANGE procedures are coded using the approach EXTERNAL

| Body Part Character 4 | Approach Character 5 | Device Character 6 | Qualifier Character 7 |
|---|---|---|---|
| Y Lower Bone | X External | Ø Drainage Device<br>Y Other Device | Z No Qualifier |

Non-OR All body part, approach, device, and qualifier values

**Ø Medical and Surgical**
**Q Lower Bones**
**5 Destruction** Definition: Physical eradication of all or a portion of a body part by the direct use of energy, force, or a destructive agent

Explanation: None of the body part is physically taken out

| Body Part Character 4 | Approach Character 5 | Device Character 6 | Qualifier Character 7 |
|---|---|---|---|
| **Ø Lumbar Vertebra**<br>Spinous process<br>Transverse process<br>Vertebral arch<br>Vertebral body<br>Vertebral foramen<br>Vertebral lamina<br>Vertebral pedicle<br>**1 Sacrum**<br>**2 Pelvic Bone, Right**<br>Iliac crest<br>Ilium<br>Ischium<br>Pubis<br>**3 Pelvic Bone, Left**<br>*See 2 Pelvic Bone, Right*<br>**4 Acetabulum, Right**<br>**5 Acetabulum, Left**<br>**6 Upper Femur, Right**<br>Femoral head<br>Greater trochanter<br>Lesser trochanter<br>Neck of femur<br>**7 Upper Femur, Left**<br>*See 6 Upper Femur, Right*<br>**8 Femoral Shaft, Right**<br>Body of femur<br>**9 Femoral Shaft, Left**<br>*See 8 Femoral Shaft, Right*<br>**B Lower Femur, Right**<br>Lateral condyle of femur<br>Lateral epicondyle of femur<br>Medial condyle of femur<br>Medial epicondyle of femur<br>**C Lower Femur, Left**<br>*See B Lower Femur, Right*<br>**D Patella, Right**<br>**F Patella, Left**<br>**G Tibia, Right**<br>Lateral condyle of tibia<br>Medial condyle of tibia<br>Medial malleolus<br>**H Tibia, Left**<br>*See G Tibia, Right*<br>**J Fibula, Right**<br>Body of fibula<br>Head of fibula<br>Lateral malleolus<br>**K Fibula, Left**<br>*See J Fibula, Right*<br>**L Tarsal, Right**<br>Calcaneus<br>Cuboid bone<br>Intermediate cuneiform bone<br>Lateral cuneiform bone<br>Medial cuneiform bone<br>Navicular bone<br>Talus bone<br>**M Tarsal, Left**<br>*See L Tarsal, Right*<br>**N Metatarsal, Right**<br>**P Metatarsal, Left**<br>**Q Toe Phalanx, Right**<br>**R Toe Phalanx, Left**<br>**S Coccyx** | Ø Open<br>3 Percutaneous<br>4 Percutaneous Endoscopic | Z No Device | Z No Qualifier |

**Ø Medical and Surgical**
**Q Lower Bones**
**8 Division**

Definition: Cutting into a body part, without draining fluids and/or gases from the body part, in order to separate or transect a body part
Explanation: All or a portion of the body part is separated into two or more portions

| Body Part Character 4 | Approach Character 5 | Device Character 6 | Qualifier Character 7 |
|---|---|---|---|
| **Ø Lumbar Vertebra**<br>Spinous process<br>Transverse process<br>Vertebral arch<br>Vertebral body<br>Vertebral foramen<br>Vertebral lamina<br>Vertebral pedicle<br>**1 Sacrum**<br>**2 Pelvic Bone, Right**<br>Iliac crest<br>Ilium<br>Ischium<br>Pubis<br>**3 Pelvic Bone, Left**<br>*See 2 Pelvic Bone, Right*<br>**4 Acetabulum, Right**<br>**5 Acetabulum, Left**<br>**6 Upper Femur, Right**<br>Femoral head<br>Greater trochanter<br>Lesser trochanter<br>Neck of femur<br>**7 Upper Femur, Left**<br>*See 6 Upper Femur, Right*<br>**8 Femoral Shaft, Right**<br>Body of femur<br>**9 Femoral Shaft, Left**<br>*See 8 Femoral Shaft, Right*<br>**B Lower Femur, Right**<br>Lateral condyle of femur<br>Lateral epicondyle of femur<br>Medial condyle of femur<br>Medial epicondyle of femur<br>**C Lower Femur, Left**<br>*See B Lower Femur, Right*<br>**D Patella, Right**<br>**F Patella, Left**<br>**G Tibia, Right**<br>Lateral condyle of tibia<br>Medial condyle of tibia<br>Medial malleolus<br>**H Tibia, Left**<br>*See G Tibia, Right*<br>**J Fibula, Right**<br>Body of fibula<br>Head of fibula<br>Lateral malleolus<br>**K Fibula, Left**<br>*See J Fibula, Right*<br>**L Tarsal, Right**<br>Calcaneus<br>Cuboid bone<br>Intermediate cuneiform bone<br>Lateral cuneiform bone<br>Medial cuneiform bone<br>Navicular bone<br>Talus bone<br>**M Tarsal, Left**<br>*See L Tarsal, Right*<br>**N Metatarsal, Right**<br>**P Metatarsal, Left**<br>**Q Toe Phalanx, Right**<br>**R Toe Phalanx, Left**<br>**S Coccyx** | **Ø Open**<br>**3 Percutaneous**<br>**4 Percutaneous Endoscopic** | **Z No Device** | **Z No Qualifier** |

**Ø Medical and Surgical**
**Q Lower Bones**
**9 Drainage**

Definition: Taking or letting out fluids and/or gases from a body part

Explanation: The qualifier DIAGNOSTIC is used to identify drainage procedures that are biopsies

| Body Part Character 4 | Body Part Character 4 | Approach Character 5 | Device Character 6 | Qualifier Character 7 |
|---|---|---|---|---|
| **Ø Lumbar Vertebra**<br>Spinous process<br>Transverse process<br>Vertebral arch<br>Vertebral body<br>Vertebral foramen<br>Vertebral lamina<br>Vertebral pedicle<br>**1 Sacrum**<br>**2 Pelvic Bone, Right**<br>Iliac crest<br>Ilium<br>Ischium<br>Pubis<br>**3 Pelvic Bone, Left**<br>*See 2 Pelvic Bone, Right*<br>**4 Acetabulum, Right**<br>**5 Acetabulum, Left**<br>**6 Upper Femur, Right**<br>Femoral head<br>Greater trochanter<br>Lesser trochanter<br>Neck of femur<br>**7 Upper Femur, Left**<br>*See 6 Upper Femur, Right*<br>**8 Femoral Shaft, Right**<br>Body of femur<br>**9 Femoral Shaft, Left**<br>*See 8 Femoral Shaft, Right*<br>**B Lower Femur, Right**<br>Lateral condyle of femur<br>Lateral epicondyle of femur<br>Medial condyle of femur<br>Medial epicondyle of femur | **C Lower Femur, Left**<br>*See B Lower Femur, Right*<br>**D Patella, Right**<br>**F Patella, Left**<br>**G Tibia, Right**<br>Lateral condyle of tibia<br>Medial condyle of tibia<br>Medial malleolus<br>**H Tibia, Left**<br>*See G Tibia, Right*<br>**J Fibula, Right**<br>Body of fibula<br>Head of fibula<br>Lateral malleolus<br>**K Fibula, Left**<br>*See J Fibula, Right*<br>**L Tarsal, Right**<br>Calcaneus<br>Cuboid bone<br>Intermediate cuneiform bone<br>Lateral cuneiform bone<br>Medial cuneiform bone<br>Navicular bone<br>Talus bone<br>**M Tarsal, Left**<br>*See L Tarsal, Right*<br>**N Metatarsal, Right**<br>**P Metatarsal, Left**<br>**Q Toe Phalanx, Right**<br>**R Toe Phalanx, Left**<br>**S Coccyx** | **Ø Open**<br>**3 Percutaneous**<br>**4 Percutaneous Endoscopic** | **Ø Drainage Device** | **Z No Qualifier** |
| **Ø Lumbar Vertebra**<br>Spinous process<br>Transverse process<br>Vertebral arch<br>Vertebral body<br>Vertebral foramen<br>Vertebral lamina<br>Vertebral pedicle<br>**1 Sacrum**<br>**2 Pelvic Bone, Right**<br>Iliac crest<br>Ilium<br>Ischium<br>Pubis<br>**3 Pelvic Bone, Left**<br>*See 2 Pelvic Bone, Right*<br>**4 Acetabulum, Right**<br>**5 Acetabulum, Left**<br>**6 Upper Femur, Right**<br>Femoral head<br>Greater trochanter<br>Lesser trochanter<br>Neck of femur<br>**7 Upper Femur, Left**<br>*See 6 Upper Femur, Right*<br>**8 Femoral Shaft, Right**<br>Body of femur<br>**9 Femoral Shaft, Left**<br>*See 8 Femoral Shaft, Right*<br>**B Lower Femur, Right**<br>Lateral condyle of femur<br>Lateral epicondyle of femur<br>Medial condyle of femur<br>Medial epicondyle of femur | **C Lower Femur, Left**<br>*See B Lower Femur, Right*<br>**D Patella, Right**<br>**F Patella, Left**<br>**G Tibia, Right**<br>Lateral condyle of tibia<br>Medial condyle of tibia<br>Medial malleolus<br>**H Tibia, Left**<br>*See G Tibia, Right*<br>**J Fibula, Right**<br>Body of fibula<br>Head of fibula<br>Lateral malleolus<br>**K Fibula, Left**<br>*See J Fibula, Right*<br>**L Tarsal, Right**<br>Calcaneus<br>Cuboid bone<br>Intermediate cuneiform bone<br>Lateral cuneiform bone<br>Medial cuneiform bone<br>Navicular bone<br>Talus bone<br>**M Tarsal, Left**<br>*See L Tarsal, Right*<br>**N Metatarsal, Right**<br>**P Metatarsal, Left**<br>**Q Toe Phalanx, Right**<br>**R Toe Phalanx, Left**<br>**S Coccyx** | **Ø Open**<br>**3 Percutaneous**<br>**4 Percutaneous Endoscopic** | **Z No Device** | **X Diagnostic**<br>**Z No Qualifier** |

**Non-OR** ØQ9[Ø,1,2,3,4,5,6,7,8,9,B,C,D,F,G,H,J,K,L,M,P,Q,R,S]3ØZ
**Non-OR** ØQ9[Ø,1,2,3,4,5,6,7,8,9,B,C,D,F,G,H,J,K,L,M,P,Q,R,S]3ZZ

**Ø Medical and Surgical**
**Q Lower Bones**
**B Excision** Definition: Cutting out or off, without replacement, a portion of a body part
Explanation: The qualifier DIAGNOSTIC is used to identify excision procedures that are biopsies

| Body Part Character 4 | | Approach Character 5 | Device Character 6 | Qualifier Character 7 |
|---|---|---|---|---|
| **Ø Lumbar Vertebra**<br>Spinous process<br>Transverse process<br>Vertebral arch<br>Vertebral body<br>Vertebral foramen<br>Vertebral lamina<br>Vertebral pedicle<br>**1 Sacrum**<br>**2 Pelvic Bone, Right**<br>Iliac crest<br>Ilium<br>Ischium<br>Pubis<br>**3 Pelvic Bone, Left**<br>*See 2 Pelvic Bone, Right*<br>**4 Acetabulum, Right**<br>**5 Acetabulum, Left**<br>**6 Upper Femur, Right**<br>Femoral head<br>Greater trochanter<br>Lesser trochanter<br>Neck of femur<br>**7 Upper Femur, Left**<br>*See 6 Upper Femur, Right*<br>**8 Femoral Shaft, Right**<br>Body of femur<br>**9 Femoral Shaft, Left**<br>*See 8 Femoral Shaft, Right*<br>**B Lower Femur, Right**<br>Lateral condyle of femur<br>Lateral epicondyle of femur<br>Medial condyle of femur<br>Medial epicondyle of femur | **C Lower Femur, Left**<br>*See B Lower Femur, Right*<br>**D Patella, Right**<br>**F Patella, Left**<br>**G Tibia, Right**<br>Lateral condyle of tibia<br>Medial condyle of tibia<br>Medial malleolus<br>**H Tibia, Left**<br>*See G Tibia, Right*<br>**J Fibula, Right**<br>Body of fibula<br>Head of fibula<br>Lateral malleolus<br>**K Fibula, Left**<br>*See J Fibula, Right*<br>**L Tarsal, Right**<br>Calcaneus<br>Cuboid bone<br>Intermediate cuneiform bone<br>Lateral cuneiform bone<br>Medial cuneiform bone<br>Navicular bone<br>Talus bone<br>**M Tarsal, Left**<br>*See L Tarsal, Right*<br>**N Metatarsal, Right**<br>**P Metatarsal, Left**<br>**Q Toe Phalanx, Right**<br>**R Toe Phalanx, Left**<br>**S Coccyx** | **Ø Open**<br>**3 Percutaneous**<br>**4 Percutaneous Endoscopic** | **Z No Device** | **X Diagnostic**<br>**Z No Qualifier** |

**Ø Medical and Surgical**
**Q Lower Bones**
**C Extirpation** Definition: Taking or cutting out solid matter from a body part

Explanation: The solid matter may be an abnormal byproduct of a biological function or a foreign body; it may be imbedded in a body part or in the lumen of a tubular body part. The solid matter may or may not have been previously broken into pieces.

| Body Part Character 4 | Approach Character 5 | Device Character 6 | Qualifier Character 7 |
|---|---|---|---|
| **Ø Lumbar Vertebra**<br>Spinous process<br>Transverse process<br>Vertebral arch<br>Vertebral body<br>Vertebral foramen<br>Vertebral lamina<br>Vertebral pedicle<br>**1 Sacrum**<br>**2 Pelvic Bone, Right**<br>Iliac crest<br>Ilium<br>Ischium<br>Pubis<br>**3 Pelvic Bone, Left**<br>*See 2 Pelvic Bone, Right*<br>**4 Acetabulum, Right**<br>**5 Acetabulum, Left**<br>**6 Upper Femur, Right**<br>Femoral head<br>Greater trochanter<br>Lesser trochanter<br>Neck of femur<br>**7 Upper Femur, Left**<br>*See 6 Upper Femur, Right*<br>**8 Femoral Shaft, Right**<br>Body of femur<br>**9 Femoral Shaft, Left**<br>*See 8 Femoral Shaft, Right*<br>**B Lower Femur, Right**<br>Lateral condyle of femur<br>Lateral epicondyle of femur<br>Medial condyle of femur<br>Medial epicondyle of femur<br>**C Lower Femur, Left**<br>*See B Lower Femur, Right*<br>**D Patella, Right**<br>**F Patella, Left**<br>**G Tibia, Right**<br>Lateral condyle of tibia<br>Medial condyle of tibia<br>Medial malleolus<br>**H Tibia, Left**<br>*See G Tibia, Right*<br>**J Fibula, Right**<br>Body of fibula<br>Head of fibula<br>Lateral malleolus<br>**K Fibula, Left**<br>*See J Fibula, Right*<br>**L Tarsal, Right**<br>Calcaneus<br>Cuboid bone<br>Intermediate cuneiform bone<br>Lateral cuneiform bone<br>Medial cuneiform bone<br>Navicular bone<br>Talus bone<br>**M Tarsal, Left**<br>*See L Tarsal, Right*<br>**N Metatarsal, Right**<br>**P Metatarsal, Left**<br>**Q Toe Phalanx, Right**<br>**R Toe Phalanx, Left**<br>**S Coccyx** | **Ø Open**<br>**3 Percutaneous**<br>**4 Percutaneous Endoscopic** | **Z** No Device | **Z** No Qualifier |

**Ø Medical and Surgical**
**Q Lower Bones**
**D Extraction** Definition: Pulling or stripping out or off all or a portion of a body part by the use of force

Explanation: The qualifier DIAGNOSTIC is used to identify extraction procedures that are biopsies

| Body Part Character 4 | Approach Character 5 | Device Character 6 | Qualifier Character 7 |
|---|---|---|---|
| **Ø Lumbar Vertebra**<br>Spinous process<br>Transverse process<br>Vertebral arch<br>Vertebral body<br>Vertebral foramen<br>Vertebral lamina<br>Vertebral pedicle<br>**1 Sacrum**<br>**2 Pelvic Bone, Right**<br>Iliac crest<br>Ilium<br>Ischium<br>Pubis<br>**3 Pelvic Bone, Left**<br>*See 2 Pelvic Bone, Right*<br>**4 Acetabulum, Right**<br>**5 Acetabulum, Left**<br>**6 Upper Femur, Right**<br>Femoral head<br>Greater trochanter<br>Lesser trochanter<br>Neck of femur<br>**7 Upper Femur, Left**<br>*See 6 Upper Femur, Right*<br>**8 Femoral Shaft, Right**<br>Body of femur<br>**9 Femoral Shaft, Left**<br>*See 8 Femoral Shaft, Right*<br>**B Lower Femur, Right**<br>Lateral condyle of femur<br>Lateral epicondyle of femur<br>Medial condyle of femur<br>Medial epicondyle of femur<br>**C Lower Femur, Left**<br>*See B Lower Femur, Right*<br>**D Patella, Right**<br>**F Patella, Left**<br>**G Tibia, Right**<br>Lateral condyle of tibia<br>Medial condyle of tibia<br>Medial malleolus<br>**H Tibia, Left**<br>*See G Tibia, Right*<br>**J Fibula, Right**<br>Body of fibula<br>Head of fibula<br>Lateral malleolus<br>**K Fibula, Left**<br>*See J Fibula, Right*<br>**L Tarsal, Right**<br>Calcaneus<br>Cuboid bone<br>Intermediate cuneiform bone<br>Lateral cuneiform bone<br>Medial cuneiform bone<br>Navicular bone<br>Talus bone<br>**M Tarsal, Left**<br>*See L Tarsal, Right*<br>**N Metatarsal, Right**<br>**P Metatarsal, Left**<br>**Q Toe Phalanx, Right**<br>**R Toe Phalanx, Left**<br>**S Coccyx** | **Ø** Open | **Z** No Device | **Z** No Qualifier |

**Ø Medical and Surgical**
**Q Lower Bones**
**H Insertion** Definition: Putting in a nonbiological appliance that monitors, assists, performs, or prevents a physiological function but does not physically take the place of a body part

Explanation: None

| Body Part Character 4 | Approach Character 5 | Device Character 6 | Qualifier Character 7 |
|---|---|---|---|
| **Ø Lumbar Vertebra**<br>Spinous process<br>Transverse process<br>Vertebral arch<br>Vertebral body<br>Vertebral foramen<br>Vertebral lamina<br>Vertebral pedicle<br>**1 Sacrum**<br>**2 Pelvic Bone, Right**<br>Iliac crest<br>Ilium<br>Ischium<br>Pubis<br>**3 Pelvic Bone, Left**<br>*See 2 Pelvic Bone, Right*<br>**4 Acetabulum, Right**<br>**5 Acetabulum, Left**<br>**D Patella, Right**<br>**F Patella, Left**<br>**L Tarsal, Right**<br>Calcaneus<br>Cuboid bone<br>Intermediate cuneiform bone<br>Lateral cuneiform bone<br>Medial cuneiform bone<br>Navicular bone<br>Talus bone<br>**M Tarsal, Left**<br>*See L Tarsal, Right*<br>**N Metatarsal, Right**<br>**P Metatarsal, Left**<br>**Q Toe Phalanx, Right**<br>**R Toe Phalanx, Left**<br>**S Coccyx** | **Ø Open**<br>**3 Percutaneous**<br>**4 Percutaneous Endoscopic** | **4 Internal Fixation Device**<br>**5 External Fixation Device** | **Z No Qualifier** |
| **6 Upper Femur, Right**<br>Femoral head<br>Greater trochanter<br>Lesser trochanter<br>Neck of femur<br>**7 Upper Femur, Left**<br>*See 6 Upper Femur, Right*<br>**8 Femoral Shaft, Right**<br>Body of femur<br>**9 Femoral Shaft, Left**<br>*See 8 Femoral Shaft, Right*<br>**B Lower Femur, Right**<br>Lateral condyle of femur<br>Lateral epicondyle of femur<br>Medial condyle of femur<br>Medial epicondyle of femur<br>**C Lower Femur, Left**<br>*See B Lower Femur, Right*<br>**G Tibia, Right**<br>Lateral condyle of tibia<br>Medial condyle of tibia<br>Medial malleolus<br>**H Tibia, Left**<br>*See G Tibia, Right*<br>**J Fibula, Right**<br>Body of fibula<br>Head of fibula<br>Lateral malleolus<br>**K Fibula, Left**<br>*See J Fibula, Right* | **Ø Open**<br>**3 Percutaneous**<br>**4 Percutaneous Endoscopic** | **4 Internal Fixation Device**<br>**5 External Fixation Device**<br>**6 Internal Fixation Device, Intramedullary**<br>**8 External Fixation Device, Limb Lengthening**<br>**B External Fixation Device, Monoplanar**<br>**C External Fixation Device, Ring**<br>**D External Fixation Device, Hybrid** | **Z No Qualifier** |
| **Y Lower Bone** | **Ø Open**<br>**3 Percutaneous**<br>**4 Percutaneous Endoscopic** | **M Bone Growth Stimulator** | **Z No Qualifier** |

**Non-OR** ØQH[6,7,8,9,B,C,G,H,J,K][Ø,3,4]8Z

**Ø Medical and Surgical**
**Q Lower Bones**
**J Inspection** Definition: Visually and/or manually exploring a body part

Explanation: Visual exploration may be performed with or without optical instrumentation. Manual exploration may be performed directly or through intervening body layers.

| Body Part Character 4 | Approach Character 5 | Device Character 6 | Qualifier Character 7 |
|---|---|---|---|
| **Y Lower Bone** | **Ø Open**<br>**3 Percutaneous**<br>**4 Percutaneous Endoscopic**<br>**X External** | **Z No Device** | **Z No Qualifier** |

**Non-OR** ØQJY[3,X]ZZ

**Ø Medical and Surgical**
**Q Lower Bones**
**N Release** Definition: Freeing a body part from an abnormal physical constraint by cutting or by the use of force
Explanation: Some of the restraining tissue may be taken out but none of the body part is taken out

| Body Part Character 4 | | Approach Character 5 | Device Character 6 | Qualifier Character 7 |
|---|---|---|---|---|
| **Ø Lumbar Vertebra**<br>Spinous process<br>Transverse process<br>Vertebral arch<br>Vertebral body<br>Vertebral foramen<br>Vertebral lamina<br>Vertebral pedicle<br>**1 Sacrum**<br>**2 Pelvic Bone, Right**<br>Iliac crest<br>Ilium<br>Ischium<br>Pubis<br>**3 Pelvic Bone, Left**<br>*See 2 Pelvic Bone, Right*<br>**4 Acetabulum, Right**<br>**5 Acetabulum, Left**<br>**6 Upper Femur, Right**<br>Femoral head<br>Greater trochanter<br>Lesser trochanter<br>Neck of femur<br>**7 Upper Femur, Left**<br>*See 6 Upper Femur, Right*<br>**8 Femoral Shaft, Right**<br>Body of femur<br>**9 Femoral Shaft, Left**<br>*See 8 Femoral Shaft, Right*<br>**B Lower Femur, Right**<br>Lateral condyle of femur<br>Lateral epicondyle of femur<br>Medial condyle of femur<br>Medial epicondyle of femur | **C Lower Femur, Left**<br>*See B Lower Femur, Right*<br>**D Patella, Right**<br>**F Patella, Left**<br>**G Tibia, Right**<br>Lateral condyle of tibia<br>Medial condyle of tibia<br>Medial malleolus<br>**H Tibia, Left**<br>*See G Tibia, Right*<br>**J Fibula, Right**<br>Body of fibula<br>Head of fibula<br>Lateral malleolus<br>**K Fibula, Left**<br>*See J Fibula, Right*<br>**L Tarsal, Right**<br>Calcaneus<br>Cuboid bone<br>Intermediate cuneiform bone<br>Lateral cuneiform bone<br>Medial cuneiform bone<br>Navicular bone<br>Talus bone<br>**M Tarsal, Left**<br>*See L Tarsal, Right*<br>**N Metatarsal, Right**<br>**P Metatarsal, Left**<br>**Q Toe Phalanx, Right**<br>**R Toe Phalanx, Left**<br>**S Coccyx** | **Ø Open**<br>**3 Percutaneous**<br>**4 Percutaneous Endoscopic** | **Z No Device** | **Z No Qualifier** |

**Ø Medical and Surgical**
**Q Lower Bones**
**P Removal** Definition: Taking out or off a device from a body part
Explanation: If a device is taken out and a similar device put in without cutting or puncturing the skin or mucous membrane, the procedure is coded to the root operation CHANGE. Otherwise, the procedure for taking out a device is coded to the root operation REMOVAL.

| Body Part Character 4 | | Approach Character 5 | Device Character 6 | Qualifier Character 7 |
|---|---|---|---|---|
| **Ø Lumbar Vertebra**<br>Spinous process<br>Transverse process<br>Vertebral arch<br>Vertebral body<br>Vertebral foramen<br>Vertebral lamina<br>Vertebral pedicle | **1 Sacrum**<br>**4 Acetabulum, Right**<br>**5 Acetabulum, Left**<br>**S Coccyx** | **Ø Open**<br>**3 Percutaneous**<br>**4 Percutaneous Endoscopic** | **4 Internal Fixation Device**<br>**7 Autologous Tissue Substitute**<br>**J Synthetic Substitute**<br>**K Nonautologous Tissue Substitute** | **Z No Qualifier** |
| **Ø Lumbar Vertebra**<br>Spinous process<br>Transverse process<br>Vertebral arch<br>Vertebral body<br>Vertebral foramen<br>Vertebral lamina<br>Vertebral pedicle | **1 Sacrum**<br>**4 Acetabulum, Right**<br>**5 Acetabulum, Left**<br>**S Coccyx** | **X External** | **4 Internal Fixation Device** | **Z No Qualifier** |

***ØQP Continued on next page***

**Non-OR** ØQP[Ø,1,4,5,S]X4Z

**Ø Medical and Surgical**
**Q Lower Bones**
**P Removal** Definition: Taking out or off a device from a body part

Explanation: If a device is taken out and a similar device put in without cutting or puncturing the skin or mucous membrane, the procedure is coded to the root operation CHANGE. Otherwise, the procedure for taking out a device is coded to the root operation REMOVAL.

***ØQP Continued***

| Body Part Character 4 | | Approach Character 5 | Device Character 6 | Qualifier Character 7 |
|---|---|---|---|---|
| **2 Pelvic Bone, Right**<br>Iliac crest<br>Ilium<br>Ischium<br>Pubis<br>**3 Pelvic Bone, Left**<br>***See*** *2 Pelvic Bone, Right*<br>**6 Upper Femur, Right**<br>Femoral head<br>Greater trochanter<br>Lesser trochanter<br>Neck of femur<br>**7 Upper Femur, Left**<br>***See*** *6 Upper Femur, Right*<br>**8 Femoral Shaft, Right**<br>Body of femur<br>**9 Femoral Shaft, Left**<br>***See*** *8 Femoral Shaft, Right*<br>**B Lower Femur, Right**<br>Lateral condyle of femur<br>Lateral epicondyle of femur<br>Medial condyle of femur<br>Medial epicondyle of femur<br>**C Lower Femur, Left**<br>***See*** *B Lower Femur, Right*<br>**D Patella, Right**<br>**F Patella, Left** | **G Tibia, Right**<br>Lateral condyle of tibia<br>Medial condyle of tibia<br>Medial malleolus<br>**H Tibia, Left**<br>***See*** *G Tibia, Right*<br>**J Fibula, Right**<br>Body of fibula<br>Head of fibula<br>Lateral malleolus<br>**K Fibula, Left**<br>***See*** *J Fibula, Right*<br>**L Tarsal, Right**<br>Calcaneus<br>Cuboid bone<br>Intermediate cuneiform bone<br>Lateral cuneiform bone<br>Medial cuneiform bone<br>Navicular bone<br>Talus bone<br>**M Tarsal, Left**<br>***See*** *L Tarsal, Right*<br>**N Metatarsal, Right**<br>**P Metatarsal, Left**<br>**Q Toe Phalanx, Right**<br>**R Toe Phalanx, Left** | **Ø Open**<br>**3 Percutaneous**<br>**4 Percutaneous Endoscopic** | **4 Internal Fixation Device**<br>**5 External Fixation Device**<br>**7 Autologous Tissue Substitute**<br>**J Synthetic Substitute**<br>**K Nonautologous Tissue Substitute** | **Z No Qualifier** |
| **2 Pelvic Bone, Right**<br>Iliac crest<br>Ilium<br>Ischium<br>Pubis<br>**3 Pelvic Bone, Left**<br>***See*** *2 Pelvic Bone, Right*<br>**6 Upper Femur, Right**<br>Femoral head<br>Greater trochanter<br>Lesser trochanter<br>Neck of femur<br>**7 Upper Femur, Left**<br>***See*** *6 Upper Femur, Right*<br>**8 Femoral Shaft, Right**<br>Body of femur<br>**9 Femoral Shaft, Left**<br>***See*** *8 Femoral Shaft, Right*<br>**B Lower Femur, Right**<br>Lateral condyle of femur<br>Lateral epicondyle of femur<br>Medial condyle of femur<br>Medial epicondyle of femur<br>**C Lower Femur, Left**<br>***See*** *B Lower Femur, Right*<br>**D Patella, Right**<br>**F Patella, Left** | **G Tibia, Right**<br>Lateral condyle of tibia<br>Medial condyle of tibia<br>Medial malleolus<br>**H Tibia, Left**<br>***See*** *G Tibia, Right*<br>**J Fibula, Right**<br>Body of fibula<br>Head of fibula<br>Lateral malleolus<br>**K Fibula, Left**<br>***See*** *J Fibula, Right*<br>**L Tarsal, Right**<br>Calcaneus<br>Cuboid bone<br>Intermediate cuneiform bone<br>Lateral cuneiform bone<br>Medial cuneiform bone<br>Navicular bone<br>Talus bone<br>**M Tarsal, Left**<br>***See*** *L Tarsal, Right*<br>**N Metatarsal, Right**<br>**P Metatarsal, Left**<br>**Q Toe Phalanx, Right**<br>**R Toe Phalanx, Left** | X External | 4 Internal Fixation Device<br>5 External Fixation Device | Z No Qualifier |
| Y Lower Bone | | Ø Open<br>3 Percutaneous<br>4 Percutaneous Endoscopic<br>X External | Ø Drainage Device<br>M Bone Growth Stimulator | Z No Qualifier |

**Non-OR** ØQP[2,3,6,7,8,9,B,C,D,F,G,H,J,K,L,M,N,P,Q,R]X[4,5]Z
**Non-OR** ØQPY3ØZ
**Non-OR** ØQPYX[Ø,M]Z

**Ø Medical and Surgical**
**Q Lower Bones**
**Q Repair**

Definition: Restoring, to the extent possible, a body part to its normal anatomic structure and function
Explanation: Used only when the method to accomplish the repair is not one of the other root operations

| Body Part Character 4 | Approach Character 5 | Device Character 6 | Qualifier Character 7 |
|---|---|---|---|
| **Ø Lumbar Vertebra**<br>Spinous process<br>Transverse process<br>Vertebral arch<br>Vertebral body<br>Vertebral foramen<br>Vertebral lamina<br>Vertebral pedicle<br>**1 Sacrum**<br>**2 Pelvic Bone, Right**<br>Iliac crest<br>Ilium<br>Ischium<br>Pubis<br>**3 Pelvic Bone, Left**<br>*See 2 Pelvic Bone, Right*<br>**4 Acetabulum, Right**<br>**5 Acetabulum, Left**<br>**6 Upper Femur, Right**<br>Femoral head<br>Greater trochanter<br>Lesser trochanter<br>Neck of femur<br>**7 Upper Femur, Left**<br>*See 6 Upper Femur, Right*<br>**8 Femoral Shaft, Right**<br>Body of femur<br>**9 Femoral Shaft, Left**<br>*See 8 Femoral Shaft, Right*<br>**B Lower Femur, Right**<br>Lateral condyle of femur<br>Lateral epicondyle of femur<br>Medial condyle of femur<br>Medial epicondyle of femur<br>**C Lower Femur, Left**<br>*See B Lower Femur, Right*<br>**D Patella, Right**<br>**F Patella, Left**<br>**G Tibia, Right**<br>Lateral condyle of tibia<br>Medial condyle of tibia<br>Medial malleolus<br>**H Tibia, Left**<br>*See G Tibia, Right*<br>**J Fibula, Right**<br>Body of fibula<br>Head of fibula<br>Lateral malleolus<br>**K Fibula, Left**<br>*See J Fibula, Right*<br>**L Tarsal, Right**<br>Calcaneus<br>Cuboid bone<br>Intermediate cuneiform bone<br>Lateral cuneiform bone<br>Medial cuneiform bone<br>Navicular bone<br>Talus bone<br>**M Tarsal, Left**<br>*See L Tarsal, Right*<br>**N Metatarsal, Right**<br>**P Metatarsal, Left**<br>**Q Toe Phalanx, Right**<br>**R Toe Phalanx, Left**<br>**S Coccyx** | **Ø Open**<br>**3 Percutaneous**<br>**4 Percutaneous Endoscopic**<br>**X External** | **Z No Device** | **Z No Qualifier** |

Non-OR ØQQ[Ø,1,2,3,4,5,6,7,8,9,B,C,D,F,G,H,J,K,L,M,N,P,Q,R,S]XZZ

**Ø Medical and Surgical**
**Q Lower Bones**
**R Replacement** Definition: Putting in or on biological or synthetic material that physically takes the place and/or function of all or a portion of a body part

Explanation: The body part may have been taken out or replaced, or may be taken out, physically eradicated, or rendered nonfunctional during the REPLACEMENT procedure. A REMOVAL procedure is coded for taking out the device used in a previous replacement procedure.

| Body Part Character 4 | Approach Character 5 | Device Character 6 | Qualifier Character 7 |
|---|---|---|---|
| **Ø Lumbar Vertebra**<br>Spinous process<br>Transverse process<br>Vertebral arch<br>Vertebral body<br>Vertebral foramen<br>Vertebral lamina<br>Vertebral pedicle<br>**1 Sacrum**<br>**2 Pelvic Bone, Right**<br>Iliac crest<br>Ilium<br>Ischium<br>Pubis<br>**3 Pelvic Bone, Left**<br>*See 2 Pelvic Bone, Right*<br>**4 Acetabulum, Right**<br>**5 Acetabulum, Left**<br>**6 Upper Femur, Right**<br>Femoral head<br>Greater trochanter<br>Lesser trochanter<br>Neck of femur<br>**7 Upper Femur, Left**<br>*See 6 Upper Femur, Right*<br>**8 Femoral Shaft, Right**<br>Body of femur<br>**9 Femoral Shaft, Left**<br>*See 8 Femoral Shaft, Right*<br>**B Lower Femur, Right**<br>Lateral condyle of femur<br>Lateral epicondyle of femur<br>Medial condyle of femur<br>Medial epicondyle of femur<br>**C Lower Femur, Left**<br>*See B Lower Femur, Right*<br>**D Patella, Right**<br>**F Patella, Left**<br>**G Tibia, Right**<br>Lateral condyle of tibia<br>Medial condyle of tibia<br>Medial malleolus<br>**H Tibia, Left**<br>*See G Tibia, Right*<br>**J Fibula, Right**<br>Body of fibula<br>Head of fibula<br>Lateral malleolus<br>**K Fibula, Left**<br>*See J Fibula, Right*<br>**L Tarsal, Right**<br>Calcaneus<br>Cuboid bone<br>Intermediate cuneiform bone<br>Lateral cuneiform bone<br>Medial cuneiform bone<br>Navicular bone<br>Talus bone<br>**M Tarsal, Left**<br>*See L Tarsal, Right*<br>**N Metatarsal, Right**<br>**P Metatarsal, Left**<br>**Q Toe Phalanx, Right**<br>**R Toe Phalanx, Left**<br>**S Coccyx** | **Ø Open**<br>**3 Percutaneous**<br>**4 Percutaneous Endoscopic** | **7 Autologous Tissue Substitute**<br>**J Synthetic Substitute**<br>**K Nonautologous Tissue Substitute** | **Z No Qualifier** |

**Ø Medical and Surgical**
**Q Lower Bones**
**S Reposition** Definition: Moving to its normal location, or other suitable location, all or a portion of a body part

Explanation: The body part is moved to a new location from an abnormal location, or from a normal location where it is not functioning correctly. The body part may or may not be cut out or off to be moved to the new location.

| Body Part Character 4 | Approach Character 5 | Device Character 6 | Qualifier Character 7 |
|---|---|---|---|
| **Ø Lumbar Vertebra** ⊞<br>Spinous process<br>Transverse process<br>Vertebral arch<br>Vertebral body<br>Vertebral foramen<br>Vertebral lamina<br>Vertebral pedicle<br>**1 Sacrum** ⊞<br>**4 Acetabulum, Right**<br>**5 Acetabulum, Left**<br>**S Coccyx** ⊞ | **Ø Open**<br>**3 Percutaneous**<br>**4 Percutaneous Endoscopic** | **4 Internal Fixation Device**<br>**Z No Device** | **Z No Qualifier** |
| **Ø Lumbar Vertebra**<br>Spinous process<br>Transverse process<br>Vertebral arch<br>Vertebral body<br>Vertebral foramen<br>Vertebral lamina<br>Vertebral pedicle<br>**1 Sacrum**<br>**4 Acetabulum, Right**<br>**5 Acetabulum, Left**<br>**S Coccyx** | **X External** | **Z No Device** | **Z No Qualifier** |
| **2 Pelvic Bone, Right**<br>Iliac crest<br>Ilium<br>Ischium<br>Pubis<br>**3 Pelvic Bone, Left**<br>*See 2 Pelvic Bone, Right*<br>**D Patella, Right**<br>**F Patella, Left**<br>**L Tarsal, Right**<br>Calcaneus<br>Cuboid bone<br>Intermediate cuneiform bone<br>Lateral cuneiform bone<br>Medial cuneiform bone<br>Navicular bone<br>Talus bone<br>**M Tarsal, Left**<br>*See L Tarsal, Right*<br>**Q Toe Phalanx, Right**<br>**R Toe Phalanx, Left** | **Ø Open**<br>**3 Percutaneous**<br>**4 Percutaneous Endoscopic** | **4 Internal Fixation Device**<br>**5 External Fixation Device**<br>**Z No Device** | **Z No Qualifier** |
| **2 Pelvic Bone, Right**<br>Iliac crest<br>Ilium<br>Ischium<br>Pubis<br>**3 Pelvic Bone, Left**<br>*See 2 Pelvic Bone, Right*<br>**D Patella, Right**<br>**F Patella, Left**<br>**L Tarsal, Right**<br>Calcaneus<br>Cuboid bone<br>Intermediate cuneiform bone<br>Lateral cuneiform bone<br>Medial cuneiform bone<br>Navicular bone<br>Talus bone<br>**M Tarsal, Left**<br>*See L Tarsal, Right*<br>**Q Toe Phalanx, Right**<br>**R Toe Phalanx, Left** | **X External** | **Z No Device** | **Z No Qualifier** |

***ØQS Continued on next page***

**Non-OR** ØQS[4,5][3,4]ZZ
**Non-OR** ØQS[Ø,1,4,5,S]XZZ
**Non-OR** ØQS[2,3,D,F,L,M,Q,R][3,4]ZZ
**Non-OR** ØQS[2,3,D,F,L,M,Q,R]XZZ

**See Appendix L for Procedure Combinations**
⊞ ØQS[Ø,1,S]3ZZ

**Ø Medical and Surgical**
**Q Lower Bones**
**S Reposition**

***ØQS Continued***

Definition: Moving to its normal location, or other suitable location, all or a portion of a body part

Explanation: The body part is moved to a new location from an abnormal location, or from a normal location where it is not functioning correctly. The body part may or may not be cut out or off to be moved to the new location.

| Body Part Character 4 | Approach Character 5 | Device Character 6 | Qualifier Character 7 |
|---|---|---|---|
| **6 Upper Femur, Right**<br>Femoral head<br>Greater trochanter<br>Lesser trochanter<br>Neck of femur<br>**7 Upper Femur, Left**<br>*See 6 Upper Femur, Right*<br>**8 Femoral Shaft, Right**<br>Body of femur<br>**9 Femoral Shaft, Left**<br>*See 8 Femoral Shaft, Right*<br>**B Lower Femur, Right**<br>Lateral condyle of femur<br>Lateral epicondyle of femur<br>Medial condyle of femur<br>Medial epicondyle of femur<br>**C Lower Femur, Left**<br>*See B Lower Femur, Right*<br>**G Tibia, Right**<br>Lateral condyle of tibia<br>Medial condyle of tibia<br>Medial malleolus<br>**H Tibia, Left**<br>*See G Tibia, Right*<br>**J Fibula, Right**<br>Body of fibula<br>Head of fibula<br>Lateral malleolus<br>**K Fibula, Left**<br>*See J Fibula, Right* | **Ø Open**<br>**3 Percutaneous**<br>**4 Percutaneous Endoscopic** | **4 Internal Fixation Device**<br>**5 External Fixation Device**<br>**6 Internal Fixation Device, Intramedullary**<br>**B External Fixation Device, Monoplanar**<br>**C External Fixation Device, Ring**<br>**D External Fixation Device, Hybrid**<br>**Z No Device** | **Z No Qualifier** |
| **6 Upper Femur, Right**<br>Femoral head<br>Greater trochanter<br>Lesser trochanter<br>Neck of femur<br>**7 Upper Femur, Left**<br>*See 6 Upper Femur, Right*<br>**8 Femoral Shaft, Right**<br>Body of femur<br>**9 Femoral Shaft, Left**<br>*See 8 Femoral Shaft, Right*<br>**B Lower Femur, Right**<br>Lateral condyle of femur<br>Lateral epicondyle of femur<br>Medial condyle of femur<br>Medial epicondyle of femur<br>**C Lower Femur, Left**<br>*See B Lower Femur, Right*<br>**G Tibia, Right**<br>Lateral condyle of tibia<br>Medial condyle of tibia<br>Medial malleolus<br>**H Tibia, Left**<br>*See G Tibia, Right*<br>**J Fibula, Right**<br>Body of fibula<br>Head of fibula<br>Lateral malleolus<br>**K Fibula, Left**<br>*See J Fibula, Right* | **X External** | **Z No Device** | **Z No Qualifier** |
| **N Metatarsal, Right**<br>**P Metatarsal, Left** | **Ø Open**<br>**3 Percutaneous**<br>**4 Percutaneous Endoscopic** | **4 Internal Fixation Device**<br>**5 External Fixation Device**<br>**Z No Device** | 2 Sesamoid Bone(s) 1st Toe<br>**Z No Qualifier** |
| **N Metatarsal, Right**<br>**P Metatarsal, Left** | **X External** | **Z No Device** | 2 Sesamoid Bone(s) 1st Toe<br>**Z No Qualifier** |

Non-OR ØQS[6,7,8,9,B,C,G,H,J,K][3,4]ZZ
Non-OR ØQS[6,7,8,9,B,C,G,H,J,K]XZZ
Non-OR ØQS[N,P][3,4]ZZ
Non-OR ØQS[N,P]XZZ

**Ø Medical and Surgical**
**Q Lower Bones**
**T Resection** Definition: Cutting out or off, without replacement, all of a body part
Explanation: None

| Body Part Character 4 | Approach Character 5 | Device Character 6 | Qualifier Character 7 |
|---|---|---|---|
| **2 Pelvic Bone, Right**<br>Iliac crest<br>Ilium<br>Ischium<br>Pubis<br>**3 Pelvic Bone, Left**<br>*See 2 Pelvic Bone, Right*<br>**4 Acetabulum, Right**<br>**5 Acetabulum, Left**<br>**6 Upper Femur, Right**<br>Femoral head<br>Greater trochanter<br>Lesser trochanter<br>Neck of femur<br>**7 Upper Femur, Left**<br>*See 6 Upper Femur, Right*<br>**8 Femoral Shaft, Right**<br>Body of femur<br>**9 Femoral Shaft, Left**<br>*See 8 Femoral Shaft, Right*<br>**B Lower Femur, Right**<br>Lateral condyle of femur<br>Lateral epicondyle of femur<br>Medial condyle of femur<br>Medial epicondyle of femur<br>**C Lower Femur, Left**<br>*See B Lower Femur, Right*<br>**D Patella, Right**<br>**F Patella, Left**<br>**G Tibia, Right**<br>Lateral condyle of tibia<br>Medial condyle of tibia<br>Medial malleolus<br>**H Tibia, Left**<br>*See G Tibia, Right*<br>**J Fibula, Right**<br>Body of fibula<br>Head of fibula<br>Lateral malleolus<br>**K Fibula, Left**<br>*See J Fibula, Right*<br>**L Tarsal, Right**<br>Calcaneus<br>Cuboid bone<br>Intermediate cuneiform bone<br>Lateral cuneiform bone<br>Medial cuneiform bone<br>Navicular bone<br>Talus bone<br>**M Tarsal, Left**<br>*See L Tarsal, Right*<br>**N Metatarsal, Right**<br>**P Metatarsal, Left**<br>**Q Toe Phalanx, Right**<br>**R Toe Phalanx, Left**<br>**S Coccyx** | **Ø Open** | **Z No Device** | **Z No Qualifier** |

**Ø Medical and Surgical**
**Q Lower Bones**
**U Supplement** Definition: Putting in or on biological or synthetic material that physically reinforces and/or augments the function of a portion of a body part
Explanation: The biological material is non-living, or is living and from the same individual. The body part may have been previously replaced, and the SUPPLEMENT procedure is performed to physically reinforce and/or augment the function of the replaced body part.

| Body Part Character 4 | Approach Character 5 | Device Character 6 | Qualifier Character 7 |
|---|---|---|---|
| **Ø Lumbar Vertebra** ⊞<br>Spinous process<br>Transverse process<br>Vertebral arch<br>Vertebral body<br>Vertebral foramen<br>Vertebral lamina<br>Vertebral pedicle<br>**1 Sacrum** ⊞<br>**2 Pelvic Bone, Right**<br>Iliac crest<br>Ilium<br>Ischium<br>Pubis<br>**3 Pelvic Bone, Left**<br>*See 2 Pelvic Bone, Right*<br>**4 Acetabulum, Right**<br>**5 Acetabulum, Left**<br>**6 Upper Femur, Right**<br>Femoral head<br>Greater trochanter<br>Lesser trochanter<br>Neck of femur<br>**7 Upper Femur, Left**<br>*See 6 Upper Femur, Right*<br>**8 Femoral Shaft, Right**<br>Body of femur<br>**9 Femoral Shaft, Left**<br>*See 8 Femoral Shaft, Right*<br>**B Lower Femur, Right**<br>Lateral condyle of femur<br>Lateral epicondyle of femur<br>Medial condyle of femur<br>Medial epicondyle of femur<br>**C Lower Femur, Left**<br>*See B Lower Femur, Right*<br>**D Patella, Right**<br>**F Patella, Left**<br>**G Tibia, Right**<br>Lateral condyle of tibia<br>Medial condyle of tibia<br>Medial malleolus<br>**H Tibia, Left**<br>*See G Tibia, Right*<br>**J Fibula, Right**<br>Body of fibula<br>Head of fibula<br>Lateral malleolus<br>**K Fibula, Left**<br>*See J Fibula, Right*<br>**L Tarsal, Right**<br>Calcaneus<br>Cuboid bone<br>Intermediate cuneiform bone<br>Lateral cuneiform bone<br>Medial cuneiform bone<br>Navicular bone<br>Talus bone<br>**M Tarsal, Left**<br>*See L Tarsal, Right*<br>**N Metatarsal, Right**<br>**P Metatarsal, Left**<br>**Q Toe Phalanx, Right**<br>**R Toe Phalanx, Left**<br>**S Coccyx** ⊞ | **Ø Open**<br>**3 Percutaneous**<br>**4 Percutaneous Endoscopic** | **7 Autologous Tissue Substitute**<br>**J Synthetic Substitute**<br>**K Nonautologous Tissue Substitute** | **Z No Qualifier** |

**See Appendix L for Procedure Combinations**
⊞ ØQU[Ø,1,S]3JZ

LC Limited Coverage NC Noncovered ⊞ Combination Member HAC associated procedure Combination Only DRG Non-OR Non-OR New/Revised in GREEN

**Ø Medical and Surgical**
**Q Lower Bones**
**W Revision**

Definition: Correcting, to the extent possible, a portion of a malfunctioning device or the position of a displaced device

Explanation: Revision can include correcting a malfunctioning or displaced device by taking out or putting in components of the device such as a screw or pin

| Body Part Character 4 | Approach Character 5 | Device Character 6 | Qualifier Character 7 |
|---|---|---|---|
| **Ø Lumbar Vertebra**<br>Spinous process<br>Transverse process<br>Vertebral arch<br>Vertebral body<br>Vertebral foramen<br>Vertebral lamina<br>Vertebral pedicle<br>**1 Sacrum**<br>**4 Acetabulum, Right**<br>**5 Acetabulum, Left**<br>**S Coccyx** | **Ø Open**<br>**3 Percutaneous**<br>**4 Percutaneous Endoscopic**<br>**X External** | **4 Internal Fixation Device**<br>**7 Autologous Tissue Substitute**<br>**J Synthetic Substitute**<br>**K Nonautologous Tissue Substitute** | **Z** No Qualifier |
| **2 Pelvic Bone, Right**<br>Iliac crest<br>Ilium<br>Ischium<br>Pubis<br>**3 Pelvic Bone, Left**<br>*See 2 Pelvic Bone, Right*<br>**6 Upper Femur, Right**<br>Femoral head<br>Greater trochanter<br>Lesser trochanter<br>Neck of femur<br>**7 Upper Femur, Left**<br>*See 6 Upper Femur, Right*<br>**8 Femoral Shaft, Right**<br>Body of femur<br>**9 Femoral Shaft, Left**<br>*See 8 Femoral Shaft, Right*<br>**B Lower Femur, Right**<br>Lateral condyle of femur<br>Lateral epicondyle of femur<br>Medial condyle of femur<br>Medial epicondyle of femur<br>**C Lower Femur, Left**<br>*See B Lower Femur, Right*<br>**D Patella, Right**<br>**F Patella, Left**<br>**G Tibia, Right**<br>Lateral condyle of tibia<br>Medial condyle of tibia<br>Medial malleolus<br>**H Tibia, Left**<br>*See G Tibia, Right*<br>**J Fibula, Right**<br>Body of fibula<br>Head of fibula<br>Lateral malleolus<br>**K Fibula, Left**<br>*See J Fibula, Right*<br>**L Tarsal, Right**<br>Calcaneus<br>Cuboid bone<br>Intermediate cuneiform bone<br>Lateral cuneiform bone<br>Medial cuneiform bone<br>Navicular bone<br>Talus bone<br>**M Tarsal, Left**<br>*See L Tarsal, Right*<br>**N Metatarsal, Right**<br>**P Metatarsal, Left**<br>**Q Toe Phalanx, Right**<br>**R Toe Phalanx, Left** | **Ø Open**<br>**3 Percutaneous**<br>**4 Percutaneous Endoscopic**<br>**X External** | **4 Internal Fixation Device**<br>**5 External Fixation Device**<br>**7 Autologous Tissue Substitute**<br>**J Synthetic Substitute**<br>**K Nonautologous Tissue Substitute** | **Z** No Qualifier |
| **Y Lower Bone** | **Ø Open**<br>**3 Percutaneous**<br>**4 Percutaneous Endoscopic**<br>**X External** | **Ø** Drainage Device<br>**M** Bone Growth Stimulator | **Z** No Qualifier |

**Non-OR** ØQW[Ø,1,4,5,S]X[4,7,J,K]Z
**Non-OR** ØQW[2,3,6,7,8,9,B,C,D,F,G,H,J,K,L,M,N,P,Q,R]X[4,5,7,J,K]Z
**Non-OR** ØQWYX[Ø,M]Z

# Upper Joints ØR2–ØRW

## Character Meanings*

This Character Meaning table is provided as a guide to assist the user in the identification of character members that may be found in this section of code tables. It **SHOULD NOT** be used to build a PCS code.

| Operation–Character 3 | Body Part–Character 4 | Approach–Character 5 | Device–Character 6 | Qualifier–Character 7 |
|---|---|---|---|---|
| 2 Change | Ø Occipital-cervical Joint | Ø Open | Ø Drainage Device OR Synthetic Substitute, Reverse Ball and Socket | Ø Anterior Approach, Anterior Column |
| 5 Destruction | 1 Cervical Vertebral Joint | 3 Percutaneous | 3 Infusion Device | 1 Posterior Approach, Posterior Column |
| 9 Drainage | 2 Cervical Vertebral Joint, 2 or more | 4 Percutaneous Endoscopic | 4 Internal Fixation Device | 6 Humeral Surface |
| B Excision | 3 Cervical Vertebral Disc | X External | 5 External Fixation Device | 7 Glenoid Surface |
| C Extirpation | 4 Cervicothoracic Vertebral Joint | | 7 Autologous Tissue Substitute | J Posterior Approach, Anterior Column |
| G Fusion | 5 Cervicothoracic Vertebral Disc | | 8 Spacer | X Diagnostic |
| H Insertion | 6 Thoracic Vertebral Joint | | A Interbody Fusion Device | Z No Qualifier |
| J Inspection | 7 Thoracic Vertebral Joint, 2 to 7 | | B Spinal Stabilization Device, Interspinous Process | |
| N Release | 8 Thoracic Vertebral Joint, 8 or more | | C Spinal Stabilization Device, Pedicle-Based | |
| P Removal | 9 Thoracic Vertebral Disc | | D Spinal Stabilization Device, Facet Replacement | |
| Q Repair | A Thoracolumbar Vertebral Joint | | J Synthetic Substitute | |
| R Replacement | B Thoracolumbar Vertebral Disc | | K Nonautologous Tissue Substitute | |
| S Reposition | C Temporomandibular Joint, Right | | Y Other Device | |
| T Resection | D Temporomandibular Joint, Left | | Z No Device | |
| U Supplement | E Sternoclavicular Joint, Right | | | |
| W Revision | F Sternoclavicular Joint, Left | | | |
| | G Acromioclavicular Joint, Right | | | |
| | H Acromioclavicular Joint, Left | | | |
| | J Shoulder Joint, Right | | | |
| | K Shoulder Joint, Left | | | |
| | L Elbow Joint, Right | | | |
| | M Elbow Joint, Left | | | |
| | N Wrist Joint, Right | | | |
| | P Wrist Joint, Left | | | |
| | Q Carpal Joint, Right | | | |
| | R Carpal Joint, Left | | | |
| | S Carpometacarpal Joint, Right | | | |
| | T Carpometacarpal Joint, Left | | | |
| | U Metacarpophalangeal Joint, Right | | | |
| | V Metacarpophalangeal Joint, Left | | | |
| | W Finger Phalangeal Joint, Right | | | |
| | X Finger Phalangeal Joint, Left | | | |
| | Y Upper Joint | | | |

* Includes synovial membrane.

**AHA Coding Clinic for table ØRG**
**2017, 2Q, 23** Decompression of spinal cord and placement of instrumentation
**2014, 3Q, 30** Spinal fusion and fixation instrumentation
**2014, 2Q, 7** Anterior cervical thoracic fusion with total discectomy
**2013, 1Q, 21-23** Spinal fusion of thoracic and lumbar vertebrae
**2013, 1Q, 29** Cervical and thoracic spinal fusion

**AHA Coding Clinic for table ØRH**
**2017, 2Q, 23** Decompression of spinal cord and placement of instrumentation
**2016, 3Q, 32** Rotator cuff repair, tenodesis, decompression, acromioplasty and coracoplasty

**AHA Coding Clinic for table ØRN**
**2016, 3Q, 32** Rotator cuff repair, tenodesis, decompression, acromioplasty and coracoplasty
**2015, 2Q, 22** Arthroscopic subacromial decompression
**2015, 2Q, 23** Arthroscopic release of shoulder joint

**AHA Coding Clinic for table ØRQ**
**2016, 1Q, 30** Thermal capsulorrhapy of shoulder

**AHA Coding Clinic for table ØRR**
**2015, 3Q, 14** Endoprosthetic replacement of humerus and tendon reattachment
**2015, 1Q, 27** Reverse total shoulder arthroplasty

**AHA Coding Clinic for table ØRS**
**2015, 2Q, 35** Application of tongs to reduce and stabilize cervical fracture
**2014, 4Q, 32** Open reduction internal fixation of fracture with debridement
**2014, 3Q, 33** Radial fracture treatment with open reduction internal fixation, and release of carpal ligament
**2013, 2Q, 39** Application of cervical tongs for reduction of cervical fracture

**AHA Coding Clinic for table ØRT**
**2014, 2Q, 7** Anterior cervical thoracic fusion with total discectomy

**AHA Coding Clinic for table ØRU**
**2015, 3Q, 26** Thumb arthroplasty with resection of trapezium

## Upper Joints

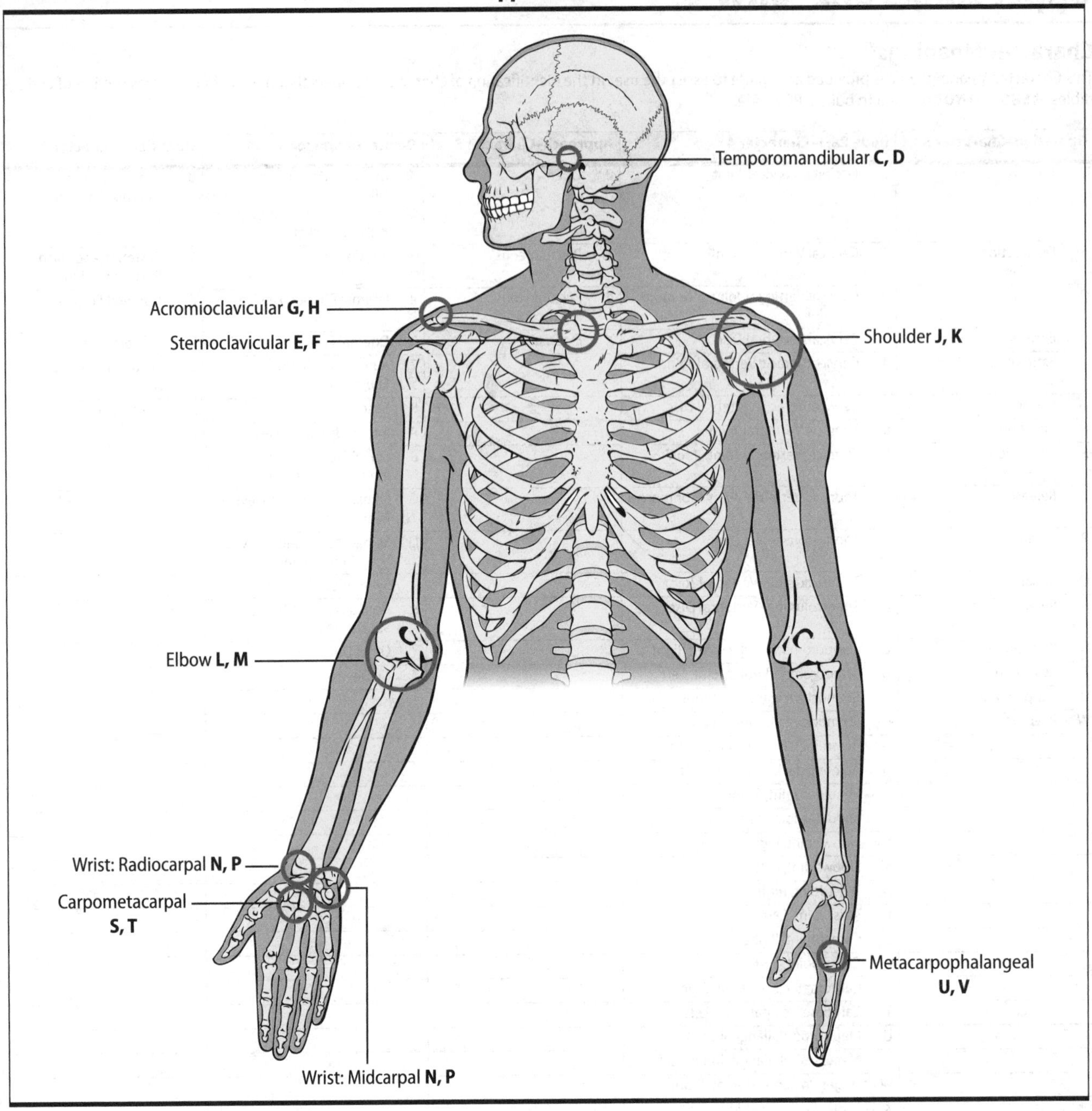
Temporomandibular C, D
Acromioclavicular G, H
Sternoclavicular E, F
Shoulder J, K
Elbow L, M
Wrist: Radiocarpal N, P
Carpometacarpal S, T
Metacarpophalangeal U, V
Wrist: Midcarpal N, P

## Hand Joints

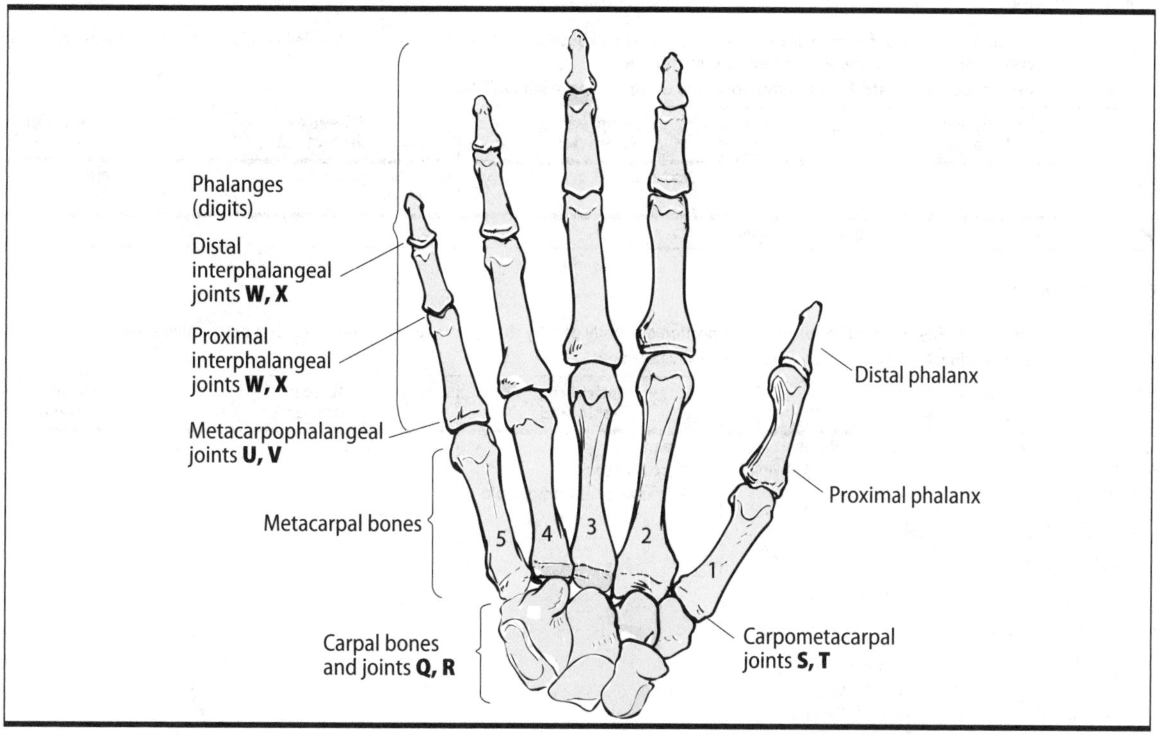
Phalanges (digits)
Distal interphalangeal joints **W, X**
Proximal interphalangeal joints **W, X**
Metacarpophalangeal joints **U, V**
Metacarpal bones
Carpal bones and joints **Q, R**
5
4
3
2
1
Distal phalanx
Proximal phalanx
Carpometacarpal joints **S, T**

## Shoulder Joints

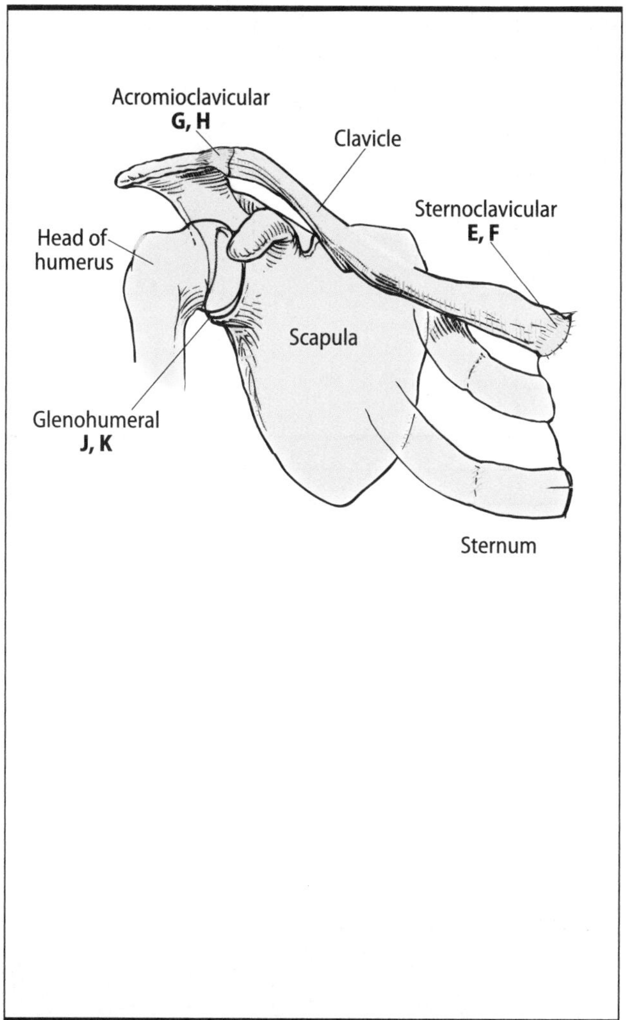
Acromioclavicular **G, H**
Clavicle
Sternoclavicular **E, F**
Head of humerus
Scapula
Glenohumeral **J, K**
Sternum

## Upper Vertebral Joints

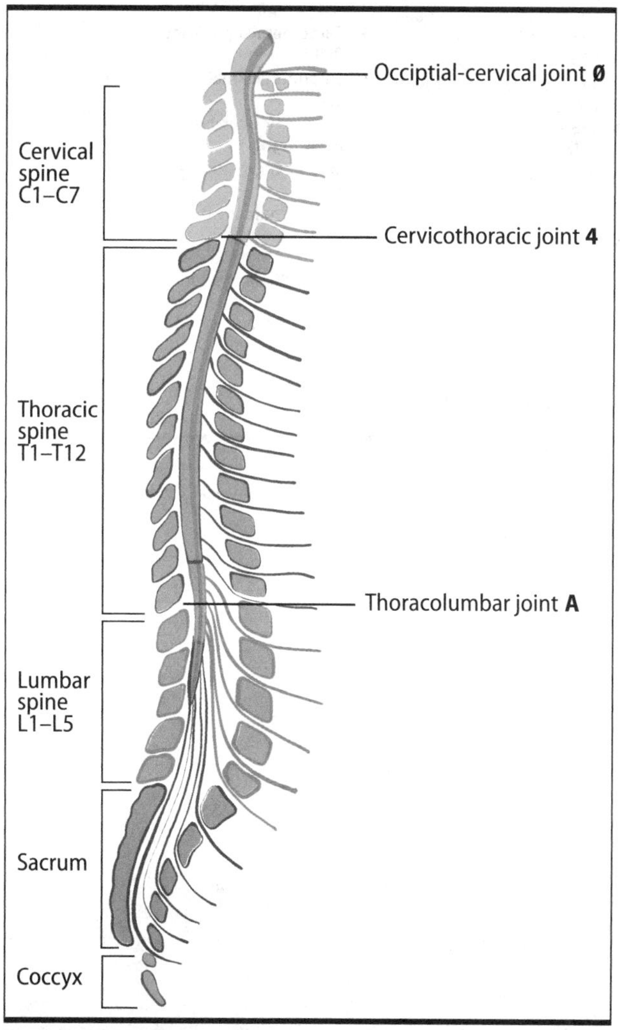
Occiptial-cervical joint **Ø**
Cervical spine C1–C7
Cervicothoracic joint **4**
Thoracic spine T1–T12
Thoracolumbar joint **A**
Lumbar spine L1–L5
Sacrum
Coccyx

**Ø Medical and Surgical**
**R Upper Joints**
**2 Change** Definition: Taking out or off a device from a body part and putting back an identical or similar device in or on the same body part without cutting or puncturing the skin or a mucous membrane

Explanation: All CHANGE procedures are coded using the approach EXTERNAL

| Body Part Character 4 | Approach Character 5 | Device Character 6 | Qualifier Character 7 |
|---|---|---|---|
| Y Upper Joint | X External | Ø Drainage Device<br>Y Other Device | Z No Qualifier |

Non-OR All body part, approach, device, and qualifier values

**Ø Medical and Surgical**
**R Upper Joints**
**5 Destruction** Definition: Physical eradication of all or a portion of a body part by the direct use of energy, force, or a destructive agent

Explanation: None of the body part is physically taken out

| Body Part Character 4 | Approach Character 5 | Device Character 6 | Qualifier Character 7 |
|---|---|---|---|
| **Ø Occipital-cervical Joint**<br>**1 Cervical Vertebral Joint**<br>Atlantoaxial joint<br>Cervical facet joint<br>**3 Cervical Vertebral Disc**<br>**4 Cervicothoracic Vertebral Joint**<br>Cervicothoracic facet joint<br>**5 Cervicothoracic Vertebral Disc**<br>**6 Thoracic Vertebral Joint**<br>Costotransverse joint<br>Costovertebral joint<br>Thoracic facet joint<br>**9 Thoracic Vertebral Disc**<br>**A Thoracolumbar Vertebral Joint**<br>Thoracolumbar facet joint<br>**B Thoracolumbar Vertebral Disc**<br>**C Temporomandibular Joint, Right**<br>**D Temporomandibular Joint, Left**<br>**E Sternoclavicular Joint, Right**<br>**F Sternoclavicular Joint, Left**<br>**G Acromioclavicular Joint, Right**<br>**H Acromioclavicular Joint, Left**<br>**J Shoulder Joint, Right**<br>Glenohumeral joint<br>Glenoid ligament (labrum)<br>**K Shoulder Joint, Left**<br>*See J Shoulder Joint, Right*<br>**L Elbow Joint, Right**<br>Distal humerus, involving joint<br>Humeroradial joint<br>Humeroulnar joint<br>Proximal radioulnar joint<br>**M Elbow Joint, Left**<br>*See L Elbow Joint, Right*<br>**N Wrist Joint, Right**<br>Distal radioulnar joint<br>Radiocarpal joint<br>**P Wrist Joint, Left**<br>*See N Wrist Joint, Right*<br>**Q Carpal Joint, Right**<br>Intercarpal joint<br>Midcarpal joint<br>**R Carpal Joint, Left**<br>*See Q Carpal Joint, Right*<br>**S Carpometacarpal Joint, Right**<br>**T Carpometacarpal Joint, Left**<br>**U Metacarpophalangeal Joint, Right**<br>**V Metacarpophalangeal Joint, Left**<br>**W Finger Phalangeal Joint, Right**<br>Interphalangeal (IP) joint<br>**X Finger Phalangeal Joint, Left**<br>*See W Finger Phalangeal Joint, Right* | **Ø Open**<br>**3 Percutaneous**<br>**4 Percutaneous Endoscopic** | **Z No Device** | **Z No Qualifier** |

Non-OR ØR5[3,5,9,B][3,4]ZZ

**Ø Medical and Surgical**
**R Upper Joints**
**9 Drainage** Definition: Taking or letting out fluids and/or gases from a body part
Explanation: The qualifier DIAGNOSTIC is used to identify drainage procedures that are biopsies

| Body Part Character 4 | Approach Character 5 | Device Character 6 | Qualifier Character 7 |
|---|---|---|---|
| **Ø Occipital-cervical Joint**<br>**1 Cervical Vertebral Joint**<br>Atlantoaxial joint<br>Cervical facet joint<br>**3 Cervical Vertebral Disc**<br>**4 Cervicothoracic Vertebral Joint**<br>Cervicothoracic facet joint<br>**5 Cervicothoracic Vertebral Disc**<br>**6 Thoracic Vertebral Joint**<br>Costotransverse joint<br>Costovertebral joint<br>Thoracic facet joint<br>**9 Thoracic Vertebral Disc**<br>**A Thoracolumbar Vertebral Joint**<br>Thoracolumbar facet joint<br>**B Thoracolumbar Vertebral Disc**<br>**C Temporomandibular Joint, Right**<br>**D Temporomandibular Joint, Left**<br>**E Sternoclavicular Joint, Right**<br>**F Sternoclavicular Joint, Left**<br>**G Acromioclavicular Joint, Right**<br>**H Acromioclavicular Joint, Left**<br>**J Shoulder Joint, Right**<br>Glenohumeral joint<br>Glenoid ligament (labrum)<br>**K Shoulder Joint, Left**<br>*See J Shoulder Joint, Right*<br>**L Elbow Joint, Right**<br>Distal humerus, involving joint<br>Humeroradial joint<br>Humeroulnar joint<br>Proximal radioulnar joint<br>**M Elbow Joint, Left**<br>*See L Elbow Joint, Right*<br>**N Wrist Joint, Right**<br>Distal radioulnar joint<br>Radiocarpal joint<br>**P Wrist Joint, Left**<br>*See N Wrist Joint, Right*<br>**Q Carpal Joint, Right**<br>Intercarpal joint<br>Midcarpal joint<br>**R Carpal Joint, Left**<br>*See Q Carpal Joint, Right*<br>**S Carpometacarpal Joint, Right**<br>**T Carpometacarpal Joint, Left**<br>**U Metacarpophalangeal Joint, Right**<br>**V Metacarpophalangeal Joint, Left**<br>**W Finger Phalangeal Joint, Right**<br>Interphalangeal (IP) joint<br>**X Finger Phalangeal Joint, Left**<br>*See W Finger Phalangeal Joint, Right* | **Ø Open**<br>**3 Percutaneous**<br>**4 Percutaneous Endoscopic** | **Ø Drainage Device** | **Z No Qualifier** |
| **Ø Occipital-cervical Joint**<br>**1 Cervical Vertebral Joint**<br>Atlantoaxial joint<br>Cervical facet joint<br>**3 Cervical Vertebral Disc**<br>**4 Cervicothoracic Vertebral Joint**<br>Cervicothoracic facet joint<br>**5 Cervicothoracic Vertebral Disc**<br>**6 Thoracic Vertebral Joint**<br>Costotransverse joint<br>Costovertebral joint<br>Thoracic facet joint<br>**9 Thoracic Vertebral Disc**<br>**A Thoracolumbar Vertebral Joint**<br>Thoracolumbar facet joint<br>**B Thoracolumbar Vertebral Disc**<br>**C Temporomandibular Joint, Right**<br>**D Temporomandibular Joint, Left**<br>**E Sternoclavicular Joint, Right**<br>**F Sternoclavicular Joint, Left**<br>**G Acromioclavicular Joint, Right**<br>**H Acromioclavicular Joint, Left**<br>**J Shoulder Joint, Right**<br>Glenohumeral joint<br>Glenoid ligament (labrum)<br>**K Shoulder Joint, Left**<br>*See J Shoulder Joint, Right*<br>**L Elbow Joint, Right**<br>Distal humerus, involving joint<br>Humeroradial joint<br>Humeroulnar joint<br>Proximal radioulnar joint<br>**M Elbow Joint, Left**<br>*See L Elbow Joint, Right*<br>**N Wrist Joint, Right**<br>Distal radioulnar joint<br>Radiocarpal joint<br>**P Wrist Joint, Left**<br>*See N Wrist Joint, Right*<br>**Q Carpal Joint, Right**<br>Intercarpal joint<br>Midcarpal joint<br>**R Carpal Joint, Left**<br>*See Q Carpal Joint, Right*<br>**S Carpometacarpal Joint, Right**<br>**T Carpometacarpal Joint, Left**<br>**U Metacarpophalangeal Joint, Right**<br>**V Metacarpophalangeal Joint, Left**<br>**W Finger Phalangeal Joint, Right**<br>Interphalangeal (IP) joint<br>**X Finger Phalangeal Joint, Left**<br>*See W Finger Phalangeal Joint, Right* | **Ø Open**<br>**3 Percutaneous**<br>**4 Percutaneous Endoscopic** | **Z No Device** | **X Diagnostic**<br>**Z No Qualifier** |

**Non-OR** ØR9[Ø,1,3,4,5,6,9,A,B,E,F,G,H,J,K,L,M,N,P,Q,R,S,T,U,V,W,X][3,4]ØZ
**Non-OR** ØR9[C,D]3ØZ
**Non-OR** ØR9[Ø,1,3,4,5,6,9,A,B,E,F,G,H,J,K,L,M,N,P,Q,R,S,T,U,V,W,X][Ø,3,4]ZX
**Non-OR** ØR9[Ø,1,3,4,5,6,9,A,B,E,F,G,H,J,K,L,M,N,P,Q,R,S,T,U,V,W,X][3,4]ZZ
**Non-OR** ØR9[C,D]3ZZ

**Ø Medical and Surgical**
**R Upper Joints**
**B Excision** Definition: Cutting out or off, without replacement, a portion of a body part

Explanation: The qualifier DIAGNOSTIC is used to identify excision procedures that are biopsies

| Body Part Character 4 | | Approach Character 5 | Device Character 6 | Qualifier Character 7 |
|---|---|---|---|---|
| **Ø Occipital-cervical Joint**<br>**1 Cervical Vertebral Joint**<br>Atlantoaxial joint<br>Cervical facet joint<br>**3 Cervical Vertebral Disc**<br>**4 Cervicothoracic Vertebral Joint**<br>Cervicothoracic facet joint<br>**5 Cervicothoracic Vertebral Disc**<br>**6 Thoracic Vertebral Joint**<br>Costotransverse joint<br>Costovertebral joint<br>Thoracic facet joint<br>**9 Thoracic Vertebral Disc**<br>**A Thoracolumbar Vertebral Joint**<br>Thoracolumbar facet joint<br>**B Thoracolumbar Vertebral Disc**<br>**C Temporomandibular Joint, Right**<br>**D Temporomandibular Joint, Left**<br>**E Sternoclavicular Joint, Right**<br>**F Sternoclavicular Joint, Left**<br>**G Acromioclavicular Joint, Right**<br>**H Acromioclavicular Joint, Left**<br>**J Shoulder Joint, Right**<br>Glenohumeral joint<br>Glenoid ligament (labrum)<br>**K Shoulder Joint, Left**<br>***See*** *J Shoulder Joint, Right* | **L Elbow Joint, Right**<br>Distal humerus, involving joint<br>Humeroradial joint<br>Humeroulnar joint<br>Proximal radioulnar joint<br>**M Elbow Joint, Left**<br>***See*** *L Elbow Joint, Right*<br>**N Wrist Joint, Right**<br>Distal radioulnar joint<br>Radiocarpal joint<br>**P Wrist Joint, Left**<br>***See*** *N Wrist Joint, Right*<br>**Q Carpal Joint, Right**<br>Intercarpal joint<br>Midcarpal joint<br>**R Carpal Joint, Left**<br>***See*** *Q Carpal Joint, Right*<br>**S Carpometacarpal Joint, Right**<br>**T Carpometacarpal Joint, Left**<br>**U Metacarpophalangeal Joint, Right**<br>**V Metacarpophalangeal Joint, Left**<br>**W Finger Phalangeal Joint, Right**<br>Interphalangeal (IP) joint<br>**X Finger Phalangeal Joint, Left**<br>***See*** *W Finger Phalangeal Joint, Right* | **Ø Open**<br>**3 Percutaneous**<br>**4 Percutaneous Endoscopic** | **Z No Device** | **X Diagnostic**<br>**Z No Qualifier** |

**Non-OR** ØRB[Ø,1,3,4,5,6,9,A,B,E,F,G,H,J,K,L,M,N,P,Q,R,S,T,U,V,W,X][Ø,3,4]ZX

**Ø Medical and Surgical**
**R Upper Joints**
**C Extirpation** Definition: Taking or cutting out solid matter from a body part

Explanation: The solid matter may be an abnormal byproduct of a biological function or a foreign body; it may be imbedded in a body part or in the lumen of a tubular body part. The solid matter may or may not have been previously broken into pieces.

| Body Part Character 4 | | Approach Character 5 | Device Character 6 | Qualifier Character 7 |
|---|---|---|---|---|
| **Ø Occipital-cervical Joint**<br>**1 Cervical Vertebral Joint**<br>Atlantoaxial joint<br>Cervical facet joint<br>**3 Cervical Vertebral Disc**<br>**4 Cervicothoracic Vertebral Joint**<br>Cervicothoracic facet joint<br>**5 Cervicothoracic Vertebral Disc**<br>**6 Thoracic Vertebral Joint**<br>Costotransverse joint<br>Costovertebral joint<br>Thoracic facet joint<br>**9 Thoracic Vertebral Disc**<br>**A Thoracolumbar Vertebral Joint**<br>Thoracolumbar facet joint<br>**B Thoracolumbar Vertebral Disc**<br>**C Temporomandibular Joint, Right**<br>**D Temporomandibular Joint, Left**<br>**E Sternoclavicular Joint, Right**<br>**F Sternoclavicular Joint, Left**<br>**G Acromioclavicular Joint, Right**<br>**H Acromioclavicular Joint, Left**<br>**J Shoulder Joint, Right**<br>Glenohumeral joint<br>Glenoid ligament (labrum)<br>**K Shoulder Joint, Left**<br>*See J Shoulder Joint, Right* | **L Elbow Joint, Right**<br>Distal humerus, involving joint<br>Humeroradial joint<br>Humeroulnar joint<br>Proximal radioulnar joint<br>**M Elbow Joint, Left**<br>*See L Elbow Joint, Right*<br>**N Wrist Joint, Right**<br>Distal radioulnar joint<br>Radiocarpal joint<br>**P Wrist Joint, Left**<br>*See N Wrist Joint, Right*<br>**Q Carpal Joint, Right**<br>Intercarpal joint<br>Midcarpal joint<br>**R Carpal Joint, Left**<br>*See Q Carpal Joint, Right*<br>S Carpometacarpal Joint, Right<br>T Carpometacarpal Joint, Left<br>**U Metacarpophalangeal Joint, Right**<br>**V Metacarpophalangeal Joint, Left**<br>**W Finger Phalangeal Joint, Right**<br>Interphalangeal (IP) joint<br>**X Finger Phalangeal Joint, Left**<br>*See W Finger Phalangeal Joint, Right* | **Ø Open**<br>**3 Percutaneous**<br>**4 Percutaneous Endoscopic** | **Z No Device** | **Z No Qualifier** |

**Ø Medical and Surgical**
**R Upper Joints**
**G Fusion** Definition: Joining together portions of an articular body part rendering the articular body part immobile
Explanation: The body part is joined together by fixation device, bone graft, or other means

| Body Part Character 4 | Approach Character 5 | Device Character 6 | Qualifier Character 7 |
|---|---|---|---|
| **Ø Occipital-cervical Joint**<br>**1 Cervical Vertebral Joint**<br>Atlantoaxial joint<br>Cervical facet joint<br>**2 Cervical Vertebral Joints, 2 or more**<br>Cervical facet joint<br>**4 Cervicothoracic Vertebral Joint**<br>Cervicothoracic facet joint<br>**6 Thoracic Vertebral Joint**<br>Costotransverse joint<br>Costovertebral joint<br>Thoracic facet joint<br>**7 Thoracic Vertebral Joints, 2 to 7** ⊞<br>**8 Thoracic Vertebral Joints, 8 or more**<br>**A Thoracolumbar Vertebral Joint**<br>Thoracolumbar facet joint | **Ø Open**<br>**3 Percutaneous**<br>**4 Percutaneous Endoscopic** | **7 Autologous Tissue Substitute**<br>**J Synthetic Substitute**<br>**K Nonautologous Tissue Substitute**<br>**Z No Device** | **Ø Anterior Approach, Anterior Column**<br>**1 Posterior Approach, Posterior Column**<br>**J Posterior Approach, Anterior Column** |
| **Ø Occipital-cervical Joint**<br>**1 Cervical Vertebral Joint**<br>Atlantoaxial joint<br>Cervical facet joint<br>**2 Cervical Vertebral Joints, 2 or more**<br>Cervical facet joint<br>**4 Cervicothoracic Vertebral Joint**<br>Cervicothoracic facet joint<br>**6 Thoracic Vertebral Joint**<br>Costotransverse joint<br>Costovertebral joint<br>Thoracic facet joint<br>**7 Thoracic Vertebral Joints, 2 to 7** ⊞<br>**8 Thoracic Vertebral Joints, 8 or more**<br>**A Thoracolumbar Vertebral Joint**<br>Thoracolumbar facet joint | **Ø Open**<br>**3 Percutaneous**<br>**4 Percutaneous Endoscopic** | **A Interbody Fusion Device** | **Ø Anterior Approach, Anterior Column**<br>**J Posterior Approach, Anterior Column** |
| **C Temporomandibular Joint, Right**<br>**D Temporomandibular Joint, Left**<br>**E Sternoclavicular Joint, Right**<br>**F Sternoclavicular Joint, Left**<br>**G Acromioclavicular Joint, Right**<br>**H Acromioclavicular Joint, Left**<br>**J Shoulder Joint, Right**<br>Glenohumeral joint<br>Glenoid ligament (labrum)<br>**K Shoulder Joint, Left**<br>*See J Shoulder Joint, Right* | **Ø Open**<br>**3 Percutaneous**<br>**4 Percutaneous Endoscopic** | **4 Internal Fixation Device**<br>**7 Autologous Tissue Substitute**<br>**J Synthetic Substitute**<br>**K Nonautologous Tissue Substitute**<br>**Z No Device** | **Z No Qualifier** |
| **L Elbow Joint, Right**<br>Distal humerus, involving joint<br>Humeroradial joint<br>Humeroulnar joint<br>Proximal radioulnar joint<br>**M Elbow Joint, Left**<br>*See L Elbow Joint, Right*<br>**N Wrist Joint, Right**<br>Distal radioulnar joint<br>Radiocarpal joint<br>**P Wrist Joint, Left**<br>*See N Wrist Joint, Right*<br>**Q Carpal Joint, Right**<br>Intercarpal joint<br>Midcarpal joint<br>**R Carpal Joint, Left**<br>*See Q Carpal Joint, Right*<br>**S Carpometacarpal Joint, Right**<br>**T Carpometacarpal Joint, Left**<br>**U Metacarpophalangeal Joint, Right**<br>**V Metacarpophalangeal Joint, Left**<br>**W Finger Phalangeal Joint, Right**<br>Interphalangeal (IP) joint<br>**X Finger Phalangeal Joint, Left**<br>*See W Finger Phalangeal Joint, Right* | **Ø Open**<br>**3 Percutaneous**<br>**4 Percutaneous Endoscopic** | **4 Internal Fixation Device**<br>**5 External Fixation Device**<br>**7 Autologous Tissue Substitute**<br>**J Synthetic Substitute**<br>**K Nonautologous Tissue Substitute**<br>**Z No Device** | **Z No Qualifier** |

HAC ØRG[Ø,1,2,4,6,7,8,A][Ø,3,4][7,J,K,Z][Ø,1,J] when reported with SDx K68.11 or T81.4XXA or T84.6Ø-T84.619, T84.63-T84.7 with 7th character A

HAC ØRG[Ø,1,2,4,6,7,8,A][Ø,3,4]A[Ø,J] when reported with SDx K68.11 or T81.4XXA or T84.6Ø-T84.619, T84.63-T84.7 with 7th character A

HAC ØRG[E,F,G,H,J,K][Ø,3,4][4,7,J,K,Z]Z when reported with SDx K68.11 or T81.4XXA or T84.6Ø-T84.619, T84.63-T84.7 with 7th character A

HAC ØRG[L,M][Ø,3,4][4,5,7,J,K,Z]Z when reported with SDx K68.11 or T81.4XXA or T84.6Ø-T84.619, T84.63-T84.7 with 7th character A

**See Appendix L for Procedure Combinations**
⊞ ØRG7[Ø,3,4][7,J,K,Z][Ø,1,J]
⊞ ØRG7[Ø,3,4]A[Ø,J]

**Ø Medical and Surgical**
**R Upper Joints**
**H Insertion** Definition: Putting in a nonbiological appliance that monitors, assists, performs, or prevents a physiological function but does not physically take the place of a body part

Explanation: None

| Body Part Character 4 | Approach Character 5 | Device Character 6 | Qualifier Character 7 |
|---|---|---|---|
| **Ø Occipital-cervical Joint**<br>**1 Cervical Vertebral Joint**<br>Atlantoaxial joint<br>Cervical facet joint<br>**4 Cervicothoracic Vertebral Joint**<br>Cervicothoracic facet joint<br>**6 Thoracic Vertebral Joint**<br>Costotransverse joint<br>Costovertebral joint<br>Thoracic facet joint<br>**A Thoracolumbar Vertebral Joint**<br>Thoracolumbar facet joint | **Ø Open**<br>**3 Percutaneous**<br>**4 Percutaneous Endoscopic** | **3 Infusion Device**<br>**4 Internal Fixation Device**<br>**8 Spacer**<br>**B Spinal Stabilization Device, Interspinous Process**<br>**C Spinal Stabilization Device, Pedicle-Based**<br>**D Spinal Stabilization Device, Facet Replacement** | **Z No Qualifier** |
| **3 Cervical Vertebral Disc**<br>**5 Cervicothoracic Vertebral Disc**<br>**9 Thoracic Vertebral Disc**<br>**B Thoracolumbar Vertebral Disc** | **Ø Open**<br>**3 Percutaneous**<br>**4 Percutaneous Endoscopic** | **3 Infusion Device** | **Z No Qualifier** |
| **C Temporomandibular Joint, Right**<br>**D Temporomandibular Joint, Left**<br>**E Sternoclavicular Joint, Right**<br>**F Sternoclavicular Joint, Left**<br>**G Acromioclavicular Joint, Right**<br>**H Acromioclavicular Joint, Left**<br>**J Shoulder Joint, Right**<br>Glenohumeral joint<br>Glenoid ligament (labrum)<br>**K Shoulder Joint, Left**<br>*See J Shoulder Joint, Right* | **Ø Open**<br>**3 Percutaneous**<br>**4 Percutaneous Endoscopic** | **3 Infusion Device**<br>**4 Internal Fixation Device**<br>**8 Spacer** | **Z No Qualifier** |
| **L Elbow Joint, Right**<br>Distal humerus, involving joint<br>Humeroradial joint<br>Humeroulnar joint<br>Proximal radioulnar joint<br>**M Elbow Joint, Left**<br>*See L Elbow Joint, Right*<br>**N Wrist Joint, Right**<br>Distal radioulnar joint<br>Radiocarpal joint<br>**P Wrist Joint, Left**<br>*See N Wrist Joint, Right*<br>**Q Carpal Joint, Right**<br>Intercarpal joint<br>Midcarpal joint<br>**R Carpal Joint, Left**<br>*See Q Carpal Joint, Right*<br>**S Carpometacarpal Joint, Right**<br>**T Carpometacarpal Joint, Left**<br>**U Metacarpophalangeal Joint, Right**<br>**V Metacarpophalangeal Joint, Left**<br>**W Finger Phalangeal Joint, Right**<br>Interphalangeal (IP) joint<br>**X Finger Phalangeal Joint, Left**<br>*See W Finger Phalangeal Joint, Right* | **Ø Open**<br>**3 Percutaneous**<br>**4 Percutaneous Endoscopic** | **3 Infusion Device**<br>**4 Internal Fixation Device**<br>**5 External Fixation Device**<br>**8 Spacer** | **Z No Qualifier** |

**Non-OR** ØRH[Ø,1,4,6,A][Ø,3,4][3,8]Z
**Non-OR** ØRH[3,5,9,B][Ø,3,4]3Z
**Non-OR** ØRH[C,D][Ø,4]8Z
**Non-OR** ØRH[C,D]3[3,8]Z
**Non-OR** ØRH[E,F,G,H,J,K][Ø,3,4][3,8]Z
**Non-OR** ØRH[L,M,N,P,Q,R,S,T,U,V,W,X][Ø,3,4][3,8]Z

**Ø Medical and Surgical**
**R Upper Joints**
**J Inspection** Definition: Visually and/or manually exploring a body part

Explanation: Visual exploration may be performed with or without optical instrumentation. Manual exploration may be performed directly or through intervening body layers.

| Body Part Character 4 | Approach Character 5 | Device Character 6 | Qualifier Character 7 |
|---|---|---|---|
| **Ø** Occipital-cervical Joint<br>**1** Cervical Vertebral Joint<br>Atlantoaxial joint<br>Cervical facet joint<br>**3** Cervical Vertebral Disc<br>**4** Cervicothoracic Vertebral Joint<br>Cervicothoracic facet joint<br>**5** Cervicothoracic Vertebral Disc<br>**6** Thoracic Vertebral Joint<br>Costotransverse joint<br>Costovertebral joint<br>Thoracic facet joint<br>**9** Thoracic Vertebral Disc<br>**A** Thoracolumbar Vertebral Joint<br>Thoracolumbar facet joint<br>**B** Thoracolumbar Vertebral Disc<br>**C** Temporomandibular Joint, Right<br>**D** Temporomandibular Joint, Left<br>**E** Sternoclavicular Joint, Right<br>**F** Sternoclavicular Joint, Left<br>**G** Acromioclavicular Joint, Right<br>**H** Acromioclavicular Joint, Left<br>**J** Shoulder Joint, Right<br>Glenohumeral joint<br>Glenoid ligament (labrum)<br>**K** Shoulder Joint, Left<br>*See J Shoulder Joint, Right*<br>**L** Elbow Joint, Right<br>Distal humerus, involving joint<br>Humeroradial joint<br>Humeroulnar joint<br>Proximal radioulnar joint<br>**M** Elbow Joint, Left<br>*See L Elbow Joint, Right*<br>**N** Wrist Joint, Right<br>Distal radioulnar joint<br>Radiocarpal joint<br>**P** Wrist Joint, Left<br>*See N Wrist Joint, Right*<br>**Q** Carpal Joint, Right<br>Intercarpal joint<br>Midcarpal joint<br>**R** Carpal Joint, Left<br>*See Q Carpal Joint, Right*<br>**S** Carpometacarpal Joint, Right<br>**T** Carpometacarpal Joint, Left<br>**U** Metacarpophalangeal Joint, Right<br>**V** Metacarpophalangeal Joint, Left<br>**W** Finger Phalangeal Joint, Right<br>Interphalangeal (IP) joint<br>**X** Finger Phalangeal Joint, Left<br>*See W Finger Phalangeal Joint, Right* | **Ø** Open<br>**3** Percutaneous<br>**4** Percutaneous Endoscopic<br>**X** External | **Z** No Device | **Z** No Qualifier |

**Non-OR** ØRJ[Ø,1,3,4,5,6,9,A,B,C,D,E,F,G,H,J,K,L,M,N,P,Q,R,S,T,U,V,W,X][3,X]ZZ

**Ø Medical and Surgical**
**R Upper Joints**
**N Release**

Definition: Freeing a body part from an abnormal physical constraint by cutting or by the use of force
Explanation: Some of the restraining tissue may be taken out but none of the body part is taken out

| Body Part Character 4 | Approach Character 5 | Device Character 6 | Qualifier Character 7 |
|---|---|---|---|
| **Ø** Occipital-cervical Joint<br>**1** Cervical Vertebral Joint<br>Atlantoaxial joint<br>Cervical facet joint<br>**3** Cervical Vertebral Disc<br>**4** Cervicothoracic Vertebral Joint<br>Cervicothoracic facet joint<br>**5** Cervicothoracic Vertebral Disc<br>**6** Thoracic Vertebral Joint<br>Costotransverse joint<br>Costovertebral joint<br>Thoracic facet joint<br>**9** Thoracic Vertebral Disc<br>**A** Thoracolumbar Vertebral Joint<br>Thoracolumbar facet joint<br>**B** Thoracolumbar Vertebral Disc<br>**C** Temporomandibular Joint, Right<br>**D** Temporomandibular Joint, Left<br>**E** Sternoclavicular Joint, Right<br>**F** Sternoclavicular Joint, Left<br>**G** Acromioclavicular Joint, Right<br>**H** Acromioclavicular Joint, Left<br>**J** Shoulder Joint, Right<br>Glenohumeral joint<br>Glenoid ligament (labrum)<br>**K** Shoulder Joint, Left<br>*See J Shoulder Joint, Right*<br>**L** Elbow Joint, Right<br>Distal humerus, involving joint<br>Humeroradial joint<br>Humeroulnar joint<br>Proximal radioulnar joint<br>**M** Elbow Joint, Left<br>*See L Elbow Joint, Right*<br>**N** Wrist Joint, Right<br>Distal radioulnar joint<br>Radiocarpal joint<br>**P** Wrist Joint, Left<br>*See N Wrist Joint, Right*<br>**Q** Carpal Joint, Right<br>Intercarpal joint<br>Midcarpal joint<br>**R** Carpal Joint, Left<br>*See Q Carpal Joint, Right*<br>**S** Carpometacarpal Joint, Right<br>**T** Carpometacarpal Joint, Left<br>**U** Metacarpophalangeal Joint, Right<br>**V** Metacarpophalangeal Joint, Left<br>**W** Finger Phalangeal Joint, Right<br>Interphalangeal (IP) joint<br>**X** Finger Phalangeal Joint, Left<br>*See W Finger Phalangeal Joint, Right* | **Ø** Open<br>**3** Percutaneous<br>**4** Percutaneous Endoscopic<br>**X** External | **Z** No Device | **Z** No Qualifier |

**Non-OR** ØRN[Ø,1,3,4,5,6,9,A,B,C,D,E,F,G,H,J,K,L,M,N,P,Q,R,S,T,U,V,W,X]XZZ

**Ø Medical and Surgical**
**R Upper Joints**
**P Removal** Definition: Taking out or off a device from a body part

Explanation: If a device is taken out and a similar device put in without cutting or puncturing the skin or mucous membrane, the procedure is coded to the root operation CHANGE. Otherwise, the procedure for taking out the device is coded to the root operation REMOVAL.

| Body Part Character 4 | Approach Character 5 | Device Character 6 | Qualifier Character 7 |
|---|---|---|---|
| **Ø Occipital-cervical Joint**<br>**1 Cervical Vertebral Joint**<br>Atlantoaxial joint<br>Cervical facet joint<br>**4 Cervicothoracic Vertebral Joint**<br>Cervicothoracic facet joint<br>**6 Thoracic Vertebral Joint**<br>Costotransverse joint<br>Costovertebral joint<br>Thoracic facet joint<br>**A Thoracolumbar Vertebral Joint**<br>Thoracolumbar facet joint | **Ø Open**<br>**3 Percutaneous**<br>**4 Percutaneous Endoscopic** | **Ø Drainage Device**<br>**3 Infusion Device**<br>**4 Internal Fixation Device**<br>**7 Autologous Tissue Substitute**<br>**8 Spacer**<br>**A Interbody Fusion Device**<br>**J Synthetic Substitute**<br>**K Nonautologous Tissue Substitute** | **Z No Qualifier** |
| **Ø Occipital-cervical Joint**<br>**1 Cervical Vertebral Joint**<br>Atlantoaxial joint<br>Cervical facet joint<br>**4 Cervicothoracic Vertebral Joint**<br>Cervicothoracic facet joint<br>**6 Thoracic Vertebral Joint**<br>Costotransverse joint<br>Costovertebral joint<br>Thoracic facet joint<br>**A Thoracolumbar Vertebral Joint**<br>Thoracolumbar facet joint | **X External** | **Ø Drainage Device**<br>**3 Infusion Device**<br>**4 Internal Fixation Device** | **Z No Qualifier** |
| **3 Cervical Vertebral Disc**<br>**5 Cervicothoracic Vertebral Disc**<br>**9 Thoracic Vertebral Disc**<br>**B Thoracolumbar Vertebral Disc** | **Ø Open**<br>**3 Percutaneous**<br>**4 Percutaneous Endoscopic** | **Ø Drainage Device**<br>**3 Infusion Device**<br>**7 Autologous Tissue Substitute**<br>**J Synthetic Substitute**<br>**K Nonautologous Tissue Substitute** | **Z No Qualifier** |
| **3 Cervical Vertebral Disc**<br>**5 Cervicothoracic Vertebral Disc**<br>**9 Thoracic Vertebral Disc**<br>**B Thoracolumbar Vertebral Disc** | **X External** | **Ø Drainage Device**<br>**3 Infusion Device** | **Z No Qualifier** |
| **C Temporomandibular Joint, Right**<br>**D Temporomandibular Joint, Left**<br>**E Sternoclavicular Joint, Right**<br>**F Sternoclavicular Joint, Left**<br>**G Acromioclavicular Joint, Right**<br>**H Acromioclavicular Joint, Left**<br>**J Shoulder Joint, Right**<br>Glenohumeral joint<br>Glenoid ligament (labrum)<br>**K Shoulder Joint, Left**<br>*See J Shoulder Joint, Right* | **Ø Open**<br>**3 Percutaneous**<br>**4 Percutaneous Endoscopic** | **Ø Drainage Device**<br>**3 Infusion Device**<br>**4 Internal Fixation Device**<br>**7 Autologous Tissue Substitute**<br>**8 Spacer**<br>**J Synthetic Substitute**<br>**K Nonautologous Tissue Substitute** | **Z No Qualifier** |
| **C Temporomandibular Joint, Right**<br>**D Temporomandibular Joint, Left**<br>**E Sternoclavicular Joint, Right**<br>**F Sternoclavicular Joint, Left**<br>**G Acromioclavicular Joint, Right**<br>**H Acromioclavicular Joint, Left**<br>**J Shoulder Joint, Right**<br>Glenohumeral joint<br>Glenoid ligament (labrum)<br>**K Shoulder Joint, Left**<br>*See J Shoulder Joint, Right* | **X External** | **Ø Drainage Device**<br>**3 Infusion Device**<br>**4 Internal Fixation Device** | **Z No Qualifier** |

***ØRP Continued on next page***

**Non-OR** ØRP[Ø,1,4,6,A]3[Ø,3,8]Z
**Non-OR** ØRP[Ø,1,4,6,A][Ø,4]8Z
**Non-OR** ØRP[Ø,1,4,6,A]X[Ø,3,4]Z
**Non-OR** ØRP[3,5,9,B]3[Ø,3]Z
**Non-OR** ØRP[3,5,9,B]X[Ø,3]Z
**Non-OR** ØRP[C,D,E,F,G,H,J,K]3[Ø,3,8]Z
**Non-OR** ØRP[C,D,E,F,G,H,J,K][Ø,4]8Z
**Non-OR** ØRP[C,D]X[Ø,3]Z
**Non-OR** ØRP[E,F,G,H,J,K]X[Ø,3,4]Z

**Ø Medical and Surgical**
**R Upper Joints**
**P Removal** Definition: Taking out or off a device from a body part

Explanation: If a device is taken out and a similar device put in without cutting or puncturing the skin or mucous membrane, the procedure is coded to the root operation CHANGE. Otherwise, the procedure for taking out the device is coded to the root operation REMOVAL.

*ØRP Continued*

| Body Part Character 4 | | Approach Character 5 | Device Character 6 | Qualifier Character 7 |
|---|---|---|---|---|
| **L Elbow Joint, Right** Distal humerus, involving joint; Humeroradial joint; Humeroulnar joint; Proximal radioulnar joint<br>**M Elbow Joint, Left** *See L Elbow Joint, Right*<br>**N Wrist Joint, Right** Distal radioulnar joint; Radiocarpal joint<br>**P Wrist Joint, Left** *See N Wrist Joint, Right*<br>**Q Carpal Joint, Right** Intercarpal joint; Midcarpal joint<br>**R Carpal Joint, Left** *See Q Carpal Joint, Right* | **S Carpometacarpal Joint, Right**<br>**T Carpometacarpal Joint, Left**<br>**U Metacarpophalangeal Joint, Right**<br>**V Metacarpophalangeal Joint, Left**<br>**W Finger Phalangeal Joint, Right** Interphalangeal (IP) joint<br>**X Finger Phalangeal Joint, Left** *See W Finger Phalangeal Joint, Right* | **Ø** Open<br>**3** Percutaneous<br>**4** Percutaneous Endoscopic | **Ø** Drainage Device<br>**3** Infusion Device<br>**4** Internal Fixation Device<br>**5** External Fixation Device<br>**7** Autologous Tissue Substitute<br>**8** Spacer<br>**J** Synthetic Substitute<br>**K** Nonautologous Tissue Substitute | **Z** No Qualifier |
| **L Elbow Joint, Right** Distal humerus, involving joint; Humeroradial joint; Humeroulnar joint; Proximal radioulnar joint<br>**M Elbow Joint, Left** *See L Elbow Joint, Right*<br>**N Wrist Joint, Right** Distal radioulnar joint; Radiocarpal joint<br>**P Wrist Joint, Left** *See N Wrist Joint, Right*<br>**Q Carpal Joint, Right** Intercarpal joint; Midcarpal joint<br>**R Carpal Joint, Left** *See Q Carpal Joint, Right* | **S Carpometacarpal Joint, Right**<br>**T Carpometacarpal Joint, Left**<br>**U Metacarpophalangeal Joint, Right**<br>**V Metacarpophalangeal Joint, Left**<br>**W Finger Phalangeal Joint, Right** Interphalangeal (IP) joint<br>**X Finger Phalangeal Joint, Left** *See W Finger Phalangeal Joint, Right* | **X** External | **Ø** Drainage Device<br>**3** Infusion Device<br>**4** Internal Fixation Device<br>**5** External Fixation Device | **Z** No Qualifier |

Non-OR ØRP[L,M,N,P,Q,R,S,T,U,V,W,X]3[Ø,3,8]Z
Non-OR ØRP[L,M,N,P,Q,R,S,T,U,V,W,X][Ø,4]8Z
Non-OR ØRP[L,M,N,P,Q,R,S,T,U,V,W,X]X[Ø,3,4,5]Z

**Ø Medical and Surgical**
**R Upper Joints**
**Q Repair** Definition: Restoring, to the extent possible, a body part to its normal anatomic structure and function
Explanation: Used only when the method to accomplish the repair is not one of the other root operations

| Body Part Character 4 | | Approach Character 5 | Device Character 6 | Qualifier Character 7 |
|---|---|---|---|---|
| **Ø Occipital-cervical Joint**<br>**1 Cervical Vertebral Joint**<br>Atlantoaxial joint<br>Cervical facet joint<br>**3 Cervical Vertebral Disc**<br>**4 Cervicothoracic Vertebral Joint**<br>Cervicothoracic facet joint<br>**5 Cervicothoracic Vertebral Disc**<br>**6 Thoracic Vertebral Joint**<br>Costotransverse joint<br>Costovertebral joint<br>Thoracic facet joint<br>**9 Thoracic Vertebral Disc**<br>**A Thoracolumbar Vertebral Joint**<br>Thoracolumbar facet joint<br>**B Thoracolumbar Vertebral Disc**<br>**C Temporomandibular Joint, Right**<br>**D Temporomandibular Joint, Left**<br>**E Sternoclavicular Joint, Right**<br>**F Sternoclavicular Joint, Left**<br>**G Acromioclavicular Joint, Right**<br>**H Acromioclavicular Joint, Left**<br>**J Shoulder Joint, Right**<br>Glenohumeral joint<br>Glenoid ligament (labrum)<br>**K Shoulder Joint, Left**<br>*See J Shoulder Joint, Right* | **L Elbow Joint, Right**<br>Distal humerus, involving joint<br>Humeroradial joint<br>Humeroulnar joint<br>Proximal radioulnar joint<br>**M Elbow Joint, Left**<br>*See L Elbow Joint, Right*<br>**N Wrist Joint, Right**<br>Distal radioulnar joint<br>Radiocarpal joint<br>**P Wrist Joint, Left**<br>*See N Wrist Joint, Right*<br>**Q Carpal Joint, Right**<br>Intercarpal joint<br>Midcarpal joint<br>**R Carpal Joint, Left**<br>*See Q Carpal Joint, Right*<br>**S Carpometacarpal Joint, Right**<br>**T Carpometacarpal Joint, Left**<br>**U Metacarpophalangeal Joint, Right**<br>**V Metacarpophalangeal Joint, Left**<br>**W Finger Phalangeal Joint, Right**<br>Interphalangeal (IP) joint<br>**X Finger Phalangeal Joint, Left**<br>*See W Finger Phalangeal Joint, Right* | **Ø Open**<br>**3 Percutaneous**<br>**4 Percutaneous Endoscopic**<br>**X External** | **Z No Device** | **Z No Qualifier** |

**Non-OR** ØRQ[Ø,1,3,4,5,6,9,A,B,C,D,E,F,G,H,J,K,L,M,N,P,Q,R,S,T,U,V,W,X]XZZ
**HAC** ØRQ[E,F,G,H,J,K,L,M][Ø,3,4,X]ZZ when reported with SDx K68.11 or T81.4XXA or T84.6Ø-T84.619, T84.63-T84.7 with 7th character A

**Ø Medical and Surgical**
**R Upper Joints**
**R Replacement**

Definition: Putting in or on biological or synthetic material that physically takes the place and/or function of all or a portion of a body part

Explanation: The body part may have been taken out or replaced, or may be taken out, physically eradicated, or rendered nonfunctional during the REPLACEMENT procedure. A REMOVAL procedure is coded for taking out the device used in a previous replacement procedure.

| Body Part Character 4 | Approach Character 5 | Device Character 6 | Qualifier Character 7 |
|---|---|---|---|
| **Ø Occipital-cervical Joint**<br>**1 Cervical Vertebral Joint**<br>Atlantoaxial joint<br>Cervical facet joint<br>**3 Cervical Vertebral Disc**<br>**4 Cervicothoracic Vertebral Joint**<br>Cervicothoracic facet joint<br>**5 Cervicothoracic Vertebral Disc**<br>**6 Thoracic Vertebral Joint**<br>Costotransverse joint<br>Costovertebral joint<br>Thoracic facet joint<br>**9 Thoracic Vertebral Disc**<br>**A Thoracolumbar Vertebral Joint**<br>Thoracolumbar facet joint<br>**B Thoracolumbar Vertebral Disc**<br>**C Temporomandibular Joint, Right**<br>**D Temporomandibular Joint, Left**<br>**E Sternoclavicular Joint, Right**<br>**F Sternoclavicular Joint, Left**<br>**G Acromioclavicular Joint, Right**<br>**H Acromioclavicular Joint, Left**<br>**L Elbow Joint, Right**<br>Distal humerus, involving joint<br>Humeroradial joint<br>Humeroulnar joint<br>Proximal radioulnar joint<br>**M Elbow Joint, Left**<br>*See L Elbow Joint, Right*<br>**N Wrist Joint, Right**<br>Distal radioulnar joint<br>Radiocarpal joint<br>**P Wrist Joint, Left**<br>*See N Wrist Joint, Right*<br>**Q Carpal Joint, Right**<br>Intercarpal joint<br>Midcarpal joint<br>**R Carpal Joint, Left**<br>*See Q Carpal Joint, Right*<br>**S Carpometacarpal Joint, Right**<br>**T Carpometacarpal Joint, Left**<br>**U Metacarpophalangeal Joint, Right**<br>**V Metacarpophalangeal Joint, Left**<br>**W Finger Phalangeal Joint, Right**<br>Interphalangeal (IP) joint<br>**X Finger Phalangeal Joint, Left**<br>*See W Finger Phalangeal Joint, Right* | Ø Open | 7 Autologous Tissue Substitute<br>J Synthetic Substitute<br>K Nonautologous Tissue Substitute | Z No Qualifier |
| **J Shoulder Joint, Right**<br>Glenohumeral joint<br>Glenoid ligament (labrum)<br>**K Shoulder Joint, Left**<br>*See J Shoulder Joint, Right* | Ø Open | Ø Synthetic Substitute, Reverse Ball and Socket<br>7 Autologous Tissue Substitute<br>K Nonautologous Tissue Substitute | Z No Qualifier |
| **J Shoulder Joint, Right**<br>Glenohumeral joint<br>Glenoid ligament (labrum)<br>**K Shoulder Joint, Left**<br>*See J Shoulder Joint, Right* | Ø Open | J Synthetic Substitute | 6 Humeral Surface<br>7 Glenoid Surface<br>Z No Qualifier |

**Ø Medical and Surgical**
**R Upper Joints**
**S Reposition**

Definition: Moving to its normal location, or other suitable location, all or a portion of a body part

Explanation: The body part is moved to a new location from an abnormal location, or from a normal location where it is not functioning correctly. The body part may or may not be cut out or off to be moved to the new location.

| Body Part Character 4 | Approach Character 5 | Device Character 6 | Qualifier Character 7 |
|---|---|---|---|
| **Ø** Occipital-cervical Joint<br>**1** Cervical Vertebral Joint<br>Atlantoaxial joint<br>Cervical facet joint<br>**4** Cervicothoracic Vertebral Joint<br>Cervicothoracic facet joint<br>**6** Thoracic Vertebral Joint<br>Costotransverse joint<br>Costovertebral joint<br>Thoracic facet joint<br>**A** Thoracolumbar Vertebral Joint<br>Thoracolumbar facet joint<br>**C** Temporomandibular Joint, Right<br>**D** Temporomandibular Joint, Left<br>**E** Sternoclavicular Joint, Right<br>**F** Sternoclavicular Joint, Left<br>**G** Acromioclavicular Joint, Right<br>**H** Acromioclavicular Joint, Left<br>**J** Shoulder Joint, Right<br>Glenohumeral joint<br>Glenoid ligament (labrum)<br>**K** Shoulder Joint, Left<br>*See J Shoulder Joint, Right* | **Ø** Open<br>**3** Percutaneous<br>**4** Percutaneous Endoscopic<br>**X** External | **4** Internal Fixation Device<br>**Z** No Device | **Z** No Qualifier |
| **L** Elbow Joint, Right<br>Distal humerus, involving joint<br>Humeroradial joint<br>Humeroulnar joint<br>Proximal radioulnar joint<br>**M** Elbow Joint, Left<br>*See L Elbow Joint, Right*<br>**N** Wrist Joint, Right<br>Distal radioulnar joint<br>Radiocarpal joint<br>**P** Wrist Joint, Left<br>*See N Wrist Joint, Right*<br>**Q** Carpal Joint, Right<br>Intercarpal joint<br>Midcarpal joint<br>**R** Carpal Joint, Left<br>*See Q Carpal Joint, Right*<br>**S** Carpometacarpal Joint, Right<br>**T** Carpometacarpal Joint, Left<br>**U** Metacarpophalangeal Joint, Right<br>**V** Metacarpophalangeal Joint, Left<br>**W** Finger Phalangeal Joint, Right<br>Interphalangeal (IP) joint<br>**X** Finger Phalangeal Joint, Left<br>*See W Finger Phalangeal Joint, Right* | **Ø** Open<br>**3** Percutaneous<br>**4** Percutaneous Endoscopic<br>**X** External | **4** Internal Fixation Device<br>**5** External Fixation Device<br>**Z** No Device | **Z** No Qualifier |

**Non-OR** ØRS[Ø,1,4,6,A,C,D,E,F,G,H,J,K][3,4,X][4,Z]Z
**Non-OR** ØRS[L,M,N,P,Q,R,S,T,U,V,W,X][3,4,X][4,5,Z]Z

**Ø Medical and Surgical**
**R Upper Joints**
**T Resection** Definition: Cutting out or off, without replacement, all of a body part
Explanation: None

| Body Part Character 4 | | Approach Character 5 | Device Character 6 | Qualifier Character 7 |
|---|---|---|---|---|
| **3 Cervical Vertebral Disc**<br>**4 Cervicothoracic Vertebral Joint**<br>Cervicothoracic facet joint<br>**5 Cervicothoracic Vertebral Disc**<br>**9 Thoracic Vertebral Disc**<br>**B Thoracolumbar Vertebral Disc**<br>**C Temporomandibular Joint, Right**<br>**D Temporomandibular Joint, Left**<br>**E Sternoclavicular Joint, Right**<br>**F Sternoclavicular Joint, Left**<br>**G Acromioclavicular Joint, Right**<br>**H Acromioclavicular Joint, Left**<br>**J Shoulder Joint, Right**<br>Glenohumeral joint<br>Glenoid ligament (labrum)<br>**K Shoulder Joint, Left**<br>*See J Shoulder Joint, Right*<br>**L Elbow Joint, Right**<br>Distal humerus, involving joint<br>Humeroradial joint<br>Humeroulnar joint<br>Proximal radioulnar joint | **M Elbow Joint, Left**<br>*See L Elbow Joint, Right*<br>**N Wrist Joint, Right**<br>Distal radioulnar joint<br>Radiocarpal joint<br>**P Wrist Joint, Left**<br>*See N Wrist Joint, Right*<br>**Q Carpal Joint, Right**<br>Intercarpal joint<br>Midcarpal joint<br>**R Carpal Joint, Left**<br>*See Q Carpal Joint, Right*<br>**S Carpometacarpal Joint, Right**<br>**T Carpometacarpal Joint, Left**<br>**U Metacarpophalangeal Joint, Right**<br>**V Metacarpophalangeal Joint, Left**<br>**W Finger Phalangeal Joint, Right**<br>Interphalangeal (IP) joint<br>**X Finger Phalangeal Joint, Left**<br>*See W Finger Phalangeal Joint, Right* | **Ø Open** | **Z No Device** | **Z No Qualifier** |

**Ø Medical and Surgical**
**R Upper Joints**
**U Supplement** Definition: Putting in or on biological or synthetic material that physically reinforces and/or augments the function of a portion of a body part
Explanation: The biological material is non-living, or is living and from the same individual. The body part may have been previously replaced, and the SUPPLEMENT procedure is performed to physically reinforce and/or augment the function of the replaced body part.

| Body Part Character 4 | | Approach Character 5 | Device Character 6 | Qualifier Character 7 |
|---|---|---|---|---|
| **Ø Occipital-cervical Joint**<br>**1 Cervical Vertebral Joint**<br>Atlantoaxial joint<br>Cervical facet joint<br>**3 Cervical Vertebral Disc**<br>**4 Cervicothoracic Vertebral Joint**<br>Cervicothoracic facet joint<br>**5 Cervicothoracic Vertebral Disc**<br>**6 Thoracic Vertebral Joint**<br>Costotransverse joint<br>Costovertebral joint<br>Thoracic facet joint<br>**9 Thoracic Vertebral Disc**<br>**A Thoracolumbar Vertebral Joint**<br>Thoracolumbar facet joint<br>**B Thoracolumbar Vertebral Disc**<br>**C Temporomandibular Joint, Right**<br>**D Temporomandibular Joint, Left**<br>**E Sternoclavicular Joint, Right**<br>**F Sternoclavicular Joint, Left**<br>**G Acromioclavicular Joint, Right**<br>**H Acromioclavicular Joint, Left**<br>**J Shoulder Joint, Right**<br>Glenohumeral joint<br>Glenoid ligament (labrum)<br>**K Shoulder Joint, Left**<br>*See J Shoulder Joint, Right* | **L Elbow Joint, Right**<br>Distal humerus, involving joint<br>Humeroradial joint<br>Humeroulnar joint<br>Proximal radioulnar joint<br>**M Elbow Joint, Left**<br>*See L Elbow Joint, Right*<br>**N Wrist Joint, Right**<br>Distal radioulnar joint<br>Radiocarpal joint<br>**P Wrist Joint, Left**<br>*See N Wrist Joint, Right*<br>**Q Carpal Joint, Right**<br>Intercarpal joint<br>Midcarpal joint<br>**R Carpal Joint, Left**<br>*See Q Carpal Joint, Right*<br>**S Carpometacarpal Joint, Right**<br>**T Carpometacarpal Joint, Left**<br>**U Metacarpophalangeal Joint, Right**<br>**V Metacarpophalangeal Joint, Left**<br>**W Finger Phalangeal Joint, Right**<br>Interphalangeal (IP) joint<br>**X Finger Phalangeal Joint, Left**<br>*See W Finger Phalangeal Joint, Right* | **Ø Open**<br>**3 Percutaneous**<br>**4 Percutaneous Endoscopic** | **7 Autologous Tissue Substitute**<br>**J Synthetic Substitute**<br>**K Nonautologous Tissue Substitute** | **Z No Qualifier** |

**HAC** ØRU[E,F,G,H,J,K,L,M][Ø,3,4][7,J,K]Z when reported with SDx K68.11 or T81.4XXA or T84.6Ø-T84.619, T84.63-T84.7 with 7th character A

**Ø Medical and Surgical**
**R Upper Joints**
**W Revision** Definition: Correcting, to the extent possible, a portion of a malfunctioning device or the position of a displaced device

Explanation: Revision can include correcting a malfunctioning or displaced device by taking out or putting in components of the device such as a screw or pin

| Body Part Character 4 | Approach Character 5 | Device Character 6 | Qualifier Character 7 |
|---|---|---|---|
| **Ø Occipital-cervical Joint**<br>**1 Cervical Vertebral Joint**<br>Atlantoaxial joint<br>Cervical facet joint<br>**4 Cervicothoracic Vertebral Joint**<br>Cervicothoracic facet joint<br>**6 Thoracic Vertebral Joint**<br>Costotransverse joint<br>Costovertebral joint<br>Thoracic facet joint<br>**A Thoracolumbar Vertebral Joint**<br>Thoracolumbar facet joint | **Ø Open**<br>**3 Percutaneous**<br>**4 Percutaneous Endoscopic**<br>**X External** | **Ø Drainage Device**<br>**3 Infusion Device**<br>**4 Internal Fixation Device**<br>**7 Autologous Tissue Substitute**<br>**8 Spacer**<br>**A Interbody Fusion Device**<br>**J Synthetic Substitute**<br>**K Nonautologous Tissue Substitute** | **Z No Qualifier** |
| **3 Cervical Vertebral Disc**<br>**5 Cervicothoracic Vertebral Disc**<br>**9 Thoracic Vertebral Disc**<br>**B Thoracolumbar Vertebral Disc** | **Ø Open**<br>**3 Percutaneous**<br>**4 Percutaneous Endoscopic**<br>**X External** | **Ø Drainage Device**<br>**3 Infusion Device**<br>**7 Autologous Tissue Substitute**<br>**J Synthetic Substitute**<br>**K Nonautologous Tissue Substitute** | **Z No Qualifier** |
| **C Temporomandibular Joint, Right**<br>**D Temporomandibular Joint, Left**<br>**E Sternoclavicular Joint, Right**<br>**F Sternoclavicular Joint, Left**<br>**G Acromioclavicular Joint, Right**<br>**H Acromioclavicular Joint, Left**<br>**J Shoulder Joint, Right**<br>Glenohumeral joint<br>Glenoid ligament (labrum)<br>**K Shoulder Joint, Left**<br>*See J Shoulder Joint, Right* | **Ø Open**<br>**3 Percutaneous**<br>**4 Percutaneous Endoscopic**<br>**X External** | **Ø Drainage Device**<br>**3 Infusion Device**<br>**4 Internal Fixation Device**<br>**7 Autologous Tissue Substitute**<br>**8 Spacer**<br>**J Synthetic Substitute**<br>**K Nonautologous Tissue Substitute** | **Z No Qualifier** |
| **L Elbow Joint, Right**<br>Distal humerus, involving joint<br>Humeroradial joint<br>Humeroulnar joint<br>Proximal radioulnar joint<br>**M Elbow Joint, Left**<br>*See L Elbow Joint, Right*<br>**N Wrist Joint, Right**<br>Distal radioulnar joint<br>Radiocarpal joint<br>**P Wrist Joint, Left**<br>*See N Wrist Joint, Right*<br>**Q Carpal Joint, Right**<br>Intercarpal joint<br>Midcarpal joint<br>**R Carpal Joint, Left**<br>*See Q Carpal Joint, Right*<br>**S Carpometacarpal Joint, Right**<br>**T Carpometacarpal Joint, Left**<br>**U Metacarpophalangeal Joint, Right**<br>**V Metacarpophalangeal Joint, Left**<br>**W Finger Phalangeal Joint, Right**<br>Interphalangeal (IP) joint<br>**X Finger Phalangeal Joint, Left**<br>*See W Finger Phalangeal Joint, Right* | **Ø Open**<br>**3 Percutaneous**<br>**4 Percutaneous Endoscopic**<br>**X External** | **Ø Drainage Device**<br>**3 Infusion Device**<br>**4 Internal Fixation Device**<br>**5 External Fixation Device**<br>**7 Autologous Tissue Substitute**<br>**8 Spacer**<br>**J Synthetic Substitute**<br>**K Nonautologous Tissue Substitute** | **Z No Qualifier** |

**Non-OR** ØRW[Ø,1,4,6,A]X[Ø,3,4,7,8,A,J,K]Z
**Non-OR** ØRW[3,5,9,B]X[Ø,3,7,J,K]Z
**Non-OR** ØRW[C,D,E,F,G,H,J,K]X[Ø,3,4,7,8,J,K]Z
**Non-OR** ØRW[L,M,N,P,Q,R,S,T,U,V,W,X]X[Ø,3,4,5,7,8,J,K]Z

# Lower Joints ØS2–ØSW

## Character Meanings*

This Character Meaning table is provided as a guide to assist the user in the identification of character members that may be found in this section of code tables. It **SHOULD NOT** be used to build a PCS code.

| Operation–Character 3 | Body Part–Character 4 | Approach–Character 5 | Device–Character 6 | Qualifier–Character 7 |
|---|---|---|---|---|
| 2 Change | Ø Lumbar Vertebral Joint | Ø Open | Ø Drainage Device OR Synthetic Substitute, Polyethylene | Ø Anterior Approach, Anterior Column |
| 5 Destruction | 1 Lumbar Vertebral Joint, 2 or more | 3 Percutaneous | 1 Synthetic Substitute, Metal | 1 Posterior Approach, Posterior Column |
| 9 Drainage | 2 Lumbar Vertebral Disc | 4 Percutaneous Endoscopic | 2 Synthetic Substitute, Metal on Polyethylene | 9 Cemented |
| B Excision | 3 Lumbosacral Joint | X External | 3 Infusion Device OR Synthetic Substitute, Ceramic | A Uncemented |
| C Extirpation | 4 Lumbosacral Disc | | 4 Internal Fixation Device OR Synthetic Substitute, Ceramic on Polyethylene | C Patellar Surface |
| G Fusion | 5 Sacrococcygeal Joint | | 5 External Fixation Device | J Posterior Approach, Anterior Column |
| H Insertion | 6 Coccygeal Joint | | 6 Synthetic Substitute, Oxidized Zirconium on Polyethylene | X Diagnostic |
| J Inspection | 7 Sacroiliac Joint, Right | | 7 Autologous Tissue Substitute | Z No Qualifier |
| N Release | 8 Sacroiliac Joint, Left | | 8 Spacer | |
| P Removal | 9 Hip Joint, Right | | 9 Liner | |
| | A Hip Joint, Acetabular Surface, Right | | A Interbody Fusion Device | |
| Q Repair | B Hip Joint, Left | | B Resurfacing Device OR Spinal Stabilization Device, Interspinous Process | |
| R Replacement | C Knee Joint, Right | | C Spinal Stabilization Device, Pedicle-Based | |
| S Reposition | D Knee Joint, Left | | D Spinal Stabilization Device, Facet Replacement | |
| T Resection | E Hip Joint, Acetabular Surface, Left | | J Synthetic Substitute | |
| U Supplement | F Ankle Joint, Right | | K Nonautologous Tissue Substitute | |
| W Revision | G Ankle Joint, Left | | L Synthetic Substitute, Unicondylar | |
| | H Tarsal Joint, Right | | Y Other Device | |
| | J Tarsal Joint, Left | | Z No Device | |
| | K Tarsometatarsal Joint, Right | | | |
| | L Tarsometatarsal Joint, Left | | | |
| | M Metatarsal-Phalangeal Joint, Right | | | |
| | N Metatarsal-Phalangeal Joint, Left | | | |
| | P Toe Phalangeal Joint, Right | | | |
| | Q Toe Phalangeal Joint, Left | | | |
| | R Hip Joint, Femoral Surface, Right | | | |
| | S Hip Joint, Femoral Surface, Left | | | |
| | T Knee Joint, Femoral Surface, Right | | | |
| | U Knee Joint, Femoral Surface, Left | | | |
| | V Knee Joint, Tibial Surface, Right | | | |
| | W Knee Joint, Tibial Surface, Left | | | |
| | Y Lower Joint | | | |

* Includes synovial membrane.

**AHA Coding Clinic for table ØS9**

| | |
|---|---|
| **2017, 1Q, 50** | Dry aspiration of ankle joint |

**AHA Coding Clinic for table ØSB**

| | |
|---|---|
| **2016, 2Q, 16** | Decompressive laminectomy/foraminotomy and lumbar discectomy |
| **2016, 1Q, 20** | Metatarsophalangeal joint resection arthroplasty |
| **2015, 1Q, 34** | Arthroscopic meniscectomy with debridement and abrasion chondroplasty |
| **2014, 2Q, 6** | Posterior lumbar fusion with discectomy |

**AHA Coding Clinic for table ØSG**

| | |
|---|---|
| **2017, 2Q, 23** | Decompression of spinal cord and placement of instrumentation |
| **2014, 3Q, 30** | Spinal fusion and fixation instrumentation |
| **2014, 3Q, 36** | Lumbar interbody fusion of two vertebral levels |
| **2014, 2Q, 6** | Posterior lumbar fusion with discectomy |
| **2013, 3Q, 25** | 36Ø-degree spinal fusion |
| **2013, 2Q, 39** | Ankle fusion, osteotomy, and removal of hardware |
| **2013, 1Q, 21-23** | Spinal fusion of thoracic and lumbar vertebrae |

**AHA Coding Clinic for table ØSH**

| | |
|---|---|
| **2017, 2Q, 23** | Decompression of spinal cord and placement of instrumentation |

**AHA Coding Clinic for table ØSJ**

| | |
|---|---|
| **2017, 1Q, 50** | Dry aspiration of ankle joint |

**AHA Coding Clinic for table ØSP**

| | |
|---|---|
| **2016, 4Q, 110-112** | Removal and revision of hip and knee devices |
| **2015, 2Q, 18** | Total knee revision |
| **2015, 2Q, 19** | Revision of femoral head and acetabular liner |
| **2013, 2Q, 39** | Ankle fusion, osteotomy, and removal of hardware |

**AHA Coding Clinic for table ØSQ**

| | |
|---|---|
| **2014, 4Q, 25** | Femoroacetabular impingement and labral tear with repair |

**AHA Coding Clinic for table ØSR**

| | |
|---|---|
| **2017, 1Q, 22** | Total knee replacement and patellar component |
| **2016, 4Q, 110-111** | Partial (unicondylar) knee replacement |
| **2016, 4Q, 111-112** | Removal and revision of hip and knee devices |
| **2016, 3Q, 35** | Use of cemented versus uncemented qualifier for joint replacement |
| **2015, 3Q, 18** | Total hip replacement with acetabular reconstruction |
| **2015, 2Q, 18** | Total knee revision |
| **2015, 2Q, 19** | Revision of femoral head and acetabular liner |

**AHA Coding Clinic for table ØSS**

| | |
|---|---|
| **2016, 2Q, 31** | Periacetabular ostectomy for repair of congenital hip dysplasia |

**AHA Coding Clinic for table ØST**

| | |
|---|---|
| **2016, 1Q, 20** | Metatarsophalangeal joint resection arthroplasty |
| **2014, 4Q, 29** | Rotational osteosynthesis |

**AHA Coding Clinic for table ØSU**

| | |
|---|---|
| **2016, 4Q, 111** | Removal and revision of hip and knee devices |
| **2015, 2Q, 19** | Revision of femoral head and acetabular liner |

**AHA Coding Clinic for table ØSW**

| | |
|---|---|
| **2016, 4Q, 110-112** | Removal and revision of hip and knee devices |
| **2015, 2Q, 18** | Total knee revision |
| **2015, 2Q, 19** | Revision of femoral head and acetabular liner |

## Lower Joints

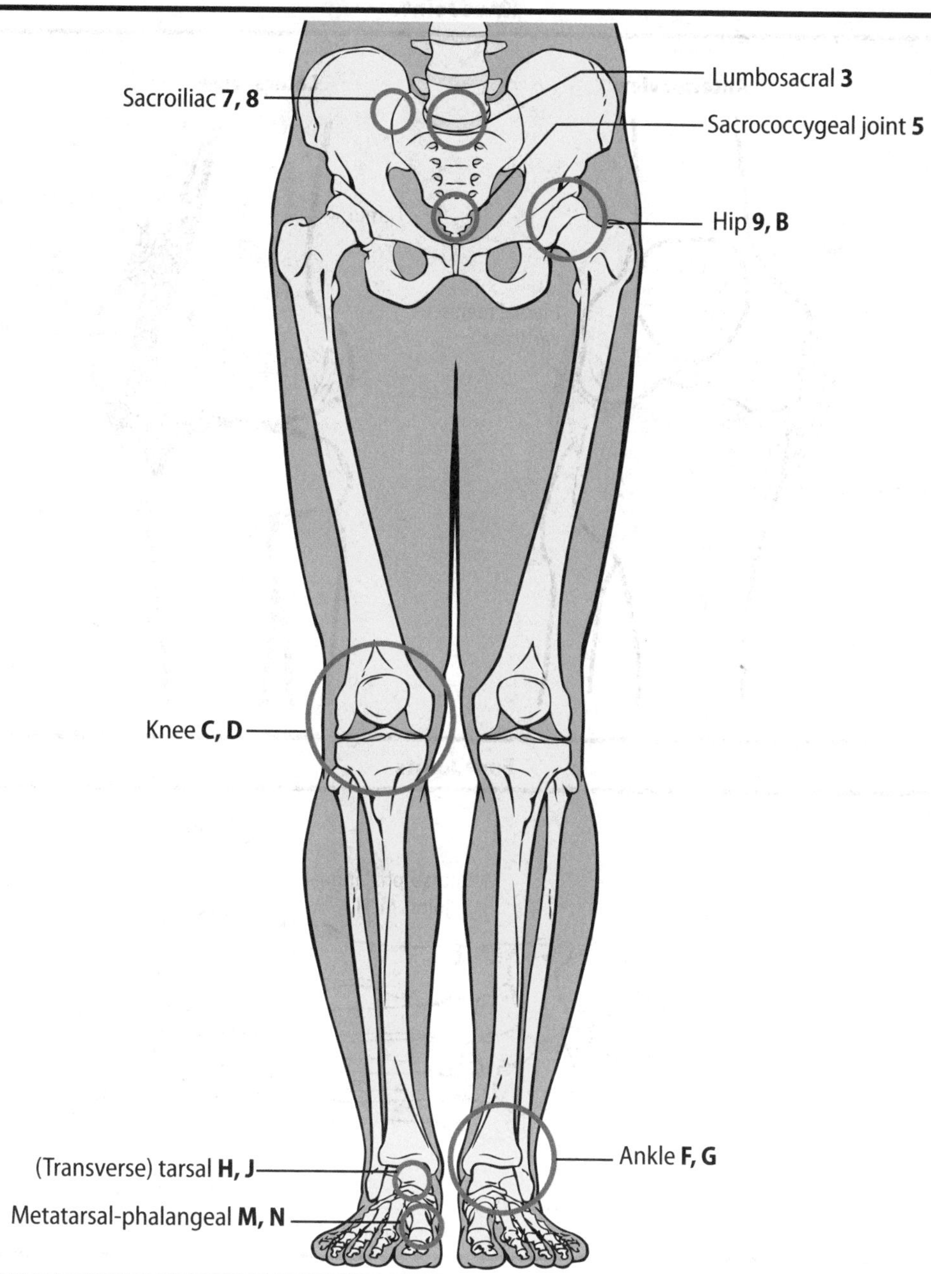
Lumbosacral 3
Sacroiliac 7, 8
Sacrococcygeal joint 5
Hip 9, B
Knee C, D
Ankle F, G
(Transverse) tarsal H, J
Metatarsal-phalangeal M, N

## Hip Joint

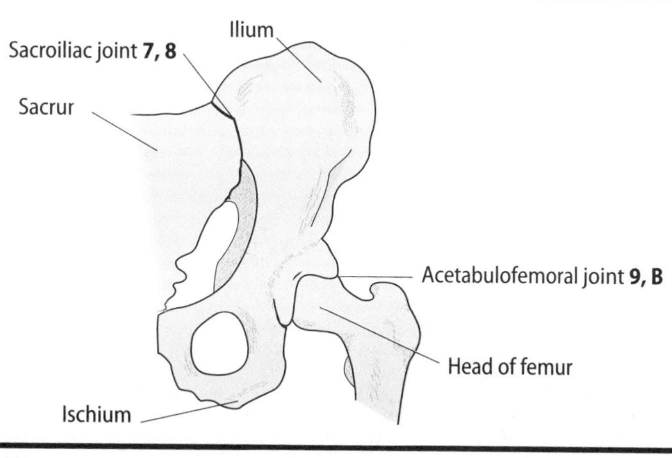
Ilium
Sacroiliac joint 7, 8
Sacrur
Acetabulofemoral joint 9, B
Head of femur
Ischium

Lower Joints

## Knee Joint

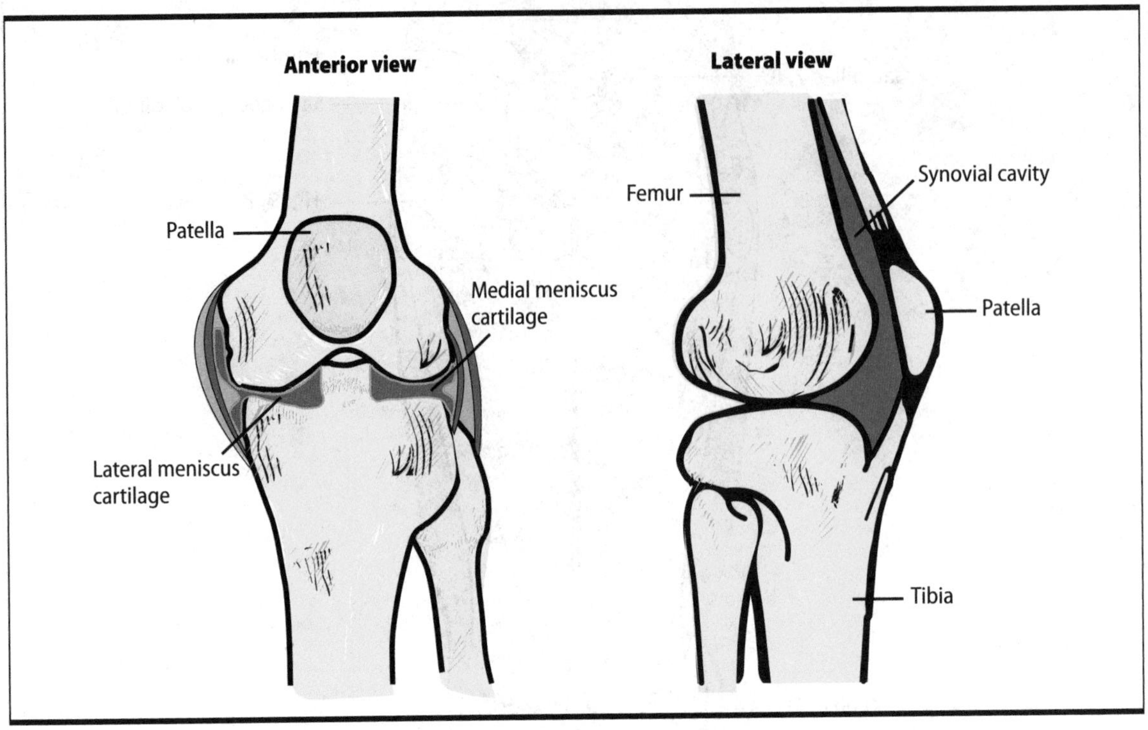
Anterior view
Lateral view
Patella
Medial meniscus cartilage
Lateral meniscus cartilage
Femur
Synovial cavity
Patella
Tibia

## Foot Joints

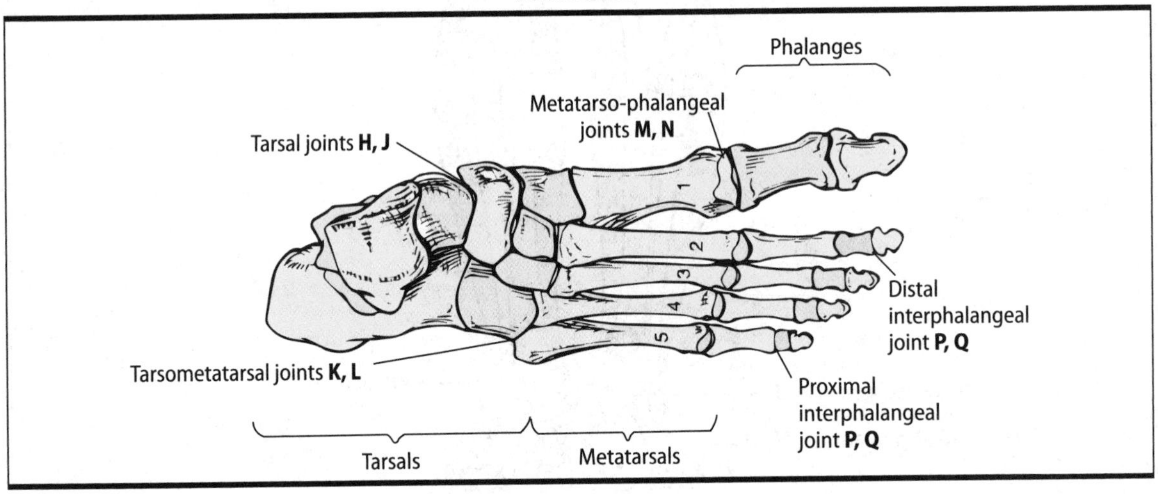
Phalanges
Metatarso-phalangeal joints **M, N**
Tarsal joints **H, J**
1
2
3
4
5
Distal interphalangeal joint **P, Q**
Tarsometatarsal joints **K, L**
Proximal interphalangeal joint **P, Q**
Tarsals
Metatarsals

**Ø Medical and Surgical**
**S Lower Joints**
**2 Change**

Definition: Taking out or off a device from a body part and putting back an identical or similar device in or on the same body part without cutting or puncturing the skin or a mucous membrane

Explanation: All CHANGE procedures are coded using the approach EXTERNAL

| Body Part Character 4 | Approach Character 5 | Device Character 6 | Qualifier Character 7 |
|---|---|---|---|
| Y Lower Joint | X External | Ø Drainage Device<br>Y Other Device | Z No Qualifier |

Non-OR All body part, approach, device, and qualifier values

**Ø Medical and Surgical**
**S Lower Joints**
**5 Destruction**

Definition: Physical eradication of all or a portion of a body part by the direct use of energy, force, or a destructive agent

Explanation: None of the body part is physically taken out

| Body Part Character 4 | Approach Character 5 | Device Character 6 | Qualifier Character 7 |
|---|---|---|---|
| **Ø Lumbar Vertebral Joint**<br>Lumbar facet joint<br>**2 Lumbar Vertebral Disc**<br>**3 Lumbosacral Joint**<br>Lumbosacral facet joint<br>**4 Lumbosacral Disc**<br>**5 Sacrococcygeal Joint**<br>Sacrococcygeal symphysis<br>**6 Coccygeal Joint**<br>**7 Sacroiliac Joint, Right**<br>**8 Sacroiliac Joint, Left**<br>**9 Hip Joint, Right**<br>Acetabulofemoral joint<br>**B Hip Joint, Left**<br>*See 9 Hip Joint, Right*<br>**C Knee Joint, Right**<br>Femoropatellar joint<br>Femorotibial joint<br>Lateral meniscus<br>Medial meniscus<br>Patellofemoral joint<br>Tibiofemoral joint<br>**D Knee Joint, Left**<br>*See C Knee Joint, Right*<br>**F Ankle Joint, Right**<br>Inferior tibiofibular joint<br>Talocrural joint<br>**G Ankle Joint, Left**<br>*See F Ankle Joint, Right*<br>**H Tarsal Joint, Right**<br>Calcaneocuboid joint<br>Cuboideonavicular joint<br>Cuneonavicular joint<br>Intercuneiform joint<br>Subtalar (talocalcaneal) joint<br>Talocalcaneal (subtalar) joint<br>Talocalcaneonavicular joint<br>**J Tarsal Joint, Left**<br>*See H Tarsal Joint, Right*<br>**K Tarsometatarsal Joint, Right**<br>**L Tarsometatarsal Joint, Left**<br>**M Metatarsal-Phalangeal Joint, Right**<br>Metatarsophalangeal (MTP) joint<br>**N Metatarsal-Phalangeal Joint, Left**<br>*See M Metatarsal-Phalangeal Joint, Right*<br>**P Toe Phalangeal Joint, Right**<br>Interphalangeal (IP) joint<br>**Q Toe Phalangeal Joint, Left**<br>*See P Toe Phalangeal Joint, Right* | **Ø Open**<br>**3 Percutaneous**<br>**4 Percutaneous Endoscopic** | **Z No Device** | **Z No Qualifier** |

**Ø Medical and Surgical**
**S Lower Joints**
**9 Drainage** Definition: Taking or letting out fluids and/or gases from a body part
Explanation: The qualifier DIAGNOSTIC is used to identify drainage procedures that are biopsies

| Body Part Character 4 | Approach Character 5 | Device Character 6 | Qualifier Character 7 |
|---|---|---|---|
| **Ø Lumbar Vertebral Joint**<br>Lumbar facet joint<br>**2 Lumbar Vertebral Disc**<br>**3 Lumbosacral Joint**<br>Lumbosacral facet joint<br>**4 Lumbosacral Disc**<br>**5 Sacrococcygeal Joint**<br>Sacrococcygeal symphysis<br>**6 Coccygeal Joint**<br>**7 Sacroiliac Joint, Right**<br>**8 Sacroiliac Joint, Left**<br>**9 Hip Joint, Right**<br>Acetabulofemoral joint<br>**B Hip Joint, Left**<br>*See 9 Hip Joint, Right*<br>**C Knee Joint, Right**<br>Femoropatellar joint<br>Femorotibial joint<br>Lateral meniscus<br>Medial meniscus<br>Patellofemoral joint<br>Tibiofemoral joint<br>**D Knee Joint, Left**<br>*See C Knee Joint, Right*<br>**F Ankle Joint, Right**<br>Inferior tibiofibular joint<br>Talocrural joint<br>**G Ankle Joint, Left**<br>*See F Ankle Joint, Right*<br>**H Tarsal Joint, Right**<br>Calcaneocuboid joint<br>Cuboideonavicular joint<br>Cuneonavicular joint<br>Intercuneiform joint<br>Subtalar (talocalcaneal) joint<br>Talocalcaneal (subtalar) joint<br>Talocalcaneonavicular joint<br>**J Tarsal Joint, Left**<br>*See H Tarsal Joint, Right*<br>**K Tarsometatarsal Joint, Right**<br>**L Tarsometatarsal Joint, Left**<br>**M Metatarsal-Phalangeal Joint, Right**<br>Metatarsophalangeal (MTP) joint<br>**N Metatarsal-Phalangeal Joint, Left**<br>*See M Metatarsal-Phalangeal Joint, Right*<br>**P Toe Phalangeal Joint, Right**<br>Interphalangeal (IP) joint<br>**Q Toe Phalangeal Joint, Left**<br>*See P Toe Phalangeal Joint, Right* | **Ø Open**<br>**3 Percutaneous**<br>**4 Percutaneous Endoscopic** | **Ø Drainage Device** | **Z No Qualifier** |
| **Ø Lumbar Vertebral Joint**<br>Lumbar facet joint<br>**2 Lumbar Vertebral Disc**<br>**3 Lumbosacral Joint**<br>Lumbosacral facet joint<br>**4 Lumbosacral Disc**<br>**5 Sacrococcygeal Joint**<br>Sacrococcygeal symphysis<br>**6 Coccygeal Joint**<br>**7 Sacroiliac Joint, Right**<br>**8 Sacroiliac Joint, Left**<br>**9 Hip Joint, Right**<br>Acetabulofemoral joint<br>**B Hip Joint, Left**<br>*See 9 Hip Joint, Right*<br>**C Knee Joint, Right**<br>Femoropatellar joint<br>Femorotibial joint<br>Lateral meniscus<br>Medial meniscus<br>Patellofemoral joint<br>Tibiofemoral joint<br>**D Knee Joint, Left**<br>*See C Knee Joint, Right*<br>**F Ankle Joint, Right**<br>Inferior tibiofibular joint<br>Talocrural joint<br>**G Ankle Joint, Left**<br>*See F Ankle Joint, Right*<br>**H Tarsal Joint, Right**<br>Calcaneocuboid joint<br>Cuboideonavicular joint<br>Cuneonavicular joint<br>Intercuneiform joint<br>Subtalar (talocalcaneal) joint<br>Talocalcaneal (subtalar) joint<br>Talocalcaneonavicular joint<br>**J Tarsal Joint, Left**<br>*See H Tarsal Joint, Right*<br>**K Tarsometatarsal Joint, Right**<br>**L Tarsometatarsal Joint, Left**<br>**M Metatarsal-Phalangeal Joint, Right**<br>Metatarsophalangeal (MTP) joint<br>**N Metatarsal-Phalangeal Joint, Left**<br>*See M Metatarsal-Phalangeal Joint, Right*<br>**P Toe Phalangeal Joint, Right**<br>Interphalangeal (IP) joint<br>**Q Toe Phalangeal Joint, Left**<br>*See P Toe Phalangeal Joint, Right* | **Ø Open**<br>**3 Percutaneous**<br>**4 Percutaneous Endoscopic** | **Z No Device** | **X Diagnostic**<br>**Z No Qualifier** |

**Non-OR** ØS9[Ø,2,3,4,5,6,7,8,9,B,C,D,F,G,H,J,K,L,M,N,P,Q][3,4]ØZ
**Non-OR** ØS9[Ø,2,3,4,5,6,7,8,9,B,C,D,F,G,H,J,K,L,M,N,P,Q][Ø,3,4]ZX
**Non-OR** ØS9[Ø,2,3,4,5,6,7,8,9,B,C,D,F,G,H,J,K,L,M,N,P,Q][3,4]ZZ

**Ø Medical and Surgical**
**S Lower Joints**
**B Excision** Definition: Cutting out or off, without replacement, a portion of a body part

Explanation: The qualifier DIAGNOSTIC is used to identify excision procedures that are biopsies

| Body Part Character 4 | | Approach Character 5 | Device Character 6 | Qualifier Character 7 |
|---|---|---|---|---|
| **Ø Lumbar Vertebral Joint** Lumbar facet joint<br>**2 Lumbar Vertebral Disc**<br>**3 Lumbosacral Joint** Lumbosacral facet joint<br>**4 Lumbosacral Disc**<br>**5 Sacrococcygeal Joint** Sacrococcygeal symphysis<br>**6 Coccygeal Joint**<br>**7 Sacroiliac Joint, Right**<br>**8 Sacroiliac Joint, Left**<br>**9 Hip Joint, Right** Acetabulofemoral joint<br>**B Hip Joint, Left** *See 9 Hip Joint, Right*<br>**C Knee Joint, Right** Femoropatellar joint, Femorotibial joint, Lateral meniscus, Medial meniscus, Patellofemoral joint, Tibiofemoral joint<br>**D Knee Joint, Left** *See C Knee Joint, Right*<br>**F Ankle Joint, Right** Inferior tibiofibular joint, Talocrural joint<br>**G Ankle Joint, Left** *See F Ankle Joint, Right* | **H Tarsal Joint, Right** Calcaneocuboid joint, Cuboideonavicular joint, Cuneonavicular joint, Intercuneiform joint, Subtalar (talocalcaneal) joint, Talocalcaneal (subtalar) joint, Talocalcaneonavicular joint<br>**J Tarsal Joint, Left** *See H Tarsal Joint, Right*<br>**K Tarsometatarsal Joint, Right**<br>**L Tarsometatarsal Joint, Left**<br>**M Metatarsal-Phalangeal Joint, Right** Metatarsophalangeal (MTP) joint<br>**N Metatarsal-Phalangeal Joint, Left** *See M Metatarsal-Phalangeal Joint, Right*<br>**P Toe Phalangeal Joint, Right** Interphalangeal (IP) joint<br>**Q Toe Phalangeal Joint, Left** *See P Toe Phalangeal Joint, Right* | **Ø Open**<br>**3 Percutaneous**<br>**4 Percutaneous Endoscopic** | **Z No Device** | **X Diagnostic**<br>**Z No Qualifier** |

**Non-OR** ØSB[Ø,2,3,4,5,6,7,8,9,B,C,D,F,G,H,J,K,L,M,N,P,Q][Ø,3,4]ZX

**Ø Medical and Surgical**
**S Lower Joints**
**C Extirpation** Definition: Taking or cutting out solid matter from a body part

Explanation: The solid matter may be an abnormal byproduct of a biological function or a foreign body; it may be imbedded in a body part or in the lumen of a tubular body part. The solid matter may or may not have been previously broken into pieces.

| Body Part Character 4 | | Approach Character 5 | Device Character 6 | Qualifier Character 7 |
|---|---|---|---|---|
| **Ø Lumbar Vertebral Joint** Lumbar facet joint<br>**2 Lumbar Vertebral Disc**<br>**3 Lumbosacral Joint** Lumbosacral facet joint<br>**4 Lumbosacral Disc**<br>**5 Sacrococcygeal Joint** Sacrococcygeal symphysis<br>**6 Coccygeal Joint**<br>**7 Sacroiliac Joint, Right**<br>**8 Sacroiliac Joint, Left**<br>**9 Hip Joint, Right** Acetabulofemoral joint<br>**B Hip Joint, Left** *See 9 Hip Joint, Right*<br>**C Knee Joint, Right** Femoropatellar joint, Femorotibial joint, Lateral meniscus, Medial meniscus, Patellofemoral joint, Tibiofemoral joint<br>**D Knee Joint, Left** *See C Knee Joint, Right*<br>**F Ankle Joint, Right** Inferior tibiofibular joint, Talocrural joint<br>**G Ankle Joint, Left** *See F Ankle Joint, Right* | **H Tarsal Joint, Right** Calcaneocuboid joint, Cuboideonavicular joint, Cuneonavicular joint, Intercuneiform joint, Subtalar (talocalcaneal) joint, Talocalcaneal (subtalar) joint, Talocalcaneonavicular joint<br>**J Tarsal Joint, Left** *See H Tarsal Joint, Right*<br>**K Tarsometatarsal Joint, Right**<br>**L Tarsometatarsal Joint, Left**<br>**M Metatarsal-Phalangeal Joint, Right** Metatarsophalangeal (MTP) joint<br>**N Metatarsal-Phalangeal Joint, Left** *See M Metatarsal-Phalangeal Joint, Right*<br>**P Toe Phalangeal Joint, Right** Interphalangeal (IP) joint<br>**Q Toe Phalangeal Joint, Left** *See P Toe Phalangeal Joint, Right* | **Ø Open**<br>**3 Percutaneous**<br>**4 Percutaneous Endoscopic** | **Z No Device** | **Z No Qualifier** |

**Ø Medical and Surgical**
**S Lower Joints**
**G Fusion**

Definition: Joining together portions of an articular body part rendering the articular body part immobile

Explanation: The body part is joined together by fixation device, bone graft, or other means

| Body Part Character 4 | Approach Character 5 | Device Character 6 | Qualifier Character 7 |
|---|---|---|---|
| **Ø Lumbar Vertebral Joint**<br>Lumbar facet joint<br>**1 Lumbar Vertebral Joints, 2 or more** ⊞<br>**3 Lumbosacral Joint**<br>Lumbosacral facet joint | **Ø Open**<br>**3 Percutaneous**<br>**4 Percutaneous Endoscopic** | **7 Autologous Tissue Substitute**<br>**J Synthetic Substitute**<br>**K Nonautologous Tissue Substitute**<br>**Z No Device** | **Ø Anterior Approach, Anterior Column**<br>**1 Posterior Approach, Posterior Column**<br>**J Posterior Approach, Anterior Column** |
| **Ø Lumbar Vertebral Joint**<br>Lumbar facet joint<br>**1 Lumbar Vertebral Joints, 2 or more** ⊞<br>**3 Lumbosacral Joint**<br>Lumbosacral facet joint | **Ø Open**<br>**3 Percutaneous**<br>**4 Percutaneous Endoscopic** | **A Interbody Fusion Device** | **Ø Anterior Approach, Anterior Column**<br>**J Posterior Approach, Anterior Column** |
| **5 Sacrococcygeal Joint**<br>Sacrococcygeal symphysis<br>**6 Coccygeal Joint**<br>**7 Sacroiliac Joint, Right**<br>**8 Sacroiliac Joint, Left** | **Ø Open**<br>**3 Percutaneous**<br>**4 Percutaneous Endoscopic** | **4 Internal Fixation Device**<br>**7 Autologous Tissue Substitute**<br>**J Synthetic Substitute**<br>**K Nonautologous Tissue Substitute**<br>**Z No Device** | **Z No Qualifier** |
| **9 Hip Joint, Right**<br>Acetabulofemoral joint<br>**B Hip Joint, Left**<br>*See 9 Hip Joint, Right*<br>**C Knee Joint, Right**<br>Femoropatellar joint<br>Femorotibial joint<br>Lateral meniscus<br>Medial meniscus<br>Patellofemoral joint<br>Tibiofemoral joint<br>**D Knee Joint, Left**<br>*See C Knee Joint, Right*<br>**F Ankle Joint, Right**<br>Inferior tibiofibular joint<br>Talocrural joint<br>**G Ankle Joint, Left**<br>*See F Ankle Joint, Right*<br>**H Tarsal Joint, Right**<br>Calcaneocuboid joint<br>Cuboideonavicular joint<br>Cuneonavicular joint<br>Intercuneiform joint<br>Subtalar (talocalcaneal) joint<br>Talocalcaneal (subtalar) joint<br>Talocalcaneonavicular joint<br>**J Tarsal Joint, Left**<br>*See H Tarsal Joint, Right*<br>**K Tarsometatarsal Joint, Right**<br>**L Tarsometatarsal Joint, Left**<br>**M Metatarsal-Phalangeal Joint, Right**<br>Metatarsophalangeal (MTP) joint<br>**N Metatarsal-Phalangeal Joint, Left**<br>*See M Metatarsal-Phalangeal Joint, Right*<br>**P Toe Phalangeal Joint, Right**<br>Interphalangeal (IP) joint<br>**Q Toe Phalangeal Joint, Left**<br>*See P Toe Phalangeal Joint, Right* | **Ø Open**<br>**3 Percutaneous**<br>**4 Percutaneous Endoscopic** | **4 Internal Fixation Device**<br>**5 External Fixation Device**<br>**7 Autologous Tissue Substitute**<br>**J Synthetic Substitute**<br>**K Nonautologous Tissue Substitute**<br>**Z No Device** | **Z No Qualifier** |

**HAC** ØSG[Ø,1,3][Ø,3,4][7,J,K,Z][Ø,1,J] when reported with SDx K68.11 or T81.4XXA or T84.6Ø-T84.619, T84.63-T84.7 with 7th character A

**HAC** ØSG[Ø,1,3][Ø,3,4]A[Ø,J] when reported with SDx K68.11 or T81.4XXA or T84.6Ø-T84.619, T84.63-T84.7 with 7th character A

**HAC** ØSG[7,8][Ø,3,4][4,7,J,K,Z]Z when reported with SDx K68.11 or T81.4XXA or T84.6Ø-T84.619, T84.63-T84.7 with 7th character A

**See Appendix L for Procedure Combinations**

⊞ ØSG1[Ø,3,4][7,J,K,Z][Ø,1,J]

⊞ ØSG1[Ø,3,4]A[Ø,J]

**Ø Medical and Surgical**
**S Lower Joints**
**H Insertion** Definition: Putting in a nonbiological appliance that monitors, assists, performs, or prevents a physiological function but does not physically take the place of a body part

Explanation: None

| Body Part Character 4 | Approach Character 5 | Device Character 6 | Qualifier Character 7 |
|---|---|---|---|
| **Ø Lumbar Vertebral Joint**<br>Lumbar facet joint<br>**3 Lumbosacral Joint**<br>Lumbosacral facet joint | **Ø Open**<br>**3 Percutaneous**<br>**4 Percutaneous Endoscopic** | **3 Infusion Device**<br>**4 Internal Fixation Device**<br>**8 Spacer**<br>**B Spinal Stabilization Device, Interspinous Process**<br>**C Spinal Stabilization Device, Pedicle-Based**<br>**D Spinal Stabilization Device, Facet Replacement** | **Z No Qualifier** |
| **2 Lumbar Vertebral Disc**<br>**4 Lumbosacral Disc** | **Ø Open**<br>**3 Percutaneous**<br>**4 Percutaneous Endoscopic** | **3 Infusion Device**<br>**8 Spacer** | **Z No Qualifier** |
| **5 Sacrococcygeal Joint**<br>Sacrococcygeal symphysis<br>**6 Coccygeal Joint**<br>**7 Sacroiliac Joint, Right**<br>**8 Sacroiliac Joint, Left** | **Ø Open**<br>**3 Percutaneous**<br>**4 Percutaneous Endoscopic** | **3 Infusion Device**<br>**4 Internal Fixation Device**<br>**8 Spacer** | **Z No Qualifier** |
| **9 Hip Joint, Right**<br>Acetabulofemoral joint<br>**B Hip Joint, Left**<br>*See 9 Hip Joint, Right*<br>**C Knee Joint, Right**<br>Femoropatellar joint<br>Femorotibial joint<br>Lateral meniscus<br>Medial meniscus<br>Patellofemoral joint<br>Tibiofemoral joint<br>**D Knee Joint, Left**<br>*See C Knee Joint, Right*<br>**F Ankle Joint, Right**<br>Inferior tibiofibular joint<br>Talocrural joint<br>**G Ankle Joint, Left**<br>*See F Ankle Joint, Right*<br>**H Tarsal Joint, Right**<br>Calcaneocuboid joint<br>Cuboideonavicular joint<br>Cuneonavicular joint<br>Intercuneiform joint<br>Subtalar (talocalcaneal) joint<br>Talocalcaneal (subtalar) joint<br>Talocalcaneonavicular joint<br>**J Tarsal Joint, Left**<br>*See H Tarsal Joint, Right*<br>**K Tarsometatarsal Joint, Right**<br>**L Tarsometatarsal Joint, Left**<br>**M Metatarsal-Phalangeal Joint, Right**<br>Metatarsophalangeal (MTP) joint<br>**N Metatarsal-Phalangeal Joint, Left**<br>*See M Metatarsal-Phalangeal Joint, Right*<br>**P Toe Phalangeal Joint, Right**<br>Interphalangeal (IP) joint<br>**Q Toe Phalangeal Joint, Left**<br>*See P Toe Phalangeal Joint, Right* | **Ø Open**<br>**3 Percutaneous**<br>**4 Percutaneous Endoscopic** | **3 Infusion Device**<br>**4 Internal Fixation Device**<br>**5 External Fixation Device**<br>**8 Spacer** | **Z No Qualifier** |

**Non-OR** ØSH[Ø,3][Ø,3,4][3,8]Z
**Non-OR** ØSH[2,4][Ø,3,4][3,8]Z
**Non-OR** ØSH[5,6,7,8][Ø,3,4][3,8]Z
**Non-OR** ØSH[9,B,C,D,F,G,H,J,K,L,M,N,P,Q][Ø,3,4][3,8]Z

**Ø Medical and Surgical**
**S Lower Joints**
**J Inspection**

Definition: Visually and/or manually exploring a body part

Explanation: Visual exploration may be performed with or without optical instrumentation. Manual exploration may be performed directly or through intervening body layers.

| Body Part Character 4 | | Approach Character 5 | Device Character 6 | Qualifier Character 7 |
|---|---|---|---|---|
| **Ø Lumbar Vertebral Joint**<br>Lumbar facet joint<br>**2 Lumbar Vertebral Disc**<br>**3 Lumbosacral Joint**<br>Lumbosacral facet joint<br>**4 Lumbosacral Disc**<br>**5 Sacrococcygeal Joint**<br>Sacrococcygeal symphysis<br>**6 Coccygeal Joint**<br>**7 Sacroiliac Joint, Right**<br>**8 Sacroiliac Joint, Left**<br>**9 Hip Joint, Right**<br>Acetabulofemoral joint<br>**B Hip Joint, Left**<br>*See 9 Hip Joint, Right*<br>**C Knee Joint, Right**<br>Femoropatellar joint<br>Femorotibial joint<br>Lateral meniscus<br>Medial meniscus<br>Patellofemoral joint<br>Tibiofemoral joint<br>**D Knee Joint, Left**<br>*See C Knee Joint, Right*<br>**F Ankle Joint, Right**<br>Inferior tibiofibular joint<br>Talocrural joint<br>**G Ankle Joint, Left**<br>*See F Ankle Joint, Right* | **H Tarsal Joint, Right**<br>Calcaneocuboid joint<br>Cuboideonavicular joint<br>Cuneonavicular joint<br>Intercuneiform joint<br>Subtalar (talocalcaneal) joint<br>Talocalcaneal (subtalar) joint<br>Talocalcaneonavicular joint<br>**J Tarsal Joint, Left**<br>*See H Tarsal Joint, Right*<br>**K Tarsometatarsal Joint, Right**<br>**L Tarsometatarsal Joint, Left**<br>**M Metatarsal-Phalangeal Joint, Right**<br>Metatarsophalangeal (MTP) joint<br>**N Metatarsal-Phalangeal Joint, Left**<br>*See M Metatarsal-Phalangeal Joint, Right*<br>**P Toe Phalangeal Joint, Right**<br>Interphalangeal (IP) joint<br>**Q Toe Phalangeal Joint, Left**<br>*See P Toe Phalangeal Joint, Right* | **Ø Open**<br>**3 Percutaneous**<br>**4 Percutaneous Endoscopic**<br>**X External** | **Z No Device** | **Z No Qualifier** |

**Non-OR** ØSJ[Ø,2,3,4,5,6,7,8,9,B,C,D,F,G,H,J,K,L,M,N,P,Q][3,X]ZZ

**Ø Medical and Surgical**
**S Lower Joints**
**N Release**

Definition: Freeing a body part from an abnormal physical constraint by cutting or by the use of force

Explanation: Some of the restraining tissue may be taken out but none of the body part is taken out

| Body Part Character 4 | | Approach Character 5 | Device Character 6 | Qualifier Character 7 |
|---|---|---|---|---|
| **Ø Lumbar Vertebral Joint**<br>Lumbar facet joint<br>**2 Lumbar Vertebral Disc**<br>**3 Lumbosacral Joint**<br>Lumbosacral facet joint<br>**4 Lumbosacral Disc**<br>**5 Sacrococcygeal Joint**<br>Sacrococcygeal symphysis<br>**6 Coccygeal Joint**<br>**7 Sacroiliac Joint, Right**<br>**8 Sacroiliac Joint, Left**<br>**9 Hip Joint, Right**<br>Acetabulofemoral joint<br>**B Hip Joint, Left**<br>*See 9 Hip Joint, Right*<br>**C Knee Joint, Right**<br>Femoropatellar joint<br>Femorotibial joint<br>Lateral meniscus<br>Medial meniscus<br>Patellofemoral joint<br>Tibiofemoral joint<br>**D Knee Joint, Left**<br>*See C Knee Joint, Right*<br>**F Ankle Joint, Right**<br>Inferior tibiofibular joint<br>Talocrural joint<br>**G Ankle Joint, Left**<br>*See F Ankle Joint, Right* | **H Tarsal Joint, Right**<br>Calcaneocuboid joint<br>Cuboideonavicular joint<br>Cuneonavicular joint<br>Intercuneiform joint<br>Subtalar (talocalcaneal) joint<br>Talocalcaneal (subtalar) joint<br>Talocalcaneonavicular joint<br>**J Tarsal Joint, Left**<br>*See H Tarsal Joint, Right*<br>**K Tarsometatarsal Joint, Right**<br>**L Tarsometatarsal Joint, Left**<br>**M Metatarsal-Phalangeal Joint, Right**<br>Metatarsophalangeal (MTP) joint<br>**N Metatarsal-Phalangeal Joint, Left**<br>*See M Metatarsal-Phalangeal Joint, Right*<br>**P Toe Phalangeal Joint, Right**<br>Interphalangeal (IP) joint<br>**Q Toe Phalangeal Joint, Left**<br>*See P Toe Phalangeal Joint, Right* | **Ø Open**<br>**3 Percutaneous**<br>**4 Percutaneous Endoscopic**<br>**X External** | **Z No Device** | **Z No Qualifier** |

**Non-OR** ØSN[Ø,2,3,4,5,6,7,8,9,B,C,D,F,G,H,J,K,L,M,N,P,Q]XZZ

**Ø Medical and Surgical**
**S Lower Joints**
**P Removal** Definition: Taking out or off a device from a body part

Explanation: If a device is taken out and a similar device put in without cutting or puncturing the skin or mucous membrane, the procedure is coded to the root operation CHANGE. Otherwise, the procedure for taking out the device is coded to the root operation REMOVAL.

| Body Part Character 4 | Approach Character 5 | Device Character 6 | Qualifier Character 7 |
|---|---|---|---|
| Ø Lumbar Vertebral Joint<br>Lumbar facet joint<br>3 Lumbosacral Joint<br>Lumbosacral facet joint | Ø Open<br>3 Percutaneous<br>4 Percutaneous Endoscopic | Ø Drainage Device<br>3 Infusion Device<br>4 Internal Fixation Device<br>7 Autologous Tissue Substitute<br>8 Spacer<br>A Interbody Fusion Device<br>J Synthetic Substitute<br>K Nonautologous Tissue Substitute | Z No Qualifier |
| Ø Lumbar Vertebral Joint<br>Lumbar facet joint<br>3 Lumbosacral Joint<br>Lumbosacral facet joint | X External | Ø Drainage Device<br>3 Infusion Device<br>4 Internal Fixation Device | Z No Qualifier |
| 2 Lumbar Vertebral Disc<br>4 Lumbosacral Disc | Ø Open<br>3 Percutaneous<br>4 Percutaneous Endoscopic | Ø Drainage Device<br>3 Infusion Device<br>7 Autologous Tissue Substitute<br>J Synthetic Substitute<br>K Nonautologous Tissue Substitute | Z No Qualifier |
| 2 Lumbar Vertebral Disc<br>4 Lumbosacral Disc | X External | Ø Drainage Device<br>3 Infusion Device | Z No Qualifier |
| 5 Sacrococcygeal Joint<br>Sacrococcygeal symphysis<br>6 Coccygeal Joint<br>7 Sacroiliac Joint, Right<br>8 Sacroiliac Joint, Left | Ø Open<br>3 Percutaneous<br>4 Percutaneous Endoscopic | Ø Drainage Device<br>3 Infusion Device<br>4 Internal Fixation Device<br>7 Autologous Tissue Substitute<br>8 Spacer<br>J Synthetic Substitute<br>K Nonautologous Tissue Substitute | Z No Qualifier |
| 5 Sacrococcygeal Joint<br>Sacrococcygeal symphysis<br>6 Coccygeal Joint<br>7 Sacroiliac Joint, Right<br>8 Sacroiliac Joint, Left | X External | Ø Drainage Device<br>3 Infusion Device<br>4 Internal Fixation Device | Z No Qualifier |
| 9 Hip Joint, Right ⊞<br>Acetabulofemoral joint<br>B Hip Joint, Left ⊞<br>*See 9 Hip Joint, Right* | Ø Open | Ø Drainage Device<br>3 Infusion Device<br>4 Internal Fixation Device<br>5 External Fixation Device<br>7 Autologous Tissue Substitute<br>8 Spacer<br>9 Liner<br>B Resurfacing Device<br>J Synthetic Substitute<br>K Nonautologous Tissue Substitute | Z No Qualifier |
| 9 Hip Joint, Right ⊞<br>Acetabulofemoral joint<br>B Hip Joint, Left ⊞<br>*See 9 Hip Joint, Right* | 3 Percutaneous<br>4 Percutaneous Endoscopic | Ø Drainage Device<br>3 Infusion Device<br>4 Internal Fixation Device<br>5 External Fixation Device<br>7 Autologous Tissue Substitute<br>8 Spacer<br>J Synthetic Substitute<br>K Nonautologous Tissue Substitute | Z No Qualifier |
| 9 Hip Joint, Right<br>Acetabulofemoral joint<br>B Hip Joint, Left<br>*See 9 Hip Joint, Right* | X External | Ø Drainage Device<br>3 Infusion Device<br>4 Internal Fixation Device<br>5 External Fixation Device | Z No Qualifier |

*ØSP Continued on next page*

| | |
|---|---|
| DRG Non-OR | ØSP[9,B]Ø8Z |
| DRG Non-OR | ØSP[9,B]48Z |
| Non-OR | ØSP[Ø,3]3[Ø,3,8]Z |
| Non-OR | ØSP[Ø,3][Ø,4]8Z |
| Non-OR | ØSP[Ø,3]X[Ø,3,4]Z |
| Non-OR | ØSP[2,4]3[Ø,3]Z |
| Non-OR | ØSP[2,4]X[Ø,3]Z |
| Non-OR | ØSP[5,6,7,8]3[Ø,3,8]Z |
| Non-OR | ØSP[5,6,7,8][Ø,4]8Z |
| Non-OR | ØSP[5,6,7,8]X[Ø,3,4]Z |
| Non-OR | ØSP[9,B]3[Ø,3,8]Z |
| Non-OR | ØSP[9,B]X[Ø,3,4,5]Z |

**See Appendix L for Procedure Combinations**

| | |
|---|---|
| Combo-only | ØSP[9,B]Ø8Z |
| Combo-only | ØSP[9,B]48Z |
| ⊞ | ØSP[9,B]Ø[9,B,J]Z |
| ⊞ | ØSP[9,B]4JZ |

ØSP Continued

**Ø Medical and Surgical**
**S Lower Joints**
**P Removal** Definition: Taking out or off a device from a body part

Explanation: If a device is taken out and a similar device put in without cutting or puncturing the skin or mucous membrane, the procedure is coded to the root operation CHANGE. Otherwise, the procedure for taking out the device is coded to the root operation REMOVAL.

| Body Part Character 4 | Approach Character 5 | Device Character 6 | Qualifier Character 7 |
|---|---|---|---|
| **A** Hip Joint, Acetabular Surface, Right ⊞<br>**E** Hip Joint, Acetabular Surface, Left ⊞<br>**R** Hip Joint, Femoral Surface, Right ⊞<br>**S** Hip Joint, Femoral Surface, Left ⊞<br>**T** Knee Joint, Femoral Surface, Right ⊞<br>Femoropatellar joint<br>Patellofemoral joint<br>**U** Knee Joint, Femoral Surface, Left ⊞<br>*See T Knee Joint, Femoral Surface, Right*<br>**V** Knee Joint, Tibial Surface, Right ⊞<br>Femorotibial joint<br>Tibiofemoral joint<br>**W** Knee Joint, Tibial Surface, Left ⊞<br>*See V Knee Joint, Tibial Surface, Right* | **Ø** Open<br>**3** Percutaneous<br>**4** Percutaneous Endoscopic | **J** Synthetic Substitute | **Z** No Qualifier |
| **C** Knee Joint, Right ⊞<br>Femoropatellar joint<br>Femorotibial joint<br>Lateral meniscus<br>Medial meniscus<br>Patellofemoral joint<br>Tibiofemoral joint<br>**D** Knee Joint, Left ⊞<br>*See C Knee Joint, Right* | **Ø** Open | **Ø** Drainage Device<br>**3** Infusion Device<br>**4** Internal Fixation Device<br>**5** External Fixation Device<br>**7** Autologous Tissue Substitute<br>**8** Spacer<br>**9** Liner<br>**K** Nonautologous Tissue Substitute | **Z** No Qualifier |
| **C** Knee Joint, Right ⊞<br>Femoropatellar joint<br>Femorotibial joint<br>Lateral meniscus<br>Medial meniscus<br>Patellofemoral joint<br>Tibiofemoral joint<br>**D** Knee Joint, Left ⊞<br>*See C Knee Joint, Right* | **Ø** Open | **J** Synthetic Substitute | **C** Patellar Surface<br>**Z** No Qualifier |
| **C** Knee Joint, Right<br>Femoropatellar joint<br>Femorotibial joint<br>Lateral meniscus<br>Medial meniscus<br>Patellofemoral joint<br>Tibiofemoral joint<br>**D** Knee Joint, Left<br>*See C Knee Joint, Right* | **3** Percutaneous<br>**4** Percutaneous Endoscopic | **Ø** Drainage Device<br>**3** Infusion Device<br>**4** Internal Fixation Device<br>**5** External Fixation Device<br>**7** Autologous Tissue Substitute<br>**8** Spacer<br>**K** Nonautologous Tissue Substitute | **Z** No Qualifier |
| **C** Knee Joint, Right ⊞<br>Femoropatellar joint<br>Femorotibial joint<br>Lateral meniscus<br>Medial meniscus<br>Patellofemoral joint<br>Tibiofemoral joint<br>**D** Knee Joint, Left ⊞<br>*See C Knee Joint, Right* | **3** Percutaneous<br>**4** Percutaneous Endoscopic | **J** Synthetic Substitute | **C** Patellar Surface<br>**Z** No Qualifier |
| **C** Knee Joint, Right<br>Femoropatellar joint<br>Femorotibial joint<br>Lateral meniscus<br>Medial meniscus<br>Patellofemoral joint<br>Tibiofemoral joint<br>**D** Knee Joint, Left<br>*See C Knee Joint, Right* | **X** External | **Ø** Drainage Device<br>**3** Infusion Device<br>**4** Internal Fixation Device<br>**5** External Fixation Device | **Z** No Qualifier |

ØSP Continued on next page

DRG Non-OR ØSP[C,D]Ø8Z
DRG Non-OR ØSP[C,D][3,4]8Z
Non-OR ØSP[C,D]3[Ø,3]Z
Non-OR ØSP[C,D]X[Ø,3,4,5]Z

**See Appendix L for Procedure Combinations**
Combo-only ØSP[C,D]Ø8Z
Combo-only ØSP[C,D][3,4]8Z
⊞ ØSP[A,E,R,S,T,U,V,W][Ø,4]JZ
⊞ ØSP[C,D]Ø9Z
⊞ ØSP[C,D]ØJ[C,Z]
⊞ ØSP[C,D]4J[C,Z]

**Ø Medical and Surgical**
**S Lower Joints**
**P Removal** Definition: Taking out or off a device from a body part

Explanation: If a device is taken out and a similar device put in without cutting or puncturing the skin or mucous membrane, the procedure is coded to the root operation CHANGE. Otherwise, the procedure for taking out the device is coded to the root operation REMOVAL.

***ØSP Continued***

| Body Part Character 4 | Approach Character 5 | Device Character 6 | Qualifier Character 7 |
|---|---|---|---|
| **F Ankle Joint, Right**<br>Inferior tibiofibular joint<br>Talocrural joint<br>**G Ankle Joint, Left**<br>*See F Ankle Joint, Right*<br>**H Tarsal Joint, Right**<br>Calcaneocuboid joint<br>Cuboideonavicular joint<br>Cuneonavicular joint<br>Intercuneiform joint<br>Subtalar (talocalcaneal) joint<br>Talocalcaneal (subtalar) joint<br>Talocalcaneonavicular joint<br>**J Tarsal Joint, Left**<br>*See H Tarsal Joint, Right*<br>**K Tarsometatarsal Joint, Right**<br>**L Tarsometatarsal Joint, Left**<br>**M Metatarsal-Phalangeal Joint, Right**<br>Metatarsophalangeal (MTP) joint<br>**N Metatarsal-Phalangeal Joint, Left**<br>*See M Metatarsal-Phalangeal Joint, Right*<br>**P Toe Phalangeal Joint, Right**<br>Interphalangeal (IP) joint<br>**Q Toe Phalangeal Joint, Left**<br>*See P Toe Phalangeal Joint, Right* | **Ø Open**<br>**3 Percutaneous**<br>**4 Percutaneous Endoscopic** | **Ø Drainage Device**<br>**3 Infusion Device**<br>**4 Internal Fixation Device**<br>**5 External Fixation Device**<br>**7 Autologous Tissue Substitute**<br>**8 Spacer**<br>**J Synthetic Substitute**<br>**K Nonautologous Tissue Substitute** | **Z No Qualifier** |
| **F Ankle Joint, Right**<br>Inferior tibiofibular joint<br>Talocrural joint<br>**G Ankle Joint, Left**<br>*See F Ankle Joint, Right*<br>**H Tarsal Joint, Right**<br>Calcaneocuboid joint<br>Cuboideonavicular joint<br>Cuneonavicular joint<br>Intercuneiform joint<br>Subtalar (talocalcaneal) joint<br>Talocalcaneal (subtalar) joint<br>Talocalcaneonavicular joint<br>**J Tarsal Joint, Left**<br>*See H Tarsal Joint, Right*<br>**K Tarsometatarsal Joint, Right**<br>**L Tarsometatarsal Joint, Left**<br>**M Metatarsal-Phalangeal Joint, Right**<br>Metatarsophalangeal (MTP) joint<br>**N Metatarsal-Phalangeal Joint, Left**<br>*See M Metatarsal-Phalangeal Joint, Right*<br>**P Toe Phalangeal Joint, Right**<br>Interphalangeal (IP) joint<br>**Q Toe Phalangeal Joint, Left**<br>*See P Toe Phalangeal Joint, Right* | **X External** | **Ø Drainage Device**<br>**3 Infusion Device**<br>**4 Internal Fixation Device**<br>**5 External Fixation Device** | **Z No Qualifier** |

**Non-OR** ØSP[F,G,H,J,K,L,M,N,P,Q]3[Ø,3,8]Z
**Non-OR** ØSP[F,G,H,J,K,L,M,N,P,Q][Ø,4]8Z
**Non-OR** ØSP[F,G,H,J,K,L,M,N,P,Q]X[Ø,3,4,5]Z

**Ø Medical and Surgical**
**S Lower Joints**
**Q Repair** Definition: Restoring, to the extent possible, a body part to its normal anatomic structure and function
Explanation: Used only when the method to accomplish the repair is not one of the other root operations

| Body Part Character 4 | Approach Character 5 | Device Character 6 | Qualifier Character 7 |
|---|---|---|---|
| **Ø Lumbar Vertebral Joint**<br>Lumbar facet joint<br>**2 Lumbar Vertebral Disc**<br>**3 Lumbosacral Joint**<br>Lumbosacral facet joint<br>**4 Lumbosacral Disc**<br>**5 Sacrococcygeal Joint**<br>Sacrococcygeal symphysis<br>**6 Coccygeal Joint**<br>**7 Sacroiliac Joint, Right**<br>**8 Sacroiliac Joint, Left**<br>**9 Hip Joint, Right**<br>Acetabulofemoral joint<br>**B Hip Joint, Left**<br>*See 9 Hip Joint, Right*<br>**C Knee Joint, Right**<br>Femoropatellar joint<br>Femorotibial joint<br>Lateral meniscus<br>Medial meniscus<br>Patellofemoral joint<br>Tibiofemoral joint<br>**D Knee Joint, Left**<br>*See C Knee Joint, Right*<br>**F Ankle Joint, Right**<br>Inferior tibiofibular joint<br>Talocrural joint<br>**G Ankle Joint, Left**<br>*See F Ankle Joint, Right*<br>**H Tarsal Joint, Right**<br>Calcaneocuboid joint<br>Cuboideonavicular joint<br>Cuneonavicular joint<br>Intercuneiform joint<br>Subtalar (talocalcaneal) joint<br>Talocalcaneal (subtalar) joint<br>Talocalcaneonavicular joint<br>**J Tarsal Joint, Left**<br>*See H Tarsal Joint, Right*<br>**K Tarsometatarsal Joint, Right**<br>**L Tarsometatarsal Joint, Left**<br>**M Metatarsal-Phalangeal Joint, Right**<br>Metatarsophalangeal (MTP) joint<br>**N Metatarsal-Phalangeal Joint, Left**<br>*See M Metatarsal-Phalangeal Joint, Right*<br>**P Toe Phalangeal Joint, Right**<br>Interphalangeal (IP) joint<br>**Q Toe Phalangeal Joint, Left**<br>*See P Toe Phalangeal Joint, Right* | **Ø Open**<br>**3 Percutaneous**<br>**4 Percutaneous Endoscopic**<br>**X External** | **Z No Device** | **Z No Qualifier** |

**Non-OR** ØSQ[Ø,2,3,4,5,6,7,8,9,B,C,D,F,G,H,J,K,L,M,N,P,Q]XZZ

**Ø Medical and Surgical**
**S Lower Joints**
**R Replacement** Definition: Putting in or on biological or synthetic material that physically takes the place and/or function of all or a portion of a body part

Explanation: The body part may have been taken out or replaced, or may be taken out, physically eradicated, or rendered nonfunctional during the REPLACEMENT procedure. A REMOVAL procedure is coded for taking out the device used in a previous replacement procedure.

| Body Part Character 4 | Approach Character 5 | Device Character 6 | Qualifier Character 7 |
|---|---|---|---|
| **Ø Lumbar Vertebral Joint**<br>Lumbar facet joint<br>**2 Lumbar Vertebral Disc** NC<br>**3 Lumbosacral Joint**<br>Lumbosacral facet joint<br>**4 Lumbosacral Disc** NC<br>**5 Sacrococcygeal Joint**<br>Sacrococcygeal symphysis<br>**6 Coccygeal Joint**<br>**7 Sacroiliac Joint, Right**<br>**8 Sacroiliac Joint, Left**<br>**H Tarsal Joint, Right**<br>Calcaneocuboid joint<br>Cuboideonavicular joint<br>Cuneonavicular joint<br>Intercuneiform joint<br>Subtalar (talocalcaneal) joint<br>Talocalcaneal (subtalar) joint<br>Talocalcaneonavicular joint<br>**J Tarsal Joint, Left**<br>*See H Tarsal Joint, Right*<br>**K Tarsometatarsal Joint, Right**<br>**L Tarsometatarsal Joint, Left**<br>**M Metatarsal-Phalangeal Joint, Right**<br>Metatarsophalangeal (MTP) joint<br>**N Metatarsal-Phalangeal Joint, Left**<br>*See M Metatarsal-Phalangeal Joint, Right*<br>**P Toe Phalangeal Joint, Right**<br>Interphalangeal (IP) joint<br>**Q Toe Phalangeal Joint, Left**<br>*See P Toe Phalangeal Joint, Right* | **Ø Open** | **7 Autologous Tissue Substitute**<br>**J Synthetic Substitute**<br>**K Nonautologous Tissue Substitute** | **Z No Qualifier** |
| **9 Hip Joint, Right** ⊞<br>Acetabulofemoral joint<br>**B Hip Joint, Left** ⊞<br>*See 9 Hip Joint, Right* | **Ø Open** | **1 Synthetic Substitute, Metal**<br>**2 Synthetic Substitute, Metal on Polyethylene**<br>**3 Synthetic Substitute, Ceramic**<br>**4 Synthetic Substitute, Ceramic on Polyethylene**<br>**6 Synthetic Substitute, Oxidized Zirconium on Polyethylene**<br>**J Synthetic Substitute** | **9 Cemented**<br>**A Uncemented**<br>**Z No Qualifier** |
| **9 Hip Joint, Right**<br>Acetabulofemoral joint<br>**B Hip Joint, Left**<br>*See 9 Hip Joint, Right* | **Ø Open** | **7 Autologous Tissue Substitute**<br>**K Nonautologous Tissue Substitute** | **Z No Qualifier** |
| **A Hip Joint, Acetabular Surface, Right** ⊞<br>**E Hip Joint, Acetabular Surface, Left** ⊞ | **Ø Open** | **Ø Synthetic Substitute, Polyethylene**<br>**1 Synthetic Substitute, Metal**<br>**3 Synthetic Substitute, Ceramic**<br>**J Synthetic Substitute** | **9 Cemented**<br>**A Uncemented**<br>**Z No Qualifier** |
| **A Hip Joint, Acetabular Surface, Right**<br>**E Hip Joint, Acetabular Surface, Left** | **Ø Open** | **7 Autologous Tissue Substitute**<br>**K Nonautologous Tissue Substitute** | **Z No Qualifier** |

***ØSR Continued on next page***

HAC ØSR[9,B]Ø[1,2,3,4,J][9,A,Z] when reported with SDx of I26.Ø2-I26.Ø9, I26.92-I26.99, or I82.4Ø1-I82.4Z9

HAC ØSR[9,B]Ø[7,K]Z when reported with SDx of I26.Ø2-I26.Ø9, I26.92-I26.99, or I82.4Ø1-I82.4Z9

HAC ØSR[A,E]Ø[Ø,1,3,J][9,A,Z] when reported with SDx of I26.Ø2-I26.Ø9, I26.92-I26.99, or I82.4Ø1-I82.4Z9

HAC ØSR[A,E]Ø[7,K]Z when reported with SDx of I26.Ø2-I26.Ø9, I26.92-I26.99, or I82.4Ø1-I82.4Z9

NC ØSR[2,4]ØJZ when beneficiary age is over 6Ø

**See Appendix L for Procedure Combinations**

⊞ ØSR[9,B]Ø[1,2,3,4,J][9,A,Z]

⊞ ØSR[A,E]Ø[Ø,1,3,J][9,A,Z]

**ØSR Continued**

**Ø Medical and Surgical**
**S Lower Joints**
**R Replacement**

Definition: Putting in or on biological or synthetic material that physically takes the place and/or function of all or a portion of a body part

Explanation: The body part may have been taken out or replaced, or may be taken out, physically eradicated, or rendered nonfunctional during the REPLACEMENT procedure. A REMOVAL procedure is coded for taking out the device used in a previous replacement procedure.

| Body Part Character 4 | Approach Character 5 | Device Character 6 | Qualifier Character 7 |
|---|---|---|---|
| **C Knee Joint, Right**<br>Femoropatellar joint<br>Femorotibial joint<br>Lateral meniscus<br>Medial meniscus<br>Patellofemoral joint<br>Tibiofemoral joint<br>**D Knee Joint, Left**<br>*See C Knee Joint, Right* | **Ø Open** | **6 Synthetic Substitute, Oxidized Zirconium on Polyethylene**<br>**J Synthetic Substitute**<br>**L Synthetic Substitute, Unicondylar** | **9 Cemented**<br>**A Uncemented**<br>**Z No Qualifier** |
| **C Knee Joint, Right** ⊞<br>Femoropatellar joint<br>Femorotibial joint<br>Lateral meniscus<br>Medial meniscus<br>Patellofemoral joint<br>Tibiofemoral joint<br>**D Knee Joint, Left** ⊞<br>*See C Knee Joint, Right* | **Ø Open** | **7 Autologous Tissue Substitute**<br>**K Nonautologous Tissue Substitute** | **Z No Qualifier** |
| **F Ankle Joint, Right**<br>Inferior tibiofibular joint<br>Talocrural joint<br>**G Ankle Joint, Left**<br>*See F Ankle Joint, Right*<br>**T Knee Joint, Femoral Surface, Right**<br>Femoropatellar joint<br>Patellofemoral joint<br>**U Knee Joint, Femoral Surface, Left**<br>*See T Knee Joint, Femoral Surface, Right*<br>**V Knee Joint, Tibial Surface, Right**<br>Femorotibial joint<br>Tibiofemoral joint<br>**W Knee Joint, Tibial Surface, Left**<br>*See V Knee Joint, Tibial Surface, Right* | **Ø Open** | **7 Autologous Tissue Substitute**<br>**K Nonautologous Tissue Substitute** | **Z No Qualifier** |
| **F Ankle Joint, Right**<br>Inferior tibiofibular joint<br>Talocrural joint<br>**G Ankle Joint, Left**<br>*See F Ankle Joint, Right*<br>**T Knee Joint, Femoral Surface, Right** ⊞<br>Femoropatellar joint<br>Patellofemoral joint<br>**U Knee Joint, Femoral Surface, Left** ⊞<br>*See T Knee Joint, Femoral Surface, Right*<br>**V Knee Joint, Tibial Surface, Right** ⊞<br>Femorotibial joint<br>Tibiofemoral joint<br>**W Knee Joint, Tibial Surface, Left** ⊞<br>*See V Knee Joint, Tibial Surface, Right* | **Ø Open** | **J Synthetic Substitute** | **9 Cemented**<br>**A Uncemented**<br>**Z No Qualifier** |
| **R Hip Joint, Femoral Surface, Right** ⊞<br>**S Hip Joint, Femoral Surface, Left** ⊞ | **Ø Open** | **1 Synthetic Substitute, Metal**<br>**3 Synthetic Substitute, Ceramic**<br>**J Synthetic Substitute** | **9 Cemented**<br>**A Uncemented**<br>**Z No Qualifier** |
| **R Hip Joint, Femoral Surface, Right**<br>**S Hip Joint, Femoral Surface, Left** | **Ø Open** | **7 Autologous Tissue Substitute**<br>**K Nonautologous Tissue Substitute** | **Z No Qualifier** |

HAC ØSR[C,D]Ø[J,L][9,A,Z] when reported with SDx of I26.Ø2-I26.Ø9, I26.92-I26.99 or I82.4Ø1-I82.4Z9

HAC ØSR[C,D]Ø[7,K]Z when reported with SDx of I26.Ø2-I26.Ø9, I26.92-I26.99 or I82.4Ø1-I82.4Z9

HAC ØSR[T,U,V,W]Ø[7,K]Z when reported with SDx of I26.Ø2-I26.Ø9, I26.92-I26.99 or I82.4Ø1-I82.4Z9

HAC ØSR[T,U,V,W]ØJ[9,A,Z] when reported with SDx of I26.Ø2-I26.Ø9, I26.92-I26.99 or I82.4Ø1-I82.4Z9

HAC ØSR[R,S]Ø[1,3,J][9,A,Z] when reported with SDx of I26.Ø2-I26.Ø9, I26.92-I26.99, or I82.4Ø1-I82.4Z9

HAC ØSR[R,S]Ø[7,K]Z when reported with SDx of I26.Ø2-I26.Ø9, I26.92-I26.99, or I82.4Ø1-I82.4Z9

**See Appendix L for Procedure Combinations**

⊞ ØSR[C,D]Ø[J,L][9,A,Z]
⊞ ØSR[T,U,V,W]ØJ[9,A,Z]
⊞ ØSR[R,S]Ø[1,3,J][9,A,Z]

**Ø Medical and Surgical**
**S Lower Joints**
**S Reposition** Definition: Moving to its normal location, or other suitable location, all or a portion of a body part

Explanation: The body part is moved to a new location from an abnormal location, or from a normal location where it is not functioning correctly. The body part may or may not be cut out or off to be moved to the new location.

| Body Part Character 4 | Approach Character 5 | Device Character 6 | Qualifier Character 7 |
|---|---|---|---|
| **Ø Lumbar Vertebral Joint**<br>Lumbar facet joint<br>**3 Lumbosacral Joint**<br>Lumbosacral facet joint<br>**5 Sacrococcygeal Joint**<br>Sacrococcygeal symphysis<br>**6 Coccygeal Joint**<br>**7 Sacroiliac Joint, Right**<br>**8 Sacroiliac Joint, Left** | **Ø Open**<br>**3 Percutaneous**<br>**4 Percutaneous Endoscopic**<br>**X External** | **4 Internal Fixation Device**<br>**Z No Device** | **Z No Qualifier** |
| **9 Hip Joint, Right**<br>Acetabulofemoral joint<br>**B Hip Joint, Left**<br>*See 9 Hip Joint, Right*<br>**C Knee Joint, Right**<br>Femoropatellar joint<br>Femorotibial joint<br>Lateral meniscus<br>Medial meniscus<br>Patellofemoral joint<br>Tibiofemoral joint<br>**D Knee Joint, Left**<br>*See C Knee Joint, Right*<br>**F Ankle Joint, Right**<br>Inferior tibiofibular joint<br>Talocrural joint<br>**G Ankle Joint, Left**<br>*See F Ankle Joint, Right*<br>**H Tarsal Joint, Right**<br>Calcaneocuboid joint<br>Cuboideonavicular joint<br>Cuneonavicular joint<br>Intercuneiform joint<br>Subtalar (talocalcaneal) joint<br>Talocalcaneal (subtalar) joint<br>Talocalcaneonavicular joint<br>**J Tarsal Joint, Left**<br>*See H Tarsal Joint, Right*<br>**K Tarsometatarsal Joint, Right**<br>**L Tarsometatarsal Joint, Left**<br>**M Metatarsal-Phalangeal Joint, Right**<br>Metatarsophalangeal (MTP) joint<br>**N Metatarsal-Phalangeal Joint, Left**<br>*See M Metatarsal-Phalangeal Joint, Right*<br>**P Toe Phalangeal Joint, Right**<br>Interphalangeal (IP) joint<br>**Q Toe Phalangeal Joint, Left**<br>*See P Toe Phalangeal Joint, Right* | **Ø Open**<br>**3 Percutaneous**<br>**4 Percutaneous Endoscopic**<br>**X External** | **4 Internal Fixation Device**<br>**5 External Fixation Device**<br>**Z No Device** | **Z No Qualifier** |

**Non-OR** ØSS[Ø,3,5,6,7,8][3,4,X][4,Z]Z
**Non-OR** ØSS[9,B,C,D,F,G,H,J,K,L,M,N,P,Q][3,4,X][4,5,Z]Z

**Ø Medical and Surgical**
**S Lower Joints**
**T Resection** Definition: Cutting out or off, without replacement, all of a body part

Explanation: None

| Body Part Character 4 | Approach Character 5 | Device Character 6 | Qualifier Character 7 |
|---|---|---|---|
| **2 Lumbar Vertebral Disc**<br>**4 Lumbosacral Disc**<br>**5 Sacrococcygeal Joint**<br>Sacrococcygeal symphysis<br>**6 Coccygeal Joint**<br>**7 Sacroiliac Joint, Right**<br>**8 Sacroiliac Joint, Left**<br>**9 Hip Joint, Right**<br>Acetabulofemoral joint<br>**B Hip Joint, Left**<br>*See 9 Hip Joint, Right*<br>**C Knee Joint, Right**<br>Femoropatellar joint<br>Femorotibial joint<br>Lateral meniscus<br>Medial meniscus<br>Patellofemoral joint<br>Tibiofemoral joint<br>**D Knee Joint, Left**<br>*See C Knee Joint, Right*<br>**F Ankle Joint, Right**<br>Inferior tibiofibular joint<br>Talocrural joint<br>**G Ankle Joint, Left**<br>*See F Ankle Joint, Right*<br>**H Tarsal Joint, Right**<br>Calcaneocuboid joint<br>Cuboideonavicular joint<br>Cuneonavicular joint<br>Intercuneiform joint<br>Subtalar (talocalcaneal) joint<br>Talocalcaneal (subtalar) joint<br>Talocalcaneonavicular joint<br>**J Tarsal Joint, Left**<br>*See H Tarsal Joint, Right*<br>**K Tarsometatarsal Joint, Right**<br>**L Tarsometatarsal Joint, Left**<br>**M Metatarsal-Phalangeal Joint, Right**<br>Metatarsophalangeal (MTP) joint<br>**N Metatarsal-Phalangeal Joint, Left**<br>*See M Metatarsal-Phalangeal Joint, Right*<br>**P Toe Phalangeal Joint, Right**<br>Interphalangeal (IP) joint<br>**Q Toe Phalangeal Joint, Left**<br>*See P Toe Phalangeal Joint, Right* | **Ø Open** | **Z No Device** | **Z No Qualifier** |

**Ø Medical and Surgical**
**S Lower Joints**
**U Supplement**

Definition: Putting in or on biological or synthetic material that physically reinforces and/or augments the function of a portion of a body part

Explanation: The biological material is non-living, or is living and from the same individual. The body part may have been previously replaced, and the SUPPLEMENT procedure is performed to physically reinforce and/or augment the function of the replaced body part.

| Body Part Character 4 | Approach Character 5 | Device Character 6 | Qualifier Character 7 |
|---|---|---|---|
| **Ø Lumbar Vertebral Joint** Lumbar facet joint<br>**2 Lumbar Vertebral Disc**<br>**3 Lumbosacral Joint** Lumbosacral facet joint<br>**4 Lumbosacral Disc**<br>**5 Sacrococcygeal Joint** Sacrococcygeal symphysis<br>**6 Coccygeal Joint**<br>**7 Sacroiliac Joint, Right**<br>**8 Sacroiliac Joint, Left**<br>**F Ankle Joint, Right** Inferior tibiofibular joint; Talocrural joint<br>**G Ankle Joint, Left** *See F Ankle Joint, Right*<br>**H Tarsal Joint, Right** Calcaneocuboid joint; Cuboideonavicular joint; Cuneonavicular joint; Intercuneiform joint; Subtalar (talocalcaneal) joint; Talocalcaneal (subtalar) joint; Talocalcaneonavicular joint<br>**J Tarsal Joint, Left** *See H Tarsal Joint, Right*<br>**K Tarsometatarsal Joint, Right**<br>**L Tarsometatarsal Joint, Left**<br>**M Metatarsal-Phalangeal Joint, Right** Metatarsophalangeal (MTP) joint<br>**N Metatarsal-Phalangeal Joint, Left** *See M Metatarsal-Phalangeal Joint, Right*<br>**P Toe Phalangeal Joint, Right** Interphalangeal (IP) joint<br>**Q Toe Phalangeal Joint, Left** *See P Toe Phalangeal Joint, Right* | **Ø Open**<br>**3 Percutaneous**<br>**4 Percutaneous Endoscopic** | **7 Autologous Tissue Substitute**<br>**J Synthetic Substitute**<br>**K Nonautologous Tissue Substitute** | **Z No Qualifier** |
| **9 Hip Joint, Right** ⊞ Acetabulofemoral joint<br>**B Hip Joint, Left** ⊞ *See 9 Hip Joint, Right* | **Ø Open** | **7 Autologous Tissue Substitute**<br>**9 Liner**<br>**B Resurfacing Device**<br>**J Synthetic Substitute**<br>**K Nonautologous Tissue Substitute** | **Z No Qualifier** |
| **9 Hip Joint, Right** Acetabulofemoral joint<br>**B Hip Joint, Left** *See 9 Hip Joint, Right* | **3 Percutaneous**<br>**4 Percutaneous Endoscopic** | **7 Autologous Tissue Substitute**<br>**J Synthetic Substitute**<br>**K Nonautologous Tissue Substitute** | **Z No Qualifier** |
| **A Hip Joint, Acetabular Surface, Right** ⊞<br>**E Hip Joint, Acetabular Surface, Left** ⊞<br>**R Hip Joint, Femoral Surface, Right** ⊞<br>**S Hip Joint, Femoral Surface, Left** ⊞ | **Ø Open** | **9 Liner**<br>**B Resurfacing Device** | **Z No Qualifier** |
| **C Knee Joint, Right** Femoropatellar joint; Femorotibial joint; Lateral meniscus; Medial meniscus; Patellofemoral joint; Tibiofemoral joint<br>**D Knee Joint, Left** *See C Knee Joint, Right* | **Ø Open** | **7 Autologous Tissue Substitute**<br>**J Synthetic Substitute**<br>**K Nonautologous Tissue Substitute** | **Z No Qualifier** |
| **C Knee Joint, Right** Femoropatellar joint; Femorotibial joint; Lateral meniscus; Medial meniscus; Patellofemoral joint; Tibiofemoral joint<br>**D Knee Joint, Left** *See C Knee Joint, Right* | **Ø Open** | **9 Liner** | **C Patellar Surface**<br>**Z No Qualifier** |

***ØSU Continued on next page***

**HAC** ØSU[9,B]ØBZ when reported with SDx of I26.Ø2-I26.Ø9, I26.92-I26.99, or I82.4Ø1-I82.4Z9

**HAC** ØSU[A,E,R,S]ØBZ when reported with SDx of I26.Ø2-I26.Ø9, I26.92-I26.99, or I82.4Ø1-I82.4Z9

**See Appendix L for Procedure Combinations**
⊞ ØSU[9,B]Ø9Z
⊞ ØSU[A,E,R,S]Ø9Z

**Ø Medical and Surgical**
**S Lower Joints**
**U Supplement**

**ØSU Continued**

Definition: Putting in or on biological or synthetic material that physically reinforces and/or augments the function of a portion of a body part

Explanation: The biological material is non-living, or is living and from the same individual. The body part may have been previously replaced, and the SUPPLEMENT procedure is performed to physically reinforce and/or augment the function of the replaced body part.

| Body Part Character 4 | Approach Character 5 | Device Character 6 | Qualifier Character 7 |
|---|---|---|---|
| **C Knee Joint, Right**<br>Femoropatellar joint<br>Femorotibial joint<br>Lateral meniscus<br>Medial meniscus<br>Patellofemoral joint<br>Tibiofemoral joint<br>**D Knee Joint, Left**<br>*See C Knee Joint, Right* | **3 Percutaneous**<br>**4 Percutaneous Endoscopic** | **7 Autologous Tissue Substitute**<br>**J Synthetic Substitute**<br>**K Nonautologous Tissue Substitute** | **Z No Qualifier** |
| **T Knee Joint, Femoral Surface, Right**<br>Femoropatellar joint<br>Patellofemoral joint<br>**U Knee Joint, Femoral Surface, Left**<br>*See T Knee Joint, Femoral Surface, Right*<br>**V Knee Joint, Tibial Surface, Right** ⊞<br>Femorotibial joint<br>Tibiofemoral joint<br>**W Knee Joint, Tibial Surface, Left** ⊞<br>*See V Knee Joint, Tibial Surface, Right* | **Ø Open** | **9 Liner** | **Z No Qualifier** |

**See Appendix L for Procedure Combinations**

⊞ ØSU[V,W]Ø9Z

**Ø Medical and Surgical**
**S Lower Joints**
**W Revision** Definition: Correcting, to the extent possible, a portion of a malfunctioning device or the position of a displaced device

Explanation: Revision can include correcting a malfunctioning or displaced device by taking out or putting in components of the device such as a screw or pin

| Body Part Character 4 | Approach Character 5 | Device Character 6 | Qualifier Character 7 |
|---|---|---|---|
| **Ø Lumbar Vertebral Joint**<br>Lumbar facet joint<br>**3 Lumbosacral Joint**<br>Lumbosacral facet joint | **Ø Open**<br>**3 Percutaneous**<br>**4 Percutaneous Endoscopic**<br>**X External** | **Ø Drainage Device**<br>**3 Infusion Device**<br>**4 Internal Fixation Device**<br>**7 Autologous Tissue Substitute**<br>**8 Spacer**<br>**A Interbody Fusion Device**<br>**J Synthetic Substitute**<br>**K Nonautologous Tissue Substitute** | **Z No Qualifier** |
| **2 Lumbar Vertebral Disc**<br>**4 Lumbosacral Disc** | **Ø Open**<br>**3 Percutaneous**<br>**4 Percutaneous Endoscopic**<br>**X External** | **Ø Drainage Device**<br>**3 Infusion Device**<br>**7 Autologous Tissue Substitute**<br>**J Synthetic Substitute**<br>**K Nonautologous Tissue Substitute** | **Z No Qualifier** |
| **5 Sacrococcygeal Joint**<br>Sacrococcygeal symphysis<br>**6 Coccygeal Joint**<br>**7 Sacroiliac Joint, Right**<br>**8 Sacroiliac Joint, Left** | **Ø Open**<br>**3 Percutaneous**<br>**4 Percutaneous Endoscopic**<br>**X External** | **Ø Drainage Device**<br>**3 Infusion Device**<br>**4 Internal Fixation Device**<br>**7 Autologous Tissue Substitute**<br>**8 Spacer**<br>**J Synthetic Substitute**<br>**K Nonautologous Tissue Substitute** | **Z No Qualifier** |
| **9 Hip Joint, Right**<br>Acetabulofemoral joint<br>**B Hip Joint, Left**<br>*See 9 Hip Joint, Right* | **Ø Open** | **Ø Drainage Device**<br>**3 Infusion Device**<br>**4 Internal Fixation Device**<br>**5 External Fixation Device**<br>**7 Autologous Tissue Substitute**<br>**8 Spacer**<br>**9 Liner**<br>**B Resurfacing Device**<br>**J Synthetic Substitute**<br>**K Nonautologous Tissue Substitute** | **Z No Qualifier** |
| **9 Hip Joint, Right**<br>Acetabulofemoral joint<br>**B Hip Joint, Left**<br>*See 9 Hip Joint, Right* | **3 Percutaneous**<br>**4 Percutaneous Endoscopic**<br>**X External** | **Ø Drainage Device**<br>**3 Infusion Device**<br>**4 Internal Fixation Device**<br>**5 External Fixation Device**<br>**7 Autologous Tissue Substitute**<br>**8 Spacer**<br>**J Synthetic Substitute**<br>**K Nonautologous Tissue Substitute** | **Z No Qualifier** |
| **A Hip Joint, Acetabular Surface, Right**<br>**E Hip Joint, Acetabular Surface, Left**<br>**R Hip Joint, Femoral Surface, Right**<br>**S Hip Joint, Femoral Surface, Left**<br>**T Knee Joint, Femoral Surface, Right**<br>Femoropatellar joint<br>Patellofemoral joint<br>**U Knee Joint, Femoral Surface, Left**<br>*See T Knee Joint, Femoral Surface, Right*<br>**V Knee Joint, Tibial Surface, Right**<br>Femorotibial joint<br>Tibiofemoral joint<br>**W Knee Joint, Tibial Surface, Left**<br>*See V Knee Joint, Tibial Surface, Right* | **Ø Open**<br>**3 Percutaneous**<br>**4 Percutaneous Endoscopic**<br>**X External** | **J Synthetic Substitute** | **Z No Qualifier** |
| **C Knee Joint, Right**<br>Femoropatellar joint<br>Femorotibial joint<br>Lateral meniscus<br>Medial meniscus<br>Patellofemoral joint<br>Tibiofemoral joint<br>**D Knee Joint, Left**<br>*See C Knee Joint, Right* | **Ø Open** | **Ø Drainage Device**<br>**3 Infusion Device**<br>**4 Internal Fixation Device**<br>**5 External Fixation Device**<br>**7 Autologous Tissue Substitute**<br>**8 Spacer**<br>**9 Liner**<br>**K Nonautologous Tissue Substitute** | **Z No Qualifier** |

***ØSW Continued on next page***

**Non-OR** ØSW[Ø,3]X[Ø,3,4,7,8,A,J,K]Z
**Non-OR** ØSW[2,4]X[Ø,3,7,J,K]Z
**Non-OR** ØSW[5,6,7,8]X[Ø,3,4,7,8,J,K]Z
**Non-OR** ØSW[9,B]X[Ø,3,4,5,7,8,J,K]Z
**Non-OR** ØSW[A,E,R,S,T,U,V,W]XJZ

**Ø Medical and Surgical**
**S Lower Joints**
**W Revision**

*ØSW Continued*

Definition: Correcting, to the extent possible, a portion of a malfunctioning device or the position of a displaced device

Explanation: Revision can include correcting a malfunctioning or displaced device by taking out or putting in components of the device such as a screw or pin

| Body Part Character 4 | Approach Character 5 | Device Character 6 | Qualifier Character 7 |
|---|---|---|---|
| **C Knee Joint, Right**<br>Femoropatellar joint<br>Femorotibial joint<br>Lateral meniscus<br>Medial meniscus<br>Patellofemoral joint<br>Tibiofemoral joint<br>**D Knee Joint, Left**<br>*See C Knee Joint, Right* | **Ø Open** | **J Synthetic Substitute** | **C Patellar Surface**<br>**Z No Qualifier** |
| **C Knee Joint, Right**<br>Femoropatellar joint<br>Femorotibial joint<br>Lateral meniscus<br>Medial meniscus<br>Patellofemoral joint<br>Tibiofemoral joint<br>**D Knee Joint, Left**<br>*See C Knee Joint, Right* | **3 Percutaneous**<br>**4 Percutaneous Endoscopic**<br>**X External** | **Ø Drainage Device**<br>**3 Infusion Device**<br>**4 Internal Fixation Device**<br>**5 External Fixation Device**<br>**7 Autologous Tissue Substitute**<br>**8 Spacer**<br>**K Nonautologous Tissue Substitute** | **Z No Qualifier** |
| **C Knee Joint, Right**<br>Femoropatellar joint<br>Femorotibial joint<br>Lateral meniscus<br>Medial meniscus<br>Patellofemoral joint<br>Tibiofemoral joint<br>**D Knee Joint, Left**<br>*See C Knee Joint, Right* | **3 Percutaneous**<br>**4 Percutaneous Endoscopic**<br>**X External** | **J Synthetic Substitute** | **C Patellar Surface**<br>**Z No Qualifier** |
| **F Ankle Joint, Right**<br>Inferior tibiofibular joint<br>Talocrural joint<br>**G Ankle Joint, Left**<br>*See F Ankle Joint, Right*<br>**H Tarsal Joint, Right**<br>Calcaneocuboid joint<br>Cuboideonavicular joint<br>Cuneonavicular joint<br>Intercuneiform joint<br>Subtalar (talocalcaneal) joint<br>Talocalcaneal (subtalar) joint<br>Talocalcaneonavicular joint<br>**J Tarsal Joint, Left**<br>*See H Tarsal Joint, Right*<br>**K Tarsometatarsal Joint, Right**<br>**L Tarsometatarsal Joint, Left**<br>**M Metatarsal-Phalangeal Joint, Right**<br>Metatarsophalangeal (MTP) joint<br>**N Metatarsal-Phalangeal Joint, Left**<br>*See M Metatarsal-Phalangeal Joint, Right*<br>**P Toe Phalangeal Joint, Right**<br>Interphalangeal (IP) joint<br>**Q Toe Phalangeal Joint, Left**<br>*See P Toe Phalangeal Joint, Right* | **Ø Open**<br>**3 Percutaneous**<br>**4 Percutaneous Endoscopic**<br>**X External** | **Ø Drainage Device**<br>**3 Infusion Device**<br>**4 Internal Fixation Device**<br>**5 External Fixation Device**<br>**7 Autologous Tissue Substitute**<br>**8 Spacer**<br>**J Synthetic Substitute**<br>**K Nonautologous Tissue Substitute** | **Z No Qualifier** |

**Non-OR** ØSW[C,D]X[Ø,3,4,5,7,8,K]Z
**Non-OR** ØSW[C,D]XJ[C,Z]
**Non-OR** ØSW[F,G,H,J,K,L,M,N,P,Q]X[Ø,3,4,5,7,8,J,K]Z

# Urinary System ØT1–ØTY

## Character Meanings

This Character Meaning table is provided as a guide to assist the user in the identification of character members that may be found in this section of code tables. It **SHOULD NOT** be used to build a PCS code.

| Operation–Character 3 | Body Part–Character 4 | Approach–Character 5 | Device–Character 6 | Qualifier–Character 7 |
|---|---|---|---|---|
| 1 Bypass | Ø Kidney, Right | Ø Open | Ø Drainage Device | Ø Allogeneic |
| 2 Change | 1 Kidney, Left | 3 Percutaneous | 2 Monitoring Device | 1 Syngeneic |
| 5 Destruction | 2 Kidneys, Bilateral | 4 Percutaneous Endoscopic | 3 Infusion Device | 2 Zooplastic |
| 7 Dilation | 3 Kidney Pelvis, Right | 7 Via Natural or Artificial Opening | 7 Autologous Tissue Substitute | 3 Kidney Pelvis, Right |
| 8 Division | 4 Kidney Pelvis, Left | 8 Via Natural or Artificial Opening Endoscopic | C Extraluminal Device | 4 Kidney Pelvis, Left |
| 9 Drainage | 5 Kidney | X External | D Intraluminal Device | 6 Ureter, Right |
| B Excision | 6 Ureter, Right | | J Synthetic Substitute | 7 Ureter, Left |
| C Extirpation | 7 Ureter, Left | | K Nonautologous Tissue Substitute | 8 Colon |
| D Extraction | 8 Ureters, Bilateral | | L Artificial Sphincter | 9 Colocutaneous |
| F Fragmentation | 9 Ureter | | M Stimulator Lead | A Ileum |
| H Insertion | B Bladder | | Y Other Device | B Bladder |
| J Inspection | C Bladder Neck | | Z No Device | C Ileocutaneous |
| L Occlusion | D Urethra | | | D Cutaneous |
| M Reattachment | | | | X Diagnostic |
| N Release | | | | Z No Qualifier |
| P Removal | | | | |
| Q Repair | | | | |
| R Replacement | | | | |
| S Reposition | | | | |
| T Resection | | | | |
| U Supplement | | | | |
| V Restriction | | | | |
| W Revision | | | | |
| Y Transplantation | | | | |

**AHA Coding Clinic for table ØT1**
**2017, 1Q, 37** Perineal urethrostomy
**2015, 3Q, 34** Redo urinary diversion surgery via left ureteral reimplantation

**AHA Coding Clinic for table ØT7**
**2016, 2Q, 27** Exchange of ureteral stents
**2015, 2Q, 8** Urinary calculi fragmentation and evacuation
**2013, 4Q, 123** Urolift® procedure

**AHA Coding Clinic for table ØTB**
**2016, 1Q, 19** Biopsy of neobladder malignancy
**2015, 3Q, 34** Excision of Mitrofanoff polyp
**2014, 2Q, 8** Ileoscopy with excision of polyp of Ileal loop urinary diversion

**AHA Coding Clinic for table ØTC**
**2016, 3Q, 23** Ureteral stone migrating into bladder
**2015, 2Q, 7** Urinary calculi fragmentation and evacuation
**2015, 2Q, 8** Urinary calculi fragmentation and evacuation
**2013, 4Q, 122** Laser lithotripsy with removal of fragments

**AHA Coding Clinic for table ØTF**
**2015, 2Q, 7** Urinary calculi fragmentation and evacuation
**2013, 4Q, 122** Extracorporeal shock wave lithotripsy
**2013, 4Q, 122** Laser lithotripsy with removal of fragments

**AHA Coding Clinic for table ØTP**
**2016, 2Q, 27** Exchange of ureteral stents

**AHA Coding Clinic for table ØTQ**
**2017, 1Q, 37** Perineal urethrostomy

**AHA Coding Clinic for table ØTS**
**2017, 1Q, 36** Dismembered pyeloplasty
**2016, 1Q, 15** Pubovaginal sling placement

**AHA Coding Clinic for table ØTT**
**2014, 3Q, 16** Hand-assisted laparoscopy nephroureterectomy

**AHA Coding Clinic for table ØTV**
**2015, 2Q, 11** Cystourethroscopic Deflux® injection

## Urinary System

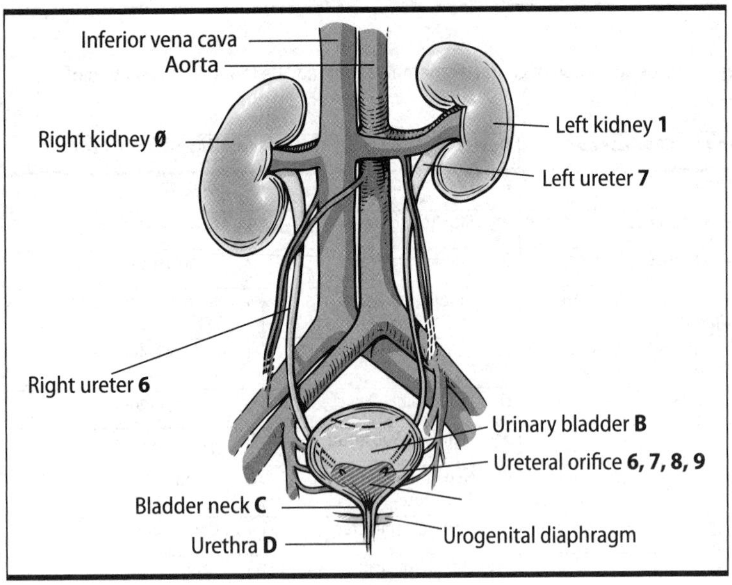
Inferior vena cava
Aorta
Right kidney Ø
Left kidney 1
Left ureter 7
Right ureter 6
Urinary bladder B
Ureteral orifice 6, 7, 8, 9
Bladder neck C
Urethra D
Urogenital diaphragm

## Kidney

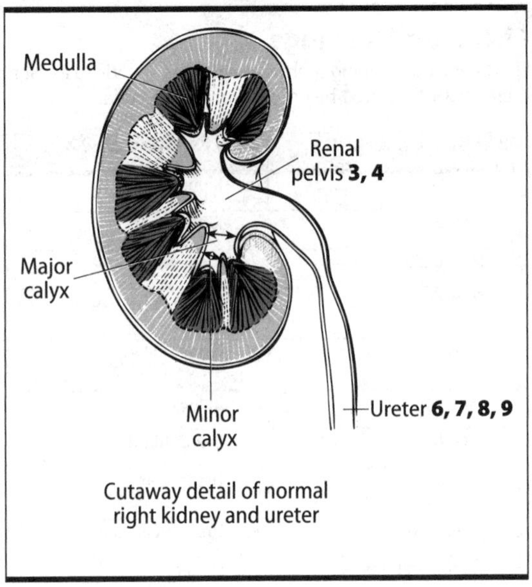
Medulla
Renal pelvis 3, 4
Major calyx
Minor calyx
Ureter 6, 7, 8, 9

Cutaway detail of normal right kidney and ureter

## Bladder

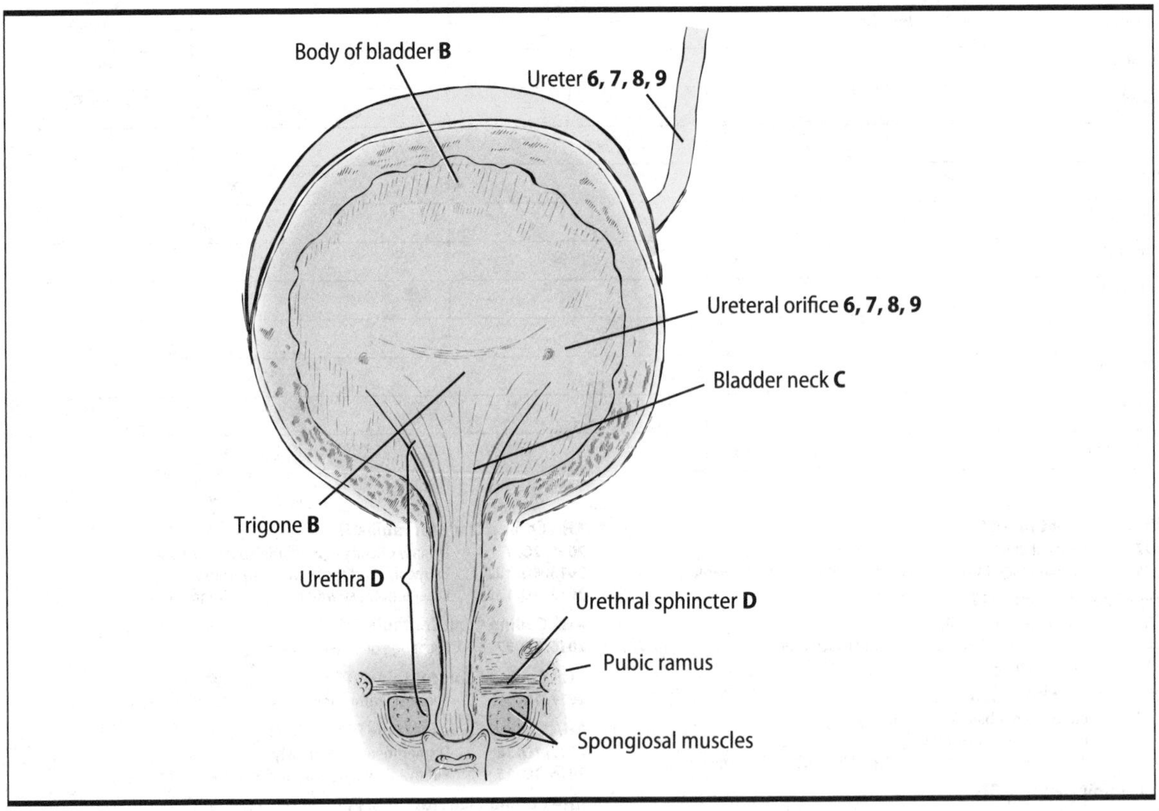
Body of bladder B
Ureter 6, 7, 8, 9
Ureteral orifice 6, 7, 8, 9
Bladder neck C
Trigone B
Urethra D
Urethral sphincter D
Pubic ramus
Spongiosal muscles

**Ø Medical and Surgical**
**T Urinary System**
**1 Bypass** Definition: Altering the route of passage of the contents of a tubular body part

Explanation: Rerouting contents of a body part to a downstream area of the normal route, to a similar route and body part, or to an abnormal route and dissimilar body part. Includes one or more anastomoses, with or without the use of a device.

| Body Part Character 4 | Approach Character 5 | Device Character 6 | Qualifier Character 7 |
|---|---|---|---|
| **3 Kidney Pelvis, Right**<br>Ureteropelvic junction (UPJ)<br>**4 Kidney Pelvis, Left**<br>*See 3 Kidney Pelvis, Right* | **Ø Open**<br>**4 Percutaneous Endoscopic** | **7 Autologous Tissue Substitute**<br>**J Synthetic Substitute**<br>**K Nonautologous Tissue Substitute**<br>**Z No Device** | **3 Kidney Pelvis, Right**<br>**4 Kidney Pelvis, Left**<br>**6 Ureter, Right**<br>**7 Ureter, Left**<br>**8 Colon**<br>**9 Colocutaneous**<br>**A Ileum**<br>**B Bladder**<br>**C Ileocutaneous**<br>**D Cutaneous** |
| **3 Kidney Pelvis, Right**<br>Ureteropelvic junction (UPJ)<br>**4 Kidney Pelvis, Left**<br>*See 3 Kidney Pelvis, Right* | **3 Percutaneous** | **J Synthetic Substitute** | **D Cutaneous** |
| **6 Ureter, Right**<br>Ureteral orifice<br>Ureterovesical orifice<br>**7 Ureter, Left**<br>*See 6 Ureter, Right*<br>**8 Ureters, Bilateral**<br>*See 6 Ureter, Right* | **Ø Open**<br>**4 Percutaneous Endoscopic** | **7 Autologous Tissue Substitute**<br>**J Synthetic Substitute**<br>**K Nonautologous Tissue Substitute**<br>**Z No Device** | **6 Ureter, Right**<br>**7 Ureter, Left**<br>**8 Colon**<br>**9 Colocutaneous**<br>**A Ileum**<br>**B Bladder**<br>**C Ileocutaneous**<br>**D Cutaneous** |
| **6 Ureter, Right**<br>Ureteral orifice<br>Ureterovesical orifice<br>**7 Ureter, Left**<br>*See 6 Ureter, Right*<br>**8 Ureters, Bilateral**<br>*See 6 Ureter, Right* | **3 Percutaneous** | **J Synthetic Substitute** | **D Cutaneous** |
| **B Bladder**<br>Trigone of bladder | **Ø Open**<br>**4 Percutaneous Endoscopic** | **7 Autologous Tissue Substitute**<br>**J Synthetic Substitute**<br>**K Nonautologous Tissue Substitute**<br>**Z No Device** | **9 Colocutaneous**<br>**C Ileocutaneous**<br>**D Cutaneous** |
| **B Bladder**<br>Trigone of bladder | **3 Percutaneous** | **J Synthetic Substitute** | **D Cutaneous** |

**Ø Medical and Surgical**
**T Urinary System**
**2 Change** Definition: Taking out or off a device from a body part and putting back an identical or similar device in or on the same body part without cutting or puncturing the skin or a mucous membrane

Explanation: All CHANGE procedures are coded using the approach EXTERNAL

| Body Part Character 4 | Approach Character 5 | Device Character 6 | Qualifier Character 7 |
|---|---|---|---|
| **5 Kidney**<br>Renal calyx<br>Renal capsule<br>Renal cortex<br>Renal segment<br>**9 Ureter**<br>Ureteral orifice<br>Ureterovesical orifice<br>**B Bladder**<br>Trigone of bladder<br>**D Urethra**<br>Bulbourethral (Cowper's) gland<br>Cowper's (bulbourethral) gland<br>External urethral sphincter<br>Internal urethral sphincter<br>Membranous urethra<br>Penile urethra<br>Prostatic urethra | **X External** | **Ø Drainage Device**<br>**Y Other Device** | **Z No Qualifier** |

**Non-OR** All body part, approach, device, and qualifier values

**Ø Medical and Surgical**
**T Urinary System**
**5 Destruction** Definition: Physical eradication of all or a portion of a body part by the direct use of energy, force, or a destructive agent

Explanation: None of the body part is physically taken out

| Body Part Character 4 | Approach Character 5 | Device Character 6 | Qualifier Character 7 |
|---|---|---|---|
| **Ø Kidney, Right**<br>Renal calyx<br>Renal capsule<br>Renal cortex<br>Renal segment<br>**1 Kidney, Left**<br>*See Ø Kidney, Right*<br>**3 Kidney Pelvis, Right**<br>Ureteropelvic junction (UPJ)<br>**4 Kidney Pelvis, Left**<br>*See 3 Kidney Pelvis, Right*<br>**6 Ureter, Right**<br>Ureteral orifice<br>Ureterovesical orifice<br>**7 Ureter, Left**<br>*See 6 Ureter, Right*<br>**B Bladder**<br>Trigone of bladder<br>**C Bladder Neck** | **Ø Open**<br>**3 Percutaneous**<br>**4 Percutaneous Endoscopic**<br>**7 Via Natural or Artificial Opening**<br>**8 Via Natural or Artificial Opening Endoscopic** | **Z No Device** | **Z No Qualifier** |
| **D Urethra**<br>Bulbourethral (Cowper's) gland<br>Cowper's (bulbourethral) gland<br>External urethral sphincter<br>Internal urethral sphincter<br>Membranous urethra<br>Penile urethra<br>Prostatic urethra | **Ø Open**<br>**3 Percutaneous**<br>**4 Percutaneous Endoscopic**<br>**7 Via Natural or Artificial Opening**<br>**8 Via Natural or Artificial Opening Endoscopic**<br>**X External** | **Z No Device** | **Z No Qualifier** |

Non-OR ØT5D[Ø,3,4,7,8,X]ZZ

**Ø Medical and Surgical**
**T Urinary System**
**7 Dilation** Definition: Expanding an orifice or the lumen of a tubular body part

Explanation: The orifice can be a natural orifice or an artificially created orifice. Accomplished by stretching a tubular body part using intraluminal pressure or by cutting part of the orifice or wall of the tubular body part.

| Body Part Character 4 | Approach Character 5 | Device Character 6 | Qualifier Character 7 |
|---|---|---|---|
| **3 Kidney Pelvis, Right**<br>Ureteropelvic junction (UPJ)<br>**4 Kidney Pelvis, Left**<br>*See 3 Kidney Pelvis, Right*<br>**6 Ureter, Right**<br>Ureteral orifice<br>Ureterovesical orifice<br>**7 Ureter, Left**<br>*See 6 Ureter, Right*<br>**8 Ureters, Bilateral**<br>*See 6 Ureter, Right*<br>**B Bladder**<br>Trigone of bladder<br>**C Bladder Neck**<br>**D Urethra**<br>Bulbourethral (Cowper's) gland<br>Cowper's (bulbourethral) gland<br>External urethral sphincter<br>Internal urethral sphincter<br>Membranous urethra<br>Penile urethra<br>Prostatic urethra | **Ø Open**<br>**3 Percutaneous**<br>**4 Percutaneous Endoscopic**<br>**7 Via Natural or Artificial Opening**<br>**8 Via Natural or Artificial Opening Endoscopic** | **D Intraluminal Device**<br>**Z No Device** | **Z No Qualifier** |

Non-OR ØT7[6,7][Ø,3,4,7,8]DZ
Non-OR ØT7[6,7][7,8]ZZ
Non-OR ØT7[8,D][Ø,3,4]DZ
Non-OR ØT7[8,B,D][7,8][D,Z]Z
Non-OR ØT7C[Ø,3,4,7,8][D,Z]Z

**Ø Medical and Surgical**
**T Urinary System**
**8 Division** Definition: Cutting into a body part, without draining fluids and/or gases from the body part, in order to separate or transect a body part

Explanation: All or a portion of the body part is separated into two or more portions

| Body Part Character 4 | Approach Character 5 | Device Character 6 | Qualifier Character 7 |
|---|---|---|---|
| **2 Kidneys, Bilateral**<br>Renal calyx<br>Renal capsule<br>Renal cortex<br>Renal segment<br>**C Bladder Neck** | **Ø Open**<br>**3 Percutaneous**<br>**4 Percutaneous Endoscopic** | **Z No Device** | **Z No Qualifier** |

**Ø Medical and Surgical**
**T Urinary System**
**9 Drainage** Definition: Taking or letting out fluids and/or gases from a body part
Explanation: The qualifier DIAGNOSTIC is used to identify drainage procedures that are biopsies

| Body Part Character 4 | Approach Character 5 | Device Character 6 | Qualifier Character 7 |
|---|---|---|---|
| **Ø Kidney, Right**<br>Renal calyx<br>Renal capsule<br>Renal cortex<br>Renal segment<br>**1 Kidney, Left**<br>*See Ø Kidney, Right*<br>**3 Kidney Pelvis, Right**<br>Ureteropelvic junction (UPJ)<br>**4 Kidney Pelvis, Left**<br>*See 3 Kidney Pelvis, Right*<br>**6 Ureter, Right**<br>Ureteral orifice<br>Ureterovesical orifice<br>**7 Ureter, Left**<br>*See 6 Ureter, Right*<br>**8 Ureters, Bilateral**<br>*See 6 Ureter, Right*<br>**B Bladder**<br>Trigone of bladder<br>**C Bladder Neck** | **Ø Open**<br>**3 Percutaneous**<br>**4 Percutaneous Endoscopic**<br>**7 Via Natural or Artificial Opening**<br>**8 Via Natural or Artificial Opening Endoscopic** | **Ø Drainage Device** | **Z No Qualifier** |
| **Ø Kidney, Right**<br>Renal calyx<br>Renal capsule<br>Renal cortex<br>Renal segment<br>**1 Kidney, Left**<br>*See Ø Kidney, Right*<br>**3 Kidney Pelvis, Right**<br>Ureteropelvic junction (UPJ)<br>**4 Kidney Pelvis, Left**<br>*See 3 Kidney Pelvis, Right*<br>**6 Ureter, Right**<br>Ureteral orifice<br>Ureterovesical orifice<br>**7 Ureter, Left**<br>*See 6 Ureter, Right*<br>**8 Ureters, Bilateral**<br>*See 6 Ureter, Right*<br>**B Bladder**<br>Trigone of bladder<br>**C Bladder Neck** | **Ø Open**<br>**3 Percutaneous**<br>**4 Percutaneous Endoscopic**<br>**7 Via Natural or Artificial Opening**<br>**8 Via Natural or Artificial Opening Endoscopic** | **Z No Device** | **X Diagnostic**<br>**Z No Qualifier** |
| **D Urethra**<br>Bulbourethral (Cowper's) gland<br>Cowper's (bulbourethral) gland<br>External urethral sphincter<br>Internal urethral sphincter<br>Membranous urethra<br>Penile urethra<br>Prostatic urethra | **Ø Open**<br>**3 Percutaneous**<br>**4 Percutaneous Endoscopic**<br>**7 Via Natural or Artificial Opening**<br>**8 Via Natural or Artificial Opening Endoscopic**<br>**X External** | **Ø Drainage Device** | **Z No Qualifier** |
| **D Urethra**<br>Bulbourethral (Cowper's) gland<br>Cowper's (bulbourethral) gland<br>External urethral sphincter<br>Internal urethral sphincter<br>Membranous urethra<br>Penile urethra<br>Prostatic urethra | **Ø Open**<br>**3 Percutaneous**<br>**4 Percutaneous Endoscopic**<br>**7 Via Natural or Artificial Opening**<br>**8 Via Natural or Artificial Opening Endoscopic**<br>**X External** | **Z No Device** | **X Diagnostic**<br>**Z No Qualifier** |

**DRG Non-OR** ØT9[3,4]3ØZ
**Non-OR** ØT9[Ø,1]3ØZ
**Non-OR** ØT9[6,7,8][Ø,3,4,7,8]ØZ
**Non-OR** ØT9[B,C][3,4,7,8]ØZ
**Non-OR** ØT9[Ø,1,3,4,6,7,8][3,4,7,8]ZX
**Non-OR** ØT9[Ø,1,3,4][3,4]ZZ
**Non-OR** ØT9[6,7,8]3ZZ
**Non-OR** ØT9[B,C][3,4,7,8]ZZ
**Non-OR** ØT9D3ØZ
**Non-OR** ØT9D[Ø,3,4,7,8,X]ZX
**Non-OR** ØT9D3ZZ

**Ø Medical and Surgical**
**T Urinary System**
**B Excision** Definition: Cutting out or off, without replacement, a portion of a body part

Explanation: The qualifier DIAGNOSTIC is used to identify excision procedures that are biopsies

| Body Part Character 4 | Approach Character 5 | Device Character 6 | Qualifier Character 7 |
|---|---|---|---|
| **Ø Kidney, Right**<br>Renal calyx<br>Renal capsule<br>Renal cortex<br>Renal segment<br>**1 Kidney, Left**<br>*See Ø Kidney, Right*<br>**3 Kidney Pelvis, Right**<br>Ureteropelvic junction (UPJ)<br>**4 Kidney Pelvis, Left**<br>*See 3 Kidney Pelvis, Right*<br>**6 Ureter, Right**<br>Ureteral orifice<br>Ureterovesical orifice<br>**7 Ureter, Left**<br>*See 6 Ureter, Right*<br>**B Bladder**<br>Trigone of bladder<br>**C Bladder Neck** | **Ø Open**<br>**3 Percutaneous**<br>**4 Percutaneous Endoscopic**<br>**7 Via Natural or Artificial Opening**<br>**8 Via Natural or Artificial Opening Endoscopic** | **Z No Device** | **X Diagnostic**<br>**Z No Qualifier** |
| **D Urethra**<br>Bulbourethral (Cowper's) gland<br>Cowper's (bulbourethral) gland<br>External urethral sphincter<br>Internal urethral sphincter<br>Membranous urethra<br>Penile urethra<br>Prostatic urethra | **Ø Open**<br>**3 Percutaneous**<br>**4 Percutaneous Endoscopic**<br>**7 Via Natural or Artificial Opening**<br>**8 Via Natural or Artificial Opening Endoscopic**<br>**X External** | **Z No Device** | **X Diagnostic**<br>**Z No Qualifier** |

**Non-OR** ØTB[Ø,1,3,4,6,7][3,4,7,8]ZX
**Non-OR** ØTBD[Ø,3,4,7,8,X]ZX

**Ø Medical and Surgical**
**T Urinary System**
**C Extirpation** Definition: Taking or cutting out solid matter from a body part

Explanation: The solid matter may be an abnormal byproduct of a biological function or a foreign body; it may be imbedded in a body part or in the lumen of a tubular body part. The solid matter may or may not have been previously broken into pieces.

| Body Part Character 4 | Approach Character 5 | Device Character 6 | Qualifier Character 7 |
|---|---|---|---|
| **Ø Kidney, Right**<br>Renal calyx<br>Renal capsule<br>Renal cortex<br>Renal segment<br>**1 Kidney, Left**<br>*See Ø Kidney, Right*<br>**3 Kidney Pelvis, Right**<br>Ureteropelvic junction (UPJ)<br>**4 Kidney Pelvis, Left**<br>*See 3 Kidney Pelvis, Right*<br>**6 Ureter, Right**<br>Ureteral orifice<br>Ureterovesical orifice<br>**7 Ureter, Left**<br>*See 6 Ureter, Right*<br>**B Bladder**<br>Trigone of bladder<br>**C Bladder Neck** | **Ø Open**<br>**3 Percutaneous**<br>**4 Percutaneous Endoscopic**<br>**7 Via Natural or Artificial Opening**<br>**8 Via Natural or Artificial Opening Endoscopic** | **Z No Device** | **Z No Qualifier** |
| **D Urethra**<br>Bulbourethral (Cowper's) gland<br>Cowper's (bulbourethral) gland<br>External urethral sphincter<br>Internal urethral sphincter<br>Membranous urethra<br>Penile urethra<br>Prostatic urethra | **Ø Open**<br>**3 Percutaneous**<br>**4 Percutaneous Endoscopic**<br>**7 Via Natural or Artificial Opening**<br>**8 Via Natural or Artificial Opening Endoscopic**<br>**X External** | **Z No Device** | **Z No Qualifier** |

**Non-OR** ØTC[B,C][7,8]ZZ
**Non-OR** ØTCD[7,8,X]ZZ

**Ø Medical and Surgical**
**T Urinary System**
**D Extraction** Definition: Pulling or stripping out or off all or a portion of a body part by the use of force

Explanation: The qualifier DIAGNOSTIC is used to identify extraction procedures that are biopsies

| Body Part Character 4 | Approach Character 5 | Device Character 6 | Qualifier Character 7 |
|---|---|---|---|
| **Ø Kidney, Right**<br>Renal calyx<br>Renal capsule<br>Renal cortex<br>Renal segment<br>**1 Kidney, Left**<br>*See Ø Kidney, Right* | **Ø Open**<br>**3 Percutaneous**<br>**4 Percutaneous Endoscopic** | **Z No Device** | **Z No Qualifier** |

**Ø Medical and Surgical**
**T Urinary System**
**F Fragmentation** Definition: Breaking solid matter in a body part into pieces

Explanation: Physical force (e.g., manual, ultrasonic) applied directly or indirectly is used to break the solid matter into pieces. The solid matter may be an abnormal byproduct of a biological function or a foreign body. The pieces of solid matter are not taken out.

| Body Part Character 4 | Approach Character 5 | Device Character 6 | Qualifier Character 7 |
|---|---|---|---|
| **3 Kidney Pelvis, Right**<br>Ureteropelvic junction (UPJ)<br>**4 Kidney Pelvis, Left**<br>*See 3 Kidney Pelvis, Right*<br>**6 Ureter, Right**<br>Ureteral orifice<br>Ureterovesical orifice<br>**7 Ureter, Left**<br>*See 6 Ureter, Right*<br>**B Bladder**<br>Trigone of bladder<br>**C Bladder Neck**<br>**D Urethra** NC<br>Bulbourethral (Cowper's) gland<br>Cowper's (bulbourethral) gland<br>External urethral sphincter<br>Internal urethral sphincter<br>Membranous urethra<br>Penile urethra<br>Prostatic urethra | **Ø Open**<br>**3 Percutaneous**<br>**4 Percutaneous Endoscopic**<br>**7 Via Natural or Artificial Opening**<br>**8 Via Natural or Artificial Opening Endoscopic**<br>**X External** | **Z No Device** | **Z No Qualifier** |

| | |
|---|---|
| **DRG Non-OR** | ØTF[3,4,6,7,B,C]XZZ |
| **Non-OR** | ØTF[3,4][Ø,7,8]ZZ |
| **Non-OR** | ØTF[6,7,B,C][Ø,3,4,7,8]ZZ |
| **Non-OR** | ØTFD[Ø,3,4,7,8,X]ZZ |
| NC | ØTFDXZZ |

**Ø Medical and Surgical**
**T Urinary System**
**H Insertion** Definition: Putting in a nonbiological appliance that monitors, assists, performs, or prevents a physiological function but does not physically take the place of a body part

Explanation: None

| Body Part Character 4 | Approach Character 5 | Device Character 6 | Qualifier Character 7 |
|---|---|---|---|
| **5 Kidney**<br>Renal calyx<br>Renal capsule<br>Renal cortex<br>Renal segment | **Ø Open**<br>**3 Percutaneous**<br>**4 Percutaneous Endoscopic**<br>**7 Via Natural or Artificial Opening**<br>**8 Via Natural or Artificial Opening Endoscopic** | **2 Monitoring Device**<br>**3 Infusion Device**<br>Y Other Device | **Z No Qualifier** |
| **9 Ureter**<br>Ureteral orifice<br>Ureterovesical orifice | **Ø Open**<br>**3 Percutaneous**<br>**4 Percutaneous Endoscopic**<br>**7 Via Natural or Artificial Opening**<br>**8 Via Natural or Artificial Opening Endoscopic** | **2 Monitoring Device**<br>**3 Infusion Device**<br>**M Stimulator Lead**<br>Y Other Device | **Z No Qualifier** |
| **B Bladder** NC<br>Trigone of bladder | **Ø Open**<br>**3 Percutaneous**<br>**4 Percutaneous Endoscopic**<br>**7 Via Natural or Artificial Opening**<br>**8 Via Natural or Artificial Opening Endoscopic** | **2 Monitoring Device**<br>**3 Infusion Device**<br>**L Artificial Sphincter**<br>**M Stimulator Lead**<br>Y Other Device | **Z No Qualifier** |
| **C Bladder Neck** | **Ø Open**<br>**3 Percutaneous**<br>**4 Percutaneous Endoscopic**<br>**7 Via Natural or Artificial Opening**<br>**8 Via Natural or Artificial Opening Endoscopic** | **L Artificial Sphincter** | **Z No Qualifier** |
| **D Urethra**<br>Bulbourethral (Cowper's) gland<br>Cowper's (bulbourethral) gland<br>External urethral sphincter<br>Internal urethral sphincter<br>Membranous urethra<br>Penile urethra<br>Prostatic urethra | **Ø Open**<br>**3 Percutaneous**<br>**4 Percutaneous Endoscopic**<br>**7 Via Natural or Artificial Opening**<br>**8 Via Natural or Artificial Opening Endoscopic** | **2 Monitoring Device**<br>**3 Infusion Device**<br>**L Artificial Sphincter**<br>Y Other Device | **Z No Qualifier** |
| **D Urethra**<br>Bulbourethral (Cowper's) gland<br>Cowper's (bulbourethral) gland<br>External urethral sphincter<br>Internal urethral sphincter<br>Membranous urethra<br>Penile urethra<br>Prostatic urethra | **X External** | **2 Monitoring Device**<br>**3 Infusion Device**<br>**L Artificial Sphincter** | **Z No Qualifier** |

**Non-OR** ØTH5Ø3Z
**Non-OR** ØTH5[3,4][3,Y]Z
**Non-OR** ØTH5[7,8][2,3,Y]Z
**Non-OR** ØTH9Ø3Z
**Non-OR** ØTH9[3,4][3,Y]Z
**Non-OR** ØTH9[7,8][2,3,Y]Z
**Non-OR** ØTHBØ3Z
**Non-OR** ØTHB[3,4][3,Y]Z
**Non-OR** ØTHB[7,8][2,3,Y]Z
**Non-OR** ØTHDØ3Z
**Non-OR** ØTHD[3,4][3,Y]Z
**Non-OR** ØTHD[7,8][2,3,Y]Z
**Non-OR** ØTHDX3Z
NC ØTHB[Ø,3,4,7,8]MZ

**Ø Medical and Surgical**
**T Urinary System**
**J Inspection** Definition: Visually and/or manually exploring a body part

Explanation: Visual exploration may be performed with or without optical instrumentation. Manual exploration may be performed directly or through intervening body layers.

| Body Part Character 4 | Approach Character 5 | Device Character 6 | Qualifier Character 7 |
|---|---|---|---|
| 5 Kidney<br>Renal calyx<br>Renal capsule<br>Renal cortex<br>Renal segment<br>9 Ureter<br>Ureteral orifice<br>Ureterovesical orifice<br>B Bladder<br>Trigone of bladder<br>D Urethra<br>Bulbourethral (Cowper's) gland<br>Cowper's (bulbourethral) gland<br>External urethral sphincter<br>Internal urethral sphincter<br>Membranous urethra<br>Penile urethra<br>Prostatic urethra | Ø Open<br>3 Percutaneous<br>4 Percutaneous Endoscopic<br>7 Via Natural or Artificial Opening<br>8 Via Natural or Artificial Opening Endoscopic<br>X External | Z No Device | Z No Qualifier |

DRG Non-OR ØTJ[5,B][3,7]ZZ
Non-OR ØTJ5[4,8,X]ZZ
Non-OR ØTJ9[3,4,7,8,X]ZZ
Non-OR ØTJB[8,X]ZZ
Non-OR ØTJD[3,4,7,8,X]ZZ

**Ø Medical and Surgical**
**T Urinary System**
**L Occlusion** Definition: Completely closing an orifice or the lumen of a tubular body part

Explanation: The orifice can be a natural orifice or an artificially created orifice

| Body Part Character 4 | Approach Character 5 | Device Character 6 | Qualifier Character 7 |
|---|---|---|---|
| 3 Kidney Pelvis, Right<br>Ureteropelvic junction (UPJ)<br>4 Kidney Pelvis, Left<br>*See 3 Kidney Pelvis, Right*<br>6 Ureter, Right<br>Ureteral orifice<br>Ureterovesical orifice<br>7 Ureter, Left<br>*See 6 Ureter, Right*<br>B Bladder<br>Trigone of bladder<br>C Bladder Neck | Ø Open<br>3 Percutaneous<br>4 Percutaneous Endoscopic | C Extraluminal Device<br>D Intraluminal Device<br>Z No Device | Z No Qualifier |
| 3 Kidney Pelvis, Right<br>Ureteropelvic junction (UPJ)<br>4 Kidney Pelvis, Left<br>*See 3 Kidney Pelvis, Right*<br>6 Ureter, Right<br>Ureteral orifice<br>Ureterovesical orifice<br>7 Ureter, Left<br>*See 6 Ureter, Right*<br>B Bladder<br>Trigone of bladder<br>C Bladder Neck | 7 Via Natural or Artificial Opening<br>8 Via Natural or Artificial Opening Endoscopic | D Intraluminal Device<br>Z No Device | Z No Qualifier |
| D Urethra<br>Bulbourethral (Cowper's) gland<br>Cowper's (bulbourethral) gland<br>External urethral sphincter<br>Internal urethral sphincter<br>Membranous urethra<br>Penile urethra<br>Prostatic urethra | Ø Open<br>3 Percutaneous<br>4 Percutaneous Endoscopic<br>X External | C Extraluminal Device<br>D Intraluminal Device<br>Z No Device | Z No Qualifier |
| D Urethra<br>Bulbourethral (Cowper's) gland<br>Cowper's (bulbourethral) gland<br>External urethral sphincter<br>Internal urethral sphincter<br>Membranous urethra<br>Penile urethra<br>Prostatic urethra | 7 Via Natural or Artificial Opening<br>8 Via Natural or Artificial Opening Endoscopic | D Intraluminal Device<br>Z No Device | Z No Qualifier |

**Ø Medical and Surgical**
**T Urinary System**
**M Reattachment** Definition: Putting back in or on all or a portion of a separated body part to its normal location or other suitable location

Explanation: Vascular circulation and nervous pathways may or may not be reestablished

| Body Part Character 4 | Approach Character 5 | Device Character 6 | Qualifier Character 7 |
|---|---|---|---|
| **Ø Kidney, Right**<br>Renal calyx<br>Renal capsule<br>Renal cortex<br>Renal segment<br>**1 Kidney, Left**<br>*See Ø Kidney, Right*<br>**2 Kidneys, Bilateral**<br>*See Ø Kidney, Right*<br>**3 Kidney Pelvis, Right**<br>Ureteropelvic junction (UPJ)<br>**4 Kidney Pelvis, Left**<br>*See 3 Kidney Pelvis, Right*<br>**6 Ureter, Right**<br>Ureteral orifice<br>Ureterovesical orifice<br>**7 Ureter, Left**<br>*See 6 Ureter, Right*<br>**8 Ureters, Bilateral**<br>*See 6 Ureter, Right*<br>**B Bladder**<br>Trigone of bladder<br>**C Bladder Neck**<br>**D Urethra**<br>Bulbourethral (Cowper's) gland<br>Cowper's (bulbourethral) gland<br>External urethral sphincter<br>Internal urethral sphincter<br>Membranous urethra<br>Penile urethra<br>Prostatic urethra | **Ø Open**<br>**4 Percutaneous Endoscopic** | **Z No Device** | **Z No Qualifier** |

**Ø Medical and Surgical**
**T Urinary System**
**N Release** Definition: Freeing a body part from an abnormal physical constraint by cutting or by the use of force

Explanation: Some of the restraining tissue may be taken out but none of the body part is taken out

| Body Part Character 4 | Approach Character 5 | Device Character 6 | Qualifier Character 7 |
|---|---|---|---|
| **Ø Kidney, Right**<br>Renal calyx<br>Renal capsule<br>Renal cortex<br>Renal segment<br>**1 Kidney, Left**<br>*See Ø Kidney, Right*<br>**3 Kidney Pelvis, Right**<br>Ureteropelvic junction (UPJ)<br>**4 Kidney Pelvis, Left**<br>*See 3 Kidney Pelvis, Right*<br>**6 Ureter, Right**<br>Ureteral orifice<br>Ureterovesical orifice<br>**7 Ureter, Left**<br>*See 6 Ureter, Right*<br>**B Bladder**<br>Trigone of bladder<br>**C Bladder Neck** | **Ø Open**<br>**3 Percutaneous**<br>**4 Percutaneous Endoscopic**<br>**7 Via Natural or Artificial Opening**<br>**8 Via Natural or Artificial Opening Endoscopic** | **Z No Device** | **Z No Qualifier** |
| **D Urethra**<br>Bulbourethral (Cowper's) gland<br>Cowper's (bulbourethral) gland<br>External urethral sphincter<br>Internal urethral sphincter<br>Membranous urethra<br>Penile urethra<br>Prostatic urethra | **Ø Open**<br>**3 Percutaneous**<br>**4 Percutaneous Endoscopic**<br>**7 Via Natural or Artificial Opening**<br>**8 Via Natural or Artificial Opening Endoscopic**<br>**X External** | **Z No Device** | **Z No Qualifier** |

**Ø Medical and Surgical**
**T Urinary System**
**P Removal** Definition: Taking out or off a device from a body part

Explanation: If a device is taken out and a similar device put in without cutting or puncturing the skin or mucous membrane, the procedure is coded to the root operation CHANGE. Otherwise, the procedure for taking out the device is coded to the root operation REMOVAL.

| Body Part Character 4 | Approach Character 5 | Device Character 6 | Qualifier Character 7 |
|---|---|---|---|
| **5 Kidney**<br>Renal calyx<br>Renal capsule<br>Renal cortex<br>Renal segment | **Ø Open**<br>**3 Percutaneous**<br>**4 Percutaneous Endoscopic**<br>**7 Via Natural or Artificial Opening**<br>**8 Via Natural or Artificial Opening Endoscopic** | **Ø Drainage Device**<br>**2 Monitoring Device**<br>**3 Infusion Device**<br>**7 Autologous Tissue Substitute**<br>**C Extraluminal Device**<br>**D Intraluminal Device**<br>**J Synthetic Substitute**<br>**K Nonautologous Tissue Substitute**<br>Y Other Device | **Z No Qualifier** |
| **5 Kidney**<br>Renal calyx<br>Renal capsule<br>Renal cortex<br>Renal segment | **X External** | **Ø Drainage Device**<br>**2 Monitoring Device**<br>**3 Infusion Device**<br>**D Intraluminal Device** | **Z No Qualifier** |
| **9 Ureter**<br>Ureteral orifice<br>Ureterovesical orifice | **Ø Open**<br>**3 Percutaneous**<br>**4 Percutaneous Endoscopic**<br>**7 Via Natural or Artificial Opening**<br>**8 Via Natural or Artificial Opening Endoscopic** | **Ø Drainage Device**<br>**2 Monitoring Device**<br>**3 Infusion Device**<br>**7 Autologous Tissue Substitute**<br>**C Extraluminal Device**<br>**D Intraluminal Device**<br>**J Synthetic Substitute**<br>**K Nonautologous Tissue Substitute**<br>**M Stimulator Lead**<br>Y Other Device | **Z No Qualifier** |
| **9 Ureter**<br>Ureteral orifice<br>Ureterovesical orifice | **X External** | **Ø Drainage Device**<br>**2 Monitoring Device**<br>**3 Infusion Device**<br>**D Intraluminal Device**<br>**M Stimulator Lead** | **Z No Qualifier** |
| **B Bladder** NC<br>Trigone of bladder | **Ø Open**<br>**3 Percutaneous**<br>**4 Percutaneous Endoscopic**<br>**7 Via Natural or Artificial Opening**<br>**8 Via Natural or Artificial Opening Endoscopic** | **Ø Drainage Device**<br>**2 Monitoring Device**<br>**3 Infusion Device**<br>**7 Autologous Tissue Substitute**<br>**C Extraluminal Device**<br>**D Intraluminal Device**<br>**J Synthetic Substitute**<br>**K Nonautologous Tissue Substitute**<br>**L Artificial Sphincter**<br>**M Stimulator Lead**<br>Y Other Device | **Z No Qualifier** |
| **B Bladder**<br>Trigone of bladder | **X External** | **Ø Drainage Device**<br>**2 Monitoring Device**<br>**3 Infusion Device**<br>**D Intraluminal Device**<br>**L Artificial Sphincter**<br>**M Stimulator Lead** | **Z No Qualifier** |
| **D Urethra**<br>Bulbourethral (Cowper's) gland<br>Cowper's (bulbourethral) gland<br>External urethral sphincter<br>Internal urethral sphincter<br>Membranous urethra<br>Penile urethra<br>Prostatic urethra | **Ø Open**<br>**3 Percutaneous**<br>**4 Percutaneous Endoscopic**<br>**7 Via Natural or Artificial Opening**<br>**8 Via Natural or Artificial Opening Endoscopic** | **Ø Drainage Device**<br>**2 Monitoring Device**<br>**3 Infusion Device**<br>**7 Autologous Tissue Substitute**<br>**C Extraluminal Device**<br>**D Intraluminal Device**<br>**J Synthetic Substitute**<br>**K Nonautologous Tissue Substitute**<br>**L Artificial Sphincter**<br>Y Other Device | **Z No Qualifier** |
| **D Urethra**<br>Bulbourethral (Cowper's) gland<br>Cowper's (bulbourethral) gland<br>External urethral sphincter<br>Internal urethral sphincter<br>Membranous urethra<br>Penile urethra<br>Prostatic urethra | **X External** | **Ø Drainage Device**<br>**2 Monitoring Device**<br>**3 Infusion Device**<br>**D Intraluminal Device**<br>**L Artificial Sphincter** | **Z No Qualifier** |

Non-OR ØTP5[3,4]YZ
Non-OR ØTP5[7,8][Ø,2,3,D,Y]Z
Non-OR ØTP5X[Ø,2,3,D]Z
Non-OR ØTP9[3,4]YZ
Non-OR ØTP9[7,8][Ø,2,3,D,Y]Z
Non-OR ØTP9X[Ø,2,3,D]Z
Non-OR ØTPB[3,4]YZ
Non-OR ØTPB[7,8][Ø,2,3,D,Y]Z
Non-OR ØTPBX[Ø,2,3,D,L]Z
Non-OR ØTPD[3,4]YZ
Non-OR ØTPD[7,8][Ø,2,3,D,Y]Z
Non-OR ØTPDX[Ø,2,3,D]Z
NC ØTPB[Ø,3,4,7,8]MZ

**Ø Medical and Surgical**
**T Urinary System**
**Q Repair**

Definition: Restoring, to the extent possible, a body part to its normal anatomic structure and function

Explanation: Used only when the method to accomplish the repair is not one of the other root operations

| Body Part Character 4 | Approach Character 5 | Device Character 6 | Qualifier Character 7 |
|---|---|---|---|
| **Ø Kidney, Right**<br>Renal calyx<br>Renal capsule<br>Renal cortex<br>Renal segment<br>**1 Kidney, Left**<br>*See Ø Kidney, Right*<br>**3 Kidney Pelvis, Right**<br>Ureteropelvic junction (UPJ)<br>**4 Kidney Pelvis, Left**<br>*See 3 Kidney Pelvis, Right*<br>**6 Ureter, Right**<br>Ureteral orifice<br>Ureterovesical orifice<br>**7 Ureter, Left**<br>*See 6 Ureter, Right*<br>**B Bladder** ⊞<br>Trigone of bladder<br>**C Bladder Neck** | **Ø Open**<br>**3 Percutaneous**<br>**4 Percutaneous Endoscopic**<br>**7 Via Natural or Artificial Opening**<br>**8 Via Natural or Artificial Opening Endoscopic** | **Z No Device** | **Z No Qualifier** |
| **D Urethra**<br>Bulbourethral (Cowper's) gland<br>Cowper's (bulbourethral) gland<br>External urethral sphincter<br>Internal urethral sphincter<br>Membranous urethra<br>Penile urethra<br>Prostatic urethra | **Ø Open**<br>**3 Percutaneous**<br>**4 Percutaneous Endoscopic**<br>**7 Via Natural or Artificial Opening**<br>**8 Via Natural or Artificial Opening Endoscopic**<br>**X External** | **Z No Device** | **Z No Qualifier** |

**See Appendix L for Procedure Combinations**
⊞ ØTQB[Ø,3,4]ZZ

**Ø Medical and Surgical**
**T Urinary System**
**R Replacement**

Definition: Putting in or on biological or synthetic material that physically takes the place and/or function of all or a portion of a body part

Explanation: The body part may have been taken out or replaced, or may be taken out, physically eradicated, or rendered nonfunctional during the REPLACEMENT procedure. A REMOVAL procedure is coded for taking out the device used in a previous replacement procedure.

| Body Part Character 4 | Approach Character 5 | Device Character 6 | Qualifier Character 7 |
|---|---|---|---|
| **3 Kidney Pelvis, Right**<br>Ureteropelvic junction (UPJ)<br>**4 Kidney Pelvis, Left**<br>*See 3 Kidney Pelvis, Right*<br>**6 Ureter, Right**<br>Ureteral orifice<br>Ureterovesical orifice<br>**7 Ureter, Left**<br>*See 6 Ureter, Right*<br>**B Bladder**<br>Trigone of bladder<br>**C Bladder Neck** | **Ø Open**<br>**4 Percutaneous Endoscopic**<br>**7 Via Natural or Artificial Opening**<br>**8 Via Natural or Artificial Opening Endoscopic** | **7 Autologous Tissue Substitute**<br>**J Synthetic Substitute**<br>**K Nonautologous Tissue Substitute** | **Z No Qualifier** |
| **D Urethra**<br>Bulbourethral (Cowper's) gland<br>Cowper's (bulbourethral) gland<br>External urethral sphincter<br>Internal urethral sphincter<br>Membranous urethra<br>Penile urethra<br>Prostatic urethra | **Ø Open**<br>**4 Percutaneous Endoscopic**<br>**7 Via Natural or Artificial Opening**<br>**8 Via Natural or Artificial Opening Endoscopic**<br>**X External** | **7 Autologous Tissue Substitute**<br>**J Synthetic Substitute**<br>**K Nonautologous Tissue Substitute** | **Z No Qualifier** |

**Ø Medical and Surgical**
**T Urinary System**
**S Reposition** Definition: Moving to its normal location, or other suitable location, all or a portion of a body part

Explanation: The body part is moved to a new location from an abnormal location, or from a normal location where it is not functioning correctly. The body part may or may not be cut out or off to be moved to the new location.

| Body Part Character 4 | Approach Character 5 | Device Character 6 | Qualifier Character 7 |
|---|---|---|---|
| **Ø Kidney, Right**<br>Renal calyx<br>Renal capsule<br>Renal cortex<br>Renal segment<br>**1 Kidney, Left**<br>*See Ø Kidney, Right*<br>**2 Kidneys, Bilateral**<br>*See Ø Kidney, Right*<br>**3 Kidney Pelvis, Right**<br>Ureteropelvic junction (UPJ)<br>**4 Kidney Pelvis, Left**<br>*See 3 Kidney Pelvis, Right*<br>**6 Ureter, Right**<br>Ureteral orifice<br>Ureterovesical orifice<br>**7 Ureter, Left**<br>*See 6 Ureter, Right*<br>**8 Ureters, Bilateral**<br>*See 6 Ureter, Right*<br>**B Bladder**<br>Trigone of bladder<br>**C Bladder Neck**<br>**D Urethra**<br>Bulbourethral (Cowper's) gland<br>Cowper's (bulbourethral) gland<br>External urethral sphincter<br>Internal urethral sphincter<br>Membranous urethra<br>Penile urethra<br>Prostatic urethra | **Ø Open**<br>**4 Percutaneous Endoscopic** | **Z No Device** | **Z No Qualifier** |

**Ø Medical and Surgical**
**T Urinary System**
**T Resection** Definition: Cutting out or off, without replacement, all of a body part

Explanation: None

| Body Part Character 4 | Approach Character 5 | Device Character 6 | Qualifier Character 7 |
|---|---|---|---|
| **Ø Kidney, Right**<br>Renal calyx<br>Renal capsule<br>Renal cortex<br>Renal segment<br>**1 Kidney, Left**<br>*See Ø Kidney, Right*<br>**2 Kidneys, Bilateral**<br>*See Ø Kidney, Right* | **Ø Open**<br>**4 Percutaneous Endoscopic** | **Z No Device** | **Z No Qualifier** |
| **3 Kidney Pelvis, Right**<br>Ureteropelvic junction (UPJ)<br>**4 Kidney Pelvis, Left**<br>*See 3 Kidney Pelvis, Right*<br>**6 Ureter, Right**<br>Ureteral orifice<br>Ureterovesical orifice<br>**7 Ureter, Left**<br>*See 6 Ureter, Right*<br>**B Bladder** ⊞<br>Trigone of bladder<br>**C Bladder Neck**<br>**D Urethra**<br>Bulbourethral (Cowper's) gland<br>Cowper's (bulbourethral) gland<br>External urethral sphincter<br>Internal urethral sphincter<br>Membranous urethra<br>Penile urethra<br>Prostatic urethra | **Ø Open**<br>**4 Percutaneous Endoscopic**<br>**7 Via Natural or Artificial Opening**<br>**8 Via Natural or Artificial Opening Endoscopic** | **Z No Device** | **Z No Qualifier** |

**DRG Non-OR** ØTTDØZZ
**Non-OR** ØTTD[4,7,8]ZZ

**See Appendix L for Procedure Combinations**
**Combo-only** ØTTDØZZ
⊞ ØTTBØZZ

**Ø Medical and Surgical**
**T Urinary System**
**U Supplement**

Definition: Putting in or on biological or synthetic material that physically reinforces and/or augments the function of a portion of a body part

Explanation: The biological material is non-living, or is living and from the same individual. The body part may have been previously replaced, and the SUPPLEMENT procedure is performed to physically reinforce and/or augment the function of the replaced body part.

| Body Part Character 4 | Approach Character 5 | Device Character 6 | Qualifier Character 7 |
|---|---|---|---|
| **3 Kidney Pelvis, Right**<br>Ureteropelvic junction (UPJ)<br>**4 Kidney Pelvis, Left**<br>*See 3 Kidney Pelvis, Right*<br>**6 Ureter, Right**<br>Ureteral orifice<br>Ureterovesical orifice<br>**7 Ureter, Left**<br>*See 6 Ureter, Right*<br>**B Bladder**<br>Trigone of bladder<br>**C Bladder Neck** | **Ø Open**<br>**4 Percutaneous Endoscopic**<br>**7 Via Natural or Artificial Opening**<br>**8 Via Natural or Artificial Opening Endoscopic** | **7 Autologous Tissue Substitute**<br>**J Synthetic Substitute**<br>**K Nonautologous Tissue Substitute** | **Z No Qualifier** |
| **D Urethra**<br>Bulbourethral (Cowper's) gland<br>Cowper's (bulbourethral) gland<br>External urethral sphincter<br>Internal urethral sphincter<br>Membranous urethra<br>Penile urethra<br>Prostatic urethra | **Ø Open**<br>**4 Percutaneous Endoscopic**<br>**7 Via Natural or Artificial Opening**<br>**8 Via Natural or Artificial Opening Endoscopic**<br>**X External** | **7 Autologous Tissue Substitute**<br>**J Synthetic Substitute**<br>**K Nonautologous Tissue Substitute** | **Z No Qualifier** |

**Ø Medical and Surgical**
**T Urinary System**
**V Restriction**

Definition: Partially closing an orifice or the lumen of a tubular body part

Explanation: The orifice can be a natural orifice or an artificially created orifice

| Body Part Character 4 | Approach Character 5 | Device Character 6 | Qualifier Character 7 |
|---|---|---|---|
| **3 Kidney Pelvis, Right**<br>Ureteropelvic junction (UPJ)<br>**4 Kidney Pelvis, Left**<br>*See 3 Kidney Pelvis, Right*<br>**6 Ureter, Right**<br>Ureteral orifice<br>Ureterovesical orifice<br>**7 Ureter, Left**<br>*See 6 Ureter, Right*<br>**B Bladder**<br>Trigone of bladder<br>**C Bladder Neck** | **Ø Open**<br>**3 Percutaneous**<br>**4 Percutaneous Endoscopic** | **C Extraluminal Device**<br>**D Intraluminal Device**<br>**Z No Device** | **Z No Qualifier** |
| **3 Kidney Pelvis, Right**<br>Ureteropelvic junction (UPJ)<br>**4 Kidney Pelvis, Left**<br>*See 3 Kidney Pelvis, Right*<br>**6 Ureter, Right**<br>Ureteral orifice<br>Ureterovesical orifice<br>**7 Ureter, Left**<br>*See 6 Ureter, Right*<br>**B Bladder**<br>Trigone of bladder<br>**C Bladder Neck** | **7 Via Natural or Artificial Opening**<br>**8 Via Natural or Artificial Opening Endoscopic** | **D Intraluminal Device**<br>**Z No Device** | **Z No Qualifier** |
| **D Urethra**<br>Bulbourethral (Cowper's) gland<br>Cowper's (bulbourethral) gland<br>External urethral sphincter<br>Internal urethral sphincter<br>Membranous urethra<br>Penile urethra<br>Prostatic urethra | **Ø Open**<br>**3 Percutaneous**<br>**4 Percutaneous Endoscopic** | **C Extraluminal Device**<br>**D Intraluminal Device**<br>**Z No Device** | **Z No Qualifier** |
| **D Urethra**<br>Bulbourethral (Cowper's) gland<br>Cowper's (bulbourethral) gland<br>External urethral sphincter<br>Internal urethral sphincter<br>Membranous urethra<br>Penile urethra<br>Prostatic urethra | **7 Via Natural or Artificial Opening**<br>**8 Via Natural or Artificial Opening Endoscopic** | **D Intraluminal Device**<br>**Z No Device** | **Z No Qualifier** |
| **D Urethra**<br>Bulbourethral (Cowper's) gland<br>Cowper's (bulbourethral) gland<br>External urethral sphincter<br>Internal urethral sphincter<br>Membranous urethra<br>Penile urethra<br>Prostatic urethra | **X External** | **Z No Device** | **Z No Qualifier** |

**Ø Medical and Surgical**
**T Urinary System**
**W Revision**

Definition: Correcting, to the extent possible, a portion of a malfunctioning device or the position of a displaced device

Explanation: Revision can include correcting a malfunctioning or displaced device by taking out or putting in components of the device such as a screw or pin

| Body Part Character 4 | Approach Character 5 | Device Character 6 | Qualifier Character 7 |
|---|---|---|---|
| **5 Kidney**<br>Renal calyx<br>Renal capsule<br>Renal cortex<br>Renal segment | **Ø** Open<br>**3** Percutaneous<br>**4** Percutaneous Endoscopic<br>**7** Via Natural or Artificial Opening<br>**8** Via Natural or Artificial Opening Endoscopic | **Ø** Drainage Device<br>**2** Monitoring Device<br>**3** Infusion Device<br>**7** Autologous Tissue Substitute<br>**C** Extraluminal Device<br>**D** Intraluminal Device<br>**J** Synthetic Substitute<br>**K** Nonautologous Tissue Substitute<br>**Y** Other Device | **Z** No Qualifier |
| **5 Kidney**<br>Renal calyx<br>Renal capsule<br>Renal cortex<br>Renal segment | **X** External | **Ø** Drainage Device<br>**2** Monitoring Device<br>**3** Infusion Device<br>**7** Autologous Tissue Substitute<br>**C** Extraluminal Device<br>**D** Intraluminal Device<br>**J** Synthetic Substitute<br>**K** Nonautologous Tissue Substitute | **Z** No Qualifier |
| **9 Ureter**<br>Ureteral orifice<br>Ureterovesical orifice | **Ø** Open<br>**3** Percutaneous<br>**4** Percutaneous Endoscopic<br>**7** Via Natural or Artificial Opening<br>**8** Via Natural or Artificial Opening Endoscopic | **Ø** Drainage Device<br>**2** Monitoring Device<br>**3** Infusion Device<br>**7** Autologous Tissue Substitute<br>**C** Extraluminal Device<br>**D** Intraluminal Device<br>**J** Synthetic Substitute<br>**K** Nonautologous Tissue Substitute<br>**M** Stimulator Lead<br>**Y** Other Device | **Z** No Qualifier |
| **9 Ureter**<br>Ureteral orifice<br>Ureterovesical orifice | **X** External | **Ø** Drainage Device<br>**2** Monitoring Device<br>**3** Infusion Device<br>**7** Autologous Tissue Substitute<br>**C** Extraluminal Device<br>**D** Intraluminal Device<br>**J** Synthetic Substitute<br>**K** Nonautologous Tissue Substitute<br>**M** Stimulator Lead | **Z** No Qualifier |
| **B Bladder**<br>Trigone of bladder | **Ø** Open<br>**3** Percutaneous<br>**4** Percutaneous Endoscopic<br>**7** Via Natural or Artificial Opening<br>**8** Via Natural or Artificial Opening Endoscopic | **Ø** Drainage Device<br>**2** Monitoring Device<br>**3** Infusion Device<br>**7** Autologous Tissue Substitute<br>**C** Extraluminal Device<br>**D** Intraluminal Device<br>**J** Synthetic Substitute<br>**K** Nonautologous Tissue Substitute<br>**L** Artificial Sphincter<br>**M** Stimulator Lead<br>**Y** Other Device | **Z** No Qualifier |
| **B Bladder**<br>Trigone of bladder | **X** External | **Ø** Drainage Device<br>**2** Monitoring Device<br>**3** Infusion Device<br>**7** Autologous Tissue Substitute<br>**C** Extraluminal Device<br>**D** Intraluminal Device<br>**J** Synthetic Substitute<br>**K** Nonautologous Tissue Substitute<br>**L** Artificial Sphincter<br>**M** Stimulator Lead | **Z** No Qualifier |

*ØTW Continued on next page*

**Non-OR** ØTW5[3,4,7,8]YZ
**Non-OR** ØTW5X[Ø,2,3,7,C,D,J,K]Z
**Non-OR** ØTW9[3,4,7,8]YZ
**Non-OR** ØTW9X[Ø,2,3,7,C,D,J,K,M]Z
**Non-OR** ØTWB[3,4,7,8]YZ
**Non-OR** ØTWBX[Ø,2,3,7,C,D,J,K,L,M]Z

**ØTW Continued**

**Ø Medical and Surgical**
**T Urinary System**
**W Revision** Definition: Correcting, to the extent possible, a portion of a malfunctioning device or the position of a displaced device

Explanation: Revision can include correcting a malfunctioning or displaced device by taking out or putting in components of the device such as a screw or pin

| Body Part Character 4 | Approach Character 5 | Device Character 6 | Qualifier Character 7 |
|---|---|---|---|
| **D Urethra**<br>Bulbourethral (Cowper's) gland<br>Cowper's (bulbourethral) gland<br>External urethral sphincter<br>Internal urethral sphincter<br>Membranous urethra<br>Penile urethra<br>Prostatic urethra | **Ø Open**<br>**3 Percutaneous**<br>**4 Percutaneous Endoscopic**<br>**7 Via Natural or Artificial Opening**<br>**8 Via Natural or Artificial Opening Endoscopic** | **Ø Drainage Device**<br>**2 Monitoring Device**<br>**3 Infusion Device**<br>**7 Autologous Tissue Substitute**<br>**C Extraluminal Device**<br>**D Intraluminal Device**<br>**J Synthetic Substitute**<br>**K Nonautologous Tissue Substitute**<br>**L Artificial Sphincter**<br>**Y Other Device** | **Z No Qualifier** |
| **D Urethra**<br>Bulbourethral (Cowper's) gland<br>Cowper's (bulbourethral) gland<br>External urethral sphincter<br>Internal urethral sphincter<br>Membranous urethra<br>Penile urethra<br>Prostatic urethra | **X External** | **Ø Drainage Device**<br>**2 Monitoring Device**<br>**3 Infusion Device**<br>**7 Autologous Tissue Substitute**<br>**C Extraluminal Device**<br>**D Intraluminal Device**<br>**J Synthetic Substitute**<br>**K Nonautologous Tissue Substitute**<br>**L Artificial Sphincter** | **Z No Qualifier** |

Non-OR ØTWD[3,4,7,8]YZ
Non-OR ØTWDX[Ø,2,3,7,C,D,J,K,L]Z

**Ø Medical and Surgical**
**T Urinary System**
**Y Transplantation** Definition: Putting in or on all or a portion of a living body part taken from another individual or animal to physically take the place and/or function of all or a portion of a similar body part

Explanation: The native body part may or may not be taken out, and the transplanted body part may take over all or a portion of its function

| Body Part Character 4 | Approach Character 5 | Device Character 6 | Qualifier Character 7 |
|---|---|---|---|
| **Ø Kidney, Right** ⊞ LC<br>Renal calyx<br>Renal capsule<br>Renal cortex<br>Renal segment<br>**1 Kidney, Left** ⊞ LC<br>*See Ø Kidney, Right* | **Ø Open** | **Z No Device** | **Ø Allogeneic**<br>**1 Syngeneic**<br>**2 Zooplastic** |

LC ØTY[Ø,1]ØZ[Ø,1,2]

**See Appendix L for Procedure Combinations**
⊞ ØTY[Ø,1]ØZ[Ø,1,2]

# Female Reproductive System ØU1–ØUY

## Character Meanings

This Character Meaning table is provided as a guide to assist the user in the identification of character members that may be found in this section of code tables. It **SHOULD NOT** be used to build a PCS code.

| Operation–Character 3 | Body Part–Character 4 | Approach–Character 5 | Device–Character 6 | Qualifier–Character 7 |
|---|---|---|---|---|
| 1 Bypass | Ø Ovary, Right | Ø Open | Ø Drainage Device | Ø Allogeneic |
| 2 Change | 1 Ovary, Left | 3 Percutaneous | 1 Radioactive Element | 1 Syngeneic |
| 5 Destruction | 2 Ovaries, Bilateral | 4 Percutaneous Endoscopic | 3 Infusion Device | 2 Zooplastic |
| 7 Dilation | 3 Ovary | 7 Via Natural or Artificial Opening | 7 Autologous Tissue Substitute | 5 Fallopian Tube, Right |
| 8 Division | 4 Uterine Supporting Structure | 8 Via Natural or Artificial Opening Endoscopic | C Extraluminal Device | 6 Fallopian Tube, Left |
| 9 Drainage | 5 Fallopian Tube, Right | F Via Natural or Artificial Opening With Percutaneous Endoscopic Assistance | D Intraluminal Device | 9 Uterus |
| B Excision | 6 Fallopian Tube, Left | X External | G Intraluminal Device, Pessary | L Supracervical |
| C Extirpation | 7 Fallopian Tubes, Bilateral | | H Contraceptive Device | X Diagnostic |
| D Extraction | 8 Fallopian Tube | | J Synthetic Substitute | Z No Qualifier |
| F Fragmentation | 9 Uterus | | K Nonautologous Tissue Substitute | |
| H Insertion | B Endometrium | | Y Other Device | |
| J Inspection | C Cervix | | Z No Device | |
| L Occlusion | D Uterus and Cervix | | | |
| M Reattachment | F Cul-de-sac | | | |
| N Release | G Vagina | | | |
| P Removal | H Vagina and Cul-de-sac | | | |
| Q Repair | J Clitoris | | | |
| S Reposition | K Hymen | | | |
| T Resection | L Vestibular Gland | | | |
| U Supplement | M Vulva | | | |
| V Restriction | N Ova | | | |
| W Revision | | | | |
| Y Transplantation | | | | |

**AHA Coding Clinic for table ØU5**
**2015, 3Q, 31** Tubal ligation for sterilization

**AHA Coding Clinic for table ØUB**
**2015, 3Q, 31** Laparoscopic partial salpingectomy for ectopic pregnancy
**2015, 3Q, 31** Tubal ligation for sterilization
**2014, 4Q, 16** Excision of multiple uterine fibroids
**2014, 3Q, 12** Excision of skin tag from labia majora

**AHA Coding Clinic for table ØUC**
**2015, 3Q, 30** Removal of cervical cerclage
**2013, 2Q, 38** Evacuation of clot post-partum

**AHA Coding Clinic for table ØUH**
**2013, 2Q, 34** Placement of intrauterine device via open approach

**AHA Coding Clinic for table ØUJ**
**2015, 1Q, 33** Robotic-assisted laparoscopic hysterectomy converted to open procedure

**AHA Coding Clinic for table ØUL**
**2015, 3Q, 31** Tubal ligation for sterilization

**AHA Coding Clinic for table ØUQ**
**2014, 4Q, 18** Obstetrical periurethral laceration
**2013, 4Q, 120** Repair of clitoral obstetric laceration

**AHA Coding Clinic for table ØUS**
**2016, 1Q, 9** Anteversion of retroverted pregnant uterus

**AHA Coding Clinic for table ØUT**
**2015, 1Q, 33** Robotic-assisted laparoscopic hysterectomy converted to open procedure
**2013, 3Q, 28** Total hysterectomy
**2013, 1Q, 24** Excision versus Resection of remaining ovarian remnant following previous excision

**AHA Coding Clinic for table ØUV**
**2015, 3Q, 30** Insertion of cervical cerclage

## Female Reproductive System

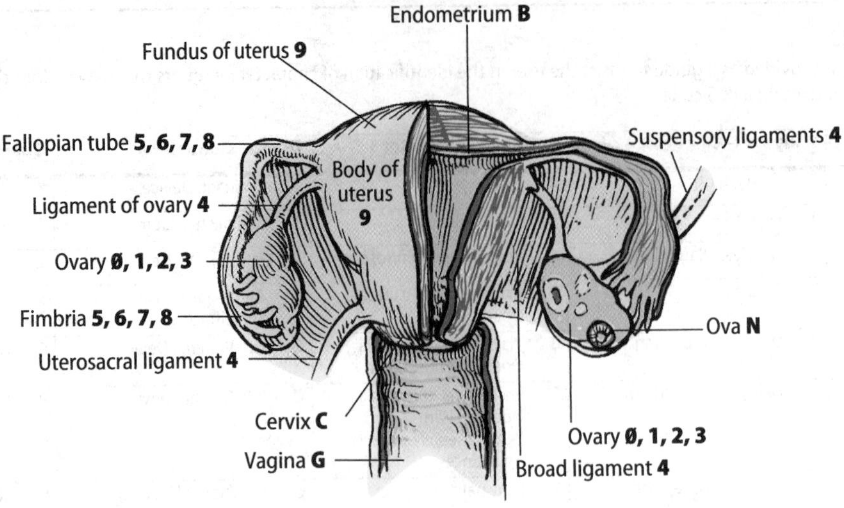
Endometrium **B**
Fundus of uterus **9**
Fallopian tube **5, 6, 7, 8**
Body of uterus **9**
Suspensory ligaments **4**
Ligament of ovary **4**
Ovary **Ø, 1, 2, 3**
Fimbria **5, 6, 7, 8**
Ova **N**
Uterosacral ligament **4**
Cervix **C**
Ovary **Ø, 1, 2, 3**
Vagina **G**
Broad ligament **4**

## Female Internal/External Structures

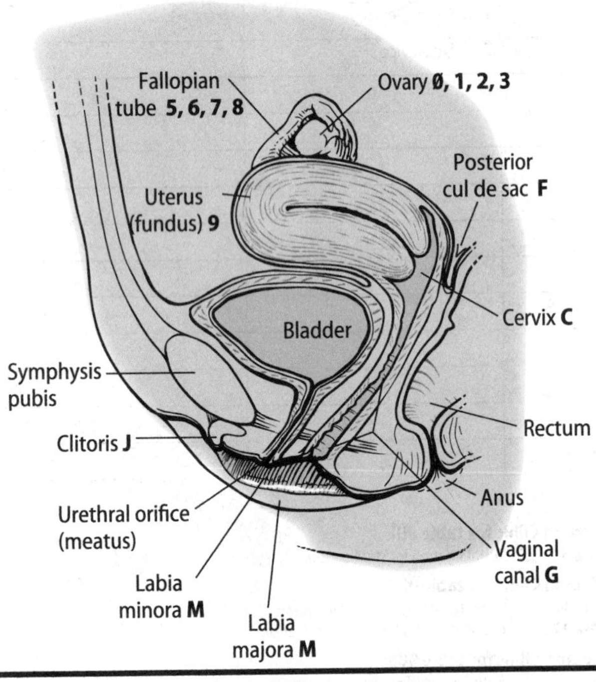
Fallopian tube **5, 6, 7, 8**
Ovary **Ø, 1, 2, 3**
Posterior cul de sac **F**
Uterus (fundus) **9**
Bladder
Cervix **C**
Symphysis pubis
Rectum
Clitoris **J**
Anus
Urethral orifice (meatus)
Vaginal canal **G**
Labia minora **M**
Labia majora **M**

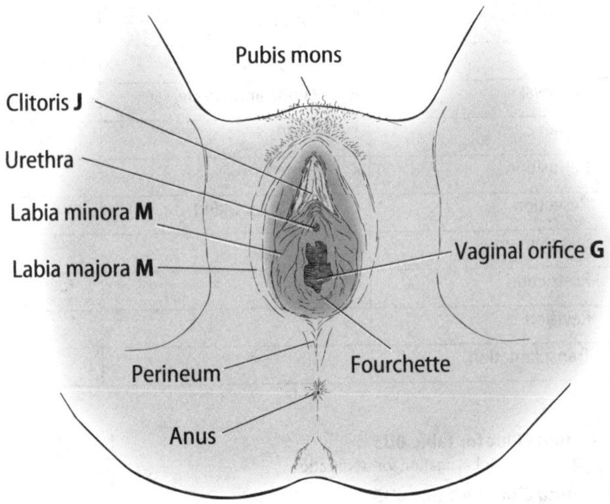
Pubis mons
Clitoris **J**
Urethra
Labia minora **M**
Vaginal orifice **G**
Labia majora **M**
Perineum
Fourchette
Anus

**Ø Medical and Surgical**
**U Female Reproductive System**
**1 Bypass** Definition: Altering the route of passage of the contents of a tubular body part

Explanation: Rerouting contents of a body part to a downstream area of the normal route, to a similar route and body part, or to an abnormal route and dissimilar body part. Includes one or more anastomoses, with or without the use of a device.

| Body Part Character 4 | Approach Character 5 | Device Character 6 | Qualifier Character 7 |
|---|---|---|---|
| 5 Fallopian Tube, Right ♀<br>Oviduct<br>Salpinx<br>Uterine tube<br>6 Fallopian Tube, Left ♀<br>*See 5 Fallopian Tube, Right* | Ø Open<br>4 Percutaneous Endoscopic | 7 Autologous Tissue Substitute<br>J Synthetic Substitute<br>K Nonautologous Tissue Substitute<br>Z No Device | 5 Fallopian Tube, Right<br>6 Fallopian Tube, Left<br>9 Uterus |

♀ All body part, approach, device, and qualifier values

**Ø Medical and Surgical**
**U Female Reproductive System**
**2 Change** Definition: Taking out or off a device from a body part and putting back an identical or similar device in or on the same body part without cutting or puncturing the skin or a mucous membrane

Explanation: All CHANGE procedures are coded using the approach EXTERNAL

| Body Part Character 4 | Approach Character 5 | Device Character 6 | Qualifier Character 7 |
|---|---|---|---|
| 3 Ovary ♀<br>8 Fallopian Tube ♀<br>M Vulva ♀<br>Labia majora<br>Labia minora | X External | Ø Drainage Device<br>Y Other Device | Z No Qualifier |
| D Uterus and Cervix ♀ | X External | Ø Drainage Device<br>H Contraceptive Device<br>Y Other Device | Z No Qualifier |
| H Vagina and Cul-de-sac ♀ | X External | Ø Drainage Device<br>G Intraluminal Device, Pessary<br>Y Other Device | Z No Qualifier |

Non-OR All body part, approach, device, and qualifier values
♀ All body part, approach, device, and qualifier values

**Ø Medical and Surgical**
**U Female Reproductive System**
**5 Destruction** Definition: Physical eradication of all or a portion of a body part by the direct use of energy, force, or a destructive agent

Explanation: None of the body part is physically taken out

| Body Part Character 4 | Approach Character 5 | Device Character 6 | Qualifier Character 7 |
|---|---|---|---|
| **Ø Ovary, Right** ♀<br>**1 Ovary, Left** ♀<br>**2 Ovaries, Bilateral** ♀<br>**4 Uterine Supporting Structure** ♀<br>Broad ligament<br>Infundibulopelvic ligament<br>Ovarian ligament<br>Round ligament of uterus | **Ø Open**<br>**3 Percutaneous**<br>**4 Percutaneous Endoscopic**<br>8 Via Natural or Artificial Opening Endoscopic | **Z No Device** | **Z No Qualifier** |
| **5 Fallopian Tube, Right** ♀<br>Oviduct<br>Salpinx<br>Uterine tube<br>**6 Fallopian Tube, Left** ♀<br>*See 5 Fallopian Tube, Right*<br>**7 Fallopian Tubes, Bilateral** NC ♀<br>**9 Uterus** ♀<br>Fundus uteri<br>Myometrium<br>Perimetrium<br>Uterine cornu<br>**B Endometrium** ♀<br>**C Cervix** ♀<br>**F Cul-de-sac** ♀ | **Ø Open**<br>**3 Percutaneous**<br>**4 Percutaneous Endoscopic**<br>**7 Via Natural or Artificial Opening**<br>**8 Via Natural or Artificial Opening Endoscopic** | **Z No Device** | **Z No Qualifier** |
| **G Vagina** ♀<br>**K Hymen** ♀ | **Ø Open**<br>**3 Percutaneous**<br>**4 Percutaneous Endoscopic**<br>**7 Via Natural or Artificial Opening**<br>**8 Via Natural or Artificial Opening Endoscopic**<br>**X External** | **Z No Device** | **Z No Qualifier** |
| **J Clitoris** ♀<br>**L Vestibular Gland** ♀<br>Bartholin's (greater vestibular) gland<br>Greater vestibular (Bartholin's) gland<br>Paraurethral (Skene's) gland<br>Skene's (paraurethral) gland<br>**M Vulva** ♀<br>Labia majora<br>Labia minora | **Ø Open**<br>**X External** | **Z No Device** | **Z No Qualifier** |

NC ØU57[Ø,3,4,7,8]ZZ with principal diagnosis code Z3Ø.2
♀ All body part, approach, device, and qualifier values

**Ø Medical and Surgical**
**U Female Reproductive System**
**7 Dilation** Definition: Expanding an orifice or the lumen of a tubular body part

Explanation: The orifice can be a natural orifice or an artificially created orifice. Accomplished by stretching a tubular body part using intraluminal pressure or by cutting part of the orifice or wall of the tubular body part.

| Body Part Character 4 | Approach Character 5 | Device Character 6 | Qualifier Character 7 |
|---|---|---|---|
| **5 Fallopian Tube, Right** ♀<br>Oviduct<br>Salpinx<br>Uterine tube<br>**6 Fallopian Tube, Left** ♀<br>*See 5 Fallopian Tube, Right*<br>**7 Fallopian Tubes, Bilateral** ♀<br>**9 Uterus** ♀<br>Fundus uteri<br>Myometrium<br>Perimetrium<br>Uterine cornu<br>**C Cervix** ♀<br>**G Vagina** ♀ | **Ø Open**<br>**3 Percutaneous**<br>**4 Percutaneous Endoscopic**<br>**7 Via Natural or Artificial Opening**<br>**8 Via Natural or Artificial Opening Endoscopic** | **D Intraluminal Device**<br>**Z No Device** | **Z No Qualifier** |
| **K Hymen** ♀ | **Ø Open**<br>**3 Percutaneous**<br>**4 Percutaneous Endoscopic**<br>**7 Via Natural or Artificial Opening**<br>**8 Via Natural or Artificial Opening Endoscopic**<br>**X External** | **D Intraluminal Device**<br>**Z No Device** | **Z No Qualifier** |

**Non-OR** ØU7C[Ø,3,4,7,8][D,Z]Z
**Non-OR** ØU7G[7,8][D,Z]Z
♀ All body part, approach, device, and qualifier values

**Ø Medical and Surgical**
**U Female Reproductive System**
**8 Division** Definition: Cutting into a body part, without draining fluids and/or gases from the body part, in order to separate or transect a body part

Explanation: All or a portion of the body part is separated into two or more portions

| Body Part Character 4 | Approach Character 5 | Device Character 6 | Qualifier Character 7 |
|---|---|---|---|
| **Ø Ovary, Right** ♀<br>**1 Ovary, Left** ♀<br>**2 Ovaries, Bilateral** ♀<br>**4 Uterine Supporting Structure** ♀<br>Broad ligament<br>Infundibulopelvic ligament<br>Ovarian ligament<br>Round ligament of uterus | **Ø Open**<br>**3 Percutaneous**<br>**4 Percutaneous Endoscopic** | **Z No Device** | **Z No Qualifier** |
| **K Hymen** ♀ | **7 Via Natural or Artificial Opening**<br>**8 Via Natural or Artificial Opening Endoscopic**<br>**X External** | **Z No Device** | **Z No Qualifier** |

**Non-OR** ØU8K[7,8,X]ZZ
♀ All body part, approach, device, and qualifier values

**Ø Medical and Surgical**
**U Female Reproductive System**
**9 Drainage** Definition: Taking or letting out fluids and/or gases from a body part
Explanation: The qualifier DIAGNOSTIC is used to identify drainage procedures that are biopsies

| Body Part Character 4 | Approach Character 5 | Device Character 6 | Qualifier Character 7 |
|---|---|---|---|
| **Ø Ovary, Right** ♀<br>**1 Ovary, Left** ♀<br>**2 Ovaries, Bilateral** ♀ | **Ø Open**<br>**3 Percutaneous**<br>**4 Percutaneous Endoscopic**<br>8 Via Natural or Artificial Opening Endoscopic | **Ø Drainage Device** | **Z No Qualifier** |
| **Ø Ovary, Right** ♀<br>**1 Ovary, Left** ♀<br>**2 Ovaries, Bilateral** ♀ | **Ø Open**<br>**3 Percutaneous**<br>**4 Percutaneous Endoscopic**<br>8 Via Natural or Artificial Opening Endoscopic | **Z No Device** | **X Diagnostic**<br>**Z No Qualifier** |
| **Ø Ovary, Right** ♀<br>**1 Ovary, Left** ♀<br>**2 Ovaries, Bilateral** ♀ | **X External** | **Z No Device** | **Z No Qualifier** |
| **4 Uterine Supporting Structure** ♀<br>Broad ligament<br>Infundibulopelvic ligament<br>Ovarian ligament<br>Round ligament of uterus | **Ø Open**<br>**3 Percutaneous**<br>**4 Percutaneous Endoscopic**<br>8 Via Natural or Artificial Opening Endoscopic | **Ø Drainage Device** | **Z No Qualifier** |
| **4 Uterine Supporting Structure** ♀<br>Broad ligament<br>Infundibulopelvic ligament<br>Ovarian ligament<br>Round ligament of uterus | **Ø Open**<br>**3 Percutaneous**<br>**4 Percutaneous Endoscopic**<br>8 Via Natural or Artificial Opening Endoscopic | **Z No Device** | **X Diagnostic**<br>**Z No Qualifier** |
| **5 Fallopian Tube, Right** ♀<br>Oviduct<br>Salpinx<br>Uterine tube<br>**6 Fallopian Tube, Left** ♀<br>*See 5 Fallopian Tube, Right*<br>**7 Fallopian Tubes, Bilateral** ♀<br>**9 Uterus** ♀<br>Fundus uteri<br>Myometrium<br>Perimetrium<br>Uterine cornu<br>**C Cervix** ♀<br>**F Cul-de-sac** ♀ | **Ø Open**<br>**3 Percutaneous**<br>**4 Percutaneous Endoscopic**<br>**7 Via Natural or Artificial Opening**<br>**8 Via Natural or Artificial Opening Endoscopic** | **Ø Drainage Device** | **Z No Qualifier** |
| **5 Fallopian Tube, Right** ♀<br>Oviduct<br>Salpinx<br>Uterine tube<br>**6 Fallopian Tube, Left** ♀<br>*See 5 Fallopian Tube, Right*<br>**7 Fallopian Tubes, Bilateral** ♀<br>**9 Uterus** ♀<br>Fundus uteri<br>Myometrium<br>Perimetrium<br>Uterine cornu<br>**C Cervix** ♀<br>**F Cul-de-sac** ♀ | **Ø Open**<br>**3 Percutaneous**<br>**4 Percutaneous Endoscopic**<br>**7 Via Natural or Artificial Opening**<br>**8 Via Natural or Artificial Opening Endoscopic** | **Z No Device** | **X Diagnostic**<br>**Z No Qualifier** |

***ØU9 Continued on next page***

**Non-OR** ØU9[Ø,1,2][3,8]ØZ
**Non-OR** ØU9[Ø,1,2][3,8]ZZ
**Non-OR** ØU9[Ø,1,2]8ZX
**Non-OR** ØU94[3,8]ØZ
**Non-OR** ØU94[3,8]ZZ
**Non-OR** ØU948ZX
**Non-OR** ØU9[5,6,7,9,C]3ØZ
**Non-OR** ØU9F[3,4]ØZ
**Non-OR** ØU9[5,6,7][3,4,7,8]ZZ
**Non-OR** ØU9[9,C]3ZZ
**Non-OR** ØU9F[3,4]ZZ
♀ All body part, approach, device, and qualifier values

**Ø Medical and Surgical**
**U Female Reproductive System**
**9 Drainage** Definition: Taking or letting out fluids and/or gases from a body part
Explanation: The qualifier DIAGNOSTIC is used to identify drainage procedures that are biopsies

*ØU9 Continued*

| Body Part Character 4 | Approach Character 5 | Device Character 6 | Qualifier Character 7 |
|---|---|---|---|
| G Vagina ♀<br>K Hymen ♀ | Ø Open<br>3 Percutaneous<br>4 Percutaneous Endoscopic<br>7 Via Natural or Artificial Opening<br>8 Via Natural or Artificial Opening Endoscopic<br>X External | Ø Drainage Device | Z No Qualifier |
| G Vagina ♀<br>K Hymen ♀ | Ø Open<br>3 Percutaneous<br>4 Percutaneous Endoscopic<br>7 Via Natural or Artificial Opening<br>8 Via Natural or Artificial Opening Endoscopic<br>X External | Z No Device | X Diagnostic<br>Z No Qualifier |
| J Clitoris ♀<br>L Vestibular Gland ♀<br>Bartholin's (greater vestibular) gland<br>Greater vestibular (Bartholin's) gland<br>Paraurethral (Skene's) gland<br>Skene's (paraurethral) gland<br>M Vulva ♀<br>Labia majora<br>Labia minora | Ø Open<br>X External | Ø Drainage Device | Z No Qualifier |
| J Clitoris ♀<br>L Vestibular Gland ♀<br>Bartholin's (greater vestibular) gland<br>Greater vestibular (Bartholin's) gland<br>Paraurethral (Skene's) gland<br>Skene's (paraurethral) gland<br>M Vulva ♀<br>Labia majora<br>Labia minora | Ø Open<br>X External | Z No Device | X Diagnostic<br>Z No Qualifier |

Non-OR ØU9G3ØZ
Non-OR ØU9K[Ø,3,4,7,8,X]ØZ
Non-OR ØU9G3ZZ
Non-OR ØU9K[Ø,3,4,7,8,X]ZZ
Non-OR ØU9L[Ø,X]ØZ
Non-OR ØU9L[Ø,X]ZZ
♀ All body part, approach, device, and qualifier values

Female Reproductive System

**Ø Medical and Surgical**
**U Female Reproductive System**
**B Excision** Definition: Cutting out or off, without replacement, a portion of a body part

Explanation: The qualifier DIAGNOSTIC is used to identify excision procedures that are biopsies

| Body Part Character 4 | Approach Character 5 | Device Character 6 | Qualifier Character 7 |
|---|---|---|---|
| **Ø Ovary, Right** ♀<br>**1 Ovary, Left** ♀<br>**2 Ovaries, Bilateral** ♀<br>**4 Uterine Supporting Structure** ♀<br>Broad ligament<br>Infundibulopelvic ligament<br>Ovarian ligament<br>Round ligament of uterus<br>**5 Fallopian Tube, Right** ♀<br>Oviduct<br>Salpinx<br>Uterine tube<br>**6 Fallopian Tube, Left** ♀<br>*See 5 Fallopian Tube, Right*<br>**7 Fallopian Tubes, Bilateral** ♀<br>**9 Uterus** ♀<br>Fundus uteri<br>Myometrium<br>Perimetrium<br>Uterine cornu<br>**C Cervix** ♀<br>**F Cul-de-sac** ♀ | **Ø Open**<br>**3 Percutaneous**<br>**4 Percutaneous Endoscopic**<br>**7 Via Natural or Artificial Opening**<br>**8 Via Natural or Artificial Opening Endoscopic** | **Z No Device** | **X Diagnostic**<br>**Z No Qualifier** |
| **G Vagina** ♀<br>**K Hymen** ♀ | **Ø Open**<br>**3 Percutaneous**<br>**4 Percutaneous Endoscopic**<br>**7 Via Natural or Artificial Opening**<br>**8 Via Natural or Artificial Opening Endoscopic**<br>**X External** | **Z No Device** | **X Diagnostic**<br>**Z No Qualifier** |
| **J Clitoris** ♀<br>**L Vestibular Gland** ♀<br>Bartholin's (greater vestibular) gland<br>Greater vestibular (Bartholin's) gland<br>Paraurethral (Skene's) gland<br>Skene's (paraurethral) gland<br>**M Vulva** ♀<br>Labia majora<br>Labia minora | **Ø Open**<br>**X External** | **Z No Device** | **X Diagnostic**<br>**Z No Qualifier** |

♀ All body part, approach, device, and qualifier values



ØUB–ØUB

**Ø Medical and Surgical**
**U Female Reproductive System**
**C Extirpation** Definition: Taking or cutting out solid matter from a body part

Explanation: The solid matter may be an abnormal byproduct of a biological function or a foreign body; it may be imbedded in a body part or in the lumen of a tubular body part. The solid matter may or may not have been previously broken into pieces.

| Body Part Character 4 | Approach Character 5 | Device Character 6 | Qualifier Character 7 |
|---|---|---|---|
| **Ø Ovary, Right** ♀<br>**1 Ovary, Left** ♀<br>**2 Ovaries, Bilateral** ♀<br>**4 Uterine Supporting Structure** ♀<br>Broad ligament<br>Infundibulopelvic ligament<br>Ovarian ligament<br>Round ligament of uterus | **Ø Open**<br>**3 Percutaneous**<br>**4 Percutaneous Endoscopic**<br>**8 Via Natural or Artificial Opening Endoscopic** | **Z No Device** | **Z No Qualifier** |
| **5 Fallopian Tube, Right** ♀<br>Oviduct<br>Salpinx<br>Uterine tube<br>**6 Fallopian Tube, Left** ♀<br>*See 5 Fallopian Tube, Right*<br>**7 Fallopian Tubes, Bilateral** ♀<br>**9 Uterus** ♀<br>Fundus uteri<br>Myometrium<br>Perimetrium<br>Uterine cornu<br>**B Endometrium** ♀<br>**C Cervix** ♀<br>**F Cul-de-sac** ♀ | **Ø Open**<br>**3 Percutaneous**<br>**4 Percutaneous Endoscopic**<br>**7 Via Natural or Artificial Opening**<br>**8 Via Natural or Artificial Opening Endoscopic** | **Z No Device** | **Z No Qualifier** |
| **G Vagina** ♀<br>**K Hymen** ♀ | **Ø Open**<br>**3 Percutaneous**<br>**4 Percutaneous Endoscopic**<br>**7 Via Natural or Artificial Opening**<br>**8 Via Natural or Artificial Opening Endoscopic**<br>**X External** | **Z No Device** | **Z No Qualifier** |
| **J Clitoris** ♀<br>**L Vestibular Gland** ♀<br>Bartholin's (greater vestibular) gland<br>Greater vestibular (Bartholin's) gland<br>Paraurethral (Skene's) gland<br>Skene's (paraurethral) gland<br>**M Vulva** ♀<br>Labia majora<br>Labia minora | **Ø Open**<br>**X External** | **Z No Device** | **Z No Qualifier** |

**Non-OR** ØUC9[7,8]ZZ
**Non-OR** ØUCG[7,8,X]ZZ
**Non-OR** ØUCK[Ø,3,4,7,8,X]ZZ
**Non-OR** ØUCMXZZ

♀ All body part, approach, device, and qualifier values

**Ø Medical and Surgical**
**U Female Reproductive System**
**D Extraction** Definition: Pulling or stripping out or off all or a portion of a body part by the use of force

Explanation: The qualifier DIAGNOSTIC is used to identify extraction procedures that are biopsies

| Body Part Character 4 | Approach Character 5 | Device Character 6 | Qualifier Character 7 |
|---|---|---|---|
| **B** Endometrium ♀ | **7** Via Natural or Artificial Opening<br>**8** Via Natural or Artificial Opening Endoscopic | **Z** No Device | **X** Diagnostic<br>**Z** No Qualifier |
| **N** Ova ♀ | **Ø** Open<br>**3** Percutaneous<br>**4** Percutaneous Endoscopic | **Z** No Device | **Z** No Qualifier |

♀ All body part, approach, device, and qualifier values

**Ø Medical and Surgical**
**U Female Reproductive System**
**F Fragmentation** Definition: Breaking solid matter in a body part into pieces

Explanation: Physical force (e.g., manual, ultrasonic) applied directly or indirectly is used to break the solid matter into pieces. The solid matter may be an abnormal byproduct of a biological function or a foreign body. The pieces of solid matter are not taken out.

| Body Part Character 4 | Approach Character 5 | Device Character 6 | Qualifier Character 7 |
|---|---|---|---|
| **5 Fallopian Tube, Right** NC ♀<br>Oviduct<br>Salpinx<br>Uterine tube<br>**6 Fallopian Tube, Left** NC ♀<br>*See 5 Fallopian Tube, Right*<br>**7 Fallopian Tubes, Bilateral** NC ♀<br>**9 Uterus** NC ♀<br>Fundus uteri<br>Myometrium<br>Perimetrium<br>Uterine cornu | **Ø Open**<br>**3 Percutaneous**<br>**4 Percutaneous Endoscopic**<br>**7 Via Natural or Artificial Opening**<br>**8 Via Natural or Artificial Opening Endoscopic**<br>**X External** | **Z No Device** | **Z No Qualifier** |

**Non-OR** ØUF[5,6,7,9]XZZ
NC ØUF[5,6,7,9]XZZ
♀ All body part, approach, device, and qualifier values

**Ø Medical and Surgical**
**U Female Reproductive System**
**H Insertion** Definition: Putting in a nonbiological appliance that monitors, assists, performs, or prevents a physiological function but does not physically take the place of a body part

Explanation: None

| Body Part Character 4 | Approach Character 5 | Device Character 6 | Qualifier Character 7 |
|---|---|---|---|
| **3 Ovary** ♀ | **Ø Open**<br>**3 Percutaneous**<br>**4 Percutaneous Endoscopic** | **3 Infusion Device**<br>**Y Other Device** | **Z No Qualifier** |
| 3 Ovary ♀ | 7 Via Natural or Artificial Opening<br>8 Via Natural or Artificial Opening Endoscopic | Y Other Device | Z No Qualifier |
| **8 Fallopian Tube** ♀<br>**D Uterus and Cervix** ♀<br>**H Vagina and Cul-de-sac** ♀ | **Ø Open**<br>**3 Percutaneous**<br>**4 Percutaneous Endoscopic**<br>**7 Via Natural or Artificial Opening**<br>**8 Via Natural or Artificial Opening Endoscopic** | **3 Infusion Device**<br>**Y Other Device** | **Z No Qualifier** |
| **9 Uterus** ♀<br>Fundus uteri<br>Myometrium<br>Perimetrium<br>Uterine cornu | Ø Open<br>**7 Via Natural or Artificial Opening**<br>**8 Via Natural or Artificial Opening Endoscopic** | **H Contraceptive Device** | **Z No Qualifier** |
| **C Cervix** ♀ | **Ø Open**<br>**3 Percutaneous**<br>**4 Percutaneous Endoscopic** | **1 Radioactive Element** | **Z No Qualifier** |
| **C Cervix** ♀ | **7 Via Natural or Artificial Opening**<br>**8 Via Natural or Artificial Opening Endoscopic** | **1 Radioactive Element**<br>**H Contraceptive Device** | **Z No Qualifier** |
| **F Cul-de-sac** ♀ | **7 Via Natural or Artificial Opening**<br>**8 Via Natural or Artificial Opening Endoscopic** | **G Intraluminal Device, Pessary** | **Z No Qualifier** |
| **G Vagina** ♀ | **Ø Open**<br>**3 Percutaneous**<br>**4 Percutaneous Endoscopic**<br>**X External** | **1 Radioactive Element** | **Z No Qualifier** |
| **G Vagina** ♀ | **7 Via Natural or Artificial Opening**<br>**8 Via Natural or Artificial Opening Endoscopic** | **1 Radioactive Element**<br>**G Intraluminal Device, Pessary** | **Z No Qualifier** |

**Non-OR** ØUH3[Ø,3,4][3,Y]Z
**Non-OR** ØUH3[7,8]YZ
**Non-OR** ØUH[8,D][Ø,3,4,7,8][3,Y]Z
**Non-OR** ØUHH[3,4]YZ
**Non-OR** ØUHH[7,8][3,Y]Z
**Non-OR** ØUH9[Ø,7,8]HZ
**Non-OR** ØUHC[7,8]HZ
**Non-OR** ØUHF[7,8]GZ
**Non-OR** ØUHG[7,8]GZ
♀ All body part, approach, device, and qualifier values

**Ø Medical and Surgical**
**U Female Reproductive System**
**J Inspection** Definition: Visually and/or manually exploring a body part

Explanation: Visual exploration may be performed with or without optical instrumentation. Manual exploration may be performed directly or through intervening body layers.

| Body Part Character 4 | Approach Character 5 | Device Character 6 | Qualifier Character 7 |
|---|---|---|---|
| 3 Ovary ♀ | Ø Open<br>3 Percutaneous<br>4 Percutaneous Endoscopic<br>8 Via Natural or Artificial Opening Endoscopic<br>X External | Z No Device | Z No Qualifier |
| 8 Fallopian Tube ♀<br>D Uterus and Cervix ♀<br>H Vagina and Cul-de-sac ♀ | Ø Open<br>3 Percutaneous<br>4 Percutaneous Endoscopic<br>7 Via Natural or Artificial Opening<br>8 Via Natural or Artificial Opening Endoscopic<br>X External | Z No Device | Z No Qualifier |
| M Vulva ♀<br>Labia majora<br>Labia minora | Ø Open<br>X External | Z No Device | Z No Qualifier |

Non-OR ØUJ3[3,8,X]ZZ
Non-OR ØUJ[8,D,H][3,7,8,X]ZZ
Non-OR ØUJMXZZ

♀ All body part, approach, device, and qualifier values

**Ø Medical and Surgical**
**U Female Reproductive System**
**L Occlusion** Definition: Completely closing an orifice or the lumen of a tubular body part

Explanation: The orifice can be a natural orifice or an artificially created orifice

| Body Part Character 4 | Approach Character 5 | Device Character 6 | Qualifier Character 7 |
|---|---|---|---|
| 5 Fallopian Tube, Right ♀<br>Oviduct<br>Salpinx<br>Uterine tube<br>6 Fallopian Tube, Left ♀<br>*See 5 Fallopian Tube, Right*<br>7 Fallopian Tubes, Bilateral NC ♀ | Ø Open<br>3 Percutaneous<br>4 Percutaneous Endoscopic | C Extraluminal Device<br>D Intraluminal Device<br>Z No Device | Z No Qualifier |
| 5 Fallopian Tube, Right ♀<br>Oviduct<br>Salpinx<br>Uterine tube<br>6 Fallopian Tube, Left ♀<br>*See 5 Fallopian Tube, Right*<br>7 Fallopian Tubes, Bilateral NC ♀ | 7 Via Natural or Artificial Opening<br>8 Via Natural or Artificial Opening Endoscopic | D Intraluminal Device<br>Z No Device | Z No Qualifier |
| F Cul-de-sac ♀<br>G Vagina ♀ | 7 Via Natural or Artificial Opening<br>8 Via Natural or Artificial Opening Endoscopic | D Intraluminal Device<br>Z No Device | Z No Qualifier |

NC ØUL7[Ø,3,4][C,D,Z]Z with prinicpal diagnosis Z3Ø.2
NC ØUL7[7,8][D,Z]Z with prinicpal diagnosis Z3Ø.2

♀ All body part, approach, device, and qualifier values

**Ø Medical and Surgical**
**U Female Reproductive System**
**M Reattachment** Definition: Putting back in or on all or a portion of a separated body part to its normal location or other suitable location
Explanation: Vascular circulation and nervous pathways may or may not be reestablished

| Body Part Character 4 | Approach Character 5 | Device Character 6 | Qualifier Character 7 |
|---|---|---|---|
| **Ø Ovary, Right** ♀<br>**1 Ovary, Left** ♀<br>**2 Ovaries, Bilateral** ♀<br>**4 Uterine Supporting Structure** ♀<br>Broad ligament<br>Infundibulopelvic ligament<br>Ovarian ligament<br>Round ligament of uterus<br>**5 Fallopian Tube, Right** ♀<br>Oviduct<br>Salpinx<br>Uterine tube<br>**6 Fallopian Tube, Left** ♀<br>*See 5 Fallopian Tube, Right*<br>**7 Fallopian Tubes, Bilateral** ♀<br>**9 Uterus** ♀<br>Fundus uteri<br>Myometrium<br>Perimetrium<br>Uterine cornu<br>**C Cervix** ♀<br>**F Cul-de-sac** ♀<br>**G Vagina** ♀ | **Ø Open**<br>**4 Percutaneous Endoscopic** | **Z No Device** | **Z No Qualifier** |
| **J Clitoris** ♀<br>**M Vulva** ♀<br>Labia majora<br>Labia minora | **X External** | **Z No Device** | **Z No Qualifier** |
| **K Hymen** ♀ | **Ø Open**<br>**4 Percutaneous Endoscopic**<br>**X External** | **Z No Device** | **Z No Qualifier** |

♀ All body part, approach, device, and qualifier values

**Ø Medical and Surgical**
**U Female Reproductive System**
**N Release** Definition: Freeing a body part from an abnormal physical constraint by cutting or by the use of force
Explanation: Some of the restraining tissue may be taken out but none of the body part is taken out

| Body Part Character 4 | Approach Character 5 | Device Character 6 | Qualifier Character 7 |
|---|---|---|---|
| **Ø Ovary, Right** ♀<br>**1 Ovary, Left** ♀<br>**2 Ovaries, Bilateral** ♀<br>**4 Uterine Supporting Structure** ♀<br>Broad ligament<br>Infundibulopelvic ligament<br>Ovarian ligament<br>Round ligament of uterus | **Ø Open**<br>**3 Percutaneous**<br>**4 Percutaneous Endoscopic**<br>8 Via Natural or Artificial Opening Endoscopic | **Z No Device** | **Z No Qualifier** |
| **5 Fallopian Tube, Right** ♀<br>Oviduct<br>Salpinx<br>Uterine tube<br>**6 Fallopian Tube, Left** ♀<br>*See 5 Fallopian Tube, Right*<br>**7 Fallopian Tubes, Bilateral** ♀<br>**9 Uterus** ♀<br>Fundus uteri<br>Myometrium<br>Perimetrium<br>Uterine cornu<br>**C Cervix** ♀<br>**F Cul-de-sac** ♀ | **Ø Open**<br>**3 Percutaneous**<br>**4 Percutaneous Endoscopic**<br>**7 Via Natural or Artificial Opening**<br>**8 Via Natural or Artificial Opening Endoscopic** | **Z No Device** | **Z No Qualifier** |
| **G Vagina** ♀<br>**K Hymen** ♀ | **Ø Open**<br>**3 Percutaneous**<br>**4 Percutaneous Endoscopic**<br>**7 Via Natural or Artificial Opening**<br>**8 Via Natural or Artificial Opening Endoscopic**<br>**X External** | **Z No Device** | **Z No Qualifier** |
| **J Clitoris** ♀<br>**L Vestibular Gland** ♀<br>Bartholin's (greater vestibular) gland<br>Greater vestibular (Bartholin's) gland<br>Paraurethral (Skene's) gland<br>Skene's (paraurethral) gland<br>**M Vulva** ♀<br>Labia majora<br>Labia minora | **Ø Open**<br>**X External** | **Z No Device** | **Z No Qualifier** |

♀ All body part, approach, device, and qualifier values

**Ø Medical and Surgical**
**U Female Reproductive System**
**P Removal** Definition: Taking out or off a device from a body part

Explanation: If a device is taken out and a similar device put in without cutting or puncturing the skin or mucous membrane, the procedure is coded to the root operation CHANGE. Otherwise, the procedure for taking out the device is coded to the root operation REMOVAL.

| Body Part Character 4 | Approach Character 5 | Device Character 6 | Qualifier Character 7 |
|---|---|---|---|
| 3 Ovary ♀ | Ø Open<br>3 Percutaneous<br>4 Percutaneous Endoscopic | Ø Drainage Device<br>3 Infusion Device<br>Y Other Device | Z No Qualifier |
| 3 Ovary ♀ | 7 Via Natural or Artificial Opening<br>8 Via Natural or Artificial Opening Endoscopic | Y Other Device | Z No Qualifier |
| 3 Ovary ♀ | X External | Ø Drainage Device<br>3 Infusion Device | Z No Qualifier |
| 8 Fallopian Tube ♀ | Ø Open<br>3 Percutaneous<br>4 Percutaneous Endoscopic<br>7 Via Natural or Artificial Opening<br>8 Via Natural or Artificial Opening Endoscopic | Ø Drainage Device<br>3 Infusion Device<br>7 Autologous Tissue Substitute<br>C Extraluminal Device<br>D Intraluminal Device<br>J Synthetic Substitute<br>K Nonautologous Tissue Substitute<br>Y Other Device | Z No Qualifier |
| 8 Fallopian Tube ♀ | X External | Ø Drainage Device<br>3 Infusion Device<br>D Intraluminal Device | Z No Qualifier |
| D Uterus and Cervix ♀ | Ø Open<br>3 Percutaneous<br>4 Percutaneous Endoscopic<br>7 Via Natural or Artificial Opening<br>8 Via Natural or Artificial Opening Endoscopic | Ø Drainage Device<br>1 Radioactive Element<br>3 Infusion Device<br>7 Autologous Tissue Substitute<br>C Extraluminal Device<br>D Intraluminal Device<br>H Contraceptive Device<br>J Synthetic Substitute<br>K Nonautologous Tissue Substitute<br>Y Other Device | Z No Qualifier |
| D Uterus and Cervix ♀ | X External | Ø Drainage Device<br>3 Infusion Device<br>D Intraluminal Device<br>H Contraceptive Device | Z No Qualifier |
| H Vagina and Cul-de-sac ♀ | Ø Open<br>3 Percutaneous<br>4 Percutaneous Endoscopic<br>7 Via Natural or Artificial Opening<br>8 Via Natural or Artificial Opening Endoscopic | Ø Drainage Device<br>1 Radioactive Element<br>3 Infusion Device<br>7 Autologous Tissue Substitute<br>D Intraluminal Device<br>J Synthetic Substitute<br>K Nonautologous Tissue Substitute<br>Y Other Device | Z No Qualifier |
| H Vagina and Cul-de-sac ♀ | X External | Ø Drainage Device<br>1 Radioactive Element<br>3 Infusion Device<br>D Intraluminal Device | Z No Qualifier |
| M Vulva ♀<br>Labia majora<br>Labia minora | Ø Open | Ø Drainage Device<br>7 Autologous Tissue Substitute<br>J Synthetic Substitute<br>K Nonautologous Tissue Substitute | Z No Qualifier |
| M Vulva ♀<br>Labia majora<br>Labia minora | X External | Ø Drainage Device | Z No Qualifier |

Non-OR ØUP3[3,4]YZ
Non-OR ØUP3[7,8]YZ
Non-OR ØUP3X[Ø,3]Z
Non-OR ØUP8[3,4]YZ
Non-OR ØUP8[7,8][Ø,3,D,Y]Z
Non-OR ØUP8X[Ø,3,D]Z
Non-OR ØUPD[3,4][C,Y]Z
Non-OR ØUPD[7,8][Ø,3,C,D,H,Y]Z
Non-OR ØUPDX[Ø,3,D,H]Z
Non-OR ØUPH[3,4]YZ
Non-OR ØUPH[7,8][Ø,3,D,Y]Z
Non-OR ØUPHX[Ø,1,3,D]Z
Non-OR ØUPMXØZ
♀ All body part, approach, device, and qualifier values

**Ø Medical and Surgical**
**U Female Reproductive System**
**Q Repair** Definition: Restoring, to the extent possible, a body part to its normal anatomic structure and function
Explanation: Used only when the method to accomplish the repair is not one of the other root operations

| Body Part Character 4 | Approach Character 5 | Device Character 6 | Qualifier Character 7 |
|---|---|---|---|
| **Ø Ovary, Right** ♀<br>**1 Ovary, Left** ♀<br>**2 Ovaries, Bilateral** ♀<br>**4 Uterine Supporting Structure** ♀<br>Broad ligament<br>Infundibulopelvic ligament<br>Ovarian ligament<br>Round ligament of uterus | **Ø Open**<br>**3 Percutaneous**<br>**4 Percutaneous Endoscopic**<br>**8 Via Natural or Artificial Opening Endoscopic** | **Z No Device** | **Z No Qualifier** |
| **5 Fallopian Tube, Right** ♀<br>Oviduct<br>Salpinx<br>Uterine tube<br>**6 Fallopian Tube, Left** ♀<br>*See 5 Fallopian Tube, Right*<br>**7 Fallopian Tubes, Bilateral** ♀<br>**9 Uterus** ♀<br>Fundus uteri<br>Myometrium<br>Perimetrium<br>Uterine cornu<br>**C Cervix** ♀<br>**F Cul-de-sac** ♀ | **Ø Open**<br>**3 Percutaneous**<br>**4 Percutaneous Endoscopic**<br>**7 Via Natural or Artificial Opening**<br>**8 Via Natural or Artificial Opening Endoscopic** | **Z No Device** | **Z No Qualifier** |
| **G Vagina** ♀<br>**K Hymen** ♀ | **Ø Open**<br>**3 Percutaneous**<br>**4 Percutaneous Endoscopic**<br>**7 Via Natural or Artificial Opening**<br>**8 Via Natural or Artificial Opening Endoscopic**<br>**X External** | **Z No Device** | **Z No Qualifier** |
| **J Clitoris** ♀<br>**L Vestibular Gland** ♀<br>Bartholin's (greater vestibular) gland<br>Greater vestibular (Bartholin's) gland<br>Paraurethral (Skene's) gland<br>Skene's (paraurethral) gland<br>**M Vulva** ♀<br>Labia majora<br>Labia minora | **Ø Open**<br>**X External** | **Z No Device** | **Z No Qualifier** |

Non-OR ØUQG[7,X]ZZ
Non-OR ØUQKXZZ
Non-OR ØUQMXZZ
♀ All body part, approach, device, and qualifier values

**Ø Medical and Surgical**
**U Female Reproductive System**
**S Reposition** Definition: Moving to its normal location, or other suitable location, all or a portion of a body part
Explanation: The body part is moved to a new location from an abnormal location, or from a normal location where it is not functioning correctly. The body part may or may not be cut out or off to be moved to the new location.

| Body Part Character 4 | Approach Character 5 | Device Character 6 | Qualifier Character 7 |
|---|---|---|---|
| **Ø Ovary, Right** ♀<br>**1 Ovary, Left** ♀<br>**2 Ovaries, Bilateral** ♀<br>**4 Uterine Supporting Structure** ♀<br>Broad ligament<br>Infundibulopelvic ligament<br>Ovarian ligament<br>Round ligament of uterus<br>**5 Fallopian Tube, Right** ♀<br>Oviduct<br>Salpinx<br>Uterine tube<br>**6 Fallopian Tube, Left** ♀<br>*See 5 Fallopian Tube, Right*<br>**7 Fallopian Tubes, Bilateral** ♀<br>**C Cervix** ♀<br>**F Cul-de-sac** ♀ | **Ø Open**<br>**4 Percutaneous Endoscopic**<br>**8 Via Natural or Artificial Opening Endoscopic** | **Z No Device** | **Z No Qualifier** |
| **9 Uterus** ♀<br>Fundus uteri<br>Myometrium<br>Perimetrium<br>Uterine cornu<br>**G Vagina** ♀ | **Ø Open**<br>**4 Percutaneous Endoscopic**<br>**7 Via Natural or Artificial Opening**<br>**8 Via Natural or Artificial Opening Endoscopic**<br>**X External** | **Z No Device** | **Z No Qualifier** |

Non-OR ØUS9XZZ
♀ All body part, approach, device, and qualifier values

**Ø Medical and Surgical**
**U Female Reproductive System**
**T Resection** Definition: Cutting out or off, without replacement, all of a body part
Explanation: None

| Body Part Character 4 | Approach Character 5 | Device Character 6 | Qualifier Character 7 |
|---|---|---|---|
| **Ø Ovary, Right** ♀<br>**1 Ovary, Left** ♀<br>**2 Ovaries, Bilateral** ⊞♀<br>**5 Fallopian Tube, Right** ♀<br>Oviduct<br>Salpinx<br>Uterine tube<br>**6 Fallopian Tube, Left** ♀<br>*See 5 Fallopian Tube, Right*<br>**7 Fallopian Tubes, Bilateral** ⊞♀ | **Ø Open**<br>**4 Percutaneous Endoscopic**<br>**7 Via Natural or Artificial Opening**<br>**8 Via Natural or Artificial Opening Endoscopic**<br>**F Via Natural or Artificial Opening With Percutaneous Endoscopic Assistance** | **Z No Device** | **Z No Qualifier** |
| **4 Uterine Supporting Structure** ⊞♀<br>Broad ligament<br>Infundibulopelvic ligament<br>Ovarian ligament<br>Round ligament of uterus<br>**C Cervix** ⊞♀<br>**F Cul-de-sac** ♀<br>**G Vagina** ⊞♀ | **Ø Open**<br>**4 Percutaneous Endoscopic**<br>**7 Via Natural or Artificial Opening**<br>**8 Via Natural or Artificial Opening Endoscopic** | **Z No Device** | **Z No Qualifier** |
| **9 Uterus** ⊞♀<br>Fundus uteri<br>Myometrium<br>Perimetrium<br>Uterine cornu | **Ø Open**<br>**4 Percutaneous Endoscopic**<br>**7 Via Natural or Artificial Opening**<br>**8 Via Natural or Artificial Opening Endoscopic**<br>**F Via Natural or Artificial Opening With Percutaneous Endoscopic Assistance** | **Z No Device** | **L Supracervical**<br>**Z No Qualifier** |
| **J Clitoris** ♀<br>**L Vestibular Gland** ♀<br>Bartholin's (greater vestibular) gland<br>Greater vestibular (Bartholin's) gland<br>Paraurethral (Skene's) gland<br>Skene's (paraurethral) gland<br>**M Vulva** ⊞♀<br>Labia majora<br>Labia minora | **Ø Open**<br>**X External** | **Z No Device** | **Z No Qualifier** |
| **K Hymen** ♀ | **Ø Open**<br>**4 Percutaneous Endoscopic**<br>**7 Via Natural or Artificial Opening**<br>**8 Via Natural or Artificial Opening Endoscopic**<br>**X External** | **Z No Device** | **Z No Device** |

**See Appendix L for Procedure Combinations**
⊞ ØUT[2,7]ØZZ
⊞ ØUT[4,C][Ø,4,7,8]ZZ
⊞ ØUTGØZZ
⊞ ØUT9[Ø,4,7,8,F]ZZ
⊞ ØUTM[Ø,X]ZZ

♀ All body part, approach, device, and qualifier values

**Ø Medical and Surgical**
**U Female Reproductive System**
**U Supplement** Definition: Putting in or on biological or synthetic material that physically reinforces and/or augments the function of a portion of a body part

Explanation: The biological material is non-living, or is living and from the same individual. The body part may have been previously replaced, and the SUPPLEMENT procedure is performed to physically reinforce and/or augment the function of the replaced body part.

| Body Part Character 4 | Approach Character 5 | Device Character 6 | Qualifier Character 7 |
|---|---|---|---|
| **4 Uterine Supporting Structure** ♀<br>Broad ligament<br>Infundibulopelvic ligament<br>Ovarian ligament<br>Round ligament of uterus | **Ø Open**<br>**4 Percutaneous Endoscopic** | **7 Autologous Tissue Substitute**<br>**J Synthetic Substitute**<br>**K Nonautologous Tissue Substitute** | **Z No Qualifier** |
| **5 Fallopian Tube, Right** ♀<br>Oviduct<br>Salpinx<br>Uterine tube<br>**6 Fallopian Tube, Left** ♀<br>*See 5 Fallopian Tube, Right*<br>**7 Fallopian Tubes, Bilateral** ♀<br>**F Cul-de-sac** ♀ | **Ø Open**<br>**4 Percutaneous Endoscopic**<br>**7 Via Natural or Artificial Opening**<br>**8 Via Natural or Artificial Opening Endoscopic** | **7 Autologous Tissue Substitute**<br>**J Synthetic Substitute**<br>**K Nonautologous Tissue Substitute** | **Z No Qualifier** |
| **G Vagina** ♀<br>**K Hymen** ♀ | **Ø Open**<br>**4 Percutaneous Endoscopic**<br>**7 Via Natural or Artificial Opening**<br>**8 Via Natural or Artificial Opening Endoscopic**<br>**X External** | **7 Autologous Tissue Substitute**<br>**J Synthetic Substitute**<br>**K Nonautologous Tissue Substitute** | **Z No Qualifier** |
| **J Clitoris** ♀<br>**M Vulva** ♀<br>Labia majora<br>Labia minora | **Ø Open**<br>**X External** | **7 Autologous Tissue Substitute**<br>**J Synthetic Substitute**<br>**K Nonautologous Tissue Substitute** | **Z No Qualifier** |

♀ All body part, approach, device, and qualifier values

**Ø Medical and Surgical**
**U Female Reproductive System**
**V Restriction** Definition: Partially closing an orifice or the lumen of a tubular body part

Explanation: The orifice can be a natural orifice or an artificially created orifice

| Body Part Character 4 | Approach Character 5 | Device Character 6 | Qualifier Character 7 |
|---|---|---|---|
| **C Cervix** ♀ | **Ø Open**<br>**3 Percutaneous**<br>**4 Percutaneous Endoscopic** | **C Extraluminal Device**<br>**D Intraluminal Device**<br>**Z No Device** | **Z No Qualifier** |
| **C Cervix** ♀ | **7 Via Natural or Artificial Opening**<br>**8 Via Natural or Artificial Opening Endoscopic** | **D Intraluminal Device**<br>**Z No Device** | **Z No Qualifier** |

♀ All body part, approach, device, and qualifier values

**Ø Medical and Surgical**
**U Female Reproductive System**
**W Revision** Definition: Correcting, to the extent possible, a portion of a malfunctioning device or the position of a displaced device

Explanation: Revision can include correcting a malfunctioning or displaced device by taking out or putting in components of the device such as a screw or pin

| Body Part Character 4 | Approach Character 5 | Device Character 6 | Qualifier Character 7 |
|---|---|---|---|
| 3 Ovary ♀ | Ø Open<br>3 Percutaneous<br>4 Percutaneous Endoscopic | Ø Drainage Device<br>3 Infusion Device<br>Y Other Device | Z No Qualifier |
| 3 Ovary ♀ | 7 Via Natural or Artificial Opening<br>8 Via Natural or Artificial Opening Endoscopic | Y Other Device | Z No Qualifier |
| 3 Ovary ♀ | X External | Ø Drainage Device<br>3 Infusion Device | Z No Qualifier |
| 8 Fallopian Tube ♀ | Ø Open<br>3 Percutaneous<br>4 Percutaneous Endoscopic<br>7 Via Natural or Artificial Opening<br>8 Via Natural or Artificial Opening Endoscopic | Ø Drainage Device<br>3 Infusion Device<br>7 Autologous Tissue Substitute<br>C Extraluminal Device<br>D Intraluminal Device<br>J Synthetic Substitute<br>K Nonautologous Tissue Substitute<br>Y Other Device | Z No Qualifier |
| 8 Fallopian Tube ♀ | X External | Ø Drainage Device<br>3 Infusion Device<br>7 Autologous Tissue Substitute<br>C Extraluminal Device<br>D Intraluminal Device<br>J Synthetic Substitute<br>K Nonautologous Tissue Substitute | Z No Qualifier |
| D Uterus and Cervix ♀ | Ø Open<br>3 Percutaneous<br>4 Percutaneous Endoscopic<br>7 Via Natural or Artificial Opening<br>8 Via Natural or Artificial Opening Endoscopic | Ø Drainage Device<br>1 Radioactive Element<br>3 Infusion Device<br>7 Autologous Tissue Substitute<br>C Extraluminal Device<br>D Intraluminal Device<br>H Contraceptive Device<br>J Synthetic Substitute<br>K Nonautologous Tissue Substitute<br>Y Other Device | Z No Qualifier |
| D Uterus and Cervix ♀ | X External | Ø Drainage Device<br>3 Infusion Device<br>7 Autologous Tissue Substitute<br>C Extraluminal Device<br>D Intraluminal Device<br>H Contraceptive Device<br>J Synthetic Substitute<br>K Nonautologous Tissue Substitute | Z No Qualifier |
| H Vagina and Cul-de-sac ♀ | Ø Open<br>3 Percutaneous<br>4 Percutaneous Endoscopic<br>7 Via Natural or Artificial Opening<br>8 Via Natural or Artificial Opening Endoscopic | Ø Drainage Device<br>1 Radioactive Element<br>3 Infusion Device<br>7 Autologous Tissue Substitute<br>D Intraluminal Device<br>J Synthetic Substitute<br>K Nonautologous Tissue Substitute<br>Y Other Device | Z No Qualifier |
| H Vagina and Cul-de-sac ♀ | X External | Ø Drainage Device<br>3 Infusion Device<br>7 Autologous Tissue Substitute<br>D Intraluminal Device<br>J Synthetic Substitute<br>K Nonautologous Tissue Substitute | Z No Qualifier |
| M Vulva ♀<br>Labia majora<br>Labia minora | Ø Open<br>X External | Ø Drainage Device<br>7 Autologous Tissue Substitute<br>J Synthetic Substitute<br>K Nonautologous Tissue Substitute | Z No Qualifier |

Non-OR ØUW3[3,4]YZ
Non-OR ØUW3[7,8]YZ
Non-OR ØUW3X[Ø,3]Z
Non-OR ØUW8[3,4,7,8]YZ
Non-OR ØUW8X[Ø,3,7,C,D,J,K]Z
Non-OR ØUWD[3,4,7,8]YZ
Non-OR ØUWDX[Ø,3,7,C,D,H,J,K]Z
Non-OR ØUWH[3,4,7,8]YZ
Non-OR ØUWHX[Ø,3,7,D,J,K]Z
Non-OR ØUWMX[Ø,7,J,K]Z
♀ All body part, approach, device, and qualifier values

**Ø Medical and Surgical**
**U Female Reproductive System**
**Y Transplantation** Definition: Putting in or on all or a portion of a living body part taken from another individual or animal to physically take the place and/or function of all or a portion of a similar body part

Explanation: The native body part may or may not be taken out, and the transplanted body part may take over all or a portion of its function

| Body Part Character 4 | Approach Character 5 | Device Character 6 | Qualifier Character 7 |
|---|---|---|---|
| Ø Ovary, Right ♀<br>1 Ovary, Left ♀ | Ø Open | Z No Device | Ø Allogeneic<br>1 Syngeneic<br>2 Zooplastic |

♀ All body part, approach, device, and qualifier values

# Male Reproductive System ØV1–ØVW



## Character Meaning

This Character Meaning table is provided as a guide to assist the user in the identification of character members that may be found in this section of code tables. It **SHOULD NOT** be used to build a PCS code.

| Operation–Character 3 | Body Part–Character 4 | Approach–Character 5 | Device–Character 6 | Qualifier–Character 7 |
|---|---|---|---|---|
| 1 Bypass | Ø Prostate | Ø Open | Ø Drainage Device | J Epididymis, Right |
| 2 Change | 1 Seminal Vesicle, Right | 3 Percutaneous | 1 Radioactive Element | K Epididymis, Left |
| 5 Destruction | 2 Seminal Vesicle, Left | 4 Percutaneous Endoscopic | 3 Infusion Device | N Vas Deferens, Right |
| 7 Dilation | 3 Seminal Vesicles, Bilateral | 7 Via Natural or Artificial Opening | 7 Autologous Tissue Substitute | P Vas Deferens, Left |
| 9 Drainage | 4 Prostate and Seminal Vesicles | 8 Via Natural or Artificial Opening Endoscopic | C Extraluminal Device | X Diagnostic |
| B Excision | 5 Scrotum | X External | D Intraluminal Device | Z No Qualifier |
| C Extirpation | 6 Tunica Vaginalis, Right | | J Synthetic Substitute | |
| H Insertion | 7 Tunica Vaginalis, Left | | K Nonautologous Tissue Substitute | |
| J Inspection | 8 Scrotum and Tunica Vaginalis | | Y Other Device | |
| L Occlusion | 9 Testis, Right | | Z No Device | |
| M Reattachment | B Testis, Left | | | |
| N Release | C Testes, Bilateral | | | |
| P Removal | D Testis | | | |
| Q Repair | F Spermatic Cord, Right | | | |
| R Replacement | G Spermatic Cord, Left | | | |
| S Reposition | H Spermatic Cords, Bilateral | | | |
| T Resection | J Epididymis, Right | | | |
| U Supplement | K Epididymis, Left | | | |
| W Revision | L Epididymis, Bilateral | | | |
| | M Epididymis and Spermatic Cord | | | |
| | N Vas Deferens, Right | | | |
| | P Vas Deferens, Left | | | |
| | Q Vas Deferens, Bilateral | | | |
| | R Vas Deferens | | | |
| | S Penis | | | |
| | T Prepuce | | | |

**AHA Coding Clinic for table ØVB**
**2016, 1Q, 23** Transurethral resection of ejaculatory ducts
**2014, 4Q, 33** Radical prostatectomy

**AHA Coding Clinic for table ØVP**
**2016, 2Q, 28** Removal of multi-component inflatable penile prosthesis with placement of new malleable device

**AHA Coding Clinic for table ØVT**
**2014, 4Q, 33** Radical prostatectomy

**AHA Coding Clinic for table ØVU**
**2016, 2Q, 28** Removal of multi-component inflatable penile prosthesis with placement of new malleable device
**2015, 3Q, 25** Placement of inflatable penile prosthesis

## Male Reproductive System

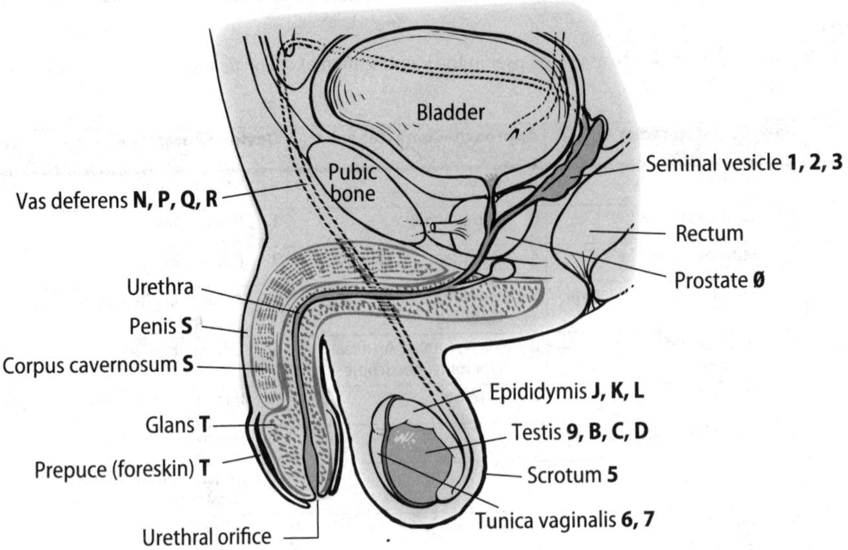
Bladder
Pubic bone
Vas deferens N, P, Q, R
Seminal vesicle 1, 2, 3
Rectum
Prostate Ø
Urethra
Penis S
Corpus cavernosum S
Glans T
Prepuce (foreskin) T
Urethral orifice
Epididymis J, K, L
Testis 9, B, C, D
Scrotum 5
Tunica vaginalis 6, 7

## Penis

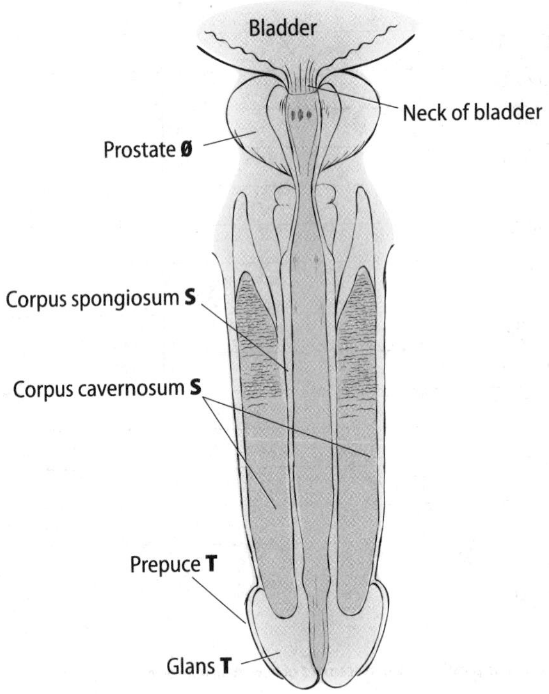
Bladder
Neck of bladder
Prostate Ø
Corpus spongiosum S
Corpus cavernosum S
Prepuce T
Glans T

**Ø Medical and Surgical**
**V Male Reproductive System**
**1 Bypass** Definition: Altering the route of passage of the contents of a tubular body part

Explanation: Rerouting contents of a body part to a downstream area of the normal route, to a similar route and body part, or to an abnormal route and dissimilar body part. Includes one or more anastomoses, with or without the use of a device.

| Body Part<br>Character 4 | Approach<br>Character 5 | Device<br>Character 6 | Qualifier<br>Character 7 |
|---|---|---|---|
| **N** Vas Deferens, Right ♂<br>Ductus deferens<br>Ejaculatory duct<br>**P** Vas Deferens, Left ♂<br>*See N Vas Deferens, Right*<br>**Q** Vas Deferens, Bilateral ♂<br>*See N Vas Deferens, Right* | **Ø** Open<br>**4** Percutaneous Endoscopic | **7** Autologous Tissue Substitute<br>**J** Synthetic Substitute<br>**K** Nonautologous Tissue Substitute<br>**Z** No Device | **J** Epididymis, Right<br>**K** Epididymis, Left<br>**N** Vas Deferens, Right<br>**P** Vas Deferens, Left |

♂ All body part, approach, device, and qualifier values

**Ø Medical and Surgical**
**V Male Reproductive System**
**2 Change** Definition: Taking out or off a device from a body part and putting back an identical or similar device in or on the same body part without cutting or puncturing the skin or a mucous membrane

Explanation: All CHANGE procedures are coded using the approach EXTERNAL

| Body Part<br>Character 4 | Approach<br>Character 5 | Device<br>Character 6 | Qualifier<br>Character 7 |
|---|---|---|---|
| **4** Prostate and Seminal Vesicles ♂<br>**8** Scrotum and Tunica Vaginalis ♂<br>**D** Testis ♂<br>**M** Epididymis and Spermatic Cord ♂<br>**R** Vas Deferens ♂<br>Ductus deferens<br>Ejaculatory duct<br>**S** Penis ♂<br>Corpus cavernosum<br>Corpus spongiosum | **X** External | **Ø** Drainage Device<br>**Y** Other Device | **Z** No Qualifier |

Non-OR All body part, approach, device, and qualifier values

♂ All body part, approach, device, and qualifier values

**Ø Medical and Surgical**
**V Male Reproductive System**
**5 Destruction** Definition: Physical eradication of all or a portion of a body part by the direct use of energy, force, or a destructive agent

Explanation: None of the body part is physically taken out

| Body Part<br>Character 4 | Approach<br>Character 5 | Device<br>Character 6 | Qualifier<br>Character 7 |
|---|---|---|---|
| **Ø** Prostate ♂ | **Ø** Open<br>**3** Percutaneous<br>**4** Percutaneous Endoscopic<br>**7** Via Natural or Artificial Opening<br>**8** Via Natural or Artificial Opening Endoscopic | **Z** No Device | **Z** No Qualifier |
| **1** Seminal Vesicle, Right ♂<br>**2** Seminal Vesicle, Left ♂<br>**3** Seminal Vesicles, Bilateral ♂<br>**6** Tunica Vaginalis, Right ♂<br>**7** Tunica Vaginalis, Left ♂<br>**9** Testis, Right ♂<br>**B** Testis, Left ♂<br>**C** Testes, Bilateral ♂ | **Ø** Open<br>**3** Percutaneous<br>**4** Percutaneous Endoscopic | **Z** No Device | **Z** No Qualifier |
| **5** Scrotum ♂<br>**S** Penis ♂<br>Corpus cavernosum<br>Corpus spongiosum<br>**T** Prepuce ♂<br>Foreskin<br>Glans penis | **Ø** Open<br>**3** Percutaneous<br>**4** Percutaneous Endoscopic<br>**X** External | **Z** No Device | **Z** No Qualifier |
| **F** Spermatic Cord, Right ♂<br>**G** Spermatic Cord, Left ♂<br>**H** Spermatic Cords, Bilateral ♂<br>**J** Epididymis, Right ♂<br>**K** Epididymis, Left ♂<br>**L** Epididymis, Bilateral ♂<br>**N** Vas Deferens, Right NC ♂<br>Ductus deferens<br>Ejaculatory duct<br>**P** Vas Deferens, Left NC ♂<br>*See N Vas Deferens, Right*<br>**Q** Vas Deferens, Bilateral NC ♂<br>*See N Vas Deferens, Right* | **Ø** Open<br>**3** Percutaneous<br>**4** Percutaneous Endoscopic<br>**8** Via Natural or Artificial Opening Endoscopic | **Z** No Device | **Z** No Qualifier |

Non-OR ØV5[N,P,Q][Ø,3,4,8]ZZ
Non-OR ØV55[Ø,3,4,X]ZZ

NC ØV5[N,P,Q][Ø,3,4]ZZ with principal diagnosis code Z3Ø.2
♂ All body part, approach, device, and qualifier values

**Ø Medical and Surgical**
**V Male Reproductive System**
**7 Dilation** Definition: Expanding an orifice or the lumen of a tubular body part

Explanation: The orifice can be a natural orifice or an artificially created orifice. Accomplished by stretching a tubular body part using intraluminal pressure or by cutting part of the orifice or wall of the tubular body part.

| Body Part Character 4 | Approach Character 5 | Device Character 6 | Qualifier Character 7 |
|---|---|---|---|
| N Vas Deferens, Right ♂<br>Ductus deferens<br>Ejaculatory duct<br>P Vas Deferens, Left ♂<br>*See N Vas Deferens, Right*<br>Q Vas Deferens, Bilateral ♂<br>*See N Vas Deferens, Right* | Ø Open<br>3 Percutaneous<br>4 Percutaneous Endoscopic | D Intraluminal Device<br>Z No Device | Z No Qualifier |

♂ All body part, approach, device, and qualifier values

**Ø Medical and Surgical**
**V Male Reproductive System**
**9 Drainage** Definition: Taking or letting out fluids and/or gases from a body part

Explanation: The qualifier DIAGNOSTIC is used to identify drainage procedures that are biopsies

| Body Part Character 4 | Approach Character 5 | Device Character 6 | Qualifier Character 7 |
|---|---|---|---|
| Ø Prostate ♂ | Ø Open<br>3 Percutaneous<br>4 Percutaneous Endoscopic<br>7 Via Natural or Artificial Opening<br>8 Via Natural or Artificial Opening Endoscopic | Ø Drainage Device | Z No Qualifier |
| Ø Prostate ♂ | Ø Open<br>3 Percutaneous<br>4 Percutaneous Endoscopic<br>7 Via Natural or Artificial Opening<br>8 Via Natural or Artificial Opening Endoscopic | Z No Device | X Diagnostic<br>Z No Qualifier |
| 1 Seminal Vesicle, Right ♂<br>2 Seminal Vesicle, Left ♂<br>3 Seminal Vesicles, Bilateral ♂<br>6 Tunica Vaginalis, Right ♂<br>7 Tunica Vaginalis, Left ♂<br>9 Testis, Right ♂<br>B Testis, Left ♂<br>C Testes, Bilateral ♂<br>F Spermatic Cord, Right ♂<br>G Spermatic Cord, Left ♂<br>H Spermatic Cords, Bilateral ♂<br>J Epididymis, Right ♂<br>K Epididymis, Left ♂<br>L Epididymis, Bilateral ♂<br>N Vas Deferens, Right ♂<br>Ductus deferens<br>Ejaculatory duct<br>P Vas Deferens, Left ♂<br>*See N Vas Deferens, Right*<br>Q Vas Deferens, Bilateral ♂<br>*See N Vas Deferens, Right* | Ø Open<br>3 Percutaneous<br>4 Percutaneous Endoscopic | Ø Drainage Device | Z No Qualifier |

***ØV9 Continued on next page***

Non-OR ØV9Ø[3,4]ØZ
Non-OR ØV9Ø[3,4]Z[X,Z]
Non-OR ØV9Ø[7,8]ZX
Non-OR ØV9[1,2,3,9,B,C][3,4]ØZ
Non-OR ØV9[6,7,F,G,H,N,P,Q][Ø,3,4]ØZ
Non-OR ØV9[J,K,L]3ØZ

♂ All body part, approach, device, and qualifier values

**Ø Medical and Surgical**
**V Male Reproductive System**
**9 Drainage** Definition: Taking or letting out fluids and/or gases from a body part
Explanation: The qualifier DIAGNOSTIC is used to identify drainage procedures that are biopsies

*ØV9 Continued*

| Body Part Character 4 | Approach Character 5 | Device Character 6 | Qualifier Character 7 |
|---|---|---|---|
| **1 Seminal Vesicle, Right** ♂<br>**2 Seminal Vesicle, Left** ♂<br>**3 Seminal Vesicles, Bilateral** ♂<br>**6 Tunica Vaginalis, Right** ♂<br>**7 Tunica Vaginalis, Left** ♂<br>**9 Testis, Right** ♂<br>**B Testis, Left** ♂<br>**C Testes, Bilateral** ♂<br>**F Spermatic Cord, Right** ♂<br>**G Spermatic Cord, Left** ♂<br>**H Spermatic Cords, Bilateral** ♂<br>**J Epididymis, Right** ♂<br>**K Epididymis, Left** ♂<br>**L Epididymis, Bilateral** ♂<br>**N Vas Deferens, Right** ♂<br>Ductus deferens<br>Ejaculatory duct<br>**P Vas Deferens, Left** ♂<br>*See N Vas Deferens, Right*<br>**Q Vas Deferens, Bilateral** ♂<br>*See N Vas Deferens, Right* | **Ø Open**<br>**3 Percutaneous**<br>**4 Percutaneous Endoscopic** | **Z No Device** | **X Diagnostic**<br>**Z No Qualifier** |
| **5 Scrotum** ♂<br>**S Penis** ♂<br>Corpus cavernosum<br>Corpus spongiosum<br>**T Prepuce** ♂<br>Foreskin<br>Glans penis | **Ø Open**<br>**3 Percutaneous**<br>**4 Percutaneous Endoscopic**<br>**X External** | **Ø Drainage Device** | **Z No Qualifier** |
| **5 Scrotum** ♂<br>**S Penis** ♂<br>Corpus cavernosum<br>Corpus spongiosum<br>**T Prepuce** ♂<br>Foreskin<br>Glans penis | **Ø Open**<br>**3 Percutaneous**<br>**4 Percutaneous Endoscopic**<br>**X External** | **Z No Device** | **X Diagnostic**<br>**Z No Qualifier** |

**Non-OR** ØV9[1,2,3,9,B,C][3,4]Z[X,Z]
**Non-OR** ØV9[6,7,F,G,H,J,K,L,N,P,Q][Ø,3,4]ZX
**Non-OR** ØV9[6,7,F,G,H,N,P,Q][Ø,3,4]ZZ
**Non-OR** ØV9[J,K,L]3ZZ
**Non-OR** ØV95[Ø,3,4,X]ØZ
**Non-OR** ØV9[S,T]3ØZ
**Non-OR** ØV95[Ø,3,4,X]Z[X,Z]
**Non-OR** ØV9[S,T]3ZZ

♂ All body part, approach, device, and qualifier values

**Ø Medical and Surgical**
**V Male Reproductive System**
**B Excision** Definition: Cutting out or off, without replacement, a portion of a body part
Explanation: The qualifier DIAGNOSTIC is used to identify excision procedures that are biopsies

| Body Part Character 4 | Approach Character 5 | Device Character 6 | Qualifier Character 7 |
|---|---|---|---|
| **Ø Prostate** ♂ | **Ø Open**<br>**3 Percutaneous**<br>**4 Percutaneous Endoscopic**<br>**7 Via Natural or Artificial Opening**<br>**8 Via Natural or Artificial Opening Endoscopic** | **Z No Device** | **X Diagnostic**<br>**Z No Qualifier** |
| **1 Seminal Vesicle, Right** ♂<br>**2 Seminal Vesicle, Left** ♂<br>**3 Seminal Vesicles, Bilateral** ♂<br>**6 Tunica Vaginalis, Right** ♂<br>**7 Tunica Vaginalis, Left** ♂<br>**9 Testis, Right** ♂<br>**B Testis, Left** ♂<br>**C Testes, Bilateral** ♂ | **Ø Open**<br>**3 Percutaneous**<br>**4 Percutaneous Endoscopic** | **Z No Device** | **X Diagnostic**<br>**Z No Qualifier** |
| **5 Scrotum** ♂<br>**S Penis** ♂<br>Corpus cavernosum<br>Corpus spongiosum<br>**T Prepuce** ♂<br>Foreskin<br>Glans penis | **Ø Open**<br>**3 Percutaneous**<br>**4 Percutaneous Endoscopic**<br>**X External** | **Z No Device** | **X Diagnostic**<br>**Z No Qualifier** |
| **F Spermatic Cord, Right** ♂<br>**G Spermatic Cord, Left** ♂<br>**H Spermatic Cords, Bilateral** ♂<br>**J Epididymis, Right** ♂<br>**K Epididymis, Left** ♂<br>**L Epididymis, Bilateral** ♂<br>**N Vas Deferens, Right** NC ♂<br>Ductus deferens<br>Ejaculatory duct<br>**P Vas Deferens, Left** NC ♂<br>*See N Vas Deferens, Right*<br>**Q Vas Deferens, Bilateral** NC ♂<br>*See N Vas Deferens, Right* | **Ø Open**<br>**3 Percutaneous**<br>**4 Percutaneous Endoscopic**<br>**8 Via Natural or Artificial Opening Endoscopic** | **Z No Device** | **X Diagnostic**<br>**Z No Qualifier** |

**Non-OR** ØVBØ[3,4,7,8]ZX
**Non-OR** ØVB[1,2,3,9,B,C][3,4]ZX
**Non-OR** ØVB[6,7][Ø,3,4]ZX
**Non-OR** ØVB5[Ø,3,4,X]Z[X,Z]
**Non-OR** ØVB[F,G,H,J,K,L][Ø,3,4,8]ZX
**Non-OR** ØVB[N,P,Q][Ø,3,4,8]Z[X,Z]
NC ØVB[N,P,Q][Ø,3,4]ZZ with principal diagnosis code Z3Ø.2
♂ All body part, approach, device, and qualifier values

**Ø Medical and Surgical**
**V Male Reproductive System**
**C Extirpation** Definition: Taking or cutting out solid matter from a body part

Explanation: The solid matter may be an abnormal byproduct of a biological function or a foreign body; it may be imbedded in a body part or in the lumen of a tubular body part. The solid matter may or may not have been previously broken into pieces.

| Body Part Character 4 | Approach Character 5 | Device Character 6 | Qualifier Character 7 |
|---|---|---|---|
| **Ø** Prostate ♂ | **Ø** Open<br>**3** Percutaneous<br>**4** Percutaneous Endoscopic<br>**7** Via Natural or Artificial Opening<br>**8** Via Natural or Artificial Opening Endoscopic | **Z** No Device | **Z** No Qualifier |
| **1** Seminal Vesicle, Right ♂<br>**2** Seminal Vesicle, Left ♂<br>**3** Seminal Vesicles, Bilateral ♂<br>**6** Tunica Vaginalis, Right ♂<br>**7** Tunica Vaginalis, Left ♂<br>**9** Testis, Right ♂<br>**B** Testis, Left ♂<br>**C** Testes, Bilateral ♂<br>**F** Spermatic Cord, Right ♂<br>**G** Spermatic Cord, Left ♂<br>**H** Spermatic Cords, Bilateral ♂<br>**J** Epididymis, Right ♂<br>**K** Epididymis, Left ♂<br>**L** Epididymis, Bilateral ♂<br>**N** Vas Deferens, Right ♂<br>Ductus deferens<br>Ejaculatory duct<br>**P** Vas Deferens, Left ♂<br>*See N Vas Deferens, Right*<br>**Q** Vas Deferens, Bilateral ♂<br>*See N Vas Deferens, Right* | **Ø** Open<br>**3** Percutaneous<br>**4** Percutaneous Endoscopic | **Z** No Device | **Z** No Qualifier |
| **5** Scrotum ♂<br>**S** Penis ♂<br>Corpus cavernosum<br>Corpus spongiosum<br>**T** Prepuce ♂<br>Foreskin<br>Glans penis | **Ø** Open<br>**3** Percutaneous<br>**4** Percutaneous Endoscopic<br>**X** External | **Z** No Device | **Z** No Qualifier |

Non-OR ØVC[6,7,N,P,Q][Ø,3,4]ZZ
Non-OR ØVC5[Ø,3,4,X]ZZ
Non-OR ØVCSXZZ
♂ All body part, approach, device, and qualifier values

**Ø Medical and Surgical**
**V Male Reproductive System**
**H Insertion** Definition: Putting in a nonbiological appliance that monitors, assists, performs, or prevents a physiological function but does not physically take the place of a body part

Explanation: None

| Body Part Character 4 | Approach Character 5 | Device Character 6 | Qualifier Character 7 |
|---|---|---|---|
| Ø Prostate ♂ | Ø Open<br>3 Percutaneous<br>4 Percutaneous Endoscopic<br>7 Via Natural or Artificial Opening<br>8 Via Natural or Artificial Opening Endoscopic | 1 Radioactive Element | Z No Qualifier |
| 4 Prostate and Seminal Vesicles ♂<br>8 Scrotum and Tunica Vaginalis ♂<br>D Testis ♂<br>M Epididymis and Spermatic Cord ♂<br>R Vas Deferens ♂<br>Ductus deferens<br>Ejaculatory duct | Ø Open<br>3 Percutaneous<br>4 Percutaneous Endoscopic<br>7 Via Natural or Artificial Opening<br>8 Via Natural or Artificial Opening Endoscopic | 3 Infusion Device<br>Y Other Device | Z No Qualifier |
| S Penis ♂<br>Corpus cavernosum<br>Corpus spongiosum | Ø Open<br>3 Percutaneous<br>4 Percutaneous Endoscopic | 3 Infusion Device<br>Y Other Device | Z No Qualifier |
| S Penis ♂<br>Corpus cavernosum<br>Corpus spongiosum | 7 Via Natural or Artificial Opening<br>8 Via Natural or Artificial Opening Endoscopic | Y Other Device | Z No Qualifier |
| S Penis ♂<br>Corpus cavernosum<br>Corpus spongiosum | X External | 3 Infusion Device | Z No Qualifier |

Non-OR ØVH[4,8,D,M,R][Ø,3,4,7,8][3,Y]Z
Non-OR ØVHS[Ø,3,4][3,Y]Z
Non-OR ØVHS[7,8]YZ
Non-OR ØVHSX3Z
♂ All body part, approach, device, and qualifier values

**Ø Medical and Surgical**
**V Male Reproductive System**
**J Inspection** Definition: Visually and/or manually exploring a body part

Explanation: Visual exploration may be performed with or without optical instrumentation. Manual exploration may be performed directly or through intervening body layers.

| Body Part Character 4 | Approach Character 5 | Device Character 6 | Qualifier Character 7 |
|---|---|---|---|
| 4 Prostate and Seminal Vesicles ♂<br>8 Scrotum and Tunica Vaginalis ♂<br>D Testis ♂<br>M Epididymis and Spermatic Cord ♂<br>R Vas Deferens ♂<br>Ductus deferens<br>Ejaculatory duct<br>S Penis ♂<br>Corpus cavernosum<br>Corpus spongiosum | Ø Open<br>3 Percutaneous<br>4 Percutaneous Endoscopic<br>X External | Z No Device | Z No Qualifier |

Non-OR ØVJ[4,D,M,R][3,X]ZZ
Non-OR ØVJ[8,S][Ø,3,4,X]ZZ
♂ All body part, approach, device, and qualifier values

**Ø Medical and Surgical**
**V Male Reproductive System**
**L Occlusion** Definition: Completely closing an orifice or the lumen of a tubular body part

Explanation: The orifice can be a natural orifice or an artificially created orifice

| Body Part Character 4 | Approach Character 5 | Device Character 6 | Qualifier Character 7 |
|---|---|---|---|
| F Spermatic Cord, Right NC ♂<br>G Spermatic Cord, Left NC ♂<br>H Spermatic Cords, Bilateral NC ♂<br>N Vas Deferens, Right NC ♂<br>Ductus deferens<br>Ejaculatory duct<br>P Vas Deferens, Left NC ♂<br>*See N Vas Deferens, Right*<br>Q Vas Deferens, Bilateral NC ♂<br>*See N Vas Deferens, Right* | Ø Open<br>3 Percutaneous<br>4 Percutaneous Endoscopic<br>8 Via Natural or Artificial Opening Endoscopic | C Extraluminal Device<br>D Intraluminal Device<br>Z No Device | Z No Qualifier |

Non-OR ØVL[F,G,H][Ø,3,4,8][C,D,Z]Z
Non-OR ØVL[N,P,Q][Ø,3,4,8][C,Z]Z
NC ØVL[F,G,H][Ø,3,4][C,D,Z]Z with principal diagnosis code Z3Ø.2
NC ØVL[N,P,Q][Ø,3,4][C,Z]Z with principal diagnosis code Z3Ø.2
♂ All body part, approach, device, and qualifier values

**Ø Medical and Surgical**
**V Male Reproductive System**
**M Reattachment** Definition: Putting back in or on all or a portion of a separated body part to its normal location or other suitable location
Explanation: Vascular circulation and nervous pathways may or may not be reestablished

| Body Part Character 4 | Approach Character 5 | Device Character 6 | Qualifier Character 7 |
|---|---|---|---|
| **5 Scrotum** ♂<br>**S Penis** ♂<br>Corpus cavernosum<br>Corpus spongiosum | **X External** | **Z No Device** | **Z No Qualifier** |
| **6 Tunica Vaginalis, Right** ♂<br>**7 Tunica Vaginalis, Left** ♂<br>**9 Testis, Right** ♂<br>**B Testis, Left** ♂<br>**C Testes, Bilateral** ♂<br>**F Spermatic Cord, Right** ♂<br>**G Spermatic Cord, Left** ♂<br>**H Spermatic Cords, Bilateral** ♂ | **Ø Open**<br>**4 Percutaneous Endoscopic** | **Z No Device** | **Z No Qualifier** |

♂ All body part, approach, device, and qualifier values

**Ø Medical and Surgical**
**V Male Reproductive System**
**N Release** Definition: Freeing a body part from an abnormal physical constraint by cutting or by the use of force
Explanation: Some of the restraining tissue may be taken out but none of the body part is taken out

| Body Part Character 4 | Approach Character 5 | Device Character 6 | Qualifier Character 7 |
|---|---|---|---|
| **Ø Prostate** ♂ | **Ø Open**<br>**3 Percutaneous**<br>**4 Percutaneous Endoscopic**<br>**7 Via Natural or Artificial Opening**<br>**8 Via Natural or Artificial Opening Endoscopic** | **Z No Device** | **Z No Qualifier** |
| **1 Seminal Vesicle, Right** ♂<br>**2 Seminal Vesicle, Left** ♂<br>**3 Seminal Vesicles, Bilateral** ♂<br>**6 Tunica Vaginalis, Right** ♂<br>**7 Tunica Vaginalis, Left** ♂<br>**9 Testis, Right** ♂<br>**B Testis, Left** ♂<br>**C Testes, Bilateral** ♂ | **Ø Open**<br>**3 Percutaneous**<br>**4 Percutaneous Endoscopic** | **Z No Device** | **Z No Qualifier** |
| **5 Scrotum** ♂<br>**S Penis** ♂<br>Corpus cavernosum<br>Corpus spongiosum<br>**T Prepuce** ♂<br>Foreskin<br>Glans penis | **Ø Open**<br>**3 Percutaneous**<br>**4 Percutaneous Endoscopic**<br>**X External** | **Z No Device** | **Z No Qualifier** |
| **F Spermatic Cord, Right** ♂<br>**G Spermatic Cord, Left** ♂<br>**H Spermatic Cords, Bilateral** ♂<br>**J Epididymis, Right** ♂<br>**K Epididymis, Left** ♂<br>**L Epididymis, Bilateral** ♂<br>**N Vas Deferens, Right** ♂<br>Ductus deferens<br>Ejaculatory duct<br>**P Vas Deferens, Left** ♂<br>*See N Vas Deferens, Right*<br>**Q Vas Deferens, Bilateral** ♂<br>*See N Vas Deferens, Right* | **Ø Open**<br>**3 Percutaneous**<br>**4 Percutaneous Endoscopic**<br>8 Via Natural or Artificial Opening Endoscopic | **Z No Device** | **Z No Qualifier** |

**Non-OR** ØVN[9,B,C][Ø,3,4]ZZ
**Non-OR** ØVNT[Ø,3,4,X]ZZ
♂ All body part, approach, device, and qualifier values

**Ø Medical and Surgical**
**V Male Reproductive System**
**P Removal** Definition: Taking out or off a device from a body part

Explanation: If a device is taken out and a similar device put in without cutting or puncturing the skin or mucous membrane, the procedure is coded to the root operation CHANGE. Otherwise, the procedure for taking out the device is coded to the root operation REMOVAL.

| Body Part Character 4 | Approach Character 5 | Device Character 6 | Qualifier Character 7 |
|---|---|---|---|
| 4 Prostate and Seminal Vesicles ♂ | Ø Open<br>3 Percutaneous<br>4 Percutaneous Endoscopic<br>7 Via Natural or Artificial Opening<br>8 Via Natural or Artificial Opening Endoscopic | Ø Drainage Device<br>1 Radioactive Element<br>3 Infusion Device<br>7 Autologous Tissue Substitute<br>J Synthetic Substitute<br>K Nonautologous Tissue Substitute<br>Y Other Device | Z No Qualifier |
| 4 Prostate and Seminal Vesicles ♂ | X External | Ø Drainage Device<br>1 Radioactive Element<br>3 Infusion Device | Z No Qualifier |
| 8 Scrotum and Tunica Vaginalis ♂<br>D Testis ♂<br>S Penis ♂<br>Corpus cavernosum<br>Corpus spongiosum | Ø Open<br>3 Percutaneous<br>4 Percutaneous Endoscopic<br>7 Via Natural or Artificial Opening<br>8 Via Natural or Artificial Opening Endoscopic | Ø Drainage Device<br>3 Infusion Device<br>7 Autologous Tissue Substitute<br>J Synthetic Substitute<br>K Nonautologous Tissue Substitute<br>Y Other Device | Z No Qualifier |
| 8 Scrotum and Tunica Vaginalis ♂<br>D Testis ♂<br>S Penis ♂<br>Corpus cavernosum<br>Corpus spongiosum | X External | Ø Drainage Device<br>3 Infusion Device | Z No Qualifier |
| M Epididymis and Spermatic Cord ♂ | Ø Open<br>3 Percutaneous<br>4 Percutaneous Endoscopic<br>7 Via Natural or Artificial Opening<br>8 Via Natural or Artificial Opening Endoscopic | Ø Drainage Device<br>3 Infusion Device<br>7 Autologous Tissue Substitute<br>C Extraluminal Device<br>J Synthetic Substitute<br>K Nonautologous Tissue Substitute<br>Y Other Device | Z No Qualifier |
| M Epididymis and Spermatic Cord ♂ | X External | Ø Drainage Device<br>3 Infusion Device | Z No Qualifier |
| R Vas Deferens ♂<br>Ductus deferens<br>Ejaculatory duct | Ø Open<br>3 Percutaneous<br>4 Percutaneous Endoscopic<br>7 Via Natural or Artificial Opening<br>8 Via Natural or Artificial Opening Endoscopic | Ø Drainage Device<br>3 Infusion Device<br>7 Autologous Tissue Substitute<br>C Extraluminal Device<br>D Intraluminal Device<br>J Synthetic Substitute<br>K Nonautologous Tissue Substitute<br>Y Other Device | Z No Qualifier |
| R Vas Deferens ♂<br>Ductus deferens<br>Ejaculatory duct | X External | Ø Drainage Device<br>3 Infusion Device<br>D Intraluminal Device | Z No Qualifier |

Non-OR ØVP4[3,4]YZ
Non-OR ØVP4[7,8][Ø,3,Y]Z
Non-OR ØVP4X[Ø,1,3]Z
Non-OR ØVP8[Ø,3,4,7,8][Ø,3,7,J,K,Y]Z
Non-OR ØVP[D,S][3,4]YZ
Non-OR ØVP[D,S][7,8][Ø,3,Y]Z
Non-OR ØVP[8,D,S]X[Ø,3]Z
Non-OR ØVPM[3,4]YZ
Non-OR ØVPM[7,8][Ø,3,Y]Z
Non-OR ØVPMX[Ø,3]Z
Non-OR ØVPR[Ø,3,4][Ø,3,7,C,J,K,Y]Z
Non-OR ØVPR[7,8][Ø,3,7,C,D,J,K,Y]Z
Non-OR ØVPRX[Ø,3,D]Z
♂ All body part, approach, device, and qualifier values

**Ø Medical and Surgical**
**V Male Reproductive System**
**Q Repair** Definition: Restoring, to the extent possible, a body part to its normal anatomic structure and function
Explanation: Used only when the method to accomplish the repair is not one of the other root operations

| Body Part Character 4 | Approach Character 5 | Device Character 6 | Qualifier Character 7 |
|---|---|---|---|
| Ø Prostate ♂ | Ø Open<br>3 Percutaneous<br>4 Percutaneous Endoscopic<br>7 Via Natural or Artificial Opening<br>8 Via Natural or Artificial Opening Endoscopic | Z No Device | Z No Qualifier |
| 1 Seminal Vesicle, Right ♂<br>2 Seminal Vesicle, Left ♂<br>3 Seminal Vesicles, Bilateral ♂<br>6 Tunica Vaginalis, Right ♂<br>7 Tunica Vaginalis, Left ♂<br>9 Testis, Right ♂<br>B Testis, Left ♂<br>C Testes, Bilateral ♂ | Ø Open<br>3 Percutaneous<br>4 Percutaneous Endoscopic | Z No Device | Z No Qualifier |
| 5 Scrotum ♂<br>S Penis ♂<br>Corpus cavernosum<br>Corpus spongiosum<br>T Prepuce ♂<br>Foreskin<br>Glans penis | Ø Open<br>3 Percutaneous<br>4 Percutaneous Endoscopic<br>X External | Z No Device | Z No Qualifier |
| F Spermatic Cord, Right ♂<br>G Spermatic Cord, Left ♂<br>H Spermatic Cords, Bilateral ♂<br>J Epididymis, Right ♂<br>K Epididymis, Left ♂<br>L Epididymis, Bilateral ♂<br>N Vas Deferens, Right ♂<br>Ductus deferens<br>Ejaculatory duct<br>P Vas Deferens, Left ♂<br>*See N Vas Deferens, Right*<br>Q Vas Deferens, Bilateral ♂<br>*See N Vas Deferens, Right* | Ø Open<br>3 Percutaneous<br>4 Percutaneous Endoscopic<br>8 Via Natural or Artificial Opening Endoscopic | Z No Device | Z No Qualifier |

Non-OR ØVQ[6,7][Ø,3,4]ZZ
Non-OR ØVQ5[Ø,3,4,X]ZZ
♂ All body part, approach, device, and qualifier values

**Ø Medical and Surgical**
**V Male Reproductive System**
**R Replacement** Definition: Putting in or on biological or synthetic material that physically takes the place and/or function of all or a portion of a body part
Explanation: The body part may have been taken out or replaced, or may be taken out, physically eradicated, or rendered nonfunctional during the REPLACEMENT procedure. A REMOVAL procedure is coded for taking out the device used in a previous replacement procedure.

| Body Part Character 4 | Approach Character 5 | Device Character 6 | Qualifier Character 7 |
|---|---|---|---|
| 9 Testis, Right ♂<br>B Testis, Left ♂<br>C Testes, Bilateral ♂ | Ø Open | J Synthetic Substitute | Z No Qualifier |

♂ All body part, approach, device, and qualifier values

**Ø Medical and Surgical**
**V Male Reproductive System**
**S Reposition** Definition: Moving to its normal location, or other suitable location, all or a portion of a body part
Explanation: The body part is moved to a new location from an abnormal location, or from a normal location where it is not functioning correctly. The body part may or may not be cut out or off to be moved to the new location.

| Body Part Character 4 | Approach Character 5 | Device Character 6 | Qualifier Character 7 |
|---|---|---|---|
| 9 Testis, Right ♂<br>B Testis, Left ♂<br>C Testes, Bilateral ♂<br>F Spermatic Cord, Right ♂<br>G Spermatic Cord, Left ♂<br>H Spermatic Cords, Bilateral ♂ | Ø Open<br>3 Percutaneous<br>4 Percutaneous Endoscopic<br>8 Via Natural or Artificial Opening Endoscopic | Z No Device | Z No Qualifier |

♂ All body part, approach, device, and qualifier values

**Ø Medical and Surgical**
**V Male Reproductive System**
**T Resection** Definition: Cutting out or off, without replacement, all of a body part
Explanation: None

| Body Part<br>Character 4 | Approach<br>Character 5 | Device<br>Character 6 | Qualifier<br>Character 7 |
|---|---|---|---|
| **Ø** Prostate ⊞ ♂ | **Ø** Open<br>**4** Percutaneous Endoscopic<br>**7** Via Natural or Artificial Opening<br>**8** Via Natural or Artificial Opening Endoscopic | **Z** No Device | **Z** No Qualifier |
| **1** Seminal Vesicle, Right ♂<br>**2** Seminal Vesicle, Left ♂<br>**3** Seminal Vesicles, Bilateral ⊞ ♂<br>**6** Tunica Vaginalis, Right ♂<br>**7** Tunica Vaginalis, Left ♂<br>**9** Testis, Right ♂<br>**B** Testis, Left ♂<br>**C** Testes, Bilateral ♂<br>**F** Spermatic Cord, Right ♂<br>**G** Spermatic Cord, Left ♂<br>**H** Spermatic Cords, Bilateral ♂<br>**J** Epididymis, Right ♂<br>**K** Epididymis, Left ♂<br>**L** Epididymis, Bilateral ♂<br>**N** Vas Deferens, Right NC ♂<br>Ductus deferens<br>Ejaculatory duct<br>**P** Vas Deferens, Left NC ♂<br>*See* *N Vas Deferens, Right*<br>**Q** Vas Deferens, Bilateral NC ♂<br>*See* *N Vas Deferens, Right* | **Ø** Open<br>**4** Percutaneous Endoscopic | **Z** No Device | **Z** No Qualifier |
| **5** Scrotum ♂<br>**S** Penis ♂<br>Corpus cavernosum<br>Corpus spongiosum<br>**T** Prepuce ♂<br>Foreskin<br>Glans penis | **Ø** Open<br>**4** Percutaneous Endoscopic<br>**X** External | **Z** No Device | **Z** No Qualifier |

**Non-OR** ØVT[N,P,Q][Ø,4]ZZ
**Non-OR** ØVT[5,T][Ø,4,X]ZZ
NC ØVT[N,P,Q][Ø,4]ZZ with prinicpal diagnosis code Z3Ø.2
♂ All body part, approach, device, and qualifier values

**See Appendix L for Procedure Combinations**
⊞ ØVTØ[Ø,4,7,8]ZZ
⊞ ØVT3[Ø,4]ZZ

**Ø Medical and Surgical**
**V Male Reproductive System**
**U Supplement** Definition: Putting in or on biological or synthetic material that physically reinforces and/or augments the function of a portion of a body part

Explanation: The biological material is non-living, or is living and from the same individual. The body part may have been previously replaced, and the SUPPLEMENT procedure is performed to physically reinforce and/or augment the function of the replaced body part.

| Body Part Character 4 | Approach Character 5 | Device Character 6 | Qualifier Character 7 |
|---|---|---|---|
| **1 Seminal Vesicle, Right** ♂<br>**2 Seminal Vesicle, Left** ♂<br>**3 Seminal Vesicles, Bilateral** ♂<br>**6 Tunica Vaginalis, Right** ♂<br>**7 Tunica Vaginalis, Left** ♂<br>**F Spermatic Cord, Right** ♂<br>**G Spermatic Cord, Left** ♂<br>**H Spermatic Cords, Bilateral** ♂<br>**J Epididymis, Right** ♂<br>**K Epididymis, Left** ♂<br>**L Epididymis, Bilateral** ♂<br>**N Vas Deferens, Right** ♂<br>Ductus deferens<br>Ejaculatory duct<br>**P Vas Deferens, Left** ♂<br>*See N Vas Deferens, Right*<br>**Q Vas Deferens, Bilateral** ♂<br>*See N Vas Deferens, Right* | **Ø Open**<br>**4 Percutaneous Endoscopic**<br>**8 Via Natural or Artificial Opening Endoscopic** | **7 Autologous Tissue Substitute**<br>**J Synthetic Substitute**<br>**K Nonautologous Tissue Substitute** | **Z No Qualifier** |
| **5 Scrotum** ♂<br>**S Penis** ♂<br>Corpus cavernosum<br>Corpus spongiosum<br>**T Prepuce** ♂<br>Foreskin<br>Glans penis | **Ø Open**<br>**4 Percutaneous Endoscopic**<br>**X External** | **7 Autologous Tissue Substitute**<br>**J Synthetic Substitute**<br>**K Nonautologous Tissue Substitute** | **Z No Qualifier** |
| **9 Testis, Right** ♂<br>**B Testis, Left** ♂<br>**C Testes, Bilateral** ♂ | **Ø Open** | **7 Autologous Tissue Substitute**<br>**J Synthetic Substitute**<br>**K Nonautologous Tissue Substitute** | **Z No Qualifier** |

**Non-OR** ØVUSX[7,J,K]Z
♂ All body part, approach, device, and qualifier values

**Ø Medical and Surgical**
**V Male Reproductive System**
**W Revision** Definition: Correcting, to the extent possible, a portion of a malfunctioning device or the position of a displaced device

Explanation: Revision can include correcting a malfunctioning or displaced device by taking out or putting in components of the device such as a screw or pin

| Body Part Character 4 | Approach Character 5 | Device Character 6 | Qualifier Character 7 |
|---|---|---|---|
| **4** Prostate and Seminal Vesicles ♂<br>**8** Scrotum and Tunica Vaginalis ♂<br>**D** Testis ♂<br>**S** Penis ♂<br>Corpus cavernosum<br>Corpus spongiosum | **Ø** Open<br>**3** Percutaneous<br>**4** Percutaneous Endoscopic<br>**7** Via Natural or Artificial Opening<br>**8** Via Natural or Artificial Opening Endoscopic | **Ø** Drainage Device<br>**3** Infusion Device<br>**7** Autologous Tissue Substitute<br>**J** Synthetic Substitute<br>**K** Nonautologous Tissue Substitute<br>**Y** Other Device | **Z** No Qualifier |
| **4** Prostate and Seminal Vesicles ♂<br>**8** Scrotum and Tunica Vaginalis ♂<br>**D** Testis ♂<br>**S** Penis ♂<br>Corpus cavernosum<br>Corpus spongiosum | **X** External | **Ø** Drainage Device<br>**3** Infusion Device<br>**7** Autologous Tissue Substitute<br>**J** Synthetic Substitute<br>**K** Nonautologous Tissue Substitute | **Z** No Qualifier |
| **M** Epididymis and Spermatic Cord ♂ | **Ø** Open<br>**3** Percutaneous<br>**4** Percutaneous Endoscopic<br>**7** Via Natural or Artificial Opening<br>**8** Via Natural or Artificial Opening Endoscopic | **Ø** Drainage Device<br>**3** Infusion Device<br>**7** Autologous Tissue Substitute<br>**C** Extraluminal Device<br>**J** Synthetic Substitute<br>**K** Nonautologous Tissue Substitute<br>**Y** Other Device | **Z** No Qualifier |
| **M** Epididymis and Spermatic Cord ♂ | **X** External | **Ø** Drainage Device<br>**3** Infusion Device<br>**7** Autologous Tissue Substitute<br>**C** Extraluminal Device<br>**J** Synthetic Substitute<br>**K** Nonautologous Tissue Substitute | **Z** No Qualifier |
| **R** Vas Deferens ♂<br>Ductus deferens<br>Ejaculatory duct | **Ø** Open<br>**3** Percutaneous<br>**4** Percutaneous Endoscopic<br>**7** Via Natural or Artificial Opening<br>**8** Via Natural or Artificial Opening Endoscopic | **Ø** Drainage Device<br>**3** Infusion Device<br>**7** Autologous Tissue Substitute<br>**C** Extraluminal Device<br>**D** Intraluminal Device<br>**J** Synthetic Substitute<br>**K** Nonautologous Tissue Substitute<br>**Y** Other Device | **Z** No Qualifier |
| **R** Vas Deferens ♂<br>Ductus deferens<br>Ejaculatory duct | **X** External | **Ø** Drainage Device<br>**3** Infusion Device<br>**7** Autologous Tissue Substitute<br>**C** Extraluminal Device<br>**D** Intraluminal Device<br>**J** Synthetic Substitute<br>**K** Nonautologous Tissue Substitute | **Z** No Qualifier |

**Non-OR** ØVW[4,D,S][3,4,7,8]YZ
**Non-OR** ØVW8[Ø,3,4,7,8][Ø,3,7,J,K,Y]Z
**Non-OR** ØVW[4,8,D,S]X[Ø,3,7,J,K]Z
**Non-OR** ØVWM[3,4,7,8]YZ
**Non-OR** ØVWMX[Ø,3,7,C,J,K]Z
**Non-OR** ØVWR[Ø,3,4,7,8][Ø,3,7,C,D,J,K,Y]Z
**Non-OR** ØVWRX[Ø,3,7,C,D,J,K]Z
♂ All body part, approach, device, and qualifier values

# Anatomical Regions, General ØWØ–ØWY

## Character Meanings

This Character Meaning table is provided as a guide to assist the user in the identification of character members that may be found in this section of code tables. It **SHOULD NOT** be used to build a PCS code.

| Operation–Character 3 | | Body Region–Character 4 | | Approach–Character 5 | | Device–Character 6 | | Qualifier–Character 7 | |
|---|---|---|---|---|---|---|---|---|---|
| Ø | Alteration | Ø | Head | Ø | Open | Ø | Drainage Device | Ø | Vagina OR Allogeneic |
| 1 | Bypass | 1 | Cranial Cavity | 3 | Percutaneous | 1 | Radioactive Element | 1 | Penis OR Syngeneic |
| 2 | Change | 2 | Face | 4 | Percutaneous Endoscopic | 3 | Infusion Device | 2 | Stoma |
| 3 | Control | 3 | Oral Cavity and Throat | 7 | Via Natural or Artificial Opening | 7 | Autologous Tissue Substitute | 4 | Cutaneous |
| 4 | Creation | 4 | Upper Jaw | 8 | Via Natural or Artificial Opening Endoscopic | J | Synthetic Substitute | 9 | Pleural Cavity, Right |
| 8 | Division | 5 | Lower Jaw | X | External | K | Nonautologous Tissue Substitute | B | Pleural Cavity, Left |
| 9 | Drainage | 6 | Neck | | | Y | Other Device | G | Peritoneal Cavity |
| B | Excision | 8 | Chest Wall | | | Z | No Device | J | Pelvic Cavity |
| C | Extirpation | 9 | Pleural Cavity, Right | | | | | X | Diagnostic |
| F | Fragmentation | B | Pleural Cavity, Left | | | | | Y | Lower Vein |
| H | Insertion | C | Mediastinum | | | | | Z | No Qualifier |
| J | Inspection | D | Pericardial Cavity | | | | | | |
| M | Reattachment | F | Abdominal Wall | | | | | | |
| P | Removal | G | Peritoneal Cavity | | | | | | |
| Q | Repair | H | Retroperitoneum | | | | | | |
| U | Supplement | J | Pelvic Cavity | | | | | | |
| W | Revision | K | Upper Back | | | | | | |
| Y | Transplantation | L | Lower Back | | | | | | |
| | | M | Perineum, Male | | | | | | |
| | | N | Perineum, Female | | | | | | |
| | | P | Gastrointestinal Tract | | | | | | |
| | | Q | Respiratory Tract | | | | | | |
| | | R | Genitourinary Tract | | | | | | |

**AHA Coding Clinic for table ØWØ**
**2015, 1Q, 31** Bilateral browpexy

**AHA Coding Clinic for table ØW1**
**2015, 2Q, 36** Insertion of infusion device into peritoneal cavity
**2013, 4Q, 126-127** Creation of percutaneous cutaneoperitoneal fistula

**AHA Coding Clinic for table ØW3**
**2016, 4Q, 99-100** Root operation Control
**2014, 4Q, 44** Bakri balloon for control of postpartum hemorrhage
**2013, 3Q, 23** Control of intraoperative bleeding

**AHA Coding Clinic for table ØW4**
**2016, 4Q, 101** Root operation Creation

**AHA Coding Clinic for table ØW9**
**2017, 2Q, 16** Incision and drainage of floor of mouth

**AHA Coding Clinic for table ØWB**
**2017, 2Q, 16** Excision of floor of mouth
**2016, 1Q, 21** Excision of urachal mass
**2013, 4Q, 119** Excision of inclusion cyst of perineum

**AHA Coding Clinic for table ØWC**
**2017, 2Q, 16** Excision of floor of mouth

**AHA Coding Clinic for table ØWH**
**2016, 2Q, 14** Insertion of peritoneal totally implantable venous access device
**2015, 2Q, 36** Insertion of infusion device into peritoneal cavity

**AHA Coding Clinic for table ØWJ**
**2013, 2Q, 36** Insertion of ventriculoperitoneal shunt with laparoscopic assistance

**AHA Coding Clinic for table ØWQ**
**2016, 3Q, 3-7** Stoma creation & takedown procedures
**2014, 4Q, 38** Abdominoplasty and abdominal wall plication for hernia repair
**2014, 3Q, 28** Ileostomy takedown and parastomal hernia repair

**AHA Coding Clinic for table ØWU**
**2016, 3Q, 40** Omentoplasty
**2015, 2Q, 29** Placement of Ioban™ antimicrobial drape over surgical wound
**2014, 4Q, 39** Abdominal component release with placement of mesh for hernia repair
**2012, 4Q, 101** Rib resection with reconstruction of anterior chest wall

**AHA Coding Clinic for table ØWW**
**2015, 2Q, 9** Revision of ventriculoperitoneal (VP) shunt

**AHA Coding Clinic for table ØWY**
**2016, 4Q, 112-113** Transplantation

**Ø Medical and Surgical**
**W Anatomical Regions, General**
**Ø Alteration** Definition: Modifying the anatomic structure of a body part without affecting the function of the body part
Explanation: Principal purpose is to improve appearance

| Body Part Character 4 | Approach Character 5 | Device Character 6 | Qualifier Character 7 |
|---|---|---|---|
| **Ø** Head<br>**2** Face<br>**4** Upper Jaw<br>**5** Lower Jaw<br>**6** Neck<br>**8** Chest Wall<br>**F** Abdominal Wall<br>**K** Upper Back<br>**L** Lower Back<br>**M** Perineum, Male ♂<br>**N** Perineum, Female ♀ | **Ø** Open<br>**3** Percutaneous<br>**4** Percutaneous Endoscopic | **7** Autologous Tissue Substitute<br>**J** Synthetic Substitute<br>**K** Nonautologous Tissue Substitute<br>**Z** No Device | **Z** No Qualifier |

♂ ØWØM[Ø,3,4][7,J,K,Z]Z
♀ ØWØN[Ø,3,4][7,J,K,Z]Z

**Ø Medical and Surgical**
**W Anatomical Regions, General**
**1 Bypass** Definition: Altering the route of passage of the contents of a tubular body part
Explanation: Rerouting contents of a body part to a downstream area of the normal route, to a similar route and body part, or to an abnormal route and dissimilar body part. Includes one or more anastomoses, with or without the use of a device.

| Body Part Character 4 | Approach Character 5 | Device Character 6 | Qualifier Character 7 |
|---|---|---|---|
| **1** Cranial Cavity | **Ø** Open | **J** Synthetic Substitute | **9** Pleural Cavity, Right<br>**B** Pleural Cavity, Left<br>**G** Peritoneal Cavity<br>**J** Pelvic Cavity |
| **9** Pleural Cavity, Right<br>**B** Pleural Cavity, Left<br>**G** Peritoneal Cavity<br>**J** Pelvic Cavity<br>Retropubic space | **Ø** Open<br>**4** Percutaneous Endoscopic | **J** Synthetic Substitute | **4** Cutaneous<br>**9** Pleural Cavity, Right<br>**B** Pleural Cavity, Left<br>**G** Peritoneal Cavity<br>**J** Pelvic Cavity<br>**Y** Lower Vein |
| **9** Pleural Cavity, Right<br>**B** Pleural Cavity, Left<br>**G** Peritoneal Cavity<br>**J** Pelvic Cavity<br>Retropubic space | **3** Percutaneous | **J** Synthetic Substitute | **4** Cutaneous |

**Non-OR** ØW1[9,B][Ø,4]J[4,G,Y]
**Non-OR** ØW1G[Ø,4]J[9,B,G,J]
**Non-OR** ØW1J[Ø,4]J[4,Y]
**Non-OR** ØW1[9,B,J]3J4

**Ø Medical and Surgical**
**W Anatomical Regions, General**
**2 Change** Definition: Taking out or off a device from a body part and putting back an identical or similar device in or on the same body part without cutting or puncturing the skin or a mucous membrane
Explanation: All CHANGE procedures are coded using the approach EXTERNAL

| Body Part Character 4 | Approach Character 5 | Device Character 6 | Qualifier Character 7 |
|---|---|---|---|
| **Ø** Head<br>**1** Cranial Cavity<br>**2** Face<br>**4** Upper Jaw<br>**5** Lower Jaw<br>**6** Neck<br>**8** Chest Wall<br>**9** Pleural Cavity, Right<br>**B** Pleural Cavity, Left<br>**C** Mediastinum<br>**D** Pericardial Cavity<br>**F** Abdominal Wall<br>**G** Peritoneal Cavity<br>**H** Retroperitoneum<br>Retroperitoneal space<br>**J** Pelvic Cavity<br>Retropubic space<br>**K** Upper Back<br>**L** Lower Back<br>**M** Perineum, Male ♂<br>**N** Perineum, Female ♀ | **X** External | **Ø** Drainage Device<br>**Y** Other Device | **Z** No Qualifier |

**Non-OR** All body part, approach, device, and qualifier values
♂ ØW2MX[Ø,Y]Z
♀ ØW2NX[Ø,Y]Z

**Ø Medical and Surgical**
**W Anatomical Regions, General**
**3 Control** Definition: Stopping, or attempting to stop, postprocedural or other acute bleeding

Explanation: The site of the bleeding is coded as an anatomical region and not to a specific body part

| Body Part Character 4 | Approach Character 5 | Device Character 6 | Qualifier Character 7 |
|---|---|---|---|
| **Ø** Head<br>**1** Cranial Cavity<br>**2** Face<br>**4** Upper Jaw<br>**5** Lower Jaw<br>**6** Neck<br>**8** Chest Wall<br>**9** Pleural Cavity, Right<br>**B** Pleural Cavity, Left<br>**C** Mediastinum<br>**D** Pericardial Cavity<br>**F** Abdominal Wall<br>**G** Peritoneal Cavity<br>**H** Retroperitoneum<br>Retroperitoneal space<br>**J** Pelvic Cavity<br>Retropubic space<br>**K** Upper Back<br>**L** Lower Back<br>**M** Perineum, Male ♂<br>**N** Perineum, Female ♀ | **Ø** Open<br>**3** Percutaneous<br>**4** Percutaneous Endoscopic | **Z** No Device | **Z** No Qualifier |
| **3** Oral Cavity and Throat | **Ø** Open<br>**3** Percutaneous<br>**4** Percutaneous Endoscopic<br>**7** Via Natural or Artificial Opening<br>**8** Via Natural or Artificial Opening Endoscopic<br>**X** External | **Z** No Device | **Z** No Qualifier |
| **P** Gastrointestinal Tract<br>**Q** Respiratory Tract<br>**R** Genitourinary Tract | **Ø** Open<br>**3** Percutaneous<br>**4** Percutaneous Endoscopic<br>**7** Via Natural or Artificial Opening<br>**8** Via Natural or Artificial Opening Endoscopic | **Z** No Device | **Z** No Qualifier |

Non-OR ØW3GØZZ
Non-OR ØW3P8ZZ
♂ ØW3M[Ø,3,4]ZZ
♀ ØW3N[Ø,3,4]ZZ

**Ø Medical and Surgical**
**W Anatomical Regions, General**
**4 Creation** Definition: Putting in or on biological or synthetic material to form a new body part that to the extent possible replicates the anatomic structure or function of an absent body part

Explanation: Used for gender reassignment surgery and corrective procedures in individuals with congenital anomalies

| Body Part Character 4 | Approach Character 5 | Device Character 6 | Qualifier Character 7 |
|---|---|---|---|
| **M** Perineum, Male ♂ | **Ø** Open | **7** Autologous Tissue Substitute<br>**J** Synthetic Substitute<br>**K** Nonautologous Tissue Substitute<br>**Z** No Device | **Ø** Vagina |
| **N** Perineum, Female ♀ | **Ø** Open | **7** Autologous Tissue Substitute<br>**J** Synthetic Substitute<br>**K** Nonautologous Tissue Substitute<br>**Z** No Device | **1** Penis |

♂ ØW4MØ[7,J,K,Z]Ø
♀ ØW4NØ[7,J,K,Z]1

**Ø Medical and Surgical**
**W Anatomical Regions, General**
**8 Division** Definition: Cutting into a body part, without draining fluids and/or gases from the body part, in order to separate or transect a body part

Explanation: All or a portion of the body part is separated into two or more portions

| Body Part Character 4 | Approach Character 5 | Device Character 6 | Qualifier Character 7 |
|---|---|---|---|
| **N** Perineum, Female ♀ | **X** External | **Z** No Device | **Z** No Qualifier |

Non-OR ØW8NXZZ
♀ ØW8NXZZ

**Ø Medical and Surgical**
**W Anatomical Regions, General**
**9 Drainage** Definition: Taking or letting out fluids and/or gases from a body part
Explanation: The qualifier DIAGNOSTIC is used to identify drainage procedures that are biopsies

| Body Part Character 4 | Approach Character 5 | Device Character 6 | Qualifier Character 7 |
|---|---|---|---|
| **Ø** Head<br>**1** Cranial Cavity<br>**2** Face<br>**3** Oral Cavity and Throat<br>**4** Upper Jaw<br>**5** Lower Jaw<br>**6** Neck<br>**8** Chest Wall<br>**9** Pleural Cavity, Right<br>**B** Pleural Cavity, Left<br>**C** Mediastinum<br>**D** Pericardial Cavity<br>**F** Abdominal Wall<br>**G** Peritoneal Cavity<br>**H** Retroperitoneum<br>Retroperitoneal space<br>**J** Pelvic Cavity<br>Retropubic space<br>**K** Upper Back<br>**L** Lower Back<br>**M** Perineum, Male ♂<br>**N** Perineum, Female ♀ | **Ø** Open<br>**3** Percutaneous<br>**4** Percutaneous Endoscopic | **Ø** Drainage Device | **Z** No Qualifier |
| **Ø** Head<br>**1** Cranial Cavity<br>**2** Face<br>**3** Oral Cavity and Throat<br>**4** Upper Jaw<br>**5** Lower Jaw<br>**6** Neck<br>**8** Chest Wall<br>**9** Pleural Cavity, Right<br>**B** Pleural Cavity, Left<br>**C** Mediastinum<br>**D** Pericardial Cavity<br>**F** Abdominal Wall<br>**G** Peritoneal Cavity<br>**H** Retroperitoneum<br>Retroperitoneal space<br>**J** Pelvic Cavity<br>Retropubic space<br>**K** Upper Back<br>**L** Lower Back<br>**M** Perineum, Male ♂<br>**N** Perineum, Female ♀ | **Ø** Open<br>**3** Percutaneous<br>**4** Percutaneous Endoscopic | **Z** No Device | **X** Diagnostic<br>**Z** No Qualifier |

**DRG Non-OR** ØW9H3ØZ
**DRG Non-OR** ØW9H3ZZ
**Non-OR** ØW9[Ø,8,9,B,K,L,M]ØØZ
**Non-OR** ØW9[Ø,1,2,3,4,5,6,8,9,B,C,D,F,G,J,K,L,M,N]3ØZ
**Non-OR** ØW9[Ø,1,8,D,F,G,K,L,M]4ØZ
**Non-OR** ØW9[Ø,2,3,4,5,6,8,9,B,K,L,M,N]ØZX
**Non-OR** ØW9[Ø,1,2,3,4,5,6,8,9,B,C,D,G,K,L,M,N]3ZX
**Non-OR** ØW9[Ø,1,2,3,4,5,6,8,9,B,C,D,K,L,M,N]4ZX
**Non-OR** ØW9[Ø,8,9,B,K,L,M]ØZZ
**Non-OR** ØW9[Ø,1,2,3,4,5,6,8,9,B,C,D,F,G,J,K,L,M,N]3ZZ
**Non-OR** ØW9[Ø,1,8,D,F,G,K,L,M]4ZZ
♂ ØW9M[Ø,3,4]ØZ
♂ ØW9M[Ø,3,4]Z[X,Z]
♀ ØW9N[Ø,3,4]ØZ
♀ ØW9N[Ø,3]Z[X,Z]
♀ ØW9N4ZZ

**Ø Medical and Surgical**
**W Anatomical Regions, General**
**B Excision** Definition: Cutting out or off, without replacement, a portion of a body part
Explanation: The qualifier DIAGNOSTIC is used to identify excision procedures that are biopsies

| Body Part Character 4 | Approach Character 5 | Device Character 6 | Qualifier Character 7 |
|---|---|---|---|
| Ø Head<br>2 Face<br>3 Oral Cavity and Throat<br>4 Upper Jaw<br>5 Lower Jaw<br>8 Chest Wall<br>K Upper Back<br>L Lower Back<br>M Perineum, Male ♂<br>N Perineum, Female ♀ | Ø Open<br>3 Percutaneous<br>4 Percutaneous Endoscopic<br>X External | Z No Device | X Diagnostic<br>Z No Qualifier |
| 6 Neck<br>F Abdominal Wall | Ø Open<br>3 Percutaneous<br>4 Percutaneous Endoscopic | Z No Device | X Diagnostic<br>Z No Qualifier |
| 6 Neck<br>F Abdominal Wall | X External | Z No Device | 2 Stoma<br>X Diagnostic<br>Z No Qualifier |
| C Mediastinum<br>H Retroperitoneum<br>Retroperitoneal space | Ø Open<br>3 Percutaneous<br>4 Percutaneous Endoscopic | Z No Device | X Diagnostic<br>Z No Qualifier |

**Non-OR** ØWB[Ø,2,4,5,8,K,L,M][Ø,3,4,X]ZX
**Non-OR** ØWB6[Ø,3,4]ZX
**Non-OR** ØWB6XZX
**Non-OR** ØWB[C,H][3,4]ZX
♂ ØWBM[Ø,3,4,X]Z[X,Z]
♀ ØWBN[Ø,3,4,X]Z[X,Z]

**Ø Medical and Surgical**
**W Anatomical Regions, General**
**C Extirpation** Definition: Taking or cutting out solid matter from a body part
Explanation: The solid matter may be an abnormal byproduct of a biological function or a foreign body; it may be imbedded in a body part or in the lumen of a tubular body part. The solid matter may or may not have been previously broken into pieces.

| Body Part Character 4 | Approach Character 5 | Device Character 6 | Qualifier Character 7 |
|---|---|---|---|
| 1 Cranial Cavity<br>3 Oral Cavity and Throat<br>9 Pleural Cavity, Right<br>B Pleural Cavity, Left<br>C Mediastinum<br>D Pericardial Cavity<br>G Peritoneal Cavity<br>H Retroperitoneum<br>J Pelvic Cavity<br>Retropubic space | Ø Open<br>3 Percutaneous<br>4 Percutaneous Endoscopic<br>X External | Z No Device | Z No Qualifier |
| P Gastrointestinal Tract<br>Q Respiratory Tract<br>R Genitourinary Tract | Ø Open<br>3 Percutaneous<br>4 Percutaneous Endoscopic<br>7 Via Natural or Artificial Opening<br>8 Via Natural or Artificial Opening Endoscopic<br>X External | Z No Device | Z No Qualifier |

**Non-OR** ØWC[1,3]XZZ
**Non-OR** ØWC[9,B][Ø,3,4,X]ZZ
**Non-OR** ØWC[C,D,G,J]XZZ
**Non-OR** ØWC[P,R][7,8,X]ZZ
**Non-OR** ØWCQ[Ø,3,4,X]ZZ

**Ø Medical and Surgical**
**W Anatomical Regions, General**
**F Fragmentation** Definition: Breaking solid matter in a body part into pieces

Explanation: Physical force (e.g., manual, ultrasonic) applied directly or indirectly is used to break the solid matter into pieces. The solid matter may be an abnormal byproduct of a biological function or a foreign body. The pieces of solid matter are not taken out.

| Body Part Character 4 | Approach Character 5 | Device Character 6 | Qualifier Character 7 |
|---|---|---|---|
| 1 Cranial Cavity NC<br>3 Oral Cavity and Throat NC<br>9 Pleural Cavity, Right NC<br>B Pleural Cavity, Left NC<br>C Mediastinum NC<br>D Pericardial Cavity<br>G Peritoneal Cavity NC<br>J Pelvic Cavity NC<br>Retropubic space | Ø Open<br>3 Percutaneous<br>4 Percutaneous Endoscopic<br>X External | Z No Device | Z No Qualifier |
| P Gastrointestinal Tract NC<br>Q Respiratory Tract NC<br>R Genitourinary Tract | Ø Open<br>3 Percutaneous<br>4 Percutaneous Endoscopic<br>7 Via Natural or Artificial Opening<br>8 Via Natural or Artificial Opening Endoscopic<br>X External | Z No Device | Z No Qualifier |

DRG Non-OR ØWFRXZZ
Non-OR ØWF[1,3,9,B,C,G]XZZ
Non-OR ØWFJ[Ø,3,4,X]ZZ
Non-OR ØWFP[Ø,3,4,7,8,X]ZZ
Non-OR ØWFQXZZ
Non-OR ØWFR[Ø,3,4,7,8]ZZ
NC ØWF[1,3,9,B,C,G,J]XZZ
NC ØWF[P,Q]XZZ

**Ø Medical and Surgical**
**W Anatomical Regions, General**
**H Insertion** Definition: Putting in a nonbiological appliance that monitors, assists, performs, or prevents a physiological function but does not physically take the place of a body part

Explanation: None

| Body Part Character 4 | Approach Character 5 | Device Character 6 | Qualifier Character 7 |
|---|---|---|---|
| Ø Head<br>1 Cranial Cavity<br>2 Face<br>3 Oral Cavity and Throat<br>4 Upper Jaw<br>5 Lower Jaw<br>6 Neck<br>8 Chest Wall<br>9 Pleural Cavity, Right<br>B Pleural Cavity, Left<br>C Mediastinum<br>D Pericardial Cavity<br>F Abdominal Wall<br>G Peritoneal Cavity<br>H Retroperitoneum<br>Retroperitoneal space<br>J Pelvic Cavity<br>Retropubic space<br>K Upper Back<br>L Lower Back<br>M Perineum, Male<br>N Perineum, Female ♀ | Ø Open<br>3 Percutaneous<br>4 Percutaneous Endoscopic | 1 Radioactive Element<br>3 Infusion Device<br>Y Other Device | Z No Qualifier |
| P Gastrointestinal Tract<br>Q Respiratory Tract<br>R Genitourinary Tract | Ø Open<br>3 Percutaneous<br>4 Percutaneous Endoscopic<br>7 Via Natural or Artificial Opening<br>8 Via Natural or Artificial Opening Endoscopic | 1 Radioactive Element<br>3 Infusion Device<br>Y Other Device | Z No Qualifier |

DRG Non-OR ØWH[Ø,2,4,5,6,K,L,M][Ø,3,4][3,Y]Z
Non-OR ØWH1[Ø,3,4]3Z
Non-OR ØWH[8,9,B][Ø,3,4][3,Y]Z
Non-OR ØWHPØYZ
Non-OR ØWHP[3,4,7,8][3,Y]Z
Non-OR ØWHQ[Ø,7,8][3,Y]Z
Non-OR ØWHR[Ø,3,4,7,8][3,Y]Z
♀ ØWHN[Ø,3,4][3,Y]Z

**Ø Medical and Surgical**
**W Anatomical Regions, General**
**J Inspection** Definition: Visually and/or manually exploring a body part

Explanation: Visual exploration may be performed with or without optical instrumentation. Manual exploration may be performed directly or through intervening body layers.

| Body Part Character 4 | Approach Character 5 | Device Character 6 | Qualifier Character 7 |
|---|---|---|---|
| Ø Head<br>2 Face<br>3 Oral Cavity and Throat<br>4 Upper Jaw<br>5 Lower Jaw<br>6 Neck<br>8 Chest Wall<br>F Abdominal Wall<br>K Upper Back<br>L Lower Back<br>M Perineum, Male ♂<br>N Perineum, Female ♀ | Ø Open<br>3 Percutaneous<br>4 Percutaneous Endoscopic<br>X External | Z No Device | Z No Qualifier |
| 1 Cranial Cavity<br>9 Pleural Cavity, Right<br>B Pleural Cavity, Left<br>C Mediastinum<br>D Pericardial Cavity<br>G Peritoneal Cavity<br>H Retroperitoneum<br>Retroperitoneal space<br>J Pelvic Cavity<br>Retropubic space | Ø Open<br>3 Percutaneous<br>4 Percutaneous Endoscopic | Z No Device | Z No Qualifier |
| P Gastrointestinal Tract<br>Q Respiratory Tract<br>R Genitourinary Tract | Ø Open<br>3 Percutaneous<br>4 Percutaneous Endoscopic<br>7 Via Natural or Artificial Opening<br>8 Via Natural or Artificial Opening Endoscopic | Z No Device | Z No Qualifier |

DRG Non-OR ØWJ[Ø,2,4,5,K,L]ØZZ
DRG Non-OR ØWJF3ZZ
DRG Non-OR ØWJM[Ø,4]ZZ
DRG Non-OR ØWJ[1,G,H,J]3ZZ
DRG Non-OR ØWJ[P,R][3,7,8]ZZ
Non-OR ØWJ[Ø,2,4,5,K,L][3,4,X]ZZ
Non-OR ØWJ3[Ø,3,4,X]ZZ
Non-OR ØWJ[6,8,M,N][3,X]ZZ
Non-OR ØWJFXZZ
Non-OR ØWJ[9,B,C]3ZZ
Non-OR ØWJD[Ø,3]ZZ
Non-OR ØWJQ[3,7,8]ZZ
♂ ØWJM[Ø,3,4,X]ZZ
♀ ØWJN[Ø,3,4,X]ZZ

**Ø Medical and Surgical**
**W Anatomical Regions, General**
**M Reattachment** Definition: Putting back in or on all or a portion of a separated body part to its normal location or other suitable location

Explanation: Vascular circulation and nervous pathways may or may not be reestablished

| Body Part Character 4 | Approach Character 5 | Device Character 6 | Qualifier Character 7 |
|---|---|---|---|
| 2 Face<br>4 Upper Jaw<br>5 Lower Jaw<br>6 Neck<br>8 Chest Wall<br>F Abdominal Wall<br>K Upper Back<br>L Lower Back<br>M Perineum, Male ♂<br>N Perineum, Female ♀ | Ø Open | Z No Device | Z No Qualifier |

♂ ØWMMØZZ
♀ ØWMNØZZ

**Ø Medical and Surgical**
**W Anatomical Regions, General**
**P Removal** Definition: Taking out or off a device from a body part

Explanation: If a device is taken out and a similar device put in without cutting or puncturing the skin or mucous membrane, the procedure is coded to the root operation CHANGE. Otherwise, the procedure for taking out the device is coded to the root operation REMOVAL.

| Body Part Character 4 | Approach Character 5 | Device Character 6 | Qualifier Character 7 |
|---|---|---|---|
| Ø Head<br>2 Face<br>4 Upper Jaw<br>5 Lower Jaw<br>6 Neck<br>8 Chest Wall<br>C Mediastinum<br>F Abdominal Wall<br>K Upper Back<br>L Lower Back<br>M Perineum, Male ♂<br>N Perineum, Female ♀ | Ø Open<br>3 Percutaneous<br>4 Percutaneous Endoscopic<br>X External | Ø Drainage Device<br>1 Radioactive Element<br>3 Infusion Device<br>7 Autologous Tissue Substitute<br>J Synthetic Substitute<br>K Nonautologous Tissue Substitute<br>Y Other Device | Z No Qualifier |
| 1 Cranial Cavity<br>9 Pleural Cavity, Right<br>B Pleural Cavity, Left<br>G Peritoneal Cavity<br>J Pelvic Cavity<br>Retropubic space | Ø Open<br>3 Percutaneous<br>4 Percutaneous Endoscopic | Ø Drainage Device<br>1 Radioactive Element<br>3 Infusion Device<br>J Synthetic Substitute<br>Y Other Device | Z No Qualifier |
| 1 Cranial Cavity<br>9 Pleural Cavity, Right<br>B Pleural Cavity, Left<br>G Peritoneal Cavity<br>J Pelvic Cavity<br>Retropubic space | X External | Ø Drainage Device<br>1 Radioactive Element<br>3 Infusion Device | Z No Qualifier |
| D Pericardial Cavity<br>H Retroperitoneum<br>Retroperitoneal space | Ø Open<br>3 Percutaneous<br>4 Percutaneous Endoscopic | Ø Drainage Device<br>1 Radioactive Element<br>3 Infusion Device<br>Y Other Device | Z No Qualifier |
| D Pericardial Cavity<br>H Retroperitoneum<br>Retroperitoneal space | X External | Ø Drainage Device<br>1 Radioactive Element<br>3 Infusion Device | Z No Qualifier |
| P Gastrointestinal Tract<br>Q Respiratory Tract<br>R Genitourinary Tract | Ø Open<br>3 Percutaneous<br>4 Percutaneous Endoscopic<br>7 Via Natural or Artificial Opening<br>8 Via Natural or Artificial Opening Endoscopic<br>X External | 1 Radioactive Element<br>3 Infusion Device<br>Y Other Device | Z No Qualifier |

Non-OR ØWP[Ø,2,4,5,6,8][Ø,3,4,X][Ø,1,3,7,J,K,Y]Z
Non-OR ØWP[C,F]X[Ø,1,3,7,J,K,Y]Z
Non-OR ØWP[K,L][Ø,3,4,X][Ø,1,3,7,J,K,Y]Z
Non-OR ØWPM[Ø,3,4][Ø,1,3,J,Y]Z
Non-OR ØWPMX[Ø,1,3,Y]Z
Non-OR ØWPNX[Ø,1,3,7,J,K,Y]Z
Non-OR ØWP1[Ø,3,4]3Z
Non-OR ØWP[9,B,J][Ø,3,4][Ø,1,3,J,Y]Z
Non-OR ØWP[1,9,B,G,J]X[Ø,1,3]Z
Non-OR ØWP[D,H]X[Ø,1,3]Z
Non-OR ØWPP[3,4,7,8,X][1,3,Y]Z
Non-OR ØWPQ73Z
Non-OR ØWPQ8[3,Y]Z
Non-OR ØWPQ[Ø,X][1,3,Y]Z
Non-OR ØWPR[Ø,3,4,7,8,X][1,3,Y]Z

♂ ØWPM[Ø,3,4,X][Ø,1,3,7,J,K,Y]Z
♀ ØWPN[Ø,3,4,X][Ø,1,3,7,J,K,Y]Z

**Ø Medical and Surgical**
**W Anatomical Regions, General**
**Q Repair** Definition: Restoring, to the extent possible, a body part to its normal anatomic structure and function
Explanation: Used only when the method to accomplish the repair is not one of the other root operations

| Body Part Character 4 | Approach Character 5 | Device Character 6 | Qualifier Character 7 |
|---|---|---|---|
| Ø Head<br>2 Face<br>3 Oral Cavity and Throat<br>4 Upper Jaw<br>5 Lower Jaw<br>8 Chest Wall<br>K Upper Back<br>L Lower Back<br>M Perineum, Male ♂<br>N Perineum, Female ♀ | Ø Open<br>3 Percutaneous<br>4 Percutaneous Endoscopic<br>X External | Z No Device | Z No Qualifier |
| 6 Neck<br>F Abdominal Wall | Ø Open<br>3 Percutaneous<br>4 Percutaneous Endoscopic | Z No Device | Z No Qualifier |
| 6 Neck<br>F Abdominal Wall ⊞ | X External | Z No Device | 2 Stoma<br>Z No Qualifier |
| C Mediastinum | Ø Open<br>3 Percutaneous<br>4 Percutaneous Endoscopic | Z No Device | Z No Qualifier |

Non-OR ØWQNXZZ
♂ ØWQM[Ø,3,4,X]ZZ
♀ ØWQN[Ø,3,4,X]ZZ

See Appendix L for Procedure Combinations
⊞ ØWQFXZ[2,Z]

**Ø Medical and Surgical**
**W Anatomical Regions, General**
**U Supplement** Definition: Putting in or on biological or synthetic material that physically reinforces and/or augments the function of a portion of a body part
Explanation: The biological material is non-living, or is living and from the same individual. The body part may have been previously replaced, and the SUPPLEMENT procedure is performed to physically reinforce and/or augment the function of the replaced body part.

| Body Part Character 4 | Approach Character 5 | Device Character 6 | Qualifier Character 7 |
|---|---|---|---|
| Ø Head<br>2 Face<br>4 Upper Jaw<br>5 Lower Jaw<br>6 Neck<br>8 Chest Wall<br>C Mediastinum<br>F Abdominal Wall<br>K Upper Back<br>L Lower Back<br>M Perineum, Male ♂<br>N Perineum, Female ♀ | Ø Open<br>4 Percutaneous Endoscopic | 7 Autologous Tissue Substitute<br>J Synthetic Substitute<br>K Nonautologous Tissue Substitute | Z No Qualifier |

♂ ØWUM[Ø,4][7,J,K]Z
♀ ØWUN[Ø,4][7,J,K]Z

**Ø Medical and Surgical**
**W Anatomical Regions, General**
**W Revision** Definition: Correcting, to the extent possible, a portion of a malfunctioning device or the position of a displaced device

Explanation: Revision can include correcting a malfunctioning or displaced device by taking out or putting in components of the device such as a screw or pin

| Body Part Character 4 | Approach Character 5 | Device Character 6 | Qualifier Character 7 |
|---|---|---|---|
| Ø Head<br>2 Face<br>4 Upper Jaw<br>5 Lower Jaw<br>6 Neck<br>8 Chest Wall<br>C Mediastinum<br>F Abdominal Wall<br>K Upper Back<br>L Lower Back<br>M Perineum, Male ♂<br>N Perineum, Female ♀ | Ø Open<br>3 Percutaneous<br>4 Percutaneous Endoscopic<br>X External | Ø Drainage Device<br>1 Radioactive Element<br>3 Infusion Device<br>7 Autologous Tissue Substitute<br>J Synthetic Substitute<br>K Nonautologous Tissue Substitute<br>Y Other Device | Z No Qualifier |
| 1 Cranial Cavity<br>9 Pleural Cavity, Right<br>B Pleural Cavity, Left<br>G Peritoneal Cavity<br>J Pelvic Cavity<br>Retropubic space | Ø Open<br>3 Percutaneous<br>4 Percutaneous Endoscopic<br>X External | Ø Drainage Device<br>1 Radioactive Element<br>3 Infusion Device<br>J Synthetic Substitute<br>Y Other Device | Z No Qualifier |
| D Pericardial Cavity<br>H Retroperitoneum<br>Retroperitoneal space | Ø Open<br>3 Percutaneous<br>4 Percutaneous Endoscopic<br>X External | Ø Drainage Device<br>1 Radioactive Element<br>3 Infusion Device<br>Y Other Device | Z No Qualifier |
| P Gastrointestinal Tract<br>Q Respiratory Tract<br>R Genitourinary Tract | Ø Open<br>3 Percutaneous<br>4 Percutaneous Endoscopic<br>7 Via Natural or Artificial Opening<br>8 Via Natural or Artificial Opening Endoscopic<br>X External | 1 Radioactive Element<br>3 Infusion Device<br>Y Other Device | Z No Qualifier |

DRG Non-OR ØWW[Ø,2,4,5,6,K,L][Ø,3,4][Ø,1,3,7,J,K,Y]Z
DRG Non-OR ØWWM[Ø,3,4][Ø,1,3,J,Y]Z
Non-OR ØWW[Ø,2,4,5,6,C,F,K,L,M,N]X[Ø,1,3,7,J,K,Y]Z
Non-OR ØWW8[Ø,3,4,X][Ø,1,3,7,J,K,Y]Z
Non-OR ØWW[1,G,J]X[Ø,1,3,J,Y]Z
Non-OR ØWW[9,B][Ø,3,4,X][Ø,1,3,J,Y]Z
Non-OR ØWW[D,H]X[Ø,1,3,Y]Z
Non-OR ØWWP[3,4,7,8,X][1,3,Y]Z
Non-OR ØWWQ[Ø,X][1,3,Y]Z
Non-OR ØWWR[Ø,3,4,7,8,X][1,3,Y]Z

♂ ØWWM[Ø,3,4,X][Ø,1,3,7,K,Y]Z
♀ ØWWN[Ø,3,4,X][Ø,1,3,7,K,Y]Z

**Ø Medical and Surgical**
**W Anatomical Regions, General**
**Y Transplantation** Definition: Putting in or on all or a portion of a living body part taken from another individual or animal to physically take the place and/or function of all or a portion of a similar body part

Explanation: The native body part may or may not be taken out, and the transplanted body part may take over all or a portion of its function

| Body Part Character 4 | Approach Character 5 | Device Character 6 | Qualifier Character 7 |
|---|---|---|---|
| 2 Face | Ø Open | Z No Device | Ø Allogeneic<br>1 Syngeneic |

# Anatomical Regions, Upper Extremities ØXØ–ØXY

## Character Meanings

This Character Meaning table is provided as a guide to assist the user in the identification of character members that may be found in this section of code tables. It **SHOULD NOT** be used to build a PCS code.

| Operation–Character 3 | Body Part–Character 4 | Approach–Character 5 | Device–Character 6 | Qualifier–Character 7 |
|---|---|---|---|---|
| Ø Alteration | Ø Forequarter, Right | Ø Open | Ø Drainage Device | Ø Complete OR Allogeneic |
| 2 Change | 1 Forequarter, Left | 3 Percutaneous | 1 Radioactive Element | 1 High OR Syngeneic |
| 3 Control | 2 Shoulder Region, Right | 4 Percutaneous Endoscopic | 3 Infusion Device | 2 Mid |
| 6 Detachment | 3 Shoulder Region, Left | X External | 7 Autologous Tissue Substitute | 3 Low |
| 9 Drainage | 4 Axilla, Right | | J Synthetic Substitute | 4 Complete 1st Ray |
| B Excision | 5 Axilla, Left | | K Nonautologous Tissue Substitute | 5 Complete 2nd Ray |
| H Insertion | 6 Upper Extremity, Right | | Y Other Device | 6 Complete 3rd Ray |
| J Inspection | 7 Upper Extremity, Left | | Z No Device | 7 Complete 4th Ray |
| M Reattachment | 8 Upper Arm, Right | | | 8 Complete 5th Ray |
| P Removal | 9 Upper Arm, Left | | | 9 Partial 1st Ray |
| Q Repair | B Elbow Region, Right | | | B Partial 2nd Ray |
| R Replacement | C Elbow Region, Left | | | C Partial 3rd Ray |
| U Supplement | D Lower Arm, Right | | | D Partial 4th Ray |
| W Revision | F Lower Arm, Left | | | F Partial 5th Ray |
| X Transfer | G Wrist Region, Right | | | L Thumb, Right |
| Y Transplantation | H Wrist Region, Left | | | M Thumb, Left |
| | J Hand, Right | | | N Toe, Right |
| | K Hand, Left | | | P Toe, Left |
| | L Thumb, Right | | | X Diagnostic |
| | M Thumb, Left | | | Z No Qualifier |
| | N Index Finger, Right | | | |
| | P Index Finger, Left | | | |
| | Q Middle Finger, Right | | | |
| | R Middle Finger, Left | | | |
| | S Ring Finger, Right | | | |
| | T Ring Finger, Left | | | |
| | V Little Finger, Right | | | |
| | W Little Finger, Left | | | |

**AHA Coding Clinic for table ØX3**
**2016, 4Q, 99** Root operation Control
**2015, 1Q, 35** Evacuation of hematoma for control of postprocedural bleeding
**2013, 3Q, 23** Control of intraoperative bleeding

**AHA Coding Clinic for table ØX6**
**2017, 2Q, 3-4** Qualifiers for the root operation detachment
**2017, 2Q, 18** Removal of polydactyl digits
**2017, 1Q, 52** Further distal phalangeal amputation
**2016, 3Q, 33** Traumatic amputation of fingers with further revision amputation

**AHA Coding Clinic for table ØXH**
**2017, 2Q, 20** Exchange of intramedullary antibiotic impregnated spacer

**AHA Coding Clinic for table ØXP**
**2017, 2Q, 20** Exchange of intramedullary antibiotic impregnated spacer

**AHA Coding Clinic for table ØXY**
**2016, 4Q, 112-113** Transplantation

# Detachment Qualifier Description

| Qualifier Definition | Upper Arm | Lower Arm |
|---|---|---|
| 1 **High:** Amputation at the proximal portion of the shaft of the: | Humerus | Radius/Ulna |
| 2 **Mid:** Amputation at the middle portion of the shaft of the: | Humerus | Radius/Ulna |
| 3 **Low:** Amputation at the distal portion of the shaft of the: | Humerus | Radius/Ulna |

| Qualifier Definition | Hand |
|---|---|
| Ø Complete 1st through 5th Rays<br>Ray: digit of hand or foot with corresponding metacarpus or metatarsus | Through carpo-metacarpal joint, **Wrist** |
| 4 Complete 1st Ray | Through carpo-metacarpal joint, **Thumb** |
| 5 Complete 2nd Ray | Through carpo-metacarpal joint, **Index Finger** |
| 6 Complete 3rd Ray | Through carpo-metacarpal joint, **Middle Finger** |
| 7 Complete 4th Ray | Through carpo-metacarpal joint, **Ring Finger** |
| 8 Complete 5th Ray | Through carpo-metacarpal joint, **Little Finger** |
| 9 Partial 1st Ray | Anywhere along shaft or head of metacarpal bone, **Thumb** |
| B Partial 2nd Ray | Anywhere along shaft or head of metacarpal bone, **Index Finger** |
| C Partial 3rd Ray | Anywhere along shaft or head of metacarpal bone, **Middle Finger** |
| D Partial 4th Ray | Anywhere along shaft or head of metacarpal bone, **Ring Finger** |
| F Partial 5th Ray | Anywhere along shaft or head of metacarpal bone, **Little Finger** |

| Qualifier Definition | Thumb/Finger |
|---|---|
| Ø Complete | At the metacarpophalangeal joint |
| 1 High | Anywhere along the proximal phalanx |
| 2 Mid | Through the proximal interphalangeal joint or anywhere along the middle phalanx |
| 3 Low | Through the distal interphalangeal joint or anywhere along the distal phalanx |

**Ø Medical and Surgical**
**X Anatomical Regions, Upper Extremities**
**Ø Alteration** Definition: Modifying the anatomic structure of a body part without affecting the function of the body part
Explanation: Principal purpose is to improve appearance

| Body Part Character 4 | Approach Character 5 | Device Character 6 | Qualifier Character 7 |
|---|---|---|---|
| 2 Shoulder Region, Right<br>3 Shoulder Region, Left<br>4 Axilla, Right<br>5 Axilla, Left<br>6 Upper Extremity, Right<br>7 Upper Extremity, Left<br>8 Upper Arm, Right<br>9 Upper Arm, Left<br>B Elbow Region, Right<br>C Elbow Region, Left<br>D Lower Arm, Right<br>F Lower Arm, Left<br>G Wrist Region, Right<br>H Wrist Region, Left | Ø Open<br>3 Percutaneous<br>4 Percutaneous Endoscopic | 7 Autologous Tissue Substitute<br>J Synthetic Substitute<br>K Nonautologous Tissue Substitute<br>Z No Device | Z No Qualifier |

**Ø Medical and Surgical**
**X Anatomical Regions, Upper Extremities**
**2 Change** Definition: Taking out or off a device from a body part and putting back an identical or similar device in or on the same body part without cutting or puncturing the skin or a mucous membrane
Explanation: All CHANGE procedures are coded using the approach EXTERNAL

| Body Part Character 4 | Approach Character 5 | Device Character 6 | Qualifier Character 7 |
|---|---|---|---|
| 6 Upper Extremity, Right<br>7 Upper Extremity, Left | X External | Ø Drainage Device<br>Y Other Device | Z No Qualifier |

Non-OR All body part, approach, device, and qualifier values

**Ø Medical and Surgical**
**X Anatomical Regions, Upper Extremities**
**3 Control** Definition: Stopping, or attempting to stop, postprocedural or other acute bleeding
Explanation: The site of the bleeding is coded as an anatomical region and not to a specific body part

| Body Part Character 4 | Approach Character 5 | Device Character 6 | Qualifier Character 7 |
|---|---|---|---|
| 2 Shoulder Region, Right<br>3 Shoulder Region, Left<br>4 Axilla, Right<br>5 Axilla, Left<br>6 Upper Extremity, Right<br>7 Upper Extremity, Left<br>8 Upper Arm, Right<br>9 Upper Arm, Left<br>B Elbow Region, Right<br>C Elbow Region, Left<br>D Lower Arm, Right<br>F Lower Arm, Left<br>G Wrist Region, Right<br>H Wrist Region, Left<br>J Hand, Right<br>K Hand, Left | Ø Open<br>3 Percutaneous<br>4 Percutaneous Endoscopic | Z No Device | Z No Qualifier |

**Ø Medical and Surgical**
**X Anatomical Regions, Upper Extremities**
**6 Detachment** Definition: Cutting off all or a portion of the upper or lower extremities

Explanation: The body part value is the site of the detachment, with a qualifier if applicable to further specify the level where the extremity was detached

| Body Part Character 4 | Approach Character 5 | Device Character 6 | Qualifier Character 7 |
|---|---|---|---|
| Ø Forequarter, Right<br>1 Forequarter, Left<br>2 Shoulder Region, Right<br>3 Shoulder Region, Left<br>B Elbow Region, Right<br>C Elbow Region, Left | Ø Open | Z No Device | Z No Qualifier |
| 8 Upper Arm, Right<br>9 Upper Arm, Left<br>D Lower Arm, Right<br>F Lower Arm, Left | Ø Open | Z No Device | 1 High<br>2 Mid<br>3 Low |
| J Hand, Right<br>K Hand, Left | Ø Open | Z No Device | Ø Complete<br>4 Complete 1st Ray<br>5 Complete 2nd Ray<br>6 Complete 3rd Ray<br>7 Complete 4th Ray<br>8 Complete 5th Ray<br>9 Partial 1st Ray<br>B Partial 2nd Ray<br>C Partial 3rd Ray<br>D Partial 4th Ray<br>F Partial 5th Ray |
| L Thumb, Right<br>M Thumb, Left<br>N Index Finger, Right<br>P Index Finger, Left<br>Q Middle Finger, Right<br>R Middle Finger, Left<br>S Ring Finger, Right<br>T Ring Finger, Left<br>V Little Finger, Right<br>W Little Finger, Left | Ø Open | Z No Device | Ø Complete<br>1 High<br>2 Mid<br>3 Low |

**Ø Medical and Surgical**
**X Anatomical Regions, Upper Extremities**
**9 Drainage** Definition: Taking or letting out fluids and/or gases from a body part
Explanation: The qualifier DIAGNOSTIC is used to identify drainage procedures that are biopsies

| Body Part Character 4 | Approach Character 5 | Device Character 6 | Qualifier Character 7 |
|---|---|---|---|
| 2 Shoulder Region, Right<br>3 Shoulder Region, Left<br>4 Axilla, Right<br>5 Axilla, Left<br>6 Upper Extremity, Right<br>7 Upper Extremity, Left<br>8 Upper Arm, Right<br>9 Upper Arm, Left<br>B Elbow Region, Right<br>C Elbow Region, Left<br>D Lower Arm, Right<br>F Lower Arm, Left<br>G Wrist Region, Right<br>H Wrist Region, Left<br>J Hand, Right<br>K Hand, Left | Ø Open<br>3 Percutaneous<br>4 Percutaneous Endoscopic | Ø Drainage Device | Z No Qualifier |
| 2 Shoulder Region, Right<br>3 Shoulder Region, Left<br>4 Axilla, Right<br>5 Axilla, Left<br>6 Upper Extremity, Right<br>7 Upper Extremity, Left<br>8 Upper Arm, Right<br>9 Upper Arm, Left<br>B Elbow Region, Right<br>C Elbow Region, Left<br>D Lower Arm, Right<br>F Lower Arm, Left<br>G Wrist Region, Right<br>H Wrist Region, Left<br>J Hand, Right<br>K Hand, Left | Ø Open<br>3 Percutaneous<br>4 Percutaneous Endoscopic | Z No Device | X Diagnostic<br>Z No Qualifier |

**Non-OR** All body part, approach, device, and qualifier values

**Ø Medical and Surgical**
**X Anatomical Regions, Upper Extremities**
**B Excision** Definition: Cutting out or off, without replacement, a portion of a body part
Explanation: The qualifier DIAGNOSTIC is used to identify excision procedures that are biopsies

| Body Part Character 4 | Approach Character 5 | Device Character 6 | Qualifier Character 7 |
|---|---|---|---|
| 2 Shoulder Region, Right<br>3 Shoulder Region, Left<br>4 Axilla, Right<br>5 Axilla, Left<br>6 Upper Extremity, Right<br>7 Upper Extremity, Left<br>8 Upper Arm, Right<br>9 Upper Arm, Left<br>B Elbow Region, Right<br>C Elbow Region, Left<br>D Lower Arm, Right<br>F Lower Arm, Left<br>G Wrist Region, Right<br>H Wrist Region, Left<br>J Hand, Right<br>K Hand, Left | Ø Open<br>3 Percutaneous<br>4 Percutaneous Endoscopic | Z No Device | X Diagnostic<br>Z No Qualifier |

**Non-OR** ØXB[2,3,4,5,6,7,8,9,B,C,D,F,G,H,J,K][Ø,3,4]ZX

**Ø Medical and Surgical**
**X Anatomical Regions, Upper Extremities**
**H Insertion** Definition: Putting in a nonbiological appliance that monitors, assists, performs, or prevents a physiological function but does not physically take the place of a body part

Explanation: None

| Body Part Character 4 | Approach Character 5 | Device Character 6 | Qualifier Character 7 |
|---|---|---|---|
| 2 Shoulder Region, Right<br>3 Shoulder Region, Left<br>4 Axilla, Right<br>5 Axilla, Left<br>6 Upper Extremity, Right<br>7 Upper Extremity, Left<br>8 Upper Arm, Right<br>9 Upper Arm, Left<br>B Elbow Region, Right<br>C Elbow Region, Left<br>D Lower Arm, Right<br>F Lower Arm, Left<br>G Wrist Region, Right<br>H Wrist Region, Left<br>J Hand, Right<br>K Hand, Left | Ø Open<br>3 Percutaneous<br>4 Percutaneous Endoscopic | 1 Radioactive Element<br>3 Infusion Device<br>Y Other Device | Z No Qualifier |

DRG Non-OR ØXH[2,3,4,5,6,7,8,9,B,C,D,F,G,H,J,K][Ø,3,4][3,Y]Z

**Ø Medical and Surgical**
**X Anatomical Regions, Upper Extremities**
**J Inspection** Definition: Visually and/or manually exploring a body part

Explanation: Visual exploration may be performed with or without optical instrumentation. Manual exploration may be performed directly or through intervening body layers.

| Body Part Character 4 | Approach Character 5 | Device Character 6 | Qualifier Character 7 |
|---|---|---|---|
| 2 Shoulder Region, Right<br>3 Shoulder Region, Left<br>4 Axilla, Right<br>5 Axilla, Left<br>6 Upper Extremity, Right<br>7 Upper Extremity, Left<br>8 Upper Arm, Right<br>9 Upper Arm, Left<br>B Elbow Region, Right<br>C Elbow Region, Left<br>D Lower Arm, Right<br>F Lower Arm, Left<br>G Wrist Region, Right<br>H Wrist Region, Left<br>J Hand, Right<br>K Hand, Left | Ø Open<br>3 Percutaneous<br>4 Percutaneous Endoscopic<br>X External | Z No Device | Z No Qualifier |

DRG Non-OR ØXJ[2,3,4,5,6,7,8,9,B,C,D,F,G,H,J,K]ØZZ
Non-OR ØXJ[2,3,4,5,6,7,8,9,B,C,D,F,G,H][3,4,X]ZZ
Non-OR ØXJ[J,K][3,X]ZZ

**Ø Medical and Surgical**
**X Anatomical Regions, Upper Extremities**
**M Reattachment** Definition: Putting back in or on all or a portion of a separated body part to its normal location or other suitable location

Explanation: Vascular circulation and nervous pathways may or may not be reestablished

| Body Part Character 4 | Approach Character 5 | Device Character 6 | Qualifier Character 7 |
|---|---|---|---|
| Ø Forequarter, Right<br>1 Forequarter, Left<br>2 Shoulder Region, Right<br>3 Shoulder Region, Left<br>4 Axilla, Right<br>5 Axilla, Left<br>6 Upper Extremity, Right<br>7 Upper Extremity, Left<br>8 Upper Arm, Right<br>9 Upper Arm, Left<br>B Elbow Region, Right<br>C Elbow Region, Left<br>D Lower Arm, Right<br>F Lower Arm, Left<br>G Wrist Region, Right<br>H Wrist Region, Left<br>J Hand, Right<br>K Hand, Left<br>L Thumb, Right<br>M Thumb, Left<br>N Index Finger, Right<br>P Index Finger, Left<br>Q Middle Finger, Right<br>R Middle Finger, Left<br>S Ring Finger, Right<br>T Ring Finger, Left<br>V Little Finger, Right<br>W Little Finger, Left | Ø Open | Z No Device | Z No Qualifier |

**Ø Medical and Surgical**
**X Anatomical Regions, Upper Extremities**
**P Removal** Definition: Taking out or off a device from a body part

Explanation: If a device is taken out and a similar device put in without cutting or puncturing the skin or mucous membrane, the procedure is coded to the root operation CHANGE. Otherwise, the procedure for taking out the device is coded to the root operation REMOVAL.

| Body Part Character 4 | Approach Character 5 | Device Character 6 | Qualifier Character 7 |
|---|---|---|---|
| 6 Upper Extremity, Right<br>7 Upper Extremity, Left | Ø Open<br>3 Percutaneous<br>4 Percutaneous Endoscopic<br>X External | Ø Drainage Device<br>1 Radioactive Element<br>3 Infusion Device<br>7 Autologous Tissue Substitute<br>J Synthetic Substitute<br>K Nonautologous Tissue Substitute<br>Y Other Device | Z No Qualifier |

**Non-OR** All body part, approach, device, and qualifier values

**Ø Medical and Surgical**
**X Anatomical Regions, Upper Extremities**
**Q Repair** Definition: Restoring, to the extent possible, a body part to its normal anatomic structure and function
Explanation: Used only when the method to accomplish the repair is not one of the other root operations

| Body Part Character 4 | Approach Character 5 | Device Character 6 | Qualifier Character 7 |
|---|---|---|---|
| 2 Shoulder Region, Right<br>3 Shoulder Region, Left<br>4 Axilla, Right<br>5 Axilla, Left<br>6 Upper Extremity, Right<br>7 Upper Extremity, Left<br>8 Upper Arm, Right<br>9 Upper Arm, Left<br>B Elbow Region, Right<br>C Elbow Region, Left<br>D Lower Arm, Right<br>F Lower Arm, Left<br>G Wrist Region, Right<br>H Wrist Region, Left<br>J Hand, Right<br>K Hand, Left<br>L Thumb, Right<br>M Thumb, Left<br>N Index Finger, Right<br>P Index Finger, Left<br>Q Middle Finger, Right<br>R Middle Finger, Left<br>S Ring Finger, Right<br>T Ring Finger, Left<br>V Little Finger, Right<br>W Little Finger, Left | Ø Open<br>3 Percutaneous<br>4 Percutaneous Endoscopic<br>X External | Z No Device | Z No Qualifier |

**Ø Medical and Surgical**
**X Anatomical Regions, Upper Extremities**
**R Replacement** Definition: Putting in or on biological or synthetic material that physically takes the place and/or function of all or a portion of a body part
Explanation: The body part may have been taken out or replaced, or may be taken out, physically eradicated, or rendered nonfunctional during the REPLACEMENT procedure. A REMOVAL procedure is coded for taking out the device used in a previous replacement procedure.

| Body Part Character 4 | Approach Character 5 | Device Character 6 | Qualifier Character 7 |
|---|---|---|---|
| L Thumb, Right<br>M Thumb, Left | Ø Open<br>4 Percutaneous Endoscopic | 7 Autologous Tissue Substitute | N Toe, Right<br>P Toe, Left |

**Ø Medical and Surgical**
**X Anatomical Regions, Upper Extremities**
**U Supplement** Definition: Putting in or on biological or synthetic material that physically reinforces and/or augments the function of a portion of a body part

Explanation: The biological material is non-living, or is living and from the same individual. The body part may have been previously replaced, and the SUPPLEMENT procedure is performed to physically reinforce and/or augment the function of the replaced body part.

| Body Part Character 4 | Approach Character 5 | Device Character 6 | Qualifier Character 7 |
|---|---|---|---|
| 2 Shoulder Region, Right<br>3 Shoulder Region, Left<br>4 Axilla, Right<br>5 Axilla, Left<br>6 Upper Extremity, Right<br>7 Upper Extremity, Left<br>8 Upper Arm, Right<br>9 Upper Arm, Left<br>B Elbow Region, Right<br>C Elbow Region, Left<br>D Lower Arm, Right<br>F Lower Arm, Left<br>G Wrist Region, Right<br>H Wrist Region, Left<br>J Hand, Right<br>K Hand, Left<br>L Thumb, Right<br>M Thumb, Left<br>N Index Finger, Right<br>P Index Finger, Left<br>Q Middle Finger, Right<br>R Middle Finger, Left<br>S Ring Finger, Right<br>T Ring Finger, Left<br>V Little Finger, Right<br>W Little Finger, Left | Ø Open<br>4 Percutaneous Endoscopic | 7 Autologous Tissue Substitute<br>J Synthetic Substitute<br>K Nonautologous Tissue Substitute | Z No Qualifier |

**Ø Medical and Surgical**
**X Anatomical Regions, Upper Extremities**
**W Revision** Definition: Correcting, to the extent possible, a portion of a malfunctioning device or the position of a displaced device

Explanation: Revision can include correcting a malfunctioning or displaced device by taking out or putting in components of the device such as a screw or pin

| Body Part Character 4 | Approach Character 5 | Device Character 6 | Qualifier Character 7 |
|---|---|---|---|
| 6 Upper Extremity, Right<br>7 Upper Extremity, Left | Ø Open<br>3 Percutaneous<br>4 Percutaneous Endoscopic<br>X External | Ø Drainage Device<br>3 Infusion Device<br>7 Autologous Tissue Substitute<br>J Synthetic Substitute<br>K Nonautologous Tissue Substitute<br>Y Other Device | Z No Qualifier |

DRG Non-OR ØXW[6,7][Ø,3,4][Ø,3,7,J,K,Y]Z
Non-OR ØXW[6,7]X[Ø,3,7,J,K,Y]Z

**Ø Medical and Surgical**
**X Anatomical Regions, Upper Extremities**
**X Transfer** Definition: Moving, without taking out, all or a portion of a body part to another location to take over the function of all or a portion of a body part

Explanation: The body part transferred remains connected to its vascular and nervous supply

| Body Part Character 4 | Approach Character 5 | Device Character 6 | Qualifier Character 7 |
|---|---|---|---|
| N Index Finger, Right | Ø Open | Z No Device | L Thumb, Right |
| P Index Finger, Left | Ø Open | Z No Device | M Thumb, Left |

**Ø Medical and Surgical**
**X Anatomical Regions, Upper Extremities**
**Y Transplantation** Definition: Putting in or on all or a portion of a living body part taken from another individual or animal to physically take the place and/or function of all or a portion of a similar body part

Explanation: The native body part may or may not be taken out, and the transplanted body part may take over all or a portion of its function

| Body Part Character 4 | Approach Character 5 | Device Character 6 | Qualifier Character 7 |
|---|---|---|---|
| J Hand, Right<br>K Hand, Left | Ø Open | Z No Device | Ø Allogeneic<br>1 Syngeneic |

# Anatomical Regions, Lower Extremities ØYØ–ØYW

## Character Meanings

This Character Meaning table is provided as a guide to assist the user in the identification of character members that may be found in this section of code tables. It **SHOULD NOT** be used to build a PCS code.

| Operation–Character 3 | Body Part–Character 4 | Approach–Character 5 | Device–Character 6 | Qualifier–Character 7 |
|---|---|---|---|---|
| Ø Alteration | Ø Buttock, Right | Ø Open | Ø Drainage Device | Ø Complete |
| 2 Change | 1 Buttock, Left | 3 Percutaneous | 1 Radioactive Element | 1 High |
| 3 Control | 2 Hindquarter, Right | 4 Percutaneous Endoscopic | 3 Infusion Device | 2 Mid |
| 6 Detachment | 3 Hindquarter, Left | X External | 7 Autologous Tissue Substitute | 3 Low |
| 9 Drainage | 4 Hindquarter, Bilateral | | J Synthetic Substitute | 4 Complete 1st Ray |
| B Excision | 5 Inguinal Region, Right | | K Nonautologous Tissue Substitute | 5 Complete 2nd Ray |
| H Insertion | 6 Inguinal Region, Left | | Y Other Device | 6 Complete 3rd Ray |
| J Inspection | 7 Femoral Region, Right | | Z No Device | 7 Complete 4th Ray |
| M Reattachment | 8 Femoral Region, Left | | | 8 Complete 5th Ray |
| P Removal | 9 Lower Extremity, Right | | | 9 Partial 1st Ray |
| Q Repair | A Inguinal Region, Bilateral | | | B Partial 2nd Ray |
| U Supplement | B Lower Extremity, Left | | | C Partial 3rd Ray |
| W Revision | C Upper Leg, Right | | | D Partial 4th Ray |
| | D Upper Leg, Left | | | F Partial 5th Ray |
| | E Femoral Region, Bilateral | | | X Diagnostic |
| | F Knee Region, Right | | | Z No Qualifier |
| | G Knee Region, Left | | | |
| | H Lower Leg, Right | | | |
| | J Lower Leg, Left | | | |
| | K Ankle Region, Right | | | |
| | L Ankle Region, Left | | | |
| | M Foot, Right | | | |
| | N Foot, Left | | | |
| | P 1st Toe, Right | | | |
| | Q 1st Toe, Left | | | |
| | R 2nd Toe, Right | | | |
| | S 2nd Toe, Left | | | |
| | T 3rd Toe, Right | | | |
| | U 3rd Toe, Left | | | |
| | V 4th Toe, Right | | | |
| | W 4th Toe, Left | | | |
| | X 5th Toe, Right | | | |
| | Y 5th Toe, Left | | | |

**AHA Coding Clinic for table ØY3**

**2016, 4Q, 99** Root operation Control
**2013, 3Q, 23** Control of intraoperative bleeding

**AHA Coding Clinic for table ØY6**

**2017, 2Q, 3-4** Qualifiers for the root operation detachment
**2017, 1Q, 22** Chopart amputation of foot
**2015, 2Q, 28** Partial amputation of hallux at interphalangeal Joint
**2015, 1Q, 28** Mid-foot amputation

**AHA Coding Clinic for table ØY9**

**2015, 1Q, 22** Incision and drainage of abscess of femoropopliteal bypass site
**2015, 1Q, 22** Incision and drainage of groin abscess

## Detachment Qualifier Descriptions

| Qualifier Definition | Upper Leg | Lower Leg |
|---|---|---|
| 1 **High:** Amputation at the proximal portion of the shaft of the: | Femur | Tibia/Fibula |
| 2 **Mid:** Amputation at the middle portion of the shaft of the: | Femur | Tibia/Fibula |
| 3 **Low:** Amputation at the distal portion of the shaft of the: | Femur | Tibia/Fibula |

| Qualifier Definition | Foot |
|---|---|
| Ø Complete 1st through 5th Rays<br>Ray: digit of hand or foot with corresponding metacarpus or metatarsus | Through tarso-metatarsal Joint, **Ankle** |
| 4 Complete 1st Ray | Through tarso-metatarsal joint, **Great Toe** |
| 5 Complete 2nd Ray | Through tarso-metatarsal joint, **2nd Toe** |
| 6 Complete 3rd Ray | Through tarso-metatarsal joint, **3rd Toe** |
| 7 Complete 4th Ray | Through tarso-metatarsal joint, **4th Toe** |
| 8 Complete 5th Ray | Through tarso-metatarsal joint, **Little Toe** |
| 9 Partial 1st Ray | Anywhere along shaft or head of metatarsal bone, **Great Toe** |
| B Partial 2nd Ray | Anywhere along shaft or head of metatarsal bone, **2nd Toe** |
| C Partial 3rd Ray | Anywhere along shaft or head of metatarsal bone, **3rd Toe** |
| D Partial 4th Ray | Anywhere along shaft or head of metatarsal bone, **4th Toe** |
| F Partial 5th Ray | Anywhere along shaft or head of metatarsal bone, **Little Toe** |

| Qualifier Definition | Toe |
|---|---|
| Ø Complete | At the metatarsal-phalangeal joint |
| 1 High | Anywhere along the proximal phalanx |
| 2 Mid | Through the proximal interphalangeal joint or anywhere along the middle phalanx |
| 3 Low | Through the distal interphalangeal joint or anywhere along the distal phalanx |

**Ø Medical and Surgical**
**Y Anatomical Regions, Lower Extremities**
**Ø Alteration** Definition: Modifying the anatomic structure of a body part without affecting the function of the body part
Explanation: Principal purpose is to improve appearance

| Body Part Character 4 | Approach Character 5 | Device Character 6 | Qualifier Character 7 |
|---|---|---|---|
| **Ø** Buttock, Right<br>**1** Buttock, Left<br>**9** Lower Extremity, Right<br>**B** Lower Extremity, Left<br>**C** Upper Leg, Right<br>**D** Upper Leg, Left<br>**F** Knee Region, Right<br>**G** Knee Region, Left<br>**H** Lower Leg, Right<br>**J** Lower Leg, Left<br>**K** Ankle Region, Right<br>**L** Ankle Region, Left | **Ø** Open<br>**3** Percutaneous<br>**4** Percutaneous Endoscopic | **7** Autologous Tissue Substitute<br>**J** Synthetic Substitute<br>**K** Nonautologous Tissue Substitute<br>**Z** No Device | **Z** No Qualifier |

**Ø Medical and Surgical**
**Y Anatomical Regions, Lower Extremities**
**2 Change** Definition: Taking out or off a device from a body part and putting back an identical or similar device in or on the same body part without cutting or puncturing the skin or a mucous membrane
Explanation: All CHANGE procedures are coded using the approach EXTERNAL

| Body Part Character 4 | Approach Character 5 | Device Character 6 | Qualifier Character 7 |
|---|---|---|---|
| **9** Lower Extremity, Right<br>**B** Lower Extremity, Left | **X** External | **Ø** Drainage Device<br>**Y** Other Device | **Z** No Qualifier |
| **Non-OR** All body part, approach, device, and qualifier values | | | |

**Ø Medical and Surgical**
**Y Anatomical Regions, Lower Extremities**
**3 Control** Definition: Stopping, or attempting to stop, postprocedural or other acute bleeding
Explanation: The site of the bleeding is coded as an anatomical region and not to a specific body part

| Body Part Character 4 | Approach Character 5 | Device Character 6 | Qualifier Character 7 |
|---|---|---|---|
| **Ø** Buttock, Right<br>**1** Buttock, Left<br>**5** Inguinal Region, Right<br>Inguinal canal<br>Inguinal triangle<br>**6** Inguinal Region, Left<br>*See 5 Inguinal Region, Right*<br>**7** Femoral Region, Right<br>**8** Femoral Region, Left<br>**9** Lower Extremity, Right<br>**B** Lower Extremity, Left<br>**C** Upper Leg, Right<br>**D** Upper Leg, Left<br>**F** Knee Region, Right<br>**G** Knee Region, Left<br>**H** Lower Leg, Right<br>**J** Lower Leg, Left<br>**K** Ankle Region, Right<br>**L** Ankle Region, Left<br>**M** Foot, Right<br>**N** Foot, Left | **Ø** Open<br>**3** Percutaneous<br>**4** Percutaneous Endoscopic | **Z** No Device | **Z** No Qualifier |

**Ø Medical and Surgical**
**Y Anatomical Regions, Lower Extremities**
**6 Detachment** Definition: Cutting off all or a portion of the upper or lower extremities

Explanation: The body part value is the site of the detachment, with a qualifier if applicable to further specify the level where the extremity was detached

| Body Part Character 4 | Approach Character 5 | Device Character 6 | Qualifier Character 7 |
|---|---|---|---|
| **2** Hindquarter, Right<br>**3** Hindquarter, Left<br>**4** Hindquarter, Bilateral<br>**7** Femoral Region, Right<br>**8** Femoral Region, Left<br>**F** Knee Region, Right<br>**G** Knee Region, Left | **Ø** Open | **Z** No Device | **Z** No Qualifier |
| **C** Upper Leg, Right<br>**D** Upper Leg, Left<br>**H** Lower Leg, Right<br>**J** Lower Leg, Left | **Ø** Open | **Z** No Device | **1** High<br>**2** Mid<br>**3** Low |
| **M** Foot, Right<br>**N** Foot, Left | **Ø** Open | **Z** No Device | **Ø** Complete<br>**4** Complete 1st Ray<br>**5** Complete 2nd Ray<br>**6** Complete 3rd Ray<br>**7** Complete 4th Ray<br>**8** Complete 5th Ray<br>**9** Partial 1st Ray<br>**B** Partial 2nd Ray<br>**C** Partial 3rd Ray<br>**D** Partial 4th Ray<br>**F** Partial 5th Ray |
| **P** 1st Toe, Right<br>Hallux<br>**Q** 1st Toe, Left<br>*See 1st Toe, Right*<br>**R** 2nd Toe, Right<br>**S** 2nd Toe, Left<br>**T** 3rd Toe, Right<br>**U** 3rd Toe, Left<br>**V** 4th Toe, Right<br>**W** 4th Toe, Left<br>**X** 5th Toe, Right<br>**Y** 5th Toe, Left | **Ø** Open | **Z** No Device | **Ø** Complete<br>**1** High<br>**2** Mid<br>**3** Low |

**Ø Medical and Surgical**
**Y Anatomical Regions, Lower Extremities**
**9 Drainage** Definition: Taking or letting out fluids and/or gases from a body part
Explanation: The qualifier DIAGNOSTIC is used to identify drainage procedures that are biopsies

| Body Part Character 4 | Approach Character 5 | Device Character 6 | Qualifier Character 7 |
|---|---|---|---|
| **Ø** Buttock, Right<br>**1** Buttock, Left<br>**5** Inguinal Region, Right<br>Inguinal canal<br>Inguinal triangle<br>**6** Inguinal Region, Left<br>*See 5 Inguinal Region, Right*<br>**7** Femoral Region, Right<br>**8** Femoral Region, Left<br>**9** Lower Extremity, Right<br>**B** Lower Extremity, Left<br>**C** Upper Leg, Right<br>**D** Upper Leg, Left<br>**F** Knee Region, Right<br>**G** Knee Region, Left<br>**H** Lower Leg, Right<br>**J** Lower Leg, Left<br>**K** Ankle Region, Right<br>**L** Ankle Region, Left<br>**M** Foot, Right<br>**N** Foot, Left | **Ø** Open<br>**3** Percutaneous<br>**4** Percutaneous Endoscopic | **Ø** Drainage Device | **Z** No Qualifier |
| **Ø** Buttock, Right<br>**1** Buttock, Left<br>**5** Inguinal Region, Right<br>Inguinal canal<br>Inguinal triangle<br>**6** Inguinal Region, Left<br>*See 5 Inguinal Region, Right*<br>**7** Femoral Region, Right<br>**8** Femoral Region, Left<br>**9** Lower Extremity, Right<br>**B** Lower Extremity, Left<br>**C** Upper Leg, Right<br>**D** Upper Leg, Left<br>**F** Knee Region, Right<br>**G** Knee Region, Left<br>**H** Lower Leg, Right<br>**J** Lower Leg, Left<br>**K** Ankle Region, Right<br>**L** Ankle Region, Left<br>**M** Foot, Right<br>**N** Foot, Left | **Ø** Open<br>**3** Percutaneous<br>**4** Percutaneous Endoscopic | **Z** No Device | **X** Diagnostic<br>**Z** No Qualifier |

**DRG Non-OR** ØY9[5,6]3ØZ
**DRG Non-OR** ØY9[5,6]3ZZ
**Non-OR** ØY9[Ø,1,7,8,9,B,C,D,F,G,H,J,K,L,M,N][Ø,3,4]ØZ
**Non-OR** ØY9[Ø,1,7,8,9,B,C,D,F,G,H,J,K,L,M,N][Ø,3,4]Z[X,Z]

**Ø Medical and Surgical**
**Y Anatomical Regions, Lower Extremities**
**B Excision** Definition: Cutting out or off, without replacement, a portion of a body part
Explanation: The qualifier DIAGNOSTIC is used to identify excision procedures that are biopsies

| Body Part Character 4 | Approach Character 5 | Device Character 6 | Qualifier Character 7 |
|---|---|---|---|
| Ø Buttock, Right<br>1 Buttock, Left<br>5 Inguinal Region, Right<br>Inguinal canal<br>Inguinal triangle<br>6 Inguinal Region, Left<br>*See 5 Inguinal Region, Right*<br>7 Femoral Region, Right<br>8 Femoral Region, Left<br>9 Lower Extremity, Right<br>B Lower Extremity, Left<br>C Upper Leg, Right<br>D Upper Leg, Left<br>F Knee Region, Right<br>G Knee Region, Left<br>H Lower Leg, Right<br>J Lower Leg, Left<br>K Ankle Region, Right<br>L Ankle Region, Left<br>M Foot, Right<br>N Foot, Left | Ø Open<br>3 Percutaneous<br>4 Percutaneous Endoscopic | Z No Device | X Diagnostic<br>Z No Qualifier |

Non-OR ØYB[Ø,1,9,B,C,D,F,G,H,J,K,L,M,N][Ø,3,4]ZX

**Ø Medical and Surgical**
**Y Anatomical Regions, Lower Extremities**
**H Insertion** Definition: Putting in a nonbiological appliance that monitors, assists, performs, or prevents a physiological function but does not physically take the place of a body part
Explanation: None

| Body Part Character 4 | Approach Character 5 | Device Character 6 | Qualifier Character 7 |
|---|---|---|---|
| Ø Buttock, Right<br>1 Buttock, Left<br>5 Inguinal Region, Right<br>Inguinal canal<br>Inguinal triangle<br>6 Inguinal Region, Left<br>*See 5 Inguinal Region, Right*<br>7 Femoral Region, Right<br>8 Femoral Region, Left<br>9 Lower Extremity, Right<br>B Lower Extremity, Left<br>C Upper Leg, Right<br>D Upper Leg, Left<br>F Knee Region, Right<br>G Knee Region, Left<br>H Lower Leg, Right<br>J Lower Leg, Left<br>K Ankle Region, Right<br>L Ankle Region, Left<br>M Foot, Right<br>N Foot, Left | Ø Open<br>3 Percutaneous<br>4 Percutaneous Endoscopic | 1 Radioactive Element<br>3 Infusion Device<br>Y Other Device | Z No Qualifier |

DRG Non-OR ØYH[Ø,1,5,6,7,8,9,B,C,D,F,G,H,J,K,L,M,N][Ø,3,4][3,Y]Z

**Ø Medical and Surgical**
**Y Anatomical Regions, Lower Extremities**
**J Inspection** Definition: Visually and/or manually exploring a body part

Explanation: Visual exploration may be performed with or without optical instrumentation. Manual exploration may be performed directly or through intervening body layers.

| Body Part Character 4 | Approach Character 5 | Device Character 6 | Qualifier Character 7 |
|---|---|---|---|
| **Ø Buttock, Right**<br>**1 Buttock, Left**<br>**5 Inguinal Region, Right**<br>Inguinal canal<br>Inguinal triangle<br>**6 Inguinal Region, Left**<br>*See 5 Inguinal Region, Right*<br>**7 Femoral Region, Right**<br>**8 Femoral Region, Left**<br>**9 Lower Extremity, Right**<br>**A Inguinal Region, Bilateral**<br>*See 5 Inguinal Region, Right*<br>**B Lower Extremity, Left**<br>**C Upper Leg, Right**<br>**D Upper Leg, Left**<br>**E Femoral Region, Bilateral**<br>**F Knee Region, Right**<br>**G Knee Region, Left**<br>**H Lower Leg, Right**<br>**J Lower Leg, Left**<br>**K Ankle Region, Right**<br>**L Ankle Region, Left**<br>**M Foot, Right**<br>**N Foot, Left** | **Ø Open**<br>**3 Percutaneous**<br>**4 Percutaneous Endoscopic**<br>**X External** | **Z No Device** | **Z No Qualifier** |

**DRG Non-OR** ØYJ[Ø,1,8,9,B,C,D,E,F,G,H,J,K,L,M,N]ØZZ
**DRG Non-OR** ØYJ[5,6,7,8,A,E]3ZZ
**Non-OR** ØYJ[Ø,1,9,B,C,D,F,G,H,J,K,L,M,N][3,4,X]ZZ
**Non-OR** ØYJ[5,6,7,8,A,E]XZZ

**Ø Medical and Surgical**
**Y Anatomical Regions, Lower Extremities**
**M Reattachment** Definition: Putting back in or on all or a portion of a separated body part to its normal location or other suitable location
Explanation: Vascular circulation and nervous pathways may or may not be reestablished

| Body Part Character 4 | Approach Character 5 | Device Character 6 | Qualifier Character 7 |
|---|---|---|---|
| **Ø** Buttock, Right<br>**1** Buttock, Left<br>**2** Hindquarter, Right<br>**3** Hindquarter, Left<br>**4** Hindquarter, Bilateral<br>**5** Inguinal Region, Right<br>Inguinal canal<br>Inguinal triangle<br>**6** Inguinal Region, Left<br>*See 5 Inguinal Region, Right*<br>**7** Femoral Region, Right<br>**8** Femoral Region, Left<br>**9** Lower Extremity, Right<br>**B** Lower Extremity, Left<br>**C** Upper Leg, Right<br>**D** Upper Leg, Left<br>**F** Knee Region, Right<br>**G** Knee Region, Left<br>**H** Lower Leg, Right<br>**J** Lower Leg, Left<br>**K** Ankle Region, Right<br>**L** Ankle Region, Left<br>**M** Foot, Right<br>**N** Foot, Left<br>**P** 1st Toe, Right<br>Hallux<br>**Q** 1st Toe, Left<br>*See 1st Toe, Right*<br>**R** 2nd Toe, Right<br>**S** 2nd Toe, Left<br>**T** 3rd Toe, Right<br>**U** 3rd Toe, Left<br>**V** 4th Toe, Right<br>**W** 4th Toe, Left<br>**X** 5th Toe, Right<br>**Y** 5th Toe, Left | **Ø** Open | **Z** No Device | **Z** No Qualifier |

**Ø Medical and Surgical**
**Y Anatomical Regions, Lower Extremities**
**P Removal** Definition: Taking out or off a device from a body part
Explanation: If a device is taken out and a similar device put in without cutting or puncturing the skin or mucous membrane, the procedure is coded to the root operation CHANGE. Otherwise, the procedure for taking out the device is coded to the root operation REMOVAL.

| Body Part Character 4 | Approach Character 5 | Device Character 6 | Qualifier Character 7 |
|---|---|---|---|
| **9** Lower Extremity, Right<br>**B** Lower Extremity, Left | **Ø** Open<br>**3** Percutaneous<br>**4** Percutaneous Endoscopic<br>**X** External | **Ø** Drainage Device<br>**1** Radioactive Element<br>**3** Infusion Device<br>**7** Autologous Tissue Substitute<br>**J** Synthetic Substitute<br>**K** Nonautologous Tissue Substitute<br>**Y** Other Device | **Z** No Qualifier |

Non-OR All body part, approach, device, and qualifier values

**Ø Medical and Surgical**
**Y Anatomical Regions, Lower Extremities**
**Q Repair** Definition: Restoring, to the extent possible, a body part to its normal anatomic structure and function
Explanation: Used only when the method to accomplish the repair is not one of the other root operations

| Body Part Character 4 | Approach Character 5 | Device Character 6 | Qualifier Character 7 |
|---|---|---|---|
| **Ø** Buttock, Right<br>**1** Buttock, Left<br>**5** Inguinal Region, Right<br>Inguinal canal<br>Inguinal triangle<br>**6** Inguinal Region, Left<br>*See 5 Inguinal Region, Right*<br>**7** Femoral Region, Right<br>**8** Femoral Region, Left<br>**9** Lower Extremity, Right<br>**A** Inguinal Region, Bilateral<br>*See 5 Inguinal Region, Right*<br>**B** Lower Extremity, Left<br>**C** Upper Leg, Right<br>**D** Upper Leg, Left<br>**E** Femoral Region, Bilateral<br>**F** Knee Region, Right<br>**G** Knee Region, Left<br>**H** Lower Leg, Right<br>**J** Lower Leg, Left<br>**K** Ankle Region, Right<br>**L** Ankle Region, Left<br>**M** Foot, Right<br>**N** Foot, Left<br>**P** 1st Toe, Right<br>Hallux<br>**Q** 1st Toe, Left<br>*See 1st Toe, Right*<br>**R** 2nd Toe, Right<br>**S** 2nd Toe, Left<br>**T** 3rd Toe, Right<br>**U** 3rd Toe, Left<br>**V** 4th Toe, Right<br>**W** 4th Toe, Left<br>**X** 5th Toe, Right<br>**Y** 5th Toe, Left | **Ø** Open<br>**3** Percutaneous<br>**4** Percutaneous Endoscopic<br>**X** External | **Z** No Device | **Z** No Qualifier |

**Non-OR** ØYQ[5,6,7,8,A,E]XZZ

**Ø Medical and Surgical**
**Y Anatomical Regions, Lower Extremities**
**U Supplement** Definition: Putting in or on biological or synthetic material that physically reinforces and/or augments the function of a portion of a body part

Explanation: The biological material is non-living, or is living and from the same individual. The body part may have been previously replaced, and the SUPPLEMENT procedure is performed to physically reinforce and/or augment the function of the replaced body part.

| Body Part Character 4 | Approach Character 5 | Device Character 6 | Qualifier Character 7 |
|---|---|---|---|
| **Ø Buttock, Right**<br>**1 Buttock, Left**<br>**5 Inguinal Region, Right**<br>Inguinal canal<br>Inguinal triangle<br>**6 Inguinal Region, Left**<br>*See 5 Inguinal Region, Right*<br>**7 Femoral Region, Right**<br>**8 Femoral Region, Left**<br>**9 Lower Extremity, Right**<br>**A Inguinal Region, Bilateral**<br>*See 5 Inguinal Region, Right*<br>**B Lower Extremity, Left**<br>**C Upper Leg, Right**<br>**D Upper Leg, Left**<br>**E Femoral Region, Bilateral**<br>**F Knee Region, Right**<br>**G Knee Region, Left**<br>**H Lower Leg, Right**<br>**J Lower Leg, Left**<br>**K Ankle Region, Right**<br>**L Ankle Region, Left**<br>**M Foot, Right**<br>**N Foot, Left**<br>**P 1st Toe, Right**<br>Hallux<br>**Q 1st Toe, Left**<br>*See 1st Toe, Right*<br>**R 2nd Toe, Right**<br>**S 2nd Toe, Left**<br>**T 3rd Toe, Right**<br>**U 3rd Toe, Left**<br>**V 4th Toe, Right**<br>**W 4th Toe, Left**<br>**X 5th Toe, Right**<br>**Y 5th Toe, Left** | **Ø Open**<br>**4 Percutaneous Endoscopic** | **7 Autologous Tissue Substitute**<br>**J Synthetic Substitute**<br>**K Nonautologous Tissue Substitute** | **Z No Qualifier** |

**Ø Medical and Surgical**
**Y Anatomical Regions, Lower Extremities**
**W Revision** Definition: Correcting, to the extent possible, a portion of a malfunctioning device or the position of a displaced device

Explanation: Revision can include correcting a malfunctioning or displaced device by taking out or putting in components of the device such as a screw or pin

| Body Part Character 4 | Approach Character 5 | Device Character 6 | Qualifier Character 7 |
|---|---|---|---|
| **9 Lower Extremity, Right**<br>**B Lower Extremity, Left** | **Ø Open**<br>**3 Percutaneous**<br>**4 Percutaneous Endoscopic**<br>**X External** | **Ø Drainage Device**<br>**3 Infusion Device**<br>**7 Autologous Tissue Substitute**<br>**J Synthetic Substitute**<br>**K Nonautologous Tissue Substitute**<br>**Y Other Device** | **Z No Qualifier** |

DRG Non-OR ØYW[9,B][Ø,3,4][Ø,3,7,J,K,Y]Z
Non-OR ØYW[9,B]X[Ø,3,7,J,K,Y]Z

# Obstetrics 1Ø2–1ØY



## Character Meanings

This Character Meaning table is provided as a guide to assist the user in the identification of character members that may be found in this section of code tables. It **SHOULD NOT** be used to build a PCS code.

### Ø: Pregnancy

| Operation–Character 3 | Body Part–Character 4 | Approach–Character 5 | Device–Character 6 | Qualifier–Character 7 |
|---|---|---|---|---|
| 2 Change | Ø Products of Conception | Ø Open | 3 Monitoring Electrode | Ø Classical |
| 9 Drainage | 1 Products of Conception, Retained | 3 Percutaneous | Y Other Device | 1 Low Cervical |
| A Abortion | 2 Products of Conception, Ectopic | 4 Percutaneous Endoscopic | Z No Device | 2 Extraperitoneal |
| D Extraction | | 7 Via Natural or Artificial Opening | | 3 Low Forceps |
| E Delivery | | 8 Via Natural or Artificial Opening Endoscopic | | 4 Mid Forceps |
| H Insertion | | X External | | 5 High Forceps |
| J Inspection | | | | 6 Vacuum |
| P Removal | | | | 7 Internal Version |
| Q Repair | | | | 8 Other |
| S Reposition | | | | 9 Fetal Blood OR Manual |
| T Resection | | | | A Fetal Cerebrospinal Fluid |
| Y Transplantation | | | | B Fetal Fluid, Other |
| | | | | C Amniotic Fluid, Therapeutic |
| | | | | D Fluid, Other |
| | | | | E Nervous System |
| | | | | F Cardiovascular System |
| | | | | G Lymphatics & Hemic |
| | | | | H Eye |
| | | | | J Ear, Nose & Sinus |
| | | | | K Respiratory System |
| | | | | L Mouth & Throat |
| | | | | M Gastrointestinal System |
| | | | | N Hepatobiliary & Pancreas |
| | | | | P Endocrine System |
| | | | | Q Skin |
| | | | | R Musculoskeletal System |
| | | | | S Urinary System |
| | | | | T Female Reproductive System |
| | | | | U Amniotic Fluid, Diagnostic |
| | | | | V Male Reproductive System |
| | | | | W Laminaria |
| | | | | X Abortifacient |
| | | | | Y Other Body System |
| | | | | Z No Qualifier |

**AHA Coding Clinic for table 1Ø9**
**2014, 3Q, 12** Fetoscopic laser photocoagulation and laser microseptostomy for twin-twin transfusion syndrome
**2014, 2Q, 9** Pitocin administration to augment labor

**AHA Coding Clinic for table 1ØD**
**2016, 1Q, 9** Vaginal delivery assisted by vacuum and low forceps extraction
**2014, 4Q, 43** Cesarean delivery assisted by vacuum extraction
**2014, 4Q, 43** Vacuum dilation and curettage for blighted ovum

**AHA Coding Clinic for table 1ØE**
**2016, 2Q, 34** Assisted vaginal delivery
**2014, 4Q, 17** RH (D) alloimmunization (sensitization)
**2014, 2Q, 9** Pitocin administration to augment labor

**AHA Coding Clinic for table 1ØH**
**2013, 2Q, 36** Intrauterine pressure monitor

**AHA Coding Clinic for table 1ØQ**
**2014, 3Q, 12** Fetoscopic laser photocoagulation and laser microseptostomy for twin-twin transfusion syndrome

**AHA Coding Clinic for table 1ØT**
**2015, 3Q, 31** Laparoscopic partial salpingectomy for ectopic pregnancy

**1 Obstetrics**
**Ø Pregnancy**
**2 Change**

Definition: Taking out or off a device from a body part and putting back an identical or similar device in or on the same body part without cutting or puncturing the skin or a mucous membrane

Explanation: None

| Body Part Character 4 | Approach Character 5 | Device Character 6 | Qualifier Character 7 |
|---|---|---|---|
| Ø Products of Conception ♀ | 7 Via Natural or Artificial Opening | 3 Monitoring Electrode<br>Y Other Device | Z No Qualifier |

Non-OR All body part, approach, device, and qualifier values
♀ All body part, approach, device, and qualifier values

**1 Obstetrics**
**Ø Pregnancy**
**9 Drainage**

Definition: Taking or letting out fluids and/or gases from a body part

Explanation: None

| Body Part Character 4 | Approach Character 5 | Device Character 6 | Qualifier Character 7 |
|---|---|---|---|
| Ø Products of Conception ♀ | Ø Open<br>3 Percutaneous<br>4 Percutaneous Endoscopic<br>7 Via Natural or Artificial Opening<br>8 Via Natural or Artificial Opening Endoscopic | Z No Device | 9 Fetal Blood<br>A Fetal Cerebrospinal Fluid<br>B Fetal Fluid, Other<br>C Amniotic Fluid, Therapeutic<br>D Fluid, Other<br>U Amniotic Fluid, Diagnostic |

Non-OR All body part, approach, device, and qualifier values
♀ All body part, approach, device, and qualifier values

**1 Obstetrics**
**Ø Pregnancy**
**A Abortion**

Definition: Artificially terminating a pregnancy

Explanation: None

| Body Part Character 4 | Approach Character 5 | Device Character 6 | Qualifier Character 7 |
|---|---|---|---|
| Ø Products of Conception ♀ | Ø Open<br>3 Percutaneous<br>4 Percutaneous Endoscopic<br>8 Via Natural or Artificial Opening Endoscopic | Z No Device | Z No Qualifier |
| Ø Products of Conception ♀ | 7 Via Natural or Artificial Opening | Z No Device | 6 Vacuum<br>W Laminaria<br>X Abortifacient<br>Z No Qualifier |

DRG Non-OR 1ØAØ7Z6
Non-OR 1ØAØ7Z[W,X]
♀ All body part, approach, device, and qualifier values

**1 Obstetrics**
**Ø Pregnancy**
**D Extraction**

Definition: Pulling or stripping out or off all or a portion of a body part by the use of force

Explanation: None

| Body Part Character 4 | Approach Character 5 | Device Character 6 | Qualifier Character 7 |
|---|---|---|---|
| Ø Products of Conception ♀ | Ø Open | Z No Device | Ø Classical<br>1 Low Cervical<br>2 Extraperitoneal |
| Ø Products of Conception ♀ | 7 Via Natural or Artificial Opening | Z No Device | 3 Low Forceps<br>4 Mid Forceps<br>5 High Forceps<br>6 Vacuum<br>7 Internal Version<br>8 Other |
| 1 Products of Conception, Retained ♀ | 7 Via Natural or Artificial Opening<br>8 Via Natural or Artificial Opening Endoscopic | Z No Device | 9 Manual<br>Z No Qualifier |
| 2 Products of Conception, Ectopic ♀ | 7 Via Natural or Artificial Opening<br>8 Via Natural or Artificial Opening Endoscopic | Z No Device | Z No Qualifier |

DRG Non-OR 1ØDØ7Z[3,4,5,6,7,8]
♀ All body part, approach, device, and qualifier values

**1 Obstetrics**
**Ø Pregnancy**
**E Delivery**

Definition: Assisting the passage of the products of conception from the genital canal
Explanation: None

| Body Part Character 4 | Approach Character 5 | Device Character 6 | Qualifier Character 7 |
|---|---|---|---|
| Ø Products of Conception ♀ | X External | Z No Device | Z No Qualifier |

DRG Non-OR 1ØEØXZZ
♀ All body part, approach, device, and qualifier values

**1 Obstetrics**
**Ø Pregnancy**
**H Insertion**

Definition: Putting in a nonbiological appliance that monitors, assists, performs, or prevents a physiological function but does not physically take the place of a body part
Explanation: None

| Body Part Character 4 | Approach Character 5 | Device Character 6 | Qualifier Character 7 |
|---|---|---|---|
| Ø Products of Conception ♀ | Ø Open<br>7 Via Natural or Artificial Opening | 3 Monitoring Electrode<br>Y Other Device | Z No Qualifier |

Non-OR 1ØHØ7[3,Y]Z
♀ All body part, approach, device, and qualifier values

**1 Obstetrics**
**Ø Pregnancy**
**J Inspection**

Definition: Visually and/or manually exploring a body part
Explanation: Visual exploration may be performed with or without optical instrumentation. Manual exploration may be performed directly or through intervening body layers.

| Body Part Character 4 | Approach Character 5 | Device Character 6 | Qualifier Character 7 |
|---|---|---|---|
| Ø Products of Conception ♀<br>1 Products of Conception, Retained ♀<br>2 Products of Conception, Ectopic ♀ | Ø Open<br>3 Percutaneous<br>4 Percutaneous Endoscopic<br>7 Via Natural or Artificial Opening<br>8 Via Natural or Artificial Opening Endoscopic<br>X External | Z No Device | Z No Qualifier |

Non-OR All body part, approach, device, and qualifier values
♀ All body part, approach, device, and qualifier values

**1 Obstetrics**
**Ø Pregnancy**
**P Removal**

Definition: Taking out or off a device from a body part, region or orifice
Explanation: If a device is taken out and a similar device put in without cutting or puncturing the skin or mucous membrane, the procedure is coded to the root operation CHANGE. Otherwise, the procedure for taking out a device is coded to the root operation REMOVAL.

| Body Part Character 4 | Approach Character 5 | Device Character 6 | Qualifier Character 7 |
|---|---|---|---|
| Ø Products of Conception ♀ | Ø Open<br>7 Via Natural or Artificial Opening | 3 Monitoring Electrode<br>Y Other Device | Z No Qualifier |

♀ All body part, approach, device, and qualifier values

**1 Obstetrics**
**Ø Pregnancy**
**Q Repair**

Definition: Restoring, to the extent possible, a body part to its normal anatomic structure and function
Explanation: Used only when the method to accomplish the repair is not one of the other root operations

| Body Part Character 4 | Approach Character 5 | Device Character 6 | Qualifier Character 7 |
|---|---|---|---|
| Ø Products of Conception ♀ | Ø Open<br>3 Percutaneous<br>4 Percutaneous Endoscopic<br>7 Via Natural or Artificial Opening<br>8 Via Natural or Artificial Opening Endoscopic | Y Other Device<br>Z No Device | E Nervous System<br>F Cardiovascular System<br>G Lymphatics and Hemic<br>H Eye<br>J Ear, Nose and Sinus<br>K Respiratory System<br>L Mouth and Throat<br>M Gastrointestinal System<br>N Hepatobiliary and Pancreas<br>P Endocrine System<br>Q Skin<br>R Musculoskeletal System<br>S Urinary System<br>T Female Reproductive System<br>V Male Reproductive System<br>Y Other Body System |

♀ All body part, approach, device, and qualifier values

**1 Obstetrics**
**Ø Pregnancy**
**S Reposition**

Definition: Moving to its normal location, or other suitable location, all or a portion of a body part

Explanation: The body part is moved to a new location from an abnormal location, or from a normal location where it is not functioning correctly. The body part may or may not be cut out or off to be moved to the new location.

| Body Part Character 4 | Approach Character 5 | Device Character 6 | Qualifier Character 7 |
|---|---|---|---|
| Ø Products of Conception ♀ | 7 Via Natural or Artificial Opening<br>X External | Z No Device | Z No Qualifier |
| 2 Products of Conception, Ectopic ♀ | Ø Open<br>3 Percutaneous<br>4 Percutaneous Endoscopic<br>7 Via Natural or Artificial Opening<br>8 Via Natural or Artificial Opening Endoscopic | Z No Device | Z No Qualifier |

DRG Non-OR 1ØSØ7ZZ
Non-OR 1ØSØXZZ

♀ All body part, approach, device, and qualifier values

**1 Obstetrics**
**Ø Pregnancy**
**T Resection**

Definition: Cutting out or off, without replacement, all of a body part

Explanation: None

| Body Part Character 4 | Approach Character 5 | Device Character 6 | Qualifier Character 7 |
|---|---|---|---|
| 2 Products of Conception, Ectopic ♀ | Ø Open<br>3 Percutaneous<br>4 Percutaneous Endoscopic<br>7 Via Natural or Artificial Opening<br>8 Via Natural or Artificial Opening Endoscopic | Z No Device | Z No Qualifier |

♀ All body part, approach, device, and qualifier values

**1 Obstetrics**
**Ø Pregnancy**
**Y Transplantation**

Definition: Putting in or on all or a portion of a living body part taken from another individual or animal to physically take the place and/or function of all or a portion of a similar body part

Explanation: The native body part may or may not be taken out, and the transplanted body part may take over all or a portion of its function

| Body Part Character 4 | Approach Character 5 | Device Character 6 | Qualifier Character 7 |
|---|---|---|---|
| Ø Products of Conception ♀ | 3 Percutaneous<br>4 Percutaneous Endoscopic<br>7 Via Natural or Artificial Opening | Z No Device | E Nervous System<br>F Cardiovascular System<br>G Lymphatics and Hemic<br>H Eye<br>J Ear, Nose and Sinus<br>K Respiratory System<br>L Mouth and Throat<br>M Gastrointestinal System<br>N Hepatobiliary and Pancreas<br>P Endocrine System<br>Q Skin<br>R Musculoskeletal System<br>S Urinary System<br>T Female Reproductive System<br>V Male Reproductive System<br>Y Other Body System |

♀ All body part, approach, device, and qualifier values

# Placement 2WØ–2Y5

## Character Meanings

This Character Meaning table is provided as a guide to assist the user in the identification of character members that may be found in this section of code tables. It **SHOULD NOT** be used to build a PCS code.

### W: Anatomical Regions

| Operation–Character 3 | Body Region–Character 4 | Approach–Character 5 | Device–Character 6 | Qualifier–Character 7 |
|---|---|---|---|---|
| Ø Change | Ø Head | X External | Ø Traction Apparatus | Z No Qualifier |
| 1 Compression | 1 Face | | 1 Splint | |
| 2 Dressing | 2 Neck | | 2 Cast | |
| 3 Immobilization | 3 Abdominal Wall | | 3 Brace | |
| 4 Packing | 4 Chest Wall | | 4 Bandage | |
| 5 Removal | 5 Back | | 5 Packing Material | |
| 6 Traction | 6 Inguinal Region, Right | | 6 Pressure Dressing | |
| | 7 Inguinal Region, Left | | 7 Intermittent Pressure Device | |
| | 8 Upper Extremity, Right | | 9 Wire | |
| | 9 Upper Extremity, Left | | Y Other Device | |
| | A Upper Arm, Right | | Z No Device | |
| | B Upper Arm, Left | | | |
| | C Lower Arm, Right | | | |
| | D Lower Arm, Left | | | |
| | E Hand, Right | | | |
| | F Hand, Left | | | |
| | G Thumb, Right | | | |
| | H Thumb, Left | | | |
| | J Finger, Right | | | |
| | K Finger, Left | | | |
| | L Lower Extremity, Right | | | |
| | M Lower Extremity, Left | | | |
| | N Upper Leg, Right | | | |
| | P Upper Leg, Left | | | |
| | Q Lower Leg, Right | | | |
| | R Lower Leg, Left | | | |
| | S Foot, Right | | | |
| | T Foot, Left | | | |
| | U Toe, Right | | | |
| | V Toe, Left | | | |

### Y: Anatomical Orifices

| Operation–Character 3 | Body Orifice–Character 4 | Approach–Character 5 | Device–Character 6 | Qualifier–Character 7 |
|---|---|---|---|---|
| Ø Change | Ø Mouth and Pharynx | X External | 5 Packing Material | Z No Qualifier |
| 4 Packing | 1 Nasal | | | |
| 5 Removal | 2 Ear | | | |
| | 3 Anorectal | | | |
| | 4 Female Genital Tract | | | |
| | 5 Urethra | | | |

**AHA Coding Clinic for table 2W6**
**2015, 2Q, 35** Application of tongs to reduce and stabilize cervical fracture
**2013, 2Q, 39** Application of cervical tongs for reduction of cervical fracture

**2 Placement**
**W Anatomical Regions**
**Ø Change** Definition: Taking out or off a device from a body part and putting back an identical or similar device in or on the same body part without cutting or puncturing the skin or a mucous membrane

| Body Region Character 4 | Approach Character 5 | Device Character 6 | Qualifier Character 7 |
|---|---|---|---|
| Ø Head<br>2 Neck<br>3 Abdominal Wall<br>4 Chest Wall<br>5 Back<br>6 Inguinal Region, Right<br>7 Inguinal Region, Left<br>8 Upper Extremity, Right<br>9 Upper Extremity, Left<br>A Upper Arm, Right<br>B Upper Arm, Left<br>C Lower Arm, Right<br>D Lower Arm, Left<br>E Hand, Right<br>F Hand, Left<br>G Thumb, Right<br>H Thumb, Left<br>J Finger, Right<br>K Finger, Left<br>L Lower Extremity, Right<br>M Lower Extremity, Left<br>N Upper Leg, Right<br>P Upper Leg, Left<br>Q Lower Leg, Right<br>R Lower Leg, Left<br>S Foot, Right<br>T Foot, Left<br>U Toe, Right<br>V Toe, Left | X External | Ø Traction Apparatus<br>1 Splint<br>2 Cast<br>3 Brace<br>4 Bandage<br>5 Packing Material<br>6 Pressure Dressing<br>7 Intermittent Pressure Device<br>Y Other Device | Z No Qualifier |
| 1 Face | X External | Ø Traction Apparatus<br>1 Splint<br>2 Cast<br>3 Brace<br>4 Bandage<br>5 Packing Material<br>6 Pressure Dressing<br>7 Intermittent Pressure Device<br>9 Wire<br>Y Other Device | Z No Qualifier |

**2 Placement**
**W Anatomical Regions**
**1 Compression** Definition: Putting pressure on a body region

| Body Region Character 4 | Approach Character 5 | Device Character 6 | Qualifier Character 7 |
|---|---|---|---|
| **Ø** Head | **X** External | **6** Pressure Dressing | **Z** No Qualifier |
| **1** Face | | **7** Intermittent Pressure Device | |
| **2** Neck | | | |
| **3** Abdominal Wall | | | |
| **4** Chest Wall | | | |
| **5** Back | | | |
| **6** Inguinal Region, Right | | | |
| **7** Inguinal Region, Left | | | |
| **8** Upper Extremity, Right | | | |
| **9** Upper Extremity, Left | | | |
| **A** Upper Arm, Right | | | |
| **B** Upper Arm, Left | | | |
| **C** Lower Arm, Right | | | |
| **D** Lower Arm, Left | | | |
| **E** Hand, Right | | | |
| **F** Hand, Left | | | |
| **G** Thumb, Right | | | |
| **H** Thumb, Left | | | |
| **J** Finger, Right | | | |
| **K** Finger, Left | | | |
| **L** Lower Extremity, Right | | | |
| **M** Lower Extremity, Left | | | |
| **N** Upper Leg, Right | | | |
| **P** Upper Leg, Left | | | |
| **Q** Lower Leg, Right | | | |
| **R** Lower Leg, Left | | | |
| **S** Foot, Right | | | |
| **T** Foot, Left | | | |
| **U** Toe, Right | | | |
| **V** Toe, Left | | | |

**2 Placement**
**W Anatomical Regions**
**2 Dressing** Definition: Putting material on a body region for protection

| Body Region Character 4 | Approach Character 5 | Device Character 6 | Qualifier Character 7 |
|---|---|---|---|
| **Ø** Head | **X** External | **4** Bandage | **Z** No Qualifier |
| **1** Face | | | |
| **2** Neck | | | |
| **3** Abdominal Wall | | | |
| **4** Chest Wall | | | |
| **5** Back | | | |
| **6** Inguinal Region, Right | | | |
| **7** Inguinal Region, Left | | | |
| **8** Upper Extremity, Right | | | |
| **9** Upper Extremity, Left | | | |
| **A** Upper Arm, Right | | | |
| **B** Upper Arm, Left | | | |
| **C** Lower Arm, Right | | | |
| **D** Lower Arm, Left | | | |
| **E** Hand, Right | | | |
| **F** Hand, Left | | | |
| **G** Thumb, Right | | | |
| **H** Thumb, Left | | | |
| **J** Finger, Right | | | |
| **K** Finger, Left | | | |
| **L** Lower Extremity, Right | | | |
| **M** Lower Extremity, Left | | | |
| **N** Upper Leg, Right | | | |
| **P** Upper Leg, Left | | | |
| **Q** Lower Leg, Right | | | |
| **R** Lower Leg, Left | | | |
| **S** Foot, Right | | | |
| **T** Foot, Left | | | |
| **U** Toe, Right | | | |
| **V** Toe, Left | | | |

**2 Placement**
**W Anatomical Regions**
**3 Immobilization** Definition: Limiting or preventing motion of a body region

| Body Region Character 4 | Approach Character 5 | Device Character 6 | Qualifier Character 7 |
|---|---|---|---|
| Ø Head<br>2 Neck<br>3 Abdominal Wall<br>4 Chest Wall<br>5 Back<br>6 Inguinal Region, Right<br>7 Inguinal Region, Left<br>8 Upper Extremity, Right<br>9 Upper Extremity, Left<br>A Upper Arm, Right<br>B Upper Arm, Left<br>C Lower Arm, Right<br>D Lower Arm, Left<br>E Hand, Right<br>F Hand, Left<br>G Thumb, Right<br>H Thumb, Left<br>J Finger, Right<br>K Finger, Left<br>L Lower Extremity, Right<br>M Lower Extremity, Left<br>N Upper Leg, Right<br>P Upper Leg, Left<br>Q Lower Leg, Right<br>R Lower Leg, Left<br>S Foot, Right<br>T Foot, Left<br>U Toe, Right<br>V Toe, Left | X External | 1 Splint<br>2 Cast<br>3 Brace<br>Y Other Device | Z No Qualifier |
| 1 Face | X External | 1 Splint<br>2 Cast<br>3 Brace<br>9 Wire<br>Y Other Device | Z No Qualifier |

**2 Placement**
**W Anatomical Regions**
**4 Packing** Definition: Putting material in a body region or orifice

| Body Region Character 4 | Approach Character 5 | Device Character 6 | Qualifier Character 7 |
|---|---|---|---|
| Ø Head<br>1 Face<br>2 Neck<br>3 Abdominal Wall<br>4 Chest Wall<br>5 Back<br>6 Inguinal Region, Right<br>7 Inguinal Region, Left<br>8 Upper Extremity, Right<br>9 Upper Extremity, Left<br>A Upper Arm, Right<br>B Upper Arm, Left<br>C Lower Arm, Right<br>D Lower Arm, Left<br>E Hand, Right<br>F Hand, Left<br>G Thumb, Right<br>H Thumb, Left<br>J Finger, Right<br>K Finger, Left<br>L Lower Extremity, Right<br>M Lower Extremity, Left<br>N Upper Leg, Right<br>P Upper Leg, Left<br>Q Lower Leg, Right<br>R Lower Leg, Left<br>S Foot, Right<br>T Foot, Left<br>U Toe, Right<br>V Toe, Left | X External | 5 Packing Material | Z No Qualifier |

**2 Placement**
**W Anatomical Regions**
**5 Removal** Definition: Taking out or off a device from a body part

| Body Region Character 4 | Approach Character 5 | Device Character 6 | Qualifier Character 7 |
|---|---|---|---|
| Ø Head<br>2 Neck<br>3 Abdominal Wall<br>4 Chest Wall<br>5 Back<br>6 Inguinal Region, Right<br>7 Inguinal Region, Left<br>8 Upper Extremity, Right<br>9 Upper Extremity, Left<br>A Upper Arm, Right<br>B Upper Arm, Left<br>C Lower Arm, Right<br>D Lower Arm, Left<br>E Hand, Right<br>F Hand, Left<br>G Thumb, Right<br>H Thumb, Left<br>J Finger, Right<br>K Finger, Left<br>L Lower Extremity, Right<br>M Lower Extremity, Left<br>N Upper Leg, Right<br>P Upper Leg, Left<br>Q Lower Leg, Right<br>R Lower Leg, Left<br>S Foot, Right<br>T Foot, Left<br>U Toe, Right<br>V Toe, Left | X External | Ø Traction Apparatus<br>1 Splint<br>2 Cast<br>3 Brace<br>4 Bandage<br>5 Packing Material<br>6 Pressure Dressing<br>7 Intermittent Pressure Device<br>Y Other Device | Z No Qualifier |
| 1 Face | X External | Ø Traction Apparatus<br>1 Splint<br>2 Cast<br>3 Brace<br>4 Bandage<br>5 Packing Material<br>6 Pressure Dressing<br>7 Intermittent Pressure Device<br>9 Wire<br>Y Other Device | Z No Qualifier |

**2 Placement**
**W Anatomical Regions**
**6 Traction** Definition: Exerting a pulling force on a body region in a distal direction

| Body Region Character 4 | Approach Character 5 | Device Character 6 | Qualifier Character 7 |
|---|---|---|---|
| Ø Head<br>1 Face<br>2 Neck<br>3 Abdominal Wall<br>4 Chest Wall<br>5 Back<br>6 Inguinal Region, Right<br>7 Inguinal Region, Left<br>8 Upper Extremity, Right<br>9 Upper Extremity, Left<br>A Upper Arm, Right<br>B Upper Arm, Left<br>C Lower Arm, Right<br>D Lower Arm, Left<br>E Hand, Right<br>F Hand, Left<br>G Thumb, Right<br>H Thumb, Left<br>J Finger, Right<br>K Finger, Left<br>L Lower Extremity, Right<br>M Lower Extremity, Left<br>N Upper Leg, Right<br>P Upper Leg, Left<br>Q Lower Leg, Right<br>R Lower Leg, Left<br>S Foot, Right<br>T Foot, Left<br>U Toe, Right<br>V Toe, Left | X External | Ø Traction Apparatus<br>Z No Device | Z No Qualifier |

**2 Placement**
**Y Anatomical Orifices**
**Ø Change** Definition: Taking out or off a device from a body part and putting back an identical or similar device in or on the same body part without cutting or puncturing the skin or a mucous membrane

| Body Region Character 4 | Approach Character 5 | Device Character 6 | Qualifier Character 7 |
|---|---|---|---|
| Ø Mouth and Pharynx<br>1 Nasal<br>2 Ear<br>3 Anorectal<br>4 Female Genital Tract ♀<br>5 Urethra | X External | 5 Packing Material | Z No Qualifier |

♀ 2YØ4X5Z

**2 Placement**
**Y Anatomical Orifices**
**4 Packing** Definition: Putting material in a body region or orifice

| Body Region Character 4 | Approach Character 5 | Device Character 6 | Qualifier Character 7 |
|---|---|---|---|
| Ø Mouth and Pharynx<br>1 Nasal<br>2 Ear<br>3 Anorectal<br>4 Female Genital Tract ♀<br>5 Urethra | X External | 5 Packing Material | Z No Qualifier |

♀ 2Y44X5Z

**2 Placement**
**Y Anatomical Orifices**
**5 Removal** Definition: Taking out or off a device from a body part

| Body Region Character 4 | Approach Character 5 | Device Character 6 | Qualifier Character 7 |
|---|---|---|---|
| Ø Mouth and Pharynx<br>1 Nasal<br>2 Ear<br>3 Anorectal<br>4 Female Genital Tract ♀<br>5 Urethra | X External | 5 Packing Material | Z No Qualifier |

♀ 2Y54XPZ

# Administration 3Ø2–3E1



## Character Meanings

This Character Meaning table is provided as a guide to assist the user in the identification of character members that may be found in this section of code tables. It **SHOULD NOT** be used to build a PCS code.

### Ø: Circulatory

| Operation–Character 3 | Body System/Region – Character 4 | Approach–Character 5 | Substance–Character 6 | Qualifier–Character 7 |
|---|---|---|---|---|
| 2 Transfusion | 3 Peripheral Vein | Ø Open | A Stem Cells, Embryonic | Ø Autologous |
| | 4 Central Vein | 3 Percutaneous | B 4-Factor Prothrombin Complex Concentrate | 1 Nonautologous |
| | 5 Peripheral Artery | 7 Via Natural or Artificial Opening | G Bone Marrow | 2 Allogeneic, Related |
| | 6 Central Artery | | H Whole Blood | 3 Allogeneic, Unrelated |
| | 7 Products of Conception, Circulatory | | J Serum Albumin | 4 Allogeneic, Unspecified |
| | 8 Vein | | K Frozen Plasma | Z No Qualifier |
| | | | L Fresh Plasma | |
| | | | M Plasma Cryoprecipitate | |
| | | | N Red Blood Cells | |
| | | | P Frozen Red Cells | |
| | | | Q White Cells | |
| | | | R Platelets | |
| | | | S Globulin | |
| | | | T Fibrinogen | |
| | | | V Antihemophilic Factors | |
| | | | W Factor IX | |
| | | | X Stem Cells, Cord Blood | |
| | | | Y Stem Cells, Hematopoietic | |

### C: Indwelling Device

| Operation–Character 3 | Body System/Region – Character 4 | Approach–Character 5 | Substance–Character 6 | Qualifier–Character 7 |
|---|---|---|---|---|
| 1 Irrigation | Z None | X External | 8 Irrigating Substance | Z No Qualifier |

*Continued on next page*

## E: Physiological Systems and Anatomical Regions

***Administration Character Meanings Continued***

| Operation–Character 3 | Body System/Region–Character 4 | Approach–Character 5 | Substance–Character 6 | Qualifier–Character 7 |
|---|---|---|---|---|
| Ø Introduction | Ø Skin and Mucous Membranes | Ø Open | Ø Antineoplastic | Ø Autologous OR Influenza Vaccine |
| 1 Irrigation | 1 Subcutaneous Tissue | 3 Percutaneous | 1 Thrombolytic | 1 Nonautologous |
| | 2 Muscle | 4 Percutaneous Endoscopic | 2 Anti-infective | 2 High-dose Interleukin-2 |
| | 3 Peripheral Vein | 7 Via Natural or Artificial Opening | 3 Anti-inflammatory | 3 Low-dose Interleukin-2 |
| | 4 Central Vein | 8 Via Natural or Artificial Opening Endoscopic | 4 Serum, Toxoid and Vaccine | 4 Liquid Brachytherapy Radioisotope |
| | 5 Peripheral Artery | X External | 5 Adhesion Barrier | 5 Other Antineoplastic |
| | 6 Central Artery | | 6 Nutritional Substance | 6 Recombinant Human-activated Protein C |
| | 7 Coronary Artery | | 7 Electrolytic and Water Balance Substance | 7 Other Thrombolytic |
| | 8 Heart | | 8 Irrigating Substance | 8 Oxazolidinones |
| | 9 Nose | | 9 Dialysate | 9 Other Anti-infective |
| | A Bone Marrow | | A Stem Cells, Embryonic | A Anti-infective Envelope |
| | B Ear | | B Anesthetic Agent | B Recombinant Bone Morphogenetic Protein |
| | C Eye | | E Stem Cells, Somatic | C Other Substance |
| | D Mouth and Pharynx | | F Intracirculatory Anesthetic | D Nitric Oxide |
| | E Products of Conception | | G Other Therapeutic Substance | F Other Gas |
| | F Respiratory Tract | | H Radioactive Substance | G Insulin |
| | G Upper GI | | K Other Diagnostic Substance | H Human B-type Natriuretic Peptide |
| | H Lower GI | | L Sperm | J Other Hormone |
| | J Biliary and Pancreatic Tract | | M Pigment | K Immunostimulator |
| | K Genitourinary Tract | | N Analgesics, Hypnotics, Sedatives | L Immunosuppressive |
| | L Pleural Cavity | | P Platelet Inhibitor | M Monoclonal Antibody |
| | M Peritoneal Cavity | | Q Fertilized Ovum | N Blood Brain Barrier Disruption |
| | N Male Reproductive | | R Antiarrhythmic | P Clofarabine |
| | P Female Reproductive | | S Gas | Q Glucarpidase |
| | Q Cranial Cavity and Brain | | T Destructive Agent | X Diagnostic |
| | R Spinal Canal | | U Pancreatic Islet Cells | Z No Qualifier |
| | S Epidural Space | | V Hormone | |
| | T Peripheral Nerves and Plexi | | W Immunotherapeutic | |
| | U Joints | | X Vasopressor | |
| | V Bones | | | |
| | W Lymphatics | | | |
| | X Cranial Nerves | | | |
| | Y Pericardial Cavity | | | |

**AHA Coding Clinic for table 3Ø2**

**2016, 4Q, 113** Bone marrow and stem cell transfusion (Transplantation)

**AHA Coding Clinic for table 3EØ**

**2017, 2Q, 14** Infusion of tPA into pleural cavity
**2017, 1Q, 37** Injection of glue into enteric fistula tract
**2016, 4Q, 113-114** Substances applied to cranial cavity and brain
**2016, 3Q, 29** Closure of bilateral alveolar clefts
**2016, 1Q, 20** Metatarsophalangeal joint resection arthroplasty
**2015, 3Q, 24** Esophagogastroduodenoscopy with epinephrine injection for control of bleeding
**2015, 3Q, 29** Placement of adhesion barrier
**2015, 2Q, 29** Insertion of nasogastric tube for drainage and feeding
**2015, 2Q, 31** Thoracoscopic talc pleurodesis
**2015, 1Q, 31** Intrathecal chemotherapy
**2015, 1Q, 38** Chemoembolization of the hepatic artery
**2014, 4Q, 16** Administration of RH (D) immunoglobulin
**2014, 4Q, 17** RH (D) alloimmunization (sensitization)
**2014, 4Q, 19** Ultrasound accelerated thrombolysis
**2014, 4Q, 34** Resection of brain malignancy with implantation of chemotherapeutic wafer
**2014, 4Q, 38** Placement of saline and seprafilm solution into abdominal cavity
**2014, 3Q, 26** Coil embolization of gastroduodenal artery with chemoembolization of hepatic artery
**2014, 2Q, 8** Medical induction of labor with Cervidil tampon insertion
**2014, 2Q, 10** Prophylactic Neulasta injection for infection prevention
**2013, 4Q, 124** Administration of tPA for stroke treatment prior to transfer
**2013, 1Q, 27** Injection of sclerosing agent into an esophageal varix

**3 Administration**
**Ø Circulatory**
**2 Transfusion** Definition: Putting in blood or blood products

| Body System/Region<br>Character 4 | Approach<br>Character 5 | Substance<br>Character 6 | Qualifier<br>Character 7 |
|---|---|---|---|
| 3 Peripheral Vein NC<br>4 Central Vein NC | Ø Open<br>3 Percutaneous | A Stem Cells, Embryonic | Z No Qualifier |
| 3 Peripheral Vein NC<br>4 Central Vein NC | Ø Open<br>3 Percutaneous | G Bone Marrow<br>X Stem Cells, Cord Blood<br>Y Stem Cells, Hematopoietic | Ø Autologous<br>2 Allogeneic, Related<br>3 Allogeneic, Unrelated<br>4 Allogeneic, Unspecified |
| 3 Peripheral Vein<br>4 Central Vein | Ø Open<br>3 Percutaneous | H Whole Blood<br>J Serum Albumin<br>K Frozen Plasma<br>L Fresh Plasma<br>M Plasma Cryoprecipitate<br>N Red Blood Cells<br>P Frozen Red Cells<br>Q White Cells<br>R Platelets<br>S Globulin<br>T Fibrinogen<br>V Antihemophilic Factors<br>W Factor IX | Ø Autologous<br>1 Nonautologous |
| 5 Peripheral Artery NC<br>6 Central Artery NC | Ø Open<br>3 Percutaneous | G Bone Marrow<br>H Whole Blood<br>J Serum Albumin<br>K Frozen Plasma<br>L Fresh Plasma<br>M Plasma Cryoprecipitate<br>N Red Blood Cells<br>P Frozen Red Cells<br>Q White Cells<br>R Platelets<br>S Globulin<br>T Fibrinogen<br>V Antihemophilic Factors<br>W Factor IX<br>X Stem Cells, Cord Blood<br>Y Stem Cells, Hematopoietic | Ø Autologous<br>1 Nonautologous |
| 7 Products of Conception, Circulatory ♀ | 3 Percutaneous<br>7 Via Natural or Artificial Opening | H Whole Blood<br>J Serum Albumin<br>K Frozen Plasma<br>L Fresh Plasma<br>M Plasma Cryoprecipitate<br>N Red Blood Cells<br>P Frozen Red Cells<br>Q White Cells<br>R Platelets<br>S Globulin<br>T Fibrinogen<br>V Antihemophilic Factors<br>W Factor IX | 1 Nonautologous |
| 8 Vein | Ø Open<br>3 Percutaneous | B 4-Factor Prothrombin Complex Concentrate | 1 Nonautologous |

**Valid OR** 3Ø2[3,4]ØAZ
**Valid OR** 3Ø2[3,4]Ø[G,X,Y][Ø,2,3,4]
**Valid OR** 3Ø2[3,4]3[G,X,Y][2,3,4]
**Valid OR** 3Ø2[5,6]Ø[G,X,Y][Ø,1]
NC 3Ø2[3,4][Ø,3]AZ Only when reported with PDx or SDx of C91.ØØ, C92.ØØ, C92.1Ø, C92.11, C92.4Ø, C92.5Ø, C92.6Ø, C92.AØ, C93.ØØ, C94.ØØ, C95.ØØ
NC 3Ø2[3,4][Ø,3][G,Y]Ø Only when reported with PDx or SDx of C91.ØØ, C92.ØØ, C92.1Ø, C92.11, C92.4Ø, C92.5Ø, C92.6Ø, C92.AØ, C93.ØØ, C94.ØØ, C95.ØØ
NC 3Ø2[3,4][Ø,3][G,Y][2,3,4]
NC 3Ø2[5,6][Ø,3][G,Y]Ø Only when reported with PDx or SDx of C91.ØØ, C92.ØØ, C92.1Ø, C92.11, C92.4Ø, C92.5Ø, C92.6Ø, C92.AØ, C93.ØØ, C94.ØØ, C95.ØØ
NC 3Ø2[5,6][Ø,3][G,Y]1 Only when reported with PDx or SDx of C9Ø.ØØ or C9Ø.Ø1
♀ 3Ø27[3,7][H,J,K,L,M,N,P,Q,R,S,T,V,W]1

**3 Administration**
**C Indwelling Device**
**1 Irrigation** Definition: Putting in or on a cleansing substance

| Body System/Region<br>Character 4 | Approach<br>Character 5 | Substance<br>Character 6 | Qualifier<br>Character 7 |
|---|---|---|---|
| Z None | X External | 8 Irrigating Substance | Z No Qualifier |

**3 Administration**
**E Physiological Systems and Anatomical Regions**
**Ø Introduction** Definition: Putting in or on a therapeutic, diagnostic, nutritional, physiological, or prophylactic substance except blood or blood products

| Body System/Region Character 4 | Approach Character 5 | Substance Character 6 | Qualifier Character 7 |
|---|---|---|---|
| Ø Skin and Mucous Membranes | X External | Ø Antineoplastic | 5 Other Antineoplastic<br>M Monoclonal Antibody |
| Ø Skin and Mucous Membranes | X External | 2 Anti-infective | 8 Oxazolidinones<br>9 Other Anti-infective |
| Ø Skin and Mucous Membranes | X External | 3 Anti-inflammatory<br>4 Serum, Toxoid and Vaccine<br>B Anesthetic Agent<br>K Other Diagnostic Substance<br>M Pigment<br>N Analgesics, Hypnotics, Sedatives<br>T Destructive Agent | Z No Qualifier |
| Ø Skin and Mucous Membranes | X External | G Other Therapeutic Substance | C Other Substance |
| 1 Subcutaneous Tissue | Ø Open | 2 Anti-infective | A Anti-Infective Envelope |
| 1 Subcutaneous Tissue | 3 Percutaneous | Ø Antineoplastic | 5 Other Antineoplastic<br>M Monoclonal Antibody |
| 1 Subcutaneous Tissue | 3 Percutaneous | 2 Anti-infective | 8 Oxazolidinones<br>9 Other Anti-infective<br>A Anti-Infective Envelope |
| 1 Subcutaneous Tissue | 3 Percutaneous | 3 Anti-inflammatory<br>6 Nutritional Substance<br>7 Electrolytic and Water Balance Substance<br>B Anesthetic Agent<br>H Radioactive Substance<br>K Other Diagnostic Substance<br>N Analgesics, Hypnotics, Sedatives<br>T Destructive Agent | Z No Qualifier |
| 1 Subcutaneous Tissue | 3 Percutaneous | 4 Serum, Toxoid and Vaccine | Ø Influenza Vaccine<br>Z No Qualifier |
| 1 Subcutaneous Tissue | 3 Percutaneous | G Other Therapeutic Substance | C Other Substance |
| 1 Subcutaneous Tissue | 3 Percutaneous | V Hormone | G Insulin<br>J Other Hormone |
| 2 Muscle | 3 Percutaneous | Ø Antineoplastic | 5 Other Antineoplastic<br>M Monoclonal Antibody |
| 2 Muscle | 3 Percutaneous | 2 Anti-infective | 8 Oxazolidinones<br>9 Other Anti-infective |
| 2 Muscle | 3 Percutaneous | 3 Anti-inflammatory<br>4 Serum, Toxoid and Vaccine<br>6 Nutritional Substance<br>7 Electrolytic and Water Balance Substance<br>B Anesthetic Agent<br>H Radioactive Substance<br>K Other Diagnostic Substance<br>N Analgesics, Hypnotics, Sedatives<br>T Destructive Agent | Z No Qualifier |
| 2 Muscle | 3 Percutaneous | G Other Therapeutic Substance | C Other Substance |
| 3 Peripheral Vein | Ø Open | Ø Antineoplastic | 2 High-dose Interleukin-2<br>3 Low-dose Interleukin-2<br>5 Other Antineoplastic<br>M Monoclonal Antibody<br>P Clofarabine |
| 3 Peripheral Vein | Ø Open | 1 Thrombolytic | 6 Recombinant Human-activated Protein C<br>7 Other Thrombolytic |
| 3 Peripheral Vein | Ø Open | 2 Anti-infective | 8 Oxazolidinones<br>9 Other Anti-infective |

***3EØ Continued on next page***

DRG Non-OR 3EØ3ØØ2
DRG Non-OR 3EØ3Ø17

**3 Administration**
**E Physiological Systems and Anatomical Regions**
**Ø Introduction** Definition: Putting in or on a therapeutic, diagnostic, nutritional, physiological, or prophylactic substance except blood or blood products

*3EØ Continued*

| Body System/Region Character 4 | Approach Character 5 | Substance Character 6 | Qualifier Character 7 |
|---|---|---|---|
| 3 Peripheral Vein | Ø Open | 3 Anti-inflammatory<br>4 Serum, Toxoid and Vaccine<br>6 Nutritional Substance<br>7 Electrolytic and Water Balance Substance<br>F Intracirculatory Anesthetic<br>H Radioactive Substance<br>K Other Diagnostic Substance<br>N Analgesics, Hypnotics, Sedatives<br>P Platelet Inhibitor<br>R Antiarrhythmic<br>T Destructive Agent<br>X Vasopressor | Z No Qualifier |
| 3 Peripheral Vein | Ø Open | G Other Therapeutic Substance | C Other Substance<br>N Blood Brain Barrier Disruption |
| 3 Peripheral Vein | Ø Open | U Pancreatic Islet Cells | Ø Autologous<br>1 Nonautologous |
| 3 Peripheral Vein | Ø Open | V Hormone | G Insulin<br>H Human B-type Natriuretic Peptide<br>J Other Hormone |
| 3 Peripheral Vein | Ø Open | W Immunotherapeutic | K Immunostimulator<br>L Immunosuppressive |
| 3 Peripheral Vein | 3 Percutaneous | Ø Antineoplastic | 2 High-dose Interleukin-2<br>3 Low-dose Interleukin-2<br>5 Other Antineoplastic<br>M Monoclonal Antibody<br>P Clofarabine |
| 3 Peripheral Vein | 3 Percutaneous | 1 Thrombolytic | 6 Recombinant Human- activated Protein C<br>7 Other Thrombolytic |
| 3 Peripheral Vein | 3 Percutaneous | 2 Anti-infective | 8 Oxazolidinones<br>9 Other Anti-infective |
| 3 Peripheral Vein | 3 Percutaneous | 3 Anti-inflammatory<br>4 Serum, Toxoid and Vaccine<br>6 Nutritional Substance<br>7 Electrolytic and Water Balance Substance<br>F Intracirculatory Anesthetic<br>H Radioactive Substance<br>K Other Diagnostic Substance<br>N Analgesics, Hypnotics, Sedatives<br>P Platelet Inhibitor<br>R Antiarrhythmic<br>T Destructive Agent<br>X Vasopressor | Z No Qualifier |
| 3 Peripheral Vein | 3 Percutaneous | G Other Therapeutic Substance | C Other Substance<br>N Blood Brain Barrier Disruption<br>Q Glucarpidase |
| 3 Peripheral Vein | 3 Percutaneous | U Pancreatic Islet Cells | Ø Autologous<br>1 Nonautologous |
| 3 Peripheral Vein | 3 Percutaneous | V Hormone | G Insulin<br>H Human B-type Natriuretic Peptide<br>J Other Hormone |
| 3 Peripheral Vein | 3 Percutaneous | W Immunotherapeutic | K Immunostimulator<br>L Immunosuppressive |
| 4 Central Vein | Ø Open | Ø Antineoplastic | 2 High-dose Interleukin-2<br>3 Low-dose Interleukin-2<br>5 Other Antineoplastic<br>M Monoclonal Antibody<br>P Clofarabine |

*3EØ Continued on next page*

| | | | |
|---|---|---|---|
| Valid OR | 3EØ3ØTZ | DRG Non-OR | 3EØ3317 |
| DRG Non-OR | 3EØ3ØU[Ø,1] | DRG Non-OR | 3EØ33U[Ø,1] |
| DRG Non-OR | 3EØ33Ø2 | DRG Non-OR | 3EØ4ØØ2 |

3EØ Continued

**3 Administration**
**E Physiological Systems and Anatomical Regions**
**Ø Introduction** Definition: Putting in or on a therapeutic, diagnostic, nutritional, physiological, or prophylactic substance except blood or blood products

| Body System/Region Character 4 | Approach Character 5 | Substance Character 6 | Qualifier Character 7 |
|---|---|---|---|
| 4 Central Vein | Ø Open | 1 Thrombolytic | 6 Recombinant Human- activated Protein C<br>7 Other Thrombolytic |
| 4 Central Vein | Ø Open | 2 Anti-infective | 8 Oxazolidinones<br>9 Other Anti-infective |
| 4 Central Vein | Ø Open | 3 Anti-inflammatory<br>4 Serum, Toxoid and Vaccine<br>6 Nutritional Substance<br>7 Electrolytic and Water Balance Substance<br>F Intracirculatory Anesthetic<br>H Radioactive Substance<br>K Other Diagnostic Substance<br>N Analgesics, Hypnotics, Sedatives<br>P Platelet Inhibitor<br>R Antiarrhythmic<br>T Destructive Agent<br>X Vasopressor | Z No Qualifier |
| 4 Central Vein | Ø Open | G Other Therapeutic Substance | C Other Substance<br>N Blood Brain Barrier Disruption |
| 4 Central Vein | Ø Open | V Hormone | G Insulin<br>H Human B-type Natriuretic Peptide<br>J Other Hormone |
| 4 Central Vein | Ø Open | W Immunotherapeutic | K Immunostimulator<br>L Immunosuppressive |
| 4 Central Vein | 3 Percutaneous | Ø Antineoplastic | 2 High-dose Interleukin-2<br>3 Low-dose Interleukin-2<br>5 Other Antineoplastic<br>M Monoclonal Antibody<br>P Clofarabine |
| 4 Central Vein | 3 Percutaneous | 1 Thrombolytic | 6 Recombinant Human- activated Protein C<br>7 Other Thrombolytic |
| 4 Central Vein | 3 Percutaneous | 2 Anti-infective | 8 Oxazolidinones<br>9 Other Anti-infective |
| 4 Central Vein | 3 Percutaneous | 3 Anti-inflammatory<br>4 Serum, Toxoid and Vaccine<br>6 Nutritional Substance<br>7 Electrolytic and Water Balance Substance<br>F Intracirculatory Anesthetic<br>H Radioactive Substance<br>K Other Diagnostic Substance<br>N Analgesics, Hypnotics, Sedatives<br>P Platelet Inhibitor<br>R Antiarrhythmic<br>T Destructive Agent<br>X Vasopressor | Z No Qualifier |
| 4 Central Vein | 3 Percutaneous | G Other Therapeutic Substance | C Other Substance<br>N Blood Brain Barrier Disruption<br>Q Glucarpidase |
| 4 Central Vein | 3 Percutaneous | V Hormone | G Insulin<br>H Human B-type Natriuretic Peptide<br>J Other Hormone |
| 4 Central Vein | 3 Percutaneous | W Immunotherapeutic | K Immunostimulator<br>L Immunosuppressive |
| 5 Peripheral Artery<br>6 Central Artery | Ø Open<br>3 Percutaneous | Ø Antineoplastic | 2 High-dose Interleukin-2<br>3 Low-dose Interleukin-2<br>5 Other Antineoplastic<br>M Monoclonal Antibody<br>P Clofarabine |

3EØ Continued on next page

Valid OR 3EØ4ØTZ
DRG Non-OR 3EØ4Ø17
DRG Non-OR 3EØ43Ø2
DRG Non-OR 3EØ4317
DRG Non-OR 3EØ[5,6][Ø,3]Ø2

**3 Administration**
**E Physiological Systems and Anatomical Regions**
**Ø Introduction** Definition: Putting in or on a therapeutic, diagnostic, nutritional, physiological, or prophylactic substance except blood or blood products

*3EØ Continued*

| Body System/Region Character 4 | Approach Character 5 | Substance Character 6 | Qualifier Character 7 |
|---|---|---|---|
| 5 Peripheral Artery<br>6 Central Artery | Ø Open<br>3 Percutaneous | 1 Thrombolytic | 6 Recombinant Human- activated Protein C<br>7 Other Thrombolytic |
| 5 Peripheral Artery<br>6 Central Artery | Ø Open<br>3 Percutaneous | 2 Anti-infective | 8 Oxazolidinones<br>9 Other Anti-infective |
| 5 Peripheral Artery<br>6 Central Artery | Ø Open<br>3 Percutaneous | 3 Anti-inflammatory<br>4 Serum, Toxoid and Vaccine<br>6 Nutritional Substance<br>7 Electrolytic and Water Balance Substance<br>F Intracirculatory Anesthetic<br>H Radioactive Substance<br>K Other Diagnostic Substance<br>N Analgesics, Hypnotics, Sedatives<br>P Platelet Inhibitor<br>R Antiarrhythmic<br>T Destructive Agent<br>X Vasopressor | Z No Qualifier |
| 5 Peripheral Artery<br>6 Central Artery | Ø Open<br>3 Percutaneous | G Other Therapeutic Substance | C Other Substance<br>N Blood Brain Barrier Disruption |
| 5 Peripheral Artery<br>6 Central Artery | Ø Open<br>3 Percutaneous | V Hormone | G Insulin<br>H Human B-type Natriuretic Peptide<br>J Other Hormone |
| 5 Peripheral Artery<br>6 Central Artery | Ø Open<br>3 Percutaneous | W Immunotherapeutic | K Immunostimulator<br>L Immunosuppressive |
| 7 Coronary Artery<br>8 Heart | Ø Open<br>3 Percutaneous | 1 Thrombolytic | 6 Recombinant Human- activated Protein C<br>7 Other Thrombolytic |
| 7 Coronary Artery<br>8 Heart | Ø Open<br>3 Percutaneous | G Other Therapeutic Substance | C Other Substance |
| 7 Coronary Artery<br>8 Heart | Ø Open<br>3 Percutaneous | K Other Diagnostic Substance<br>P Platelet Inhibitor | Z No Qualifier |
| 7 Coronary Artery<br>8 Heart | 4 Percutaneous Endoscopic | G Other Therapeutic Substance | C Other Substance |
| 9 Nose | 3 Percutaneous<br>7 Via Natural or Artificial Opening<br>X External | Ø Antineoplastic | 5 Other Antineoplastic<br>M Monoclonal Antibody |
| 9 Nose | 3 Percutaneous<br>7 Via Natural or Artificial Opening<br>X External | 2 Anti-infective | 8 Oxazolidinones<br>9 Other Anti-infective |
| 9 Nose | 3 Percutaneous<br>7 Via Natural or Artificial Opening<br>X External | 3 Anti-inflammatory<br>4 Serum, Toxoid and Vaccine<br>B Anesthetic Agent<br>H Radioactive Substance<br>K Other Diagnostic Substance<br>N Analgesics, Hypnotics, Sedatives<br>T Destructive Agent | Z No Qualifier |
| 9 Nose | 3 Percutaneous<br>7 Via Natural or Artificial Opening<br>X External | G Other Therapeutic Substance | C Other Substance |
| A Bone Marrow | 3 Percutaneous | Ø Antineoplastic | 5 Other Antineoplastic<br>M Monoclonal Antibody |
| A Bone Marrow | 3 Percutaneous | G Other Therapeutic Substance | C Other Substance |
| B Ear | 3 Percutaneous<br>7 Via Natural or Artificial Opening<br>X External | Ø Antineoplastic | 4 Liquid Brachytherapy Radioisotope<br>5 Other Antineoplastic<br>M Monoclonal Antibody |
| B Ear | 3 Percutaneous<br>7 Via Natural or Artificial Opening<br>X External | 2 Anti-infective | 8 Oxazolidinones<br>9 Other Anti-infective |

*3EØ Continued on next page*

DRG Non-OR 3EØ[5,6][Ø,3]17
DRG Non-OR 3EØ8[Ø,3]17

**3EØ Continued**

**3 Administration**
**E Physiological Systems and Anatomical Regions**
**Ø Introduction** Definition: Putting in or on a therapeutic, diagnostic, nutritional, physiological, or prophylactic substance except blood or blood products

| Body System/Region Character 4 | Approach Character 5 | Substance Character 6 | Qualifier Character 7 |
|---|---|---|---|
| B Ear | 3 Percutaneous<br>7 Via Natural or Artificial Opening<br>X External | 3 Anti-inflammatory<br>B Anesthetic Agent<br>H Radioactive Substance<br>K Other Diagnostic Substance<br>N Analgesics, Hypnotics, Sedatives<br>T Destructive Agent | Z No Qualifier |
| B Ear | 3 Percutaneous<br>7 Via Natural or Artificial Opening<br>X External | G Other Therapeutic Substance | C Other Substance |
| C Eye | 3 Percutaneous<br>7 Via Natural or Artificial Opening<br>X External | Ø Antineoplastic | 4 Liquid Brachytherapy Radioisotope<br>5 Other Antineoplastic<br>M Monoclonal Antibody |
| C Eye | 3 Percutaneous<br>7 Via Natural or Artificial Opening<br>X External | 2 Anti-infective | 8 Oxazolidinones<br>9 Other Anti-infective |
| C Eye | 3 Percutaneous<br>7 Via Natural or Artificial Opening<br>X External | 3 Anti-inflammatory<br>B Anesthetic Agent<br>H Radioactive Substance<br>K Other Diagnostic Substance<br>M Pigment<br>N Analgesics, Hypnotics, Sedatives<br>T Destructive Agent | Z No Qualifier |
| C Eye | 3 Percutaneous<br>7 Via Natural or Artificial Opening<br>X External | G Other Therapeutic Substance | C Other Substance |
| C Eye | 3 Percutaneous<br>7 Via Natural or Artificial Opening<br>X External | S Gas | F Other Gas |
| D Mouth and Pharynx | 3 Percutaneous<br>7 Via Natural or Artificial Opening<br>X External | Ø Antineoplastic | 4 Liquid Brachytherapy Radioisotope<br>5 Other Antineoplastic<br>M Monoclonal Antibody |
| D Mouth and Pharynx | 3 Percutaneous<br>7 Via Natural or Artificial Opening<br>X External | 2 Anti-infective | 8 Oxazolidinones<br>9 Other Anti-infective |
| D Mouth and Pharynx | 3 Percutaneous<br>7 Via Natural or Artificial Opening<br>X External | 3 Anti-inflammatory<br>4 Serum, Toxoid and Vaccine<br>6 Nutritional Substance<br>7 Electrolytic and Water Balance Substance<br>B Anesthetic Agent<br>H Radioactive Substance<br>K Other Diagnostic Substance<br>N Analgesics, Hypnotics, Sedatives<br>R Antiarrhythmic<br>T Destructive Agent | Z No Qualifier |
| D Mouth and Pharynx | 3 Percutaneous<br>7 Via Natural or Artificial Opening<br>X External | G Other Therapeutic Substance | C Other Substance |
| E Products of Conception ♀<br>G Upper GI<br>H Lower GI<br>K Genitourinary Tract<br>N Male Reproductive ♂ | 3 Percutaneous<br>7 Via Natural or Artificial Opening<br>8 Via Natural or Artificial Opening Endoscopic | Ø Antineoplastic | 4 Liquid Brachytherapy Radioisotope<br>5 Other Antineoplastic<br>M Monoclonal Antibody |
| E Products of Conception ♀<br>G Upper GI<br>H Lower GI<br>K Genitourinary Tract<br>N Male Reproductive ♂ | 3 Percutaneous<br>7 Via Natural or Artificial Opening<br>8 Via Natural or Artificial Opening Endoscopic | 2 Anti-infective | 8 Oxazolidinones<br>9 Other Anti-infective |

3EØ Continued on next page

♂ 3EØN[3,7,8]Ø[4,5,M]
♂ 3EØN[3,7,8]2[8,9]
♀ 3EØE[3,7,8]Ø[4,5,M]
♀ 3EØE[3,7,8]2[8,9]

**3 Administration**
**E Physiological Systems and Anatomical Regions**
**Ø Introduction** Definition: Putting in or on a therapeutic, diagnostic, nutritional, physiological, or prophylactic substance except blood or blood products

*3EØ Continued*

| Body System/Region Character 4 | Approach Character 5 | Substance Character 6 | Qualifier Character 7 |
|---|---|---|---|
| E Products of Conception ♀<br>G Upper GI<br>H Lower GI<br>K Genitourinary Tract<br>N Male Reproductive ♂ | 3 Percutaneous<br>7 Via Natural or Artificial Opening<br>8 Via Natural or Artificial Opening Endoscopic | 3 Anti-inflammatory<br>6 Nutritional Substance<br>7 Electrolytic and Water Balance Substance<br>B Anesthetic Agent<br>H Radioactive Substance<br>K Other Diagnostic Substance<br>N Analgesics, Hypnotics, Sedatives<br>T Destructive Agent | Z No Qualifier |
| E Products of Conception ♀<br>G Upper GI<br>H Lower GI<br>K Genitourinary Tract<br>N Male Reproductive ♂ | 3 Percutaneous<br>7 Via Natural or Artificial Opening<br>8 Via Natural or Artificial Opening Endoscopic | G Other Therapeutic Substance | C Other Substance |
| E Products of Conception ♀<br>G Upper GI<br>H Lower GI<br>K Genitourinary Tract<br>N Male Reproductive ♂ | 3 Percutaneous<br>7 Via Natural or Artificial Opening<br>8 Via Natural or Artificial Opening Endoscopic | S Gas | F Other Gas |
| E Products of Conception<br>G Upper GI<br>H Lower GI<br>K Genitourinary Tract<br>N Male Reproductive | 4 Percutaneous Endoscopic | G Other Therapeutic Substance | C Other Substance |
| F Respiratory Tract | 3 Percutaneous<br>7 Via Natural or Artificial Opening<br>8 Via Natural or Artificial Opening Endoscopic | Ø Antineoplastic | 4 Liquid Brachytherapy Radioisotope<br>5 Other Antineoplastic<br>M Monoclonal Antibody |
| F Respiratory Tract | 3 Percutaneous<br>7 Via Natural or Artificial Opening<br>8 Via Natural or Artificial Opening Endoscopic | 2 Anti-infective | 8 Oxazolidinones<br>9 Other Anti-infective |
| F Respiratory Tract | 3 Percutaneous<br>7 Via Natural or Artificial Opening<br>8 Via Natural or Artificial Opening Endoscopic | 3 Anti-inflammatory<br>6 Nutritional Substance<br>7 Electrolytic and Water Balance Substance<br>B Anesthetic Agent<br>H Radioactive Substance<br>K Other Diagnostic Substance<br>N Analgesics, Hypnotics, Sedatives<br>T Destructive Agent | Z No Qualifier |
| F Respiratory Tract | 3 Percutaneous<br>7 Via Natural or Artificial Opening<br>8 Via Natural or Artificial Opening Endoscopic | G Other Therapeutic Substance | C Other Substance |
| F Respiratory Tract | 3 Percutaneous<br>7 Via Natural or Artificial Opening<br>8 Via Natural or Artificial Opening Endoscopic | S Gas | D Nitric Oxide<br>F Other Gas |
| F Respiratory Tract | 4 Percutaneous Endoscopic | G Other Therapeutic Substance | C Other Substance |
| J Biliary and Pancreatic Tract | 3 Percutaneous<br>7 Via Natural or Artificial Opening<br>8 Via Natural or Artificial Opening Endoscopic | Ø Antineoplastic | 4 Liquid Brachytherapy Radioisotope<br>5 Other Antineoplastic<br>M Monoclonal Antibody |

*3EØ Continued on next page*

♂ 3EØN[3,7,8][3,6,7,B,H,K,N,T]Z
♂ 3EØN[3,7,8]GC
♂ 3EØN[3,7,8]SF
♀ 3EØE[3,7,8][3,6,7,B,H,K,N,T]Z
♀ 3EØE[3,7,8]GC
♀ 3EØE[3,7,8]SF

3EØ Continued

**3 Administration**
**E Physiological Systems and Anatomical Regions**
**Ø Introduction** Definition: Putting in or on a therapeutic, diagnostic, nutritional, physiological, or prophylactic substance except blood or blood products

| Body System/Region Character 4 | Approach Character 5 | Substance Character 6 | Qualifier Character 7 |
|---|---|---|---|
| J Biliary and Pancreatic Tract | 3 Percutaneous<br>7 Via Natural or Artificial Opening<br>8 Via Natural or Artificial Opening Endoscopic | 2 Anti-infective | 8 Oxazolidinones<br>9 Other Anti-infective |
| J Biliary and Pancreatic Tract | 3 Percutaneous<br>7 Via Natural or Artificial Opening<br>8 Via Natural or Artificial Opening Endoscopic | 3 Anti-inflammatory<br>6 Nutritional Substance<br>7 Electrolytic and Water Balance Substance<br>B Anesthetic Agent<br>H Radioactive Substance<br>K Other Diagnostic Substance<br>N Analgesics, Hypnotics, Sedatives<br>T Destructive Agent | Z No Qualifier |
| J Biliary and Pancreatic Tract | 3 Percutaneous<br>7 Via Natural or Artificial Opening<br>8 Via Natural or Artificial Opening Endoscopic | G Other Therapeutic Substance | C Other Substance |
| J Biliary and Pancreatic Tract | 3 Percutaneous<br>7 Via Natural or Artificial Opening<br>8 Via Natural or Artificial Opening Endoscopic | S Gas | F Other Gas |
| J Biliary and Pancreatic Tract | 3 Percutaneous<br>7 Via Natural or Artificial Opening<br>8 Via Natural or Artificial Opening Endoscopic | U Pancreatic Islet Cells | Ø Autologous<br>1 Nonautologous |
| J Biliary and Pancreatic Tract | 4 Percutaneous Endoscopic | G Other Therapeutic Substance | C Other Substance |
| L Pleural Cavity<br>M Peritoneal Cavity | Ø Open | 5 Adhesion Barrier | Z No Qualifier |
| L Pleural Cavity<br>M Peritoneal Cavity | 3 Percutaneous | Ø Antineoplastic | 4 Liquid Brachytherapy Radioisotope<br>5 Other Antineoplastic<br>M Monoclonal Antibody |
| L Pleural Cavity<br>M Peritoneal Cavity | 3 Percutaneous | 2 Anti-infective | 8 Oxazolidinones<br>9 Other Anti-infective |
| L Pleural Cavity<br>M Peritoneal Cavity | 3 Percutaneous | 3 Anti-inflammatory<br>5 Adhesion Barrier<br>6 Nutritional Substance<br>7 Electrolytic and Water Balance Substance<br>B Anesthetic Agent<br>H Radioactive Substance<br>K Other Diagnostic Substance<br>N Analgesics, Hypnotics, Sedatives<br>T Destructive Agent | Z No Qualifier |
| L Pleural Cavity<br>M Peritoneal Cavity | 3 Percutaneous | G Other Therapeutic Substance | C Other Substance |
| L Pleural Cavity<br>M Peritoneal Cavity | 3 Percutaneous | S Gas | F Other Gas |
| L Pleural Cavity<br>M Peritoneal Cavity | 4 Percutaneous Endoscopic | 5 Adhesion Barrier | Z No Qualifier |
| L Pleural Cavity<br>M Peritoneal Cavity | 4 Percutaneous Endoscopic | G Other Therapeutic Substance | C Other Substance |
| L Pleural Cavity<br>M Peritoneal Cavity | 7 Via Natural or Artificial Opening | Ø Antineoplastic | 4 Liquid Brachytherapy Radioisotope<br>5 Other Antineoplastic<br>M Monoclonal Antibody |
| L Pleural Cavity<br>M Peritoneal Cavity | 7 Via Natural or Artificial Opening | S Gas | F Other Gas |
| P Female Reproductive ♀ | Ø Open | 5 Adhesion Barrier | Z No Qualifier |
| P Female Reproductive ♀ | 3 Percutaneous | Ø Antineoplastic | 4 Liquid Brachytherapy Radioisotope<br>5 Other Antineoplastic<br>M Monoclonal Antibody |
| P Female Reproductive ♀ | 3 Percutaneous | 2 Anti-infective | 8 Oxazolidinones<br>9 Other Anti-infective |

3EØ Continued on next page

DRG Non-OR 3EØJ[3,7,8]U[Ø,1]
♀ All approach, substance, and qualifier values for body system/region (character 4) with this icon

**3 Administration**
**E Physiological Systems and Anatomical Regions**
**Ø Introduction** Definition: Putting in or on a therapeutic, diagnostic, nutritional, physiological, or prophylactic substance except blood or blood products

3EØ Continued

| Body System/Region Character 4 | Approach Character 5 | Substance Character 6 | Qualifier Character 7 |
|---|---|---|---|
| P Female Reproductive ♀ | 3 Percutaneous | 3 Anti-inflammatory<br>5 Adhesion Barrier<br>6 Nutritional Substance<br>7 Electrolytic and Water Balance Substance<br>B Anesthetic Agent<br>H Radioactive Substance<br>K Other Diagnostic Substance<br>L Sperm<br>N Analgesics, Hypnotics, Sedatives<br>T Destructive Agent<br>V Hormone | Z No Qualifier |
| P Female Reproductive ♀ | 3 Percutaneous | G Other Therapeutic Substance | C Other Substance |
| P Female Reproductive ♀ | 3 Percutaneous | Q Fertilized Ovum | Ø Autologous<br>1 Nonautologous |
| P Female Reproductive ♀ | 3 Percutaneous | S Gas | F Other Gas |
| P Female Reproductive | 4 Percutaneous Endoscopic | 5 Adhesion Barrier | Z No Qualifier |
| P Female Reproductive | 4 Percutaneous Endoscopic | G Other Therapeutic Substance | C Other Substance |
| P Female Reproductive ♀ | 7 Via Natural or Artificial Opening | Ø Antineoplastic | 4 Liquid Brachytherapy Radioisotope<br>5 Other Antineoplastic<br>M Monoclonal Antibody |
| P Female Reproductive ♀ | 7 Via Natural or Artificial Opening | 2 Anti-infective | 8 Oxazolidinones<br>9 Other Anti-infective |
| P Female Reproductive ♀ | 7 Via Natural or Artificial Opening | 3 Anti-inflammatory<br>6 Nutritional Substance<br>7 Electrolytic and Water Balance Substance<br>B Anesthetic Agent<br>H Radioactive Substance<br>K Other Diagnostic Substance<br>L Sperm<br>N Analgesics, Hypnotics, Sedatives<br>T Destructive Agent<br>V Hormone | Z No Qualifier |
| P Female Reproductive | 7 Via Natural or Artificial Opening | G Other Therapeutic Substance | C Other Substance |
| P Female Reproductive | 7 Via Natural or Artificial Opening | Q Fertilized Ovum | Ø Autologous<br>1 Nonautologous |
| P Female Reproductive | 7 Via Natural or Artificial Opening | S Gas | F Other Gas |
| P Female Reproductive | 8 Via Natural or Artificial Opening Endoscopic | Ø Antineoplastic | 4 Liquid Brachytherapy Radioisotope<br>5 Other Antineoplastic<br>M Monoclonal Antibody |
| P Female Reproductive | 8 Via Natural or Artificial Opening Endoscopic | 2 Anti-infective | 8 Oxazolidinones<br>9 Other Anit-infection |
| P Female Reproductive | 8 Via Natural or Artificial Opening Endoscopic | 3 Anti-inflammatory<br>6 Nutritional Substance<br>7 Electrolytic and Water Balance Substance<br>B Anesthetic Agent<br>H Radioactive Substance<br>K Other Diagnostic Substance<br>N Analgesics, Hypnotics, Sedative<br>T Destructive Agent | Z No Qualifier |
| P Female Reproductive | 8 Via Natural or Artificial Opening Endoscopic | G Other Therapeutic Substance | C Other Substance |
| P Female Reproductive | 8 Via Natural or Artificial Opening Endoscopic | S Gas | F Other Gas |
| Q Cranial Cavity and Brain | Ø Open<br>3 Percutaneous | Ø Antineoplastic | 4 Liquid Brachytherapy Radioisotope<br>5 Other Antineoplastic<br>M Monoclonal Antibody |
| Q Cranial Cavity and Brain | Ø Open<br>3 Percutaneous | 2 Anti-infective | 8 Oxazolidinones<br>9 Other Anti-infective |

3EØ Continued on next page

**Valid OR** 3EØP3Q[Ø,1]
**Valid OR** 3EØP7Q[Ø,1]
**DRG Non-OR** 3EØQ[Ø,3]Ø5
♀ All approach, substance, and qualifier values for body system/region (character 4) with this icon

*3EØ Continued*

**3 Administration**
**E Physiological Systems and Anatomical Regions**
**Ø Introduction** Definition: Putting in or on a therapeutic, diagnostic, nutritional, physiological, or prophylactic substance except blood or blood products

| Body System/Region Character 4 | Approach Character 5 | Substance Character 6 | Qualifier Character 7 |
|---|---|---|---|
| Q Cranial Cavity and Brain | Ø Open<br>3 Percutaneous | 3 Anti-inflammatory<br>6 Nutritional Substance<br>7 Electrolytic and Water Balance Substance<br>A Stem Cells, Embryonic<br>B Anesthetic Agent<br>H Radioactive Substance<br>K Other Diagnostic Substance<br>N Analgesics, Hypnotics, Sedatives<br>T Destructive Agent | Z No Qualifier |
| Q Cranial Cavity and Brain | Ø Open<br>3 Percutaneous | E Stem Cells, Somatic | Ø Autologous<br>1 Nonautologous |
| Q Cranial Cavity and Brain | Ø Open<br>3 Percutaneous | G Other Therapeutic Substance | C Other Substance |
| Q Cranial Cavity and Brain | Ø Open<br>3 Percutaneous | S Gas | F Other Gas |
| Q Cranial Cavity and Brain | 7 Via Natural or Artificial Opening | Ø Antineoplastic | 4 Liquid Brachytherapy Radioisotope<br>5 Other Antineoplastic<br>M Monoclonal Antibody |
| Q Cranial Cavity and Brain | 7 Via Natural or Artificial Opening | S Gas | F Other Gas |
| R Spinal Canal | Ø Open | A Stem Cells, Embryonic | Z No Qualifier |
| R Spinal Canal | Ø Open | E Stem Cells, Somatic | Ø Autologous<br>1 Nonautologous |
| R Spinal Canal | 3 Percutaneous | Ø Antineoplastic | 2 High-dose Interleukin-2<br>3 Low-dose Interleukin-2<br>4 Liquid Brachytherapy Radioisotope<br>5 Other Antineoplastic<br>M Monoclonal Antibody |
| R Spinal Canal | 3 Percutaneous | 2 Anti-infective | 8 Oxazolidinones<br>9 Other Anti-infective |
| R Spinal Canal | 3 Percutaneous | 3 Anti-inflammatory<br>6 Nutritional Substance<br>7 Electrolytic and Water Balance Substance<br>A Stem Cells, Embryonic<br>B Anesthetic Agent<br>H Radioactive Substance<br>K Other Diagnostic Substance<br>N Analgesics, Hypnotics, Sedatives<br>T Destructive Agent | Z No Qualifier |
| R Spinal Canal | 3 Percutaneous | E Stem Cells, Somatic | Ø Autologous<br>1 Nonautologous |
| R Spinal Canal | 3 Percutaneous | G Other Therapeutic Substance | C Other Substance |
| R Spinal Canal | 3 Percutaneous | S Gas | F Other Gas |
| R Spinal Canal | 7 Via Natural or Artificial Opening | S Gas | F Other Gas |
| S Epidural Space | 3 Percutaneous | Ø Antineoplastic | 2 High-dose Interleukin-2<br>3 Low-dose Interleukin-2<br>4 Liquid Brachytherapy Radioisotope<br>5 Other Antineoplastic<br>M Monoclonal Antibody |
| S Epidural Space | 3 Percutaneous | 2 Anti-infective | 8 Oxazolidinones<br>9 Other Anti-infective |
| S Epidural Space | 3 Percutaneous | 3 Anti-inflammatory<br>6 Nutritional Substance<br>7 Electrolytic and Water Balance Substance<br>B Anesthetic Agent<br>H Radioactive Substance<br>K Other Diagnostic Substance<br>N Analgesics, Hypnotics, Sedatives<br>T Destructive Agent | Z No Qualifier |

*3EØ Continued on next page*

DRG Non-OR 3EØQ7Ø5
DRG Non-OR 3EØR3Ø2
DRG Non-OR 3EØS3Ø2

**3 Administration**
**E Physiological Systems and Anatomical Regions**
**0 Introduction** Definition: Putting in or on a therapeutic, diagnostic, nutritional, physiological, or prophylactic substance except blood or blood products

*3E0 Continued*

| Body System/Region Character 4 | Approach Character 5 | Substance Character 6 | Qualifier Character 7 |
|---|---|---|---|
| S Epidural Space | 3 Percutaneous | G Other Therapeutic Substance | C Other Substance |
| S Epidural Space | 3 Percutaneous | S Gas | F Other Gas |
| S Epidural Space | 7 Via Natural or Artificial Opening | S Gas | F Other Gas |
| T Peripheral Nerves and Plexi<br>X Cranial Nerves | 3 Percutaneous | 3 Anti-inflammatory<br>B Anesthetic Agent<br>T Destructive Agent | Z No Qualifier |
| T Peripheral Nerves and Plexi<br>X Cranial Nerves | 3 Percutaneous | G Other Therapeutic Substance | C Other Substance |
| U Joints | 0 Open | 2 Anti-infective | 8 Oxazolidinones<br>9 Other Anti-infective |
| U Joints | 0 Open | G Other Therapeutic Substance | B Recombinant Bone Morphogenetic Protein |
| U Joints | 3 Percutaneous | 0 Antineoplastic | 4 Liquid Brachytherapy Radioisotope<br>5 Other Antineoplastic<br>M Monoclonal Antibody |
| U Joints | 3 Percutaneous | 2 Anti-infective | 8 Oxazolidinones<br>9 Other Anti-infective |
| U Joints | 3 Percutaneous | 3 Anti-inflammatory<br>6 Nutritional Substance<br>7 Electrolytic and Water Balance Substance<br>B Anesthetic Agent<br>H Radioactive Substance<br>K Other Diagnostic Substance<br>N Analgesics, Hypnotics, Sedatives<br>T Destructive Agent | Z No Qualifier |
| U Joints | 3 Percutaneous | G Other Therapeutic Substance | B Recombinant Bone Morphogenetic Protein<br>C Other Substance |
| U Joints | 3 Percutaneous | S Gas | F Other Gas |
| U Joints | 4 Percutaneous Endoscopic | G Other Therapeutic Substance | C Other Substance |
| V Bones | 0 Open | G Other Therapeutic Substance | B Recombinant Bone Morphogenetic Protein |
| V Bones | 3 Percutaneous | 0 Antineoplastic | 5 Other Antineoplastic<br>M Monoclonal Antibody |
| V Bones | 3 Percutaneous | 2 Anti-infective | 8 Oxazolidinones<br>9 Other Anti-infective |
| V Bones | 3 Percutaneous | 3 Anti-inflammatory<br>6 Nutritional Substance<br>7 Electrolytic and Water Balance Substance<br>B Anesthetic Agent<br>H Radioactive Substance<br>K Other Diagnostic Substance<br>N Analgesics, Hypnotics, Sedatives<br>T Destructive Agent | Z No Qualifier |
| V Bones | 3 Percutaneous | G Other Therapeutic Substance | B Recombinant Bone Morphogenetic Protein<br>C Other Substance |
| W Lymphatics | 3 Percutaneous | 0 Antineoplastic | 5 Other Antineoplastic<br>M Monoclonal Antibody |
| W Lymphatics | 3 Percutaneous | 2 Anti-infective | 8 Oxazolidinones<br>9 Other Anti-infective |
| W Lymphatics | 3 Percutaneous | 3 Anti-inflammatory<br>6 Nutritional Substance<br>7 Electrolytic and Water Balance Substance<br>B Anesthetic Agent<br>H Radioactive Substance<br>K Other Diagnostic Substance<br>N Analgesics, Hypnotics, Sedatives<br>T Destructive Agent | Z No Qualifier |

*3E0 Continued on next page*

*3EØ Continued*

**3 Administration**
**E Physiological Systems and Anatomical Regions**
**Ø Introduction** Definition: Putting in or on a therapeutic, diagnostic, nutritional, physiological, or prophylactic substance except blood or blood products

| Body System/Region Character 4 | Approach Character 5 | Substance Character 6 | Qualifier Character 7 |
|---|---|---|---|
| W Lymphatics | 3 Percutaneous | G Other Therapeutic Substance | C Other Substance |
| Y Pericardial Cavity | 3 Percutaneous | Ø Antineoplastic | 4 Liquid Brachytherapy Radioisotope<br>5 Other Antineoplastic<br>M Monoclonal Antibody |
| Y Pericardial Cavity | 3 Percutaneous | 2 Anti-infective | 8 Oxazolidinones<br>9 Other Anti-infective |
| Y Pericardial Cavity | 3 Percutaneous | 3 Anti-inflammatory<br>6 Nutritional Substance<br>7 Electrolytic and Water Balance Substance<br>B Anesthetic Agent<br>H Radioactive Substance<br>K Other Diagnostic Substance<br>N Analgesics, Hypnotics, Sedatives<br>T Destructive Agent | Z No Qualifier |
| Y Pericardial Cavity | 3 Percutaneous | G Other Therapeutic Substance | C Other Substance |
| Y Pericardial Cavity | 3 Percutaneous | S Gas | F Other Gas |
| Y Pericardial Cavity | 4 Percutaneous Endoscopic | G Other Therapeutic Substance | C Other Substance |
| Y Pericardial Cavity | 7 Via Natural or Artificial Opening | Ø Antineoplastic | 4 Liquid Brachytherapy Radioisotope<br>5 Other Antineoplastic<br>M Monoclonal Antibody |
| Y Pericardial Cavity | 7 Via Natural or Artificial Opening | S Gas | F Other Gas |

**3 Administration**
**E Physiological Systems and Anatomical Regions**
**1 Irrigation** Definition: Putting in or on a cleansing substance

| Body System/Region Character 4 | Approach Character 5 | Substance Character 6 | Qualifier Character 7 |
|---|---|---|---|
| Ø Skin and Mucous Membranes<br>C Eye | 3 Percutaneous<br>X External | 8 Irrigating Substance | X Diagnostic<br>Z No Qualifier |
| 9 Nose<br>B Ear<br>F Respiratory Tract<br>G Upper GI<br>H Lower GI<br>J Biliary and Pancreatic Tract<br>K Genitourinary Tract<br>N Male Reproductive ♂<br>P Female Reproductive ♀ | 3 Percutaneous<br>7 Via Natural or Artificial Opening<br>8 Via Natural or Artificial Opening Endoscopic | 8 Irrigating Substance | X Diagnostic<br>Z No Qualifier |
| L Pleural Cavity<br>Q Cranial Cavity and Brain<br>R Spinal Canal<br>S Epidural Space<br>U Joints<br>Y Pericardial Cavity | 3 Percutaneous | 8 Irrigating Substance | X Diagnostic<br>Z No Qualifier |
| M Peritoneal Cavity | 3 Percutaneous | 8 Irrigating Substance | X Diagnostic<br>Z No Qualifier |
| M Peritoneal Cavity | 3 Percutaneous | 9 Dialysate | Z No Qualifier |

♂ 3E1N[3,7,8]8XZ
♀ 3E1P[3,7,8]8XZ

# Measurement and Monitoring 4AØ–4BØ

## Character Meanings

This Character Meaning table is provided as a guide to assist the user in the identification of character members that may be found in this section of code tables. It **SHOULD NOT** be used to build a PCS code.

### A: Physiological Systems

| Operation–Character 3 | Body System–Character 4 | Approach–Character 5 | Function/Device–Character 6 | Qualifier–Character 7 |
|---|---|---|---|---|
| Ø Measurement | Ø Central Nervous | Ø Open | Ø Acuity | Ø Central |
| 1 Monitoring | 1 Peripheral Nervous | 3 Percutaneous | 1 Capacity | 1 Peripheral |
| | 2 Cardiac | 4 Percutaneous Endoscopic | 2 Conductivity | 2 Portal |
| | 3 Arterial | 7 Via Natural or Artificial Opening | 3 Contractility | 3 Pulmonary |
| | 4 Venous | 8 Via Natural or Artificial Opening Endoscopic | 4 Electrical Activity | 4 Stress |
| | 5 Circulatory | X External | 5 Flow | 5 Ambulatory |
| | 6 Lymphatic | | 6 Metabolism | 6 Right Heart |
| | 7 Visual | | 7 Mobility | 7 Left Heart |
| | 8 Olfactory | | 8 Motility | 8 Bilateral |
| | 9 Respiratory | | 9 Output | 9 Sensory |
| | B Gastrointestinal | | B Pressure | A Guidance |
| | C Biliary | | C Rate | B Motor |
| | D Urinary | | D Resistance | C Coronary |
| | F Musculoskeletal | | F Rhythm | D Intracranial |
| | G Skin and Breast | | G Secretion | F Other Thoracic |
| | H Products of Conception, Cardiac | | H Sound | G Intraoperative |
| | J Products of Conception, Nervous | | J Pulse | H Indocyanine Green Dye |
| | Z None | | K Temperature | Z No Qualifier |
| | | | L Volume | |
| | | | M Total Activity | |
| | | | N Sampling and Pressure | |
| | | | P Action Currents | |
| | | | Q Sleep | |
| | | | R Saturation | |
| | | | S Vascular Perfusion | |

### B: Physiological Devices

| Operation–Character 3 | Body System–Character 4 | Approach–Character 5 | Function/Device–Character 6 | Qualifier–Character 7 |
|---|---|---|---|---|
| Ø Measurement | Ø Central Nervous | X External | S Pacemaker | Z No Qualifier |
| | 1 Peripheral Nervous | | T Defibrillator | |
| | 2 Cardiac | | V Stimulator | |
| | 9 Respiratory | | | |
| | F Musculoskeletal | | | |

**AHA Coding Clinic for table 4AØ**

**2016, 3Q, 37** Fractional flow reserve
**2015, 3Q, 29** Approach value for esophageal electrophysiology study

**AHA Coding Clinic for table 4A1**

**2016, 4Q, 114** Fluorescence vascular angiography
**2016, 2Q, 29** Decompressive craniectomy with cryopreservation and storage of bone flap
**2016, 2Q, 33** Monitoring of arterial pressure & pulse
**2015, 3Q, 35** Swan Ganz catheterization
**2015, 2Q, 14** Intraoperative EMG monitoring via endotracheal tube
**2015, 1Q, 26** Intraoperative monitoring using Sentio MMG®
**2014, 4Q, 28** Removal and replacement of displaced growing rods

**4 Measurement and Monitoring**
**A Physiological Systems**
**Ø Measurement** Definition: Determining the level of a physiological or physical function at a point in time

| Body System Character 4 | Approach Character 5 | Function/Device Character 6 | Qualifier Character 7 |
|---|---|---|---|
| Ø Central Nervous | Ø Open | 2 Conductivity<br>4 Electrical Activity<br>B Pressure | Z No Qualifier |
| Ø Central Nervous | 3 Percutaneous<br>7 Via Natural or Artificial Opening<br>8 Via Natural or Artificial Opening Endoscopic | 4 Electrical Activity | Z No Qualifier |
| Ø Central Nervous | 3 Percutaneous<br>7 Via Natural or Artificial Opening<br>8 Via Natural or Artificial Opening Endoscopic | B Pressure<br>K Temperature<br>R Saturation | D Intracranial |
| Ø Central Nervous | X External | 2 Conductivity<br>4 Electrical Activity | Z No Qualifier |
| 1 Peripheral Nervous | Ø Open<br>3 Percutaneous<br>7 Via Natural or Artificial Opening<br>8 Via Natural or Artificial Opening Endoscopic<br>X External | 2 Conductivity | 9 Sensory<br>B Motor |
| 1 Peripheral Nervous | Ø Open<br>3 Percutaneous<br>7 Via Natural or Artificial Opening<br>8 Via Natural or Artificial Opening Endoscopic<br>X External | 4 Electrical Activity | Z No Qualifier |
| 2 Cardiac | Ø Open<br>3 Percutaneous<br>7 Via Natural or Artificial Opening<br>8 Via Natural or Artificial Opening Endoscopic | 4 Electrical Activity<br>9 Output<br>C Rate<br>F Rhythm<br>H Sound<br>P Action Currents | Z No Qualifier |
| 2 Cardiac | Ø Open<br>3 Percutaneous<br>7 Via Natural or Artificial Opening<br>8 Via Natural or Artificial Opening Endoscopic | N Sampling and Pressure | 6 Right Heart<br>7 Left Heart<br>8 Bilateral |
| 2 Cardiac | X External | 4 Electrical Activity | A Guidance<br>Z No Qualifier |
| 2 Cardiac | X External | 9 Output<br>C Rate<br>F Rhythm<br>H Sound<br>P Action Currents | Z No Qualifier |
| 2 Cardiac | X External | M Total Activity | 4 Stress |
| 3 Arterial | Ø Open<br>3 Percutaneous | 5 Flow<br>J Pulse | 1 Peripheral<br>3 Pulmonary<br>C Coronary |
| 3 Arterial | Ø Open<br>3 Percutaneous | B Pressure | 1 Peripheral<br>3 Pulmonary<br>C Coronary<br>F Other Thoracic |
| 3 Arterial | Ø Open<br>3 Percutaneous | H Sound<br>R Saturation | 1 Peripheral |
| 3 Arterial | X External | 5 Flow<br>B Pressure<br>H Sound<br>J Pulse<br>R Saturation | 1 Peripheral |

*4AØ Continued on next page*

DRG Non-OR 4AØ2[3,7,8]FZ
DRG Non-OR 4AØ2[Ø,3,7,8]N[6,7,8]

**4 Measurement and Monitoring**
**A Physiological Systems**
**Ø Measurement** Definition: Determining the level of a physiological or physical function at a point in time

*4AØ Continued*

| Body System Character 4 | Approach Character 5 | Function/Device Character 6 | Qualifier Character 7 |
|---|---|---|---|
| **4** Venous | **Ø** Open<br>**3** Percutaneous | **5** Flow<br>**B** Pressure<br>**J** Pulse | **Ø** Central<br>**1** Peripheral<br>**2** Portal<br>**3** Pulmonary |
| **4** Venous | **Ø** Open<br>**3** Percutaneous | **R** Saturation | **1** Peripheral |
| **4** Venous | **X** External | **5** Flow<br>**B** Pressure<br>**J** Pulse<br>**R** Saturation | **1** Peripheral |
| **5** Circulatory | **X** External | **L** Volume | **Z** No Qualifier |
| **6** Lymphatic | **Ø** Open<br>**3** Percutaneous<br>**7** Via Natural or Artificial Opening<br>**8** Via Natural or Artificial Opening Endoscopic | **5** Flow<br>**B** Pressure | **Z** No Qualifier |
| **7** Visual | **X** External | **Ø** Acuity<br>**7** Mobility<br>**B** Pressure | **Z** No Qualifier |
| **8** Olfactory | **X** External | **Ø** Acuity | **Z** No Qualifier |
| **9** Respiratory | **7** Via Natural or Artificial Opening<br>**8** Via Natural or Artificial Opening Endoscopic<br>**X** External | **1** Capacity<br>**5** Flow<br>**C** Rate<br>**D** Resistance<br>**L** Volume<br>**M** Total Activity | **Z** No Qualifier |
| **B** Gastrointestinal | **7** Via Natural or Artificial Opening<br>**8** Via Natural or Artificial Opening Endoscopic | **8** Motility<br>**B** Pressure<br>**G** Secretion | **Z** No Qualifier |
| **C** Biliary | **3** Percutaneous<br>**4** Percutaneous Endoscopic<br>**7** Via Natural or Artificial Opening<br>**8** Via Natural or Artificial Opening Endoscopic | **5** Flow<br>**B** Pressure | **Z** No Qualifier |
| **D** Urinary | **7** Via Natural or Artificial Opening<br>**8** Via Natural or Artificial Opening Endoscopic | **3** Contractility<br>**5** Flow<br>**B** Pressure<br>**D** Resistance<br>**L** Volume | **Z** No Qualifier |
| **F** Musculoskeletal | **3** Percutaneous<br>**X** External | **3** Contractility | **Z** No Qualifier |
| **H** Products of Conception, Cardiac ♀ | **7** Via Natural or Artificial Opening<br>**8** Via Natural or Artificial Opening Endoscopic<br>**X** External | **4** Electrical Activity<br>**C** Rate<br>**F** Rhythm<br>**H** Sound | **Z** No Qualifier |
| **J** Products of Conception, Nervous ♀ | **7** Via Natural or Artificial Opening<br>**8** Via Natural or Artificial Opening Endoscopic<br>**X** External | **2** Conductivity<br>**4** Electrical Activity<br>**B** Pressure | **Z** No Qualifier |
| **Z** None | **7** Via Natural or Artificial Opening | **6** Metabolism<br>**K** Temperature | **Z** No Qualifier |
| **Z** None | **X** External | **6** Metabolism<br>**K** Temperature<br>**Q** Sleep | **Z** No Qualifier |

**Valid OR** 4AØ6Ø[5,B]Z
**Valid OR** 4AØC4[5,B]Z
♀ 4AØH[7,8,X][4,C,F,H]Z
♀ 4AØJ[7,8,X][2,4,B]Z

**4 Measurement and Monitoring**
**A Physiological Systems**
**1 Monitoring** Definition: Determining the level of a physiological or physical function repetitively over a period of time

| Body System Character 4 | Approach Character 5 | Function/Device Character 6 | Qualifier Character 7 |
|---|---|---|---|
| Ø Central Nervous | Ø Open | 2 Conductivity<br>B Pressure | Z No Qualifier |
| Ø Central Nervous | Ø Open | 4 Electrical Activity | G Intraoperative<br>Z No Qualifier |
| Ø Central Nervous | 3 Percutaneous<br>7 Via Natural or Artificial Opening<br>8 Via Natural or Artificial Opening Endoscopic | 4 Electrical Activity | G Intraoperative<br>Z No Qualifier |
| Ø Central Nervous | 3 Percutaneous<br>7 Via Natural or Artificial Opening<br>8 Via Natural or Artificial Opening Endoscopic | B Pressure<br>K Temperature<br>R Saturation | D Intracranial |
| Ø Central Nervous | X External | 2 Conductivity | Z No Qualifier |
| Ø Central Nervous | X External | 4 Electrical Activity | G Intraoperative<br>Z No Qualifier |
| 1 Peripheral Nervous | Ø Open<br>3 Percutaneous<br>7 Via Natural or Artificial Opening<br>8 Via Natural or Artificial Opening Endoscopic<br>X External | 2 Conductivity | 9 Sensory<br>B Motor |
| 1 Peripheral Nervous | Ø Open<br>3 Percutaneous<br>7 Via Natural or Artificial Opening<br>8 Via Natural or Artificial Opening Endoscopic<br>X External | 4 Electrical Activity | G Intraoperative<br>Z No Qualifier |
| 2 Cardiac | Ø Open<br>3 Percutaneous<br>7 Via Natural or Artificial Opening<br>8 Via Natural or Artificial Opening Endoscopic | 4 Electrical Activity<br>9 Output<br>C Rate<br>F Rhythm<br>H Sound | Z No Qualifier |
| 2 Cardiac | X External | 4 Electrical Activity | 5 Ambulatory<br>Z No Qualifier |
| 2 Cardiac | X External | 9 Output<br>C Rate<br>F Rhythm<br>H Sound | Z No Qualifier |
| 2 Cardiac | X External | M Total Activity | 4 Stress |
| 2 Cardiac | X External | S Vascular Perfusion | H Indocyanine Green Dye |
| 3 Arterial | Ø Open<br>3 Percutaneous | 5 Flow<br>B Pressure<br>J Pulse | 1 Peripheral<br>3 Pulmonary<br>C Coronary |
| 3 Arterial | Ø Open<br>3 Percutaneous | H Sound<br>R Saturation | 1 Peripheral |
| 3 Arterial | X External | 5 Flow<br>B Pressure<br>H Sound<br>J Pulse<br>R Saturation | 1 Peripheral |
| 4 Venous | Ø Open<br>3 Percutaneous | 5 Flow<br>B Pressure<br>J Pulse | Ø Central<br>1 Peripheral<br>2 Portal<br>3 Pulmonary |
| 4 Venous | Ø Open<br>3 Percutaneous | R Saturation | Ø Central<br>2 Portal<br>3 Pulmonary |
| 4 Venous | X External | 5 Flow<br>B Pressure<br>J Pulse | 1 Peripheral |
| 6 Lymphatic | Ø Open<br>3 Percutaneous<br>7 Via Natural or Artificial Opening<br>8 Via Natural or Artificial Opening Endoscopic | 5 Flow<br>B Pressure | Z No Qualifier |

*4A1 Continued on next page*

**Valid OR** 4A160[5,B]Z

**4 Measurement and Monitoring**
**A Physiological Systems**
**1 Monitoring** Definition: Determining the level of a physiological or physical function repetitively over a period of time

*4A1 Continued*

| Body System Character 4 | Approach Character 5 | Function/Device Character 6 | Qualifier Character 7 |
|---|---|---|---|
| 9 Respiratory | 7 Via Natural or Artificial Opening<br>X External | 1 Capacity<br>5 Flow<br>C Rate<br>D Resistance<br>L Volume | Z No Qualifier |
| B Gastrointestinal | 7 Via Natural or Artificial Opening<br>8 Via Natural or Artificial Opening Endoscopic | 8 Motility<br>B Pressure<br>G Secretion | Z No Qualifier |
| B Gastrointestinal | X External | S Vascular Perfusion | H Indocyanine Green Dye |
| D Urinary | 7 Via Natural or Artificial Opening<br>8 Via Natural or Artificial Opening Endoscopic | 3 Contractility<br>5 Flow<br>B Pressure<br>D Resistance<br>L Volume | Z No Qualifier |
| G Skin and Breast | X External | S Vascular Perfusion | H Indocyanine Green Dye |
| H Products of Conception, Cardiac ♀ | 7 Via Natural or Artificial Opening<br>8 Via Natural or Artificial Opening Endoscopic<br>X External | 4 Electrical Activity<br>C Rate<br>F Rhythm<br>H Sound | Z No Qualifier |
| J Products of Conception, Nervous ♀ | 7 Via Natural or Artificial Opening<br>8 Via Natural or Artificial Opening Endoscopic<br>X External | 2 Conductivity<br>4 Electrical Activity<br>B Pressure | Z No Qualifier |
| Z None | 7 Via Natural or Artificial Opening | K Temperature | Z No Qualifier |
| Z None | X External | K Temperature<br>Q Sleep | Z No Qualifier |

♀ 4A1H[7,8,X][4,C,F,H]Z
♀ 4A1J[7,8,X][2,4,B]Z

**4 Measurement and Monitoring**
**B Physiological Devices**
**Ø Measurement** Definition: Determining the level of a physiological or physical function at a point in time

| Body System Character 4 | Approach Character 5 | Function/Device Character 6 | Qualifier Character 7 |
|---|---|---|---|
| Ø Central Nervous<br>1 Peripheral Nervous<br>F Musculoskeletal | X External | V Stimulator | Z No Qualifier |
| 2 Cardiac | X External | S Pacemaker<br>T Defibrillator | Z No Qualifier |
| 9 Respiratory | X External | S Pacemaker | Z No Qualifier |

# Extracorporeal or Systemic Assistance and Performance 5AØ–5A2

## Character Meanings

This Character Meaning table is provided as a guide to assist the user in the identification of character members that may be found in this section of code tables. It **SHOULD NOT** be used to build a PCS code.

### A: Physiological Systems

| Operation–Character 3 | Body System–Character 4 | Duration–Character 5 | Function–Character 6 | Qualifier–Character 7 |
|---|---|---|---|---|
| Ø Assistance | 2 Cardiac | Ø Single | Ø Filtration | Ø Balloon Pump |
| 1 Performance | 5 Circulatory | 1 Intermittent | 1 Output | 1 Hyperbaric |
| 2 Restoration | 9 Respiratory | 2 Continuous | 2 Oxygenation | 2 Manual |
| | C Biliary | 3 Less than 24 Consecutive Hours | 3 Pacing | 3 Membrane |
| | D Urinary | 4 24-96 Consecutive Hours | 4 Rhythm | 4 Nonmechanical |
| | | 5 Greater than 96 Consecutive Hours | 5 Ventilation | 5 Pulsatile Compression |
| | | 6 Multiple | | 6 Other Pump |
| | | 7 Intermittent, Less than 6 Hours per Day | | 7 Continuous Positive Airway Pressure |
| | | 8 Prolonged Intermittent, 6-18 hours per Day | | 8 Intermittent Positive Airway Pressure |
| | | 9 Continuous, Greater than 18 hours per Day | | 9 Continuous Negative Airway Pressure |
| | | | | B Intermittent Negative Airway Pressure |
| | | | | C Supersaturated |
| | | | | D Impeller Pump |
| | | | | Z No Qualifier |

**AHA Coding Clinic for table 5AØ**

**2017, 1Q, 10-11** External heart assist device
**2017, 1Q, 29** Newborn resuscitation using positive pressure ventilation
**2017, 1Q, 29** Newborn noninvasive ventilation
**2016, 4Q, 137-139** Heart assist device systems
**2014, 4Q, 9** Mechanical ventilation
**2014, 3Q, 19** Ablation of ventricular tachycardia with Impella® support
**2013, 3Q, 18** Heart transplant surgery

**AHA Coding Clinic for table 5A1**

**2017, 1Q, 19** Norwood Sano procedure
**2016, 1Q, 27** Aortocoronary bypass graft utilizing Y-graft
**2016, 1Q, 28** Extracorporeal liver assist device
**2016, 1Q, 29** Duration of hemodialysis
**2015, 4Q, 22-24** Congenital heart corrective procedures
**2014, 4Q, 3-10** Mechanical ventilation
**2014, 4Q, 11-15** Sequencing of mechanical ventilation with other procedures
**2014, 3Q, 16** Repair of Tetralogy of Fallot
**2014, 3Q, 20** MAZE procedure performed with coronary artery bypass graft
**2014, 1Q, 10** Repair of thoracic aortic aneurysm & coronary artery bypass graft
**2013, 3Q, 18** Heart transplant surgery

**5 Extracorporeal or Systemic Assistance and Performance**
**A Physiological Systems**
**Ø Assistance** Definition: Taking over a portion of a physiological function by extracorporeal means

| Body System Character 4 | Duration Character 5 | Function Character 6 | Qualifier Character 7 |
|---|---|---|---|
| 2 Cardiac | 1 Intermittent<br>2 Continuous | 1 Output | Ø Balloon Pump<br>5 Pulsatile Compression<br>6 Other Pump<br>D Impeller Pump |
| 5 Circulatory | 1 Intermittent<br>2 Continuous | 2 Oxygenation | 1 Hyperbaric<br>C Supersaturated |
| 9 Respiratory | 2 Continuous | Ø Filtration | Z No Qualifier |
| 9 Respiratory | 3 Less than 24 Consecutive Hours<br>4 24-96 Consecutive Hours<br>5 Greater than 96 Consecutive Hours | 5 Ventilation | 7 Continuous Positive Airway Pressure<br>8 Intermittent Positive Airway Pressure<br>9 Continuous Negative Airway Pressure<br>B Intermittent Negative Airway Pressure<br>Z No Qualifier |

**Valid OR** 5AØ2[1,2]1[Ø,6,D]

**5 Extracorporeal or Systemic Assistance and Performance**
**A Physiological Systems**
**1 Performance** Definition: Completely taking over a physiological function by extracorporeal means

| Body System Character 4 | Duration Character 5 | Function Character 6 | Qualifier Character 7 |
|---|---|---|---|
| 2 Cardiac | Ø Single | 1 Output | 2 Manual |
| 2 Cardiac | 1 Intermittent | 3 Pacing | Z No Qualifier |
| 2 Cardiac | 2 Continuous | 1 Output<br>3 Pacing | Z No Qualifier |
| 5 Circulatory | 2 Continuous | 2 Oxygenation | 3 Membrane |
| 9 Respiratory | Ø Single | 5 Ventilation | 4 Nonmechanical |
| 9 Respiratory | 3 Less than 24 Consecutive Hours<br>4 24-96 Consecutive Hours<br>5 Greater than 96 Consecutive Hours | 5 Ventilation | Z No Qualifier |
| C Biliary | Ø Single<br>6 Multiple | Ø Filtration | Z No Qualifier |
| D Urinary | 7 Intermittent, Less than 6 Hours per day<br>8 Prolonged Intermittent, 6-18 Hours per day<br>9 Continuous, Greater than 18 Hours per day | Ø Filtration | Z No Qualifier |

**Valid OR** 5A15223
**DRG Non-OR** 5A19[3,4,5]5Z
**Note:** For code 5A1955Z, length of stay must be > 4 consecutive days.

**5 Extracorporeal or Systemic Assistance and Performance**
**A Physiological Systems**
**2 Restoration** Definition: Returning, or attempting to return, a physiological function to its original state by extracorporeal means.

| Body System Character 4 | Duration Character 5 | Function Character 6 | Qualifier Character 7 |
|---|---|---|---|
| 2 Cardiac | Ø Single | 4 Rhythm | Z No Qualifier |

# Extracorporeal or Systemic Therapies 6AØ–6AB

## Character Meanings

This Character Meaning table is provided as a guide to assist the user in the identification of character members that may be found in this section of code tables. It **SHOULD NOT** be used to build a PCS code.

### A: Physiological Systems

| Operation–Character 3 | Body System–Character 4 | Duration–Character 5 | Qualifier–Character 6 | Qualifier–Character 7 |
|---|---|---|---|---|
| Ø Atmospheric Control | Ø Skin | Ø Single | B Donor Organ | Ø Erythrocytes |
| 1 Decompression | 1 Urinary | 1 Multiple | Z No Qualifier | 1 Leukocytes |
| 2 Electromagnetic Therapy | 2 Central Nervous | | | 2 Platelets |
| 3 Hyperthermia | 3 Musculoskeletal | | | 3 Plasma |
| 4 Hypothermia | 5 Circulatory | | | 4 Head and Neck Vessels |
| 5 Pheresis | B Respiratory System | | | 5 Heart |
| 6 Phototherapy | F Hepatobiliary System and Pancreas | | | 6 Peripheral Vessels |
| 7 Ultrasound Therapy | T Urinary System | | | 7 Other Vessels |
| 8 Ultraviolet Light Therapy | Z None | | | T Stem Cells, Cord Blood |
| 9 Shock Wave Therapy | | | | V Stem Cells, Hematopoietic |
| B Perfusion | | | | Z No Qualifier |

**AHA Coding Clinic for table 6A7**
**2014, 4Q, 19** Ultrasound accelerated thrombolysis

**AHA Coding Clinic for table 6AB**
**2016, 4Q, 115** Donor organ perfusion

**6 Extracorporeal or Systemic Therapies**
**A Physiological Systems**
**Ø Atmospheric Control** Definition: Extracorporeal control of atmospheric pressure and composition

| Body System Character 4 | Duration Character 5 | Qualifier Character 6 | Qualifier Character 7 |
|---|---|---|---|
| Z None | Ø Single<br>1 Multiple | Z No Qualifier | Z No Qualifier |

**6 Extracorporeal or Systemic Therapies**
**A Physiological Systems**
**1 Decompression** Definition: Extracorporeal elimination of undissolved gas from body fluids

| Body System Character 4 | Duration Character 5 | Qualifier Character 6 | Qualifier Character 7 |
|---|---|---|---|
| 5 Circulatory | Ø Single<br>1 Multiple | Z No Qualifier | Z No Qualifier |

**6 Extracorporeal or Systemic Therapies**
**A Physiological Systems**
**2 Electromagnetic Therapy** Definition: Extracorporeal treatment by electromagnetic rays

| Body System Character 4 | Duration Character 5 | Qualifier Character 6 | Qualifier Character 7 |
|---|---|---|---|
| 1 Urinary<br>2 Central Nervous | Ø Single<br>1 Multiple | Z No Qualifier | Z No Qualifier |

**6 Extracorporeal or Systemic Therapies**
**A Physiological Systems**
**3 Hyperthermia** Definition: Extracorporeal raising of body temperature

| Body System Character 4 | Duration Character 5 | Qualifier Character 6 | Qualifier Character 7 |
|---|---|---|---|
| Z None | Ø Single<br>1 Multiple | Z No Qualifier | Z No Qualifier |

**6 Extracorporeal or Systemic Therapies**
**A Physiological Systems**
**4 Hypothermia** Definition: Extracorporeal lowering of body temperature

| Body System Character 4 | Duration Character 5 | Qualifier Character 6 | Qualifier Character 7 |
|---|---|---|---|
| Z None | Ø Single<br>1 Multiple | Z No Qualifier | Z No Qualifier |

**6 Extracorporeal or Systemic Therapies**
**A Physiological Systems**
**5 Pheresis** Definition: Extracorporeal separation of blood products

| Body System Character 4 | Duration Character 5 | Qualifier Character 6 | Qualifier Character 7 |
|---|---|---|---|
| 5 Circulatory | Ø Single<br>1 Multiple | Z No Qualifier | Ø Erythrocytes<br>1 Leukocytes<br>2 Platelets<br>3 Plasma<br>T Stem Cells, Cord Blood<br>V Stem Cells, Hematopoietic |

**6 Extracorporeal or Systemic Therapies**
**A Physiological Systems**
**6 Phototherapy** Definition: Extracorporeal treatment by light rays

| Body System Character 4 | Duration Character 5 | Qualifier Character 6 | Qualifier Character 7 |
|---|---|---|---|
| Ø Skin<br>5 Circulatory | Ø Single<br>1 Multiple | Z No Qualifier | Z No Qualifier |

**6 Extracorporeal or Systemic Therapies**
**A Physiological Systems**
**7 Ultrasound Therapy** Definition: Extracorporeal treatment by ultrasound

| Body System Character 4 | Duration Character 5 | Qualifier Character 6 | Qualifier Character 7 |
|---|---|---|---|
| 5 Circulatory | Ø Single<br>1 Multiple | Z No Qualifier | 4 Head and Neck Vessels<br>5 Heart<br>6 Peripheral Vessels<br>7 Other Vessels<br>Z No Qualifier |

**6 Extracorporeal or Systemic Therapies**
**A Physiological Systems**
**8 Ultraviolet Light Therapy** Definition: Extracorporeal treatment by ultraviolet light

| Body System Character 4 | Duration Character 5 | Qualifier Character 6 | Qualifier Character 7 |
|---|---|---|---|
| Ø Skin | Ø Single<br>1 Multiple | Z No Qualifier | Z No Qualifier |

**6 Extracorporeal or Systemic Therapies**
**A Physiological Systems**
**9 Shock Wave Therapy** Definition: Extracorporeal treatment by shock waves

| Body System Character 4 | Duration Character 5 | Qualifier Character 6 | Qualifier Character 7 |
|---|---|---|---|
| 3 Musculoskeletal | Ø Single<br>1 Multiple | Z No Qualifier | Z No Qualifier |

**6 Extracorporeal or Systemic Therapies**
**A Physiological Systems**
**B Perfusion** Definition: Extracorporeal treatment by diffusion of therapeutic fluid

| Body System Character 4 | Duration Character 5 | Qualifier Character 6 | Qualifier Character 7 |
|---|---|---|---|
| 5 Circulatory<br>B Respiratory System<br>F Hepatobiliary System and Pancreas<br>T Urinary System | Ø Single | B Donor Organ | Z No Qualifier |

# Osteopathic 7WØ

## Character Meanings

This Character Meaning table is provided as a guide to assist the user in the identification of character members that may be found in this section of code tables. It **SHOULD NOT** be used to build a PCS code.

### W: Anatomical Regions

| Operation–Character 3 | Body Region–Character 4 | Approach–Character 5 | Method–Character 6 | Qualifier–Character 7 |
|---|---|---|---|---|
| Ø Treatment | Ø Head | X External | Ø Articulatory-Raising | Z None |
| | 1 Cervical | | 1 Fascial Release | |
| | 2 Thoracic | | 2 General Mobilization | |
| | 3 Lumbar | | 3 High Velocity-Low Amplitude | |
| | 4 Sacrum | | 4 Indirect | |
| | 5 Pelvis | | 5 Low Velocity-High Amplitude | |
| | 6 Lower Extremities | | 6 Lymphatic Pump | |
| | 7 Upper Extremities | | 7 Muscle Energy-Isometric | |
| | 8 Rib Cage | | 8 Muscle Energy-Isotonic | |
| | 9 Abdomen | | 9 Other Method | |

**7 Osteopathic**
**W Anatomical Regions**
**Ø Treatment** Definition: Manual treatment to eliminate or alleviate somatic dysfunction and related disorders

| Body Region Character 4 | Approach Character 5 | Method Character 6 | Qualifier Character 7 |
|---|---|---|---|
| **Ø** Head<br>**1** Cervical<br>**2** Thoracic<br>**3** Lumbar<br>**4** Sacrum<br>**5** Pelvis<br>**6** Lower Extremities<br>**7** Upper Extremities<br>**8** Rib Cage<br>**9** Abdomen | **X** External | **Ø** Articulatory-Raising<br>**1** Fascial Release<br>**2** General Mobilization<br>**3** High Velocity-Low Amplitude<br>**4** Indirect<br>**5** Low Velocity-High Amplitude<br>**6** Lymphatic Pump<br>**7** Muscle Energy-Isometric<br>**8** Muscle Energy-Isotonic<br>**9** Other Method | **Z** None |

# Other Procedures 8CØ–8EØ

## Character Meanings

This Character Meaning table is provided as a guide to assist the user in the identification of character members that may be found in this section of code tables. It **SHOULD NOT** be used to build a PCS code.

### C: Indwelling Devices

| Operation–Character 3 | Body Region–Character 4 | Approach–Character 5 | Method–Character 6 | Qualifier–Character 7 |
|---|---|---|---|---|
| Ø Other procedures | 1 Nervous System | X External | 6 Collection | J Cerebrospinal Fluid |
| | 2 Circulatory System | | | K Blood |
| | | | | L Other Fluid |

### E: Physiological Systems and Anatomical Regions

| Operation–Character 3 | Body Region–Character 4 | Approach–Character 5 | Method–Character 6 | Qualifier–Character 7 |
|---|---|---|---|---|
| Ø Other Procedures | 1 Nervous System | Ø Open | Ø Acupuncture | Ø Anesthesia |
| | 2 Circulatory System | 3 Percutaneous | 1 Therapeutic Massage | 1 In Vitro Fertilization |
| | 9 Head and Neck Region | 4 Percutaneous Endoscopic | 6 Collection | 2 Breast Milk |
| | H Integumentary System and Breast | 7 Via Natural or Artificial Opening | B Computer Assisted Procedure | 3 Sperm |
| | K Musculoskeletal System | 8 Via Natural or Artificial Opening Endoscopic | C Robotic Assisted Procedure | 4 Yoga Therapy |
| | U Female Reproductive System | X External | D Near Infrared Spectroscopy | 5 Meditation |
| | V Male Reproductive System | | Y Other Method | 6 Isolation |
| | W Trunk Region | | | 7 Examination |
| | X Upper Extremity | | | 8 Suture Removal |
| | Y Lower Extremity | | | 9 Piercing |
| | Z None | | | C Prostate |
| | | | | D Rectum |
| | | | | F With Fluoroscopy |
| | | | | G With Computerized Tomography |
| | | | | H With Magnetic Resonance Imaging |
| | | | | Z No Qualifier |

**AHA Coding Clinic for table 8EØ**

**2015, 1Q, 33** Robotic-assisted laparoscopic hysterectomy converted to open procedure
**2014, 4Q, 33** Radical prostatectomy

**8 Other Procedures**
**C Indwelling Device**
**Ø Other Procedures** Definition: Methodologies which attempt to remediate or cure a disorder or disease

| Body Region Character 4 | Approach Character 5 | Method Character 6 | Qualifier Character 7 |
|---|---|---|---|
| **1** Nervous System | **X** External | **6** Collection | **J** Cerebrospinal Fluid<br>**L** Other Fluid |
| **2** Circulatory System | **X** External | **6** Collection | **K** Blood<br>**L** Other Fluid |

**8 Other Procedures**
**E Physiological Systems and Anatomical Regions**
**Ø Other Procedures** Definition: Methodologies which attempt to remediate or cure a disorder or disease

| Body Region Character 4 | Approach Character 5 | Method Character 6 | Qualifier Character 7 |
|---|---|---|---|
| 1 Nervous System<br>U Female Reproductive System ♀ | X External | Y Other Method | 7 Examination |
| 2 Circulatory System | 3 Percutaneous | D Near Infrared Spectroscopy | Z No Qualifier |
| 9 Head and Neck Region<br>W Trunk Region | Ø Open<br>3 Percutaneous<br>4 Percutaneous Endoscopic<br>7 Via Natural or Artificial Opening<br>8 Via Natural or Artificial Opening Endoscopic | C Robotic Assisted Procedure | Z No Qualifier |
| 9 Head and Neck Region<br>W Trunk Region | X External | B Computer Assisted Procedure | F With Fluoroscopy<br>G With Computerized Tomography<br>H With Magnetic Resonance Imaging<br>Z No Qualifier |
| 9 Head and Neck Region<br>W Trunk Region | X External | C Robotic Assisted Procedure | Z No Qualifier |
| 9 Head and Neck Region<br>W Trunk Region | X External | Y Other Method | 8 Suture Removal |
| H Integumentary System and Breast | 3 Percutaneous | Ø Acupuncture | Ø Anesthesia<br>Z No Qualifier |
| H Integumentary System and Breast ♀ | X External | 6 Collection | 2 Breast Milk |
| H Integumentary System and Breast | X External | Y Other Method | 9 Piercing |
| K Musculoskeletal System | X External | 1 Therapeutic Massage | Z No Qualifier |
| K Musculoskeletal System | X External | Y Other Method | 7 Examination |
| V Male Reproductive System ♂ | X External | 1 Therapeutic Massage | C Prostate<br>D Rectum |
| V Male Reproductive System ♂ | X External | 6 Collection | 3 Sperm |
| X Upper Extremity<br>Y Lower Extremity | Ø Open<br>3 Percutaneous<br>4 Percutaneous Endoscopic | C Robotic Assisted Procedure | Z No Qualifier |
| X Upper Extremity<br>Y Lower Extremity | X External | B Computer Assisted Procedure | F With Fluoroscopy<br>G With Computerized Tomography<br>H With Magnetic Resonance Imaging<br>Z No Qualifier |
| X Upper Extremity<br>Y Lower Extremity | X External | C Robotic Assisted Procedure | Z No Qualifier |
| X Upper Extremity<br>Y Lower Extremity | X External | Y Other Method | 8 Suture Removal |
| Z None | X External | Y Other Method | 1 In Vitro Fertilization<br>4 Yoga Therapy<br>5 Meditation<br>6 Isolation |

♂ 8EØVXIC
♂ 8EØVX63
♀ 8EØUXY7
♀ 8EØHX62

# Chiropractic 9WB

## Character Meanings

This Character Meaning table is provided as a guide to assist the user in the identification of character members that may be found in this section of code tables. It **SHOULD NOT** be used to build a PCS code.

### W: Anatomical Regions

| Operation–Character 3 | Body Region–Character 4 | Approach–Character 5 | Method–Character 6 | Qualifier–Character 7 |
|---|---|---|---|---|
| B Manipulation | Ø Head | X External | B Non-Manual | Z None |
| | 1 Cervical | | C Indirect Visceral | |
| | 2 Thoracic | | D Extra-Articular | |
| | 3 Lumbar | | F Direct Visceral | |
| | 4 Sacrum | | G Long Lever Specific Contact | |
| | 5 Pelvis | | H Short Lever Specific Contact | |
| | 6 Lower Extremities | | J Long and Short Lever Specific Contact | |
| | 7 Upper Extremities | | K Mechanically Assisted | |
| | 8 Rib Cage | | L Other Method | |
| | 9 Abdomen | | | |

**9 Chiropractic**
**W Anatomical Regions**
**B Manipulation** Definition: Manual procedure that involves a directed thrust to move a joint past the physiological range of motion, without exceeding the anatomical limit

| Body Region Character 4 | Approach Character 5 | Method Character 6 | Qualifier Character 7 |
|---|---|---|---|
| **Ø** Head<br>**1** Cervical<br>**2** Thoracic<br>**3** Lumbar<br>**4** Sacrum<br>**5** Pelvis<br>**6** Lower Extremities<br>**7** Upper Extremities<br>**8** Rib Cage<br>**9** Abdomen | **X** External | **B** Non-Manual<br>**C** Indirect Visceral<br>**D** Extra-Articular<br>**F** Direct Visceral<br>**G** Long Lever Specific Contact<br>**H** Short Lever Specific Contact<br>**J** Long and Short Lever Specific Contact<br>**K** Mechanically Assisted<br>**L** Other Method | **Z** None |

# Imaging BØØ–BY4

## Character Meanings

This Character Meaning table is provided as a guide to assist the user in the identification of character members that may be found in this section of code tables. It **SHOULD NOT** be used to build a PCS code.

| Body System–Character 2 | Type–Character 3 | Body Part–Character 4 | Contrast–Character 5 | Qualifier–Character 6 | Qualifier–Character 7 |
|---|---|---|---|---|---|
| Ø Central Nervous System | Ø Plain Radiography | See next page | Ø High Osmolar | Ø Unenhanced and Enhanced | Ø Intraoperative |
| 2 Heart | 1 Fluoroscopy | | 1 Low Osmolar | 1 Laser | 1 Densitometry |
| 3 Upper Arteries | 2 Computerized Tomography (CT Scan) | | Y Other Contrast | 2 Intravascular Optical Coherence | 3 Intravascular |
| 4 Lower Arteries | 3 Magnetic Resonance Imaging (MRI) | | Z None | Z None | 4 Transesophageal |
| 5 Veins | 4 Ultrasonography | | | | A Guidance |
| 7 Lymphatic System | | | | | Z None |
| 8 Eye | | | | | |
| 9 Ear, Nose, Mouth and Throat | | | | | |
| B Respiratory System | | | | | |
| D Gastrointestinal System | | | | | |
| F Hepatobiliary System and Pancreas | | | | | |
| G Endocrine System | | | | | |
| H Skin, Subcutaneous Tissue and Breast | | | | | |
| L Connective Tissue | | | | | |
| N Skull and Facial Bones | | | | | |
| P Non-Axial Upper Bones | | | | | |
| Q Non-Axial Lower Bones | | | | | |
| R Axial Skeleton, Except Skull and Facial Bones | | | | | |
| T Urinary System | | | | | |
| U Female Reproductive System | | | | | |
| V Male Reproductive System | | | | | |
| W Anatomical Regions | | | | | |
| Y Fetus and Obstetrical | | | | | |

*Continued on next page*

# Body Part—Character 4 Meanings

Continued from previous page

| Body System–Character 2 | Meanings– Character 4 | |
|---|---|---|
| Ø Central Nervous System | Ø Brain<br>7 Cisterna<br>8 Cerebral Ventricle(s) | 9 Sella Turcica/Pituitary Gland<br>B Spinal Cord<br>C Acoustic Nerves |
| 2 Heart | Ø Coronary Artery, Single<br>1 Coronary Arteries, Multiple<br>2 Coronary Artery Bypass Graft, Single<br>3 Coronary Artery Bypass Grafts, Multiple<br>4 Heart, Right<br>5 Heart, Left<br>6 Heart, Right and Left | 7 Internal Mammary Bypass Graft, Right<br>8 Internal Mammary Bypass Graft, Left<br>B Heart with Aorta<br>C Pericardium<br>D Pediatric Heart<br>F Bypass Graft, Other |
| 3 Upper Arteries | Ø Thoracic Aorta<br>1 Brachiocephalic-Subclavian Artery, Right<br>2 Subclavian Artery, Left<br>3 Common Carotid Artery, Right<br>4 Common Carotid Artery, Left<br>5 Common Carotid Arteries, Bilateral<br>6 Internal Carotid Artery, Right<br>7 Internal Carotid Artery, Left<br>8 Internal Carotid Arteries, Bilateral<br>9 External Carotid Artery, Right<br>B External Carotid Artery, Left<br>C External Carotid Arteries, Bilateral<br>D Vertebral Artery, Right<br>F Vertebral Artery, Left | G Vertebral Arteries, Bilateral<br>H Upper Extremity Arteries, Right<br>J Upper Extremity Arteries, Left<br>K Upper Extremity Arteries, Bilateral<br>L Intercostal and Bronchial Arteries<br>M Spinal Arteries<br>N Upper Arteries, Other<br>P Thoraco-Abdominal Aorta<br>Q Cervico-Cerebral Arch<br>R Intracranial Arteries<br>S Pulmonary Artery, Right<br>T Pulmonary Artery, Left<br>U Pulmonary Trunk<br>V Ophthalmic Arteries |
| 4 Lower Arteries | Ø Abdominal Aorta<br>1 Celiac Artery<br>2 Hepatic Artery<br>3 Splenic Arteries<br>4 Superior Mesenteric Artery<br>5 Inferior Mesenteric Artery<br>6 Renal Artery, Right<br>7 Renal Artery, Left<br>8 Renal Arteries, Bilateral<br>9 Lumbar Arteries<br>B Intra-Abdominal Arteries, Other | C Pelvic Arteries<br>D Aorta and Bilateral Lower Extremity Arteries<br>F Lower Extremity Arteries, Right<br>G Lower Extremity Arteries, Left<br>H Lower Extremity Arteries, Bilateral<br>J Lower Arteries, Other<br>K Celiac and Mesenteric Arteries<br>L Femoral Artery<br>M Renal Artery Transplant<br>N Penile Arteries |
| 5 Veins | Ø Epidural Veins<br>1 Cerebral and Cerebellar Veins<br>2 Intracranial Sinuses<br>3 Jugular Veins, Right<br>4 Jugular Veins, Left<br>5 Jugular Veins, Bilateral<br>6 Subclavian Vein, Right<br>7 Subclavian Vein, Left<br>8 Superior Vena Cava<br>9 Inferior Vena Cava<br>B Lower Extremity Veins, Right<br>C Lower Extremity Veins, Left<br>D Lower Extremity Veins, Bilateral<br>F Pelvic (Iliac) Veins, Right | G Pelvic (Iliac) Veins, Left<br>H Pelvic (Iliac) Veins, Bilateral<br>J Renal Vein, Right<br>K Renal Vein, Left<br>L Renal Veins, Bilateral<br>M Upper Extremity Veins, Right<br>N Upper Extremity Veins, Left<br>P Upper Extremity Veins, Bilateral<br>Q Pulmonary Vein, Right<br>R Pulmonary Vein, Left<br>S Pulmonary Veins, Bilateral<br>T Portal and Splanchnic Veins<br>V Veins, Other<br>W Dialysis Shunt/Fistula |
| 7 Lymphatic System | Ø Abdominal/Retroperitoneal Lymphatics, Unilateral<br>1 Abdominal/Retroperitoneal Lymphatics, Bilateral<br>4 Lymphatics, Head and Neck<br>5 Upper Extremity Lymphatics, Right<br>6 Upper Extremity Lymphatics, Left | 7 Upper Extremity Lymphatics, Bilateral<br>8 Lower Extremity Lymphatics, Right<br>9 Lower Extremity Lymphatics, Left<br>B Lower Extremity Lymphatics, Bilateral<br>C Lymphatics, Pelvic |
| 8 Eye | Ø Lacrimal Duct, Right<br>1 Lacrimal Duct, Left<br>2 Lacrimal Ducts, Bilateral<br>3 Optic Foramina, Right | 4 Optic Foramina, Left<br>5 Eye, Right<br>6 Eye, Left<br>7 Eyes, Bilateral |
| 9 Ear, Nose, Mouth and Throat | Ø Ear<br>2 Paranasal Sinuses<br>4 Parotid Gland, Right<br>5 Parotid Gland, Left<br>6 Parotid Glands, Bilateral<br>7 Submandibular Gland, Right<br>8 Submandibular Gland, Left<br>9 Submandibular Glands, Bilateral | B Salivary Gland, Right<br>C Salivary Gland, Left<br>D Salivary Glands, Bilateral<br>F Nasopharynx/Oropharynx<br>G Pharynx and Epiglottis<br>H Mastoids<br>J Larynx |
| B Respiratory System | 2 Lung, Right<br>3 Lung, Left<br>4 Lungs, Bilateral<br>6 Diaphragm<br>7 Tracheobronchial Tree, Right<br>8 Tracheobronchial Tree, Left | 9 Tracheobronchial Trees, Bilateral<br>B Pleura<br>C Mediastinum<br>D Upper Airways<br>F Trachea/Airways<br>G Lung Apices |

Continued on next page

Continued from previous page

| Body System–Character 2 | Meanings– Character 4 | |
|---|---|---|
| D Gastrointestinal System | 1 Esophagus<br>2 Stomach<br>3 Small Bowel<br>4 Colon<br>5 Upper GI<br>6 Upper GI and Small Bowel | 7 Gastrointestinal Tract<br>8 Appendix<br>9 Duodenum<br>B Mouth/Oropharynx<br>C Rectum |
| F Hepatobiliary System and Pancreas | Ø Bile Ducts<br>1 Biliary and Pancreatic Ducts<br>2 Gallbladder<br>3 Gallbladder and Bile Ducts<br>4 Gallbladder, Bile Ducts and Pancreatic Ducts | 5 Liver<br>6 Liver and Spleen<br>7 Pancreas<br>8 Pancreatic Ducts<br>C Hepatobiliary System, All |
| G Endocrine System | Ø Adrenal Gland, Right<br>1 Adrenal Gland, Left<br>2 Adrenal Glands, Bilateral | 3 Parathyroid Glands<br>4 Thyroid Gland |
| H Skin, Subcutaneous Tissue and Breast | Ø Breast, Right<br>1 Breast, Left<br>2 Breasts, Bilateral<br>3 Single Mammary Duct, Right<br>4 Single Mammary Duct, Left<br>5 Multiple Mammary Ducts, Right<br>6 Multiple Mammary Ducts, Left<br>7 Extremity, Upper<br>8 Extremity, Lower | 9 Abdominal Wall<br>B Chest Wall<br>C Head and Neck<br>D Subcutaneous Tissue, Head/Neck<br>F Subcutaneous Tissue, Upper Extremity<br>G Subcutaneous Tissue, Thorax<br>H Subcutaneous Tissue, Abdomen and Pelvis<br>J Subcutaneous Tissue, Lower Extremity |
| L Connective Tissue | Ø Connective Tissue, Upper Extremity<br>1 Connective Tissue, Lower Extremity | 2 Tendons, Upper Extremity<br>3 Tendons, Lower Extremity |
| N Skull and Facial Bones | Ø Skull<br>1 Orbit, Right<br>2 Orbit, Left<br>3 Orbits, Bilateral<br>4 Nasal Bones<br>5 Facial Bones<br>6 Mandible<br>7 Temporomandibular Joint, Right<br>8 Temporomandibular Joint, Left | 9 Temporomandibular Joints, Bilateral<br>B Zygomatic Arch, Right<br>C Zygomatic Arch, Left<br>D Zygomatic Arches, Bilateral<br>F Temporal Bones<br>G Tooth, Single<br>H Teeth, Multiple<br>J Teeth, All |
| P Non-Axial Upper Bones | Ø Sternoclavicular Joint, Right<br>1 Sternoclavicular Joint, Left<br>2 Sternoclavicular Joints, Bilateral<br>3 Acromioclavicular Joints, Bilateral<br>4 Clavicle, Right<br>5 Clavicle, Left<br>6 Scapula, Right<br>7 Scapula, Left<br>8 Shoulder, Right<br>9 Shoulder, Left<br>A Humerus, Right<br>B Humerus, Left<br>C Hand/Finger Joint, Right<br>D Hand/Finger Joint, Left<br>E Upper Arm, Right<br>F Upper Arm, Left<br>G Elbow, Right | H Elbow, Left<br>J Forearm, Right<br>K Forearm, Left<br>L Wrist, Right<br>M Wrist, Left<br>N Hand, Right<br>P Hand, Left<br>Q Hands and Wrists, Bilateral<br>R Finger(s), Right<br>S Finger(s), Left<br>T Upper Extremity, Right<br>U Upper Extremity, Left<br>V Upper Extremities, Bilateral<br>W Thorax<br>X Ribs, Right<br>Y Ribs, Left |
| Q Non-Axial Lower Bones | Ø Hip, Right<br>1 Hip, Left<br>2 Hips, Bilateral<br>3 Femur, Right<br>4 Femur, Left<br>7 Knee, Right<br>8 Knee, Left<br>9 Knees, Bilateral<br>B Tibia/Fibula, Right<br>C Tibia/Fibula, Left<br>D Lower Leg, Right<br>F Lower Leg, Left<br>G Ankle, Right | H Ankle, Left<br>J Calcaneus, Right<br>K Calcaneus, Left<br>L Foot, Right<br>M Foot, Left<br>P Toe(s), Right<br>Q Toe(s), Left<br>R Lower Extremity, Right<br>S Lower Extremity, Left<br>V Patella, Right<br>W Patella, Left<br>X Foot/Toe Joint, Right<br>Y Foot/Toe Joint, Left |
| R Axial Skeleton, Except Skull and Facial Bones | Ø Cervical Spine<br>1 Cervical Disc(s)<br>2 Thoracic Disc(s)<br>3 Lumbar Disc(s)<br>4 Cervical Facet Joint(s)<br>5 Thoracic Facet Joint(s)<br>6 Lumbar Facet Joint(s)<br>7 Thoracic Spine | 8 Thoracolumbar Joint<br>9 Lumbar Spine<br>B Lumbosacral Joint<br>C Pelvis<br>D Sacroiliac Joints<br>F Sacrum and Coccyx<br>G Whole Spine<br>H Sternum |

Continued on next page

*Continued from previous page*

| Body System–Character 2 | Meanings– Character 4 | |
|---|---|---|
| T Urinary System | Ø Bladder<br>1 Kidney, Right<br>2 Kidney, Left<br>3 Kidneys, Bilateral<br>4 Kidneys, Ureters and Bladder<br>5 Urethra<br>6 Ureter, Right<br>7 Ureter, Left | 8 Ureters, Bilateral<br>9 Kidney Transplant<br>B Bladder and Urethra<br>C Ileal Diversion Loop<br>D Kidney, Ureter and Bladder, Right<br>F Kidney, Ureter and Bladder, Left<br>G Ileal Loop, Ureters and Kidneys<br>J Kidneys and Bladder |
| U Female Reproductive System | Ø Fallopian Tube, Right<br>1 Fallopian Tube, Left<br>2 Fallopian Tubes, Bilateral<br>3 Ovary, Right<br>4 Ovary, Left<br>5 Ovaries, Bilateral | 6 Uterus<br>8 Uterus and Fallopian Tubes<br>9 Vagina<br>B Pregnant Uterus<br>C Uterus and Ovaries |
| V Male Reproductive System | Ø Corpora Cavernosa<br>1 Epididymis, Right<br>2 Epididymis, Left<br>3 Prostate<br>4 Scrotum<br>5 Testicle, Right | 6 Testicle, Left<br>7 Testicles, Bilateral<br>8 Vasa Vasorum<br>9 Prostate and Seminal Vesicles<br>B Penis |
| W Anatomical Regions | Ø Abdomen<br>1 Abdomen and Pelvis<br>3 Chest<br>4 Chest and Abdomen<br>5 Chest, Abdomen and Pelvis<br>8 Head<br>9 Head and Neck<br>B Long Bones, All<br>C Lower Extremity | F Neck<br>G Pelvic Region<br>H Retroperitoneum<br>J Upper Extremity<br>K Whole Body<br>L Whole Skeleton<br>M Whole Body, Infant<br>P Brachial Plexus |
| Y Fetus and Obstetrical | Ø Fetal Head<br>1 Fetal Heart<br>2 Fetal Thorax<br>3 Fetal Abdomen<br>4 Fetal Spine<br>5 Fetal Extremities<br>6 Whole Fetus<br>7 Fetal Umbilical Cord | 8 Placenta<br>9 First Trimester, Single Fetus<br>B First Trimester, Multiple Gestation<br>C Second Trimester, Single Fetus<br>D Second Trimester, Multiple Gestation<br>F Third Trimester, Single Fetus<br>G Third Trimester, Multiple Gestation |

**AHA Coding Clinic for table B21**
**2016, 3Q, 36** Type of contrast medium for angiography (high osmolar, low osmolar, and other)

**AHA Coding Clinic for table B41**
**2015, 3Q, 9** Aborted endovascular stenting of superficial femoral artery

**AHA Coding Clinic for table B51**
**2015, 4Q, 30** Vascular access devices

**AHA Coding Clinic for table BF4**
**2014, 3Q, 15** Drainage of pancreatic pseudocyst

**B Imaging**
**0 Central Nervous System**
**0 Plain Radiography** Definition: Planar display of an image developed from the capture of external ionizing radiation on photographic or photoconductive plate

| Body Part Character 4 | Contrast Character 5 | Qualifier Character 6 | Qualifier Character 7 |
|---|---|---|---|
| B Spinal Cord | 0 High Osmolar<br>1 Low Osmolar<br>Y Other Contrast<br>Z None | Z None | Z None |

**B Imaging**
**0 Central Nervous System**
**1 Fluoroscopy** Definition: Single plane or bi-plane real time display of an image developed from the capture of external ionizing radioation on a fluorescent screen. The image may also be stored by either digital or analog means.

| Body Part Character 4 | Contrast Character 5 | Qualifier Character 6 | Qualifier Character 7 |
|---|---|---|---|
| B Spinal Cord | 0 High Osmolar<br>1 Low Osmolar<br>Y Other Contrast<br>Z None | Z None | Z None |

**B Imaging**
**0 Central Nervous System**
**2 Computerized Tomography (CT Scan)** Definition: Computer reformatted digital display of multiplanar images developed from the capture of multiple exposures of external ionizing radiation

| Body Part Character 4 | Contrast Character 5 | Qualifier Character 6 | Qualifier Character 7 |
|---|---|---|---|
| 0 Brain<br>7 Cisterna<br>8 Cerebral Ventricle(s)<br>9 Sella Turcica/Pituitary Gland<br>B Spinal Cord | 0 High Osmolar<br>1 Low Osmolar<br>Y Other Contrast | 0 Unenhanced and Enhanced<br>Z None | Z None |
| 0 Brain<br>7 Cisterna<br>8 Cerebral Ventricle(s)<br>9 Sella Turcica/Pituitary Gland<br>B Spinal Cord | Z None | Z None | Z None |

**B Imaging**
**0 Central Nervous System**
**3 Magnetic Resonance Imaging (MRI)** Definition: Computer reformatted digital display of multiplanar images developed from the capture of radio-frequency signals emitted by nuclei in a body site excited within a magnetic field

| Body Part Character 4 | Contrast Character 5 | Qualifier Character 6 | Qualifier Character 7 |
|---|---|---|---|
| 0 Brain<br>9 Sella Turcica/Pituitary Gland<br>B Spinal Cord<br>C Acoustic Nerves | Y Other Contrast | 0 Unenhanced and Enhanced<br>Z None | Z None |
| 0 Brain<br>9 Sella Turcica/Pituitary Gland<br>B Spinal Cord<br>C Acoustic Nerves | Z None | Z None | Z None |

**B Imaging**
**0 Central Nervous System**
**4 Ultrasonography** Definition: Real time display of images of anatomy or flow information developed from the capture of relected and attenuated high frequency sound waves

| Body Part Character 4 | Contrast Character 5 | Qualifier Character 6 | Qualifier Character 7 |
|---|---|---|---|
| 0 Brain<br>B Spinal Cord | Z None | Z None | Z None |

**B Imaging**
**2 Heart**
**Ø Plain Radiography** Definition: Planar display of an image developed from the capture of external ionizing radiation on photographic or photoconductive plate

| Body Part Character 4 | Contrast Character 5 | Qualifier Character 6 | Qualifier Character 7 |
|---|---|---|---|
| Ø Coronary Artery, Single<br>1 Coronary Arteries, Multiple<br>2 Coronary Artery Bypass Graft, Single<br>3 Coronary Artery Bypass Grafts, Multiple<br>4 Heart, Right<br>5 Heart, Left<br>6 Heart, Right and Left<br>7 Internal Mammary Bypass Graft, Right<br>8 Internal Mammary Bypass Graft, Left<br>F Bypass Graft, Other | Ø High Osmolar<br>1 Low Osmolar<br>Y Other Contrast | Z None | Z None |

DRG Non-OR All body part, contrast, and qualifier values

**B Imaging**
**2 Heart**
**1 Fluoroscopy** Definition: Single plane or bi-plane real time display of an image developed from the capture of external ionizing radioation on a fluorescent screen. The image may also be stored by either digital or analog means.

| Body Part Character 4 | Contrast Character 5 | Qualifier Character 6 | Qualifier Character 7 |
|---|---|---|---|
| Ø Coronary Artery, Single<br>1 Coronary Arteries, Multiple<br>2 Coronary Artery Bypass Graft, Single<br>3 Coronary Artery Bypass Grafts, Multiple | Ø High Osmolar<br>1 Low Osmolar<br>Y Other Contrast | 1 Laser | Ø Intraoperative |
| Ø Coronary Artery, Single<br>1 Coronary Arteries, Multiple<br>2 Coronary Artery Bypass Graft, Single<br>3 Coronary Artery Bypass Grafts, Multiple | Ø High Osmolar<br>1 Low Osmolar<br>Y Other Contrast | Z None | Z None |
| 4 Heart, Right<br>5 Heart, Left<br>6 Heart, Right and Left<br>7 Internal Mammary Bypass Graft, Right<br>8 Internal Mammary Bypass Graft, Left<br>F Bypass Graft, Other | Ø High Osmolar<br>1 Low Osmolar<br>Y Other Contrast | Z None | Z None |

DRG Non-OR All body part, contrast, and qualifier values

**B Imaging**
**2 Heart**
**2 Computerized Tomography (CT Scan)** Definition: Computer reformatted digital display of multiplanar images developed from the capture of multiple exposures of external ionizing radiation

| Body Part Character 4 | Contrast Character 5 | Qualifier Character 6 | Qualifier Character 7 |
|---|---|---|---|
| 1 Coronary Arteries, Multiple<br>3 Coronary Artery Bypass Grafts, Multiple<br>6 Heart, Right and Left | Ø High Osmolar<br>1 Low Osmolar<br>Y Other Contrast | Ø Unenhanced and Enhanced<br>Z None | Z None |
| 1 Coronary Arteries, Multiple<br>3 Coronary Artery Bypass Grafts, Multiple<br>6 Heart, Right and Left | Z None | 2 Intravascular Optical Coherence<br>Z None | Z None |

**B Imaging**
**2 Heart**
**3 Magnetic Resonance Imaging (MRI)** Definition: Computer reformatted digital display of multiplanar images developed from the capture of radio-frequency signals emitted by nuclei in a body site excited within a magnetic field

| Body Part Character 4 | Contrast Character 5 | Qualifier Character 6 | Qualifier Character 7 |
|---|---|---|---|
| 1 Coronary Arteries, Multiple<br>3 Coronary Artery Bypass Grafts, Multiple<br>6 Heart, Right and Left | Y Other Contrast | Ø Unenhanced and Enhanced<br>Z None | Z None |
| 1 Coronary Arteries, Multiple<br>3 Coronary Artery Bypass Grafts, Multiple<br>6 Heart, Right and Left | Z None | Z None | Z None |

**B Imaging**
**2 Heart**
**4 Ultrasonography** Definition: Real time display of images of anatomy or flow information developed from the capture of relected and attenuated high frequency sound waves

| Body Part Character 4 | Contrast Character 5 | Qualifier Character 6 | Qualifier Character 7 |
|---|---|---|---|
| Ø Coronary Artery, Single<br>1 Coronary Arteries, Multiple<br>4 Heart, Right<br>5 Heart, Left<br>6 Heart, Right and Left<br>B Heart with Aorta<br>C Pericardium<br>D Pediatric Heart | Y Other Contrast | Z None | Z None |
| Ø Coronary Artery, Single<br>1 Coronary Arteries, Multiple<br>4 Heart, Right<br>5 Heart, Left<br>6 Heart, Right and Left<br>B Heart with Aorta<br>C Pericardium<br>D Pediatric Heart | Z None | Z None | 3 Intravascular<br>4 Transesophageal<br>Z None |

**B Imaging**
**3 Upper Arteries**
**Ø Plain Radiography** Definition: Planar display of an image developed from the capture of external ionizing radiation on photographic or photoconductive plate

| Body Part Character 4 | Contrast Character 5 | Qualifier Character 6 | Qualifier Character 7 |
|---|---|---|---|
| Ø Thoracic Aorta<br>1 Brachiocephalic-Subclavian Artery, Right<br>2 Subclavian Artery, Left<br>3 Common Carotid Artery, Right<br>4 Common Carotid Artery, Left<br>5 Common Carotid Arteries, Bilateral<br>6 Internal Carotid Artery, Right<br>7 Internal Carotid Artery, Left<br>8 Internal Carotid Arteries, Bilateral<br>9 External Carotid Artery, Right<br>B External Carotid Artery, Left<br>C External Carotid Arteries, Bilateral<br>D Vertebral Artery, Right<br>F Vertebral Artery, Left<br>G Vertebral Arteries, Bilateral<br>H Upper Extremity Arteries, Right<br>J Upper Extremity Arteries, Left<br>K Upper Extremity Arteries, Bilateral<br>L Intercostal and Bronchial Arteries<br>M Spinal Arteries<br>N Upper Arteries, Other<br>P Thoraco-Abdominal Aorta<br>Q Cervico-Cerebral Arch<br>R Intracranial Arteries<br>S Pulmonary Artery, Right<br>T Pulmonary Artery, Left | Ø High Osmolar<br>1 Low Osmolar<br>Y Other Contrast<br>Z None | Z None | Z None |

**B Imaging**
**3 Upper Arteries**
**1 Fluoroscopy** Definition: Single plane or bi-plane real time display of an image developed from the capture of external ionizing radiation on a fluorescent screen. The image may also be stored by either digital or analog means.

| Body Part Character 4 | Contrast Character 5 | Qualifier Character 6 | Qualifier Character 7 |
|---|---|---|---|
| Ø Thoracic Aorta<br>1 Brachiocephalic-Subclavian Artery, Right<br>2 Subclavian Artery, Left<br>3 Common Carotid Artery, Right<br>4 Common Carotid Artery, Left<br>5 Common Carotid Arteries, Bilateral<br>6 Internal Carotid Artery, Right<br>7 Internal Carotid Artery, Left<br>8 Internal Carotid Arteries, Bilateral<br>9 External Carotid Artery, Right<br>B External Carotid Artery, Left<br>C External Carotid Arteries, Bilateral<br>D Vertebral Artery, Right<br>F Vertebral Artery, Left<br>G Vertebral Arteries, Bilateral<br>H Upper Extremity Arteries, Right<br>J Upper Extremity Arteries, Left<br>K Upper Extremity Arteries, Bilateral<br>L Intercostal and Bronchial Arteries<br>M Spinal Arteries<br>N Upper Arteries, Other<br>P Thoraco-Abdominal Aorta<br>Q Cervico-Cerebral Arch<br>R Intracranial Arteries<br>S Pulmonary Artery, Right<br>T Pulmonary Artery, Left<br>U Pulmonary Trunk | Ø High Osmolar<br>1 Low Osmolar<br>Y Other Contrast | 1 Laser | Ø Intraoperative |
| Ø Thoracic Aorta<br>1 Brachiocephalic-Subclavian Artery, Right<br>2 Subclavian Artery, Left<br>3 Common Carotid Artery, Right<br>4 Common Carotid Artery, Left<br>5 Common Carotid Arteries, Bilateral<br>6 Internal Carotid Artery, Right<br>7 Internal Carotid Artery, Left<br>8 Internal Carotid Arteries, Bilateral<br>9 External Carotid Artery, Right<br>B External Carotid Artery, Left<br>C External Carotid Arteries, Bilateral<br>D Vertebral Artery, Right<br>F Vertebral Artery, Left<br>G Vertebral Arteries, Bilateral<br>H Upper Extremity Arteries, Right<br>J Upper Extremity Arteries, Left<br>K Upper Extremity Arteries, Bilateral<br>L Intercostal and Bronchial Arteries<br>M Spinal Arteries<br>N Upper Arteries, Other<br>P Thoraco-Abdominal Aorta<br>Q Cervico-Cerebral Arch<br>R Intracranial Arteries<br>S Pulmonary Artery, Right<br>T Pulmonary Artery, Left<br>U Pulmonary Trunk | Ø High Osmolar<br>1 Low Osmolar<br>Y Other Contrast | Z None | Z None |

*B31 Continued on next page*

**B Imaging**
**3 Upper Arteries**
**1 Fluoroscopy**

*B31 Continued*

Definition: Single plane or bi-plane real time display of an image developed from the capture of external ionizing radiation on a fluorescent screen. The image may also be stored by either digital or analog means.

| Body Part Character 4 | Contrast Character 5 | Qualifier Character 6 | Qualifier Character 7 |
|---|---|---|---|
| Ø Thoracic Aorta<br>1 Brachiocephalic-Subclavian Artery, Right<br>2 Subclavian Artery, Left<br>3 Common Carotid Artery, Right<br>4 Common Carotid Artery, Left<br>5 Common Carotid Arteries, Bilateral<br>6 Internal Carotid Artery, Right<br>7 Internal Carotid Artery, Left<br>8 Internal Carotid Arteries, Bilateral<br>9 External Carotid Artery, Right<br>B External Carotid Artery, Left<br>C External Carotid Arteries, Bilateral<br>D Vertebral Artery, Right<br>F Vertebral Artery, Left<br>G Vertebral Arteries, Bilateral<br>H Upper Extremity Arteries, Right<br>J Upper Extremity Arteries, Left<br>K Upper Extremity Arteries, Bilateral<br>L Intercostal and Bronchial Arteries<br>M Spinal Arteries<br>N Upper Arteries, Other<br>P Thoraco-Abdominal Aorta<br>Q Cervico-Cerebral Arch<br>R Intracranial Arteries<br>S Pulmonary Artery, Right<br>T Pulmonary Artery, Left<br>U Pulmonary Trunk | Z None | Z None | Z None |

**B Imaging**
**3 Upper Arteries**
**2 Computerized Tomography (CT Scan)**

Definition: Computer reformatted digital display of multiplanar images developed from the capture of multiple exposures of external ionizing radiation

| Body Part Character 4 | Contrast Character 5 | Qualifier Character 6 | Qualifier Character 7 |
|---|---|---|---|
| Ø Thoracic Aorta<br>5 Common Carotid Arteries, Bilateral<br>8 Internal Carotid Arteries, Bilateral<br>G Vertebral Arteries, Bilateral<br>R Intracranial Arteries<br>S Pulmonary Artery, Right<br>T Pulmonary Artery, Left | Ø High Osmolar<br>1 Low Osmolar<br>Y Other Contrast | Z None | Z None |
| Ø Thoracic Aorta<br>5 Common Carotid Arteries, Bilateral<br>8 Internal Carotid Arteries, Bilateral<br>G Vertebral Arteries, Bilateral<br>R Intracranial Arteries<br>S Pulmonary Artery, Right<br>T Pulmonary Artery, Left | Z None | 2 Intravascular Optical Coherence<br>Z None | Z None |

**B Imaging**
**3 Upper Arteries**
**3 Magnetic Resonance Imaging (MRI)** Definition: Computer reformatted digital display of multiplanar images developed from the capture of radio-frequency signals emitted by nuclei in a body site excited within a magnetic field

| Body Part Character 4 | Contrast Character 5 | Qualifier Character 6 | Qualifier Character 7 |
|---|---|---|---|
| Ø Thoracic Aorta<br>5 Common Carotid Arteries, Bilateral<br>8 Internal Carotid Arteries, Bilateral<br>G Vertebral Arteries, Bilateral<br>H Upper Extremity Arteries, Right<br>J Upper Extremity Arteries, Left<br>K Upper Extremity Arteries, Bilateral<br>M Spinal Arteries<br>Q Cervico-Cerebral Arch<br>R Intracranial Arteries | Y Other Contrast | Ø Unenhanced and Enhanced<br>Z None | Z None |
| Ø Thoracic Aorta<br>5 Common Carotid Arteries, Bilateral<br>8 Internal Carotid Arteries, Bilateral<br>G Vertebral Arteries, Bilateral<br>H Upper Extremity Arteries, Right<br>J Upper Extremity Arteries, Left<br>K Upper Extremity Arteries, Bilateral<br>M Spinal Arteries<br>Q Cervico-Cerebral Arch<br>R Intracranial Arteries | Z None | Z None | Z None |

**B Imaging**
**3 Upper Arteries**
**4 Ultrasonography** Definition: Real time display of images of anatomy or flow information developed from the capture of relected and attenuated high frequency sound waves

| Body Part Character 4 | Contrast Character 5 | Qualifier Character 6 | Qualifier Character 7 |
|---|---|---|---|
| Ø Thoracic Aorta<br>1 Brachiocephalic-Subclavian Artery, Right<br>2 Subclavian Artery, Left<br>3 Common Carotid Artery, Right<br>4 Common Carotid Artery, Left<br>5 Common Carotid Arteries, Bilateral<br>6 Internal Carotid Artery, Right<br>7 Internal Carotid Artery, Left<br>8 Internal Carotid Arteries, Bilateral<br>H Upper Extremity Arteries, Right<br>J Upper Extremity Arteries, Left<br>K Upper Extremity Arteries, Bilateral<br>R Intracranial Arteries<br>S Pulmonary Artery, Right<br>T Pulmonary Artery, Left<br>V Ophthalmic Arteries | Z None | Z None | 3 Intravascular<br>Z None |

**B Imaging**
**4 Lower Arteries**
**Ø Plain Radiography** Definition: Planar display of an image developed from the capture of external ionizing radiation on photographic or photoconductive plate

| Body Part Character 4 | Contrast Character 5 | Qualifier Character 6 | Qualifier Character 7 |
|---|---|---|---|
| Ø Abdominal Aorta<br>2 Hepatic Artery<br>3 Splenic Arteries<br>4 Superior Mesenteric Artery<br>5 Inferior Mesenteric Artery<br>6 Renal Artery, Right<br>7 Renal Artery, Left<br>8 Renal Arteries, Bilateral<br>9 Lumbar Arteries<br>B Intra-Abdominal Arteries, Other<br>C Pelvic Arteries<br>D Aorta and Bilateral Lower Extremity Arteries<br>F Lower Extremity Arteries, Right<br>G Lower Extremity Arteries, Left<br>J Lower Arteries, Other<br>M Renal Artery Transplant | Ø High Osmolar<br>1 Low Osmolar<br>Y Other Contrast | Z None | Z None |

**B Imaging**
**4 Lower Arteries**
**1 Fluoroscopy** Definition: Single plane or bi-plane real time display of an image developed from the capture of external ionizing radiation on a fluorescent screen. The image may also be stored by either digital or analog means.

| Body Part Character 4 | Contrast Character 5 | Qualifier Character 6 | Qualifier Character 7 |
|---|---|---|---|
| Ø Abdominal Aorta<br>2 Hepatic Artery<br>3 Splenic Arteries<br>4 Superior Mesenteric Artery<br>5 Inferior Mesenteric Artery<br>6 Renal Artery, Right<br>7 Renal Artery, Left<br>8 Renal Arteries, Bilateral<br>9 Lumbar Arteries<br>B Intra-Abdominal Arteries, Other<br>C Pelvic Arteries<br>D Aorta and Bilateral Lower Extremity Arteries<br>F Lower Extremity Arteries, Right<br>G Lower Extremity Arteries, Left<br>J Lower Arteries, Other | Ø High Osmolar<br>1 Low Osmolar<br>Y Other Contrast | 1 Laser | Ø Intraoperative |
| Ø Abdominal Aorta<br>2 Hepatic Artery<br>3 Splenic Arteries<br>4 Superior Mesenteric Artery<br>5 Inferior Mesenteric Artery<br>6 Renal Artery, Right<br>7 Renal Artery, Left<br>8 Renal Arteries, Bilateral<br>9 Lumbar Arteries<br>B Intra-Abdominal Arteries, Other<br>C Pelvic Arteries<br>D Aorta and Bilateral Lower Extremity Arteries<br>F Lower Extremity Arteries, Right<br>G Lower Extremity Arteries, Left<br>J Lower Arteries, Other | Ø High Osmolar<br>1 Low Osmolar<br>Y Other Contrast | Z None | Z None |
| Ø Abdominal Aorta<br>2 Hepatic Artery<br>3 Splenic Arteries<br>4 Superior Mesenteric Artery<br>5 Inferior Mesenteric Artery<br>6 Renal Artery, Right<br>7 Renal Artery, Left<br>8 Renal Arteries, Bilateral<br>9 Lumbar Arteries<br>B Intra-Abdominal Arteries, Other<br>C Pelvic Arteries<br>D Aorta and Bilateral Lower Extremity Arteries<br>F Lower Extremity Arteries, Right<br>G Lower Extremity Arteries, Left<br>J Lower Arteries, Other | Z None | Z None | Z None |

**B Imaging**
**4 Lower Arteries**
**2 Computerized Tomography (CT Scan)** Definition: Computer reformatted digital display of multiplanar images developed from the capture of multiple exposures of external ionizing radiation

| Body Part Character 4 | Contrast Character 5 | Qualifier Character 6 | Qualifier Character 7 |
|---|---|---|---|
| Ø Abdominal Aorta<br>1 Celiac Artery<br>4 Superior Mesenteric Artery<br>8 Renal Arteries, Bilateral<br>C Pelvic Arteries<br>F Lower Extremity Arteries, Right<br>G Lower Extremity Arteries, Left<br>H Lower Extremity Arteries, Bilateral<br>M Renal Artery Transplant | Ø High Osmolar<br>1 Low Osmolar<br>Y Other Contrast | Z None | Z None |
| Ø Abdominal Aorta<br>1 Celiac Artery<br>4 Superior Mesenteric Artery<br>8 Renal Arteries, Bilateral<br>C Pelvic Arteries<br>F Lower Extremity Arteries, Right<br>G Lower Extremity Arteries, Left<br>H Lower Extremity Arteries, Bilateral<br>M Renal Artery Transplant | Z None | 2 Intravascular Optical Coherence<br>Z None | Z None |

**B Imaging**
**4 Lower Arteries**
**3 Magnetic Resonance Imaging (MRI)** Definition: Computer reformatted digital display of multiplanar images developed from the capture of radio-frequency signals emitted by nuclei in a body site excited within a magnetic field

| Body Part Character 4 | Contrast Character 5 | Qualifier Character 6 | Qualifier Character 7 |
|---|---|---|---|
| Ø Abdominal Aorta<br>1 Celiac Artery<br>4 Superior Mesenteric Artery<br>8 Renal Arteries, Bilateral<br>C Pelvic Arteries<br>F Lower Extremity Arteries, Right<br>G Lower Extremity Arteries, Left<br>H Lower Extremity Arteries, Bilateral | Y Other Contrast | Ø Unenhanced and Enhanced<br>Z None | Z None |
| Ø Abdominal Aorta<br>1 Celiac Artery<br>4 Superior Mesenteric Artery<br>8 Renal Arteries, Bilateral<br>C Pelvic Arteries<br>F Lower Extremity Arteries, Right<br>G Lower Extremity Arteries, Left<br>H Lower Extremity Arteries, Bilateral | Z None | Z None | Z None |

**B Imaging**
**4 Lower Arteries**
**4 Ultrasonography** Definition: Real time display of images of anatomy or flow information developed from the capture of relected and attenuated high frequency sound waves

| Body Part Character 4 | Contrast Character 5 | Qualifier Character 6 | Qualifier Character 7 |
|---|---|---|---|
| Ø Abdominal Aorta<br>4 Superior Mesenteric Artery<br>5 Inferior Mesenteric Artery<br>6 Renal Artery, Right<br>7 Renal Artery, Left<br>8 Renal Arteries, Bilateral<br>B Intra-Abdominal Arteries, Other<br>F Lower Extremity Arteries, Right<br>G Lower Extremity Arteries, Left<br>H Lower Extremity Arteries, Bilateral<br>K Celiac and Mesenteric Arteries<br>L Femoral Artery<br>N Penile Arteries | Z None | Z None | 3 Intravascular<br>Z None |

**B Imaging**
**5 Veins**
**Ø Plain Radiography** Definition: Planar display of an image developed from the capture of external ionizing radiation on photographic or photoconductive plate

| Body Part Character 4 | Contrast Character 5 | Qualifier Character 6 | Qualifier Character 7 |
|---|---|---|---|
| **Ø** Epidural Veins<br>**1** Cerebral and Cerebellar Veins<br>**2** Intracranial Sinuses<br>**3** Jugular Veins, Right<br>**4** Jugular Veins, Left<br>**5** Jugular Veins, Bilateral<br>**6** Subclavian Vein, Right<br>**7** Subclavian Vein, Left<br>**8** Superior Vena Cava<br>**9** Inferior Vena Cava<br>**B** Lower Extremity Veins, Right<br>**C** Lower Extremity Veins, Left<br>**D** Lower Extremity Veins, Bilateral<br>**F** Pelvic (Iliac) Veins, Right<br>**G** Pelvic (Iliac) Veins, Left<br>**H** Pelvic (Iliac) Veins, Bilateral<br>**J** Renal Vein, Right<br>**K** Renal Vein, Left<br>**L** Renal Veins, Bilateral<br>**M** Upper Extremity Veins, Right<br>**N** Upper Extremity Veins, Left<br>**P** Upper Extremity Veins, Bilateral<br>**Q** Pulmonary Vein, Right<br>**R** Pulmonary Vein, Left<br>**S** Pulmonary Veins, Bilateral<br>**T** Portal and Splanchnic Veins<br>**V** Veins, Other<br>**W** Dialysis Shunt/Fistula | **Ø** High Osmolar<br>**1** Low Osmolar<br>**Y** Other Contrast | **Z** None | **Z** None |

**B Imaging**
**5 Veins**
**1 Fluoroscopy** Definition: Single plane or bi-plane real time display of an image developed from the capture of external ionizing radioation on a fluorescent screen. The image may also be stored by either digital or analog means.

| Body Part Character 4 | Contrast Character 5 | Qualifier Character 6 | Qualifier Character 7 |
|---|---|---|---|
| **Ø** Epidural Veins<br>**1** Cerebral and Cerebellar Veins<br>**2** Intracranial Sinuses<br>**3** Jugular Veins, Right<br>**4** Jugular Veins, Left<br>**5** Jugular Veins, Bilateral<br>**6** Subclavian Vein, Right<br>**7** Subclavian Vein, Left<br>**8** Superior Vena Cava<br>**9** Inferior Vena Cava<br>**B** Lower Extremity Veins, Right<br>**C** Lower Extremity Veins, Left<br>**D** Lower Extremity Veins, Bilateral<br>**F** Pelvic (Iliac) Veins, Right<br>**G** Pelvic (Iliac) Veins, Left<br>**H** Pelvic (Iliac) Veins, Bilateral<br>**J** Renal Vein, Right<br>**K** Renal Vein, Left<br>**L** Renal Veins, Bilateral<br>**M** Upper Extremity Veins, Right<br>**N** Upper Extremity Veins, Left<br>**P** Upper Extremity Veins, Bilateral<br>**Q** Pulmonary Vein, Right<br>**R** Pulmonary Vein, Left<br>**S** Pulmonary Veins, Bilateral<br>**T** Portal and Splanchnic Veins<br>**V** Veins, Other<br>**W** Dialysis Shunt/Fistula | **Ø** High Osmolar<br>**1** Low Osmolar<br>**Y** Other Contrast<br>**Z** None | **Z** None | **A** Guidance<br>**Z** None |

**B Imaging**
**5 Veins**
**2 Computerized Tomography (CT Scan)** Definition: Computer reformatted digital display of multiplanar images developed from the capture of multiple exposures of external ionizing radiation

| Body Part Character 4 | Contrast Character 5 | Qualifier Character 6 | Qualifier Character 7 |
|---|---|---|---|
| 2 Intracranial Sinuses<br>8 Superior Vena Cava<br>9 Inferior Vena Cava<br>F Pelvic (Iliac) Veins, Right<br>G Pelvic (Iliac) Veins, Left<br>H Pelvic (Iliac) Veins, Bilateral<br>J Renal Vein, Right<br>K Renal Vein, Left<br>L Renal Veins, Bilateral<br>Q Pulmonary Vein, Right<br>R Pulmonary Vein, Left<br>S Pulmonary Veins, Bilateral<br>T Portal and Splanchnic Veins | Ø High Osmolar<br>1 Low Osmolar<br>Y Other Contrast | Ø Unenhanced and Enhanced<br>Z None | Z None |
| 2 Intracranial Sinuses<br>8 Superior Vena Cava<br>9 Inferior Vena Cava<br>F Pelvic (Iliac) Veins, Right<br>G Pelvic (Iliac) Veins, Left<br>H Pelvic (Iliac) Veins, Bilateral<br>J Renal Vein, Right<br>K Renal Vein, Left<br>L Renal Veins, Bilateral<br>Q Pulmonary Vein, Right<br>R Pulmonary Vein, Left<br>S Pulmonary Veins, Bilateral<br>T Portal and Splanchnic Veins | Z None | 2 Intravascular Optical Coherence<br>Z None | Z None |

**B Imaging**
**5 Veins**
**3 Magnetic Resonance Imaging (MRI)** Definition: Computer reformatted digital display of multiplanar images developed from the capture of radio-frequency signals emitted by nuclei in a body site excited within a magnetic field

| Body Part Character 4 | Contrast Character 5 | Qualifier Character 6 | Qualifier Character 7 |
|---|---|---|---|
| 1 Cerebral and Cerebellar Veins<br>2 Intracranial Sinuses<br>5 Jugular Veins, Bilateral<br>8 Superior Vena Cava<br>9 Inferior Vena Cava<br>B Lower Extremity Veins, Right<br>C Lower Extremity Veins, Left<br>D Lower Extremity Veins, Bilateral<br>H Pelvic (Iliac) Veins, Bilateral<br>L Renal Veins, Bilateral<br>M Upper Extremity Veins, Right<br>N Upper Extremity Veins, Left<br>P Upper Extremity Veins, Bilateral<br>S Pulmonary Veins, Bilateral<br>T Portal and Splanchnic Veins<br>V Veins, Other | Y Other Contrast | Ø Unenhanced and Enhanced<br>Z None | Z None |
| 1 Cerebral and Cerebellar Veins<br>2 Intracranial Sinuses<br>5 Jugular Veins, Bilateral<br>8 Superior Vena Cava<br>9 Inferior Vena Cava<br>B Lower Extremity Veins, Right<br>C Lower Extremity Veins, Left<br>D Lower Extremity Veins, Bilateral<br>H Pelvic (Iliac) Veins, Bilateral<br>L Renal Veins, Bilateral<br>M Upper Extremity Veins, Right<br>N Upper Extremity Veins, Left<br>P Upper Extremity Veins, Bilateral<br>S Pulmonary Veins, Bilateral<br>T Portal and Splanchnic Veins<br>V Veins, Other | Z None | Z None | Z None |

**B Imaging**
**5 Veins**
**4 Ultrasonography** Definition: Real time display of images of anatomy or flow information developed from the capture of relected and attenuated high frequency sound waves

| Body Part Character 4 | Contrast Character 5 | Qualifier Character 6 | Qualifier Character 7 |
|---|---|---|---|
| 3 Jugular Veins, Right<br>4 Jugular Veins, Left<br>6 Subclavian Vein, Right<br>7 Subclavian Vein, Left<br>8 Superior Vena Cava<br>9 Inferior Vena Cava<br>B Lower Extremity Veins, Right<br>C Lower Extremity Veins, Left<br>D Lower Extremity Veins, Bilateral<br>J Renal Vein, Right<br>K Renal Vein, Left<br>L Renal Veins, Bilateral<br>M Upper Extremity Veins, Right<br>N Upper Extremity Veins, Left<br>P Upper Extremity Veins, Bilateral<br>T Portal and Splanchnic Veins | Z None | Z None | 3 Intravascular<br>A Guidance<br>Z None |

**B Imaging**
**7 Lymphatic System**
**Ø Plain Radiography** Definition: Planar display of an image developed from the capture of external ionizing radiation on photographic or photoconductive plate

| Body Part Character 4 | Contrast Character 5 | Qualifier Character 6 | Qualifier Character 7 |
|---|---|---|---|
| Ø Abdominal/Retroperitoneal Lymphatics, Unilateral<br>1 Abdominal/Retroperitoneal Lymphatics, Bilateral<br>4 Lymphatics, Head and Neck<br>5 Upper Extremity Lymphatics, Right<br>6 Upper Extremity Lymphatics, Left<br>7 Upper Extremity Lymphatics, Bilateral<br>8 Lower Extremity Lymphatics, Right<br>9 Lower Extremity Lymphatics, Left<br>B Lower Extremity Lymphatics, Bilateral<br>C Lymphatics, Pelvic | Ø High Osmolar<br>1 Low Osmolar<br>Y Other Contrast | Z None | Z None |

**B Imaging**
**8 Eye**
**Ø Plain Radiography** Definition: Planar display of an image developed from the capture of external ionizing radiation on photographic or photoconductive plate

| Body Part Character 4 | Contrast Character 5 | Qualifier Character 6 | Qualifier Character 7 |
|---|---|---|---|
| Ø Lacrimal Duct, Right<br>1 Lacrimal Duct, Left<br>2 Lacrimal Ducts, Bilateral | Ø High Osmolar<br>1 Low Osmolar<br>Y Other Contrast | Z None | Z None |
| 3 Optic Foramina, Right<br>4 Optic Foramina, Left<br>5 Eye, Right<br>6 Eye, Left<br>7 Eyes, Bilateral | Z None | Z None | Z None |

**B Imaging**
**8 Eye**
**2 Computerized Tomography (CT Scan)** Definition: Computer reformatted digital display of multiplanar images developed from the capture of multiple exposures of external ionizing radiation

| Body Part Character 4 | Contrast Character 5 | Qualifier Character 6 | Qualifier Character 7 |
|---|---|---|---|
| 5 Eye, Right<br>6 Eye, Left<br>7 Eyes, Bilateral | Ø High Osmolar<br>1 Low Osmolar<br>Y Other Contrast | Ø Unenhanced and Enhanced<br>Z None | Z None |
| 5 Eye, Right<br>6 Eye, Left<br>7 Eyes, Bilateral | Z None | Z None | Z None |

**B Imaging**
**8 Eye**
**3 Magnetic Resonance Imaging (MRI)** Definition: Computer reformatted digital display of multiplanar images developed from the capture of radio-frequency signals emitted by nuclei in a body site excited within a magnetic field

| Body Part Character 4 | Contrast Character 5 | Qualifier Character 6 | Qualifier Character 7 |
|---|---|---|---|
| 5 Eye, Right<br>6 Eye, Left<br>7 Eyes, Bilateral | Y Other Contrast | Ø Unenhanced and Enhanced<br>Z None | Z None |
| 5 Eye, Right<br>6 Eye, Left<br>7 Eyes, Bilateral | Z None | Z None | Z None |

**B Imaging**
**8 Eye**
**4 Ultrasonography** Definition: Real time display of images of anatomy or flow information developed from the capture of relected and attenuated high frequency sound waves

| Body Part Character 4 | Contrast Character 5 | Qualifier Character 6 | Qualifier Character 7 |
|---|---|---|---|
| 5 Eye, Right<br>6 Eye, Left<br>7 Eyes, Bilateral | Z None | Z None | Z None |

**B Imaging**
**9 Ear, Nose, Mouth and Throat**
**Ø Plain Radiography** Definition: Planar display of an image developed from the capture of external ionizing radiation on photographic or photoconductive plate

| Body Part Character 4 | Contrast Character 5 | Qualifier Character 6 | Qualifier Character 7 |
|---|---|---|---|
| 2 Paranasal Sinuses<br>F Nasopharynx/Oropharynx<br>H Mastoids | Z None | Z None | Z None |
| 4 Parotid Gland, Right<br>5 Parotid Gland, Left<br>6 Parotid Glands, Bilateral<br>7 Submandibular Gland, Right<br>8 Submandibular Gland, Left<br>9 Submandibular Glands, Bilateral<br>B Salivary Gland, Right<br>C Salivary Gland, Left<br>D Salivary Glands, Bilateral | Ø High Osmolar<br>1 Low Osmolar<br>Y Other Contrast | Z None | Z None |

**B Imaging**
**9 Ear, Nose, Mouth and Throat**
**1 Fluoroscopy** Definition: Single plane or bi-plane real time display of an image developed from the capture of external ionizing radioation on a fluorescent screen. The image may also be stored by either digital or analog means.

| Body Part Character 4 | Contrast Character 5 | Qualifier Character 6 | Qualifier Character 7 |
|---|---|---|---|
| G Pharynx and Epiglottis<br>J Larynx | Y Other Contrast<br>Z None | Z None | Z None |

**B Imaging**
**9 Ear, Nose, Mouth and Throat**
**2 Computerized Tomography (CT Scan)** Definition: Computer reformatted digital display of multiplanar images developed from the capture of multiple exposures of external ionizing radiation

| Body Part Character 4 | Contrast Character 5 | Qualifier Character 6 | Qualifier Character 7 |
|---|---|---|---|
| Ø Ear<br>2 Paranasal Sinuses<br>6 Parotid Glands, Bilateral<br>9 Submandibular Glands, Bilateral<br>D Salivary Glands, Bilateral<br>F Nasopharynx/Oropharynx<br>J Larynx | Ø High Osmolar<br>1 Low Osmolar<br>Y Other Contrast | Ø Unenhanced and Enhanced<br>Z None | Z None |
| Ø Ear<br>2 Paranasal Sinuses<br>6 Parotid Glands, Bilateral<br>9 Submandibular Glands, Bilateral<br>D Salivary Glands, Bilateral<br>F Nasopharynx/Oropharynx<br>J Larynx | Z None | Z None | Z None |

**B Imaging**
**9 Ear, Nose, Mouth and Throat**
**3 Magnetic Resonance Imaging (MRI)** Definition: Computer reformatted digital display of multiplanar images developed from the capture of radio-frequency signals emitted by nuclei in a body site excited within a magnetic field

| Body Part Character 4 | Contrast Character 5 | Qualifier Character 6 | Qualifier Character 7 |
|---|---|---|---|
| Ø Ear<br>2 Paranasal Sinuses<br>6 Parotid Glands, Bilateral<br>9 Submandibular Glands, Bilateral<br>D Salivary Glands, Bilateral<br>F Nasopharynx/Oropharynx<br>J Larynx | Y Other Contrast | Ø Unenhanced and Enhanced<br>Z None | Z None |
| Ø Ear<br>2 Paranasal Sinuses<br>6 Parotid Glands, Bilateral<br>9 Submandibular Glands, Bilateral<br>D Salivary Glands, Bilateral<br>F Nasopharynx/Oropharynx<br>J Larynx | Z None | Z None | Z None |

**B Imaging**
**B Respiratory System**
**Ø Plain Radiography** Definition: Planar display of an image developed from the capture of external ionizing radiation on photographic or photoconductive plate

| Body Part Character 4 | Contrast Character 5 | Qualifier Character 6 | Qualifier Character 7 |
|---|---|---|---|
| 7 Tracheobronchial Tree, Right<br>8 Tracheobronchial Tree, Left<br>9 Tracheobronchial Trees, Bilateral | Y Other Contrast | Z None | Z None |
| D Upper Airways | Z None | Z None | Z None |

**B Imaging**
**B Respiratory System**
**1 Fluoroscopy** Definition: Single plane or bi-plane real time display of an image developed from the capture of external ionizing radioation on a fluorescent screen. The image may also be stored by either digital or analog means.

| Body Part Character 4 | Contrast Character 5 | Qualifier Character 6 | Qualifier Character 7 |
|---|---|---|---|
| 2 Lung, Right<br>3 Lung, Left<br>4 Lungs, Bilateral<br>6 Diaphragm<br>C Mediastinum<br>D Upper Airways | Z None | Z None | Z None |
| 7 Tracheobronchial Tree, Right<br>8 Tracheobronchial Tree, Left<br>9 Tracheobronchial Trees, Bilateral | Y Other Contrast | Z None | Z None |

**B Imaging**
**B Respiratory System**
**2 Computerized Tomography (CT Scan)** Definition: Computer reformatted digital display of multiplanar images developed from the capture of multiple exposures of external ionizing radiation

| Body Part Character 4 | Contrast Character 5 | Qualifier Character 6 | Qualifier Character 7 |
|---|---|---|---|
| 4 Lungs, Bilateral<br>7 Tracheobronchial Tree, Right<br>8 Tracheobronchial Tree, Left<br>9 Tracheobronchial Trees, Bilateral<br>F Trachea/Airways | Ø High Osmolar<br>1 Low Osmolar<br>Y Other Contrast | Ø Unenhanced and Enhanced<br>Z None | Z None |
| 4 Lungs, Bilateral<br>7 Tracheobronchial Tree, Right<br>8 Tracheobronchial Tree, Left<br>9 Tracheobronchial Trees, Bilateral<br>F Trachea/Airways | Z None | Z None | Z None |

**B Imaging**
**B Respiratory System**
**3 Magnetic Resonance Imaging (MRI)** Definition: Computer reformatted digital display of multiplanar images developed from the capture of radio-frequency signals emitted by nuclei in a body site excited within a magnetic field

| Body Part Character 4 | Contrast Character 5 | Qualifier Character 6 | Qualifier Character 7 |
|---|---|---|---|
| G Lung Apices | Y Other Contrast | Ø Unenhanced and Enhanced<br>Z None | Z None |
| G Lung Apices | Z None | Z None | Z None |

**B Imaging**
**B Respiratory System**
**4 Ultrasonography** Definition: Real time display of images of anatomy or flow information developed from the capture of relected and attenuated high frequency sound waves

| Body Part Character 4 | Contrast Character 5 | Qualifier Character 6 | Qualifier Character 7 |
|---|---|---|---|
| B Pleura<br>C Mediastinum | Z None | Z None | Z None |

**B Imaging**
**D Gastrointestinal System**
**1 Fluoroscopy** Definition: Single plane or bi-plane real time display of an image developed from the capture of external ionizing radioation on a fluorescent screen. The image may also be stored by either digital or analog means.

| Body Part Character 4 | Contrast Character 5 | Qualifier Character 6 | Qualifier Character 7 |
|---|---|---|---|
| 1 Esophagus<br>2 Stomach<br>3 Small Bowel<br>4 Colon<br>5 Upper GI<br>6 Upper GI and Small Bowel<br>9 Duodenum<br>B Mouth/Oropharynx | Y Other Contrast<br>Z None | Z None | Z None |

**B Imaging**
**D Gastrointestinal System**
**2 Computerized Tomography (CT Scan)** Definition: Computer reformatted digital display of multiplanar images developed from the capture of multiple exposures of external ionizing radiation

| Body Part Character 4 | Contrast Character 5 | Qualifier Character 6 | Qualifier Character 7 |
|---|---|---|---|
| 4 Colon | Ø High Osmolar<br>1 Low Osmolar<br>Y Other Contrast | Ø Unenhanced and Enhanced<br>Z None | Z None |
| 4 Colon | Z None | Z None | Z None |

**B Imaging**
**D Gastrointestinal System**
**4 Ultrasonography** Definition: Real time display of images of anatomy or flow information developed from the capture of relected and attenuated high frequency sound waves

| Body Part Character 4 | Contrast Character 5 | Qualifier Character 6 | Qualifier Character 7 |
|---|---|---|---|
| 1 Esophagus<br>2 Stomach<br>7 Gastrointestinal Tract<br>8 Appendix<br>9 Duodenum<br>C Rectum | Z None | Z None | Z None |

**B Imaging**
**F Hepatobiliary System and Pancreas**
**Ø Plain Radiography** Definition: Planar display of an image developed from the capture of external ionizing radiation on photographic or photoconductive plate

| Body Part Character 4 | Contrast Character 5 | Qualifier Character 6 | Qualifier Character 7 |
|---|---|---|---|
| Ø Bile Ducts<br>3 Gallbladder and Bile Ducts<br>C Hepatobiliary System, All | Ø High Osmolar<br>1 Low Osmolar<br>Y Other Contrast | Z None | Z None |

**B Imaging**
**F Hepatobiliary System and Pancreas**
**1 Fluoroscopy** Definition: Single plane or bi-plane real time display of an image developed from the capture of external ionizing radioation on a fluorescent screen. The image may also be stored by either digital or analog means.

| Body Part Character 4 | Contrast Character 5 | Qualifier Character 6 | Qualifier Character 7 |
|---|---|---|---|
| Ø Bile Ducts<br>1 Biliary and Pancreatic Ducts<br>2 Gallbladder<br>3 Gallbladder and Bile Ducts<br>4 Gallbladder, Bile Ducts and Pancreatic Ducts<br>8 Pancreatic Ducts | Ø High Osmolar<br>1 Low Osmolar<br>Y Other Contrast | Z None | Z None |

**B Imaging**
**F Hepatobiliary System and Pancreas**
**2 Computerized Tomography (CT Scan)** Definition: Computer reformatted digital display of multiplanar images developed from the capture of multiple exposures of external ionizing radiation

| Body Part Character 4 | Contrast Character 5 | Qualifier Character 6 | Qualifier Character 7 |
|---|---|---|---|
| 5 Liver<br>6 Liver and Spleen<br>7 Pancreas<br>C Hepatobiliary System, All | Ø High Osmolar<br>1 Low Osmolar<br>Y Other Contrast | Ø Unenhanced and Enhanced<br>Z None | Z None |
| 5 Liver<br>6 Liver and Spleen<br>7 Pancreas<br>C Hepatobiliary System, All | Z None | Z None | Z None |

**B Imaging**
**F Hepatobiliary System and Pancreas**
**3 Magnetic Resonance Imaging (MRI)** Definition: Computer reformatted digital display of multiplanar images developed from the capture of radio-frequency signals emitted by nuclei in a body site excited within a magnetic field

| Body Part Character 4 | Contrast Character 5 | Qualifier Character 6 | Qualifier Character 7 |
|---|---|---|---|
| 5 Liver<br>6 Liver and Spleen<br>7 Pancreas | Y Other Contrast | Ø Unenhanced and Enhanced<br>Z None | Z None |
| 5 Liver<br>6 Liver and Spleen<br>7 Pancreas | Z None | Z None | Z None |

**B Imaging**
**F Hepatobiliary System and Pancreas**
**4 Ultrasonography** Definition: Real time display of images of anatomy or flow information developed from the capture of relected and attenuated high frequency sound waves

| Body Part Character 4 | Contrast Character 5 | Qualifier Character 6 | Qualifier Character 7 |
|---|---|---|---|
| Ø Bile Ducts<br>2 Gallbladder<br>3 Gallbladder and Bile Ducts<br>5 Liver<br>6 Liver and Spleen<br>7 Pancreas<br>C Hepatobiliary System, All | Z None | Z None | Z None |

**B Imaging**
**G Endocrine System**
**2 Computerized Tomography (CT Scan)** Definition: Computer reformatted digital display of multiplanar images developed from the capture of multiple exposures of external ionizing radiation

| Body Part Character 4 | Contrast Character 5 | Qualifier Character 6 | Qualifier Character 7 |
|---|---|---|---|
| 2 Adrenal Glands, Bilateral<br>3 Parathyroid Glands<br>4 Thyroid Gland | Ø High Osmolar<br>1 Low Osmolar<br>Y Other Contrast | Ø Unenhanced and Enhanced<br>Z None | Z None |
| 2 Adrenal Glands, Bilateral<br>3 Parathyroid Glands<br>4 Thyroid Gland | Z None | Z None | Z None |

**B Imaging**
**G Endocrine System**
**3 Magnetic Resonance Imaging (MRI)** Definition: Computer reformatted digital display of multiplanar images developed from the capture of radio-frequency signals emitted by nuclei in a body site excited within a magnetic field

| Body Part Character 4 | Contrast Character 5 | Qualifier Character 6 | Qualifier Character 7 |
|---|---|---|---|
| 2 Adrenal Glands, Bilateral<br>3 Parathyroid Glands<br>4 Thyroid Gland | Y Other Contrast | Ø Unenhanced and Enhanced<br>Z None | Z None |
| 2 Adrenal Glands, Bilateral<br>3 Parathyroid Glands<br>4 Thyroid Gland | Z None | Z None | Z None |

**B Imaging**
**G Endocrine System**
**4 Ultrasonography** Definition: Real time display of images of anatomy or flow information developed from the capture of relected and attenuated high frequency sound waves

| Body Part Character 4 | Contrast Character 5 | Qualifier Character 6 | Qualifier Character 7 |
|---|---|---|---|
| Ø Adrenal Gland, Right<br>1 Adrenal Gland, Left<br>2 Adrenal Glands, Bilateral<br>3 Parathyroid Glands<br>4 Thyroid Gland | Z None | Z None | Z None |

**B Imaging**
**H Skin, Subcutaneous Tissue and Breast**
**Ø Plain Radiography** Definition: Planar display of an image developed from the capture of external ionizing radiation on photographic or photoconductive plate

| Body Part Character 4 | Contrast Character 5 | Qualifier Character 6 | Qualifier Character 7 |
|---|---|---|---|
| Ø Breast, Right<br>1 Breast, Left<br>2 Breasts, Bilateral | Z None | Z None | Z None |
| 3 Single Mammary Duct, Right<br>4 Single Mammary Duct, Left<br>5 Multiple Mammary Ducts, Right<br>6 Multiple Mammary Ducts, Left | Ø High Osmolar<br>1 Low Osmolar<br>Y Other Contrast<br>Z None | Z None | Z None |

**B Imaging**
**H Skin, Subcutaneous Tissue and Breast**
**3 Magnetic Resonance Imaging (MRI)** Definition: Computer reformatted digital display of multiplanar images developed from the capture of radio-frequency signals emitted by nuclei in a body site excited within a magnetic field

| Body Part Character 4 | Contrast Character 5 | Qualifier Character 6 | Qualifier Character 7 |
|---|---|---|---|
| Ø Breast, Right<br>1 Breast, Left<br>2 Breasts, Bilateral<br>D Subcutaneous Tissue, Head/Neck<br>F Subcutaneous Tissue, Upper Extremity<br>G Subcutaneous Tissue, Thorax<br>H Subcutaneous Tissue, Abdomen and Pelvis<br>J Subcutaneous Tissue, Lower Extremity | Y Other Contrast | Ø Unenhanced and Enhanced<br>Z None | Z None |
| Ø Breast, Right<br>1 Breast, Left<br>2 Breasts, Bilateral<br>D Subcutaneous Tissue, Head/Neck<br>F Subcutaneous Tissue, Upper Extremity<br>G Subcutaneous Tissue, Thorax<br>H Subcutaneous Tissue, Abdomen and Pelvis<br>J Subcutaneous Tissue, Lower Extremity | Z None | Z None | Z None |

**B Imaging**
**H Skin, Subcutaneous Tissue and Breast**
**4 Ultrasonography** Definition: Real time display of images of anatomy or flow information developed from the capture of relected and attenuated high frequency sound waves

| Body Part Character 4 | Contrast Character 5 | Qualifier Character 6 | Qualifier Character 7 |
|---|---|---|---|
| **Ø** Breast, Right<br>**1** Breast, Left<br>**2** Breasts, Bilateral<br>**7** Extremity, Upper<br>**8** Extremity, Lower<br>**9** Abdominal Wall<br>**B** Chest Wall<br>**C** Head and Neck | **Z** None | **Z** None | **Z** None |

**B Imaging**
**L Connective Tissue**
**3 Magnetic Resonance Imaging (MRI)** Definition: Computer reformatted digital display of multiplanar images developed from the capture of radio-frequency signals emitted by nuclei in a body site excited within a magnetic field

| Body Part Character 4 | Contrast Character 5 | Qualifier Character 6 | Qualifier Character 7 |
|---|---|---|---|
| **Ø** Connective Tissue, Upper Extremity<br>**1** Connective Tissue, Lower Extremity<br>**2** Tendons, Upper Extremity<br>**3** Tendons, Lower Extremity | **Y** Other Contrast | **Ø** Unenhanced and Enhanced<br>**Z** None | **Z** None |
| **Ø** Connective Tissue, Upper Extremity<br>**1** Connective Tissue, Lower Extremity<br>**2** Tendons, Upper Extremity<br>**3** Tendons, Lower Extremity | **Z** None | **Z** None | **Z** None |

**B Imaging**
**L Connective Tissue**
**4 Ultrasonography** Definition: Real time display of images of anatomy or flow information developed from the capture of relected and attenuated high frequency sound waves

| Body Part Character 4 | Contrast Character 5 | Qualifier Character 6 | Qualifier Character 7 |
|---|---|---|---|
| **Ø** Connective Tissue, Upper Extremity<br>**1** Connective Tissue, Lower Extremity<br>**2** Tendons, Upper Extremity<br>**3** Tendons, Lower Extremity | **Z** None | **Z** None | **Z** None |

**B Imaging**
**N Skull and Facial Bones**
**Ø Plain Radiography** Definition: Planar display of an image developed from the capture of external ionizing radiation on photographic or photoconductive plate

| Body Part Character 4 | Contrast Character 5 | Qualifier Character 6 | Qualifier Character 7 |
|---|---|---|---|
| **Ø** Skull<br>**1** Orbit, Right<br>**2** Orbit, Left<br>**3** Orbits, Bilateral<br>**4** Nasal Bones<br>**5** Facial Bones<br>**6** Mandible<br>**B** Zygomatic Arch, Right<br>**C** Zygomatic Arch, Left<br>**D** Zygomatic Arches, Bilateral<br>**G** Tooth, Single<br>**H** Teeth, Multiple<br>**J** Teeth, All | **Z** None | **Z** None | **Z** None |
| **7** Temporomandibular Joint, Right<br>**8** Temporomandibular Joint, Left<br>**9** Temporomandibular Joints, Bilateral | **Ø** High Osmolar<br>**1** Low Osmolar<br>**Y** Other Contrast<br>**Z** None | **Z** None | **Z** None |

**B Imaging**
**N Skull and Facial Bones**
**1 Fluoroscopy** Definition: Single plane or bi-plane real time display of an image developed from the capture of external ionizing radioation on a fluorescent screen. The image may also be stored by either digital or analog means.

| Body Part Character 4 | Contrast Character 5 | Qualifier Character 6 | Qualifier Character 7 |
|---|---|---|---|
| 7 Temporomandibular Joint, Right<br>8 Temporomandibular Joint, Left<br>9 Temporomandibular Joints, Bilateral | Ø High Osmolar<br>1 Low Osmolar<br>Y Other Contrast<br>Z None | Z None | Z None |

**B Imaging**
**N Skull and Facial Bones**
**2 Computerized Tomography (CT Scan)** Definition: Computer reformatted digital display of multiplanar images developed from the capture of multiple exposures of external ionizing radiation

| Body Part Character 4 | Contrast Character 5 | Qualifier Character 6 | Qualifier Character 7 |
|---|---|---|---|
| Ø Skull<br>3 Orbits, Bilateral<br>5 Facial Bones<br>6 Mandible<br>9 Temporomandibular Joints, Bilateral<br>F Temporal Bones | Ø High Osmolar<br>1 Low Osmolar<br>Y Other Contrast<br>Z None | Z None | Z None |

**B Imaging**
**N Skull and Facial Bones**
**3 Magnetic Resonance Imaging (MRI)** Definition: Computer reformatted digital display of multiplanar images developed from the capture of radio-frequency signals emitted by nuclei in a body site excited within a magnetic field

| Body Part Character 4 | Contrast Character 5 | Qualifier Character 6 | Qualifier Character 7 |
|---|---|---|---|
| 9 Temporomandibular Joints, Bilateral | Y Other Contrast<br>Z None | Z None | Z None |

**B Imaging**
**P Non-Axial Upper Bones**
**Ø Plain Radiography** Definition: Planar display of an image developed from the capture of external ionizing radiation on photographic or photoconductive plate

| Body Part Character 4 | Contrast Character 5 | Qualifier Character 6 | Qualifier Character 7 |
|---|---|---|---|
| Ø Sternoclavicular Joint, Right<br>1 Sternoclavicular Joint, Left<br>2 Sternoclavicular Joints, Bilateral<br>3 Acromioclavicular Joints, Bilateral<br>4 Clavicle, Right<br>5 Clavicle, Left<br>6 Scapula, Right<br>7 Scapula, Left<br>A Humerus, Right<br>B Humerus, Left<br>E Upper Arm, Right<br>F Upper Arm, Left<br>J Forearm, Right<br>K Forearm, Left<br>N Hand, Right<br>P Hand, Left<br>R Finger(s), Right<br>S Finger(s), Left<br>X Ribs, Right<br>Y Ribs, Left | Z None | Z None | Z None |
| 8 Shoulder, Right<br>9 Shoulder, Left<br>C Hand/Finger Joint, Right<br>D Hand/Finger Joint, Left<br>G Elbow, Right<br>H Elbow, Left<br>L Wrist, Right<br>M Wrist, Left | Ø High Osmolar<br>1 Low Osmolar<br>Y Other Contrast<br>Z None | Z None | Z None |

**B Imaging**
**P Non-Axial Upper Bones**
**1 Fluoroscopy** Definition: Single plane or bi-plane real time display of an image developed from the capture of external ionizing radioation on a fluorescent screen. The image may also be stored by either digital or analog means.

| Body Part Character 4 | Contrast Character 5 | Qualifier Character 6 | Qualifier Character 7 |
|---|---|---|---|
| Ø Sternoclavicular Joint, Right<br>1 Sternoclavicular Joint, Left<br>2 Sternoclavicular Joints, Bilateral<br>3 Acromioclavicular Joints, Bilateral<br>4 Clavicle, Right<br>5 Clavicle, Left<br>6 Scapula, Right<br>7 Scapula, Left<br>A Humerus, Right<br>B Humerus, Left<br>E Upper Arm, Right<br>F Upper Arm, Left<br>J Forearm, Right<br>K Forearm, Left<br>N Hand, Right<br>P Hand, Left<br>R Finger(s), Right<br>S Finger(s), Left<br>X Ribs, Right<br>Y Ribs, Left | Z None | Z None | Z None |
| 8 Shoulder, Right<br>9 Shoulder, Left<br>L Wrist, Right<br>M Wrist, Left | Ø High Osmolar<br>1 Low Osmolar<br>Y Other Contrast<br>Z None | Z None | Z None |
| C Hand/Finger Joint, Right<br>D Hand/Finger Joint, Left<br>G Elbow, Right<br>H Elbow, Left | Ø High Osmolar<br>1 Low Osmolar<br>Y Other Contrast | Z None | Z None |

**B Imaging**
**P Non-Axial Upper Bones**
**2 Computerized Tomography (CT Scan)** Definition: Computer reformatted digital display of multiplanar images developed from the capture of multiple exposures of external ionizing radiation

| Body Part Character 4 | Contrast Character 5 | Qualifier Character 6 | Qualifier Character 7 |
|---|---|---|---|
| Ø Sternoclavicular Joint, Right<br>1 Sternoclavicular Joint, Left<br>W Thorax | Ø High Osmolar<br>1 Low Osmolar<br>Y Other Contrast | Z None | Z None |
| 2 Sternoclavicular Joints, Bilateral<br>3 Acromioclavicular Joints, Bilateral<br>4 Clavicle, Right<br>5 Clavicle, Left<br>6 Scapula, Right<br>7 Scapula, Left<br>8 Shoulder, Right<br>9 Shoulder, Left<br>A Humerus, Right<br>B Humerus, Left<br>E Upper Arm, Right<br>F Upper Arm, Left<br>G Elbow, Right<br>H Elbow, Left<br>J Forearm, Right<br>K Forearm, Left<br>L Wrist, Right<br>M Wrist, Left<br>N Hand, Right<br>P Hand, Left<br>Q Hands and Wrists, Bilateral<br>R Finger(s), Right<br>S Finger(s), Left<br>T Upper Extremity, Right<br>U Upper Extremity, Left<br>V Upper Extremities, Bilateral<br>X Ribs, Right<br>Y Ribs, Left | Ø High Osmolar<br>1 Low Osmolar<br>Y Other Contrast<br>Z None | Z None | Z None |
| C Hand/Finger Joint, Right<br>D Hand/Finger Joint, Left | Z None | Z None | Z None |

**B Imaging**
**P Non-Axial Upper Bones**
**3 Magnetic Resonance Imaging (MRI)** Definition: Computer reformatted digital display of multiplanar images developed from the capture of radio-frequency signals emitted by nuclei in a body site excited within a magnetic field

| Body Part Character 4 | Contrast Character 5 | Qualifier Character 6 | Qualifier Character 7 |
|---|---|---|---|
| **8** Shoulder, Right<br>**9** Shoulder, Left<br>**C** Hand/Finger Joint, Right<br>**D** Hand/Finger Joint, Left<br>**E** Upper Arm, Right<br>**F** Upper Arm, Left<br>**G** Elbow, Right<br>**H** Elbow, Left<br>**J** Forearm, Right<br>**K** Forearm, Left<br>**L** Wrist, Right<br>**M** Wrist, Left | **Y** Other Contrast | **Ø** Unenhanced and Enhanced<br>**Z** None | **Z** None |
| **8** Shoulder, Right<br>**9** Shoulder, Left<br>**C** Hand/Finger Joint, Right<br>**D** Hand/Finger Joint, Left<br>**E** Upper Arm, Right<br>**F** Upper Arm, Left<br>**G** Elbow, Right<br>**H** Elbow, Left<br>**J** Forearm, Right<br>**K** Forearm, Left<br>**L** Wrist, Right<br>**M** Wrist, Left | **Z** None | **Z** None | **Z** None |

**B Imaging**
**P Non-Axial Upper Bones**
**4 Ultrasonography** Definition: Real time display of images of anatomy or flow information developed from the capture of relected and attenuated high frequency sound waves

| Body Part Character 4 | Contrast Character 5 | Qualifier Character 6 | Qualifier Character 7 |
|---|---|---|---|
| **8** Shoulder, Right<br>**9** Shoulder, Left<br>**G** Elbow, Right<br>**H** Elbow, Left<br>**L** Wrist, Right<br>**M** Wrist, Left<br>**N** Hand, Right<br>**P** Hand, Left | **Z** None | **Z** None | **1** Densitometry<br>**Z** None |

**B Imaging**
**Q Non-Axial Lower Bones**
**Ø Plain Radiography** Definition: Planar display of an image developed from the capture of external ionizing radiation on photographic or photoconductive plate

| Body Part Character 4 | Contrast Character 5 | Qualifier Character 6 | Qualifier Character 7 |
|---|---|---|---|
| **Ø** Hip, Right<br>**1** Hip, Left | **Ø** High Osmolar<br>**1** Low Osmolar<br>**Y** Other Contrast | **Z** None | **Z** None |
| **Ø** Hip, Right<br>**1** Hip, Left | **Z** None | **Z** None | **1** Densitometry<br>**Z** None |
| **3** Femur, Right<br>**4** Femur, Left | **Z** None | **Z** None | **1** Densitometry<br>**Z** None |
| **7** Knee, Right<br>**8** Knee, Left<br>**G** Ankle, Right<br>**H** Ankle, Left | **Ø** High Osmolar<br>**1** Low Osmolar<br>**Y** Other Contrast<br>**Z** None | **Z** None | **Z** None |
| **D** Lower Leg, Right<br>**F** Lower Leg, Left<br>**J** Calcaneus, Right<br>**K** Calcaneus, Left<br>**L** Foot, Right<br>**M** Foot, Left<br>**P** Toe(s), Right<br>**Q** Toe(s), Left<br>**V** Patella, Right<br>**W** Patella, Left | **Z** None | **Z** None | **Z** None |
| **X** Foot/Toe Joint, Right<br>**Y** Foot/Toe Joint, Left | **Ø** High Osmolar<br>**1** Low Osmolar<br>**Y** Other Contrast | **Z** None | **Z** None |

**B Imaging**
**Q Non-Axial Lower Bones**
**1 Fluoroscopy** Definition: Single plane or bi-plane real time display of an image developed from the capture of external ionizing radioation on a fluorescent screen. The image may also be stored by either digital or analog means.

| Body Part Character 4 | Contrast Character 5 | Qualifier Character 6 | Qualifier Character 7 |
|---|---|---|---|
| **Ø** Hip, Right<br>**1** Hip, Left<br>**7** Knee, Right<br>**8** Knee, Left<br>**G** Ankle, Right<br>**H** Ankle, Left<br>**X** Foot/Toe Joint, Right<br>**Y** Foot/Toe Joint, Left | **Ø** High Osmolar<br>**1** Low Osmolar<br>**Y** Other Contrast<br>**Z** None | **Z** None | **Z** None |
| **3** Femur, Right<br>**4** Femur, Left<br>**D** Lower Leg, Right<br>**F** Lower Leg, Left<br>**J** Calcaneus, Right<br>**K** Calcaneus, Left<br>**L** Foot, Right<br>**M** Foot, Left<br>**P** Toe(s), Right<br>**Q** Toe(s), Left<br>**V** Patella, Right<br>**W** Patella, Left | **Z** None | **Z** None | **Z** None |

**B Imaging**
**Q Non-Axial Lower Bones**
**2 Computerized Tomography (CT Scan)** Definition: Computer reformatted digital display of multiplanar images developed from the capture of multiple exposures of external ionizing radiation

| Body Part Character 4 | Contrast Character 5 | Qualifier Character 6 | Qualifier Character 7 |
|---|---|---|---|
| **Ø** Hip, Right<br>**1** Hip, Left<br>**3** Femur, Right<br>**4** Femur, Left<br>**7** Knee, Right<br>**8** Knee, Left<br>**D** Lower Leg, Right<br>**F** Lower Leg, Left<br>**G** Ankle, Right<br>**H** Ankle, Left<br>**J** Calcaneus, Right<br>**K** Calcaneus, Left<br>**L** Foot, Right<br>**M** Foot, Left<br>**P** Toe(s), Right<br>**Q** Toe(s), Left<br>**R** Lower Extremity, Right<br>**S** Lower Extremity, Left<br>**V** Patella, Right<br>**W** Patella, Left<br>**X** Foot/Toe Joint, Right<br>**Y** Foot/Toe Joint, Left | **Ø** High Osmolar<br>**1** Low Osmolar<br>**Y** Other Contrast<br>**Z** None | **Z** None | **Z** None |
| **B** Tibia/Fibula, Right<br>**C** Tibia/Fibula, Left | **Ø** High Osmolar<br>**1** Low Osmolar<br>**Y** Other Contrast | **Z** None | **Z** None |

**B Imaging**
**Q Non-Axial Lower Bones**
**3 Magnetic Resonance Imaging (MRI)** Definition: Computer reformatted digital display of multiplanar images developed from the capture of radio-frequency signals emitted by nuclei in a body site excited within a magnetic field

| Body Part Character 4 | Contrast Character 5 | Qualifier Character 6 | Qualifier Character 7 |
|---|---|---|---|
| Ø Hip, Right<br>1 Hip, Left<br>3 Femur, Right<br>4 Femur, Left<br>7 Knee, Right<br>8 Knee, Left<br>D Lower Leg, Right<br>F Lower Leg, Left<br>G Ankle, Right<br>H Ankle, Left<br>J Calcaneus, Right<br>K Calcaneus, Left<br>L Foot, Right<br>M Foot, Left<br>P Toe(s), Right<br>Q Toe(s), Left<br>V Patella, Right<br>W Patella, Left | Y Other Contrast | Ø Unenhanced and Enhanced<br>Z None | Z None |
| Ø Hip, Right<br>1 Hip, Left<br>3 Femur, Right<br>4 Femur, Left<br>7 Knee, Right<br>8 Knee, Left<br>D Lower Leg, Right<br>F Lower Leg, Left<br>G Ankle, Right<br>H Ankle, Left<br>J Calcaneus, Right<br>K Calcaneus, Left<br>L Foot, Right<br>M Foot, Left<br>P Toe(s), Right<br>Q Toe(s), Left<br>V Patella, Right<br>W Patella, Left | Z None | Z None | Z None |

**B Imaging**
**Q Non-Axial Lower Bones**
**4 Ultrasonography** Definition: Real time display of images of anatomy or flow information developed from the capture of relected and attenuated high frequency sound waves

| Body Part Character 4 | Contrast Character 5 | Qualifier Character 6 | Qualifier Character 7 |
|---|---|---|---|
| Ø Hip, Right<br>1 Hip, Left<br>2 Hips, Bilateral<br>7 Knee, Right<br>8 Knee, Left<br>9 Knees, Bilateral | Z None | Z None | Z None |

**B Imaging**
**R Axial Skeleton, Except Skull and Facial Bones**
**Ø Plain Radiography** Definition: Planar display of an image developed from the capture of external ionizing radiation on photographic or photoconductive plate

| Body Part Character 4 | Contrast Character 5 | Qualifier Character 6 | Qualifier Character 7 |
|---|---|---|---|
| **Ø** Cervical Spine<br>**7** Thoracic Spine<br>**9** Lumbar Spine<br>**G** Whole Spine | **Z** None | **Z** None | **1** Densitometry<br>**Z** None |
| **1** Cervical Disc(s)<br>**2** Thoracic Disc(s)<br>**3** Lumbar Disc(s)<br>**4** Cervical Facet Joint(s)<br>**5** Thoracic Facet Joint(s)<br>**6** Lumbar Facet Joint(s)<br>**D** Sacroiliac Joints | **Ø** High Osmolar<br>**1** Low Osmolar<br>**Y** Other Contrast<br>**Z** None | **Z** None | **Z** None |
| **8** Thoracolumbar Joint<br>**B** Lumbosacral Joint<br>**C** Pelvis<br>**F** Sacrum and Coccyx<br>**H** Sternum | **Z** None | **Z** None | **Z** None |

**B Imaging**
**R Axial Skeleton, Except Skull and Facial Bones**
**1 Fluoroscopy** Definition: Single plane or bi-plane real time display of an image developed from the capture of external ionizing radioation on a fluorescent screen. The image may also be stored by either digital or analog means.

| Body Part Character 4 | Contrast Character 5 | Qualifier Character 6 | Qualifier Character 7 |
|---|---|---|---|
| **Ø** Cervical Spine<br>**1** Cervical Disc(s)<br>**2** Thoracic Disc(s)<br>**3** Lumbar Disc(s)<br>**4** Cervical Facet Joint(s)<br>**5** Thoracic Facet Joint(s)<br>**6** Lumbar Facet Joint(s)<br>**7** Thoracic Spine<br>**8** Thoracolumbar Joint<br>**9** Lumbar Spine<br>**B** Lumbosacral Joint<br>**C** Pelvis<br>**D** Sacroiliac Joints<br>**F** Sacrum and Coccyx<br>**G** Whole Spine<br>**H** Sternum | **Ø** High Osmolar<br>**1** Low Osmolar<br>**Y** Other Contrast<br>**Z** None | **Z** None | **Z** None |

**B Imaging**
**R Axial Skeleton, Except Skull and Facial Bones**
**2 Computerized Tomography (CT Scan)** Definition: Computer reformatted digital display of multiplanar images developed from the capture of multiple exposures of external ionizing radiation

| Body Part Character 4 | Contrast Character 5 | Qualifier Character 6 | Qualifier Character 7 |
|---|---|---|---|
| **Ø** Cervical Spine<br>**7** Thoracic Spine<br>**9** Lumbar Spine<br>**C** Pelvis<br>**D** Sacroiliac Joints<br>**F** Sacrum and Coccyx | **Ø** High Osmolar<br>**1** Low Osmolar<br>**Y** Other Contrast<br>**Z** None | **Z** None | **Z** None |

**B Imaging**
**R Axial Skeleton, Except Skull and Facial Bones**
**3 Magnetic Resonance Imaging (MRI)** Definition: Computer reformatted digital display of multiplanar images developed from the capture of radio-frequency signals emitted by nuclei in a body site excited within a magnetic field

| Body Part Character 4 | Contrast Character 5 | Qualifier Character 6 | Qualifier Character 7 |
|---|---|---|---|
| Ø Cervical Spine<br>1 Cervical Disc(s)<br>2 Thoracic Disc(s)<br>3 Lumbar Disc(s)<br>7 Thoracic Spine<br>9 Lumbar Spine<br>C Pelvis<br>F Sacrum and Coccyx | Y Other Contrast | Ø Unenhanced and Enhanced<br>Z None | Z None |
| Ø Cervical Spine<br>1 Cervical Disc(s)<br>2 Thoracic Disc(s)<br>3 Lumbar Disc(s)<br>7 Thoracic Spine<br>9 Lumbar Spine<br>C Pelvis<br>F Sacrum and Coccyx | Z None | Z None | Z None |

**B Imaging**
**R Axial Skeleton, Except Skull and Facial Bones**
**4 Ultrasonography** Definition: Real time display of images of anatomy or flow information developed from the capture of relected and attenuated high frequency sound waves

| Body Part Character 4 | Contrast Character 5 | Qualifier Character 6 | Qualifier Character 7 |
|---|---|---|---|
| Ø Cervical Spine<br>7 Thoracic Spine<br>9 Lumbar Spine<br>F Sacrum and Coccyx | Z None | Z None | Z None |

**B Imaging**
**T Urinary System**
**Ø Plain Radiography** Definition: Planar display of an image developed from the capture of external ionizing radiation on photographic or photoconductive plate

| Body Part Character 4 | Contrast Character 5 | Qualifier Character 6 | Qualifier Character 7 |
|---|---|---|---|
| Ø Bladder<br>1 Kidney, Right<br>2 Kidney, Left<br>3 Kidneys, Bilateral<br>4 Kidneys, Ureters and Bladder<br>5 Urethra<br>6 Ureter, Right<br>7 Ureter, Left<br>8 Ureters, Bilateral<br>B Bladder and Urethra<br>C Ileal Diversion Loop | Ø High Osmolar<br>1 Low Osmolar<br>Y Other Contrast<br>Z None | Z None | Z None |

**B Imaging**
**T Urinary System**
**1 Fluoroscopy** Definition: Single plane or bi-plane real time display of an image developed from the capture of external ionizing radioation on a fluorescent screen. The image may also be stored by either digital or analog means.

| Body Part Character 4 | Contrast Character 5 | Qualifier Character 6 | Qualifier Character 7 |
|---|---|---|---|
| Ø Bladder<br>1 Kidney, Right<br>2 Kidney, Left<br>3 Kidneys, Bilateral<br>4 Kidneys, Ureters and Bladder<br>5 Urethra<br>6 Ureter, Right<br>7 Ureter, Left<br>B Bladder and Urethra<br>C Ileal Diversion Loop<br>D Kidney, Ureter and Bladder, Right<br>F Kidney, Ureter and Bladder, Left<br>G Ileal Loop, Ureters and Kidneys | Ø High Osmolar<br>1 Low Osmolar<br>Y Other Contrast<br>Z None | Z None | Z None |

**B Imaging**
**T Urinary System**
**2 Computerized Tomography (CT Scan)** Definition: Computer reformatted digital display of multiplanar images developed from the capture of multiple exposures of external ionizing radiation

| Body Part Character 4 | Contrast Character 5 | Qualifier Character 6 | Qualifier Character 7 |
|---|---|---|---|
| Ø Bladder<br>1 Kidney, Right<br>2 Kidney, Left<br>3 Kidneys, Bilateral<br>9 Kidney Transplant | Ø High Osmolar<br>1 Low Osmolar<br>Y Other Contrast | Ø Unenhanced and Enhanced<br>Z None | Z None |
| Ø Bladder<br>1 Kidney, Right<br>2 Kidney, Left<br>3 Kidneys, Bilateral<br>9 Kidney Transplant | Z None | Z None | Z None |

**B Imaging**
**T Urinary System**
**3 Magnetic Resonance Imaging (MRI)** Definition: Computer reformatted digital display of multiplanar images developed from the capture of radio-frequency signals emitted by nuclei in a body site excited within a magnetic field

| Body Part Character 4 | Contrast Character 5 | Qualifier Character 6 | Qualifier Character 7 |
|---|---|---|---|
| Ø Bladder<br>1 Kidney, Right<br>2 Kidney, Left<br>3 Kidneys, Bilateral<br>9 Kidney Transplant | Y Other Contrast | Ø Unenhanced and Enhanced<br>Z None | Z None |
| Ø Bladder<br>1 Kidney, Right<br>2 Kidney, Left<br>3 Kidneys, Bilateral<br>9 Kidney Transplant | Z None | Z None | Z None |

**B Imaging**
**T Urinary System**
**4 Ultrasonography** Definition: Real time display of images of anatomy or flow information developed from the capture of relected and attenuated high frequency sound waves

| Body Part Character 4 | Contrast Character 5 | Qualifier Character 6 | Qualifier Character 7 |
|---|---|---|---|
| Ø Bladder<br>1 Kidney, Right<br>2 Kidney, Left<br>3 Kidneys, Bilateral<br>5 Urethra<br>6 Ureter, Right<br>7 Ureter, Left<br>8 Ureters, Bilateral<br>9 Kidney Transplant<br>J Kidneys and Bladder | Z None | Z None | Z None |

**B Imaging**
**U Female Reproductive System**
**Ø Plain Radiography** Definition: Planar display of an image developed from the capture of external ionizing radiation on photographic or photoconductive plate

| Body Part Character 4 | Contrast Character 5 | Qualifier Character 6 | Qualifier Character 7 |
|---|---|---|---|
| Ø Fallopian Tube, Right ♀<br>1 Fallopian Tube, Left ♀<br>2 Fallopian Tubes, Bilateral ♀<br>6 Uterus ♀<br>8 Uterus and Fallopian Tubes ♀<br>9 Vagina ♀ | Ø High Osmolar<br>1 Low Osmolar<br>Y Other Contrast | Z None | Z None |

♀ All body part, contrast, and qualifier values

**B Imaging**
**U Female Reproductive System**
**1 Fluoroscopy** Definition: Single plane or bi-plane real time display of an image developed from the capture of external ionizing radioation on a fluorescent screen. The image may also be stored by either digital or analog means.

| Body Part Character 4 | Contrast Character 5 | Qualifier Character 6 | Qualifier Character 7 |
|---|---|---|---|
| Ø Fallopian Tube, Right ♀<br>1 Fallopian Tube, Left ♀<br>2 Fallopian Tubes, Bilateral ♀<br>6 Uterus ♀<br>8 Uterus and Fallopian Tubes ♀<br>9 Vagina ♀ | Ø High Osmolar<br>1 Low Osmolar<br>Y Other Contrast<br>Z None | Z None | Z None |

♀ All body part, contrast, and qualifier values

**B Imaging**
**U Female Reproductive System**
**3 Magnetic Resonance Imaging (MRI)** Definition: Computer reformatted digital display of multiplanar images developed from the capture of radio-frequency signals emitted by nuclei in a body site excited within a magnetic field

| Body Part Character 4 | Contrast Character 5 | Qualifier Character 6 | Qualifier Character 7 |
|---|---|---|---|
| 3 Ovary, Right ♀<br>4 Ovary, Left ♀<br>5 Ovaries, Bilateral ♀<br>6 Uterus ♀<br>9 Vagina ♀<br>B Pregnant Uterus ♀<br>C Uterus and Ovaries ♀ | Y Other Contrast | Ø Unenhanced and Enhanced<br>Z None | Z None |
| 3 Ovary, Right ♀<br>4 Ovary, Left ♀<br>5 Ovaries, Bilateral ♀<br>6 Uterus ♀<br>9 Vagina ♀<br>B Pregnant Uterus ♀<br>C Uterus and Ovaries ♀ | Z None | Z None | Z None |

♀ All body part, contrast, and qualifier values

**B Imaging**
**U Female Reproductive System**
**4 Ultrasonography** Definition: Real time display of images of anatomy or flow information developed from the capture of relected and attenuated high frequency sound waves

| Body Part Character 4 | Contrast Character 5 | Qualifier Character 6 | Qualifier Character 7 |
|---|---|---|---|
| Ø Fallopian Tube, Right ♀<br>1 Fallopian Tube, Left ♀<br>2 Fallopian Tubes, Bilateral ♀<br>3 Ovary, Right ♀<br>4 Ovary, Left ♀<br>5 Ovaries, Bilateral ♀<br>6 Uterus ♀<br>C Uterus and Ovaries ♀ | Y Other Contrast<br>Z None | Z None | Z None |

♀ All body part, contrast, and qualifier values

**B Imaging**
**V Male Reproductive System**
**Ø Plain Radiography** Definition: Planar display of an image developed from the capture of external ionizing radiation on photographic or photoconductive plate

| Body Part Character 4 | Contrast Character 5 | Qualifier Character 6 | Qualifier Character 7 |
|---|---|---|---|
| Ø Corpora Cavernosa ♂<br>1 Epididymis, Right ♂<br>2 Epididymis, Left ♂<br>3 Prostate ♂<br>5 Testicle, Right ♂<br>6 Testicle, Left ♂<br>8 Vasa Vasorum ♂ | Ø High Osmolar<br>1 Low Osmolar<br>Y Other Contrast | Z None | Z None |

♂ All body part, contrast, and qualifier values

**B Imaging**
**V Male Reproductive System**
**1 Fluoroscopy** Definition: Single plane or bi-plane real time display of an image developed from the capture of external ionizing radioation on a fluorescent screen. The image may also be stored by either digital or analog means.

| Body Part Character 4 | Contrast Character 5 | Qualifier Character 6 | Qualifier Character 7 |
|---|---|---|---|
| Ø Corpora Cavernosa ♂<br>8 Vasa Vasorum ♂ | Ø High Osmolar<br>1 Low Osmolar<br>Y Other Contrast<br>Z None | Z None | Z None |

♂ All body part, contrast, and qualifier values

**B Imaging**
**V Male Reproductive System**
**2 Computerized Tomography (CT Scan)** Definition: Computer reformatted digital display of multiplanar images developed from the capture of multiple exposures of external ionizing radiation

| Body Part Character 4 | Contrast Character 5 | Qualifier Character 6 | Qualifier Character 7 |
|---|---|---|---|
| 3 Prostate ♂ | Ø High Osmolar<br>1 Low Osmolar<br>Y Other Contrast | Ø Unenhanced and Enhanced<br>Z None | Z None |
| 3 Prostate ♂ | Z None | Z None | Z None |

♂ BV23[Ø,Y][Ø,Z]Z
♂ BV231ZZ

**B Imaging**
**V Male Reproductive System**
**3 Magnetic Resonance Imaging (MRI)** Definition: Computer reformatted digital display of multiplanar images developed from the capture of radio-frequency signals emitted by nuclei in a body site excited within a magnetic field

| Body Part Character 4 | Contrast Character 5 | Qualifier Character 6 | Qualifier Character 7 |
|---|---|---|---|
| Ø Corpora Cavernosa ♂<br>3 Prostate ♂<br>4 Scrotum ♂<br>5 Testicle, Right ♂<br>6 Testicle, Left ♂<br>7 Testicles, Bilateral ♂ | Y Other Contrast | Ø Unenhanced and Enhanced<br>Z None | Z None |
| Ø Corpora Cavernosa ♂<br>3 Prostate ♂<br>4 Scrotum ♂<br>5 Testicle, Right ♂<br>6 Testicle, Left ♂<br>7 Testicles, Bilateral ♂ | Z None | Z None | Z None |

♂ All body part, contrast, and qualifier values

**B Imaging**
**V Male Reproductive System**
**4 Ultrasonography** Definition: Real time display of images of anatomy or flow information developed from the capture of relected and attenuated high frequency sound waves

| Body Part Character 4 | Contrast Character 5 | Qualifier Character 6 | Qualifier Character 7 |
|---|---|---|---|
| 4 Scrotum ♂<br>9 Prostate and Seminal Vesicles ♂<br>B Penis ♂ | Z None | Z None | Z None |

♂ All body part, contrast, and qualifier values

**B Imaging**
**W Anatomical Regions**
**Ø Plain Radiography** Definition: Planar display of an image developed from the capture of external ionizing radiation on photographic or photoconductive plate

| Body Part Character 4 | Contrast Character 5 | Qualifier Character 6 | Qualifier Character 7 |
|---|---|---|---|
| Ø Abdomen<br>1 Abdomen and Pelvis<br>3 Chest<br>B Long Bones, All<br>C Lower Extremity<br>J Upper Extremity<br>K Whole Body<br>L Whole Skeleton<br>M Whole Body, Infant | Z None | Z None | Z None |

**B Imaging**
**W Anatomical Regions**
**1 Fluoroscopy** Definition: Single plane or bi-plane real time display of an image developed from the capture of external ionizing radioation on a fluorescent screen. The image may also be stored by either digital or analog means.

| Body Part Character 4 | Contrast Character 5 | Qualifier Character 6 | Qualifier Character 7 |
|---|---|---|---|
| 1 Abdomen and Pelvis<br>9 Head and Neck<br>C Lower Extremity<br>J Upper Extremity | Ø High Osmolar<br>1 Low Osmolar<br>Y Other Contrast<br>Z None | Z None | Z None |

**B Imaging**
**W Anatomical Regions**
**2 Computerized Tomography (CT Scan)** Definition: Computer reformatted digital display of multiplanar images developed from the capture of multiple exposures of external ionizing radiation

| Body Part Character 4 | Contrast Character 5 | Qualifier Character 6 | Qualifier Character 7 |
|---|---|---|---|
| Ø Abdomen<br>1 Abdomen and Pelvis<br>4 Chest and Abdomen<br>5 Chest, Abdomen and Pelvis<br>8 Head<br>9 Head and Neck<br>F Neck<br>G Pelvic Region | Ø High Osmolar<br>1 Low Osmolar<br>Y Other Contrast | Ø Unenhanced and Enhanced<br>Z None | Z None |
| Ø Abdomen<br>1 Abdomen and Pelvis<br>4 Chest and Abdomen<br>5 Chest, Abdomen and Pelvis<br>8 Head<br>9 Head and Neck<br>F Neck<br>G Pelvic Region | Z None | Z None | Z None |

**B Imaging**
**W Anatomical Regions**
**3 Magnetic Resonance Imaging (MRI)** Definition: Computer reformatted digital display of multiplanar images developed from the capture of radio-frequency signals emitted by nuclei in a body site excited within a magnetic field

| Body Part Character 4 | Contrast Character 5 | Qualifier Character 6 | Qualifier Character 7 |
|---|---|---|---|
| Ø Abdomen<br>8 Head<br>F Neck<br>G Pelvic Region<br>H Retroperitoneum<br>P Brachial Plexus | Y Other Contrast | Ø Unenhanced and Enhanced<br>Z None | Z None |
| Ø Abdomen<br>8 Head<br>F Neck<br>G Pelvic Region<br>H Retroperitoneum<br>P Brachial Plexus | Z None | Z None | Z None |
| 3 Chest | Y Other Contrast | Ø Unenhanced and Enhanced<br>Z None | Z None |

**B Imaging**
**W Anatomical Regions**
**4 Ultrasonography** Definition: Real time display of images of anatomy or flow information developed from the capture of relected and attenuated high frequency sound waves

| Body Part Character 4 | Contrast Character 5 | Qualifier Character 6 | Qualifier Character 7 |
|---|---|---|---|
| Ø Abdomen<br>1 Abdomen and Pelvis<br>F Neck<br>G Pelvic Region | Z None | Z None | Z None |

**B Imaging**
**Y Fetus and Obstetrical**
**3 Magnetic Resonance Imaging (MRI)** Definition: Computer reformatted digital display of multiplanar images developed from the capture of radio-frequency signals emitted by nuclei in a body site excited within a magnetic field

| Body Part Character 4 | Contrast Character 5 | Qualifier Character 6 | Qualifier Character 7 |
|---|---|---|---|
| **Ø** Fetal Head ♀<br>**1** Fetal Heart ♀<br>**2** Fetal Thorax ♀<br>**3** Fetal Abdomen ♀<br>**4** Fetal Spine ♀<br>**5** Fetal Extremities ♀<br>**6** Whole Fetus ♀ | **Y** Other Contrast | **Ø** Unenhanced and Enhanced<br>**Z** None | **Z** None |
| **Ø** Fetal Head ♀<br>**1** Fetal Heart ♀<br>**2** Fetal Thorax ♀<br>**3** Fetal Abdomen ♀<br>**4** Fetal Spine ♀<br>**5** Fetal Extremities ♀<br>**6** Whole Fetus ♀ | **Z** None | **Z** None | **Z** None |

♀ BY3[Ø,1,2,3,5,6]Y[Ø,Z]Z
♀ BY34YZZ
♀ BY3[Ø,1,2,3,4,5,6]ZZZ

**B Imaging**
**Y Fetus and Obstetrical**
**4 Ultrasonography** Definition: Real time display of images of anatomy or flow information developed from the capture of relected and attenuated high frequency sound waves

| Body Part Character 4 | Contrast Character 5 | Qualifier Character 6 | Qualifier Character 7 |
|---|---|---|---|
| **7** Fetal Umbilical Cord ♀<br>**8** Placenta ♀<br>**9** First Trimester, Single Fetus ♀<br>**B** First Trimester, Multiple Gestation ♀<br>**C** Second Trimester, Single Fetus ♀<br>**D** Second Trimester, Multiple Gestation ♀<br>**F** Third Trimester, Single Fetus ♀<br>**G** Third Trimester, Multiple Gestation ♀ | **Z** None | **Z** None | **Z** None |

♀ All body part, contrast, and qualifier values

# Nuclear Medicine CØ1–CW7

## Character Meanings

This Character Meaning table is provided as a guide to assist the user in the identification of character members that may be found in this section of code tables. It **SHOULD NOT** be used to build a PCS code.

| Body System–Character 2 | Type–Character 3 | Meaning–Character 4 | Radionuclide–Character 5 | Qualifier–Character 6 | Qualifier–Character 7 |
|---|---|---|---|---|---|
| Ø Central Nervous System | 1 Planar Nuclear Medicine Imaging | See below | 1 Technetium 99m (Tc-99m) | Z None | Z None |
| 2 Heart | 2 Tomographic (Tomo) Nuclear Medicine Imaging | | 7 Cobalt 58 (Co-58) | | |
| 5 Veins | 3 Positron Emission Tomographic (PET) Imaging | | 8 Samarium 153 (Sm-153) | | |
| 7 Lymphatic and Hematologic System | 4 Nonimaging Nuclear Medicine Uptake | | 9 Krypton (Kr-81m) | | |
| 8 Eye | 5 Nonimaging Nuclear Medicine Probe | | B Carbon 11 (C-11) | | |
| 9 Ear, Nose, Mouth and Throat | 6 Nonimaging Nuclear Medicine Assay | | C Cobalt 57 (Co-57) | | |
| B Respiratory System | 7 Systemic Nuclear Medicine Therapy | | D Indium 111 (In-111) | | |
| D Gastrointestinal System | | | F Iodine 123 (I-123) | | |
| F Hepatobiliary System and Pancreas | | | G Iodine 131 (I-131) | | |
| G Endocrine System | | | H Iodine 125 (I-125) | | |
| H Skin, Subcutaneous Tissue and Breast | | | K Fluorine 18 (F-18) | | |
| P Musculoskeletal System | | | L Gallium 67 (Ga-67) | | |
| T Urinary System | | | M Oxygen 15 (O-15) | | |
| V Male Reproductive System | | | N Phosphorus 32 (P-32) | | |
| W Anatomical Regions | | | P Strontium 89 (Sr-89) | | |
| | | | Q Rubidium 82 (Rb-82) | | |
| | | | R Nitrogen 13 (N-13) | | |
| | | | S Thallium 2Ø1 (Tl-2Ø1) | | |
| | | | T Xenon 127 (Xe-127) | | |
| | | | V Xenon 133 (Xe-133) | | |
| | | | W Chromium (Cr-51) | | |
| | | | Y Other Radionuclide | | |
| | | | Z None | | |

## Body Part—Character 4 Meanings

| Body System– Character 2 | Meanings– Character 4 |
|---|---|
| Ø Central Nervous System | Ø Brain<br>5 Cerebrospinal Fluid<br>Y Central Nervous System |
| 2 Heart | 6 Heart, Right and Left<br>G Myocardium<br>Y Heart |
| 5 Veins | B Lower Extremity Veins, Right<br>C Lower Extremity Veins, Left<br>D Lower Extremity Veins, Bilateral<br>N Upper Extremity Veins, Right<br>P Upper Extremity Veins, Left<br>Q Upper Extremity Veins, Bilateral<br>R Central Veins<br>Y Veins |

*Continued on next page*

Nuclear Medicine

*Continued from previous page*

| Body System– Character 2 | Meanings– Character 4 |
|---|---|
| 7 Lymphatic and Hematologic System | Ø Bone Marrow<br>2 Spleen<br>3 Blood<br>5 Lymphatics, Head and Neck<br>D Lymphatics, Pelvic<br>J Lymphatics, Head<br>K Lymphatics, Neck<br>L Lymphatics, Upper Chest<br>M Lymphatics, Trunk<br>N Lymphatics, Upper Extremity<br>P Lymphatics, Lower Extremity<br>Y Lymphatic and Hematologic System |
| 8 Eye | 9 Lacrimal Ducts, Bilateral<br>Y Eye |
| 9 Ear, Nose, Mouth and Throat | B Salivary Glands, Bilateral<br>Y Ear, Nose, Mouth and Throat |
| B Respiratory System | 2 Lungs and Bronchi<br>Y Respiratory System |
| D Gastrointestinal System | 5 Upper Gastrointestinal Tract<br>7 Gastrointestinal Tract<br>Y Digestive System |
| F Hepatobiliary System and Pancreas | 4 Gallbladder<br>5 Liver<br>6 Liver and Spleen<br>C Hepatobiliary System, All<br>Y Hepatobiliary System and Pancreas |
| G Endocrine System | 1 Parathyroid Glands<br>2 Thyroid Gland<br>4 Adrenal Glands, Bilateral<br>Y Endocrine System |
| H Skin, Subcutaneous Tissue and Breast | Ø Breast, Right<br>1 Breast, Left<br>2 Breasts, Bilateral<br>Y Skin, Subcutaneous Tissue and Breast |
| P Musculoskeletal System | 1 Skull<br>2 Cervical Spine<br>3 Skull and Cervical Spine<br>4 Thorax<br>5 Spine<br>6 Pelvis<br>7 Spine and Pelvis<br>8 Upper Extremity, Right<br>9 Upper Extremity, Left<br>B Upper Extremities, Bilateral<br>C Lower Extremity, Right<br>D Lower Extremity, Left<br>F Lower Extremities, Bilateral<br>G Thoracic Spine<br>H Lumbar Spine<br>J Thoracolumbar Spine<br>N Upper Extremities<br>P Lower Extremities<br>Y Musculoskeletal System, Other<br>Z Musculoskeletal System, All |
| T Urinary System | 3 Kidneys, Ureters and Bladder<br>H Bladder and Ureters<br>Y Urinary System |
| V Male Reproductive System | 9 Testicles, Bilateral<br>Y Male Reproductive System |
| W Anatomical Regions | Ø Abdomen<br>1 Abdomen and Pelvis<br>3 Chest<br>4 Chest and Abdomen<br>6 Chest and Neck<br>B Head and Neck<br>D Lower Extremity<br>G Thyroid<br>J Pelvic Region<br>M Upper Extremity<br>N Whole Body<br>Y Anatomical Regions, Multiple<br>Z Anatomical Region, Other |

**C Nuclear Medicine**
**Ø Central Nervous System**
**1 Planar Nuclear Medicine Imaging**

Definition: Introduction of radioactive materials into the body for single plane display of images developed from the capture of radioactive emissions

| Body Part Character 4 | Radionuclide Character 5 | Qualifier Character 6 | Qualifier Character 7 |
|---|---|---|---|
| Ø Brain | 1 Technetium 99m (Tc-99m)<br>Y Other Radionuclide | Z None | Z None |
| 5 Cerebrospinal Fluid | D Indium 111 (In-111)<br>Y Other Radionuclide | Z None | Z None |
| Y Central Nervous System | Y Other Radionuclide | Z None | Z None |

**C Nuclear Medicine**
**Ø Central Nervous System**
**2 Tomographic (Tomo) Nuclear Medicine Imaging**

Definition: Introduction of radioactive materials into the body for three dimensional display of images developed from the capture of radioactive emissions

| Body Part Character 4 | Radionuclide Character 5 | Qualifier Character 6 | Qualifier Character 7 |
|---|---|---|---|
| Ø Brain | 1 Technetium 99m (Tc-99m)<br>F Iodine 123 (I-123)<br>S Thallium 201 (Tl-201)<br>Y Other Radionuclide | Z None | Z None |
| 5 Cerebrospinal Fluid | D Indium 111 (In-111)<br>Y Other Radionuclide | Z None | Z None |
| Y Central Nervous System | Y Other Radionuclide | Z None | Z None |

**C Nuclear Medicine**
**Ø Central Nervous System**
**3 Positron Emission Tomographic (PET) Imaging**

Definition: Introduction of radioactive materials into the body for three dimensional display of images developed from the simultaneous capture, 180 degrees apart, of radioactive emissions

| Body Part Character 4 | Radionuclide Character 5 | Qualifier Character 6 | Qualifier Character 7 |
|---|---|---|---|
| Ø Brain | B Carbon 11 (C-11)<br>K Fluorine 18 (F-18)<br>M Oxygen 15 (O-15)<br>Y Other Radionuclide | Z None | Z None |
| Y Central Nervous System | Y Other Radionuclide | Z None | Z None |

**C Nuclear Medicine**
**Ø Central Nervous System**
**5 Nonimaging Nuclear Medicine Probe**

Definition: Introduction of radioactive materials into the body for the study of distribution and fate of certain substances by the detection of radioactive emissions; or, alternatively, measurement of absorption of radioactive emissions from an external source

| Body Part Character 4 | Radionuclide Character 5 | Qualifier Character 6 | Qualifier Character 7 |
|---|---|---|---|
| Ø Brain | V Xenon 133 (Xe-133)<br>Y Other Radionuclide | Z None | Z None |
| Y Central Nervous System | Y Other Radionuclide | Z None | Z None |

**C Nuclear Medicine**
**2 Heart**
**1 Planar Nuclear Medicine Imaging**

Definition: Introduction of radioactive materials into the body for single plane display of images developed from the capture of radioactive emissions

| Body Part Character 4 | Radionuclide Character 5 | Qualifier Character 6 | Qualifier Character 7 |
|---|---|---|---|
| 6 Heart, Right and Left | 1 Technetium 99m (Tc-99m)<br>Y Other Radionuclide | Z None | Z None |
| G Myocardium | 1 Technetium 99m (Tc-99m)<br>D Indium 111 (In-111)<br>S Thallium 201 (Tl-201)<br>Y Other Radionuclide<br>Z None | Z None | Z None |
| Y Heart | Y Other Radionuclide | Z None | Z None |

**C Nuclear Medicine**
**2 Heart**
**2 Tomographic (Tomo) Nuclear Medicine Imaging** Definition: Introduction of radioactive materials into the body for three dimensional display of images developed from the capture of radioactive emissions

| Body Part Character 4 | Radionuclide Character 5 | Qualifier Character 6 | Qualifier Character 7 |
|---|---|---|---|
| 6 Heart, Right and Left | 1 Technetium 99m (Tc-99m)<br>Y Other Radionuclide | Z None | Z None |
| G Myocardium | 1 Technetium 99m (Tc-99m)<br>D Indium 111 (In-111)<br>K Fluorine 18 (F-18)<br>S Thallium 201 (Tl-201)<br>Y Other Radionuclide<br>Z None | Z None | Z None |
| Y Heart | Y Other Radionuclide | Z None | Z None |

**C Nuclear Medicine**
**2 Heart**
**3 Positron Emission Tomographic (PET) Imaging** Definition: Introduction of radioactive materials into the body for three dimensional display of images developed from the simultaneous capture, 180 degrees apart, of radioactive emissions

| Body Part Character 4 | Radionuclide Character 5 | Qualifier Character 6 | Qualifier Character 7 |
|---|---|---|---|
| G Myocardium | K Fluorine 18 (F-18)<br>M Oxygen 15 (O-15)<br>Q Rubidium 82 (Rb-82)<br>R Nitrogen 13 (N-13)<br>Y Other Radionuclide | Z None | Z None |
| Y Heart | Y Other Radionuclide | Z None | Z None |

**C Nuclear Medicine**
**2 Heart**
**5 Nonimaging Nuclear Medicine Probe** Definition: Introduction of radioactive materials into the body for the study of distribution and fate of certain substances by the detection of radioactive emissions; or, alternatively, measurement of absorption of radioactive emissions from an external source

| Body Part Character 4 | Radionuclide Character 5 | Qualifier Character 6 | Qualifier Character 7 |
|---|---|---|---|
| 6 Heart, Right and Left | 1 Technetium 99m (Tc-99m)<br>Y Other Radionuclide | Z None | Z None |
| Y Heart | Y Other Radionuclide | Z None | Z None |

**C Nuclear Medicine**
**5 Veins**
**1 Planar Nuclear Medicine Imaging** Definition: Introduction of radioactive materials into the body for single plane display of images developed from the capture of radioactive emissions

| Body Part Character 4 | Radionuclide Character 5 | Qualifier Character 6 | Qualifier Character 7 |
|---|---|---|---|
| B Lower Extremity Veins, Right<br>C Lower Extremity Veins, Left<br>D Lower Extremity Veins, Bilateral<br>N Upper Extremity Veins, Right<br>P Upper Extremity Veins, Left<br>Q Upper Extremity Veins, Bilateral<br>R Central Veins | 1 Technetium 99m (Tc-99m)<br>Y Other Radionuclide | Z None | Z None |
| Y Veins | Y Other Radionuclide | Z None | Z None |

**C Nuclear Medicine**
**7 Lymphatic and Hematologic System**
**1 Planar Nuclear Medicine Imaging** Definition: Introduction of radioactive materials into the body for single plane display of images developed from the capture of radioactive emissions

| Body Part Character 4 | Radionuclide Character 5 | Qualifier Character 6 | Qualifier Character 7 |
|---|---|---|---|
| Ø Bone Marrow | 1 Technetium 99m (Tc-99m)<br>D Indium 111 (In-111)<br>Y Other Radionuclide | Z None | Z None |
| 2 Spleen<br>5 Lymphatics, Head and Neck<br>D Lymphatics, Pelvic<br>J Lymphatics, Head<br>K Lymphatics, Neck<br>L Lymphatics, Upper Chest<br>M Lymphatics, Trunk<br>N Lymphatics, Upper Extremity<br>P Lymphatics, Lower Extremity | 1 Technetium 99m (Tc-99m)<br>Y Other Radionuclide | Z None | Z None |
| 3 Blood | D Indium 111 (In-111)<br>Y Other Radionuclide | Z None | Z None |
| Y Lymphatic and Hematologic System | Y Other Radionuclide | Z None | Z None |

**C Nuclear Medicine**
**7 Lymphatic and Hematologic System**
**2 Tomographic (Tomo) Nuclear Medicine Imaging** Definition: Introduction of radioactive materials into the body for three dimensional display of images developed from the capture of radioactive emissions

| Body Part Character 4 | Radionuclide Character 5 | Qualifier Character 6 | Qualifier Character 7 |
|---|---|---|---|
| 2 Spleen | 1 Technetium 99m (Tc-99m)<br>Y Other Radionuclide | Z None | Z None |
| Y Lymphatic and Hematologic System | Y Other Radionuclide | Z None | Z None |

**C Nuclear Medicine**
**7 Lymphatic and Hematologic System**
**5 Nonimaging Nuclear Medicine Probe** Definition: Introduction of radioactive materials into the body for the study of distribution and fate of certain substances by the detection of radioactive emissions; or, alternatively, measurement of absorption of radioactive emissions from an external source

| Body Part Character 4 | Radionuclide Character 5 | Qualifier Character 6 | Qualifier Character 7 |
|---|---|---|---|
| 5 Lymphatics, Head and Neck<br>D Lymphatics, Pelvic<br>J Lymphatics, Head<br>K Lymphatics, Neck<br>L Lymphatics, Upper Chest<br>M Lymphatics, Trunk<br>N Lymphatics, Upper Extremity<br>P Lymphatics, Lower Extremity | 1 Technetium 99m (Tc-99m)<br>Y Other Radionuclide | Z None | Z None |
| Y Lymphatic and Hematologic System | Y Other Radionuclide | Z None | Z None |

**C Nuclear Medicine**
**7 Lymphatic and Hematologic System**
**6 Nonimaging Nuclear Medicine Assay** Definition: Introduction of radioactive materials into the body for the study of body fluids and blood elements, by the detection of radioactive emissions

| Body Part Character 4 | Radionuclide Character 5 | Qualifier Character 6 | Qualifier Character 7 |
|---|---|---|---|
| 3 Blood | 1 Technetium 99m (Tc-99m)<br>7 Cobalt 58 (Co-58)<br>C Cobalt 57 (Co-57)<br>D Indium 111 (In-111)<br>H Iodine 125 (I-125)<br>W Chromium (Cr-51)<br>Y Other Radionuclide | Z None | Z None |
| Y Lymphatic and Hematologic System | Y Other Radionuclide | Z None | Z None |

**C Nuclear Medicine**
**8 Eye**
**1 Planar Nuclear Medicine Imaging**

Definition: Introduction of radioactive materials into the body for single plane display of images developed from the capture of radioactive emissions

| Body Part Character 4 | Radionuclide Character 5 | Qualifier Character 6 | Qualifier Character 7 |
|---|---|---|---|
| 9 Lacrimal Ducts, Bilateral | 1 Technetium 99m (Tc-99m)<br>Y Other Radionuclide | Z None | Z None |
| Y Eye | Y Other Radionuclide | Z None | Z None |

**C Nuclear Medicine**
**9 Ear, Nose, Mouth and Throat**
**1 Planar Nuclear Medicine Imaging**

Definition: Introduction of radioactive materials into the body for single plane display of images developed from the capture of radioactive emissions

| Body Part Character 4 | Radionuclide Character 5 | Qualifier Character 6 | Qualifier Character 7 |
|---|---|---|---|
| B Salivary Glands, Bilateral | 1 Technetium 99m (Tc-99m)<br>Y Other Radionuclide | Z None | Z None |
| Y Ear, Nose, Mouth and Throat | Y Other Radionuclide | Z None | Z None |

**C Nuclear Medicine**
**B Respiratory System**
**1 Planar Nuclear Medicine Imaging**

Definition: Introduction of radioactive materials into the body for single plane display of images developed from the capture of radioactive emissions

| Body Part Character 4 | Radionuclide Character 5 | Qualifier Character 6 | Qualifier Character 7 |
|---|---|---|---|
| 2 Lungs and Bronchi | 1 Technetium 99m (Tc-99m)<br>9 Krypton (Kr-81m)<br>T Xenon 127 (Xe-127)<br>V Xenon 133 (Xe-133)<br>Y Other Radionuclide | Z None | Z None |
| Y Respiratory System | Y Other Radionuclide | Z None | Z None |

**C Nuclear Medicine**
**B Respiratory System**
**2 Tomographic (Tomo) Nuclear Medicine Imaging**

Definition: Introduction of radioactive materials into the body for three dimensional display of images developed from the capture of radioactive emissions

| Body Part Character 4 | Radionuclide Character 5 | Qualifier Character 6 | Qualifier Character 7 |
|---|---|---|---|
| 2 Lungs and Bronchi | 1 Technetium 99m (Tc-99m)<br>9 Krypton (Kr-81m)<br>Y Other Radionuclide | Z None | Z None |
| Y Respiratory System | Y Other Radionuclide | Z None | Z None |

**C Nuclear Medicine**
**B Respiratory System**
**3 Positron Emission Tomographic (PET) Imaging**

Definition: Introduction of radioactive materials into the body for three dimensional display of images developed from the simultaneous capture, 180 degrees apart, of radioactive emissions

| Body Part Character 4 | Radionuclide Character 5 | Qualifier Character 6 | Qualifier Character 7 |
|---|---|---|---|
| 2 Lungs and Bronchi | K Fluorine 18 (F-18)<br>Y Other Radionuclide | Z None | Z None |
| Y Respiratory System | Y Other Radionuclide | Z None | Z None |

**C Nuclear Medicine**
**D Gastrointestinal System**
**1 Planar Nuclear Medicine Imaging**

Definition: Introduction of radioactive materials into the body for single plane display of images developed from the capture of radioactive emissions

| Body Part Character 4 | Radionuclide Character 5 | Qualifier Character 6 | Qualifier Character 7 |
|---|---|---|---|
| 5 Upper Gastrointestinal Tract<br>7 Gastrointestinal Tract | 1 Technetium 99m (Tc-99m)<br>D Indium 111 (In-111)<br>Y Other Radionuclide | Z None | Z None |
| Y Digestive System | Y Other Radionuclide | Z None | Z None |

**C Nuclear Medicine**
**D Gastrointestinal System**
**2 Tomographic (Tomo) Nuclear Medicine Imaging** Definition: Introduction of radioactive materials into the body for three dimensional display of images developed from the capture of radioactive emissions

| Body Part Character 4 | Radionuclide Character 5 | Qualifier Character 6 | Qualifier Character 7 |
|---|---|---|---|
| 7 Gastrointestinal Tract | 1 Technetium 99m (Tc-99m)<br>D Indium 111 (In-111)<br>Y Other Radionuclide | Z None | Z None |
| Y Digestive System | Y Other Radionuclide | Z None | Z None |

**C Nuclear Medicine**
**F Hepatobiliary System and Pancreas**
**1 Planar Nuclear Medicine Imaging** Definition: Introduction of radioactive materials into the body for single plane display of images developed from the capture of radioactive emissions

| Body Part Character 4 | Radionuclide Character 5 | Qualifier Character 6 | Qualifier Character 7 |
|---|---|---|---|
| 4 Gallbladder<br>5 Liver<br>6 Liver and Spleen<br>C Hepatobiliary System, All | 1 Technetium 99m (Tc-99m)<br>Y Other Radionuclide | Z None | Z None |
| Y Hepatobiliary System and Pancreas | Y Other Radionuclide | Z None | Z None |

**C Nuclear Medicine**
**F Hepatobiliary System and Pancreas**
**2 Tomographic (Tomo) Nuclear Medicine Imaging** Definition: Introduction of radioactive materials into the body for three dimensional display of images developed from the capture of radioactive emissions

| Body Part Character 4 | Radionuclide Character 5 | Qualifier Character 6 | Qualifier Character 7 |
|---|---|---|---|
| 4 Gallbladder<br>5 Liver<br>6 Liver and Spleen | 1 Technetium 99m (Tc-99m)<br>Y Other Radionuclide | Z None | Z None |
| Y Hepatobiliary System and Pancreas | Y Other Radionuclide | Z None | Z None |

**C Nuclear Medicine**
**G Endocrine System**
**1 Planar Nuclear Medicine Imaging** Definition: Introduction of radioactive materials into the body for single plane display of images developed from the capture of radioactive emissions

| Body Part Character 4 | Radionuclide Character 5 | Qualifier Character 6 | Qualifier Character 7 |
|---|---|---|---|
| 1 Parathyroid Glands | 1 Technetium 99m (Tc-99m)<br>S Thallium 201 (Tl-201)<br>Y Other Radionuclide | Z None | Z None |
| 2 Thyroid Gland | 1 Technetium 99m (Tc-99m)<br>F Iodine 123 (I-123)<br>G Iodine 131 (I-131)<br>Y Other Radionuclide | Z None | Z None |
| 4 Adrenal Glands, Bilateral | G Iodine 131 (I-131)<br>Y Other Radionuclide | Z None | Z None |
| Y Endocrine System | Y Other Radionuclide | Z None | Z None |

**C Nuclear Medicine**
**G Endocrine System**
**2 Tomographic (Tomo) Nuclear Medicine Imaging** Definition: Introduction of radioactive materials into the body for three dimensional display of images developed from the capture of radioactive emissions

| Body Part Character 4 | Radionuclide Character 5 | Qualifier Character 6 | Qualifier Character 7 |
|---|---|---|---|
| 1 Parathyroid Glands | 1 Technetium 99m (Tc-99m)<br>S Thallium 201 (Tl-201)<br>Y Other Radionuclide | Z None | Z None |
| Y Endocrine System | Y Other Radionuclide | Z None | Z None |

**C Nuclear Medicine**
**G Endocrine System**
**4 Nonimaging Nuclear Medicine Uptake**

Definition: Introduction of radioactive materials into the body for measurements of organ function, from the detection of radioactive emmissions

| Body Part Character 4 | Radionuclide Character 5 | Qualifier Character 6 | Qualifier Character 7 |
|---|---|---|---|
| 2 Thyroid Gland | 1 Technetium 99m (Tc-99m)<br>F Iodine 123 (I-123)<br>G Iodine 131 (I-131)<br>Y Other Radionuclide | Z None | Z None |
| Y Endocrine System | Y Other Radionuclide | Z None | Z None |

**C Nuclear Medicine**
**H Skin, Subcutaneous Tissue and Breast**
**1 Planar Nuclear Medicine Imaging**

Definition: Introduction of radioactive materials into the body for single plane display of images developed from the capture of radioactive emissions

| Body Part Character 4 | Radionuclide Character 5 | Qualifier Character 6 | Qualifier Character 7 |
|---|---|---|---|
| Ø Breast, Right<br>1 Breast, Left<br>2 Breasts, Bilateral | 1 Technetium 99m (Tc-99m)<br>S Thallium 201 (Tl-201)<br>Y Other Radionuclide | Z None | Z None |
| Y Skin, Subcutaneous Tissue and Breast | Y Other Radionuclide | Z None | Z None |

**C Nuclear Medicine**
**H Skin, Subcutaneous Tissue and Breast**
**2 Tomographic (Tomo) Nuclear Medicine Imaging**

Definition: Introduction of radioactive materials into the body for three dimensional display of images developed from the capture of radioactive emissions

| Body Part Character 4 | Radionuclide Character 5 | Qualifier Character 6 | Qualifier Character 7 |
|---|---|---|---|
| Ø Breast, Right<br>1 Breast, Left<br>2 Breasts, Bilateral | 1 Technetium 99m (Tc-99m)<br>S Thallium 201 (Tl-201)<br>Y Other Radionuclide | Z None | Z None |
| Y Skin, Subcutaneous Tissue and Breast | Y Other Radionuclide | Z None | Z None |

**C Nuclear Medicine**
**P Musculoskeletal System**
**1 Planar Nuclear Medicine Imaging**

Definition: Introduction of radioactive materials into the body for single plane display of images developed from the capture of radioactive emissions

| Body Part Character 4 | Radionuclide Character 5 | Qualifier Character 6 | Qualifier Character 7 |
|---|---|---|---|
| 1 Skull<br>4 Thorax<br>5 Spine<br>6 Pelvis<br>7 Spine and Pelvis<br>8 Upper Extremity, Right<br>9 Upper Extremity, Left<br>B Upper Extremities, Bilateral<br>C Lower Extremity, Right<br>D Lower Extremity, Left<br>F Lower Extremities, Bilateral<br>Z Musculoskeletal System, All | 1 Technetium 99m (Tc-99m)<br>Y Other Radionuclide | Z None | Z None |
| Y Musculoskeletal System, Other | Y Other Radionuclide | Z None | Z None |

**C Nuclear Medicine**
**P Musculoskeletal System**
**2 Tomographic (Tomo) Nuclear Medicine Imaging** Definition: Introduction of radioactive materials into the body for three dimensional display of images developed from the capture of radioactive emissions

| Body Part Character 4 | Radionuclide Character 5 | Qualifier Character 6 | Qualifier Character 7 |
|---|---|---|---|
| 1 Skull<br>2 Cervical Spine<br>3 Skull and Cervical Spine<br>4 Thorax<br>6 Pelvis<br>7 Spine and Pelvis<br>8 Upper Extremity, Right<br>9 Upper Extremity, Left<br>B Upper Extremities, Bilateral<br>C Lower Extremity, Right<br>D Lower Extremity, Left<br>F Lower Extremities, Bilateral<br>G Thoracic Spine<br>H Lumbar Spine<br>J Thoracolumbar Spine | 1 Technetium 99m (Tc-99m)<br>Y Other Radionuclide | Z None | Z None |
| Y Musculoskeletal System, Other | Y Other Radionuclide | Z None | Z None |

**C Nuclear Medicine**
**P Musculoskeletal System**
**5 Nonimaging Nuclear Medicine Probe** Definition: Introduction of radioactive materials into the body for the study of distribution and fate of certain substances by the detection of radioactive emissions; or, alternatively, measurement of absorption of radioactive emissions from an external source

| Body Part Character 4 | Radionuclide Character 5 | Qualifier Character 6 | Qualifier Character 7 |
|---|---|---|---|
| 5 Spine<br>N Upper Extremities<br>P Lower Extremities | Z None | Z None | Z None |
| Y Musculoskeletal System, Other | Y Other Radionuclide | Z None | Z None |

**C Nuclear Medicine**
**T Urinary System**
**1 Planar Nuclear Medicine Imaging** Definition: Introduction of radioactive materials into the body for single plane display of images developed from the capture of radioactive emissions

| Body Part Character 4 | Radionuclide Character 5 | Qualifier Character 6 | Qualifier Character 7 |
|---|---|---|---|
| 3 Kidneys, Ureters and Bladder | 1 Technetium 99m (Tc-99m)<br>F Iodine 123 (I-123)<br>G Iodine 131 (I-131)<br>Y Other Radionuclide | Z None | Z None |
| H Bladder and Ureters | 1 Technetium 99m (Tc-99m)<br>Y Other Radionuclide | Z None | Z None |
| Y Urinary System | Y Other Radionuclide | Z None | Z None |

**C Nuclear Medicine**
**T Urinary System**
**2 Tomographic (Tomo) Nuclear Medicine Imaging** Definition: Introduction of radioactive materials into the body for three dimensional display of images developed from the capture of radioactive emissions

| Body Part Character 4 | Radionuclide Character 5 | Qualifier Character 6 | Qualifier Character 7 |
|---|---|---|---|
| 3 Kidneys, Ureters and Bladder | 1 Technetium 99m (Tc-99m)<br>Y Other Radionuclide | Z None | Z None |
| Y Urinary System | Y Other Radionuclide | Z None | Z None |

**C Nuclear Medicine**
**T Urinary System**
**6 Nonimaging Nuclear Medicine Assay** Definition: Introduction of radioactive materials into the body for the study of body fluids and blood elements, by the detection of radioactive emissions

| Body Part Character 4 | Radionuclide Character 5 | Qualifier Character 6 | Qualifier Character 7 |
|---|---|---|---|
| 3 Kidneys, Ureters and Bladder | 1 Technetium 99m (Tc-99m)<br>F Iodine 123 (I-123)<br>G Iodine 131 (I-131)<br>H Iodine 125 (I-125)<br>Y Other Radionuclide | Z None | Z None |
| Y Urinary System | Y Other Radionuclide | Z None | Z None |

**C Nuclear Medicine**
**V Male Reproductive System**
**1 Planar Nuclear Medicine Imaging**

Definition: Introduction of radioactive materials into the body for single plane display of images developed from the capture of radioactive emissions

| Body Part Character 4 | Radionuclide Character 5 | Qualifier Character 6 | Qualifier Character 7 |
|---|---|---|---|
| 9 Testicles, Bilateral ♂ | 1 Technetium 99m (Tc-99m)<br>Y Other Radionuclide | Z None | Z None |
| Y Male Reproductive System ♂ | Y Other Radionuclide | Z None | Z None |

♂ All body part, radionuclide, and qualifier values

**C Nuclear Medicine**
**W Anatomical Regions**
**1 Planar Nuclear Medicine Imaging**

Definition: Introduction of radioactive materials into the body for single plane display of images developed from the capture of radioactive emissions

| Body Part Character 4 | Radionuclide Character 5 | Qualifier Character 6 | Qualifier Character 7 |
|---|---|---|---|
| Ø Abdomen<br>1 Abdomen and Pelvis<br>4 Chest and Abdomen<br>6 Chest and Neck<br>B Head and Neck<br>D Lower Extremity<br>J Pelvic Region<br>M Upper Extremity<br>N Whole Body | 1 Technetium 99m (Tc-99m)<br>D Indium 111 (In-111)<br>F Iodine 123 (I-123)<br>G Iodine 131 (I-131)<br>L Gallium 67 (Ga-67)<br>S Thallium 201 (Tl-201)<br>Y Other Radionuclide | Z None | Z None |
| 3 Chest | 1 Technetium 99m (Tc-99m)<br>D Indium 111 (In-111)<br>F Iodine 123 (I-123)<br>G Iodine 131 (I-131)<br>K Fluorine 18 (F-18)<br>L Gallium 67 (Ga-67)<br>S Thallium 201 (Tl-201)<br>Y Other Radionuclide | Z None | Z None |
| Y Anatomical Regions, Multiple | Y Other Radionuclide | Z None | Z None |
| Z Anatomical Region, Other | Z None | Z None | Z None |

**C Nuclear Medicine**
**W Anatomical Regions**
**2 Tomographic (Tomo) Nuclear Medicine Imaging**

Definition: Introduction of radioactive materials into the body for three dimensional display of images developed from the capture of radioactive emissions

| Body Part Character 4 | Radionuclide Character 5 | Qualifier Character 6 | Qualifier Character 7 |
|---|---|---|---|
| Ø Abdomen<br>1 Abdomen and Pelvis<br>3 Chest<br>4 Chest and Abdomen<br>6 Chest and Neck<br>B Head and Neck<br>D Lower Extremity<br>J Pelvic Region<br>M Upper Extremity | 1 Technetium 99m (Tc-99m)<br>D Indium 111 (In-111)<br>F Iodine 123 (I-123)<br>G Iodine 131 (I-131)<br>K Fluorine 18 (F-18)<br>L Gallium 67 (Ga-67)<br>S Thallium 201 (Tl-201)<br>Y Other Radionuclide | Z None | Z None |
| Y Anatomical Regions, Multiple | Y Other Radionuclide | Z None | Z None |

**C Nuclear Medicine**
**W Anatomical Regions**
**3 Positron Emission Tomographic (PET) Imaging**

Definition: Introduction of radioactive materials into the body for three dimensional display of images developed from the simultaneous capture, 180 degrees apart, of radioactive emissions

| Body Part Character 4 | Radionuclide Character 5 | Qualifier Character 6 | Qualifier Character 7 |
|---|---|---|---|
| N Whole Body | Y Other Radionuclide | Z None | Z None |

**C Nuclear Medicine**
**W Anatomical Regions**
**5 Nonimaging Nuclear Medicine Probe** Definition: Introduction of radioactive materials into the body for the study of distribution and fate of certain substances by the detection of radioactive emissions; or, alternatively, measurement of absorption of radioactive emissions from an external source

| Body Part Character 4 | Radionuclide Character 5 | Qualifier Character 6 | Qualifier Character 7 |
|---|---|---|---|
| Ø Abdomen<br>1 Abdomen and Pelvis<br>3 Chest<br>4 Chest and Abdomen<br>6 Chest and Neck<br>B Head and Neck<br>D Lower Extremity<br>J Pelvic Region<br>M Upper Extremity | 1 Technetium 99m (Tc-99m)<br>D Indium 111 (In-111)<br>Y Other Radionuclide | Z None | Z None |

**C Nuclear Medicine**
**W Anatomical Regions**
**7 Systemic Nuclear Medicine Therapy** Definition: Introduction of unsealed radioactive materials into the body for treatment

| Body Part Character 4 | Radionuclide Character 5 | Qualifier Character 6 | Qualifier Character 7 |
|---|---|---|---|
| Ø Abdomen<br>3 Chest | N Phosphorus 32 (P-32)<br>Y Other Radionuclide | Z None | Z None |
| G Thyroid | G Iodine 131 (I-131)<br>Y Other Radionuclide | Z None | Z None |
| N Whole Body | 8 Samarium 153 (Sm-153)<br>G Iodine 131 (I-131)<br>N Phosphorus 32 (P-32)<br>P Strontium 89 (Sr-89)<br>Y Other Radionuclide | Z None | Z None |
| Y Anatomical Regions, Multiple | Y Other Radionuclide | Z None | Z None |

# Radiation Therapy DØØ–DWY

## Character Meanings

This Character Meaning table is provided as a guide to assist the user in the identification of character members that may be found in this section of code tables. It **SHOULD NOT** be used to build a PCS code.

| Body System–Character 2 | Modality–Character 3 | Meanings–Character 4 | Modality-Qualifier Character 5 | Isotope–Character 6 | Qualifier–Character 7 |
|---|---|---|---|---|---|
| Ø Central and Peripheral Nervous System | Ø Beam Radiation | See below | Ø Photons <1 MeV | 7 Cesium 137 (Cs-137) | Ø Intraoperative |
| 7 Lymphatic and Hematologic System | 1 Brachytherapy | | 1 Photons 1 - 1Ø MeV | 8 Iridium 192 (Ir-192) | Z None |
| 8 Eye | 2 Stereotactic Radiosurgery | | 2 Photons >1Ø MeV | 9 Iodine 125 (I-125) | |
| 9 Ear, Nose, Mouth and Throat | Y Other Radiation | | 3 Electrons | B Palladium 1Ø3 (Pd-1Ø3) | |
| B Respiratory System | | | 4 Heavy Particles (Protons, Ions) | C Californium 252 (Cf-252) | |
| D Gastrointestinal System | | | 5 Neutrons | D Iodine 131 (I-131) | |
| F Hepatobiliary System and Pancreas | | | 6 Neutron Capture | F Phosphorus 32 (P-32) | |
| G Endocrine System | | | 7 Contact Radiation | G Strontium 89 (Sr-89) | |
| H Skin | | | 8 Hyperthermia | H Strontium 9Ø (Sr-9Ø) | |
| M Breast | | | 9 High Dose Rate (HDR) | Y Other Isotope | |
| P Musculoskeletal System | | | B Low Dose Rate (LDR) | Z None | |
| T Urinary System | | | C Intraoperative Radiation Therapy (IORT) | | |
| U Female Reproductive System | | | D Stereotactic Other Photon Radiosurgery | | |
| V Male Reproductive System | | | F Plaque Radiation | | |
| W Anatomical Regions | | | G Isotope Administration | | |
| | | | H Stereotactic Particulate Radiosurgery | | |
| | | | J Stereotactic Gamma Beam Radiosurgery | | |
| | | | K Laser Interstitial Thermal Therapy | | |

## Treatment Site—Character 4 Meanings

| Body System–Character 2 | Treatment Site–Character 4 |
|---|---|
| Ø Central and Peripheral Nervous System | Ø Brain<br>1 Brain Stem<br>6 Spinal Cord<br>7 Peripheral Nerve |
| 7 Lymphatic and Hematologic System | Ø Bone Marrow<br>1 Thymus<br>2 Spleen<br>3 Lymphatics, Neck<br>4 Lymphatics, Axillary<br>5 Lymphatics, Thorax<br>6 Lymphatics, Abdomen<br>7 Lymphatics, Pelvis<br>8 Lymphatics, Inguinal |
| 8 Eye | Ø Eye |

*Continued on next page*

*Continued from previous page*

| Body System– Character 2 | Treatment Site– Character 4 |
|---|---|
| 9 Ear, Nose, Mouth and Throat | Ø Ear<br>1 Nose<br>3 Hypopharynx<br>4 Mouth<br>5 Tongue<br>6 Salivary Glands<br>7 Sinuses<br>8 Hard Palate<br>9 Soft Palate<br>B Larynx<br>C Pharynx<br>D Nasopharynx<br>F Oropharynx |
| B Respiratory System | Ø Trachea<br>1 Bronchus<br>2 Lung<br>5 Pleura<br>6 Mediastinum<br>7 Chest Wall<br>8 Diaphragm |
| D Gastrointestinal System | Ø Esophagus<br>1 Stomach<br>2 Duodenum<br>3 Jejunum<br>4 Ileum<br>5 Colon<br>7 Rectum<br>8 Anus |
| F Hepatobiliary System and Pancreas | Ø Liver<br>1 Gallbladder<br>2 Bile Ducts<br>3 Pancreas |
| G Endocrine System | Ø Pituitary Gland<br>1 Pineal Body<br>2 Adrenal Glands<br>4 Parathyroid Glands<br>5 Thyroid |
| H Skin | 2 Skin, Face<br>3 Skin, Neck<br>4 Skin, Arm<br>5 Skin, Hand<br>6 Skin, Chest<br>7 Skin, Back<br>8 Skin, Abdomen<br>9 Skin, Buttock<br>B Skin, Leg<br>C Skin, Foot |
| M Breast | Ø Breast, Left<br>1 Breast, Right |
| P Musculoskeletal System | Ø Skull<br>2 Maxilla<br>3 Mandible<br>4 Sternum<br>5 Rib(s)<br>6 Humerus<br>7 Radius/Ulna<br>8 Pelvic Bones<br>9 Femur<br>B Tibia/Fibula<br>C Other Bone |
| T Urinary System | Ø Kidney<br>1 Ureter<br>2 Bladder<br>3 Urethra |
| U Female Reproductive System | Ø Ovary<br>1 Cervix<br>2 Uterus |
| V Male Reproductive System | Ø Prostate<br>1 Testis |
| W Anatomical Regions | 1 Head and Neck<br>2 Chest<br>3 Abdomen<br>4 Hemibody<br>5 Whole Body<br>6 Pelvic Region |

**D Radiation Therapy**
**Ø Central and Peripheral Nervous System**
**Ø Beam Radiation**

| Treatment Site Character 4 | Modality Qualifier Character 5 | Isotope Character 6 | Qualifier Character 7 |
|---|---|---|---|
| **Ø** Brain<br>**1** Brain Stem<br>**6** Spinal Cord<br>**7** Peripheral Nerve | **Ø** Photons <1 MeV<br>**1** Photons 1- 10 MeV<br>**2** Photons >10 MeV<br>**4** Heavy Particles (Protons, Ions)<br>**5** Neutrons<br>**6** Neutron Capture | **Z** None | **Z** None |
| **Ø** Brain<br>**1** Brain Stem<br>**6** Spinal Cord<br>**7** Peripheral Nerve | **3** Electrons | **Z** None | **Ø** Intraoperative<br>**Z** None |

**D Radiation Therapy**
**Ø Central and Peripheral Nervous System**
**1 Brachytherapy**

| Treatment Site Character 4 | Modality Qualifier Character 5 | Isotope Character 6 | Qualifier Character 7 |
|---|---|---|---|
| **Ø** Brain<br>**1** Brain Stem<br>**6** Spinal Cord<br>**7** Peripheral Nerve | **9** High Dose Rate (HDR)<br>**B** Low Dose Rate (LDR) | **7** Cesium 137 (Cs-137)<br>**8** Iridium 192 (Ir-192)<br>**9** Iodine 125 (I-125)<br>**B** Palladium 103 (Pd-103)<br>**C** Californium 252 (Cf-252)<br>**Y** Other Isotope | **Z** None |

**D Radiation Therapy**
**Ø Central and Peripheral Nervous System**
**2 Stereotactic Radiosurgery**

| Treatment Site Character 4 | Modality Qualifier Character 5 | Isotope Character 6 | Qualifier Character 7 |
|---|---|---|---|
| **Ø** Brain<br>**1** Brain Stem<br>**6** Spinal Cord<br>**7** Peripheral Nerve | **D** Stereotactic Other Photon Radiosurgery<br>**H** Stereotactic Particulate Radiosurgery<br>**J** Stereotactic Gamma Beam Radiosurgery | **Z** None | **Z** None |

**DRG Non-OR** All treatment site, modality, isotope, and qualifier values

**D Radiation Therapy**
**Ø Central and Peripheral Nervous System**
**Y Other Radiation**

| Treatment Site Character 4 | Modality Qualifier Character 5 | Isotope Character 6 | Qualifier Character 7 |
|---|---|---|---|
| **Ø** Brain<br>**1** Brain Stem<br>**6** Spinal Cord<br>**7** Peripheral Nerve | **7** Contact Radiation<br>**8** Hyperthermia<br>**F** Plaque Radiation<br>**K** Laser Interstitial Thermal Therapy | **Z** None | **Z** None |

**Valid OR** DØY[Ø,1,6,7]KZZ

**D Radiation Therapy**
**7 Lymphatic and Hematologic System**
**Ø Beam Radiation**

| Treatment Site Character 4 | Modality Qualifier Character 5 | Isotope Character 6 | Qualifier Character 7 |
|---|---|---|---|
| Ø Bone Marrow<br>1 Thymus<br>2 Spleen<br>3 Lymphatics, Neck<br>4 Lymphatics, Axillary<br>5 Lymphatics, Thorax<br>6 Lymphatics, Abdomen<br>7 Lymphatics, Pelvis<br>8 Lymphatics, Inguinal | Ø Photons <1 MeV<br>1 Photons 1-10 MeV<br>2 Photons >10 MeV<br>4 Heavy Particles (Protons, Ions)<br>5 Neutrons<br>6 Neutron Capture | Z None | Z None |
| Ø Bone Marrow<br>1 Thymus<br>2 Spleen<br>3 Lymphatics, Neck<br>4 Lymphatics, Axillary<br>5 Lymphatics, Thorax<br>6 Lymphatics, Abdomen<br>7 Lymphatics, Pelvis<br>8 Lymphatics, Inguinal | 3 Electrons | Z None | Ø Intraoperative<br>Z None |

**D Radiation Therapy**
**7 Lymphatic and Hematologic System**
**1 Brachytherapy**

| Treatment Site Character 4 | Modality Qualifier Character 5 | Isotope Character 6 | Qualifier Character 7 |
|---|---|---|---|
| Ø Bone Marrow<br>1 Thymus<br>2 Spleen<br>3 Lymphatics, Neck<br>4 Lymphatics, Axillary<br>5 Lymphatics, Thorax<br>6 Lymphatics, Abdomen<br>7 Lymphatics, Pelvis<br>8 Lymphatics, Inguinal | 9 High Dose Rate (HDR)<br>B Low Dose Rate (LDR) | 7 Cesium 137 (Cs-137)<br>8 Iridium 192 (Ir-192)<br>9 Iodine 125 (I-125)<br>B Palladium 103 (Pd-103)<br>C Californium 252 (Cf-252)<br>Y Other Isotope | Z None |

**D Radiation Therapy**
**7 Lymphatic and Hematologic System**
**2 Stereotactic Radiosurgery**

| Treatment Site Character 4 | Modality Qualifier Character 5 | Isotope Character 6 | Qualifier Character 7 |
|---|---|---|---|
| Ø Bone Marrow<br>1 Thymus<br>2 Spleen<br>3 Lymphatics, Neck<br>4 Lymphatics, Axillary<br>5 Lymphatics, Thorax<br>6 Lymphatics, Abdomen<br>7 Lymphatics, Pelvis<br>8 Lymphatics, Inguinal | D Stereotactic Other Photon Radiosurgery<br>H Stereotactic Particulate Radiosurgery<br>J Stereotactic Gamma Beam Radiosurgery | Z None | Z None |

DRG Non-OR All treatment site, modality, isotope, and qualifier values

**D Radiation Therapy**
**7 Lymphatic and Hematologic System**
**Y Other Radiation**

| Treatment Site Character 4 | Modality Qualifier Character 5 | Isotope Character 6 | Qualifier Character 7 |
|---|---|---|---|
| Ø Bone Marrow<br>1 Thymus<br>2 Spleen<br>3 Lymphatics, Neck<br>4 Lymphatics, Axillary<br>5 Lymphatics, Thorax<br>6 Lymphatics, Abdomen<br>7 Lymphatics, Pelvis<br>8 Lymphatics, Inguinal | 8 Hyperthermia<br>F Plaque Radiation | Z None | Z None |

**D Radiation Therapy**
**8 Eye**
**Ø Beam Radiation**

| Treatment Site Character 4 | Modality Qualifier Character 5 | Isotope Character 6 | Qualifier Character 7 |
|---|---|---|---|
| Ø Eye | Ø Photons <1 MeV<br>1 Photons 1- 10 MeV<br>2 Photons >10 MeV<br>4 Heavy Particles (Protons, Ions)<br>5 Neutrons<br>6 Neutron Capture | Z None | Z None |
| Ø Eye | 3 Electrons | Z None | Ø Intraoperative<br>Z None |

**D Radiation Therapy**
**8 Eye**
**1 Brachytherapy**

| Treatment Site Character 4 | Modality Qualifier Character 5 | Isotope Character 6 | Qualifier Character 7 |
|---|---|---|---|
| Ø Eye | 9 High Dose Rate (HDR)<br>B Low Dose Rate (LDR) | 7 Cesium 137 (Cs-137)<br>8 Iridium 192 (Ir-192)<br>9 Iodine 125 (I-125)<br>B Palladium 103 (Pd-103)<br>C Californium 252 (Cf-252)<br>Y Other Isotope | Z None |

**D Radiation Therapy**
**8 Eye**
**2 Stereotactic Radiosurgery**

| Treatment Site Character 4 | Modality Qualifier Character 5 | Isotope Character 6 | Qualifier Character 7 |
|---|---|---|---|
| Ø Eye | D Stereotactic Other Photon Radiosurgery<br>H Stereotactic Particulate Radiosurgery<br>J Stereotactic Gamma Beam Radiosurgery | Z None | Z None |

DRG Non-OR All treatment site, modality, isotope, and qualifier values

**D Radiation Therapy**
**8 Eye**
**Y Other Radiation**

| Treatment Site Character 4 | Modality Qualifier Character 5 | Isotope Character 6 | Qualifier Character 7 |
|---|---|---|---|
| Ø Eye | 7 Contact Radiation<br>8 Hyperthermia<br>F Plaque Radiation | Z None | Z None |

**D Radiation Therapy**
**9 Ear, Nose, Mouth and Throat**
**Ø Beam Radiation**

| Treatment Site Character 4 | Modality Qualifier Character 5 | Isotope Character 6 | Qualifier Character 7 |
|---|---|---|---|
| Ø Ear<br>1 Nose<br>3 Hypopharynx<br>4 Mouth<br>5 Tongue<br>6 Salivary Glands<br>7 Sinuses<br>8 Hard Palate<br>9 Soft Palate<br>B Larynx<br>D Nasopharynx<br>F Oropharynx | Ø Photons <1 MeV<br>1 Photons 1- 10 MeV<br>2 Photons >10 MeV<br>4 Heavy Particles (Protons, Ions)<br>5 Neutrons<br>6 Neutron Capture | Z None | Z None |
| Ø Ear<br>1 Nose<br>3 Hypopharynx<br>4 Mouth<br>5 Tongue<br>6 Salivary Glands<br>7 Sinuses<br>8 Hard Palate<br>9 Soft Palate<br>B Larynx<br>D Nasopharynx<br>F Oropharynx | 3 Electrons | Z None | Ø Intraoperative<br>Z None |

**D Radiation Therapy**
**9 Ear, Nose, Mouth and Throat**
**1 Brachytherapy**

| Treatment Site Character 4 | Modality Qualifier Character 5 | Isotope Character 6 | Qualifier Character 7 |
|---|---|---|---|
| Ø Ear<br>1 Nose<br>3 Hypopharynx<br>4 Mouth<br>5 Tongue<br>6 Salivary Glands<br>7 Sinuses<br>8 Hard Palate<br>9 Soft Palate<br>B Larynx<br>D Nasopharynx<br>F Oropharynx | 9 High Dose Rate (HDR)<br>B Low Dose Rate (LDR) | 7 Cesium 137 (Cs-137)<br>8 Iridium 192 (Ir-192)<br>9 Iodine 125 (I-125)<br>B Palladium 103 (Pd-103)<br>C Californium 252 (Cf-252)<br>Y Other Isotope | Z None |

**D Radiation Therapy**
**9 Ear, Nose, Mouth and Throat**
**2 Stereotactic Radiosurgery**

| Treatment Site Character 4 | Modality Qualifier Character 5 | Isotope Character 6 | Qualifier Character 7 |
|---|---|---|---|
| Ø Ear<br>1 Nose<br>4 Mouth<br>5 Tongue<br>6 Salivary Glands<br>7 Sinuses<br>8 Hard Palate<br>9 Soft Palate<br>B Larynx<br>C Pharynx<br>D Nasopharynx | D Stereotactic Other Photon Radiosurgery<br>H Stereotactic Particulate Radiosurgery<br>J Stereotactic Gamma Beam Radiosurgery | Z None | Z None |

DRG Non-OR All treatment site, modality, isotope, and qualifier values

**D Radiation Therapy**
**9 Ear, Nose, Mouth and Throat**
**Y Other Radiation**

| Treatment Site Character 4 | Modality Qualifier Character 5 | Isotope Character 6 | Qualifier Character 7 |
|---|---|---|---|
| Ø Ear<br>1 Nose<br>5 Tongue<br>6 Salivary Glands<br>7 Sinuses<br>8 Hard Palate<br>9 Soft Palate | 7 Contact Radiation<br>8 Hyperthermia<br>F Plaque Radiation | Z None | Z None |
| 3 Hypopharynx<br>F Oropharynx | 7 Contact Radiation<br>8 Hyperthermia | Z None | Z None |
| 4 Mouth<br>B Larynx<br>D Nasopharynx | 7 Contact Radiation<br>8 Hyperthermia<br>C Intraoperative Radiation Therapy (IORT)<br>F Plaque Radiation | Z None | Z None |
| C Pharynx | C Intraoperative Radiation Therapy (IORT)<br>F Plaque Radiation | Z None | Z None |

**D Radiation Therapy**
**B Respiratory System**
**Ø Beam Radiation**

| Treatment Site Character 4 | Modality Qualifier Character 5 | Isotope Character 6 | Qualifier Character 7 |
|---|---|---|---|
| Ø Trachea<br>1 Bronchus<br>2 Lung<br>5 Pleura<br>6 Mediastinum<br>7 Chest Wall<br>8 Diaphragm | Ø Photons <1 MeV<br>1 Photons 1- 10 MeV<br>2 Photons >10 MeV<br>4 Heavy Particles (Protons, Ions)<br>5 Neutrons<br>6 Neutron Capture | Z None | Z None |
| Ø Trachea<br>1 Bronchus<br>2 Lung<br>5 Pleura<br>6 Mediastinum<br>7 Chest Wall<br>8 Diaphragm | 3 Electrons | Z None | Ø Intraoperative<br>Z None |

**D Radiation Therapy**
**B Respiratory System**
**1 Brachytherapy**

| Treatment Site Character 4 | Modality Qualifier Character 5 | Isotope Character 6 | Qualifier Character 7 |
|---|---|---|---|
| Ø Trachea<br>1 Bronchus<br>2 Lung<br>5 Pleura<br>6 Mediastinum<br>7 Chest Wall<br>8 Diaphragm | 9 High Dose Rate (HDR)<br>B Low Dose Rate (LDR) | 7 Cesium 137 (Cs-137)<br>8 Iridium 192 (Ir-192)<br>9 Iodine 125 (I-125)<br>B Palladium 103 (Pd-103)<br>C Californium 252 (Cf-252)<br>Y Other Isotope | Z None |

**D Radiation Therapy**
**B Respiratory System**
**2 Stereotactic Radiosurgery**

| Treatment Site Character 4 | Modality Qualifier Character 5 | Isotope Character 6 | Qualifier Character 7 |
|---|---|---|---|
| Ø Trachea<br>1 Bronchus<br>2 Lung<br>5 Pleura<br>6 Mediastinum<br>7 Chest Wall<br>8 Diaphragm | D Stereotactic Other Photon Radiosurgery<br>H Stereotactic Particulate Radiosurgery<br>J Stereotactic Gamma Beam Radiosurgery | Z None | Z None |

DRG Non-OR All treatment site, modality, isotope, and qualifier values

**D Radiation Therapy**
**B Respiratory System**
**Y Other Radiation**

| Treatment Site Character 4 | Modality Qualifier Character 5 | Isotope Character 6 | Qualifier Character 7 |
|---|---|---|---|
| Ø Trachea<br>1 Bronchus<br>2 Lung<br>5 Pleura<br>6 Mediastinum<br>7 Chest Wall<br>8 Diaphragm | 7 Contact Radiation<br>8 Hyperthermia<br>F Plaque Radiation<br>K Laser Interstitial Thermal Therapy | Z None | Z None |

Valid OR DBY[Ø,1,2,5,6,7,8]KZZ

**D Radiation Therapy**
**D Gastrointestinal System**
**Ø Beam Radiation**

| Treatment Site Character 4 | Modality Qualifier Character 5 | Isotope Character 6 | Qualifier Character 7 |
|---|---|---|---|
| Ø Esophagus<br>1 Stomach<br>2 Duodenum<br>3 Jejunum<br>4 Ileum<br>5 Colon<br>7 Rectum | Ø Photons <1 MeV<br>1 Photons 1- 10 MeV<br>2 Photons >10 MeV<br>4 Heavy Particles (Protons, Ions)<br>5 Neutrons<br>6 Neutron Capture | Z None | Z None |
| Ø Esophagus<br>1 Stomach<br>2 Duodenum<br>3 Jejunum<br>4 Ileum<br>5 Colon<br>7 Rectum | 3 Electrons | Z None | Ø Intraoperative<br>Z None |

**D Radiation Therapy**
**D Gastrointestinal System**
**1 Brachytherapy**

| Treatment Site Character 4 | Modality Qualifier Character 5 | Isotope Character 6 | Qualifier Character 7 |
|---|---|---|---|
| Ø Esophagus<br>1 Stomach<br>2 Duodenum<br>3 Jejunum<br>4 Ileum<br>5 Colon<br>7 Rectum | 9 High Dose Rate (HDR)<br>B Low Dose Rate (LDR) | 7 Cesium 137 (Cs-137)<br>8 Iridium 192 (Ir-192)<br>9 Iodine 125 (I-125)<br>B Palladium 103 (Pd-103)<br>C Californium 252 (Cf-252)<br>Y Other Isotope | Z None |

**D Radiation Therapy**
**D Gastrointestinal System**
**2 Stereotactic Radiosurgery**

| Treatment Site Character 4 | Modality Qualifier Character 5 | Isotope Character 6 | Qualifier Character 7 |
|---|---|---|---|
| Ø Esophagus<br>1 Stomach<br>2 Duodenum<br>3 Jejunum<br>4 Ileum<br>5 Colon<br>7 Rectum | D Stereotactic Other Photon Radiosurgery<br>H Stereotactic Particulate Radiosurgery<br>J Stereotactic Gamma Beam Radiosurgery | Z None | Z None |

DRG Non-OR All treatment site, modality, isotope, and qualifier values

**D Radiation therapy**
**D Gastrointestinal System**
**Y Other Radiation**

| Treatment Site Character 4 | Modality Qualifier Character 5 | Isotope Character 6 | Qualifier Character 7 |
|---|---|---|---|
| Ø Esophagus | 7 Contact Radiation<br>8 Hyperthermia<br>F Plaque Radiation<br>K Laser Interstitial Thermal Therapy | Z None | Z None |
| 1 Stomach<br>2 Duodenum<br>3 Jejunum<br>4 Ileum<br>5 Colon<br>7 Rectum | 7 Contact Radiation<br>8 Hyperthermia<br>C Intraoperative Radiation Therapy (IORT)<br>F Plaque Radiation<br>K Laser Interstitial Thermal Therapy | Z None | Z None |
| 8 Anus | C Intraoperative Radiation Therapy (IORT)<br>F Plaque Radiation<br>K Laser Interstitial Thermal Therapy | Z None | Z None |

Valid OR DDYØKZZ
Valid OR DDY[1,2,3,4,5,7]KZZ
Valid OR DDY8KZZ

**D Radiation Therapy**
**F Hepatobiliary System and Pancreas**
**Ø Beam Radiation**

| Treatment Site Character 4 | Modality Qualifier Character 5 | Isotope Character 6 | Qualifier Character 7 |
|---|---|---|---|
| Ø Liver<br>1 Gallbladder<br>2 Bile Ducts<br>3 Pancreas | Ø Photons <1 MeV<br>1 Photons 1- 10 MeV<br>2 Photons >10 MeV<br>4 Heavy Particles (Protons, Ions)<br>5 Neutrons<br>6 Neutron Capture | Z None | Z None |
| Ø Liver<br>1 Gallbladder<br>2 Bile Ducts<br>3 Pancreas | 3 Electrons | Z None | Ø Intraoperative<br>Z None |

**D Radiation Therapy**
**F Hepatobiliary System and Pancreas**
**1 Brachytherapy**

| Treatment Site Character 4 | Modality Qualifier Character 5 | Isotope Character 6 | Qualifier Character 7 |
|---|---|---|---|
| Ø Liver<br>1 Gallbladder<br>2 Bile Ducts<br>3 Pancreas | 9 High Dose Rate (HDR)<br>B Low Dose Rate (LDR) | 7 Cesium 137 (Cs-137)<br>8 Iridium 192 (Ir-192)<br>9 Iodine 125 (I-125)<br>B Palladium 103 (Pd-103)<br>C Californium 252 (Cf-252)<br>Y Other Isotope | Z None |

**D Radiation Therapy**
**F Hepatobiliary System and Pancreas**
**2 Stereotactic Radiosurgery**

| Treatment Site Character 4 | Modality Qualifier Character 5 | Isotope Character 6 | Qualifier Character 7 |
|---|---|---|---|
| Ø Liver<br>1 Gallbladder<br>2 Bile Ducts<br>3 Pancreas | D Stereotactic Other Photon Radiosurgery<br>H Stereotactic Particulate Radiosurgery<br>J Stereotactic Gamma Beam Radiosurgery | Z None | Z None |

DRG Non-OR All treatment site, modality, isotope, and qualifier values

Radiation Therapy

DDY–DF2

**D Radiation Therapy**
**F Hepatobiliary System and Pancreas**
**Y Other Radiation**

| Treatment Site Character 4 | Modality Qualifier Character 5 | Isotope Character 6 | Qualifier Character 7 |
|---|---|---|---|
| Ø Liver<br>1 Gallbladder<br>2 Bile Ducts<br>3 Pancreas | 7 Contact Radiation<br>8 Hyperthermia<br>C Intraoperative Radiation Therapy (IORT)<br>F Plaque Radiation<br>K Laser Interstitial Thermal Therapy | Z None | Z None |

Valid OR DFY[Ø,1,2,3]KZZ

**D Radiation Therapy**
**G Endocrine System**
**Ø Beam Radiation**

| Treatment Site Character 4 | Modality Qualifier Character 5 | Isotope Character 6 | Qualifier Character 7 |
|---|---|---|---|
| Ø Pituitary Gland<br>1 Pineal Body<br>2 Adrenal Glands<br>4 Parathyroid Glands<br>5 Thyroid | Ø Photons <1 MeV<br>1 Photons 1- 10 MeV<br>2 Photons >10 MeV<br>5 Neutrons<br>6 Neutron Capture | Z None | Z None |
| Ø Pituitary Gland<br>1 Pineal Body<br>2 Adrenal Glands<br>4 Parathyroid Glands<br>5 Thyroid | 3 Electrons | Z None | Ø Intraoperative<br>Z None |

**D Radiation Therapy**
**G Endocrine System**
**1 Brachytherapy**

| Treatment Site Character 4 | Modality Qualifier Character 5 | Isotope Character 6 | Qualifier Character 7 |
|---|---|---|---|
| Ø Pituitary Gland<br>1 Pineal Body<br>2 Adrenal Glands<br>4 Parathyroid Glands<br>5 Thyroid | 9 High Dose Rate (HDR)<br>B Low Dose Rate (LDR) | 7 Cesium 137 (Cs-137)<br>8 Iridium 192 (Ir-192)<br>9 Iodine 125 (I-125)<br>B Palladium 103 (Pd-103)<br>C Californium 252 (Cf-252)<br>Y Other Isotope | Z None |

**D Radiation Therapy**
**G Endocrine System**
**2 Stereotactic Radiosurgery**

| Treatment Site Character 4 | Modality Qualifier Character 5 | Isotope Character 6 | Qualifier Character 7 |
|---|---|---|---|
| Ø Pituitary Gland<br>1 Pineal Body<br>2 Adrenal Glands<br>4 Parathyroid Glands<br>5 Thyroid | D Stereotactic Other Photon Radiosurgery<br>H Stereotactic Particulate Radiosurgery<br>J Stereotactic Gamma Beam Radiosurgery | Z None | Z None |

DRG Non-OR All treatment site, modality, isotope, and qualifier values

**D Radiation therapy**
**G Endocrine System**
**Y Other Radiation**

| Treatment Site Character 4 | Modality Qualifier Character 5 | Isotope Character 6 | Qualifier Character 7 |
|---|---|---|---|
| Ø Pituitary Gland<br>1 Pineal Body<br>2 Adrenal Glands<br>4 Parathyroid Glands<br>5 Thyroid | 7 Contact Radiation<br>8 Hyperthermia<br>F Plaque Radiation<br>K Laser Interstitial Thermal Therapy | Z None | Z None |

Valid OR DGY[Ø,1,2,4,5]KZZ

**D Radiation Therapy**
**H Skin**
**Ø Beam Radiation**

| Treatment Site Character 4 | Modality Qualifier Character 5 | Isotope Character 6 | Qualifier Character 7 |
|---|---|---|---|
| 2 Skin, Face<br>3 Skin, Neck<br>4 Skin, Arm<br>6 Skin, Chest<br>7 Skin, Back<br>8 Skin, Abdomen<br>9 Skin, Buttock<br>B Skin, Leg | Ø Photons <1 MeV<br>1 Photons 1- 10 MeV<br>2 Photons >10 MeV<br>4 Heavy Particles (Protons, Ions)<br>5 Neutrons<br>6 Neutron Capture | Z None | Z None |
| 2 Skin, Face<br>3 Skin, Neck<br>4 Skin, Arm<br>6 Skin, Chest<br>7 Skin, Back<br>8 Skin, Abdomen<br>9 Skin, Buttock<br>B Skin, Leg | 3 Electrons | Z None | Ø Intraoperative<br>Z None |

**D Radiation Therapy**
**H Skin**
**Y Other Radiation**

| Treatment Site Character 4 | Modality Qualifier Character 5 | Isotope Character 6 | Qualifier Character 7 |
|---|---|---|---|
| 2 Skin, Face<br>3 Skin, Neck<br>4 Skin, Arm<br>6 Skin, Chest<br>7 Skin, Back<br>8 Skin, Abdomen<br>9 Skin, Buttock<br>B Skin, Leg | 7 Contact Radiation<br>8 Hyperthermia<br>F Plaque Radiation | Z None | Z None |
| 5 Skin, Hand<br>C Skin, Foot | F Plaque Radiation | Z None | Z None |

**D Radiation Therapy**
**M Breast**
**Ø Beam Radiation**

| Treatment Site Character 4 | Modality Qualifier Character 5 | Isotope Character 6 | Qualifier Character 7 |
|---|---|---|---|
| Ø Breast, Left<br>1 Breast, Right | Ø Photons <1 MeV<br>1 Photons 1- 10 MeV<br>2 Photons >10 MeV<br>4 Heavy Particles (Protons, Ions)<br>5 Neutrons<br>6 Neutron Capture | Z None | Z None |
| Ø Breast, Left<br>1 Breast, Right | 3 Electrons | Z None | Ø Intraoperative<br>Z None |

**D Radiation Therapy**
**M Breast**
**1 Brachytherapy**

| Treatment Site Character 4 | Modality Qualifier Character 5 | Isotope Character 6 | Qualifier Character 7 |
|---|---|---|---|
| Ø Breast, Left<br>1 Breast, Right | 9 High Dose Rate (HDR)<br>B Low Dose Rate (LDR) | 7 Cesium 137 (Cs-137)<br>8 Iridium 192 (Ir-192)<br>9 Iodine 125 (I-125)<br>B Palladium 103 (Pd-103)<br>C Californium 252 (Cf-252)<br>Y Other Isotope | Z None |

**D Radiation Therapy**
**M Breast**
**2 Stereotactic Radiosurgery**

| Treatment Site Character 4 | Modality Qualifier Character 5 | Isotope Character 6 | Qualifier Character 7 |
|---|---|---|---|
| Ø Breast, Left<br>1 Breast, Right | D Stereotactic Other Photon Radiosurgery<br>H Stereotactic Particulate Radiosurgery<br>J Stereotactic Gamma Beam Radiosurgery | Z None | Z None |

DRG Non-OR All treatment site, modality, isotope, and qualifier values

**D Radiation Therapy**
**M Breast**
**Y Other Radiation**

| Treatment Site Character 4 | Modality Qualifier Character 5 | Isotope Character 6 | Qualifier Character 7 |
|---|---|---|---|
| Ø Breast, Left<br>1 Breast, Right | 7 Contact Radiation<br>8 Hyperthermia<br>F Plaque Radiation<br>K Laser Interstitial Thermal Therapy | Z None | Z None |

Valid OR DMY[Ø,1]KZZ

**D Radiation Therapy**
**P Musculoskeletal System**
**Ø Beam Radiation**

| Treatment Site Character 4 | Modality Qualifier Character 5 | Isotope Character 6 | Qualifier Character 7 |
|---|---|---|---|
| Ø Skull<br>2 Maxilla<br>3 Mandible<br>4 Sternum<br>5 Rib(s)<br>6 Humerus<br>7 Radius/Ulna<br>8 Pelvic Bones<br>9 Femur<br>B Tibia/Fibula<br>C Other Bone | Ø Photons <1 MeV<br>1 Photons 1- 10 MeV<br>2 Photons >10 MeV<br>4 Heavy Particles (Protons, Ions)<br>5 Neutrons<br>6 Neutron Capture | Z None | Z None |
| Ø Skull<br>2 Maxilla<br>3 Mandible<br>4 Sternum<br>5 Rib(s)<br>6 Humerus<br>7 Radius/Ulna<br>8 Pelvic Bones<br>9 Femur<br>B Tibia/Fibula<br>C Other Bone | 3 Electrons | Z None | Ø Intraoperative<br>Z None |

**D Radiation Therapy**
**P Musculoskeletal System**
**Y Other Radiation**

| Treatment Site Character 4 | Modality Qualifier Character 5 | Isotope Character 6 | Qualifier Character 7 |
|---|---|---|---|
| Ø Skull<br>2 Maxilla<br>3 Mandible<br>4 Sternum<br>5 Rib(s)<br>6 Humerus<br>7 Radius/Ulna<br>8 Pelvic Bones<br>9 Femur<br>B Tibia/Fibula<br>C Other Bone | 7 Contact Radiation<br>8 Hyperthermia<br>F Plaque Radiation | Z None | Z None |

**D Radiation Therapy**
**T Urinary System**
**Ø Beam Radiation**

| Treatment Site Character 4 | Modality Qualifier Character 5 | Isotope Character 6 | Qualifier Character 7 |
|---|---|---|---|
| Ø Kidney<br>1 Ureter<br>2 Bladder<br>3 Urethra | Ø Photons <1 MeV<br>1 Photons 1- 10 MeV<br>2 Photons >10 MeV<br>4 Heavy Particles (Protons, Ions)<br>5 Neutrons<br>6 Neutron Capture | Z None | Z None |
| Ø Kidney<br>1 Ureter<br>2 Bladder<br>3 Urethra | 3 Electrons | Z None | Ø Intraoperative<br>Z None |

**D Radiation Therapy**
**T Urinary System**
**1 Brachytherapy**

| Treatment Site Character 4 | Modality Qualifier Character 5 | Isotope Character 6 | Qualifier Character 7 |
|---|---|---|---|
| Ø Kidney<br>1 Ureter<br>2 Bladder<br>3 Urethra | 9 High Dose Rate (HDR)<br>B Low Dose Rate (LDR) | 7 Cesium 137 (Cs-137)<br>8 Iridium 192 (Ir-192)<br>9 Iodine 125 (I-125)<br>B Palladium 103 (Pd-103)<br>C Californium 252 (Cf-252)<br>Y Other Isotope | Z None |

**D Radiation Therapy**
**T Urinary System**
**2 Stereotactic Radiosurgery**

| Treatment Site Character 4 | Modality Qualifier Character 5 | Isotope Character 6 | Qualifier Character 7 |
|---|---|---|---|
| Ø Kidney<br>1 Ureter<br>2 Bladder<br>3 Urethra | D Stereotactic Other Photon Radiosurgery<br>H Stereotactic Particulate Radiosurgery<br>J Stereotactic Gamma Beam Radiosurgery | Z None | Z None |

DRG Non-OR All treatment site, modality, isotope, and qualifier values

**D Radiation Therapy**
**T Urinary System**
**Y Other Radiation**

| Treatment Site Character 4 | Modality Qualifier Character 5 | Isotope Character 6 | Qualifier Character 7 |
|---|---|---|---|
| Ø Kidney<br>1 Ureter<br>2 Bladder<br>3 Urethra | 7 Contact Radiation<br>8 Hyperthermia<br>C Intraoperative Radiation Therapy (IORT)<br>F Plaque Radiation | Z None | Z None |

**D Radiation Therapy**
**U Female Reproductive System**
**Ø Beam Radiation**

| Treatment Site Character 4 | Modality Qualifier Character 5 | Isotope Character 6 | Qualifier Character 7 |
|---|---|---|---|
| Ø Ovary ♀<br>1 Cervix ♀<br>2 Uterus ♀ | Ø Photons <1 MeV<br>1 Photons 1- 10 MeV<br>2 Photons >10 MeV<br>4 Heavy Particles (Protons, Ions)<br>5 Neutrons<br>6 Neutron Capture | Z None | Z None |
| Ø Ovary ♀<br>1 Cervix ♀<br>2 Uterus ♀ | 3 Electrons | Z None | Ø Intraoperative<br>Z None |

♀ All treatment site, modality, isotope, and qualifier values

**D Radiation Therapy**
**U Female Reproductive System**
**1 Brachytherapy**

| Treatment Site Character 4 | Modality Qualifier Character 5 | Isotope Character 6 | Qualifier Character 7 |
|---|---|---|---|
| Ø Ovary ♀<br>1 Cervix ♀<br>2 Uterus ♀ | 9 High Dose Rate (HDR)<br>B Low Dose Rate (LDR) | 7 Cesium 137 (Cs-137)<br>8 Iridium 192 (Ir-192)<br>9 Iodine 125 (I-125)<br>B Palladium 103 (Pd-103)<br>C Californium 252 (Cf-252)<br>Y Other Isotope | Z None |

♀ All treatment site, modality, isotope, and qualifier values

**D Radiation Therapy**
**U Female Reproductive System**
**2 Stereotactic Radiosurgery**

| Treatment Site Character 4 | Modality Qualifier Character 5 | Isotope Character 6 | Qualifier Character 7 |
|---|---|---|---|
| Ø Ovary ♀<br>1 Cervix ♀<br>2 Uterus ♀ | D Stereotactic Other Photon Radiosurgery<br>H Stereotactic Particulate Radiosurgery<br>J Stereotactic Gamma Beam Radiosurgery | Z None | Z None |

DRG Non-OR All treatment site, modality, isotope, and qualifier values
♀ All treatment site, modality, isotope, and qualifier values

**D Radiation Therapy**
**U Female Reproductive System**
**Y Other Radiation**

| Treatment Site Character 4 | Modality Qualifier Character 5 | Isotope Character 6 | Qualifier Character 7 |
|---|---|---|---|
| Ø Ovary ♀<br>1 Cervix ♀<br>2 Uterus ♀ | 7 Contact Radiation<br>8 Hyperthermia<br>C Intraoperative Radiation Therapy (IORT)<br>F Plaque Radiation | Z None | Z None |

♀ All treatment site, modality, isotope, and qualifier values

**D Radiation Therapy**
**V Male Reproductive System**
**Ø Beam Radiation**

| Treatment Site Character 4 | Modality Qualifier Character 5 | Isotope Character 6 | Qualifier Character 7 |
|---|---|---|---|
| Ø Prostate ♂<br>1 Testis ♂ | Ø Photons <1 MeV<br>1 Photons 1 - 10 MeV<br>2 Photons >10 MeV<br>4 Heavy Particles (Protons, Ions)<br>5 Neutrons<br>6 Neutron Capture | Z None | Z None |
| Ø Prostate ♂<br>1 Testis ♂ | 3 Electrons | Z None | Ø Intraoperative<br>Z None |

♂ All treatment site, modality, isotope, and qualifier values

**D Radiation Therapy**
**V Male Reproductive System**
**1 Brachytherapy**

| Treatment Site Character 4 | Modality Qualifier Character 5 | Isotope Character 6 | Qualifier Character 7 |
|---|---|---|---|
| Ø Prostate ♂<br>1 Testis ♂ | 9 High Dose Rate (HDR)<br>B Low Dose Rate (LDR) | 7 Cesium 137 (Cs-137)<br>8 Iridium 192 (Ir-192)<br>9 Iodine 125 (I-125)<br>B Palladium 103 (Pd-103)<br>C Californium 252 (Cf-252)<br>Y Other Isotope | Z None |

♂ All treatment site, modality, isotope, and qualifier values

**D Radiation Therapy**
**V Male Reproductive System**
**2 Stereotactic Radiosurgery**

| Treatment Site Character 4 | Modality Qualifier Character 5 | Isotope Character 6 | Qualifier Character 7 |
|---|---|---|---|
| Ø Prostate ♂<br>1 Testis ♂ | D Stereotactic Other Photon Radiosurgery<br>H Stereotactic Particulate Radiosurgery<br>J Stereotactic Gamma Beam Radiosurgery | Z None | Z None |

DRG Non-OR All treatment site, modality, isotope, and qualifier values
♂ All treatment site, modality, isotope, and qualifier values

**D Radiation Therapy**
**V Male Reproductive System**
**Y Other Radiation**

| Treatment Site Character 4 | Modality Qualifier Character 5 | Isotope Character 6 | Qualifier Character 7 |
|---|---|---|---|
| Ø Prostate ♂ | 7 Contact Radiation<br>8 Hyperthermia<br>C Intraoperative Radiation Therapy (IORT)<br>F Plaque Radiation<br>K Laser Interstitial Thermal Therapy | Z None | Z None |
| 1 Testis ♂ | 7 Contact Radiation<br>8 Hyperthermia<br>F Plaque Radiation | Z None | Z None |

Valid OR DVYØKZZ
♂ All treatment site, modality, isotope, and qualifier values

**D Radiation Therapy**
**W Anatomical Regions**
**Ø Beam Radiation**

| Treatment Site Character 4 | Modality Qualifier Character 5 | Isotope Character 6 | Qualifier Character 7 |
|---|---|---|---|
| 1 Head and Neck<br>2 Chest<br>3 Abdomen<br>4 Hemibody<br>5 Whole Body<br>6 Pelvic Region | Ø Photons <1 MeV<br>1 Photons 1- 10 MeV<br>2 Photons >10 MeV<br>4 Heavy Particles (Protons, Ions)<br>5 Neutrons<br>6 Neutron Capture | Z None | Z None |
| 1 Head and Neck<br>2 Chest<br>3 Abdomen<br>4 Hemibody<br>5 Whole Body<br>6 Pelvic Region | 3 Electrons | Z None | Ø Intraoperative<br>Z None |

**D Radiation Therapy**
**W Anatomical Regions**
**1 Brachytherapy**

| Treatment Site Character 4 | Modality Qualifier Character 5 | Isotope Character 6 | Qualifier Character 7 |
|---|---|---|---|
| 1 Head and Neck<br>2 Chest<br>3 Abdomen<br>6 Pelvic Region | 9 High Dose Rate (HDR)<br>B Low Dose Rate (LDR) | 7 Cesium 137 (Cs-137)<br>8 Iridium 192 (Ir-192)<br>9 Iodine 125 (I-125)<br>B Palladium 103 (Pd-103)<br>C Californium 252 (Cf-252)<br>Y Other Isotope | Z None |

**D Radiation Therapy**
**W Anatomical Regions**
**2 Stereotactic Radiosurgery**

| Treatment Site Character 4 | Modality Qualifier Character 5 | Isotope Character 6 | Qualifier Character 7 |
|---|---|---|---|
| 1 Head and Neck<br>2 Chest<br>3 Abdomen<br>6 Pelvic Region | D Stereotactic Other Photon Radiosurgery<br>H Stereotactic Particulate Radiosurgery<br>J Stereotactic Gamma Beam Radiosurgery | Z None | Z None |

DRG Non-OR All treatment site, modality, isotope, and qualifier values

**D Radiation Therapy**
**W Anatomical Regions**
**Y Other Radiation**

| Treatment Site Character 4 | Modality Qualifier Character 5 | Isotope Character 6 | Qualifier Character 7 |
|---|---|---|---|
| 1 Head and Neck<br>2 Chest<br>3 Abdomen<br>4 Hemibody<br>6 Pelvic Region | 7 Contact Radiation<br>8 Hyperthermia<br>F Plaque Radiation | Z None | Z None |
| 5 Whole Body | 7 Contact Radiation<br>8 Hyperthermia<br>F Plaque Radiation | Z None | Z None |
| 5 Whole Body | G Isotope Administration | D Iodine 131 (I-131)<br>F Phosphorus 32 (P-32)<br>G Strontium 89 (Sr-89)<br>H Strontium 90 (Sr-90)<br>Y Other Isotope | Z None |

# Physical Rehabilitation and Diagnostic Audiology FØØ–F15

## Character Meanings

This Character Meaning table is provided as a guide to assist the user in the identification of character members that may be found in this section of code tables. It **SHOULD NOT** be used to build a PCS code.

### Ø: Rehabilitation

| Type–Character 3 | Body System–Body Region–Character 4 | Type Qualifier–Character 5 | Equipment – Character 6 | Qualifier–Character 7 |
|---|---|---|---|---|
| Ø Speech Assessment | Ø Neurological System - Head and Neck | See next page | 1 Audiometer | Z None |
| 1 Motor and/or Nerve Function Assessment | 1 Neurological System - Upper Back / Upper Extremity | | 2 Sound Field / Booth | |
| 2 Activities of Daily Living Assessment | 2 Neurological System - Lower Back / Lower Extremity | | 4 Electroacoustic Immitance/ Acoustic Reflex | |
| 6 Speech Treatment | 3 Neurological System - Whole Body | | 5 Hearing Aid Selection / Fitting / Test | |
| 7 Motor Treatment | 4 Circulatory System - Head and Neck | | 7 Electrophysiologic | |
| 8 Activities of Daily Living Treatment | 5 Circulatory System - Upper Back / Upper Extremity | | 8 Vestibular / Balance | |
| 9 Hearing Treatment | 6 Circulatory System - Lower Back / Lower Extremity | | 9 Cochlear Implant | |
| B Cochlear Implant Treatment | 7 Circulatory System - Whole Body | | B Physical Agents | |
| C Vestibular Treatment | 8 Respiratory System - Head and Neck | | C Mechanical | |
| D Device Fitting | 9 Respiratory System - Upper Back / Upper Extremity | | D Electrotherapeutic | |
| F Caregiver Training | B Respiratory System - Lower Back / Lower Extremity | | E Orthosis | |
| | C Respiratory System - Whole Body | | F Assistive, Adaptive, Supportive or Protective | |
| | D Integumentary System - Head and Neck | | G Aerobic Endurance and Conditioning | |
| | F Integumentary System - Upper Back / Upper Extremity | | H Mechanical or Electromechanical | |
| | G Integumentary System - Lower Back / Lower Extremity | | J Somatosensory | |
| | H Integumentary System - Whole Body | | K Audiovisual | |
| | J Musculoskeletal System - Head and Neck | | L Assistive Listening | |
| | K Musculoskeletal System - Upper Back / Upper Extremity | | M Augmentative / Alternative Communication | |
| | L Musculoskeletal System - Lower Back / Lower Extremity | | N Biosensory Feedback | |
| | M Musculoskeletal System - Whole Body | | P Computer | |
| | N Genitourinary System | | Q Speech Analysis | |
| | Z None | | S Voice Analysis | |
| | | | T Aerodynamic Function | |
| | | | U Prosthesis | |
| | | | V Speech Prosthesis | |
| | | | W Swallowing | |
| | | | X Cerumen Management | |
| | | | Y Other Equipment | |
| | | | Z None | |

*Continued on next page*

**Ø: Rehabilitation**

*Continued from previous page*

**Type Qualifier—Character 5 Meanings**

| Type–Character 3 | Type Qualifier–Character 5 | |
|---|---|---|
| Ø Speech Assessment | Ø Filtered Speech<br>1 Speech Threshold<br>2 Speech/Word Recognition<br>3 Staggered Spondaic Word<br>4 Sensorineural Acuity Level<br>5 Synthetic Sentence Identification<br>6 Speech and/or Language Screening<br>7 Nonspoken Language<br>8 Receptive/Expressive Language<br>9 Articulation/Phonology<br>B Motor Speech<br>C Aphasia<br>D Fluency<br>F Voice<br>G Communicative/Cognitive Integration Skills<br>H Bedside Swallowing and Oral Function | J Instrumental Swallowing and Oral Function<br>K Orofacial Myofunctional<br>L Augmentative/Alternative Communication System<br>M Voice Prosthetic<br>N Non-invasive Instrumental Status<br>P Oral Peripheral Mechanism<br>Q Performance Intensity Phonetically Balanced Speech Discrimination<br>R Brief Tone Stimuli<br>S Distorted Speech<br>T Dichotic Stimuli<br>V Temporal Ordering of Stimuli<br>W Masking Patterns<br>X Other Specified Central Auditory Processing |
| 1 Motor and/or Nerve Function Assessment | Ø Muscle Performance<br>1 Integumentary Integrity<br>2 Visual Motor Integration<br>3 Coordination/Dexterity<br>4 Motor Function<br>5 Range of Motion and Joint Integrity<br>6 Sensory Awareness/Processing/Integrity | 7 Facial Nerve Function<br>9 Somatosensory Evoked Potentials<br>B Bed Mobility<br>C Transfer<br>D Gait and/or Balance<br>F Wheelchair Mobility<br>G Reflex Integrity |
| 2 Activities of Daily Living Assessment | Ø Bathing/Showering<br>1 Dressing<br>2 Feeding/Eating<br>3 Grooming/Personal Hygiene<br>4 Home Management<br>5 Perceptual Processing<br>6 Psychosocial Skills<br>7 Aerobic Capacity and Endurance<br>8 Anthropometric Characteristics | 9 Cranial Nerve Integrity<br>B Environmental, Home and Work Barriers<br>C Ergonomics and Body Mechanics<br>D Neuromotor Development<br>F Pain<br>G Ventilation, Respiration and Circulation<br>H Vocational Activities and Functional Community or Work Reintegration Skills |
| 6 Speech Treatment | Ø Nonspoken Language<br>1 Speech-Language Pathology and Related Disorders Counseling<br>2 Speech-Language Pathology and Related Disorders Prevention<br>3 Aphasia<br>4 Articulation/Phonology<br>5 Aural Rehabilitation | 6 Communicative/Cognitive Integration Skills<br>7 Fluency<br>8 Motor Speech<br>9 Orofacial Myofunctional<br>B Receptive/Expressive Language<br>C Voice<br>D Swallowing Dysfunction |
| 7 Motor Treatment | Ø Range of Motion and Joint Mobility<br>1 Muscle Performance<br>2 Coordination/Dexterity<br>3 Motor Function<br>4 Wheelchair Mobility | 5 Bed Mobility<br>6 Therapeutic Exercise<br>7 Manual Therapy Techniques<br>8 Transfer Training<br>9 Gait Training/Functional Ambulation |
| 8 Activities of Daily Living Treatment | Ø Bathing/Showering Techniques<br>1 Dressing Techniques<br>2 Grooming/Personal Hygiene<br>3 Feeding/Eating<br>4 Home Management | 5 Wound Management<br>6 Psychosocial Skills<br>7 Vocational Activities and Functional Community or Work Reintegration Skills |
| 9 Hearing Treatment | Ø Hearing and Related Disorders Counseling<br>1 Hearing and Related Disorders Prevention<br>2 Auditory Processing<br>3 Cerumen Management | |
| B Cochlear Implant Treatment | Ø Cochlear Implant Rehabilitation | |
| C Vestibular Treatment | Ø Vestibular<br>1 Perceptual Processing | 2 Visual Motor Integration<br>3 Postural Control |
| D Device Fitting | Ø Tinnitus Masker<br>1 Monaural Hearing Aid<br>2 Binaural Hearing Aid<br>3 Augmentative/Alternative Communication System<br>4 Voice Prosthetic | 5 Assistive Listening Device<br>6 Dynamic Orthosis<br>7 Static Orthosis<br>8 Prosthesis<br>9 Assistive, Adaptive, Supportive or Protective Devices |
| F Caregiver Training | Ø Bathing/Showering Technique<br>1 Dressing<br>2 Feeding and Eating<br>3 Grooming/Personal Hygiene<br>4 Bed Mobility<br>5 Transfer<br>6 Wheelchair Mobility<br>7 Therapeutic Exercise<br>8 Airway Clearance Techniques<br>9 Wound Management | B Vocational Activities and Functional Community or Work Reintegration Skills<br>C Gait Training/Functional Ambulation<br>D Application, Proper Use and Care of Assistive, Adaptive, Supportive or Protective Devices<br>F Application, Proper Use and Care of Orthoses<br>G Application, Proper Use and Care of Prosthesis<br>H Home Management<br>J Communication Skills |

**1: Diagnostic Audiology**

| Type–Character 3 | Body System–Body Region–Character 4 | Meanings–Character 5 | Equipment–Character 6 | Qualifer–Character 7 |
|---|---|---|---|---|
| 3 Hearing Assessment | Z None | See below | Ø Occupational Hearing | Z None |
| 4 Hearing Aid Assessment | | | 1 Audiometer | |
| 5 Vestibular Assessment | | | 2 Sound Field / Booth | |
| | | | 3 Tympanometer | |
| | | | 4 Electroacoustic Immitance / Acoustic Reflex | |
| | | | 5 Hearing Aid Selection / Fitting / Test | |
| | | | 6 Otoacoustic Emission (OAE) | |
| | | | 7 Electrophysiologic | |
| | | | 8 Vestibular / Balance | |
| | | | 9 Cochlear Implant | |
| | | | K Audiovisual | |
| | | | L Assistive Listening | |
| | | | P Computer | |
| | | | Y Other Equipment | |
| | | | Z None | |

**1: Diagnostic Audiology**
**Type Qualifier—Character 5 Meanings**

| Type–Character 3 | Type Qualifier–Character 5 |
|---|---|
| 3 Hearing Assessment | Ø Hearing Screening<br>1 Pure Tone Audiometry, Air<br>2 Pure Tone Audiometry, Air and Bone<br>3 Bekesy Audiometry<br>4 Conditioned Play Audiometry<br>5 Select Picture Audiometry<br>6 Visual Reinforcement Audiometry<br>7 Alternate Binaural or Monaural Loudness Balance<br>8 Tone Decay<br>9 Short Increment Sensitivity Index<br>B Stenger<br>C Pure Tone Stenger<br>D Tympanometry<br>F Eustachian Tube Function<br>G Acoustic Reflex Patterns<br>H Acoustic Reflex Threshold<br>J Acoustic Reflex Decay<br>K Electrocochleography<br>L Auditory Evoked Potentials<br>M Evoked Otoacoustic Emissions, Screening<br>N Evoked Otoacoustic Emissions, Diagnostic<br>P Aural Rehabilitation Status<br>Q Auditory Processing |
| 4 Hearing Aid Assessment | Ø Cochlear Implant<br>1 Ear Canal Probe Microphone<br>2 Monaural Hearing Aid<br>3 Binaural Hearing Aid<br>4 Assistive Listening System/Device Selection<br>5 Sensory Aids<br>6 Binaural Electroacoustic Hearing Aid Check<br>7 Ear Protector Attentuation<br>8 Monaural Electroacoustic Hearing Aid Check |
| 5 Vestibular Assessment | Ø Bithermal, Bionaural Caloric Irrigation<br>1 Bithermal, Monaural Caloric Irrigation<br>2 Unithermal Binaural Screen<br>3 Oscillating Tracking<br>4 Sinusoidal Vertical Axis Rotational<br>5 Dix-Hallpike Dynamic<br>6 Computerized Dynamic Posturography<br>7 Tinnitus Masker |

**F Physical Rehabilitation and Diagnostic Audiology**
**Ø Rehabilitation**
**Ø Speech Assessment** Definition: Measurement of speech and related functions

| Body System/Region Character 4 | Type Qualifier Character 5 | Equipment Character 6 | Qualifier Character 7 |
|---|---|---|---|
| 3 Neurological System - Whole Body | G Communicative/Cognitive Integration Skills | K Audiovisual<br>M Augmentative / Alternative Communication<br>P Computer<br>Y Other Equipment<br>Z None | Z None |
| Z None | Ø Filtered Speech<br>3 Staggered Spondaic Word<br>Q Performance Intensity Phonetically Balanced Speech Discrimination<br>R Brief Tone Stimuli<br>S Distorted Speech<br>T Dichotic Stimuli<br>V Temporal Ordering of Stimuli<br>W Masking Patterns | 1 Audiometer<br>2 Sound Field / Booth<br>K Audiovisual<br>Z None | Z None |
| Z None | 1 Speech Threshold<br>2 Speech/Word Recognition | 1 Audiometer<br>2 Sound Field / Booth<br>9 Cochlear Implant<br>K Audiovisual<br>Z None | Z None |
| Z None | 4 Sensorineural Acuity Level | 1 Audiometer<br>2 Sound Field / Booth<br>Z None | Z None |
| Z None | 5 Synthetic Sentence Identification | 1 Audiometer<br>2 Sound Field / Booth<br>9 Cochlear Implant<br>K Audiovisual | Z None |
| Z None | 6 Speech and/or Language Screening<br>7 Nonspoken Language<br>8 Receptive/Expressive Language<br>C Aphasia<br>G Communicative/Cognitive Integration Skills<br>L Augmentative/Alternative Communication System | K Audiovisual<br>M Augmentative / Alternative Communication<br>P Computer<br>Y Other Equipment<br>Z None | Z None |
| Z None | 9 Articulation/Phonology | K Audiovisual<br>P Computer<br>Q Speech Analysis<br>Y Other Equipment<br>Z None | Z None |
| Z None | B Motor Speech | K Audiovisual<br>N Biosensory Feedback<br>P Computer<br>Q Speech Analysis<br>T Aerodynamic Function<br>Y Other Equipment<br>Z None | Z None |
| Z None | D Fluency | K Audiovisual<br>N Biosensory Feedback<br>P Computer<br>Q Speech Analysis<br>S Voice Analysis<br>T Aerodynamic Function<br>Y Other Equipment<br>Z None | Z None |
| Z None | F Voice | K Audiovisual<br>N Biosensory Feedback<br>P Computer<br>S Voice Analysis<br>T Aerodynamic Function<br>Y Other Equipment<br>Z None | Z None |

***FØØ Continued on next page***

DRG Non-OR All body system/region, type qualifier, equipment, and qualifier values

**F Physical Rehabilitation and Diagnostic Audiology**
**Ø Rehabilitation**
**Ø Speech Assessment** Definition: Measurement of speech and related functions

*FØØ Continued*

| Body System/Region Character 4 | Type Qualifier Character 5 | Equipment Character 6 | Qualifier Character 7 |
|---|---|---|---|
| Z None | H Bedside Swallowing and Oral Function<br>P Oral Peripheral Mechanism | Y Other Equipment<br>Z None | Z None |
| Z None | J Instrumental Swallowing and Oral Function | T Aerodynamic Function<br>W Swallowing<br>Y Other Equipment | Z None |
| Z None | K Orofacial Myofunctional | K Audiovisual<br>P Computer<br>Y Other Equipment<br>Z None | Z None |
| Z None | M Voice Prosthetic | K Audiovisual<br>P Computer<br>S Voice Analysis<br>V Speech Prosthesis<br>Y Other Equipment<br>Z None | Z None |
| Z None | N Non-invasive Instrumental Status | N Biosensory Feedback<br>P Computer<br>Q Speech Analysis<br>S Voice Analysis<br>T Aerodynamic Function<br>Y Other Equipment | Z None |
| Z None | X Other Specified Central Auditory Processing | Z None | Z None |

DRG Non-OR All body system/region, type qualifier, equipment, and qualifier values

**F Physical Rehabilitation and Diagnostic Audiology**
**Ø Rehabilitation**
**1 Motor and/or Nerve Function Assessment** Definition: Measurement of motor, nerve, and related functions

| Body System/Region Character 4 | Type Qualifier Character 5 | Equipment Character 6 | Qualifier Character 7 |
|---|---|---|---|
| Ø Neurological System - Head and Neck<br>1 Neurological System - Upper Back/ Upper Extremity<br>2 Neurological System - Lower Back/ Lower Extremity<br>3 Neurological System - Whole Body | Ø Muscle Performance | E Orthosis<br>F Assistive, Adaptive, Supportive or Protective<br>U Prosthesis<br>Y Other Equipment<br>Z None | Z None |
| Ø Neurological System - Head and Neck<br>1 Neurological System - Upper Back/ Upper Extremity<br>2 Neurological System - Lower Back/ Lower Extremity<br>3 Neurological System - Whole Body | 1 Integumentary Integrity<br>3 Coordination/Dexterity<br>4 Motor Function<br>G Reflex Integrity | Z None | Z None |
| Ø Neurological System - Head and Neck<br>1 Neurological System - Upper Back/ Upper Extremity<br>2 Neurological System - Lower Back/ Lower Extremity<br>3 Neurological System - Whole Body | 5 Range of Motion and Joint Integrity<br>6 Sensory Awareness/Processing/ Integrity | Y Other Equipment<br>Z None | Z None |
| D Integumentary System - Head and Neck<br>F Integumentary System - Upper Back/Upper Extremity<br>G Integumentary System - Lower Back/Lower Extremity<br>H Integumentary System - Whole Body<br>J Musculoskeletal System - Head and Neck<br>K Musculoskeletal System - Upper Back/ Upper Extremity<br>L Musculoskeletal System - Lower Back/ Lower Extremity<br>M Musculoskeletal System - Whole Body | Ø Muscle Performance | E Orthosis<br>F Assistive, Adaptive, Supportive or Protective<br>U Prosthesis<br>Y Other Equipment<br>Z None | Z None |

*FØ1 Continued on next page*

DRG Non-OR All body system/region, type qualifier, equipment, and qualifier values

*FØ1 Continued*

**F Physical Rehabilitation and Diagnostic Audiology**
**Ø Rehabilitation**
**1 Motor and/or Nerve Function Assessment** Definition: Measurement of motor, nerve, and related functions

| Body System/Region Character 4 | Type Qualifier Character 5 | Equipment Character 6 | Qualifier Character 7 |
|---|---|---|---|
| D Integumentary System - Head and Neck<br>F Integumentary System - Upper Back/Upper Extremity<br>G Integumentary System - Lower Back/Lower Extremity<br>H Integumentary System - Whole Body<br>J Musculoskeletal System - Head and Neck<br>K Musculoskeletal System - Upper Back/ Upper Extremity<br>L Musculoskeletal System - Lower Back/ Lower Extremity<br>M Musculoskeletal System - Whole Body | 1 Integumentary Integrity | Z None | Z None |
| D Integumentary System - Head and Neck<br>F Integumentary System - Upper Back/Upper Extremity<br>G Integumentary System - Lower Back/Lower Extremity<br>H Integumentary System - Whole Body<br>J Musculoskeletal System - Head and Neck<br>K Musculoskeletal System - Upper Back/Upper Extremity<br>L Musculoskeletal System - Lower Back/Lower Extremity<br>M Musculoskeletal System - Whole Body | 5 Range of Motion and Joint Integrity<br>6 Sensory Awareness/Processing/ Integrity | Y Other Equipment<br>Z None | Z None |
| N Genitourinary System | Ø Muscle Performance | E Orthosis<br>F Assistive, Adaptive, Supportive or Protective<br>U Prosthesis<br>Y Other Equipment<br>Z None | Z None |
| Z None | 2 Visual Motor Integration | K Audiovisual<br>M Augmentative / Alternative Communication<br>N Biosensory Feedback<br>P Computer<br>Q Speech Analysis<br>S Voice Analysis<br>Y Other Equipment<br>Z None | Z None |
| Z None | 7 Facial Nerve Function | 7 Electrophysiologic | Z None |
| Z None | 9 Somatosensory Evoked Potentials | J Somatosensory | Z None |
| Z None | B Bed Mobility<br>C Transfer<br>F Wheelchair Mobility | E Orthosis<br>F Assistive, Adaptive, Supportive or Protective<br>U Prosthesis<br>Z None | Z None |
| Z None | D Gait and/or Balance | E Orthosis<br>F Assistive, Adaptive, Supportive or Protective<br>U Prosthesis<br>Y Other Equipment<br>Z None | Z None |

DRG Non-OR All body system/region, type qualifier, equipment, and qualifier values

**F Physical Rehabilitation and Diagnostic Audiology**
**Ø Rehabilitation**
**2 Activities of Daily Living Assessment** Definition: Measurement of functional level for activities of daily living

| Body System/Region Character 4 | Type Qualifier Character 5 | Equipment Character 6 | Qualifier Character 7 |
|---|---|---|---|
| Ø Neurological System - Head and Neck | 9 Cranial Nerve Integrity<br>D Neuromotor Development | Y Other Equipment<br>Z None | Z None |
| 1 Neurological System - Upper Back/ Upper Extremity<br>2 Neurological System - Lower Back/ Lower Extremity<br>3 Neurological System - Whole Body | D Neuromotor Development | Y Other Equipment<br>Z None | Z None |
| 4 Circulatory System - Head and Neck<br>5 Circulatory System - Upper Back/ Upper Extremity<br>6 Circulatory System - Lower Back/ Lower Extremity<br>8 Respiratory System - Head and Neck<br>9 Respiratory System - Upper Back/ Upper Extremity<br>B Respiratory System - Lower Back/ Lower Extremity | G Ventilation, Respiration and Circulation | C Mechanical<br>G Aerobic Endurance and Conditioning<br>Y Other Equipment<br>Z None | Z None |
| 7 Circulatory System - Whole Body<br>C Respiratory System - Whole Body | 7 Aerobic Capacity and Endurance | E Orthosis<br>G Aerobic Endurance and Conditioning<br>U Prosthesis<br>Y Other Equipment<br>Z None | Z None |
| 7 Circulatory System - Whole Body<br>C Respiratory System - Whole Body | G Ventilation, Respiration and Circulation | C Mechanical<br>G Aerobic Endurance and Conditioning<br>Y Other Equipment<br>Z None | Z None |
| Z None | Ø Bathing/Showering<br>1 Dressing<br>3 Grooming/Personal Hygiene<br>4 Home Management | E Orthosis<br>F Assistive, Adaptive, Supportive or Protective<br>U Prosthesis<br>Z None | Z None |
| Z None | 2 Feeding/Eating<br>8 Anthropometric Characteristics<br>F Pain | Y Other Equipment<br>Z None | Z None |
| Z None | 5 Perceptual Processing | K Audiovisual<br>M Augmentative / Alternative Communication<br>N Biosensory Feedback<br>P Computer<br>Q Speech Analysis<br>S Voice Analysis<br>Y Other Equipment<br>Z None | Z None |
| Z None | 6 Psychosocial Skills | Z None | Z None |
| Z None | B Environmental, Home and Work Barriers<br>C Ergonomics and Body Mechanics | E Orthosis<br>F Assistive, Adaptive, Supportive or Protective<br>U Prosthesis<br>Y Other Equipment<br>Z None | Z None |
| Z None | H Vocational Activities and Functional Community or Work Reintegration Skills | E Orthosis<br>F Assistive, Adaptive, Supportive or Protective<br>G Aerobic Endurance and Conditioning<br>U Prosthesis<br>Y Other Equipment<br>Z None | Z None |

DRG Non-OR All body system/region, type qualifier, equipment, and qualifier values

**F Physical Rehabilitation and Diagnostic Audiology**
**Ø Rehabilitation**
**6 Speech Treatment** Definition: Application of techniques to improve, augment, or compensate for speech and related functional impairment

| Body System/Region Character 4 | Type Qualifier Character 5 | Equipment Character 6 | Qualifier Character 7 |
|---|---|---|---|
| 3 Neurological System - Whole Body | 6 Communicative/Cognitive Integration Skills | K Audiovisual<br>M Augmentative / Alternative Communication<br>P Computer<br>Y Other Equipment<br>Z None | Z None |
| Z None | Ø Nonspoken Language<br>3 Aphasia<br>6 Communicative/Cognitive Integration Skills | K Audiovisual<br>M Augmentative / Alternative Communication<br>P Computer<br>Y Other Equipment<br>Z None | Z None |
| Z None | 1 Speech-Language Pathology and Related Disorders Counseling<br>2 Speech-Language Pathology and Related Disorders Prevention | K Audiovisual<br>Z None | Z None |
| Z None | 4 Articulation/Phonology | K Audiovisual<br>P Computer<br>Q Speech Analysis<br>T Aerodynamic Function<br>Y Other Equipment<br>Z None | Z None |
| Z None | 5 Aural Rehabilitation | K Audiovisual<br>L Assistive Listening<br>M Augmentative / Alternative Communication<br>N Biosensory Feedback<br>P Computer<br>Q Speech Analysis<br>S Voice Analysis<br>Y Other Equipment<br>Z None | Z None |
| Z None | 7 Fluency | 4 Electroacoustic Immitance / Acoustic Reflex<br>K Audiovisual<br>N Biosensory Feedback<br>Q Speech Analysis<br>S Voice Analysis<br>T Aerodynamic Function<br>Y Other Equipment<br>Z None | Z None |
| Z None | 8 Motor Speech | K Audiovisual<br>N Biosensory Feedback<br>P Computer<br>Q Speech Analysis<br>S Voice Analysis<br>T Aerodynamic Function<br>Y Other Equipment<br>Z None | Z None |
| Z None | 9 Orofacial Myofunctional | K Audiovisual<br>P Computer<br>Y Other Equipment<br>Z None | Z None |
| Z None | B Receptive/Expressive Language | K Audiovisual<br>L Assistive Listening<br>M Augmentative / Alternative Communication<br>P Computer<br>Y Other Equipment<br>Z None | Z None |

***FØ6 Continued on next page***

DRG Non-OR All body system/region, type qualifier, equipment, and qualifier values

**F06 Continued**

**F Physical Rehabilitation and Diagnostic Audiology**
**0 Rehabilitation**
**6 Speech Treatment** Definition: Application of techniques to improve, augment, or compensate for speech and related functional impairment

| Body System/Region Character 4 | Type Qualifier Character 5 | Equipment Character 6 | Qualifier Character 7 |
|---|---|---|---|
| **Z** None | **C** Voice | **K** Audiovisual<br>**N** Biosensory Feedback<br>**P** Computer<br>**S** Voice Analysis<br>**T** Aerodynamic Function<br>**V** Speech Prosthesis<br>**Y** Other Equipment<br>**Z** None | **Z** None |
| **Z** None | **D** Swallowing Dysfunction | **M** Augmentative / Alternative Communication<br>**T** Aerodynamic Function<br>**V** Speech Prosthesis<br>**Y** Other Equipment<br>**Z** None | **Z** None |

DRG Non-OR All body system/region, type qualifier, equipment, and qualifier values

**F Physical Rehabilitation and Diagnostic Audiology**
**Ø Rehabilitation**
**7 Motor Treatment** Definition: Exercise or activities to increase or facilitate motor function

| Body System/Region Character 4 | Type Qualifier Character 5 | Equipment Character 6 | Qualifier Character 7 |
|---|---|---|---|
| Ø Neurological System - Head and Neck<br>1 Neurological System - Upper Back/ Upper Extremity<br>2 Neurological System - Lower Back/ Lower Extremity<br>3 Neurological System - Whole Body<br>D Integumentary System - Head and Neck<br>F Integumentary System - Upper Back/Upper Extremity<br>G Integumentary System - Lower Back/Lower Extremity<br>H Integumentary System - Whole Body<br>J Musculoskeletal System - Head and Neck<br>K Musculoskeletal System - Upper Back/Upper Extremity<br>L Musculoskeletal System - Lower Back/Lower Extremity<br>M Musculoskeletal System - Whole Body | Ø Range of Motion and Joint Mobility<br>1 Muscle Performance<br>2 Coordination/Dexterity<br>3 Motor Function | E Orthosis<br>F Assistive, Adaptive, Supportive or Protective<br>U Prosthesis<br>Y Other Equipment<br>Z None | Z None |
| Ø Neurological System - Head and Neck<br>1 Neurological System - Upper Back/ Upper Extremity<br>2 Neurological System - Lower Back/ Lower Extremity<br>3 Neurological System - Whole Body<br>D Integumentary System - Head and Neck<br>F Integumentary System - Upper Back/Upper Extremity<br>G Integumentary System - Lower Back/Lower Extremity<br>H Integumentary System - Whole Body<br>J Musculoskeletal System - Head and Neck<br>K Musculoskeletal System - Upper Back/Upper Extremity<br>L Musculoskeletal System - Lower Back/Lower Extremity<br>M Musculoskeletal System - Whole Body | 6 Therapeutic Exercise | B Physical Agents<br>C Mechanical<br>D Electrotherapeutic<br>E Orthosis<br>F Assistive, Adaptive, Supportive or Protective<br>G Aerobic Endurance and Conditioning<br>H Mechanical or Electromechanical<br>U Prosthesis<br>Y Other Equipment<br>Z None | Z None |
| Ø Neurological System - Head and Neck<br>1 Neurological System - Upper Back/ Upper Extremity<br>2 Neurological System - Lower Back/ Lower Extremity<br>3 Neurological System - Whole Body<br>D Integumentary System - Head and Neck<br>F Integumentary System - Upper Back/Upper Extremity<br>G Integumentary System - Lower Back/Lower Extremity<br>H Integumentary System - Whole Body<br>J Musculoskeletal System - Head and Neck<br>K Musculoskeletal System - Upper Back/Upper Extremity<br>L Musculoskeletal System - Lower Back/Lower Extremity<br>M Musculoskeletal System - Whole Body | 7 Manual Therapy Techniques | Z None | Z None |

***FØ7 Continued on next page***

DRG Non-OR All body system/region, type qualifier, equipment, and qualifier values

**F Physical Rehabilitation and Diagnostic Audiology**
**Ø Rehabilitation**
**7 Motor Treatment** Definition: Exercise or activities to increase or facilitate motor function

*FØ7 Continued*

| Body System/Region Character 4 | Type Qualifier Character 5 | Equipment Character 6 | Qualifier Character 7 |
|---|---|---|---|
| 4 Circulatory System - Head and Neck<br>5 Circulatory System - Upper Back / Upper Extremity<br>6 Circulatory System - Lower Back / Lower Extremity<br>7 Circulatory System - Whole Body<br>8 Respiratory System - Head and Neck<br>9 Respiratory System - Upper Back / Upper Extremity<br>B Respiratory System -Lower Back / Lower Extremity<br>C Respiratory System -Whole Body | 6 Therapeutic Exercise | B Physical Agents<br>C Mechanical<br>D Electrotherapeutic<br>E Orthosis<br>F Assistive, Adaptive, Supportive or Protective<br>G Aerobic Endurance and Conditioning<br>H Mechanical or Electromechanical<br>U Prosthesis<br>Y Other Equipment<br>Z None | Z None |
| N Genitourinary System | 1 Muscle Performance | E Orthosis<br>F Assistive, Adaptive, Supportive or Protective<br>U Prosthesis<br>Y Other Equipment<br>Z None | Z None |
| N Genitourinary System | 6 Therapeutic Exercise | B Physical Agents<br>C Mechanical<br>D Electrotherapeutic<br>E Orthosis<br>F Assistive, Adaptive, Supportive or Protective<br>G Aerobic Endurance and Conditioning<br>H Mechanical or Electromechanical<br>U Prosthesis<br>Y Other Equipment<br>Z None | Z None |
| Z None | 4 Wheelchair Mobility | D Electrotherapeutic<br>E Orthosis<br>F Assistive, Adaptive, Supportive or Protective<br>U Prosthesis<br>Y Other Equipment<br>Z None | Z None |
| Z None | 5 Bed Mobility | C Mechanical<br>E Orthosis<br>F Assistive, Adaptive, Supportive or Protective<br>U Prosthesis<br>Y Other Equipment<br>Z None | Z None |
| Z None | 8 Transfer Training | C Mechanical<br>D Electrotherapeutic<br>E Orthosis<br>F Assistive, Adaptive, Supportive or Protective<br>U Prosthesis<br>Y Other Equipment<br>Z None | Z None |
| Z None | 9 Gait Training/Functional Ambulation | C Mechanical<br>D Electrotherapeutic<br>E Orthosis<br>F Assistive, Adaptive, Supportive or Protective<br>G Aerobic Endurance and Conditioning<br>U Prosthesis<br>Y Other Equipment<br>Z None | Z None |

DRG Non-OR All body system/region, type qualifier, equipment, and qualifier values

Physical Rehabilitation and Diagnostic Audiology

F07–F07

**F Physical Rehabilitation and Diagnostic Audiology**
**Ø Rehabilitation**
**8 Activities of Daily Living Treatment** Definition: Exercise or activities to facilitate functional competence for activities of daily living

| Body System/Region Character 4 | Type Qualifier Character 5 | Equipment Character 6 | Qualifier Character 7 |
|---|---|---|---|
| D Integumentary System - Head and Neck<br>F Integumentary System - Upper Back/Upper Extremity<br>G Integumentary System - Lower Back/Lower Extremity<br>H Integumentary System - Whole Body<br>J Musculoskeletal System - Head and Neck<br>K Musculoskeletal System - Upper Back/Upper Extremity<br>L Musculoskeletal System - Lower Back/Lower Extremity<br>M Musculoskeletal System - Whole Body | 5 Wound Management | B Physical Agents<br>C Mechanical<br>D Electrotherapeutic<br>E Orthosis<br>F Assistive, Adaptive, Supportive or Protective<br>U Prosthesis<br>Y Other Equipment<br>Z None | Z None |
| Z None | Ø Bathing/Showering Techniques<br>1 Dressing Techniques<br>2 Grooming/Personal Hygiene | E Orthosis<br>F Assistive, Adaptive, Supportive or Protective<br>U Prosthesis<br>Y Other Equipment<br>Z None | Z None |
| Z None | 3 Feeding/Eating | C Mechanical<br>D Electrotherapeutic<br>E Orthosis<br>F Assistive, Adaptive, Supportive or Protective<br>U Prosthesis<br>Y Other Equipment<br>Z None | Z None |
| Z None | 4 Home Management | D Electrotherapeutic<br>E Orthosis<br>F Assistive, Adaptive, Supportive or Protective<br>U Prosthesis<br>Y Other Equipment<br>Z None | Z None |
| Z None | 6 Psychosocial Skills | Z None | Z None |
| Z None | 7 Vocational Activities and Functional Community or Work Reintegration Skills | B Physical Agents<br>C Mechanical<br>D Electrotherapeutic<br>E Orthosis<br>F Assistive, Adaptive, Supportive or Protective<br>G Aerobic Endurance and Conditioning<br>U Prosthesis<br>Y Other Equipment<br>Z None | Z None |

DRG Non-OR All body system/region, type qualifier, equipment, and qualifier values

**F Physical Rehabilitation and Diagnostic Audiology**
**Ø Rehabilitation**
**9 Hearing Treatment** Definition: Application of techniques to improve, augment, or compensate for hearing and related functional impairment

| Body System/Region Character 4 | Type Qualifier Character 5 | Equipment Character 6 | Qualifier Character 7 |
|---|---|---|---|
| Z None | Ø Hearing and Related Disorders Counseling<br>1 Hearing and Related Disorders Prevention | K Audiovisual<br>Z None | Z None |
| Z None | 2 Auditory Processing | K Audiovisual<br>L Assistive Listening<br>P Computer<br>Y Other Equipment<br>Z None | Z None |
| Z None | 3 Cerumen Management | X Cerumen Management<br>Z None | Z None |

DRG Non-OR All body system/region, type qualifier, equipment, and qualifier values

**F Physical Rehabilitation and Diagnostic Audiology**
**Ø Rehabilitation**
**B Cochlear Implant Treatment** Definition: Application of techniques to improve the communication abilities of individuals with cochlear implant

| Body System/Region Character 4 | Type Qualifier Character 5 | Equipment Character 6 | Qualifier Character 7 |
|---|---|---|---|
| Z None | Ø Cochlear Implant Rehabilitation | 1 Audiometer<br>2 Sound Field / Booth<br>9 Cochlear Implant<br>K Audiovisual<br>P Computer<br>Y Other Equipment | Z None |

DRG Non-OR All body system/region, type qualifier, equipment, and qualifier values

**F Physical Rehabilitation and Diagnostic Audiology**
**Ø Rehabilitation**
**C Vestibular Treatment** Definition: Application of techniques to improve, augment, or compensate for vestibular and related functional impairment

| Body System/Region Character 4 | Type Qualifier Character 5 | Equipment Character 6 | Qualifier Character 7 |
|---|---|---|---|
| 3 Neurological System - Whole Body<br>H Integumentary System - Whole Body<br>M Musculoskeletal System - Whole Body | 3 Postural Control | E Orthosis<br>F Assistive, Adaptive, Supportive or Protective<br>U Prosthesis<br>Y Other Equipment<br>Z None | Z None |
| Z None | Ø Vestibular | 8 Vestibular / Balance<br>Z None | Z None |
| Z None | 1 Perceptual Processing<br>2 Visual Motor Integration | K Audiovisual<br>L Assistive Listening<br>N Biosensory Feedback<br>P Computer<br>Q Speech Analysis<br>S Voice Analysis<br>T Aerodynamic Function<br>Y Other Equipment<br>Z None | Z None |

DRG Non-OR All body system/region, type qualifier, equipment, and qualifier values

**F Physical Rehabilitation and Diagnostic Audiology**
**Ø Rehabilitation**
**D Device Fitting** Definition: Fitting of a device designed to facilitate or support achievement of a higher level of function

| Body System/Region Character 4 | Type Qualifier Character 5 | Equipment Character 6 | Qualifier Character 7 |
|---|---|---|---|
| Z None | Ø Tinnitus Masker | 5 Hearing Aid Selection / Fitting / Test<br>Z None | Z None |
| Z None | 1 Monaural Hearing Aid<br>2 Binaural Hearing Aid<br>5 Assistive Listening Device | 1 Audiometer<br>2 Sound Field / Booth<br>5 Hearing Aid Selection / Fitting / Test<br>K Audiovisual<br>L Assistive Listening<br>Z None | Z None |
| Z None | 3 Augmentative/Alternative Communication System | M Augmentative / Alternative Communication | Z None |
| Z None | 4 Voice Prosthetic | S Voice Analysis<br>V Speech Prosthesis | Z None |
| Z None | 6 Dynamic Orthosis<br>7 Static Orthosis<br>8 Prosthesis<br>9 Assistive, Adaptive,Supportive or Protective Devices | E Orthosis<br>F Assistive, Adaptive, Supportive or Protective<br>U Prosthesis<br>Z None | Z None |

DRG Non-OR FØDZØ[5,Z]Z
DRG Non-OR FØDZ[1, 2,5][1,2,5, K,L,Z]Z
DRG Non-OR FØDZ3MZ
DRG Non-OR FØDZ4[S,V]Z
DRG Non-OR FØDZ[6,7][E,F,U,Z]Z
DRG Non-OR FØDZ8[E,F,U]Z

**F Physical Rehabilitation and Diagnostic Audiology**
**Ø Rehabilitation**
**F Caregiver Training** Definition: Training in activities to support patient's optimal level of function

| Body System/Region Character 4 | Type Qualifier Character 5 | Equipment Character 6 | Qualifier Character 7 |
|---|---|---|---|
| Z None | Ø Bathing/Showering Technique<br>1 Dressing<br>2 Feeding and Eating<br>3 Grooming/Personal Hygiene<br>4 Bed Mobility<br>5 Transfer<br>6 Wheelchair Mobility<br>7 Therapeutic Exercise<br>8 Airway Clearance Techniques<br>9 Wound Management<br>B Vocational Activities and Functional Community or Work Reintegration Skills<br>C Gait Training/Functional Ambulation<br>D Application, Proper Use and Care of Devices<br>F Application, Proper Use and Care of Orthoses<br>G Application, Proper Use and Care of Prosthesis<br>H Home Management | E Orthosis<br>F Assistive, Adaptive, Supportive or Protective<br>U Prosthesis<br>Z None | Z None |
| Z None | J Communication Skills | K Audiovisual<br>L Assistive Listening<br>M Augmentative / Alternative Communication<br>P Computer<br>Z None | Z None |

DRG Non-OR All body system/region, type qualifier, equipment, and qualifier values

**F Physical Rehabilitation and Diagnostic Audiology**
**1 Diagnostic Audiology**
**3 Hearing Assessment** Definition: Measurement of hearing and related functions

| Body System/Region Character 4 | Type Qualifier Character 5 | Equipment Character 6 | Qualifier Character 7 |
|---|---|---|---|
| Z None | Ø Hearing Screening | Ø Occupational Hearing<br>1 Audiometer<br>2 Sound Field / Booth<br>3 Tympanometer<br>8 Vestibular / Balance<br>9 Cochlear Implant<br>Z None | Z None |
| Z None | 1 Pure Tone Audiometry, Air<br>2 Pure Tone Audiometry, Air and Bone | Ø Occupational Hearing<br>1 Audiometer<br>2 Sound Field / Booth<br>Z None | Z None |
| Z None | 3 Bekesy Audiometry<br>6 Visual Reinforcement Audiometry<br>9 Short Increment Sensitivity Index<br>B Stenger<br>C Pure Tone Stenger | 1 Audiometer<br>2 Sound Field / Booth<br>Z None | Z None |
| Z None | 4 Conditioned Play Audiometry<br>5 Select Picture Audiometry | 1 Audiometer<br>2 Sound Field / Booth<br>K Audiovisual<br>Z None | Z None |
| Z None | 7 Alternate Binaural or Monaural Loudness Balance | 1 Audiometer<br>K Audiovisual<br>Z None | Z None |
| Z None | 8 Tone Decay<br>D Tympanometry<br>F Eustachian Tube Function<br>G Acoustic Reflex Patterns<br>H Acoustic Reflex Threshold<br>J Acoustic Reflex Decay | 3 Tympanometer<br>4 Electroacoustic Immitance / Acoustic Reflex<br>Z None | Z None |
| Z None | K Electrocochleography<br>L Auditory Evoked Potentials | 7 Electrophysiologic<br>Z None | Z None |
| Z None | M Evoked Otoacoustic Emissions, Screening<br>N Evoked Otoacoustic Emissions, Diagnostic | 6 Otoacoustic Emission (OAE)<br>Z None | Z None |
| Z None | P Aural Rehabilitation Status | 1 Audiometer<br>2 Sound Field / Booth<br>4 Electroacoustic Immitance / Acoustic Reflex<br>9 Cochlear Implant<br>K Audiovisual<br>L Assistive Listening<br>P Computer<br>Z None | Z None |
| Z None | Q Auditory Processing | K Audiovisual<br>P Computer<br>Y Other Equipment<br>Z None | Z None |

**F Physical Rehabilitation and Diagnostic Audiology**
**1 Diagnostic Audiology**
**4 Hearing Aid Assessment** Definition: Measurement of the appropriateness and/or effectiveness of a hearing device

| Body System/Region Character 4 | Type Qualifier Character 5 | Equipment Character 6 | Qualifier Character 7 |
|---|---|---|---|
| Z None | Ø Cochlear Implant | 1 Audiometer<br>2 Sound Field / Booth<br>3 Tympanometer<br>4 Electroacoustic Immitance / Acoustic Reflex<br>5 Hearing Aid Selection / Fitting / Test<br>7 Electrophysiologic<br>9 Cochlear Implant<br>K Audiovisual<br>L Assistive Listening<br>P Computer<br>Y Other Equipment<br>Z None | Z None |
| Z None | 1 Ear Canal Probe Microphone<br>6 Binaural Electroacoustic Hearing Aid Check<br>8 Monaural Electroacoustic Hearing Aid Check | 5 Hearing Aid Selection / Fitting / Test<br>Z None | Z None |
| Z None | 2 Monaural Hearing Aid<br>3 Binaural Hearing Aid | 1 Audiometer<br>2 Sound Field / Booth<br>3 Tympanometer<br>4 Electroacoustic Immitance / Acoustic Reflex<br>5 Hearing Aid Selection / Fitting / Test<br>K Audiovisual<br>L Assistive Listening<br>P Computer<br>Z None | Z None |
| Z None | 4 Assistive Listening System/Device Selection | 1 Audiometer<br>2 Sound Field / Booth<br>3 Tympanometer<br>4 Electroacoustic Immitance / Acoustic Reflex<br>K Audiovisual<br>L Assistive Listening<br>Z None | Z None |
| Z None | 5 Sensory Aids | 1 Audiometer<br>2 Sound Field / Booth<br>3 Tympanometer<br>4 Electroacoustic Immitance / Acoustic Reflex<br>5 Hearing Aid Selection / Fitting / Test<br>K Audiovisual<br>L Assistive Listening<br>Z None | Z None |
| Z None | 7 Ear Protector Attentuation | Ø Occupational Hearing<br>Z None | Z None |

**F Physical Rehabilitation and Diagnostic Audiology**
**1 Diagnostic Audiology**
**5 Vestibular Assessment** Definition: Measurement of the vestibular system and related functions

| Body System/Region Character 4 | Type Qualifier Character 5 | Equipment Character 6 | Qualifier Character 7 |
|---|---|---|---|
| Z None | Ø Bithermal, Binaural Caloric Irrigation<br>1 Bithermal, Monaural Caloric Irrigation<br>2 Unithermal Binaural Screen<br>3 Oscillating Tracking<br>4 Sinusoidal Vertical Axis Rotational<br>5 Dix-Hallpike Dynamic<br>6 Computerized Dynamic Posturography | 8 Vestibular / Balance<br>Z None | Z None |
| Z None | 7 Tinnitus Masker | 5 Hearing Aid Selection / Fitting / Test<br>Z None | Z None |

# Mental Health GZ1–GZJ



## Character Meanings

This Character Meaning table is provided as a guide to assist the user in the identification of character members that may be found in this section of code tables. It **SHOULD NOT** be used to build a PCS code.

### Z: None

| Type–Character 3 | Type Qualifier –Character 4 | Qualifier–Character 5 | Qualifier–Character 6 | Qualifier–Character 7 |
|---|---|---|---|---|
| 1 Psychological Tests | Ø Developmental | Z None | Z None | Z None |
| | 1 Personality and Behavioral | | | |
| | 2 Intellectual and Psychoeducational | | | |
| | 3 Neuropsychological | | | |
| | 4 Neurobehavioral and Cognitive Status | | | |
| 2 Crisis Intervention | Z None | | | |
| 3 Medication Management | Z None | | | |
| 5 Individual Psychotherapy | Ø Interactive | | | |
| | 1 Behavioral | | | |
| | 2 Cognitive | | | |
| | 3 Interpersonal | | | |
| | 4 Psychoanalysis | | | |
| | 5 Psychodynamic | | | |
| | 6 Supportive | | | |
| | 8 Cognitive-Behavioral | | | |
| | 9 Psychophysiological | | | |
| 6 Counseling | Ø Educational | | | |
| | 1 Vocational | | | |
| | 3 Other Counseling | | | |
| 7 Family Psychotherapy | 2 Other Family Psychotherapy | | | |
| B Electroconvulsive Therapy | Ø Unilateral-Single Seizure | | | |
| | 1 Unilateral-Multiple Seizure | | | |
| | 2 Bilateral-Single Seizure | | | |
| | 3 Bilateral-Multiple Seizure | | | |
| | 4 Other Electroconvulsive Therapy | | | |
| C Biofeedback | 9 Other Biofeedback | | | |
| F Hypnosis | Z None | | | |
| G Narcosynthesis | Z None | | | |
| H Group Psychotherapy | Z None | | | |
| J Light Therapy | Z None | | | |

**G Mental Health**
**Z None**
**1 Psychological Tests** Definition: The administration and interpretation of standardized psychological tests and measurement instruments for the assessment of psychological function

| Type Qualifier Character 4 | Qualifier Character 5 | Qualifier Character 6 | Qualifier Character 7 |
|---|---|---|---|
| Ø Developmental<br>1 Personality and Behavioral<br>2 Intellectual and Psychoeducational<br>3 Neuropsychological<br>4 Neurobehavioral and Cognitive Status | Z None | Z None | Z None |

**G Mental Health**
**Z None**
**2 Crisis Intervention** Definition: Treatment of a traumatized, acutely disturbed or distressed individual for the purpose of short-term stabilization

| Type Qualifier Character 4 | Qualifier Character 5 | Qualifier Character 6 | Qualifier Character 7 |
|---|---|---|---|
| Z None | Z None | Z None | Z None |

**G Mental Health**
**Z None**
**3 Medication Management** Definition: Monitoring and adjusting the use of medications for the treatment of a mental health disorder

| Type Qualifier Character 4 | Qualifier Character 5 | Qualifier Character 6 | Qualifier Character 7 |
|---|---|---|---|
| Z None | Z None | Z None | Z None |

**G Mental Health**
**Z None**
**5 Individual Psychotherapy** Definition: Treatment of an individual with a mental health disorder by behavioral, cognitive, psychoanalytic, psychodynamic or psychophysiological means to improve functioning or well-being

| Type Qualifier Character 4 | Qualifier Character 5 | Qualifier Character 6 | Qualifier Character 7 |
|---|---|---|---|
| Ø Interactive<br>1 Behavioral<br>2 Cognitive<br>3 Interpersonal<br>4 Psychoanalysis<br>5 Psychodynamic<br>6 Supportive<br>8 Cognitive-Behavioral<br>9 Psychophysiological | Z None | Z None | Z None |

**G Mental Health**
**Z None**
**6 Counseling** Definition: The application of psychological methods to treat an individual with normal developmental issues and psychological problems in order to increase function, improve well-being, alleviate distress, maladjustment or resolve crises

| Type Qualifier Character 4 | Qualifier Character 5 | Qualifier Character 6 | Qualifier Character 7 |
|---|---|---|---|
| Ø Educational<br>1 Vocational<br>3 Other Counseling | Z None | Z None | Z None |

**G Mental Health**
**Z None**
**7 Family Psychotherapy** Definition: Treatment that includes one or more family members of an individual with a mental health disorder by behavioral, cognitive, psychoanalytic, psychodynamic or psychophysiological means to improve functioning or well-being

Explanation: Remediation of emotional or behavioral problems presented by one or more family members in cases where psychotherapy with more than one family member is indicated

| Type Qualifier Character 4 | Qualifier Character 5 | Qualifier Character 6 | Qualifier Character 7 |
|---|---|---|---|
| 2 Other Family Psychotherapy | Z None | Z None | Z None |

**G Mental Health**
**Z None**
**B Electroconvulsive Therapy** Definition: The application of controlled electrical voltages to treat a mental health disorder

| Type Qualifier Character 4 | Qualifier Character 5 | Qualifier Character 6 | Qualifier Character 7 |
|---|---|---|---|
| Ø Unilateral-Single Seizure<br>1 Unilateral-Multiple Seizure<br>2 Bilateral-Single Seizure<br>3 Bilateral-Multiple Seizure<br>4 Other Electroconvulsive Therapy | Z None | Z None | Z None |

**G Mental Health**
**Z None**
**C Biofeedback** Definition: Provision of information from the monitoring and regulating of physiological processes in conjunction with cognitive-behavioral techniques to improve patient functioning or well-being

| Type Qualifier Character 4 | Qualifier Character 5 | Qualifier Character 6 | Qualifier Character 7 |
|---|---|---|---|
| 9 Other Biofeedback | Z None | Z None | Z None |

**G Mental Health**
**Z None**
**F Hypnosis** Definition: Induction of a state of heightened suggestibility by auditory, visual and tactile techniques to elicit an emotional or behavioral response

| Type Qualifier Character 4 | Qualifier Character 5 | Qualifier Character 6 | Qualifier Character 7 |
|---|---|---|---|
| Z None | Z None | Z None | Z None |

**G Mental Health**
**Z None**
**G Narcosynthesis** Definition: Administration of intravenous barbiturates in order to release suppressed or repressed thoughts

| Type Qualifier Character 4 | Qualifier Character 5 | Qualifier Character 6 | Qualifier Character 7 |
|---|---|---|---|
| Z None | Z None | Z None | Z None |

**G Mental Health**
**Z None**
**H Group Psychotherapy** Definition: Treatment of two or more individuals with a mental health disorder by behavioral, cognitive, psychoanalytic, psychodynamic or psychophysiological means to improve functioning or well-being

| Type Qualifier Character 4 | Qualifier Character 5 | Qualifier Character 6 | Qualifier Character 7 |
|---|---|---|---|
| Z None | Z None | Z None | Z None |

**G Mental Health**
**Z None**
**J Light Therapy** Definition: Application of specialized light treatments to improve functioning or well-being

| Type Qualifier Character 4 | Qualifier Character 5 | Qualifier Character 6 | Qualifier Character 7 |
|---|---|---|---|
| Z None | Z None | Z None | Z None |

# Substance Abuse Treatment HZ2–HZ9

## Character Meanings

This Character Meaning table is provided as a guide to assist the user in the identification of character members that may be found in this section of code tables. It **SHOULD NOT** be used to build a PCS code.

### Z: None

| Type–Character 3 | Type Qualifier–Character 4 | Qualifier–Character 5 | Qualifier–Character 6 | Qualifier–Character 7 |
|---|---|---|---|---|
| 2 Detoxification Services | Z None | Z None | Z None | Z None |
| 3 Individual Counseling | Ø Cognitive<br>1 Behavioral<br>2 Cognitive-Behavioral<br>3 12-Step<br>4 Interpersonal<br>5 Vocational<br>6 Psychoeducation<br>7 Motivational Enhancement<br>8 Confrontational<br>9 Continuing Care<br>B Spiritual<br>C Pre/Post-Test Infectious Disease | | | |
| 4 Group Counseling | Ø Cognitive<br>1 Behavioral<br>2 Cognitive-Behavioral<br>3 12-Step<br>4 Interpersonal<br>5 Vocational<br>6 Psychoeducation<br>7 Motivational Enhancement<br>8 Confrontational<br>9 Continuing Care<br>B Spiritual<br>C Pre/Post-Test Infectious Disease | | | |
| 5 Individual Psychotherapy | Ø Cognitive<br>1 Behavioral<br>2 Cognitive-Behavioral<br>3 12-Step<br>4 Interpersonal<br>5 Interactive<br>6 Psychoeducation<br>7 Motivational Enhancement<br>8 Confrontational<br>9 Supportive<br>B Psychoanalysis<br>C Psychodynamic<br>D Psychophysiological | | | |
| 6 Family Counseling | 3 Other Family Counseling | | | |
| 8 Medication Management | Ø Nicotine Replacement<br>1 Methadone Maintenance<br>2 Levo-alpha-acetyl-methadol (LAAM)<br>3 Antabuse<br>4 Naltrexone<br>5 Naloxone<br>6 Clonidine<br>7 Bupropion<br>8 Psychiatric Medication<br>9 Other Replacement Medication | | | |
| 9 Pharmacotherapy | Ø Nicotine Replacement<br>1 Methadone Maintenance<br>2 Levo-alpha-acetyl-methadol (LAAM)<br>3 Antabuse<br>4 Naltrexone<br>5 Naloxone<br>6 Clonidine<br>7 Bupropion<br>8 Psychiatric Medication<br>9 Other Replacement Medication | | | |

**H Substance Abuse Treatment**
**Z None**
**2 Detoxification Services** Definition: Detoxification from alcohol and/or drugs

Explanation: Not a treatment modality, but helps the patient stabilize physically and psychologically until the body becomes free of drugs and the effects of alcohol

| Type Qualifier Character 4 | Qualifier Character 5 | Qualifier Character 6 | Qualifier Character 7 |
|---|---|---|---|
| Z None | Z None | Z None | Z None |

**H Substance Abuse Treatment**
**Z None**
**3 Individual Counseling** Definition: The application of psychological methods to treat an individual with addictive behavior

Explanation: Comprised of several different techniques, which apply various strategies to address drug addiction

| Type Qualifier Character 4 | Qualifier Character 5 | Qualifier Character 6 | Qualifier Character 7 |
|---|---|---|---|
| Ø Cognitive<br>1 Behavioral<br>2 Cognitive-Behavioral<br>3 12-Step<br>4 Interpersonal<br>5 Vocational<br>6 Psychoeducation<br>7 Motivational Enhancement<br>8 Confrontational<br>9 Continuing Care<br>B Spiritual<br>C Pre/Post-Test Infectious Disease | Z None | Z None | Z None |

DRG Non-OR HZ3[Ø,1,2,3,4,5,6,7,8,9,B]ZZZ

**H Substance Abuse Treatment**
**Z None**
**4 Group Counseling** Definition: The application of psychological methods to treat two or more individuals with addictive behavior

Explanation: Provides structured group counseling sessions and healing power through the connection with others

| Type Qualifier Character 4 | Qualifier Character 5 | Qualifier Character 6 | Qualifier Character 7 |
|---|---|---|---|
| Ø Cognitive<br>1 Behavioral<br>2 Cognitive-Behavioral<br>3 12-Step<br>4 Interpersonal<br>5 Vocational<br>6 Psychoeducation<br>7 Motivational Enhancement<br>8 Confrontational<br>9 Continuing Care<br>B Spiritual<br>C Pre/Post-Test Infectious Disease | Z None | Z None | Z None |

DRG Non-OR HZ4[Ø,1,2,3,4,5,6,7,8,9,B]ZZZ

**H Substance Abuse Treatment**
**Z None**
**5 Individual Psychotherapy** Definition: Treatment of an individual with addictive behavior by behavioral, cognitive, psychoanalytic, psychodynamic or psychophysiological means

| Type Qualifier Character 4 | Qualifier Character 5 | Qualifier Character 6 | Qualifier Character 7 |
|---|---|---|---|
| Ø Cognitive<br>1 Behavioral<br>2 Cognitive-Behavioral<br>3 12-Step<br>4 Interpersonal<br>5 Interactive<br>6 Psychoeducation<br>7 Motivational Enhancement<br>8 Confrontational<br>9 Supportive<br>B Psychoanalysis<br>C Psychodynamic<br>D Psychophysiological | Z None | Z None | Z None |

DRG Non-OR For all type qualifier and qualifier values

**H Substance Abuse Treatment**
**Z None**
**6 Family Counseling** Definition: The application of psychological methods that includes one or more family members to treat an individual with addictive behavior

Explanation: Provides support and education for family members of addicted individuals. Family member participation is seen as a critical area of substance abuse treatment

| Type Qualifier Character 4 | Qualifier Character 5 | Qualifier Character 6 | Qualifier Character 7 |
|---|---|---|---|
| 3 Other Family Counseling | Z None | Z None | Z None |

**H Substance Abuse Treatment**
**Z None**
**8 Medication Management** Definition: Monitoring or adjusting the use of replacement medications for the treatment of addiction

| Type Qualifier Character 4 | Qualifier Character 5 | Qualifier Character 6 | Qualifier Character 7 |
|---|---|---|---|
| Ø Nicotine Replacement<br>1 Methadone Maintenance<br>2 Levo-alpha-acetyl-methadol (LAAM)<br>3 Antabuse<br>4 Naltrexone<br>5 Naloxone<br>6 Clonidine<br>7 Bupropion<br>8 Psychiatric Medication<br>9 Other Replacement Medication | Z None | Z None | Z None |

**H Substance Abuse Treatment**
**Z None**
**9 Pharmacotherapy** Definition: The use of replacement medications for the treatment of addiction

| Type Qualifier Character 4 | Qualifier Character 5 | Qualifier Character 6 | Qualifier Character 7 |
|---|---|---|---|
| Ø Nicotine Replacement<br>1 Methadone Maintenance<br>2 Levo-alpha-acetyl-methadol (LAAM)<br>3 Antabuse<br>4 Naltrexone<br>5 Naloxone<br>6 Clonidine<br>7 Bupropion<br>8 Psychiatric Medication<br>9 Other Replacement Medication | Z None | Z None | Z None |

# New Technology X2A–XYØ

**AHA Coding Clinic for all tables in the New Technology Section**
**2015, 4Q, 8-11**

**AHA Coding Clinic for table X2A**
**2016, 4Q, 115-116** Cerebral embolic filtration

**AHA Coding Clinic for table X2C**
**2016, 4Q, 82-83** Coronary artery, number of arteries
**2015, 4Q, 8-14** New Section X codes—New Technology procedures

**AHA Coding Clinic for table X2R**
**2016, 4Q, 116** Aortic valve rapid deployment
**2015, 4Q, 8-12** New Section X codes—New Technology procedures

**AHA Coding Clinic for table XHR**
**2016, 4Q, 116** Application of wound matrix

**AHA Coding Clinic for table XNS**
**2016, 4Q, 117** Placement of magnetic growth rods

**AHA Coding Clinic for table XWØ**
**2015, 4Q, 8-15** New Section X codes—New Technology procedures

**X New Technology**
**2 Cardiovascular System**
**A Assistance** Definition: Taking over a portion of a physiological function by extracorporeal means
Explanation: None

| Body Part Character 4 | Approach Character 5 | Device/Substance/Technology Character 6 | Qualifier Character 7 |
|---|---|---|---|
| 5 Innominate Artery and Left Common Carotid Artery | 3 Percutaneous | 1 Cerebral Embolic Filtration, Dual Filter | 2 New Technology Group 2 |

**X New Technology**
**2 Cardiovascular System**
**C Extirpation** Definition: Taking or cutting out solid matter from a body part
Explanation: The solid matter may be an abnormal byproduct of a biological function or a foreign body; it may be imbedded in a body part or in the lumen of a tubular body part. The solid matter may or may not have been previously broken into pieces.

| Body Part Character 4 | Approach Character 5 | Device/Substance/Technology Character 6 | Qualifier Character 7 |
|---|---|---|---|
| Ø Coronary Artery, One Artery<br>1 Coronary Artery, Two Arteries<br>2 Coronary Artery, Three Arteries<br>3 Coronary Artery, Four or More Arteries | 3 Percutaneous | 6 Orbital Atherectomy Technology | 1 New Technology Group 1 |

Valid OR All body part, approach, device/substance/technology, and qualifier values

**X New Technology**
**2 Cardiovascular System**
**R Replacement** Definition: Putting in or on biological or synthetic material that physically takes the place and/or function of all or a portion of a body part
Explanation: The body part may have been taken out or replaced, or may be taken out, physically eradicated, or rendered nonfunctional during the REPLACEMENT procedure. A REMOVAL procedure is coded for taking out the device used in a previous replacement procedure

| Body Part Character 4 | Approach Character 5 | Device/Substance/Technology Character 6 | Qualifier Character 7 |
|---|---|---|---|
| F Aortic Valve | Ø Open<br>3 Percutaneous<br>4 Percutaneous Endoscopic | 3 Zooplastic Tissue, Rapid Deployment Technique | 2 New Technology Group 2 |

Valid OR All body part, approach, device/substance/technology, and qualifier values

**X New Technology**
**H Skin, Subcutaneous Tissue, Fascia and Breast**
**R Replacement** Definition: Putting in or on biological or synthetic material that physically takes the place and/or function of all or a portion of a body part
Explanation: The body part may have been taken out or replaced, or may be taken out, physically eradicated, or rendered nonfunctional during the REPLACEMENT procedure. A REMOVAL procedure is coded for taking out the device used in a previous replacement procedure

| Body Part Character 4 | Approach Character 5 | Device/Substance/Technology Character 6 | Qualifier Character 7 |
|---|---|---|---|
| P Skin | X External | L Skin Substitute, Porcine Liver Derived | 2 New Technology Group 2 |

Valid OR All body part, approach, device/substance/technology, and qualifier values

**X New Technology**
**K Muscles, Tendons, Bursae and Ligaments**
**Ø Introduction** Definition: Putting in or on a therapeutic, diagnostic, nutritional, physiological, or prophylactic substance except blood or blood products

Explanation: None

| Body Part Character 4 | Approach Character 5 | Device/Substance/Technology Character 6 | Qualifier Character 7 |
|---|---|---|---|
| 2 Muscle | 3 Percutaneous | Ø Concentrated Bone Marrow Aspirate | 3 New Technology Group 3 |

**X New Technology**
**N Bones**
**S Reposition** Definition: Moving to its normal location, or other suitable location, all or a portion of a body part

Explanation: The body part is moved to a new location from an abnormal location, or from a normal location where it is not functioning correctly. The body part may or may not be cut out or off to be moved to the new location.

| Body Part Character 4 | Approach Character 5 | Device/Substance/Technology Character 6 | Qualifier Character 7 |
|---|---|---|---|
| Ø Lumbar Vertebra<br>3 Cervical Vertebra<br>4 Thoracic Vertebra | Ø Open<br>3 Percutaneous | 3 Magnetically Controlled Growth Rod(s) | 2 New Technology Group 2 |

Valid OR XNS[Ø,3,4]Ø32

**X New Technology**
**R Joints**
**2 Monitoring** Definition: Determining the level of a physiological or physical function repetitively over a period of time

Explanation: None

| Body Part Character 4 | Approach Character 5 | Device/Substance/Technology Character 6 | Qualifier Character 7 |
|---|---|---|---|
| G Knee Joint, Right<br>H Knee Joint, Left | Ø Open | 2 Intraoperative Knee Replacement Sensor | 1 New Technology Group 1 |

Valid OR All body part, approach, device/substance/technology, and qualifier values

**X New Technology**
**R Joints**
**G Fusion**

Definition: Joining together portions of an articular body part rendering the articular body part immobile

Explanation: The body part is joined together by fixation device, bone graft, or other means

| Body Part Character 4 | Approach Character 5 | Device/Substance/Technology Character 6 | Qualifier Character 7 |
|---|---|---|---|
| Ø Occipital-cervical Joint | Ø Open | 9 Interbody Fusion Device, Nanotextured Surface | 2 New Technology Group 2 |
| Ø Occipital-cervical Joint | Ø Open | F Interbody Fusion Device, Radiolucent Porous | 3 New Technology Group 3 |
| 1 Cervical Vertebral Joint | Ø Open | 9 Interbody Fusion Device, Nanotextured Surface | 2 New Technology Group 2 |
| 1 Cervical Vertebral Joint | Ø Open | F Interbody Fusion Device, Radiolucent Porous | 3 New Technology Group 3 |
| 2 Cervical Vertebral Joints, 2 or more | Ø Open | 9 Interbody Fusion Device, Nanotextured Surface | 2 New Technology Group 2 |
| 2 Cervical Vertebral Joints, 2 or more | Ø Open | F Interbody Fusion Device, Radiolucent Porous | 3 New Technology Group 3 |
| 4 Cervicothoracic Vertebral Joint | Ø Open | 9 Interbody Fusion Device, Nanotextured Surface | 2 New Technology Group 2 |
| 4 Cervicothoracic Vertebral Joint | Ø Open | F Interbody Fusion Device, Radiolucent Porous | 3 New Technology Group 3 |
| 6 Thoracic Vertebral Joint | Ø Open | 9 Interbody Fusion Device, Nanotextured Surface | 2 New Technology Group 2 |
| 6 Thoracic Vertebral Joint | Ø Open | F Interbody Fusion Device, Radiolucent Porous | 3 New Technology Group 3 |
| 7 Thoracic Vertebral Joints, 2 to 7 ⊞ | Ø Open | 9 Interbody Fusion Device, Nanotextured Surface | 2 New Technology Group 2 |
| 7 Thoracic Vertebral Joints, 2 to 7 | Ø Open | F Interbody Fusion Device, Radiolucent Porous | 3 New Technology Group 3 |
| 8 Thoracic Vertebral Joints, 8 or more | Ø Open | 9 Interbody Fusion Device, Nanotextured Surface | 2 New Technology Group 2 |
| 8 Thoracic Vertebral Joints, 8 or more | Ø Open | F Interbody Fusion Device, Radiolucent Porous | 3 New Technology Group 3 |
| A Thoracolumbar Vertebral Joint | Ø Open | 9 Interbody Fusion Device, Nanotextured Surface | 2 New Technology Group 2 |
| A Thoracolumbar Vertebral Joint | Ø Open | F Interbody Fusion Device, Radiolucent Porous | 3 New Technology Group 3 |
| B Lumbar Vertebral Joint | Ø Open | 9 Interbody Fusion Device, Nanotextured Surface | 2 New Technology Group 2 |
| B Lumbar Vertebral Joint | Ø Open | F Interbody Fusion Device, Radiolucent Porous | 3 New Technology Group 3 |
| C Lumbar Vertebral Joints, 2 or more ⊞ | Ø Open | 9 Interbody Fusion Device, Nanotextured Surface | 2 New Technology Group 2 |
| C Lumbar Vertebral Joints, 2 or more | Ø Open | F Interbody Fusion Device, Radiolucent Porous | 3 New Technology Group 3 |
| D Lumbosacral Joint | Ø Open | 9 Interbody Fusion Device, Nanotextured Surface | 2 New Technology Group 2 |
| D Lumbosacral Joint | Ø Open | F Interbody Fusion Device, Radiolucent Porous | 3 New Technology Group 3 |

**Valid OR** XRG[Ø,1,2,4,6,8,A,B,D]Ø92

**HAC** XRG[Ø,1,2,4,6,7,8,A,B,C,D]Ø92 when reported with SDx K68.11 or T81.4XXA or T84.6Ø-T84.619, T84.63-T84.7 with 7th character A

**See Appendix L for Procedure Combinations**

⊞ XRG[7,C]Ø92

**X New Technology**
**W Anatomical Regions**
**Ø Introduction** Definition: Putting in or on a therapeutic, diagnostic, nutritional, physiological, or prophylactic substance except blood or blood products

Explanation: None

| Body Part Character 4 | Approach Character 5 | Device/Substance/Technology Character 6 | Qualifier Character 7 |
|---|---|---|---|
| 3 Peripheral Vein | 3 Percutaneous | 2 Ceftazidime-Avibactam Anti-infective<br>3 Idarucizumab, Dabigatran Reversal Agent<br>4 Isavuconazole Anti- infective<br>5 Blinatumomab Antineoplastic Immunotherapy | 1 New Technology Group 1 |
| 3 Peripheral Vein | 3 Percutaneous | 7 Andexanet Alfa, Factor Xa Inhibitor Reversal Agent<br>9 Defibrotide Sodium Anticoagulant | 2 New Technology Group 2 |
| 3 Peripheral Vein | 3 Percutaneous | A Bezlotoxumab Monoclonal Antibody<br>B Cytarabine and Daunorubicin Liposome Antineoplastic<br>C Engineered Autologous Chimeric Antigen Receptor T-cell Immunotherapy<br>F Other New Technology Therapeutic Substance | 3 New Technology Group 3 |
| 4 Central Vein | 3 Percutaneous | 2 Ceftazidime-Avibactam Anti-infective<br>3 Idarucizumab, Dabigatran Reversal Agent<br>4 Isavuconazole Anti- infective<br>5 Blinatumomab Antineoplastic Immunotherapy | 1 New Technology Group 1 |
| 4 Central Vein | 3 Percutaneous | 7 Andexanet Alfa, Factor Xa Inhibitor Reversal Agent<br>9 Defibrotide Sodium Anticoagulant | 2 New Technology Group 2 |
| 4 Central Vein | 3 Percutaneous | A Bezlotoxumab Monoclonal Antibody<br>B Cytarabine and Daunorubicin Liposome Antineoplastic<br>C Engineered Autologous Chimeric Antigen Receptor T-cell Immunotherapy<br>F Other New Technology Therapeutic Substance | 3 New Technology Group 3 |
| D Mouth and Pharynx | X External | 8 Uridine Triacetate | 2 New Technology Group 2 |

**X New Technology**
**Y Extracorporeal**
**Ø Introduction** Definition: Putting in or on a therapeutic, diagnostic, nutritional, physiological, or prophylactic substance except blood or blood products

Explanation: None

| Body Part Character 4 | Approach Character 5 | Device/Substance/Technology Character 6 | Qualifier Character 7 |
|---|---|---|---|
| V Vein Graft | X External | 8 Endothelial Damage Inhibitor | 3 New Technology Group 3 |

# Appendixes



## Appendix A: Components of the Medical and Surgical Approach Definitions

| ICD-10-PCS Value | Definition | Access Location | Method | Type of Instrumentation | Example |
|---|---|---|---|---|---|
| Open (Ø) | Cutting through the skin or mucous membrane and any other body layers necessary to expose the site of the procedure | Skin or mucous membrane, any other body layers | Cutting | None | Abdominal hysterectomy |
| Percutaneous (3) | Entry, by puncture or minor incision, of instrumentation through the skin or mucous membrane and any other body layers necessary to reach the site of the procedure | Skin or mucous membrane, any other body layers | Puncture or minor incision | Without visualization | Needle biopsy of liver, Liposuction |
| Percutaneous endoscopic (4) | Entry, by puncture or minor incision, of instrumentation through the skin or mucous membrane and any other body layers necessary to reach and visualize the site of the procedure | Skin or mucous membrane, any other body layers | Puncture or minor incision | With visualization | Arthroscopy, Laparoscopic cholecystectomy |
| Via natural or artificial opening (7) | Entry of instrumentation through a natural or artificial external opening to reach the site of the procedure | Natural or artificial external opening | Direct entry | Without visualization | Endotracheal tube insertion, Foley catheter placement |
| Via natural or artificial opening endoscopic (8) | Entry of instrumentation through a natural or artificial external opening to reach and visualize the site of the procedure | Natural or artificial external opening | Direct entry | With visualization | Sigmoidoscopy, EGD, ERCP |
| Via natural or artificial opening with percutaneous endoscopic assistance (F) | Entry of instrumentation through a natural or artificial external opening and entry, by puncture or minor incision, of instrumentation through the skin or mucous membrane and any other body layers necessary to aid in the performance of the procedure | Skin or mucous membrane, any other body layers | Direct entry with puncture or minor incision for instrumentation only | With visualization | Laparoscopic-assisted vaginal hysterectomy |
| External (X) | Procedures performed directly on the skin or mucous membrane and procedures performed indirectly by the application of external force through the skin or mucous membrane | Skin or mucous membrane | Direct or indirect application | None | Closed fracture reduction, Resection of tonsils |

# Appendix B: Root Operation Definitions



| Ø | Medical and Surgical | | |
|---|---|---|---|
| **ICD-10-PCS Value** | | **Definition** | |
| Ø | Alteration | Definition: | Modifying the natural anatomic structure of a body part without affecting the function of the body part |
| | | Explanation: | Principal purpose is to improve appearance |
| | | Examples: | Face lift, breast augmentation |
| 1 | Bypass | Definition: | Altering the route of passage of the contents of a tubular body part |
| | | Explanation: | Rerouting contents of a body part to a downstream area of the normal route, to a similar route and body part, or to an abnormal route and dissimilar body part. Includes one or more anastomoses, with or without the use of a device. |
| | | Examples: | Coronary artery bypass, colostomy formation |
| 2 | Change | Definition: | Taking out or off a device from a body part and putting back an identical or similar device in or on the same body part without cutting or puncturing the skin or a mucous membrane |
| | | Explanation: | All CHANGE procedures are coded using the approach EXTERNAL |
| | | Example: | Urinary catheter change, gastrostomy tube change |
| 3 | Control | Definition: | Stopping, or attempting to stop, postprocedural or other acute bleeding |
| | | Explanation: | The site of the bleeding is coded as an anatomical region and not to a specific body part |
| | | Examples: | Control of post-prostatectomy hemorrhage, control of intracranial subdural hemorrhage, control of bleeding duodenal ulcer, control of retroperitoneal hemorrhage |
| 4 | Creation | Definition: | Putting in or on biological or synthetic material to form a new body part that to the extent possible replicates the anatomic structure or function of an absent body part |
| | | Explanation: | Used for gender reassignment surgery and corrective procedures in individuals with congenital anomalies |
| | | Examples: | Creation of vagina in a male, creation of right and left atrioventricular valve from common atrioventricular valve |
| 5 | Destruction | Definition: | Physical eradication of all or a portion of a body part by the direct use of energy, force, or a destructive agent |
| | | Explanation: | None of the body part is physically taken out |
| | | Examples: | Fulguration of rectal polyp, cautery of skin lesion |
| 6 | Detachment | Definition: | Cutting off all or a portion of the upper or lower extremities |
| | | Explanation: | The body part value is the site of the detachment, with a qualifier if applicable to further specify the level where the extremity was detached |
| | | Examples: | Below knee amputation, disarticulation of shoulder |
| 7 | Dilation | Definition: | Expanding an orifice or the lumen of a tubular body part |
| | | Explanation: | The orifice can be a natural orifice or an artificially created orifice. Accomplished by stretching a tubular body part using intraluminal pressure or by cutting part of the orifice or wall of the tubular body part. |
| | | Examples: | Percutaneous transluminal angioplasty, internal urethrotomy |
| 8 | Division | Definition: | Cutting into a body part, without draining fluids and/or gases from the body part, in order to separate or transect a body part |
| | | Explanation: | All or a portion of the body part is separated into two or more portions |
| | | Examples: | Spinal cordotomy, osteotomy |
| 9 | Drainage | Definition: | Taking or letting out fluids and/or gases from a body part |
| | | Explanation: | The qualifier DIAGNOSTIC is used to identify drainage procedures that are biopsies |
| | | Examples: | Thoracentesis, incision and drainage |
| B | Excision | Definition: | Cutting out or off, without replacement, a portion of a body part |
| | | Explanation: | The qualifier DIAGNOSTIC is used to identify excision procedures that are biopsies |
| | | Examples: | Partial nephrectomy, liver biopsy |
| C | Extirpation | Definition: | Taking or cutting out solid matter from a body part |
| | | Explanation: | The solid matter may be an abnormal byproduct of a biological function or a foreign body; it may be imbedded in a body part or in the lumen of a tubular body part. The solid matter may or may not have been previously broken into pieces. |
| | | Examples: | Thrombectomy, choledocholithotomy |

*Continued on next page*

## Ø Medical and Surgical

*Continued from previous page*

| ICD-10-PCS Value | | Definition | |
|---|---|---|---|
| D | Extraction | Definition: | Pulling or stripping out or off all or a portion of a body part by the use of force |
| | | Explanation: | The qualifier DIAGNOSTIC is used to identify extractions that are biopsies |
| | | Examples: | Dilation and curettage, vein stripping |
| F | Fragmentation | Definition: | Breaking solid matter in a body part into pieces |
| | | Explanation: | Physical force (e.g., manual, ultrasonic) applied directly or indirectly is used to break the solid matter into pieces. The solid matter may be an abnormal byproduct of a biological function or a foreign body. The pieces of solid matter are not taken out. |
| | | Examples: | Extracorporeal shockwave lithotripsy, transurethral lithotripsy |
| G | Fusion | Definition: | Joining together portions of an articular body part rendering the articular body part immobile |
| | | Explanation: | The body part is joined together by fixation device, bone graft, or other means |
| | | Examples: | Spinal fusion, ankle arthrodesis |
| H | Insertion | Definition: | Putting in a nonbiological appliance that monitors, assists, performs, or prevents a physiological function but does not physically take the place of a body part |
| | | Explanation: | None |
| | | Examples: | Insertion of radioactive implant, insertion of central venous catheter |
| J | Inspection | Definition: | Visually and/or manually exploring a body part |
| | | Explanation: | Visual exploration may be performed with or without optical instrumentation. Manual exploration may be performed directly or through intervening body layers. |
| | | Examples: | Diagnostic arthroscopy, exploratory laparotomy |
| K | Map | Definition: | Locating the route of passage of electrical impulses and/or locating functional areas in a body part |
| | | Explanation: | Applicable only to the cardiac conduction mechanism and the central nervous system |
| | | Examples: | Cardiac mapping, cortical mapping |
| L | Occlusion | Definition: | Completely closing an orifice or lumen of a tubular body part |
| | | Explanation: | The orifice can be a natural orifice or an artificially created orifice |
| | | Examples: | Fallopian tube ligation, ligation of inferior vena cava |
| M | Reattachment | Definition: | Putting back in or on all or a portion of a separated body part to its normal location or other suitable location |
| | | Explanation: | Vascular circulation and nervous pathways may or may not be reestablished |
| | | Examples: | Reattachment of hand, reattachment of avulsed kidney |
| N | Release | Definition: | Freeing a body part from an abnormal physical constraint by cutting or by use of force |
| | | Explanation: | Some of the restraining tissue may be taken out but none of the body part is taken out |
| | | Examples: | Adhesiolysis, carpal tunnel release |
| P | Removal | Definition: | Taking out or off a device from a body part |
| | | Explanation: | If a device is taken out and a similar device put in without cutting or puncturing the skin or mucous membrane, the procedure is coded to the root operation CHANGE. Otherwise, the procedure for taking out a device is coded to the root operation REMOVAL. |
| | | Examples: | Drainage tube removal, cardiac pacemaker removal |
| Q | Repair | Definition: | Restoring, to the extent possible, a body part to its normal anatomic structure and function |
| | | Explanation: | Used only when the method to accomplish the repair is not one of the other root operations |
| | | Examples: | Colostomy takedown, suture of laceration |
| R | Replacement | Definition: | Putting in or on biological or synthetic material that physically takes the place and/or function of all or a portion of a body part |
| | | Explanation: | The body part may have been taken out or replaced, or may be taken out, physically eradicated, or rendered nonfunctional during the REPLACEMENT procedure. A REMOVAL procedure is coded for taking out the device used in a previous replacement procedure. |
| | | Examples: | Total hip replacement, bone graft, free skin graft |
| S | Reposition | Definition: | Moving to its normal location, or other suitable location, all or a portion of a body part |
| | | Explanation: | The body part is moved to a new location from an abnormal location, or from a normal location where it is not functioning correctly. The body part may or may not be cut out or off to be moved to the new location. |
| | | Examples: | Reposition of undescended testicle, fracture reduction |

*Continued on next page*

## Ø Medical and Surgical

*Continued from previous page*

| ICD-10-PCS Value | | Definition | |
|---|---|---|---|
| T | Resection | Definition: | Cutting out or off, without replacement, all of a body part |
| | | Explanation: | None |
| | | Examples: | Total nephrectomy, total lobectomy of lung |
| V | Restriction | Definition: | Partially closing an orifice or the lumen of a tubular body part |
| | | Explanation: | The orifice can be a natural orifice or an artificially created orifice |
| | | Examples: | Esophagogastric fundoplication, cervical cerclage |
| W | Revision | Definition: | Correcting, to the extent possible, a portion of a malfunctioning device or the position of a displaced device |
| | | Explanation: | Revision can include correcting a malfunctioning or displaced device by taking out or putting in components of the device such as a screw or pin |
| | | Examples: | Adjustment of position of pacemaker lead, recementing of hip prosthesis |
| U | Supplement | Definition: | Putting in or on biological or synthetic material that physically reinforces and/or augments the function of a portion of a body part |
| | | Explanation: | The biological material is non-living, or is living and from the same individual. The body part may have been previously replaced, and the SUPPLEMENT procedure is performed to physically reinforce and/or augment the function of the replaced body part. |
| | | Examples: | Herniorrhaphy using mesh, free nerve graft, mitral valve ring annuloplasty, put a new acetabular liner in a previous hip replacement |
| X | Transfer | Definition: | Moving, without taking out, all or a portion of a body part to another location to take over the function of all or a portion of a body part |
| | | Explanation: | The body part transferred remains connected to its vascular and nervous supply |
| | | Examples: | Tendon transfer, skin pedicle flap transfer |
| Y | Transplantation | Definition: | Putting in or on all or a portion of a living body part taken from another individual or animal to physically take the place and/or function of all or a portion of a similar body part |
| | | Explanation: | The native body part may or may not be taken out, and the transplanted body part may take over all or a portion of its function |
| | | Examples: | Kidney transplant, heart transplant |

# Root Operation Definitions for Other Sections

## 1 Obstetrics

| ICD-10-PCS Value | | Definition | |
|---|---|---|---|
| 2 | Change | Definition: | Taking out or off a device from a body part and putting back an identical or similar device in or on the same body part without cutting or puncturing the skin or a mucous membrane |
| | | Explanation: | None |
| | | Examples: | Replacement of fetal scalp electrode |
| 9 | Drainage | Definition: | Taking or letting out fluids and/or gases from a body part |
| | | Explanation: | None |
| | | Examples: | Biopsy of amniotic fluid |
| A | Abortion | Definition: | Artificially terminating a pregnancy |
| | | Explanation: | None |
| | | Examples: | Transvaginal abortion using vacuum aspiration technique |
| D | Extraction | Definition: | Pulling or stripping out or off all or a portion of a body part by the use of force |
| | | Explanation: | None |
| | | Examples: | Low-transverse C-section |
| E | Delivery | Definition: | Assisting the passage of the products of conception from the genital canal |
| | | Explanation: | None |
| | | Examples: | Manually-assisted delivery |
| H | Insertion | Definition: | Putting in a nonbiological appliance that monitors, assists, performs, or prevents a physiological function but does not physically take the place of a body part |
| | | Explanation: | None |
| | | Examples: | Placement of fetal scalp electrode |

*Continued on next page*

## 1 Obstetrics

*Continued from previous page*

| ICD-10-PCS Value | | Definition | |
|---|---|---|---|
| J | Inspection | Definition: | Visually and/or manually exploring a body part |
| | | Explanation: | Visual exploration may be performed with or without optical instrumentation. Manual exploration may be performed directly or through intervening body layers. |
| | | Examples: | Bimanual pregnancy exam |
| P | Removal | Definition: | Taking out or off a device from a body part, region or orifice |
| | | Explanation: | If a device is taken out and a similar device put in without cutting or puncturing the skin or mucous membrane, the procedure is coded to the root operation CHANGE. Otherwise, the procedure for taking out a device is coded to the root operation REMOVAL. |
| | | Examples: | Removal of fetal monitoring electrode |
| Q | Repair | Definition: | Restoring, to the extent possible, a body part to its normal anatomic structure and function |
| | | Explanation: | Used only when the method to accomplish the repair is not one of the other root operations |
| | | Examples: | In utero repair of congenital diaphragmatic hernia |
| S | Reposition | Definition: | Moving to its normal location, or other suitable location, all or a portion of a body part |
| | | Explanation: | The body part is moved to a new location from an abnormal location, or from a normal location where it is not functioning correctly. The body part may or may not be cut out or off to be moved to the new location. |
| | | Examples: | External version of fetus |
| T | Resection | Definition: | Cutting out or off, without replacement, all of a body part |
| | | Explanation: | None |
| | | Examples: | Total excision of tubal pregnancy |
| Y | Transplantation | Definition: | Putting in or on all or a portion of a living body part taken from another individual or animal to physically take the place and/or function of all or a portion of a similar body part |
| | | Explanation: | The native body part may or may not be taken out, and the transplanted body part may take over all or a portion of its function |
| | | Examples: | In utero fetal kidney transplant |

## 2 Placement

| ICD-10-PCS Value | | Definition | |
|---|---|---|---|
| Ø | Change | Definition: | Taking out or off a device from a body region and putting back an identical or similar device in or on the same body region without cutting or puncturing the skin or a mucous membrane |
| | | Examples: | Change of vaginal packing |
| 1 | Compression | Definition: | Putting pressure on a body region |
| | | Examples: | Placement of pressure dressing on abdominal wall |
| 2 | Dressing | Definition: | Putting material on a body region for protection |
| | | Examples: | Application of sterile dressing to head wound |
| 3 | Immobilization | Definition: | Limiting or preventing motion of a body region |
| | | Examples: | Placement of splint on left finger |
| 4 | Packing | Definition: | Putting material in a body region or orifice |
| | | Examples: | Placement of nasal packing |
| 5 | Removal | Definition: | Taking out or off a device from a body part |
| | | Examples: | Removal of stereotactic head frame |
| 6 | Traction | Definition: | Exerting a pulling force on a body region in a distal direction |
| | | Examples: | Lumbar traction using motorized split-traction table |

## 3 Administration

| ICD-10-PCS Value | | Definition | |
|---|---|---|---|
| Ø | Introduction | Definition: | Putting in or on a therapeutic, diagnostic, nutritional, physiological, or prophylactic substance except blood or blood products |
| | | Examples: | Nerve block injection to median nerve |
| 1 | Irrigation | Definition: | Putting in or on a cleansing substance |
| | | Examples: | Flushing of eye |
| 2 | Transfusion | Definition: | Putting in blood or blood products |
| | | Examples: | Transfusion of cell saver red cells into central venous line |

## 4 Measurement and Monitoring

| ICD-10-PCS Value | | Definition | |
|---|---|---|---|
| Ø | Measurement | Definition: | Determining the level of a physiological or physical function at a point in time |
| | | Examples: | External electrocardiogram(EKG), single reading |
| 1 | Monitoring | Definition: | Determining the level of a physiological or physical function repetitively over a period of time |
| | | Examples: | Urinary pressure monitoring |

## 5 Extracorporeal or Systemic Assistance and Performance

| ICD-10-PCS Value | | Definition | |
|---|---|---|---|
| Ø | Assistance | Definition: | Taking over a portion of a physiological function by extracorporeal means |
| | | Examples: | Hyperbaric oxygenation of wound |
| 1 | Performance | Definition: | Completely taking over a physiological function by extracorporeal means |
| | | Examples: | Cardiopulmonary bypass in conjunction with CABG |
| 2 | Restoration | Definition: | Returning, or attempting to return, a physiological function to its original state by extracorporeal means |
| | | Examples: | Attempted cardiac defibrillation, unsuccessful |

## 6 Extracorporeal or Systemic Therapies

| ICD-10-PCS Value | | Definition | |
|---|---|---|---|
| Ø | Atmospheric Control | Definition: | Extracorporeal control of atmospheric pressure and composition |
| | | Examples: | Antigen-free air conditioning, series treatment |
| 1 | Decompression | Definition: | Extracorporeal elimination of undissolved gas from body fluids |
| | | Examples: | Hyperbaric decompression treatment, single |
| 2 | Electromagnetic Therapy | Definition: | Extracorporeal treatment by electromagnetic rays |
| | | Examples: | TMS (transcranial magnetic stimulation), series treatment |
| 3 | Hyperthermia | Definition: | Extracorporeal raising of body temperature |
| | | Examples: | None |
| 4 | Hypothermia | Definition: | Extracorporeal lowering of body temperature |
| | | Examples: | Whole body hypothermia treatment for temperature imbalances, series |
| 5 | Pheresis | Definition: | Extracorporeal separation of blood products |
| | | Examples: | Therapeutic leukopheresis, single treatment |
| 6 | Phototherapy | Definition: | Extracorporeal treatment by light rays |
| | | Examples: | Phototherapy of circulatory system, series treatment |
| 7 | Ultrasound Therapy | Definition: | Extracorporeal treatment by ultrasound |
| | | Examples: | Therapeutic ultrasound of peripheral vessels, single treatment |
| 8 | Ultraviolet Light Therapy | Definition: | Extracorporeal treatment by ultraviolet light |
| | | Examples: | Ultraviolet light phototherapy, series treatment |
| 9 | Shock Wave Therapy | Definition: | Extracorporeal treatment by shock waves |
| | | Examples: | Shockwave therapy of plantar fascia, single treatment |
| B | Perfusion | Definition: | Extracorporeal treatment by diffusion of therapeutic fluid |
| | | Examples: | Perfusion of donor liver while preparing transplant patient |

## 7 Osteopathic

| ICD-10-PCS Value | | Definition | |
|---|---|---|---|
| Ø | Treatment | Definition: | Manual treatment to eliminate or alleviate somatic dysfunction and related disorders |
| | | Examples: | Fascial release of abdomen, osteopathic treatment |

## 8 Other Procedures

| ICD-10-PCS Value | | Definition | |
|---|---|---|---|
| Ø | Other Procedures | Definition: | Methodologies which attempt to remediate or cure a disorder or disease |
| | | Examples: | Acupuncture, yoga therapy |

## 9 Chiropractic

| ICD-10-PCS Value | | Definition | |
|---|---|---|---|
| B | Manipulation | Definition: | Manual procedure that involves a directed thrust to move a joint past the physiological range of motion, without exceeding the anatomical limit |
| | | Examples: | Chiropractic treatment of cervical spine, short lever specific contact |

**Note:** Sections B-H (Imaging through Substance Abuse Treatment) do not include root operations. The character 3 position represents type of procedure, therefore those definitions are not included in this appendix. See appendix I for definitions of the type (character 3) or type qualifiers (character 5) that provide details of the procedures performed.

# Appendix C: Comparison of Medical and Surgical Root Operations



**Note: the character associated with each operation appears in parentheses after its title.**

## Procedures That Take Out Some or All of a Body Part

| Root Operation | Objective of Procedure | Site of Procedure | Example |
|---|---|---|---|
| Destruction (5) | Eradicating without taking out or replacement | Some/all of a body part | Fulguration of endometrium |
| Detachment (6) | Cutting out/off without replacement | Extremity only, any level | Amputation above elbow |
| Excision (B) | Cutting out/off without replacement | Some of a body part | Breast lumpectomy |
| Extraction (D) | Pulling out or off without replacement | Some/all of a body part | Suction D&C |
| Resection (T) | Cutting out/off without replacement | All of a body part | Total mastectomy |

## Procedures That Put in/Put Back or Move Some/All of a Body Part

| Root Operation | Objective of Procedure | Site of Procedure | Example |
|---|---|---|---|
| Reattachment (M) | Putting back a detached body part | Some/all of a body part | Reattach finger |
| Reposition (S) | Moving a body part to normal or other suitable location | Some/all of a body part | Move undescended testicle |
| Transfer (X) | Moving a body part to function for a similar body part | Some/all of a body part | Skin pedicle transfer flap |
| Transplantation (Y) | Putting in a living body part from a person/animal | Some/all of a body part | Kidney transplant |

## Procedures That Take Out or Eliminate Solid Matter, Fluids, or Gases From a Body Part

| Root Operation | Objective of Procedure | Site of Procedure | Example |
|---|---|---|---|
| Drainage (9) | Taking or letting out | Fluids and/or gases from a body part | Incision and drainage |
| Extirpation (C) | Taking or cutting out | Solid matter in a body part | Thrombectomy |
| Fragmentation (F) | Breaking into pieces | Solid matter within a body part | Lithotripsy |

## Procedures That Involve Only Examination of Body Parts and Regions

| Root Operation | Objective of Procedure | Site of Procedure | Example |
|---|---|---|---|
| Inspection (J) | Visual/manual exploration | Some/all of a body part | Diagnostic cystoscopy<br>Exploratory laparoscopy |
| Map (K) | Locating electrical impulse route/functional areas | Brain/cardiac conduction mechanism | Cardiac mapping |

## Procedures That Alter the Diameter/Route of a Tubular Body Part

| Root Operation | Objective of Procedure | Site of Procedure | Example |
|---|---|---|---|
| Bypass (1) | Altering route of passage of contents | Tubular body part | Coronary artery bypass graft (CABG) |
| Dilation (7) | Expanding natural or artificially created orifice/lumen | Tubular body part | Percutaneous transluminal coronary angioplasty (PTCA) |
| Occlusion (L) | Completely closing natural or artificially created orifice/lumen | Tubular body part | Fallopian tube ligation |
| Restriction (V) | Partially closing natural or artificially created orifice/lumen | Tubular body part | Gastroesophageal fundoplication |

## Procedures That Always Involve Devices

| Root Operation | Objective of Procedure | Site of Procedure | Example |
|---|---|---|---|
| Change (2) DVC | Exchanging device w/out cutting/puncturing | In/on a body part | Gastrostomy tube change |
| Insertion (H) DVC | Putting in nonbiological device | In/on a body part | Central line insertion |
| Removal (P) DVC | Taking out device | In/on a body part | Central line removal |
| Replacement (R) DVC | Putting in device that replaces a body part | Some/all of a body part | Total hip replacement |
| Revision (W) DVC | Correcting a malfunctioning/displaced device | In/on a body part | Revision of pacemaker |
| Supplement (U) DVC | Putting in device that reinforces or augments a body part | In/on a body part | Abdominal wall herniorrhaphy using mesh |

DVC = Device involved in root operation

## Procedures Involving Cutting or Separation Only

| Root Operation | Objective of Procedure | Site of Procedure | Example |
|---|---|---|---|
| Division (8) | Cutting into/separating | A body part | Neurotomy |
| Release (N) | Freeing a body part from constraint | Around a body part | Adhesiolysis |

## Procedures That Define Other Repairs

| Root Operation | Objective of Procedure | Site of Procedure | Example |
|---|---|---|---|
| Control (3) | Stopping/attempting to stop postprocedural or other acute bleeding | Anatomical region | Post-prostatectomy bleeding control, control subdural hemorrhage, bleeding ulcer, retroperitoneal hemorrhage |
| Repair (Q) | Restoring body part to its normal structure/function | Some/all of a body part | Suture laceration |

## Procedures That Define Other Objectives

| Root Operation | Objective of Procedure | Site of Procedure | Example |
|---|---|---|---|
| Alteration (Ø) | Modifying body part for cosmetic purposes without affecting function | Some/all of a body part | Face lift |
| Creation (4) | Using biological or synthetic material to form a new body part that replicates the anatomic structure or function of a missing body part | Perineum, valve | Sex change/artificial vagina/penis, atrioventricular valve creation |
| Fusion (G) | Unification or immobilization | Joint or articular body part | Spinal fusion |

# Appendix D: Body Part Key

| Term | ICD-10-PCS Value |
|---|---|
| **Abdominal aortic plexus** | Abdominal Sympathetic Nerve |
| **Abdominal esophagus** | Esophagus, Lower |
| **Abductor hallucis muscle** | Foot Muscle, Right |
| | Foot Muscle, Left |
| **Accessory cephalic vein** | Cephalic Vein, Right |
| | Cephalic Vein, Left |
| **Accessory obturator nerve** | Lumbar Plexus |
| **Accessory phrenic nerve** | Phrenic nerve |
| **Accessory spleen** | Spleen |
| **Acetabulofemoral joint** | Hip Joint, Right |
| | Hip Joint, Left |
| **Achilles tendon** | Lower Leg Tendon, Right |
| | Lower Leg Tendon, Left |
| **Acromioclavicular ligament** | Shoulder Bursa and Ligament, Right |
| | Shoulder Bursa and Ligament, Left |
| **Acromion (process)** | Scapula, Right |
| | Scapula, Left |
| **Adductor brevis muscle** | Upper Leg Muscle, Right |
| | Upper Leg Muscle, Left |
| **Adductor hallucis muscle** | Foot Muscle, Right |
| | Foot Muscle, Left |
| **Adductor longus muscle** | Upper Leg Muscle, Right |
| | Upper Leg Muscle, Left |
| **Adductor magnus muscle** | Upper Leg Muscle, Right |
| | Upper Leg Muscle, Left |
| **Adenohypophysis** | Pituitary Gland |
| **Alar ligament of axis** | Head and Neck Bursa and Ligament |
| **Alveolar process of mandible** | Mandible, Right |
| | Mandible, Left |
| **Alveolar process of maxilla** | Maxilla |
| **Anal orifice** | Anus |
| **Anatomical snuffbox** | Lower Arm and Wrist Muscle, Right |
| | Lower Arm and Wrist Muscle, Left |
| **Angular artery** | Face Artery |
| **Angular vein** | Face Vein, Right |
| | Face Vein, Left |
| **Annular ligament** | Elbow Bursa and Ligament, Right |
| | Elbow Bursa and Ligament, Left |
| **Anorectal junction** | Rectum |
| **Ansa cervicalis** | Cervical Plexus |
| **Antebrachial fascia** | Subcutaneous Tissue and Fascia, Right Lower Arm |
| | Subcutaneous Tissue and Fascia, Left Lower Arm |
| **Anterior (pectoral) lymph node** | Lymphatic, Right Axillary |
| | Lymphatic, Left Axillary |
| **Anterior cerebral artery** | Intracranial Artery |
| **Anterior cerebral vein** | Intracranial Vein |
| **Anterior choroidal artery** | Intracranial Artery |
| **Anterior circumflex humeral artery** | Axillary Artery, Right |
| | Axillary Artery, Left |
| **Anterior communicating artery** | Intracranial Artery |

| Term | ICD-10-PCS Value |
|---|---|
| **Anterior cruciate ligament (ACL)** | Knee Bursa and Ligament, Right |
| | Knee Bursa and Ligament, Left |
| **Anterior crural nerve** | Femoral Nerve |
| **Anterior facial vein** | Face Vein, Right |
| | Face Vein, Left |
| **Anterior intercostal artery** | Internal Mammary Artery, Right |
| | Internal Mammary Artery, Left |
| **Anterior interosseous nerve** | Median Nerve |
| **Anterior lateral malleolar artery** | Anterior Tibial Artery, Right |
| | Anterior Tibial Artery, Left |
| **Anterior lingual gland** | Minor Salivary Gland |
| **Anterior medial malleolar artery** | Anterior Tibial Artery, Right |
| | Anterior Tibial Artery, Left |
| **Anterior spinal artery** | Vertebral Artery, Right |
| | Vertebral Artery, Left |
| **Anterior tibial recurrent artery** | Anterior Tibial Artery, Right |
| | Anterior Tibial Artery, Left |
| **Anterior ulnar recurrent artery** | Ulnar Artery, Right |
| | Ulnar Artery, Left |
| **Anterior vagal trunk** | Vagus Nerve |
| **Anterior vertebral muscle** | Neck Muscle, Right |
| | Neck Muscle, Left |
| **Antihelix** | External Ear, Right |
| | External Ear, Left |
| | External Ear, Bilateral |
| **Antitragus** | External Ear, Right |
| | External Ear, Left |
| | External Ear, Bilateral |
| **Antrum of Highmore** | Maxillary Sinus, Right |
| | Maxillary Sinus, Left |
| **Aortic annulus** | Aortic Valve |
| **Aortic arch** | Thoracic Aorta, Ascending/Arch |
| **Aortic intercostal artery** | Upper Artery |
| **Apical (subclavicular) lymph node** | Lymphatic, Right Axillary |
| | Lymphatic, Left Axillary |
| **Apneustic center** | Pons |
| **Aqueduct of Sylvius** | Cerebral Ventricle |
| **Aqueous humour** | Anterior Chamber, Right |
| | Anterior Chamber, Left |
| **Arachnoid mater, intracranial** | Cerebral Meninges |
| **Arachnoid mater, spinal** | Spinal Meninges |
| **Arcuate artery** | Foot Artery, Right |
| | Foot Artery, Left |
| **Areola** | Nipple, Right |
| | Nipple, Left |
| **Arterial canal (duct)** | Pulmonary Artery, Left |
| **Aryepiglottic fold** | Larynx |
| **Arytenoid cartilage** | Larynx |
| **Arytenoid muscle** | Neck Muscle, Right |
| | Neck Muscle, Left |
| **Ascending aorta** | Thoracic Aorta, Ascending/Arch |

| Term | ICD-10-PCS Value |
|---|---|
| Ascending palatine artery | Face Artery |
| Ascending pharyngeal artery | External Carotid Artery, Right |
| | External Carotid Artery, Left |
| Atlantoaxial joint | Cervical Vertebral Joint |
| Atrioventricular node | Conduction Mechanism |
| Atrium dextrum cordis | Atrium, Right |
| Atrium pulmonale | Atrium, Left |
| Auditory tube | Eustachian Tube, Right |
| | Eustachian Tube, Left |
| Auerbach's (myenteric)plexus | Abdominal Sympathetic Nerve |
| Auricle | External Ear, Right |
| | External Ear, Left |
| | External Ear, Bilateral |
| Auricularis muscle | Head Muscle |
| Axillary fascia | Subcutaneous Tissue and Fascia, Right Upper Arm |
| | Subcutaneous Tissue and Fascia, Left Upper Arm |
| Axillary nerve | Brachial Plexus |
| Bartholin's (greater vestibular) gland | Vestibular Gland |
| Basal (internal) cerebral vein | Intracranial Vein |
| Basal nuclei | Basal Ganglia |
| Base of tongue | Pharynx |
| Basilar artery | Intracranial Artery |
| Basis pontis | Pons |
| Biceps brachii muscle | Upper Arm Muscle, Right |
| | Upper Arm Muscle, Left |
| Biceps femoris muscle | Upper Leg Muscle, Right |
| | Upper Leg Muscle, Left |
| Bicipital aponeurosis | Subcutaneous Tissue and Fascia, Right Lower Arm |
| | Subcutaneous Tissue and Fascia, Left Lower Arm |
| Bicuspid valve | Mitral Valve |
| Body of femur | Femoral Shaft, Right |
| | Femoral Shaft, Left |
| Body of fibula | Fibula, Right |
| | Fibula, Left |
| Bony labyrinth | Inner Ear, Right |
| | Inner Ear, Left |
| Bony orbit | Orbit, Right |
| | Orbit, Left |
| Bony vestibule | Inner Ear, Right |
| | Inner Ear, Left |
| Botallo's duct | Pulmonary Artery, Left |
| Brachial (lateral) lymph node | Lymphatic, Right Axillary |
| | Lymphatic, Left Axillary |
| Brachialis muscle | Upper Arm Muscle, Right |
| | Upper Arm Muscle, Left |
| Brachiocephalic artery | Innominate Artery |
| Brachiocephalic trunk | Innominate Artery |
| Brachiocephalic vein | Innominate Vein, Right |
| | Innominate Vein, Left |

| Term | ICD-10-PCS Value |
|---|---|
| Brachioradialis muscle | Lower Arm and Wrist Muscle, Right |
| | Lower Arm and Wrist Muscle, Left |
| Broad ligament | Uterine Supporting Structure |
| Bronchial artery | Upper Artery |
| Bronchus intermedius | Main Bronchus, Right |
| Buccal gland | Buccal Mucosa |
| Buccinator lymph node | Lymphatic, Head |
| Buccinator muscle | Facial Muscle |
| Bulbospongiosus muscle | Perineum Muscle |
| Bulbourethral (Cowper's) gland | Urethra |
| Bundle of His | Conduction Mechanism |
| Bundle of Kent | Conduction Mechanism |
| Calcaneocuboid joint | Tarsal Joint, Right |
| | Tarsal Joint, Left |
| Calcaneocuboid ligament | Foot Bursa and Ligament, Right |
| | Foot Bursa and Ligament, Left |
| Calcaneofibular ligament | Ankle Bursa and Ligament, Right |
| | Ankle Bursa and Ligament, Left |
| Calcaneus | Tarsal, Right |
| | Tarsal, Left |
| Capitate bone | Carpal, Right |
| | Carpal, Left |
| Cardia | Esophagogastric Junction |
| Cardiac plexus | Thoracic Sympathetic Nerve |
| Cardioesophageal junction | Esophagogastric Junction |
| Caroticotympanic artery | Internal Carotid Artery, Right |
| | Internal Carotid Artery, Left |
| Carotid glomus | Carotid Body, Right |
| | Carotid Body, Left |
| | Carotid Bodies, Bilateral |
| Carotid sinus | Internal Carotid Artery, Right |
| | Internal Carotid Artery, Left |
| Carotid sinus nerve | Glossopharyngeal Nerve |
| Carpometacarpal ligament | Hand Bursa and Ligament, Right |
| | Hand Bursa and Ligament, Left |
| Cauda equina | Lumbar Spinal Cord |
| Cavernous plexus | Head and Neck Sympathetic Nerve |
| Celiac ganglion | Abdominal Sympathetic Nerve |
| Celiac (solar) plexus | Abdominal Sympathetic Nerve |
| Celiac lymph node | Lymphatic, Aortic |
| Celiac trunk | Celiac Artery |
| Central axillary lymph node | Lymphatic, Right Axillary |
| | Lymphatic, Left Axillary |
| Cerebral aqueduct (Sylvius) | Cerebral Ventricle |
| Cerebrum | Brain |
| Cervical esophagus | Esophagus, Upper |
| Cervical facet joint | Cervical Vertebral Joint |
| | Cervical Vertebral Joints, 2 or more |
| Cervical ganglion | Head and Neck Sympathetic Nerve |
| Cervical interspinous ligament | Head and Neck Bursa and Ligament |
| Cervical intertransverse ligament | Head and Neck Bursa and Ligament |

| Term | ICD-10-PCS Value |
|---|---|
| **Cervical ligamentum flavum** | Head and Neck Bursa and Ligament |
| **Cervical lymph node** | Lymphatic, Right Neck |
| | Lymphatic, Left Neck |
| **Cervicothoracic facet joint** | Cervicothoracic Vertebral Joint |
| **Choana** | Nasopharynx |
| **Chondroglossus muscle** | Tongue, Palate, Pharynx Muscle |
| **Chorda tympani** | Facial Nerve |
| **Choroid plexus** | Cerebral Ventricle |
| **Ciliary body** | Eye, Right |
| | Eye, Left |
| **Ciliary ganglion** | Head and Neck Sympathetic Nerve |
| **Circle of Willis** | Intracranial Artery |
| **Circumflex illiac artery** | Femoral Artery, Right |
| | Femoral Artery, Left |
| **Claustrum** | Basal Ganglia |
| **Coccygeal body** | Coccygeal Glomus |
| **Coccygeus muscle** | Trunk Muscle, Right |
| | Trunk Muscle, Left |
| **Cochlea** | Inner Ear, Right |
| | Inner Ear, Left |
| **Cochlear nerve** | Acoustic Nerve |
| **Columella** | Nasal Mucosa and Soft Tissue |
| **Common digital vein** | Foot Vein, Right |
| | Foot Vein, Left |
| **Common facial vein** | Face Vein, Right |
| | Face Vein, Left |
| **Common fibular nerve** | Peroneal Nerve |
| **Common hepatic artery** | Hepatic Artery |
| **Common iliac (subaortic) lymph node** | Lymphatic, Pelvis |
| **Common interosseous artery** | Ulnar Artery, Right |
| | Ulnar Artery, Left |
| **Common peroneal nerve** | Peroneal Nerve |
| **Condyloid process** | Mandible, Right |
| | Mandible, Left |
| **Conus arteriosus** | Ventricle, Right |
| **Conus medullaris** | Lumbar Spinal Cord |
| **Coracoacromial ligament** | Shoulder Bursa and Ligament, Right |
| | Shoulder Bursa and Ligament, Left |
| **Coracobrachialis muscle** | Upper Arm Muscle, Right |
| | Upper Arm Muscle, Left |
| **Coracoclavicular ligament** | Shoulder Bursa and Ligament, Right |
| | Shoulder Bursa and Ligament, Left |
| **Coracohumeral ligament** | Shoulder Bursa and Ligament, Right |
| | Shoulder Bursa and Ligament, Left |
| **Coracoid process** | Scapula, Right |
| | Scapula, Left |
| **Corniculate cartilage** | Larynx |
| **Corpus callosum** | Brain |
| **Corpus cavernosum** | Penis |
| **Corpus spongiosum** | Penis |
| **Corpus striatum** | Basal Ganglia |
| **Corrugator supercilii muscle** | Facial Muscle |

| Term | ICD-10-PCS Value |
|---|---|
| **Costocervical trunk** | Subclavian Artery, Right |
| | Subclavian Artery, Left |
| **Costoclavicular ligament** | Shoulder Bursa and Ligament, Right |
| | Shoulder Bursa and Ligament, Left |
| **Costotransverse joint** | Thoracic Vertebral Joint |
| **Costotransverse ligament** | Sternum Bursa and Ligament |
| | Rib(s) Bursa and Ligament |
| **Costovertebral joint** | Thoracic Vertebral Joint |
| **Costoxiphoid ligament** | Sternum Bursa and Ligament |
| | Rib(s) Bursa and Ligament |
| **Cowper's (bulbourethral) gland** | Urethra |
| **Cremaster muscle** | Perineum Muscle |
| **Cribriform plate** | Ethmoid Bone, Right |
| | Ethmoid Bone, Left |
| **Cricoid cartilage** | Trachea |
| **Cricothyroid artery** | Thyroid Artery, Right |
| | Thyroid Artery, Left |
| **Cricothyroid muscle** | Neck Muscle, Right |
| | Neck Muscle, Left |
| **Crural fascia** | Subcutaneous Tissue and Fascia, Right Upper Leg |
| | Subcutaneous Tissue and Fascia, Left Upper Leg |
| **Cubital lymph node** | Lymphatic, Right Upper Extremity |
| | Lymphatic, Left Upper Extremity |
| **Cubital nerve** | Ulnar Nerve |
| **Cuboid bone** | Tarsal, Right |
| | Tarsal, Left |
| **Cuboideonavicular joint** | Tarsal Joint, Right |
| | Tarsal Joint, Left |
| **Culmen** | Cerebellum |
| **Cuneiform cartilage** | Larynx |
| **Cuneonavicular joint** | Tarsal Joint, Right |
| | Tarsal Joint, Left |
| **Cuneonavicular ligament** | Foot Bursa and Ligament, Right |
| | Foot Bursa and Ligament, Left |
| **Cutaneous (transverse) cervical nerve** | Cervical Plexus |
| **Deep cervical fascia** | Subcutaneous Tissue and Fascia, Right Neck |
| | Subcutaneous Tissue and Fascia, Left Neck |
| **Deep cervical vein** | Vertebral Vein, Right |
| | Vertebral Vein, Left |
| **Deep circumflex iliac artery** | External Iliac Artery, Right |
| | External Iliac Artery, Left |
| **Deep facial vein** | Face Vein, Right |
| | Face Vein, Left |
| **Deep femoral artery** | Femoral Artery, Right |
| | Femoral Artery, Left |
| **Deep femoral (profunda femoris) vein** | Femoral Vein, Right |
| | Femoral Vein, Left |
| **Deep palmar arch** | Hand Artery, Right |
| | Hand Artery, Left |
| **Deep transverse perineal muscle** | Perineum Muscle |

| Term | ICD-10-PCS Value |
|---|---|
| **Deferential artery** | Internal Iliac Artery, Right |
| | Internal Iliac Artery, Left |
| **Deltoid fascia** | Subcutaneous Tissue and Fascia, Right Upper Arm |
| | Subcutaneous Tissue and Fascia, Left Upper Arm |
| **Deltoid ligament** | Ankle Bursa and Ligament, Right |
| | Ankle Bursa and Ligament, Left |
| **Deltoid muscle** | Shoulder Muscle, Right |
| | Shoulder Muscle, Left |
| **Deltopectoral (infraclavicular) lymph node** | Lymphatic, Right Upper Extremity |
| | Lymphatic, Left Upper Extremity |
| **Dens** | Cervical Vertebra |
| **Denticulate (dentate) ligament** | Spinal Meninges |
| **Depressor anguli oris muscle** | Facial Muscle |
| **Depressor labii inferioris muscle** | Facial Muscle |
| **Depressor septi nasi muscle** | Facial Muscle |
| **Depressor supercilii muscle** | Facial Muscle |
| **Dermis** | Skin |
| **Descending genicular artery** | Femoral Artery, Right |
| | Femoral Artery, Left |
| **Diaphragma sellae** | Dura Mater |
| **Distal humerus** | Humeral Shaft, Right |
| | Humeral Shaft, Left |
| **Distal humerus, involving joint** | Elbow Joint, Right |
| | Elbow Joint, Left |
| **Distal radioulnar joint** | Wrist Joint, Right |
| | Wrist Joint, Left |
| **Dorsal digital nerve** | Radial Nerve |
| **Dorsal metacarpal vein** | Hand Vein, Right |
| | Hand Vein, Left |
| **Dorsal metatarsal artery** | Foot Artery, Right |
| | Foot Artery, Left |
| **Dorsal metatarsal vein** | Foot Vein, Right |
| | Foot Vein, Left |
| **Dorsal scapular artery** | Subclavian Artery, Right |
| | Subclavian Artery, Left |
| **Dorsal scapular nerve** | Brachial Plexus |
| **Dorsal venous arch** | Foot Vein, Right |
| | Foot Vein, Left |
| **Dorsalis pedis artery** | Anterior Tibial Artery, Right |
| | Anterior Tibial Artery, Left |
| **Duct of Santorini** | Pancreatic Duct, Accessory |
| **Duct of Wirsung** | Pancreatic Duct |
| **Ductus deferens** | Vas Deferens, Right |
| | Vas Deferens, Left |
| | Vas Deferens, Bilateral |
| | Vas Deferens |
| **Duodenal ampulla** | Ampulla of Vater |
| **Duodenojejunal flexure** | Jejunum |
| **Dura mater, intracranial** | Dura Mater |
| **Dura mater, spinal** | Spinal Meninges |
| **Dural venous sinus** | Intracranial Vein |
| **Earlobe** | External Ear, Right |
| | External Ear, Left |
| | External Ear, Bilateral |
| **Eighth cranial nerve** | Acoustic Nerve |
| **Ejaculatory duct** | Vas Deferens, Right |
| | Vas Deferens, Left |
| | Vas Deferens, Bilateral |
| | Vas Deferens |
| **Eleventh cranial nerve** | Accessory Nerve |
| **Encephalon** | Brain |
| **Ependyma** | Cerebral Ventricle |
| **Epidermis** | Skin |
| **Epidural space, spinal** | Spinal Canal |
| **Epiploic foramen** | Peritoneum |
| **Epithalamus** | Thalamus |
| **Epitroclear lymph node** | Lymphatic, Right Upper Extremity |
| | Lymphatic, Left Upper Extremity |
| **Erector spinae muscle** | Trunk Muscle, Right |
| | Trunk Muscle, Left |
| **Esophageal artery** | Upper Artery |
| **Esophageal plexus** | Thoracic Sympathetic Nerve |
| **Ethmoidal air cell** | Ethmoid Sinus, Right |
| | Ethmoid Sinus, Left |
| **Extensor carpi radialis muscle** | Lower Arm and Wrist Muscle, Right |
| **Extensor carpi ulnaris muscle** | Lower Arm and Wrist Muscle, Left |
| **Extensor digitorum brevis muscle** | Foot Muscle, Right |
| | Foot Muscle, Left |
| **Extensor digitorum longus muscle** | Lower Leg Muscle, Right |
| | Lower Leg Muscle, Left |
| **Extensor hallucis brevis muscle** | Foot Muscle, Right |
| | Foot Muscle, Left |
| **Extensor hallucis longus muscle** | Lower Leg Muscle, Right |
| | Lower Leg Muscle, Left |
| **External anal sphincter** | Anal Sphincter |
| **External auditory meatus** | External Auditory Canal, Right |
| | External Auditory Canal, Left |
| **External maxillary artery** | Face Artery |
| **External naris** | Nasal Mucosa and Soft Tissue |
| **External oblique aponeurosis** | Subcutaneous Tissue and Fascia, Trunk |
| **External oblique muscle** | Abdomen Muscle, Right |
| | Abdomen Muscle, Left |
| **External popliteal nerve** | Peroneal Nerve |
| **External pudendal artery** | Femoral Artery, Right |
| | Femoral Artery, Left |
| **External pudenal vein** | Saphenous Vein, Right |
| | Saphenous Vein, Left |
| **External urethral sphincter** | Urethra |
| **Extradural space, intracranial** | Epidural Space, Intracranial |
| **Extradural space, spinal** | Spinal Canal |
| **Facial artery** | Face Artery |

| Term | ICD-10-PCS Value |
|---|---|
| **False vocal cord** | Larynx |
| **Falx cerebri** | Dura Mater |
| **Fascia lata** | Subcutaneous Tissue and Fascia, Right Upper Leg |
| | Subcutaneous Tissue and Fascia, Left Upper Leg |
| **Femoral head** | Upper Femur, Right |
| | Upper Femur, Left |
| **Femoral lymph node** | Lymphatic, Right Lower Extremity |
| | Lymphatic, Left Lower Extremity |
| **Femoropatellar joint** | Knee Joint, Right |
| | Knee Joint, Left |
| | Knee Joint, Femoral Surface, Right |
| | Knee Joint, Femoral Surface, Left |
| **Femorotibial joint** | Knee Joint, Right |
| | Knee Joint, Left |
| | Knee Joint, Tibial Surface, Right |
| | Knee Joint, Tibial Surface, Left |
| **Fibular artery** | Peroneal Artery, Right |
| | Peroneal Artery, Left |
| **Fibularis brevis muscle** | Lower Leg Muscle, Right |
| | Lower Leg Muscle, Left |
| **Fibularis longus muscle** | Lower Leg Muscle, Right |
| | Lower Leg Muscle, Left |
| **Fifth cranial nerve** | Trigeminal Nerve |
| **Filum terminale** | Spinal Meninges |
| **First cranial nerve** | Olfactory Nerve |
| **First intercostal nerve** | Brachial Plexus |
| **Flexor carpi radialis muscle** | Lower Arm and Wrist Muscle, Right |
| | Lower Arm and Wrist Muscle, Left |
| **Flexor carpi ulnaris muscle** | Lower Arm and Wrist Muscle, Right |
| | Lower Arm and Wrist Muscle, Left |
| **Flexor digitorum brevis muscle** | Foot Muscle, Right |
| | Foot Muscle, Left |
| **Flexor digitorum longus muscle** | Lower Leg Muscle, Right |
| | Lower Leg Muscle, Left |
| **Flexor hallucis brevis muscle** | Foot Muscle, Right |
| | Foot Muscle, Left |
| **Flexor hallucis longus muscle** | Lower Leg Muscle, Right |
| | Lower Leg Muscle, Left |
| **Flexor pollicis longus muscle** | Lower Arm and Wrist Muscle, Right |
| | Lower Arm and Wrist Muscle, Left |
| **Foramen magnum** | Occipital Bone |
| **Foramen of Monro (intraventricular)** | Cerebral Ventricle |
| **Foreskin** | Prepuce |
| **Fossa of Rosenmuller** | Nasopharynx |
| **Fourth cranial nerve** | Trochlear Nerve |
| **Fourth ventricle** | Cerebral Ventricle |
| **Fovea** | Retina, Right |
| | Retina, Left |
| **Frenulum labii inferioris** | Lower Lip |
| **Frenulum labii superioris** | Upper Lip |
| **Frenulum linguae** | Tongue |
| **Frontal lobe** | Cerebral Hemisphere |

| Term | ICD-10-PCS Value |
|---|---|
| **Frontal vein** | Face Vein, Right |
| | Face Vein, Left |
| **Fundus uteri** | Uterus |
| **Galea aponeurotica** | Subcutaneous Tissue and Fascia, Scalp |
| **Ganglion impar (ganglion of Walther)** | Sacral Sympathetic Nerve |
| **Gasserian ganglion** | Trigeminal Nerve |
| **Gastric lymph node** | Lymphatic, Aortic |
| **Gastric plexus** | Abdominal Sympathetic Nerve |
| **Gastrocnemius muscle** | Lower Leg Muscle, Right |
| | Lower Leg Muscle, Left |
| **Gastrocolic ligament** | Omentum |
| **Gastrocolic omentum** | Omentum |
| **Gastroduodenal artery** | Hepatic Artery |
| **Gastroesophageal (GE) junction** | Esophagogastric Junction |
| **Gastrohepatic omentum** | Omentum |
| **Gastrophrenic ligament** | Omentum |
| **Gastrosplenic ligament** | Omentum |
| **Gemellus muscle** | Hip Muscle, Right |
| | Hip Muscle, Left |
| **Geniculate ganglion** | Facial Nerve |
| **Geniculate nucleus** | Thalamus |
| **Genioglossus muscle** | Tongue, Palate, Pharynx Muscle |
| **Genitofemoral nerve** | Lumbar Plexus |
| **Glans penis** | Prepuce |
| **Glenohumeral joint** | Shoulder Joint, Right |
| | Shoulder Joint, Left |
| **Glenohumeral ligament** | Shoulder Bursa and Ligament, Right |
| | Shoulder Bursa and Ligament, Left |
| **Glenoid fossa (of scapula)** | Glenoid Cavity, Right |
| | Glenoid Cavity, Left |
| **Glenoid ligament (labrum)** | Shoulder Joint, Right |
| | Shoulder Joint, Left |
| **Globus pallidus** | Basal Ganglia |
| **Glossoepiglottic fold** | Epiglottis |
| **Glottis** | Larynx |
| **Gluteal lymph node** | Lymphatic, Pelvis |
| **Gluteal vein** | Hypogastric Vein, Right |
| | Hypogastric Vein, Left |
| **Gluteus maximus muscle** | Hip Muscle, Right |
| | Hip Muscle, Left |
| **Gluteus medius muscle** | Hip Muscle, Right |
| | Hip Muscle, Left |
| **Gluteus minimus muscle** | Hip Muscle, Right |
| | Hip Muscle, Left |
| **Gracilis muscle** | Upper Leg Muscle, Right |
| | Upper Leg Muscle, Left |
| **Great auricular nerve** | Cervical Plexus |
| **Great cerebral vein** | Intracranial Vein |
| **Great(er) saphenous vein** | Saphenous Vein, Right |
| | Saphenous Vein, Left |
| **Greater alar cartilage** | Nasal Mucosa and Soft Tissue |
| **Greater occipital nerve** | Cervical Nerve |
| **Greater omentum** | Omentum |

| Term | ICD-10-PCS Value |
|---|---|
| **Greater splanchnic nerve** | Thoracic Sympathetic Nerve |
| **Greater superficial petrosal nerve** | Facial Nerve |
| **Greater trochanter** | Upper Femur, Right |
| | Upper Femur, Left |
| **Greater tuberosity** | Humeral Head, Right |
| | Humeral Head, Left |
| **Greater vestibular (Bartholin's) gland** | Vestibular Gland |
| **Greater wing** | Sphenoid Bone |
| **Hallux** | 1st Toe, Right |
| | 1st Toe, Left |
| **Hamate bone** | Carpal, Right |
| | Carpal, Left |
| **Head of fibula** | Fibula, Right |
| | Fibula, Left |
| **Helix** | External Ear, Right |
| | External Ear, Left |
| | External Ear, Bilateral |
| **Hepatic artery proper** | Hepatic Artery |
| **Hepatic flexure** | Transverse Colon |
| **Hepatic lymph node** | Lymphatic, Aortic |
| **Hepatic plexus** | Abdominal Sympathetic Nerve |
| **Hepatic portal vein** | Portal Vein |
| **Hepatogastric ligament** | Omentum |
| **Hepatopancreatic ampulla** | Ampulla of Vater |
| **Humeroradial joint** | Elbow Joint, Right |
| | Elbow Joint, Left |
| **Humeroulnar joint** | Elbow Joint, Right |
| | Elbow Joint, Left |
| **Humerus, distal** | Humeral Shaft, Right |
| | Humeral Shaft, Left |
| **Hyoglossus muscle** | Tongue, Palate, Pharynx Muscle |
| **Hyoid artery** | Thyroid Artery, Right |
| | Thyroid Artery, Left |
| **Hypogastric artery** | Internal Iliac Artery, Right |
| | Internal Iliac Artery, Left |
| **Hypopharynx** | Pharynx |
| **Hypophysis** | Pituitary Gland |
| **Hypothenar muscle** | Hand Muscle, Right |
| | Hand Muscle, Left |
| **Ileal artery** | Superior Mesenteric Artery |
| **Ileocolic artery** | Superior Mesenteric Artery |
| **Ileocolic vein** | Colic Vein |
| **Iliac crest** | Pelvic Bone, Right |
| | Pelvic Bone, Left |
| **Iliac fascia** | Subcutaneous Tissue and Fascia, Right Upper Leg |
| | Subcutaneous Tissue and Fascia, Left Upper Leg |
| **Iliac lymph node** | Lymphatic, Pelvis |
| **Iliacus muscle** | Hip Muscle, Right |
| | Hip Muscle, Left |
| **Iliofemoral ligament** | Hip Bursa and Ligament, Right |
| | Hip Bursa and Ligament, Left |
| **Iliohypogastric nerve** | Lumbar Plexus |
| **Ilioinguinal nerve** | Lumbar Plexus |
| **Iliolumbar artery** | Internal Iliac Artery, Right |
| | Internal Iliac Artery, Left |
| **Iliolumbar ligament** | Lower Spine Bursa and Ligament |
| **Iliotibial tract (band)** | Subcutaneous Tissue and Fascia, Right Upper Leg |
| | Subcutaneous Tissue and Fascia, Left Upper Leg |
| **Ilium** | Pelvic Bone, Right |
| | Pelvic Bone, Left |
| **Incus** | Auditory Ossicle, Right |
| | Auditory Ossicle, Left |
| **Inferior cardiac nerve** | Thoracic Sympathetic Nerve |
| **Inferior cerebellar vein** | Intracranial Vein |
| **Inferior cerebral vein** | Intracranial Vein |
| **Inferior epigastric artery** | External Iliac Artery, Right |
| | External Iliac Artery, Left |
| **Inferior epigastric lymph node** | Lymphatic, Pelvis |
| **Inferior genicular artery** | Popliteal Artery, Right |
| | Popliteal Artery, Left |
| **Inferior gluteal artery** | Internal Iliac Artery, Right |
| | Internal Iliac Artery, Left |
| **Inferior gluteal nerve** | Sacral Plexus |
| **Inferior hypogastric plexus** | Abdominal Sympathetic Nerve |
| **Inferior labial artery** | Face Artery |
| **Inferior longitudinal muscle** | Tongue, Palate, Pharynx Muscle |
| **Inferior mesenteric ganglion** | Abdominal Sympathetic Nerve |
| **Inferior mesenteric lymph node** | Lymphatic, Mesenteric |
| **Inferior mesenteric plexus** | Abdominal Sympathetic Nerve |
| **Inferior oblique muscle** | Extraocular Muscle, Right |
| | Extraocular Muscle, Left |
| **Inferior pancreaticoduo-denal artery** | Superior Mesenteric Artery |
| **Inferior phrenic artery** | Abdominal Aorta |
| **Inferior rectus muscle** | Extraocular Muscle, Right |
| | Extraocular Muscle, Left |
| **Inferior suprarenal artery** | Renal Artery, Right |
| | Renal Artery, Left |
| **Inferior tarsal plate** | Lower Eyelid, Right |
| | Lower Eyelid, Left |
| **Inferior thyroid vein** | Innominate Vein, Right |
| | Innominate Vein, Left |
| **Inferior tibiofibular joint** | Ankle Joint, Right |
| | Ankle Joint, Left |
| **Inferior turbinate** | Nasal Turbinate |
| **Inferior ulnar collateral artery** | Brachial Artery, Right |
| | Brachial Artery, Left |
| **Inferior vesical artery** | Internal Iliac Artery, Right |
| | Internal Iliac Artery, Left |
| **Infraauricular lymph node** | Lymphatic, Head |
| **Infraclavicular (deltopectoral) lymph node** | Lymphatic, Right Upper Extremity |
| | Lymphatic, Left Upper Extremity |

| Term | ICD-10-PCS Value |
|---|---|
| **Infrahyoid muscle** | Neck Muscle, Right |
| | Neck Muscle, Left |
| **Infraparotid lymph node** | Lymphatic, Head |
| **Infraspinatus fascia** | Subcutaneous Tissue and Fascia, Right Upper Arm |
| | Subcutaneous Tissue and Fascia, Left Upper Arm |
| **Infraspinatus muscle** | Shoulder Muscle, Right |
| | Shoulder Muscle, Left |
| **Infundibulopelvic ligament** | Uterine Supporting Structure |
| **Inguinal canal** | Inguinal Region, Right |
| | Inguinal Region, Left |
| | Inguinal Region, Bilateral |
| **Inguinal triangle** | Inguinal Region, Right |
| | Inguinal Region, Left |
| | Inguinal Region, Bilateral |
| **Interatrial septum** | Atrial Septum |
| **Intercarpal joint** | Carpal Joint, Right |
| | Carpal Joint, Left |
| **Intercarpal ligament** | Hand Bursa and Ligament, Right |
| | Hand Bursa and Ligament, Left |
| **Interclavicular ligament** | Shoulder Bursa and Ligament, Right |
| | Shoulder Bursa and Ligament, Left |
| **Intercostal lymph node** | Lymphatic, Thorax |
| **Intercostal muscle** | Thorax Muscle, Right |
| | Thorax Muscle, Left |
| **Intercostal nerve** | Thoracic Nerve |
| **Intercostobrachial nerve** | Thoracic Nerve |
| **Intercuneiform joint** | Tarsal Joint, Right |
| | Tarsal Joint, Left |
| **Intercuneiform ligament** | Foot Bursa and Ligament, Right |
| | Foot Bursa and Ligament, Left |
| **Intermediate bronchus** | Main Bronchus, Right |
| **Intermediate cuneiform bone** | Tarsal, Right |
| | Tarsal, Left |
| **Internal anal sphincter** | Anal Sphincter |
| **Internal (basal) cerebral vein** | Intracranial Vein |
| **Internal carotid artery, intracranial portion** | Intracranial Artery |
| **Internal carotid plexus** | Head and Neck Sympathetic Nerve |
| **Internal iliac vein** | Hypogastric Vein, Right |
| | Hypogastric Vein, Left |
| **Internal maxillary artery** | External Carotid Artery, Right |
| | External Carotid Artery, Left |
| **Internal naris** | Nasal Mucosa and Soft Tissue |
| **Internal oblique muscle** | Abdomen Muscle, Right |
| | Abdomen Muscle, Left |
| **Internal pudendal artery** | Internal Iliac Artery, Right |
| | Internal Iliac Artery, Left |
| **Internal pudendal vein** | Hypogastric Vein, Right |
| | Hypogastric Vein, Left |

| Term | ICD-10-PCS Value |
|---|---|
| **Internal thoracic artery** | Internal Mammary Artery, Right |
| | Internal Mammary Artery, Left |
| | Subclavian Artery, Right |
| | Subclavian Artery, Left |
| **Internal urethral sphincter** | Urethra |
| **Interphalangeal (IP) joint** | Finger Phalangeal Joint, Right |
| | Finger Phalangeal Joint, Left |
| | Toe Phalangeal Joint, Right |
| | Toe Phalangeal Joint, Left |
| **Interphalangeal ligament** | Foot Bursa and Ligament, Right |
| | Foot Bursa and Ligament, Left |
| | Hand Bursa and Ligament, Right |
| | Hand Bursa and Ligament, Left |
| **Interspinalis muscle** | Trunk Muscle, Right |
| | Trunk Muscle, Left |
| **Interspinous ligament** | Head and Neck Bursa and Ligament |
| | Upper Spine Bursa and Ligament |
| | Lower Spine Bursa and Ligament |
| **Intertransversarius muscle** | Trunk Muscle, Right |
| | Trunk Muscle, Left |
| **Intertransverse ligament** | Upper Spine Bursa and Ligament |
| | Lower Spine Bursa and Ligament |
| **Interventricular foramen (Monro)** | Cerebral Ventricle |
| **Interventricular septum** | Ventricular Septum |
| **Intestinal lymphatic trunk** | Cisterna Chyli |
| **Ischiatic nerve** | Sciatic Nerve |
| **Ischiocavernosus muscle** | Perineum Muscle |
| **Ischiofemoral ligament** | Hip Bursa and Ligament, Right |
| | Hip Bursa and Ligament, Left |
| **Ischium** | Pelvic Bone, Right |
| | Pelvic Bone, Left |
| **Jejunal artery** | Superior Mesenteric Artery |
| **Jugular body** | Glomus Jugulare |
| **Jugular lymph node** | Lymphatic, Right Neck |
| | Lymphatic, Left Neck |
| **Labia majora** | Vulva |
| **Labia minora** | Vulva |
| **Labial gland** | Upper Lip |
| | Lower Lip |
| **Lacrimal canaliculus** | Lacrimal Duct, Right |
| | Lacrimal Duct, Left |
| **Lacrimal punctum** | Lacrimal Duct, Right |
| | Lacrimal Duct, Left |
| **Lacrimal sac** | Lacrimal Duct, Right |
| | Lacrimal Duct, Left |
| **Laryngopharynx** | Pharynx |
| **Lateral (brachial) lymph node** | Lymphatic, Right Axillary |
| | Lymphatic, Left Axillary |
| **Lateral canthus** | Upper Eyelid, Right |
| | Upper Eyelid, Left |
| **Lateral collateral ligament (LCL)** | Knee Bursa and Ligament, Right |
| | Knee Bursa and Ligament, Left |
| **Lateral condyle of femur** | Lower Femur, Right |
| | Lower Femur, Left |

| Term | ICD-10-PCS Value |
|---|---|
| Lateral condyle of tibia | Tibia, Right |
| | Tibia, Left |
| Lateral cuneiform bone | Tarsal, Right |
| | Tarsal, Left |
| Lateral epicondyle of femur | Lower Femur, Right |
| | Lower Femur, Left |
| Lateral epicondyle of humerus | Humeral Shaft, Right |
| | Humeral Shaft, Left |
| Lateral femoral cutaneous nerve | Lumbar Plexus |
| Lateral malleolus | Fibula, Right |
| | Fibula, Left |
| Lateral meniscus | Knee Joint, Right |
| | Knee Joint, Left |
| Lateral nasal cartilage | Nasal Mucosa and Soft Tissue |
| Lateral plantar artery | Foot Artery, Right |
| | Foot Artery, Left |
| Lateral plantar nerve | Tibial Nerve |
| Lateral rectus muscle | Extraocular Muscle, Right |
| | Extraocular Muscle, Left |
| Lateral sacral artery | Internal Iliac Artery, Right |
| | Internal Iliac Artery, Left |
| Lateral sacral vein | Hypogastric Vein, Right |
| | Hypogastric Vein, Left |
| Lateral sural cutaneous nerve | Peroneal Nerve |
| Lateral tarsal artery | Foot Artery, Right |
| | Foot Artery, Left |
| Lateral temporo-mandibular ligament | Head and Neck Bursa and Ligament |
| Lateral thoracic artery | Axillary Artery, Right |
| | Axillary Artery, Left |
| Latissimus dorsi muscle | Trunk Muscle, Right |
| | Trunk Muscle, Left |
| Least splanchnic nerve | Thoracic Sympathetic Nerve |
| Left ascending lumbar vein | Hemiazygos Vein |
| Left atrioventricular valve | Mitral Valve |
| Left auricular appendix | Atrium, Left |
| Left colic vein | Colic Vein |
| Left coronary sulcus | Heart, Left |
| Left gastric artery | Gastric Artery |
| Left gastroepiploic artery | Splenic Artery |
| Left gastroepiploic vein | Splenic Vein |
| Left inferior phrenic vein | Renal Vein, Left |
| Left inferior pulmonary vein | Pulmonary Vein, Left |
| Left jugular trunk | Thoracic Duct |
| Left lateral ventricle | Cerebral Ventricle |
| Left ovarian vein | Renal Vein, Left |
| Left second lumbar vein | Renal Vein, Left |
| Left subclavian trunk | Thoracic Duct |
| Left subcostal vein | Hemiazygos Vein |
| Left superior pulmonary vein | Pulmonary Vein, Left |
| Left suprarenal vein | Renal Vein, Left |
| Left testicular vein | Renal Vein, Left |

| Term | ICD-10-PCS Value |
|---|---|
| Leptomeninges, intracranial | Cerebral Meninges |
| Leptomeninges, spinal | Spinal Meninges |
| Lesser alar cartilage | Nasal Mucosa and Soft Tissue |
| Lesser occipital nerve | Cervical Plexus |
| Lesser omentum | Omentum |
| Lesser saphenous vein | Saphenous Vein, Right |
| | Saphenous Vein, Left |
| Lesser splanchnic nerve | Thoracic Sympathetic Nerve |
| Lesser trochanter | Upper Femur, Right |
| | Upper Femur, Left |
| Lesser tuberosity | Humeral Head, Right |
| | Humeral Head, Left |
| Lesser wing | Sphenoid Bone |
| Levator anguli oris muscle | Facial Muscle |
| Levator ani muscle | Perineum Muscle |
| Levator labii superioris alaeque nasi muscle | Facial Muscle |
| Levator labii superioris muscle | Facial Muscle |
| Levator palpebrae superioris muscle | Upper Eyelid, Right |
| | Upper Eyelid, Left |
| Levator scapulae muscle | Neck Muscle, Right |
| | Neck Muscle, Left |
| Levator veli palatini muscle | Tongue, Palate, Pharynx Muscle |
| Levatores costarum muscle | Thorax Muscle, Right |
| | Thorax Muscle, Left |
| Ligament of head of fibula | Knee Bursa and Ligament, Right |
| | Knee Bursa and Ligament, Left |
| Ligament of the lateral malleolus | Ankle Bursa and Ligament, Right |
| | Ankle Bursa and Ligament, Left |
| Ligamentum flavum | Upper Spine Bursa and Ligament |
| | Lower Spine Bursa and Ligament |
| Lingual artery | External Carotid Artery, Right |
| | External Carotid Artery, Left |
| Lingual tonsil | Pharynx |
| Locus ceruleus | Pons |
| Long thoracic nerve | Brachial Plexus |
| Lumbar artery | Abdominal Aorta |
| Lumbar facet joint | Lumbar Vertebral Joint |
| Lumbar ganglion | Lumbar Sympathetic Nerve |
| Lumbar lymph node | Lymphatic, Aortic |
| Lumbar lymphatic trunk | Cisterna Chyli |
| Lumbar splanchnic nerve | Lumbar Sympathetic Nerve |
| Lumbosacral facet joint | Lumbosacral Joint |
| Lumbosacraltrunk | Lumbar Nerve |
| Lunate bone | Carpal, Right |
| | Carpal, Left |
| Lunotriquetral ligament | Hand Bursa and Ligament, Right |
| | Hand Bursa and Ligament, Left |
| Macula | Retina, Right |
| | Retina, Left |
| Malleus | Auditory Ossicle, Right |
| | Auditory Ossicle, Left |

| Term | ICD-10-PCS Value |
|---|---|
| **Mammary duct** | Breast, Right |
| | Breast, Left |
| | Breast, Bilateral |
| **Mammary gland** | Breast, Right |
| | Breast, Left |
| | Breast, Bilateral |
| **Mammillary body** | Hypothalamus |
| **Mandibular nerve** | Trigeminal Nerve |
| **Mandibular notch** | Mandible, Right |
| | Mandible, Left |
| **Manubrium** | Sternum |
| **Masseter muscle** | Head Muscle |
| **Masseteric fascia** | Subcutaneous Tissue and Fascia, Face |
| **Mastoid (postauricular) lymph node** | Lymphatic, Right Neck |
| | Lymphatic, Left Neck |
| **Mastoid air cells** | Mastoid Sinus, Right |
| | Mastoid Sinus, Left |
| **Mastoid process** | Temporal Bone, Right |
| | Temporal Bone, Left |
| **Maxillary artery** | External Carotid Artery, Right |
| | External Carotid Artery, Left |
| **Maxillary nerve** | Trigeminal Nerve |
| **Medial canthus** | Lower Eyelid, Right |
| | Lower Eyelid, Left |
| **Medial collateral ligament (MCL)** | Knee Bursa and Ligament, Right |
| | Knee Bursa and Ligament, Left |
| **Medial condyle of femur** | Lower Femur, Right |
| | Lower Femur, Left |
| **Medial condyle of tibia** | Tibia, Right |
| | Tibia, Left |
| **Medial cuneiform bone** | Tarsal, Right |
| | Tarsal, Left |
| **Medial epicondyle of femur** | Lower Femur, Right |
| | Lower Femur, Left |
| **Medial epicondyle of humerus** | Humeral Shaft, Right |
| | Humeral Shaft, Left |
| **Medial malleolus** | Tibia, Right |
| | Tibia, Left |
| **Medial meniscus** | Knee Joint, Right |
| | Knee Joint, Left |
| **Medial plantar artery** | Foot Artery, Right |
| | Foot Artery, Left |
| **Medial plantar nerve** | Tibial Nerve |
| **Medial popliteal nerve** | Tibial Nerve |
| **Medial rectus muscle** | Extraocular Muscle, Right |
| | Extraocular Muscle, Left |
| **Medial sural cutaneous nerve** | Tibial Nerve |
| **Median antebrachial vein** | Basilic Vein, Right |
| | Basilic Vein, Left |
| **Median cubital vein** | Basilic Vein, Right |
| | Basilic Vein, Left |
| **Median sacral artery** | Abdominal Aorta |
| **Mediastinal lymph node** | Lymphatic, Thorax |

| Term | ICD-10-PCS Value |
|---|---|
| **Meissner's (submucous) plexus** | Abdominal Sympathetic Nerve |
| **Membranous urethra** | Urethra |
| **Mental foramen** | Mandible, Right |
| | Mandible, Left |
| **Mentalis muscle** | Facial Muscle |
| **Mesoappendix** | Mesentery |
| **Mesocolon** | Mesentery |
| **Metacarpal ligament** | Hand Bursa and Ligament, Right |
| | Hand Bursa and Ligament, Left |
| **Metacarpophalangeal ligament** | Hand Bursa and Ligament, Right |
| | Hand Bursa and Ligament, Left |
| **Metatarsal ligament** | Foot Bursa and Ligament, Right |
| | Foot Bursa and Ligament, Left |
| **Metatarsophalangeal ligament** | Foot Bursa and Ligament, Right |
| | Foot Bursa and Ligament, Left |
| **Metatarsophalangeal (MTP) joint** | Metatarsal-Phalangeal Joint, Right |
| | Metatarsal-Phalangeal Joint, Left |
| **Metathalamus** | Thalamus |
| **Midcarpal joint** | Carpal Joint, Right |
| | Carpal Joint, Left |
| **Middle cardiac nerve** | Thoracic Sympathetic Nerve |
| **Middle cerebral artery** | Intracranial Artery |
| **Middle cerebral vein** | Intracranial Vein |
| **Middle colic vein** | Colic Vein |
| **Middle genicular artery** | Popliteal Artery, Right |
| | Popliteal Artery, Left |
| **Middle hemorrhoidal vein** | Hypogastric Vein, Right |
| | Hypogastric Vein, Left |
| **Middle rectal artery** | Internal Iliac Artery, Right |
| | Internal Iliac Artery, Left |
| **Middle suprarenal artery** | Abdominal Aorta |
| **Middle temporal artery** | Temporal Artery, Right |
| | Temporal Artery, Left |
| **Middle turbinate** | Nasal Turbinate |
| **Mitral annulus** | Mitral Valve |
| **Molar gland** | Buccal Mucosa |
| **Musculocutaneous nerve** | Brachial Plexus |
| **Musculophrenic artery** | Internal Mammary Artery, Right |
| | Internal Mammary Artery, Left |
| **Musculospiral nerve** | Radial Nerve |
| **Myelencephalon** | Medulla Oblongata |
| **Myenteric (Auerbach's) plexus** | Abdominal Sympathetic Nerve |
| **Myometrium** | Uterus |
| **Nail bed** | Finger Nail |
| | Toe Nail |
| **Nail plate** | Finger Nail |
| | Toe Nail |
| **Nasal cavity** | Nasal Mucosa and Soft Tissue |
| **Nasal concha** | Nasal Turbinate |
| **Nasalis muscle** | Facial Muscle |
| **Nasolacrimal duct** | Lacrimal Duct, Right |
| | Lacrimal Duct, Left |

Appendix D: Body Part Key

| Term | ICD-10-PCS Value |
|---|---|
| **Navicular bone** | Tarsal, Right |
| | Tarsal, Left |
| **Neck of femur** | Upper Femur, Right |
| | Upper Femur, Left |
| **Neck of humerus (anatomical) (surgical)** | Humeral Head, Right |
| | Humeral Head, Left |
| **Nerve to the stapedius** | Facial Nerve |
| **Neurohypophysis** | Pituitary Gland |
| **Ninth cranial nerve** | Glossopharyngeal Nerve |
| **Nostril** | Nasal Mucosa and Soft Tissue |
| **Obturator artery** | Internal Iliac Artery, Right |
| | Internal Iliac Artery, Left |
| **Obturator lymph node** | Lymphatic, Pelvis |
| **Obturator muscle** | Hip Muscle, Right |
| | Hip Muscle, Left |
| **Obturator nerve** | Lumbar Plexus |
| **Obturator vein** | Hypogastric Vein, Right |
| | Hypogastric Vein, Left |
| **Obtuse margin** | Heart, Left |
| **Occipital artery** | External Carotid Artery, Right |
| | External Carotid Artery, Left |
| **Occipital lobe** | Cerebral Hemisphere |
| **Occipital lymph node** | Lymphatic, Right Neck |
| | Lymphatic, Left Neck |
| **Occipitofrontalis muscle** | Facial Muscle |
| **Odontoid process** | Cervical Vertebra |
| **Olecranon bursa** | Elbow Bursa and Ligament, Right |
| | Elbow Bursa and Ligament, Left |
| **Olecranon process** | Ulna, Right |
| | Ulna, Left |
| **Olfactory bulb** | Olfactory Nerve |
| **Ophthalmic artery** | Intracranial Artery |
| **Ophthalmic nerve** | Trigeminal Nerve |
| **Ophthalmic vein** | Intracranial Vein |
| **Optic chiasma** | Optic Nerve |
| **Optic disc** | Retina, Right |
| | Retina, Left |
| **Optic foramen** | Sphenoid Bone |
| **Orbicularis oculi muscle** | Upper Eyelid, Right |
| | Upper Eyelid, Left |
| **Orbicularis oris muscle** | Facial Muscle |
| **Orbital fascia** | Subcutaneous Tissue and Fascia, Face |
| **Orbital portion of ethmoid bone** | Orbit, Right |
| | Orbit, Left |
| **Orbital portion of frontal bone** | Orbit, Right |
| | Orbit, Left |
| **Orbital portion of lacrimal bone** | Orbit, Right |
| | Orbit, Left |
| **Orbital portion of maxilla** | Orbit, Right |
| | Orbit, Left |
| **Orbital portion of palatine bone** | Orbit, Right |
| | Orbit, Left |
| **Orbital portion of sphenoid bone** | Orbit, Right |
| | Orbit, Left |

| Term | ICD-10-PCS Value |
|---|---|
| **Orbital portion of zygomatic bone** | Orbit, Right |
| | Orbit, Left |
| **Oropharynx** | Pharynx |
| **Otic ganglion** | Head and Neck Sympathetic Nerve |
| **Oval window** | Middle Ear, Right |
| | Middle Ear, Left |
| **Ovarian artery** | Abdominal Aorta |
| **Ovarian ligament** | Uterine Supporting Structure |
| **Oviduct** | Fallopian Tube, Right |
| | Fallopian Tube, Left |
| **Palatine gland** | Buccal Mucosa |
| **Palatine tonsil** | Tonsils |
| **Palatine uvula** | Uvula |
| **Palatoglossal muscle** | Tongue, Palate, Pharynx Muscle |
| **Palatopharyngeal muscle** | Tongue, Palate, Pharynx Muscle |
| **Palmar (volar) digital vein** | Hand Vein, Right |
| | Hand Vein, Left |
| **Palmar (volar) metacarpal vein** | Hand Vein, Right |
| | Hand Vein, Left |
| **Palmar cutaneous nerve** | Median Nerve |
| | Radial Nerve |
| **Palmar fascia (aponeurosis)** | Subcutaneous Tissue and Fascia, Right Hand |
| | Subcutaneous Tissue and Fascia, Left Hand |
| **Palmar interosseous muscle** | Hand Muscle, Right |
| | Hand Muscle, Left |
| **Palmar ulnocarpal ligament** | Wrist Bursa and Ligament, Right |
| | Wrist Bursa and Ligament, Left |
| **Palmaris longus muscle** | Lower Arm and Wrist Muscle, Right |
| | Lower Arm and Wrist Muscle, Left |
| **Pancreatic artery** | Splenic Artery |
| **Pancreatic plexus** | Abdominal Sympathetic Nerve |
| **Pancreatic vein** | Splenic Vein |
| **Pancreaticosplenic lymph node** | Lymphatic, Aortic |
| **Paraaortic lymph node** | Lymphatic, Aortic |
| **Pararectal lymph node** | Lymphatic, Mesenteric |
| **Parasternal lymph node** | Lymphatic, Thorax |
| **Paratracheal lymph node** | Lymphatic, Thorax |
| **Paraurethral (Skene's) gland** | Vestibular Gland |
| **Parietal lobe** | Cerebral Hemisphere |
| **Parotid lymph node** | Lymphatic, Head |
| **Parotid plexus** | Facial Nerve |
| **Pars flaccida** | Tympanic Membrane, Right |
| | Tympanic Membrane, Left |
| **Patellar ligament** | Knee Bursa and Ligament, Right |
| | Knee Bursa and Ligament, Left |
| **Patellar tendon** | Knee Tendon, Right |
| | Knee Tendon, Left |
| **Patellofemoral joint** | Knee Joint, Right |
| | Knee Joint, Left |
| | Knee Joint, Femoral Surface, Right |
| | Knee Joint, Femoral Surface, Left |

| Term | ICD-10-PCS Value |
|---|---|
| Pectineus muscle | Upper Leg Muscle, Right |
| | Upper Leg Muscle, Left |
| Pectoral (anterior) lymph node | Lymphatic, Right Axillary |
| | Lymphatic, Left Axillary |
| Pectoral fascia | Subcutaneous Tissue and Fascia, Chest |
| Pectoralis major muscle | Thorax Muscle, Right |
| | Thorax Muscle, Left |
| Pectoralis minor muscle | Thorax Muscle, Right |
| | Thorax Muscle, Left |
| Pelvic splanchnic nerve | Abdominal Sympathetic Nerve |
| | Sacral Sympathetic Nerve |
| Penile urethra | Urethra |
| Pericardiophrenic artery | Internal Mammary Artery, Right |
| | Internal Mammary Artery, Left |
| Perimetrium | Uterus |
| Peroneus brevis muscle | Lower Leg Muscle, Right |
| | Lower Leg Muscle, Left |
| Peroneus longus muscle | Lower Leg Muscle, Right |
| | Lower Leg Muscle, Left |
| Petrous part of temporal bone | Temporal Bone, Right |
| | Temporal Bone, Left |
| Pharyngeal constrictor muscle | Tongue, Palate, Pharynx Muscle |
| Pharyngeal plexus | Vagus Nerve |
| Pharyngeal recess | Nasopharynx |
| Pharyngeal tonsil | Adenoids |
| Pharyngotympanic tube | Eustachian Tube, Right |
| | Eustachian Tube, Left |
| Pia mater, intracranial | Cerebral Meninges |
| Pia mater, spinal | Spinal Meninges |
| Pinna | External Ear, Right |
| | External Ear, Left |
| | External Ear, Bilateral |
| Piriform recess (sinus) | Pharynx |
| Piriformis muscle | Hip Muscle, Right |
| | Hip Muscle, Left |
| Pisiform bone | Carpal, Right |
| | Carpal, Left |
| Pisohamate ligament | Hand Bursa and Ligament, Right |
| | Hand Bursa and Ligament, Left |
| Pisometacarpal ligament | Hand Bursa and Ligament, Right |
| | Hand Bursa and Ligament, Left |
| Plantar digital vein | Foot Vein, Right |
| | Foot Vein, Left |
| Plantar fascia (aponeurosis) | Subcutaneous Tissue and Fascia, Right Foot |
| | Subcutaneous Tissue and Fascia, Left Foot |
| Plantar metatarsal vein | Foot Vein, Right |
| | Foot Vein, Left |
| Plantar venous arch | Foot Vein, Right |
| | Foot Vein, Left |
| Platysma muscle | Neck Muscle, Right |
| | Neck Muscle, Left |
| Plica semilunaris | Conjunctiva, Right |
| | Conjunctiva, Left |
| Pneumogastric nerve | Vagus Nerve |

| Term | ICD-10-PCS Value |
|---|---|
| Pneumotaxic center | Pons |
| Pontine tegmentum | Pons |
| Popliteal ligament | Knee Bursa and Ligament, Right |
| | Knee Bursa and Ligament, Left |
| Popliteallymph node | Lymphatic, Left Lower Extremity |
| | Lymphatic, Right Lower Extremity |
| Popliteal vein | Femoral Vein, Right |
| | Femoral Vein, Left |
| Popliteus muscle | Lower Leg Muscle, Right |
| | Lower Leg Muscle, Left |
| Postauricular (mastoid) lymph node | Lymphatic, Right Neck |
| | Lymphatic, Left Neck |
| Postcava | Inferior Vena Cava |
| Posterior (subscapular) lymph node | Lymphatic, Right Axillary |
| | Lymphatic, Left Axillary |
| Posterior auricular artery | External Carotid Artery, Right |
| | External Carotid Artery, Left |
| Posterior auricular nerve | Facial Nerve |
| Posterior auricular vein | External Jugular Vein, Right |
| | External Jugular Vein, Left |
| Posterior cerebral artery | Intracranial Artery |
| Posterior chamber | Eye, Right |
| | Eye, Left |
| Posterior circumflex humeral artery | Axillary Artery, Right |
| | Axillary Artery, Left |
| Posterior communicating artery | Intracranial Artery |
| Posterior cruciate ligament (PCL) | Knee Bursa and Ligament, Right |
| | Knee Bursa and Ligament, Left |
| Posterior facial (retromandibular) vein | Face Vein, Right |
| | Face Vein, Left |
| Posterior femoral cutaneous nerve | Sacral Plexus |
| Posterior inferior cerebellar artery (PICA) | Intracranial Artery |
| Posterior interosseous nerve | Radial Nerve |
| Posterior labial nerve | Pudendal Nerve |
| Posterior scrotal nerve | Pudendal Nerve |
| Posterior spinal artery | Vertebral Artery, Right |
| | Vertebral Artery, Left |
| Posterior tibial recurrent artery | Anterior Tibial Artery, Right |
| | Anterior Tibial Artery, Left |
| Posterior ulnar recurrent artery | Ulnar Artery, Right |
| | Ulnar Artery, Left |
| Posterior vagal trunk | Vagus Nerve |
| Preauricular lymph node | Lymphatic, Head |
| Precava | Superior Vena Cava |
| Prepatellar bursa | Knee Bursa and Ligament, Right |
| | Knee Bursa and Ligament, Left |
| Pretracheal fascia | Subcutaneous Tissue and Fascia, Right Neck |
| | Subcutaneous Tissue and Fascia, Left Neck |
| Prevertebral fascia | Subcutaneous Tissue and Fascia, Right Neck |
| | Subcutaneous Tissue and Fascia, Left Neck |

| Term | ICD-10-PCS Value |
|---|---|
| **Princeps pollicis artery** | Hand Artery, Right |
| | Hand Artery, Left |
| **Procerus muscle** | Facial Muscle |
| **Profunda brachii** | Brachial Artery, Right |
| | Brachial Artery, Left |
| **Profunda femoris (deep femoral) vein** | Femoral Vein, Right |
| | Femoral Vein, Left |
| **Pronator quadratus muscle** | Lower Arm and Wrist Muscle, Right |
| | Lower Arm and Wrist Muscle, Left |
| **Pronator teres muscle** | Lower Arm and Wrist Muscle, Right |
| | Lower Arm and Wrist Muscle, Left |
| **Prostatic urethra** | Urethra |
| **Proximal radioulnar joint** | Elbow Joint, Right |
| | Elbow Joint, Left |
| **Psoas muscle** | Hip Muscle, Right |
| | Hip Muscle, Left |
| **Pterygoid muscle** | Head Muscle |
| **Pterygoid process** | Sphenoid Bone |
| **Pterygopalatine (sphenopalatine) ganglion** | Head and Neck Sympathetic Nerve |
| **Pubis** | Pelvic Bone, Right |
| | Pelvic Bone, Left |
| **Pubofemoral ligament** | Hip Bursa and Ligament, Right |
| | Hip Bursa and Ligament, Left |
| **Pudendal nerve** | Sacral Plexus |
| **Pulmoaortic canal** | Pulmonary Artery, Left |
| **Pulmonary annulus** | Pulmonary Valve |
| **Pulmonary plexus** | Thoracic Sympathetic Nerve |
| | Vagus Nerve |
| **Pulmonic valve** | Pulmonary Valve |
| **Pulvinar** | Thalamus |
| **Pyloric antrum** | Stomach, Pylorus |
| **Pyloric canal** | Stomach, Pylorus |
| **Pyloric sphincter** | Stomach, Pylorus |
| **Pyramidalis muscle** | Abdomen Muscle, Right |
| | Abdomen Muscle, Left |
| **Quadrangular cartilage** | Nasal Septum |
| **Quadrate lobe** | Liver |
| **Quadratus femoris muscle** | Hip Muscle, Right |
| | Hip Muscle, Left |
| **Quadratus lumborum muscle** | Trunk Muscle, Right |
| | Trunk Muscle, Left |
| **Quadratus plantae muscle** | Foot Muscle, Right |
| | Foot Muscle, Left |
| **Quadriceps (femoris)** | Upper Leg Muscle, Right |
| | Upper Leg Muscle, Left |
| **Radial collateral carpal ligament** | Wrist Bursa and Ligament, Right |
| | Wrist Bursa and Ligament, Left |
| **Radial collateral ligament** | Elbow Bursa and Ligament, Right |
| | Elbow Bursa and Ligament, Left |
| **Radial notch** | Ulna, Right |
| | Ulna, Left |
| **Radial recurrent artery** | Radial Artery, Right |
| | Radial Artery, Left |

| Term | ICD-10-PCS Value |
|---|---|
| **Radial vein** | Brachial Vein, Right |
| | Brachial Vein, Left |
| **Radialis indicis** | Hand Artery, Right |
| | Hand Artery, Left |
| **Radiocarpal joint** | Wrist Joint, Right |
| | Wrist Joint, Left |
| **Radiocarpal ligament** | Wrist Bursa and Ligament, Right |
| | Wrist Bursa and Ligament, Left |
| **Radioulnar ligament** | Wrist Bursa and Ligament, Right |
| | Wrist Bursa and Ligament, Left |
| **Rectosigmoid junction** | Sigmoid Colon |
| **Rectus abdominis muscle** | Abdomen Muscle, Right |
| | Abdomen Muscle, Left |
| **Rectus femoris muscle** | Upper Leg Muscle, Right |
| | Upper Leg Muscle, Left |
| **Recurrent laryngeal nerve** | Vagus Nerve |
| **Renal calyx** | Kidney, Right |
| | Kidney, Left |
| | Kidneys, Bilateral |
| | Kidney |
| **Renal capsule** | Kidney, Right |
| | Kidney, Left |
| | Kidneys, Bilateral |
| | Kidney |
| **Renal cortex** | Kidney, Right |
| | Kidney, Left |
| | Kidneys, Bilateral |
| | Kidney |
| **Renal plexus** | Abdominal Sympathetic Nerve |
| **Renal segment** | Kidney, Right |
| | Kidney, Left |
| | Kidneys, Bilateral |
| | Kidney |
| **Renal segmental artery** | Renal Artery, Right |
| | Renal Artery, Left |
| **Retroperitoneal lymph node** | Lymphatic, Aortic |
| **Retroperitoneal space** | Retroperitoneum |
| **Retropharyngeal lymph node** | Lymphatic, Right Neck |
| | Lymphatic, Left Neck |
| **Retropubic space** | Pelvic Cavity |
| **Rhinopharynx** | Nasopharynx |
| **Rhomboid major muscle** | Trunk Muscle, Right |
| | Trunk Muscle, Left |
| **Rhomboid minor muscle** | Trunk Muscle, Right |
| | Trunk Muscle, Left |
| **Right ascending lumbar vein** | Azygos Vein |
| **Right atrioventricular valve** | Tricuspid Valve |
| **Right auricular appendix** | Atrium, Right |
| **Right colic vein** | Colic Vein |
| **Right coronary sulcus** | Heart, Right |
| **Right gastric artery** | Gastric Artery |
| **Right gastroepiploic vein** | Superior Mesenteric Vein |



Appendix D: Body Part Key

| Term | ICD-10-PCS Value |
|---|---|
| Right inferior phrenic vein | Inferior Vena Cava |
| Right inferior pulmonary vein | Pulmonary Vein, Right |
| Right jugular trunk | Lymphatic, Right Neck |
| Right lateral ventricle | Cerebral Ventricle |
| Right lymphatic duct | Lymphatic, Right Neck |
| Right ovarian vein | Inferior Vena Cava |
| Right second lumbar vein | Inferior Vena Cava |
| Right subclavian trunk | Lymphatic, Right Neck |
| Right subcostal vein | Azygos Vein |
| Right superior pulmonary vein | Pulmonary Vein, Right |
| Right suprarenal vein | Inferior Vena Cava |
| Right testicular vein | Inferior Vena Cava |
| Rima glottidis | Larynx |
| Risorius muscle | Facial Muscle |
| Round ligament of uterus | Uterine Supporting Structure |
| Round window | Inner Ear, Right |
| | Inner Ear, Left |
| Sacral ganglion | Sacral Sympathetic Nerve |
| Sacral lymph node | Lymphatic, Pelvis |
| Sacral splanchnic nerve | Sacral Sympathetic Nerve |
| Sacrococcygeal ligament | Lower Spine Bursa and Ligament |
| Sacrococcygeal symphysis | Sacrococcygeal Joint |
| Sacroiliac ligament | Lower Spine Bursa and Ligament |
| Sacrospinous ligament | Lower Spine Bursa and Ligament |
| Sacrotuberous ligament | Lower Spine Bursa and Ligament |
| Salpingopharyngeus muscle | Tongue, Palate, Pharynx Muscle |
| Salpinx | Fallopian Tube, Right |
| | Fallopian Tube, Left |
| Saphenous nerve | Femoral Nerve |
| Sartorius muscle | Upper Leg Muscle, Right |
| | Upper Leg Muscle, Left |
| Scalene muscle | Neck Muscle, Right |
| | Neck Muscle, Left |
| Scaphoid bone | Carpal, Right |
| | Carpal, Left |
| Scapholunate ligament | Hand Bursa and Ligament, Right |
| | Hand Bursa and Ligament, Left |
| Scaphotrapezium ligament | Hand Bursa and Ligament, Right |
| | Hand Bursa and Ligament, Left |
| Scarpa's (vestibular) ganglion | Acoustic Nerve |
| Sebaceous gland | Skin |
| Second cranial nerve | Optic Nerve |
| Sella turcica | Sphenoid Bone |
| Semicircular canal | Inner Ear, Right |
| | Inner Ear, Left |
| Semimembranosus muscle | Upper Leg Muscle, Right |
| | Upper Leg Muscle, Left |
| Semitendinosus muscle | Upper Leg Muscle, Right |
| | Upper Leg Muscle, Left |
| Septal cartilage | Nasal Septum |
| Serratus anterior muscle | Thorax Muscle, Right |
| | Thorax Muscle, Left |

| Term | ICD-10-PCS Value |
|---|---|
| Serratus posterior muscle | Trunk Muscle, Right |
| | Trunk Muscle, Left |
| Seventh cranial nerve | Facial Nerve |
| Short gastric artery | Splenic Artery |
| Sigmoid artery | Inferior Mesenteric Artery |
| Sigmoid flexure | Sigmoid Colon |
| Sigmoid vein | Inferior Mesenteric Vein |
| Sinoatrial node | Conduction Mechanism |
| Sinus venosus | Atrium, Right |
| Sixth cranial nerve | Abducens Nerve |
| Skene's (paraurethral) gland | Vestibular Gland |
| Small saphenous vein | Saphenous Vein, Right |
| | Saphenous Vein, Left |
| Solar (celiac) plexus | Abdominal Sympathetic Nerve |
| Soleus muscle | Lower Leg Muscle, Right |
| | Lower Leg Muscle, Left |
| Sphenomandibular ligament | Head and Neck Bursa and Ligament |
| Sphenopalatine (pterygopalatine) ganglion | Head and Neck Sympathetic Nerve |
| Spinal nerve, cervical | Cervical Nerve |
| Spinal nerve, lumbar | Lumbar Nerve |
| Spinal nerve, sacral | Sacral Nerve |
| Spinal nerve, thoracic | Thoracic Nerve |
| Spinous process | Cervical Vertebra |
| | Lumbar Vertebra |
| | Thoracic Vertebra |
| Spiral ganglion | Acoustic Nerve |
| Splenic flexure | Transverse Colon |
| Splenic plexus | Abdominal Sympathetic Nerve |
| Splenius capitis muscle | Head Muscle |
| Splenius cervicis muscle | Neck Muscle, Right |
| | Neck Muscle, Left |
| Stapes | Auditory Ossicle, Right |
| | Auditory Ossicle, Left |
| Stellate ganglion | Head and Neck Sympathetic Nerve |
| Stensen's duct | Parotid Duct, Right |
| | Parotid Duct, Left |
| Sternoclavicular ligament | Shoulder Bursa and Ligament, Right |
| | Shoulder Bursa and Ligament, Left |
| Sternocleidomastoid artery | Thyroid Artery, Right |
| | Thyroid Artery, Left |
| Sternocleidomastoid muscle | Neck Muscle, Right |
| | Neck Muscle, Left |
| Sternocostal ligament | Sternum Bursa and Ligament |
| | Rib(s) Bursa and Ligament |
| Styloglossus muscle | Tongue, Palate, Pharynx Muscle |
| Stylomandibular ligament | Head and Neck Bursa and Ligament |
| Stylopharyngeus muscle | Tongue, Palate, Pharynx Muscle |
| Subacromial bursa | Shoulder Bursa and Ligament, Right |
| | Shoulder Bursa and Ligament, Left |
| Subaortic (common iliac) lymph node | Lymphatic, Pelvis |
| Subarachnoid space, spinal | Spinal Canal |

| Term | ICD-10-PCS Value |
|---|---|
| **Subclavicular (apical) lymph node** | Lymphatic, Right Axillary |
| | Lymphatic, Left Axillary |
| **Subclavius muscle** | Thorax Muscle, Right |
| | Thorax Muscle, Left |
| **Subclavius nerve** | Brachial Plexus |
| **Subcostal artery** | Upper Artery |
| **Subcostal muscle** | Thorax Muscle, Right |
| | Thorax Muscle, Left |
| **Subcostal nerve** | Thoracic Nerve |
| **Subdural space, spinal** | Spinal Canal |
| **Submandibular ganglion** | Facial Nerve |
| | Head and Neck Sympathetic Nerve |
| **Submandibular gland** | Submaxillary Gland, Right |
| | Submaxillary Gland, Left |
| **Submandibular lymph node** | Lymphatic, Head |
| **Submaxillary ganglion** | Head and Neck Sympathetic Nerve |
| **Submaxillary lymph node** | Lymphatic, Head |
| **Submental artery** | Face Artery |
| **Submental lymph node** | Lymphatic, Head |
| **Submucous (Meissner's) plexus** | Abdominal Sympathetic Nerve |
| **Suboccipital nerve** | Cervical Nerve |
| **Suboccipital venous plexus** | Vertebral Vein, Right |
| | Vertebral Vein, Left |
| **Subparotid lymph node** | Lymphatic, Head |
| **Subscapular aponeurosis** | Subcutaneous Tissue and Fascia, Right Upper Arm |
| | Subcutaneous Tissue and Fascia, Left Upper Arm |
| **Subscapular artery** | Axillary Artery, Right |
| | Axillary Artery, Left |
| **Subscapular (posterior) lymph node** | Lymphatic, Right Axillary |
| | Lymphatic, Left Axillary |
| **Subscapularis muscle** | Shoulder Muscle, Right |
| | Shoulder Muscle, Left |
| **Substantia nigra** | Basal Ganglia |
| **Subtalar (talocalcaneal) joint** | Tarsal Joint, Right |
| | Tarsal Joint, Left |
| **Subtalar ligament** | Foot Bursa and Ligament, Right |
| | Foot Bursa and Ligament, Left |
| **Subthalamic nucleus** | Basal Ganglia |
| **Superficial circumflex iliac vein** | Saphenous Vein, Right |
| | Saphenous Vein, Left |
| **Superficial epigastric artery** | Femoral Artery, Right |
| | Femoral Artery, Left |
| **Superficial epigastric vein** | Saphenous Vein, Right |
| | Saphenous Vein, Left |
| **Superficial palmar arch** | Hand Artery, Right |
| | Hand Artery, Left |
| **Superficial palmar venous arch** | Hand Vein, Right |
| | Hand Vein, Left |
| **Superficial temporal artery** | Temporal Artery, Right |
| | Temporal Artery, Left |
| **Superficial transverse perineal muscle** | Perineum Muscle |

| Term | ICD-10-PCS Value |
|---|---|
| **Superior cardiac nerve** | Thoracic Sympathetic Nerve |
| **Superior cerebellar vein** | Intracranial Vein |
| **Superior cerebral vein** | Intracranial Vein |
| **Superior clunic (cluneal) nerve** | Lumbar Nerve |
| **Superior epigastric artery** | Internal Mammary Artery, Right |
| | Internal Mammary Artery, Left |
| **Superior genicular artery** | Popliteal Artery, Right |
| | Popliteal Artery, Left |
| **Superior gluteal artery** | Internal Iliac Artery, Right |
| | Internal Iliac Artery, Left |
| **Superior gluteal nerve** | Lumbar Plexus |
| **Superior hypogastric plexus** | Abdominal Sympathetic Nerve |
| **Superior labial artery** | Face Artery |
| **Superior laryngeal artery** | Thyroid Artery, Right |
| | Thyroid Artery, Left |
| **Superior laryngeal nerve** | Vagus Nerve |
| **Superior longitudinal muscle** | Tongue, Palate, Pharynx Muscle |
| **Superior mesenteric ganglion** | Abdominal Sympathetic Nerve |
| **Superior mesenteric lymph node** | Lymphatic, Mesenteric |
| **Superior mesenteric plexus** | Abdominal Sympathetic Nerve |
| **Superior oblique muscle** | Extraocular Muscle, Right |
| | Extraocular Muscle, Left |
| **Superior olivary nucleus** | Pons |
| **Superior rectal artery** | Inferior Mesenteric Artery |
| **Superior rectal vein** | Inferior Mesenteric Vein |
| **Superior rectus muscle** | Extraocular Muscle, Right |
| | Extraocular Muscle, Left |
| **Superior tarsal plate** | Upper Eyelid, Right |
| | Upper Eyelid, Left |
| **Superior thoracic artery** | Axillary Artery, Right |
| | Axillary Artery, Left |
| **Superior thyroid artery** | External Carotid Artery, Right |
| | External Carotid Artery, Left |
| | Thyroid Artery, Right |
| | Thyroid Artery, Left |
| **Superior turbinate** | Nasal Turbinate |
| **Superior ulnar collateral artery** | Brachial Artery, Right |
| | Brachial Artery, Left |
| **Supraclavicular nerve** | Cervical Plexus |
| **Supraclavicular (Virchow's) lymph node** | Lymphatic, Right Neck |
| | Lymphatic, Left Neck |
| **Suprahyoid lymph node** | Lymphatic, Head |
| **Suprahyoid muscle** | Neck Muscle, Right |
| | Neck Muscle, Left |
| **Suprainguinal lymph node** | Lymphatic, Pelvis |
| **Supraorbital vein** | Face Vein, Right |
| | Face Vein, Left |

| Term | ICD-10-PCS Value |
|---|---|
| Suprarenal gland | Adrenal Gland, Right |
| | Adrenal Gland, Left |
| | Adrenal Glands, Bilateral |
| | Adrenal Gland |
| Suprarenal plexus | Abdominal Sympathetic Nerve |
| Suprascapular nerve | Brachial Plexus |
| Supraspinatus fascia | Subcutaneous Tissue and Fascia, Right Upper Arm |
| | Subcutaneous Tissue and Fascia, Left Upper Arm |
| Supraspinatus muscle | Shoulder Muscle, Right |
| | Shoulder Muscle, Left |
| Supraspinous ligament | Upper Spine Bursa and Ligament |
| | Lower Spine Bursa and Ligament |
| Suprasternal notch | Sternum |
| Supratrochlear lymph node | Lymphatic, Right Upper Extremity |
| | Lymphatic, Left Upper Extremity |
| Sural artery | Popliteal Artery, Right |
| | Popliteal Artery, Left |
| Sweat gland | Skin |
| Talocalcaneal ligament | Foot Bursa and Ligament, Right |
| | Foot Bursa and Ligament, Left |
| Talocalcaneal (subtalar) joint | Tarsal Joint, Right |
| | Tarsal Joint, Left |
| Talocalcaneonavicular joint | Tarsal Joint, Right |
| | Tarsal Joint, Left |
| Talocalcaneonavicular ligament | Foot Bursa and Ligament, Right |
| | Foot Bursa and Ligament, Left |
| Talocrural joint | Ankle Joint, Right |
| | Ankle Joint, Left |
| Talofibular ligament | Ankle Bursa and Ligament, Right |
| | Ankle Bursa and Ligament, Left |
| Talus bone | Tarsal, Right |
| | Tarsal, Left |
| Tarsometatarsal ligament | Foot Bursa and Ligament, Right |
| | Foot Bursa and Ligament, Left |
| Temporal lobe | Cerebral Hemisphere |
| Temporalis muscle | Head Muscle |
| Temporoparietalis muscle | Head Muscle |
| Tensor fasciae latae muscle | Hip Muscle, Right |
| | Hip Muscle, Left |
| Tensor veli palatini muscle | Tongue, Palate, Pharynx Muscle |
| Tenth cranial nerve | Vagus Nerve |
| Tentorium cerebelli | Dura Mater |
| Teres major muscle | Shoulder Muscle, Right |
| | Shoulder Muscle, Left |
| Teres minor muscle | Shoulder Muscle, Right |
| | Shoulder Muscle, Left |
| Testicular artery | Abdominal Aorta |
| Thenar muscle | Hand Muscle, Right |
| | Hand Muscle, Left |
| Third cranial nerve | Oculomotor Nerve |
| Third occipital nerve | Cervical Nerve |
| Third ventricle | Cerebral Ventricle |
| Thoracic aortic plexus | Thoracic Sympathetic Nerve |

| Term | ICD-10-PCS Value |
|---|---|
| Thoracic esophagus | Esophagus, Middle |
| Thoracic facet joint | Thoracic Vertebral Joint |
| Thoracic ganglion | Thoracic Sympathetic Nerve |
| Thoracoacromial artery | Axillary Artery, Right |
| | Axillary Artery, Left |
| Thoracolumbar facet joint | Thoracolumbar Vertebral Joint |
| Thymus gland | Thymus |
| Thyroarytenoid muscle | Neck Muscle, Right |
| | Neck Muscle, Left |
| Thyrocervical trunk | Thyroid Artery, Right |
| | Thyroid Artery, Left |
| Thyroid cartilage | Larynx |
| Tibialis anterior muscle | Lower Leg Muscle, Right |
| | Lower Leg Muscle, Left |
| Tibialis posterior muscle | Lower Leg Muscle, Right |
| | Lower Leg Muscle, Left |
| Tibiofemoral joint | Knee Joint, Right |
| | Knee Joint, Left |
| | Knee Joint, Tibial Surface, Right |
| | Knee Joint, Tibial Surface, Left |
| Tongue, base of | Pharynx |
| Tracheobronchial lymph node | Lymphatic, Thorax |
| Tragus | External Ear, Right |
| | External Ear, Left |
| | External Ear, Bilateral |
| Transversalis fascia | Subcutaneous Tissue and Fascia, Trunk |
| Transverse acetabular ligament | Hip Bursa and Ligament, Right |
| | Hip Bursa and Ligament, Left |
| Transverse (cutaneous) cervical nerve | Cervical Plexus |
| Transverse facial artery | Temporal Artery, Right |
| | Temporal Artery, Left |
| Transverse foramen | Cervical Vertebra |
| Transverse humeral ligament | Shoulder Bursa and Ligament, Right |
| | Shoulder Bursa and Ligament, Left |
| Transverse ligament of atlas | Head and Neck Bursa and Ligament |
| Transverse process | Cervical Vertebra |
| | Thoracic Vertebra |
| | Lumbar Vertebra |
| Transverse scapular ligament | Shoulder Bursa and Ligament, Right |
| | Shoulder Bursa and Ligament, Left |
| Transverse thoracis muscle | Thorax Muscle, Right |
| | Thorax Muscle, Left |
| Transversospinalis muscle | Trunk Muscle, Right |
| | Trunk Muscle, Left |
| Transversus abdominis muscle | Abdomen Muscle, Right |
| | Abdomen Muscle, Left |
| Trapezium bone | Carpal, Right |
| | Carpal, Left |
| Trapezius muscle | Trunk Muscle, Right |
| | Trunk Muscle, Left |
| Trapezoid bone | Carpal, Right |
| | Carpal, Left |

| Term | ICD-10-PCS Value |
|---|---|
| **Triceps brachii muscle** | Upper Arm Muscle, Right |
| | Upper Arm Muscle, Left |
| **Tricuspid annulus** | Tricuspid Valve |
| **Trifacial nerve** | Trigeminal Nerve |
| **Trigone of bladder** | Bladder |
| **Triquetral bone** | Carpal, Right |
| | Carpal, Left |
| **Trochantericbursa** | Hip Bursa and Ligament, Right |
| | Hip Bursa and Ligament, Left |
| **Twelfth cranial nerve** | Hypoglossal Nerve |
| **Tympanic cavity** | Middle Ear, Right |
| | Middle Ear, Left |
| **Tympanic nerve** | Glossopharyngeal Nerve |
| **Tympanic part of temoporal bone** | Temporal Bone, Right |
| | Temporal Bone, Left |
| **Ulnar collateral carpal ligament** | Wrist Bursa and Ligament, Right |
| | Wrist Bursa and Ligament, Left |
| **Ulnar collateral ligament** | Elbow Bursa and Ligament, Right |
| | Elbow Bursa and Ligament, Left |
| **Ulnar notch** | Radius, Right |
| | Radius, Left |
| **Ulnar vein** | Brachial Vein, Right |
| | Brachial Vein, Left |
| **Umbilical artery** | Internal Iliac Artery, Right |
| | Internal Iliac Artery, Left |
| | Lower Artery |
| **Ureteral orifice** | Ureter, Right |
| | Ureter, Left |
| | Ureters, Bilateral |
| | Ureter |
| **Ureteropelvic junction (UPJ)** | Kidney Pelvis, Right |
| | Kidney Pelvis, Left |
| **Ureterovesical orifice** | Ureter, Right |
| | Ureter, Left |
| | Ureters, Bilateral |
| | Ureter |
| **Uterine artery** | Internal Iliac Artery, Right |
| | Internal Iliac Artery, Left |
| **Uterine cornu** | Uterus |
| **Uterine tube** | Fallopian Tube, Right |
| | Fallopian Tube, Left |
| **Uterine vein** | Hypogastric Vein, Right |
| | Hypogastric Vein, Left |
| **Vaginal artery** | Internal Iliac Artery, Right |
| | Internal Iliac Artery, Left |
| **Vaginal vein** | Hypogastric Vein, Right |
| | Hypogastric Vein, Left |
| **Vastus intermedius muscle** | Upper Leg Muscle, Right |
| | Upper Leg Muscle, Left |
| **Vastus lateralis muscle** | Upper Leg Muscle, Right |
| | Upper Leg Muscle, Left |
| **Vastus medialis muscle** | Upper Leg Muscle, Right |
| | Upper Leg Muscle, Left |
| **Ventricular fold** | Larynx |
| **Vermiform appendix** | Appendix |

| Term | ICD-10-PCS Value |
|---|---|
| **Vermilion border** | Upper Lip |
| | Lower Lip |
| **Vertebral arch** | Cervical Vertebra |
| | Lumbar Vertebra |
| | Thoracic Vertebra |
| **Vertebral body** | Cervical Vertebra |
| | Lumbar Vertebra |
| | Thoracic Vertebra |
| **Vertebral canal** | Spinal Canal |
| **Vertebral foramen** | Cervical Vertebra |
| | Lumbar Vertebra |
| | Thoracic Vertebra |
| **Vertebral lamina** | Cervical Vertebra |
| | Lumbar Vertebra |
| | Thoracic Vertebra |
| **Vertebral pedicle** | Cervical Vertebra |
| | Lumbar Vertebra |
| | Thoracic Vertebra |
| **Vesical vein** | Hypogastric Vein, Right |
| | Hypogastric Vein, Left |
| **Vestibular (Scarpa's) ganglion** | Acoustic Nerve |
| **Vestibular nerve** | Acoustic Nerve |
| **Vestibulocochlear nerve** | Acoustic Nerve |
| **Virchow's (supraclavicular) lymph node** | Lymphatic, Right Neck |
| | Lymphatic, Left Neck |
| **Vitreous body** | Vitreous, Right |
| | Vitreous, Left |
| **Vocal fold** | Vocal Cord, Right |
| | Vocal Cord, Left |
| **Volar (palmar) digital vein** | Hand Vein, Right |
| | Hand Vein, Left |
| **Volar (palmar) metacarpal vein** | Hand Vein, Right |
| | Hand Vein, Left |
| **Vomer bone** | Nasal Septum |
| **Vomer of nasal septum** | Nasal Bone |
| **Xiphoid process** | Sternum |
| **Zonule of Zinn** | Lens, Right |
| | Lens, Left |
| **Zygomatic process of frontal bone** | Frontal Bone |
| **Zygomatic process of temporal bone** | Temporal Bone, Right |
| | Temporal Bone, Left |
| **Zygomaticus muscle** | Facial Muscle |

# Appendix E: Body Part Definitions

| ICD-10-PCS Value | Definition |
|---|---|
| **1st Toe, Left**<br>**1st Toe, Right** | **Includes:**<br>Hallux |
| **Abdomen Muscle, Left**<br>**Abdomen Muscle, Right** | **Includes:**<br>External oblique muscle<br>Internal oblique muscle<br>Pyramidalis muscle<br>Rectus abdominis muscle<br>Transversus abdominis muscle |
| **Abdominal Aorta** | **Includes:**<br>Inferior phrenic artery<br>Lumbar artery<br>Median sacral artery<br>Middle suprarenal artery<br>Ovarian artery<br>Testicular artery |
| **Abdominal Sympathetic Nerve** | **Includes:**<br>Abdominal aortic plexus<br>Auerbach's (myenteric) plexus<br>Celiac (solar) plexus<br>Celiac ganglion<br>Gastric plexus<br>Hepatic plexus<br>Inferior hypogastric plexus<br>Inferior mesenteric ganglion<br>Inferior mesenteric plexus<br>Meissner's (submucous) plexus<br>Myenteric (Auerbach's) plexus<br>Pancreatic plexus<br>Pelvic splanchnic nerve<br>Renal plexus<br>Solar (celiac) plexus<br>Splenic plexus<br>Submucous (Meissner's) plexus<br>Superior hypogastric plexus<br>Superior mesenteric ganglion<br>Superior mesenteric plexus<br>Suprarenal plexus |
| **Abducens Nerve** | **Includes:**<br>Sixth cranial nerve |
| **Accessory Nerve** | **Includes:**<br>Eleventh cranial nerve |
| **Acoustic Nerve** | **Includes:**<br>Cochlear nerve<br>Eighth cranial nerve<br>Scarpa's (vestibular) ganglion<br>Spiral ganglion<br>Vestibular (Scarpa's) ganglion<br>Vestibular nerve<br>Vestibulocochlear nerve |
| **Adenoids** | **Includes:**<br>Pharyngeal tonsil |
| **Adrenal Gland**<br>**Adrenal Gland, Left**<br>**Adrenal Gland, Right**<br>**Adrenal Glands, Bilateral** | **Includes:**<br>Suprarenal gland |
| **Ampulla of Vater** | **Includes:**<br>Duodenal ampulla<br>Hepatopancreatic ampulla |
| **Anal Sphincter** | **Includes:**<br>External anal sphincter<br>Internal anal sphincter |

| ICD-10-PCS Value | Definition |
|---|---|
| **Ankle Bursa and Ligament, Left**<br>**Ankle Bursa and Ligament, Right** | **Includes:**<br>Calcaneofibular ligament<br>Deltoid ligament<br>Ligament of the lateral malleolus<br>Talofibular ligament |
| **Ankle Joint, Left**<br>**Ankle Joint, Right** | **Includes:**<br>Inferior tibiofibular joint<br>Talocrural joint |
| **Anterior Chamber, Left**<br>**Anterior Chamber, Right** | **Includes:**<br>Aqueous humour |
| **Anterior Tibial Artery, Left**<br>**Anterior Tibial Artery, Right** | **Includes:**<br>Anterior lateral malleolar artery<br>Anterior medial malleolar artery<br>Anterior tibial recurrent artery<br>Dorsalis pedis artery<br>Posterior tibial recurrent artery |
| **Anus** | **Includes:**<br>Anal orifice |
| **Aortic Valve** | **Includes:**<br>Aortic annulus |
| **Appendix** | **Includes:**<br>Vermiform appendix |
| **Atrial Septum** | **Includes:**<br>Interatrial septum |
| **Atrium, Left** | **Includes:**<br>Atrium pulmonale<br>Left auricular appendix |
| **Atrium, Right** | **Includes:**<br>Atrium dextrum cordis<br>Right auricular appendix<br>Sinus venosus |
| **Auditory Ossicle, Left**<br>**Auditory Ossicle, Right** | **Includes:**<br>Incus<br>Malleus<br>Stapes |
| **Axillary Artery, Left**<br>**Axillary Artery, Right** | **Includes:**<br>Anterior circumflex humeral artery<br>Lateral thoracic artery<br>Posterior circumflex humeral artery<br>Subscapular artery<br>Superior thoracic artery<br>Thoracoacromial artery |
| **Azygos Vein** | **Includes:**<br>Right ascending lumbar vein<br>Right subcostal vein |
| **Basal Ganglia** | **Includes:**<br>Basal nuclei<br>Claustrum<br>Corpus striatum<br>Globus pallidus<br>Substantia nigra<br>Subthalamic nucleus |
| **Basilic Vein, Left**<br>**Basilic Vein, Right** | **Includes:**<br>Median antebrachial vein<br>Median cubital vein |
| **Bladder** | **Includes:**<br>Trigone of bladder |
| **Brachial Artery, Left**<br>**Brachial Artery, Right** | **Includes:**<br>Inferior ulnar collateral artery<br>Profunda brachii<br>Superior ulnar collateral artery |

| ICD-10-PCS Value | Definition |
|---|---|
| **Brachial Plexus** | **Includes:**<br>Axillary nerve<br>Dorsal scapular nerve<br>First intercostal nerve<br>Long thoracic nerve<br>Musculocutaneous nerve<br>Subclavius nerve<br>Suprascapular nerve |
| **Brachial Vein, Left**<br>**Brachial Vein, Right** | **Includes:**<br>Radial vein<br>Ulnar vein |
| **Brain** | **Includes:**<br>Cerebrum<br>Corpus callosum<br>Encephalon |
| **Breast, Bilateral**<br>**Breast, Left**<br>**Breast, Right** | **Includes:**<br>Mammary duct<br>Mammary gland |
| **Buccal Mucosa** | **Includes:**<br>Buccal gland<br>Molar gland<br>Palatine gland |
| **Carotid Bodies, Bilateral**<br>**Carotid Body, Left**<br>**Carotid Body, Right** | **Includes:**<br>Carotid glomus |
| **Carpal Joint, Left**<br>**Carpal Joint, Right** | **Includes:**<br>Intercarpal joint<br>Midcarpal joint |
| **Carpal, Left**<br>**Carpal, Right** | **Includes:**<br>Capitate bone<br>Hamate bone<br>Lunate bone<br>Pisiform bone<br>Scaphoid bone<br>Trapezium bone<br>Trapezoid bone<br>Triquetral bone |
| **Celiac Artery** | **Includes:**<br>Celiac trunk |
| **Cephalic Vein, Left**<br>**Cephalic Vein, Right** | **Includes:**<br>Accessory cephalic vein |
| **Cerebellum** | **Includes:**<br>Culmen |
| **Cerebral Hemisphere** | **Includes:**<br>Frontal lobe<br>Occipital lobe<br>Parietal lobe<br>Temporal lobe |
| **Cerebral Meninges** | **Includes:**<br>Arachnoid mater, intracranial<br>Leptomeninges, intracranial<br>Pia mater, intracranial |
| **Cerebral Ventricle** | **Includes:**<br>Aqueduct of Sylvius<br>Cerebral aqueduct (Sylvius)<br>Choroid plexus<br>Ependyma<br>Foramen of Monro (intraventricular)<br>Fourth ventricle<br>Interventricular foramen (Monro)<br>Left lateral ventricle<br>Right lateral ventricle<br>Third ventricle |

| ICD-10-PCS Value | Definition |
|---|---|
| **Cervical Nerve** | **Includes:**<br>Greater occipital nerve<br>Spinal nerve, cervical<br>Suboccipital nerve<br>Third occipital nerve |
| **Cervical Plexus** | **Includes:**<br>Ansa cervicalis<br>Cutaneous (transverse) cervical nerve<br>Great auricular nerve<br>Lesser occipital nerve<br>Supraclavicular nerve<br>Transverse (cutaneous) cervical nerve |
| **Cervical Vertebra** | **Includes:**<br>Dens<br>Odontoid process<br>Spinous process<br>Transverse foramen<br>Transverse process<br>Vertebral arch<br>Vertebral body<br>Vertebral foramen<br>Vertebral lamina<br>Vertebral pedicle |
| **Cervical Vertebral Joint** | **Includes:**<br>Atlantoaxial joint<br>Cervical facet joint |
| **Cervical Vertebral Joints, 2 or more** | **Includes:**<br>Cervical facet joint |
| **Cervicothoracic Vertebral Joint** | **Includes:**<br>Cervicothoracic facet joint |
| **Cisterna Chyli** | **Includes:**<br>Intestinal lymphatic trunk<br>Lumbar lymphatic trunk |
| **Coccygeal Glomus** | **Includes:**<br>Coccygeal body |
| **Colic Vein** | **Includes:**<br>Ileocolic vein<br>Left colic vein<br>Middle colic vein<br>Right colic vein |
| **Conduction Mechanism** | **Includes:**<br>Atrioventricular node<br>Bundle of His<br>Bundle of Kent<br>Sinoatrial node |
| **Conjunctiva, Left**<br>**Conjunctiva, Right** | **Includes:**<br>Plica semilunaris |
| **Dura Mater** | **Includes:**<br>Diaphragma sellae<br>Dura mater, intracranial<br>Falx cerebri<br>Tentorium cerebelli |
| **Elbow Bursa and Ligament, Left**<br>**Elbow Bursa and Ligament, Right** | **Includes:**<br>Annular ligament<br>Olecranon bursa<br>Radial collateral ligament<br>Ulnar collateral ligament |
| **Elbow Joint, Left**<br>**Elbow Joint, Right** | **Includes:**<br>Distal humerus, involving joint<br>Humeroradial joint<br>Humeroulnar joint<br>Proximal radioulnar joint |
| **Epidural Space, Intracranial** | **Includes:**<br>Extradural space, intracranial |

| ICD-10-PCS Value | Definition |
|---|---|
| **Epiglottis** | **Includes:**<br>Glossoepiglottic fold |
| **Esophagogastric Junction** | **Includes:**<br>Cardia<br>Cardioesophageal junction<br>Gastroesophageal (GE) junction |
| **Esophagus, Lower** | **Includes:**<br>Abdominal esophagus |
| **Esophagus, Middle** | **Includes:**<br>Thoracic esophagus |
| **Esophagus, Upper** | **Includes:**<br>Cervical esophagus |
| **Ethmoid Bone, Left**<br>**Ethmoid Bone, Right** | **Includes:**<br>Cribriform plate |
| **Ethmoid Sinus, Left**<br>**Ethmoid Sinus, Right** | **Includes:**<br>Ethmoidal air cell |
| **Eustachian Tube, Left**<br>**Eustachian Tube, Right** | **Includes:**<br>Auditory tube<br>Pharyngotympanic tube |
| **External Auditory Canal, Left**<br>**External Auditory Canal, Right** | **Includes:**<br>External auditory meatus |
| **External Carotid Artery, Left**<br>**External Carotid Artery, Right** | **Includes:**<br>Ascending pharyngeal artery<br>Internal maxillary artery<br>Lingual artery<br>Maxillary artery<br>Occipital artery<br>Posterior auricular artery<br>Superior thyroid artery |
| **External Ear, Bilateral**<br>**External Ear, Left**<br>**External Ear, Right** | **Includes:**<br>Antihelix<br>Antitragus<br>Auricle<br>Earlobe<br>Helix<br>Pinna<br>Tragus |
| **External Iliac Artery, Left**<br>**External Iliac Artery, Right** | **Includes:**<br>Deep circumflex iliac artery<br>Inferior epigastric artery |
| **External Jugular Vein, Left**<br>**External Jugular Vein, Right** | **Includes:**<br>Posterior auricular vein |
| **Extraocular Muscle, Left**<br>**Extraocular Muscle, Right** | **Includes:**<br>Inferior oblique muscle<br>Inferior rectus muscle<br>Lateral rectus muscle<br>Medial rectus muscle<br>Superior oblique muscle<br>Superior rectus muscle |
| **Eye, Left**<br>**Eye, Right** | **Includes:**<br>Ciliary body<br>Posterior chamber |
| **Face Artery** | **Includes:**<br>Angular artery<br>Ascending palatine artery<br>External maxillary artery<br>Facial artery<br>Inferior labial artery<br>Submental artery<br>Superior labial artery |
| **Face Vein, Left**<br>**Face Vein, Right** | **Includes:**<br>Angular vein<br>Anterior facial vein<br>Common facial vein<br>Deep facial vein<br>Frontal vein<br>Posterior facial (retromandibular) vein<br>Supraorbital vein |
| **Facial Muscle** | **Includes:**<br>Buccinator muscle<br>Corrugator supercilii muscle<br>Depressor anguli oris muscle<br>Depressor labii inferioris muscle<br>Depressor septi nasi muscle<br>Depressor supercilii muscle<br>Levator anguli oris muscle<br>Levator labii superioris alaeque nasi muscle<br>Levator labii superioris muscle<br>Mentalis muscle<br>Nasalis muscle<br>Occipitofrontalis muscle<br>Orbicularis oris muscle<br>Procerus muscle<br>Risorius muscle<br>Zygomaticus muscle |
| **Facial Nerve** | **Includes:**<br>Chorda tympani<br>Geniculate ganglion<br>Greater superficial petrosal nerve<br>Nerve to the stapedius<br>Parotid plexus<br>Posterior auricular nerve<br>Seventh cranial nerve<br>Submandibular ganglion |
| **Fallopian Tube, Left**<br>**Fallopian Tube, Right** | **Includes:**<br>Oviduct<br>Salpinx<br>Uterine tube |
| **Femoral Artery, Left**<br>**Femoral Artery, Right** | **Includes:**<br>Circumflex iliac artery<br>Deep femoral artery<br>Descending genicular artery<br>External pudendal artery<br>Superficial epigastric artery |
| **Femoral Nerve** | **Includes:**<br>Anterior crural nerve<br>Saphenous nerve |
| **Femoral Shaft, Left**<br>**Femoral Shaft, Right** | **Includes:**<br>Body of femur |
| **Femoral Vein, Left**<br>**Femoral Vein, Right** | **Includes:**<br>Deep femoral (profunda femoris) vein<br>Popliteal vein<br>Profunda femoris (deep femoral) vein |
| **Fibula, Left**<br>**Fibula, Right** | **Includes:**<br>Body of fibula<br>Head of fibula<br>Lateral malleolus |
| **Finger Nail** | **Includes:**<br>Nail bed<br>Nail plate |

| ICD-10-PCS Value | Definition |
|---|---|
| **Finger Phalangeal Joint, Left**<br>**Finger Phalangeal Joint, Right** | **Includes:**<br>Interphalangeal (IP) joint |
| **Foot Artery, Left**<br>**Foot Artery, Right** | **Includes:**<br>Arcuate artery<br>Dorsal metatarsal artery<br>Lateral plantar artery<br>Lateral tarsal artery<br>Medial plantar artery |
| **Foot Bursa and Ligament, Left**<br>**Foot Bursa and Ligament, Right** | **Includes:**<br>Calcaneocuboid ligament<br>Cuneonavicular ligament<br>Intercuneiform ligament<br>Interphalangeal ligament<br>Metatarsal ligament<br>Metatarsophalangeal ligament<br>Subtalar ligament<br>Talocalcaneal ligament<br>Talocalcaneonavicular ligament<br>Tarsometatarsal ligament |
| **Foot Muscle, Left**<br>**Foot Muscle, Right** | **Includes:**<br>Abductor hallucis muscle<br>Adductor hallucis muscle<br>Extensor digitorum brevis muscle<br>Extensor hallucis brevis muscle<br>Flexor digitorum brevis muscle<br>Flexor hallucis brevis muscle<br>Quadratus plantae muscle |
| **Foot Vein, Left**<br>**Foot Vein, Right** | **Includes:**<br>Common digital vein<br>Dorsal metatarsal vein<br>Dorsal venous arch<br>Plantar digital vein<br>Plantar metatarsal vein<br>Plantar venous arch |
| **Frontal Bone** | **Includes:**<br>Zygomatic process of frontal bone |
| **Gastric Artery** | **Includes:**<br>Left gastric artery<br>Right gastric artery |
| **Glenoid Cavity, Left**<br>**Glenoid Cavity, Right** | **Includes:**<br>Glenoid fossa (of scapula) |
| **Glomus Jugulare** | **Includes:**<br>Jugular body |
| **Glossopharyngeal Nerve** | **Includes:**<br>Carotid sinus nerve<br>Ninth cranial nerve<br>Tympanic nerve |
| **Hand Artery, Left**<br>**Hand Artery, Right** | **Includes:**<br>Deep palmar arch<br>Princeps pollicis artery<br>Radialis indicis<br>Superficial palmar arch |
| **Hand Bursa and Ligament, Left**<br>**Hand Bursa and Ligament, Right** | **Includes:**<br>Carpometacarpal ligament<br>Intercarpal ligament<br>Interphalangeal ligament<br>Lunotriquetral ligament<br>Metacarpal ligament<br>Metacarpophalangeal ligament<br>Pisohamate ligament<br>Pisometacarpal ligament<br>Scapholunate ligament<br>Scaphotrapezium ligament |

| ICD-10-PCS Value | Definition |
|---|---|
| **Hand Muscle, Left**<br>**Hand Muscle, Right** | **Includes:**<br>Hypothenar muscle<br>Palmar interosseous muscle<br>Thenar muscle |
| **Hand Vein, Left**<br>**Hand Vein, Right** | **Includes:**<br>Dorsal metacarpal vein<br>Palmar (volar) digital vein<br>Palmar (volar) metacarpal vein<br>Superficial palmar venous arch<br>Volar (palmar) digital vein<br>Volar (palmar) metacarpal vein |
| **Head and Neck Bursa and Ligament** | **Includes:**<br>Alar ligament of axis<br>Cervical interspinous ligament<br>Cervical intertransverse ligament<br>Cervical ligamentum flavum<br>Interspinous ligament<br>Lateral temporomandibular ligament<br>Sphenomandibular ligament<br>Stylomandibular ligament<br>Transverse ligament of atlas |
| **Head and Neck Sympathetic Nerve** | **Includes:**<br>Cavernous plexus<br>Cervical ganglion<br>Ciliary ganglion<br>Internal carotid plexus<br>Otic ganglion<br>Pterygopalatine (sphenopalatine) ganglion<br>Sphenopalatine (pterygopalatine) ganglion<br>Stellate ganglion<br>Submandibular ganglion<br>Submaxillary ganglion |
| **Head Muscle** | **Includes:**<br>Auricularis muscle<br>Masseter muscle<br>Pterygoid muscle<br>Splenius capitis muscle<br>Temporalis muscle<br>Temporoparietalis muscle |
| **Heart, Left** | **Includes:**<br>Left coronary sulcus<br>Obtuse margin |
| **Heart, Right** | **Includes:**<br>Right coronary sulcus |
| **Hemiazygos Vein** | **Includes:**<br>Left ascending lumbar vein<br>Left subcostal vein |
| **Hepatic Artery** | **Includes:**<br>Common hepatic artery<br>Gastroduodenal artery<br>Hepatic artery proper |
| **Hip Bursa and Ligament, Left**<br>**Hip Bursa and Ligament, Right** | **Includes:**<br>Iliofemoral ligament<br>Ischiofemoral ligament<br>Pubofemoral ligament<br>Transverse acetabular ligament<br>Trochanteric bursa |
| **Hip Joint, Left**<br>**Hip Joint, Right** | **Includes:**<br>Acetabulofemoral joint |

| ICD-10-PCS Value | Definition |
|---|---|
| **Hip Muscle, Left**<br>**Hip Muscle, Right** | **Includes:**<br>Gemellus muscle<br>Gluteus maximus muscle<br>Gluteus medius muscle<br>Gluteus minimus muscle<br>Iliacus muscle<br>Obturator muscle<br>Piriformis muscle<br>Psoas muscle<br>Quadratus femoris muscle<br>Tensor fasciae latae muscle |
| **Humeral Head, Left**<br>**Humeral Head, Right** | **Includes:**<br>Greater tuberosity<br>Lesser tuberosity<br>Neck of humerus (anatomical)(surgical) |
| **Humeral Shaft, Left**<br>**Humeral Shaft, Right** | **Includes:**<br>Distal humerus<br>Humerus, distal<br>Lateral epicondyle of humerus<br>Medial epicondyle of humerus |
| **Hypogastric Vein, Left**<br>**Hypogastric Vein, Right** | **Includes:**<br>Gluteal vein<br>Internal iliac vein<br>Internal pudendal vein<br>Lateral sacral vein<br>Middle hemorrhoidal vein<br>Obturator vein<br>Uterine vein<br>Vaginal vein<br>Vesical vein |
| **Hypoglossal Nerve** | **Includes:**<br>Twelfth cranial nerve |
| **Hypothalamus** | **Includes:**<br>Mammillary body |
| **Inferior Mesenteric Artery** | **Includes:**<br>Sigmoid artery<br>Superior rectal artery |
| **Inferior Mesenteric Vein** | **Includes:**<br>Sigmoid vein<br>Superior rectal vein |
| **Inferior Vena Cava** | **Includes:**<br>Postcava<br>Right inferior phrenic vein<br>Right ovarian vein<br>Right second lumbar vein<br>Right suprarenal vein<br>Right testicular vein |
| **Inguinal Region, Bilateral**<br>**Inguinal Region, Left**<br>**Inguinal Region, Right** | **Includes:**<br>Inguinal canal<br>Inguinal triangle |
| **Inner Ear, Left**<br>**Inner Ear, Right** | **Includes:**<br>Bony labyrinth<br>Bony vestibule<br>Cochlea<br>Round window<br>Semicircular canal |
| **Innominate Artery** | **Includes:**<br>Brachiocephalic artery<br>Brachiocephalic trunk |
| **Innominate Vein, Left**<br>**Innominate Vein, Right** | **Includes:**<br>Brachiocephalic vein<br>Inferior thyroid vein |
| **Internal Carotid Artery, Left**<br>**Internal Carotid Artery, Right** | **Includes:**<br>Caroticotympanic artery<br>Carotid sinus |
| **Internal Iliac Artery, Left**<br>**Internal Iliac Artery, Right** | **Includes:**<br>Deferential artery<br>Hypogastric artery<br>Iliolumbar artery<br>Inferior gluteal artery<br>Inferior vesical artery<br>Internal pudendal artery<br>Lateral sacral artery<br>Middle rectal artery<br>Obturator artery<br>Superior gluteal artery<br>Umbilical artery<br>Uterine artery<br>Vaginal artery |
| **Internal Mammary Artery, Left**<br>**Internal Mammary Artery, Right** | **Includes:**<br>Anterior intercostal artery<br>Internal thoracic artery<br>Musculophrenic artery<br>Pericardiophrenic artery<br>Superior epigastric artery |
| **Intracranial Artery** | **Includes:**<br>Anterior cerebral artery<br>Anterior choroidal artery<br>Anterior communicating artery<br>Basilar artery<br>Circle of Willis<br>Internal carotid artery, intracranial portion<br>Middle cerebral artery<br>Ophthalmic artery<br>Posterior cerebral artery<br>Posterior communicating artery<br>Posterior inferior cerebellar artery (PICA) |
| **Intracranial Vein** | **Includes:**<br>Anterior cerebral vein<br>Basal (internal) cerebral vein<br>Dural venous sinus<br>Great cerebral vein<br>Inferior cerebellar vein<br>Inferior cerebral vein<br>Internal (basal) cerebral vein<br>Middle cerebral vein<br>Ophthalmic vein<br>Superior cerebellar vein<br>Superior cerebral vein |
| **Jejunum** | **Includes:**<br>Duodenojejunal flexure |
| **Kidney** | **Includes:**<br>Renal calyx<br>Renal capsule<br>Renal cortex<br>Renal segment |
| **Kidney Pelvis, Left**<br>**Kidney Pelvis, Right** | **Includes:**<br>Ureteropelvic junction (UPJ) |
| **Kidney, Left**<br>**Kidney, Right**<br>**Kidneys, Bilateral** | **Includes:**<br>Renal calyx<br>Renal capsule<br>Renal cortex<br>Renal segment |

| ICD-10-PCS Value | Definition |
|---|---|
| **Knee Bursa and Ligament, Left**<br>**Knee Bursa and Ligament, Right** | **Includes:**<br>Anterior cruciate ligament (ACL)<br>Lateral collateral ligament (LCL)<br>Ligament of head of fibula<br>Medial collateral ligament (MCL)<br>Patellar ligament<br>Popliteal ligament<br>Posterior cruciate ligament (PCL)<br>Prepatellar bursa |
| **Knee Joint, Femoral Surface, Left**<br>**Knee Joint, Femoral Surface, Right** | **Includes:**<br>Femoropatellar joint<br>Patellofemoral joint |
| **Knee Joint, Left**<br>**Knee Joint, Right** | **Includes:**<br>Femoropatellar joint<br>Femorotibial joint<br>Lateral meniscus<br>Medial meniscus<br>Patellofemoral joint<br>Tibiofemoral joint |
| **Knee Joint, Tibial Surface, Left**<br>**Knee Joint, Tibial Surface, Right** | **Includes:**<br>Femorotibial joint<br>Tibiofemoral joint |
| **Knee Tendon, Left**<br>**Knee Tendon, Right** | **Includes:**<br>Patellar tendon |
| **Lacrimal Duct, Left**<br>**Lacrimal Duct, Right** | **Includes:**<br>Lacrimal canaliculus<br>Lacrimal punctum<br>Lacrimal sac<br>Nasolacrimal duct |
| **Larynx** | **Includes:**<br>Aryepiglottic fold<br>Arytenoid cartilage<br>Corniculate cartilage<br>Cuneiform cartilage<br>False vocal cord<br>Glottis<br>Rima glottidis<br>Thyroid cartilage<br>Ventricular fold |
| **Lens, Left**<br>**Lens, Right** | **Includes:**<br>Zonule of Zinn |
| **Liver** | **Includes:**<br>Quadrate lobe |
| **Lower Arm and Wrist Muscle, Left**<br>**Lower Arm and Wrist Muscle, Right** | **Includes:**<br>Anatomical snuffbox<br>Brachioradialis muscle<br>Extensor carpi radialis muscle<br>Extensor carpi ulnaris muscle<br>Flexor carpi radialis muscle<br>Flexor carpi ulnaris muscle<br>Flexor pollicis longus muscle<br>Palmaris longus muscle<br>Pronator quadratus muscle<br>Pronator teres muscle |
| **Lower Artery** | **Includes:**<br>Umbilical artery |
| **Lower Eyelid, Left**<br>**Lower Eyelid, Right** | **Includes:**<br>Inferior tarsal plate<br>Medial canthus |
| **Lower Femur, Left**<br>**Lower Femur, Right** | **Includes:**<br>Lateral condyle of femur<br>Lateral epicondyle of femur<br>Medial condyle of femur<br>Medial epicondyle of femur |

| ICD-10-PCS Value | Definition |
|---|---|
| **Lower Leg Muscle, Left**<br>**Lower Leg Muscle, Right** | **Includes:**<br>Extensor digitorum longus muscle<br>Extensor hallucis longus muscle<br>Fibularis brevis muscle<br>Fibularis longus muscle<br>Flexor digitorum longus muscle<br>Flexor hallucis longus muscle<br>Gastrocnemius muscle<br>Peroneus brevis muscle<br>Peroneus longus muscle<br>Popliteus muscle<br>Soleus muscle<br>Tibialis anterior muscle<br>Tibialis posterior muscle |
| **Lower Leg Tendon, Left**<br>**Lower Leg Tendon, Right** | **Includes:**<br>Achilles tendon |
| **Lower Lip** | **Includes:**<br>Frenulum labii inferioris<br>Labial gland<br>Vermilion border |
| **Lower Spine Bursa and Ligament** | **Includes:**<br>Iliolumbar ligament<br>Interspinous ligament<br>Intertransverse ligament<br>Ligamentum flavum<br>Sacrococcygeal ligament<br>Sacroiliac ligament<br>Sacrospinous ligament<br>Sacrotuberous ligament<br>Supraspinous ligament |
| **Lumbar Nerve** | **Includes:**<br>Lumbosacral trunk<br>Spinal nerve, lumbar<br>Superior clunic (cluneal) nerve |
| **Lumbar Plexus** | **Includes:**<br>Accessory obturator nerve<br>Genitofemoral nerve<br>Iliohypogastric nerve<br>Ilioinguinal nerve<br>Lateral femoral cutaneous nerve<br>Obturator nerve<br>Superior gluteal nerve |
| **Lumbar Spinal Cord** | **Includes:**<br>Cauda equina<br>Conus medullaris |
| **Lumbar Sympathetic Nerve** | **Includes:**<br>Lumbar ganglion<br>Lumbar splanchnic nerve |
| **Lumbar Vertebra** | **Includes:**<br>Spinous process<br>Transverse process<br>Vertebral arch<br>Vertebral body<br>Vertebral foramen<br>Vertebral lamina<br>Vertebral pedicle |
| **Lumbar Vertebral Joint** | **Includes:**<br>Lumbar facet joint |
| **Lumbosacral Joint** | **Includes:**<br>Lumbosacral facet joint |

| ICD-10-PCS Value | Definition |
|---|---|
| **Lymphatic, Aortic** | **Includes:**<br>Celiac lymph node<br>Gastric lymph node<br>Hepatic lymph node<br>Lumbar lymph node<br>Pancreaticosplenic lymph node<br>Paraaortic lymph node<br>Retroperitoneal lymph node |
| **Lymphatic, Head** | **Includes:**<br>Buccinator lymph node<br>Infraauricular lymph node<br>Infraparotid lymph node<br>Parotid lymph node<br>Preauricular lymph node<br>Submandibular lymph node<br>Submaxillary lymph node<br>Submental lymph node<br>Subparotid lymph node<br>Suprahyoid lymph node |
| **Lymphatic, Left Axillary** | **Includes:**<br>Anterior (pectoral) lymph node<br>Apical (subclavicular) lymph node<br>Brachial (lateral) lymph node<br>Central axillary lymph node<br>Lateral (brachial) lymph node<br>Pectoral (anterior) lymph node<br>Posterior (subscapular) lymph node<br>Subclavicular (apical) lymph node<br>Subscapular (posterior) lymph node |
| **Lymphatic, Left Lower Extremity** | **Includes:**<br>Femoral lymph node<br>Popliteal lymph node |
| **Lymphatic, Left Neck** | **Includes:**<br>Cervical lymph node<br>Jugular lymph node<br>Mastoid (postauricular) lymph node<br>Occipital lymph node<br>Postauricular (mastoid) lymph node<br>Retropharyngeal lymph node<br>Supraclavicular (Virchow's) lymph node<br>Virchow's (supraclavicular) lymph node |
| **Lymphatic, Left Upper Extremity** | **Includes:**<br>Cubital lymph node<br>Deltopectoral (infraclavicular) lymph node<br>Epitrochlear lymph node<br>Infraclavicular (deltopectoral) lymph node<br>Supratrochlear lymph node |
| **Lymphatic, Mesenteric** | **Includes:**<br>Inferior mesenteric lymph node<br>Pararectal lymph node<br>Superior mesenteric lymph node |
| **Lymphatic, Pelvis** | **Includes:**<br>Common iliac (subaortic) lymph node<br>Gluteal lymph node<br>Iliac lymph node<br>Inferior epigastric lymph node<br>Obturator lymph node<br>Sacral lymph node<br>Subaortic (common iliac) lymph node<br>Suprainguinal lymph node |
| **Lymphatic, Right Axillary** | **Includes:**<br>Anterior (pectoral) lymph node<br>Apical (subclavicular) lymph node<br>Brachial (lateral) lymph node<br>Central axillary lymph node<br>Lateral (brachial) lymph node<br>Pectoral (anterior) lymph node<br>Posterior (subscapular) lymph node<br>Subclavicular (apical) lymph node<br>Subscapular (posterior) lymph node |
| **Lymphatic, Right Lower Extremity** | **Includes:**<br>Femoral lymph node<br>Popliteal lymph node |
| **Lymphatic, Right Neck** | **Includes:**<br>Cervical lymph node<br>Jugular lymph node<br>Mastoid (postauricular) lymph node<br>Occipital lymph node<br>Postauricular (mastoid) lymph node<br>Retropharyngeal lymph node<br>Right jugular trunk<br>Right lymphatic duct<br>Right subclavian trunk<br>Supraclavicular (Virchow's) lymph node<br>Virchow's (supraclavicular) lymph node |
| **Lymphatic, Right Upper Extremity** | **Includes:**<br>Cubital lymph node<br>Deltopectoral (infraclavicular) lymph node<br>Epitrochlear lymph node<br>Infraclavicular (deltopectoral) lymph node<br>Supratrochlear lymph node |
| **Lymphatic, Thorax** | **Includes:**<br>Intercostal lymph node<br>Mediastinal lymph node<br>Parasternal lymph node<br>Paratracheal lymph node<br>Tracheobronchial lymph node |
| **Main Bronchus, Right** | **Includes:**<br>Bronchus intermedius<br>Intermediate bronchus |
| **Mandible, Left**<br>**Mandible, Right** | **Includes:**<br>Alveolar process of mandible<br>Condyloid process<br>Mandibular notch<br>Mental foramen |
| **Mastoid Sinus, Left**<br>**Mastoid Sinus, Right** | **Includes:**<br>Mastoid air cells |
| **Maxilla** | **Includes:**<br>Alveolar process of maxilla |
| **Maxillary Sinus, Left**<br>**Maxillary Sinus, Right** | **Includes:**<br>Antrum of Highmore |
| **Median Nerve** | **Includes:**<br>Anterior interosseous nerve<br>Palmar cutaneous nerve |
| **Medulla Oblongata** | **Includes:**<br>Myelencephalon |
| **Mesentery** | **Includes:**<br>Mesoappendix<br>Mesocolon |

Appendix E: Body Part Definitions

| ICD-10-PCS Value | Definition |
|---|---|
| **Metatarsal-Phalangeal Joint, Left**<br>**Metatarsal-Phalangeal Joint, Right** | **Includes:**<br>Metatarsophalangeal (MTP) joint |
| **Middle Ear, Left**<br>**Middle Ear, Right** | **Includes:**<br>Oval window<br>Tympanic cavity |
| **Minor Salivary Gland** | **Includes:**<br>Anterior lingual gland |
| **Mitral Valve** | **Includes:**<br>Bicuspid valve<br>Left atrioventricular valve<br>Mitral annulus |
| **Nasal Bone** | **Includes:**<br>Vomer of nasal septum |
| **Nasal Mucosa and Soft Tissue** | **Includes:**<br>Columella<br>External naris<br>Greater alar cartilage<br>Internal naris<br>Lateral nasal cartilage<br>Lesser alar cartilage<br>Nasal cavity<br>Nostril |
| **Nasal Septum** | **Includes:**<br>Quadrangular cartilage<br>Septal cartilage<br>Vomer bone |
| **Nasal Turbinate** | **Includes:**<br>Inferior turbinate<br>Middle turbinate<br>Nasal concha<br>Superior turbinate |
| **Nasopharynx** | **Includes:**<br>Choana<br>Fossa of Rosenmuller<br>Pharyngeal recess<br>Rhinopharynx |
| **Neck Muscle, Left**<br>**Neck Muscle, Right** | **Includes:**<br>Anterior vertebral muscle<br>Arytenoid muscle<br>Cricothyroid muscle<br>Infrahyoid muscle<br>Levator scapulae muscle<br>Platysma muscle<br>Scalene muscle<br>Splenius cervicis muscle<br>Sternocleidomastoid muscle<br>Suprahyoid muscle<br>Thyroarytenoid muscle |
| **Nipple, Left**<br>**Nipple, Right** | **Includes:**<br>Areola |
| **Occipital Bone** | **Includes:**<br>Foramen magnum |
| **Oculomotor Nerve** | **Includes:**<br>Third cranial nerve |
| **Olfactory Nerve** | **Includes:**<br>First cranial nerve<br>Olfactory bulb |
| **Omentum** | **Includes:**<br>Gastrocolic ligament<br>Gastrocolic omentum<br>Gastrohepatic omentum<br>Gastrophrenic ligament<br>Gastrosplenic ligament<br>Greater Omentum<br>Hepatogastric ligament<br>Lesser Omentum |
| **Optic Nerve** | **Includes:**<br>Optic chiasma<br>Second cranial nerve |
| **Orbit, Left**<br>**Orbit, Right** | **Includes:**<br>Bony orbit<br>Orbital portion of ethmoid bone<br>Orbital portion of frontal bone<br>Orbital portion of lacrimal bone<br>Orbital portion of maxilla<br>Orbital portion of palatine bone<br>Orbital portion of sphenoid bone<br>Orbital portion of zygomatic bone |
| **Pancreatic Duct** | **Includes:**<br>Duct of Wirsung |
| **Pancreatic Duct, Accessory** | **Includes:**<br>Duct of Santorini |
| **Parotid Duct, Left**<br>**Parotid Duct, Right** | **Includes:**<br>Stensen's duct |
| **Pelvic Bone, Left**<br>**Pelvic Bone, Right** | **Includes:**<br>Iliac crest<br>Ilium<br>Ischium<br>Pubis |
| **Pelvic Cavity** | **Includes:**<br>Retropubic space |
| **Penis** | **Includes:**<br>Corpus cavernosum<br>Corpus spongiosum |
| **Perineum Muscle** | **Includes:**<br>Bulbospongiosus muscle<br>Cremaster muscle<br>Deep transverse perineal muscle<br>Ischiocavernosus muscle<br>Levator ani muscle<br>Superficial transverse perineal muscle |
| **Peritoneum** | **Includes:**<br>Epiploic foramen |
| **Peroneal Artery, Left**<br>**Peroneal Artery, Right** | **Includes:**<br>Fibular artery |
| **Peroneal Nerve** | **Includes:**<br>Common fibular nerve<br>Common peroneal nerve<br>External popliteal nerve<br>Lateral sural cutaneous nerve |
| **Pharynx** | **Includes:**<br>Base of Tongue<br>Hypopharynx<br>Laryngopharynx<br>Lingual tonsil<br>Oropharynx<br>Piriform recess (sinus)<br>Tongue, base of |
| **Phrenic Nerve** | **Includes:**<br>Accessory phrenic nerve |

| ICD-10-PCS Value | Definition |
|---|---|
| **Pituitary Gland** | **Includes:**<br>Adenohypophysis<br>Hypophysis<br>Neurohypophysis |
| **Pons** | **Includes:**<br>Apneustic center<br>Basis pontis<br>Locus ceruleus<br>Pneumotaxic center<br>Pontine tegmentum<br>Superior olivary nucleus |
| **Popliteal Artery, Left**<br>**Popliteal Artery, Right** | **Includes:**<br>Inferior genicular artery<br>Middle genicular artery<br>Superior genicular artery<br>Sural artery |
| **Portal Vein** | **Includes:**<br>Hepatic portal vein |
| **Prepuce** | **Includes:**<br>Foreskin<br>Glans penis |
| **Pudendal Nerve** | **Includes:**<br>Posterior labial nerve<br>Posterior scrotal nerve |
| **Pulmonary Artery, Left** | **Includes:**<br>Arterial canal (duct)<br>Botallo's duct<br>Pulmoaortic canal |
| **Pulmonary Valve** | **Includes:**<br>Pulmonary annulus<br>Pulmonic valve |
| **Pulmonary Vein, Left** | **Includes:**<br>Left inferior pulmonary vein<br>Left superior pulmonary vein |
| **Pulmonary Vein, Right** | **Includes:**<br>Right inferior pulmonary vein<br>Right superior pulmonary vein |
| **Radial Artery, Left**<br>**Radial Artery, Right** | **Includes:**<br>Radial recurrent artery |
| **Radial Nerve** | **Includes:**<br>Dorsal digital nerve<br>Musculospiral nerve<br>Palmar cutaneous nerve<br>Posterior interosseous nerve |
| **Radius, Left**<br>**Radius, Right** | **Includes:**<br>Ulnar notch |
| **Rectum** | **Includes:**<br>Anorectal junction |
| **Renal Artery, Left**<br>**Renal Artery, Right** | **Includes:**<br>Inferior suprarenal artery<br>Renal segmental artery |
| **Renal Vein, Left** | **Includes:**<br>Left inferior phrenic vein<br>Left ovarian vein<br>Left second lumbar vein<br>Left suprarenal vein<br>Left testicular vein |
| **Retina, Left**<br>**Retina, Right** | **Includes:**<br>Fovea<br>Macula<br>Optic disc |
| **Retroperitoneum** | **Includes:**<br>Retroperitoneal space |
| **Rib(s) Bursa and Ligament** | **Includes:**<br>Costotransverse ligament<br>Costoxiphoid ligament<br>Sternocostal ligament |
| **Sacral Nerve** | **Includes:**<br>Spinal nerve, sacral |
| **Sacral Plexus** | **Includes:**<br>Inferior gluteal nerve<br>Posterior femoral cutaneous nerve<br>Pudendal nerve |
| **Sacral Sympathetic Nerve** | **Includes:**<br>Ganglion impar (ganglion of Walther)<br>Pelvic splanchnic nerve<br>Sacral ganglion<br>Sacral splanchnic nerve |
| **Sacrococcygeal Joint** | **Includes:**<br>Sacrococcygeal symphysis |
| **Saphenous Vein, Left**<br>**Saphenous Vein, Right** | **Includes:**<br>External pudendal vein<br>Great(er) saphenous vein<br>Lesser saphenous vein<br>Small saphenous vein<br>Superficial circumflex iliac vein<br>Superficial epigastric vein |
| **Scapula, Left**<br>**Scapula, Right** | **Includes:**<br>Acromion (process)<br>Coracoid process |
| **Sciatic Nerve** | **Includes:**<br>Ischiatic nerve |
| **Shoulder Bursa and Ligament, Left**<br>**Shoulder Bursa and Ligament, Right** | **Includes:**<br>Acromioclavicular ligament<br>Coracoacromial ligament<br>Coracoclavicular ligament<br>Coracohumeral ligament<br>Costoclavicular ligament<br>Glenohumeral ligament<br>Interclavicular ligament<br>Sternoclavicular ligament<br>Subacromial bursa<br>Transverse humeral ligament<br>Transverse scapular ligament |
| **Shoulder Joint, Left**<br>**Shoulder Joint, Right** | **Includes:**<br>Glenohumeral joint<br>Glenoid ligament (labrum) |
| **Shoulder Muscle, Left**<br>**Shoulder Muscle, Right** | **Includes:**<br>Deltoid muscle<br>Infraspinatus muscle<br>Subscapularis muscle<br>Supraspinatus muscle<br>Teres major muscle<br>Teres minor muscle |
| **Sigmoid Colon** | **Includes:**<br>Rectosigmoid junction<br>Sigmoid flexure |
| **Skin** | **Includes:**<br>Dermis<br>Epidermis<br>Sebaceous gland<br>Sweat gland |
| **Sphenoid Bone** | **Includes:**<br>Greater wing<br>Lesser wing<br>Optic foramen<br>Pterygoid process<br>Sella turcica |

| ICD-10-PCS Value | Definition |
|---|---|
| **Spinal Canal** | **Includes:**<br>Epidural space, spinal<br>Extradural space, spinal<br>Subarachnoid space, spinal<br>Subdural space, spinal<br>Vertebral canal |
| **Spinal Meninges** | **Includes:**<br>Arachnoid mater, spinal<br>Denticulate (dentate) ligament<br>Dura mater, spinal<br>Filum terminale<br>Leptomeninges, spinal<br>Pia mater, spinal |
| **Spleen** | **Includes:**<br>Accessory spleen |
| **Splenic Artery** | **Includes:**<br>Left gastroepiploic artery<br>Pancreatic artery<br>Short gastric artery |
| **Splenic Vein** | **Includes:**<br>Left gastroepiploic vein<br>Pancreatic vein |
| **Sternum** | **Includes:**<br>Manubrium<br>Suprasternal notch<br>Xiphoid process |
| **Sternum Bursa and Ligament** | **Includes:**<br>Costotransverse ligament<br>Costoxiphoid ligament<br>Sternocostal ligament |
| **Stomach, Pylorus** | **Includes:**<br>Pyloric antrum<br>Pyloric canal<br>Pyloric sphincter |
| **Subclavian Artery, Left**<br>**Subclavian Artery, Right** | **Includes:**<br>Costocervical trunk<br>Dorsal scapular artery<br>Internal thoracic artery |
| **Subcutaneous Tissue and Fascia, Chest** | **Includes:**<br>Pectoral fascia |
| **Subcutaneous Tissue and Fascia, Face** | **Includes:**<br>Masseteric fascia<br>Orbital fascia |
| **Subcutaneous Tissue and Fascia, Left Foot** | **Includes:**<br>Plantar fascia (aponeurosis) |
| **Subcutaneous Tissue and Fascia, Left Hand** | **Includes:**<br>Palmar fascia (aponeurosis) |
| **Subcutaneous Tissue and Fascia, Left Lower Arm** | **Includes:**<br>Antebrachial fascia<br>Bicipital aponeurosis |
| **Subcutaneous Tissue and Fascia, Left Neck** | **Includes:**<br>Deep cervical fascia<br>Pretracheal fascia<br>Prevertebral fascia |
| **Subcutaneous Tissue and Fascia, Left Upper Arm** | **Includes:**<br>Axillary fascia<br>Deltoid fascia<br>Infraspinatus fascia<br>Subscapular aponeurosis<br>Supraspinatus fascia |
| **Subcutaneous Tissue and Fascia, Left Upper Leg** | **Includes:**<br>Crural fascia<br>Fascia lata<br>Iliac fascia<br>Iliotibial tract (band) |
| **Subcutaneous Tissue and Fascia, Right Foot** | **Includes:**<br>Plantar fascia (aponeurosis) |
| **Subcutaneous Tissue and Fascia, Right Hand** | **Includes:**<br>Palmar fascia (aponeurosis) |
| **Subcutaneous Tissue and Fascia, Right Lower Arm** | **Includes:**<br>Antebrachial fascia<br>Bicipital aponeurosis |
| **Subcutaneous Tissue and Fascia, Right Neck** | **Includes:**<br>Deep cervical fascia<br>Pretracheal fascia<br>Prevertebral fascia |
| **Subcutaneous Tissue and Fascia, Right Upper Arm** | **Includes:**<br>Axillary fascia<br>Deltoid fascia<br>Infraspinatus fascia<br>Subscapular aponeurosis<br>Supraspinatus fascia |
| **Subcutaneous Tissue and Fascia, Right Upper Leg** | **Includes:**<br>Crural fascia<br>Fascia lata<br>Iliac fascia<br>Iliotibial tract (band) |
| **Subcutaneous Tissue and Fascia, Scalp** | **Includes:**<br>Galea aponeurotica |
| **Subcutaneous Tissue and Fascia, Trunk** | **Includes:**<br>External oblique aponeurosis<br>Transversalis fascia |
| **Submaxillary Gland, Left**<br>**Submaxillary Gland, Right** | **Includes:**<br>Submandibular gland |
| **Superior Mesenteric Artery** | **Includes:**<br>Ileal artery<br>Ileocolic artery<br>Inferior pancreaticoduodenal artery<br>Jejunal artery |
| **Superior Mesenteric Vein** | **Includes:**<br>Right gastroepiploic vein |
| **Superior Vena Cava** | **Includes:**<br>Precava |
| **Tarsal Joint, Left**<br>**Tarsal Joint, Right** | **Includes:**<br>Calcaneocuboid joint<br>Cuboideonavicular joint<br>Cuneonavicular joint<br>Intercuneiform joint<br>Subtalar (talocalcaneal) joint<br>Talocalcaneal (subtalar) joint<br>Talocalcaneonavicular joint |
| **Tarsal, Left**<br>**Tarsal, Right** | **Includes:**<br>Calcaneus<br>Cuboid bone<br>Intermediate cuneiform bone<br>Lateral cuneiform bone<br>Medial cuneiform bone<br>Navicular bone<br>Talus bone |
| **Temporal Artery, Left**<br>**Temporal Artery, Right** | **Includes:**<br>Middle temporal artery<br>Superficial temporal artery<br>Transverse facial artery |
| **Temporal Bone, Left**<br>**Temporal Bone, Right** | **Includes:**<br>Mastoid process<br>Petrous part of temporal bone<br>Tympanic part of temporal bone<br>Zygomatic process of temporal bone |

| ICD-10-PCS Value | Definition |
|---|---|
| **Thalamus** | **Includes:**<br>Epithalamus<br>Geniculate nucleus<br>Metathalamus<br>Pulvinar |
| **Thoracic Aorta, Ascending/Arch** | **Includes:**<br>Aortic arch<br>Ascending aorta |
| **Thoracic Duct** | **Includes:**<br>Left jugular trunk<br>Left subclavian trunk |
| **Thoracic Nerve** | **Includes:**<br>Intercostal nerve<br>Intercostobrachial nerve<br>Spinal nerve, thoracic<br>Subcostal nerve |
| **Thoracic Sympathetic Nerve** | **Includes:**<br>Cardiac plexus<br>Esophageal plexus<br>Greater splanchnic nerve<br>Inferior cardiac nerve<br>Least splanchnic nerve<br>Lesser splanchnic nerve<br>Middle cardiac nerve<br>Pulmonary plexus<br>Superior cardiac nerve<br>Thoracic aortic plexus<br>Thoracic ganglion |
| **Thoracic Vertebra** | **Includes:**<br>Spinous process<br>Transverse process<br>Vertebral arch<br>Vertebral body<br>Vertebral foramen<br>Vertebral lamina<br>Vertebral pedicle |
| **Thoracic Vertebral Joint** | **Includes:**<br>Costotransverse joint<br>Costovertebral joint<br>Thoracic facet joint |
| **Thoracolumbar Vertebral Joint** | **Includes:**<br>Thoracolumbar facet joint |
| **Thorax Muscle, Left**<br>**Thorax Muscle, Right** | **Includes:**<br>Intercostal muscle<br>Levatores costarum muscle<br>Pectoralis major muscle<br>Pectoralis minor muscle<br>Serratus anterior muscle<br>Subclavius muscle<br>Subcostal muscle<br>Transverse thoracis muscle |
| **Thymus** | **Includes:**<br>Thymus gland |
| **Thyroid Artery, Left**<br>**Thyroid Artery, Right** | **Includes:**<br>Cricothyroid artery<br>Hyoid artery<br>Sternocleidomastoid artery<br>Superior laryngeal artery<br>Superior thyroid artery<br>Thyrocervical trunk |
| **Tibia, Left**<br>**Tibia, Right** | **Includes:**<br>Lateral condyle of tibia<br>Medial condyle of tibia<br>Medial malleolus |

| ICD-10-PCS Value | Definition |
|---|---|
| **Tibial Nerve** | **Includes:**<br>Lateral plantar nerve<br>Medial plantar nerve<br>Medial popliteal nerve<br>Medial sural cutaneous nerve |
| **Toe Nail** | **Includes:**<br>Nail bed<br>Nail plate |
| **Toe Phalangeal Joint, Left**<br>**Toe Phalangeal Joint, Right** | **Includes:**<br>Interphalangeal (IP) joint |
| **Tongue** | **Includes:**<br>Frenulum linguae |
| **Tongue, Palate, Pharynx Muscle** | **Includes:**<br>Chondroglossus muscle<br>Genioglossus muscle<br>Hyoglossus muscle<br>Inferior longitudinal muscle<br>Levator veli palatini muscle<br>Palatoglossal muscle<br>Palatopharyngeal muscle<br>Pharyngeal constrictor muscle<br>Salpingopharyngeus muscle<br>Styloglossus muscle<br>Stylopharyngeus muscle<br>Superior longitudinal muscle<br>Tensor veli palatini muscle |
| **Tonsils** | **Includes:**<br>Palatine tonsil |
| **Trachea** | **Includes:**<br>Cricoid cartilage |
| **Transverse Colon** | **Includes:**<br>Hepatic flexure<br>Splenic flexure |
| **Tricuspid Valve** | **Includes:**<br>Right atrioventricular valve<br>Tricuspid annulus |
| **Trigeminal Nerve** | **Includes:**<br>Fifth cranial nerve<br>Gasserian ganglion<br>Mandibular nerve<br>Maxillary nerve<br>Ophthalmic nerve<br>Trifacial nerve |
| **Trochlear Nerve** | **Includes:**<br>Fourth cranial nerve |
| **Trunk Muscle, Left**<br>**Trunk Muscle, Right** | **Includes:**<br>Coccygeus muscle<br>Erector spinae muscle<br>Interspinalis muscle<br>Intertransversarius muscle<br>Latissimus dorsi muscle<br>Quadratus lumborum muscle<br>Rhomboid major muscle<br>Rhomboid minor muscle<br>Serratus posterior muscle<br>Transversospinalis muscle<br>Trapezius muscle |
| **Tympanic Membrane, Left**<br>**Tympanic Membrane, Right** | **Includes:**<br>Pars flaccida |
| **Ulna, Left**<br>**Ulna, Right** | **Includes:**<br>Olecranon process<br>Radial notch |

| ICD-10-PCS Value | Definition |
|---|---|
| **Ulnar Artery, Left**<br>**Ulnar Artery, Right** | **Includes:**<br>Anterior ulnar recurrent artery<br>Common interosseous artery<br>Posterior ulnar recurrent artery |
| **Ulnar Nerve** | **Includes:**<br>Cubital nerve |
| **Upper Arm Muscle, Left**<br>**Upper Arm Muscle, Right** | **Includes:**<br>Biceps brachii muscle<br>Brachialis muscle<br>Coracobrachialis muscle<br>Triceps brachii muscle |
| **Upper Artery** | **Includes:**<br>Aortic intercostal artery<br>Bronchial artery<br>Esophageal artery<br>Subcostal artery |
| **Upper Eyelid, Left**<br>**Upper Eyelid, Right** | **Includes:**<br>Lateral canthus<br>Levator palpebrae superioris muscle<br>Orbicularis oculi muscle<br>Superior tarsal plate |
| **Upper Femur, Left**<br>**Upper Femur, Right** | **Includes:**<br>Femoral head<br>Greater trochanter<br>Lesser trochanter<br>Neck of femur |
| **Upper Leg Muscle, Left**<br>**Upper Leg Muscle, Right** | **Includes:**<br>Adductor brevis muscle<br>Adductor longus muscle<br>Adductor magnus muscle<br>Biceps femoris muscle<br>Gracilis muscle<br>Pectineus muscle<br>Quadriceps (femoris)<br>Rectus femoris muscle<br>Sartorius muscle<br>Semimembranosus muscle<br>Semitendinosus muscle<br>Vastus intermedius muscle<br>Vastus lateralis muscle<br>Vastus medialis muscle |
| **Upper Lip** | **Includes:**<br>Frenulum labii superioris<br>Labial gland<br>Vermilion border |
| **Upper Spine Bursa and Ligament** | **Includes:**<br>Interspinous ligament<br>Intertransverse ligament<br>Ligamentum flavum<br>Supraspinous ligament |
| **Ureter**<br>**Ureter, Left**<br>**Ureter, Right**<br>**Ureters, Bilateral** | **Includes:**<br>Ureteral orifice<br>Ureterovesical orifice |
| **Urethra** | **Includes:**<br>Bulbourethral (Cowper's) gland<br>Cowper's (bulbourethral) gland<br>External urethral sphincter<br>Internal urethral sphincter<br>Membranous urethra<br>Penile urethra<br>Prostatic urethra |
| **Uterine Supporting Structure** | **Includes:**<br>Broad ligament<br>Infundibulopelvic ligament<br>Ovarian ligament<br>Round ligament of uterus |

| ICD-10-PCS Value | Definition |
|---|---|
| **Uterus** | **Includes:**<br>Fundus uteri<br>Myometrium<br>Perimetrium<br>Uterine cornu |
| **Uvula** | **Includes:**<br>Palatine uvula |
| **Vagus Nerve** | **Includes:**<br>Anterior vagal trunk<br>Pharyngeal plexus<br>Pneumogastric nerve<br>Posterior vagal trunk<br>Pulmonary plexus<br>Recurrent laryngeal nerve<br>Superior laryngeal nerve<br>Tenth cranial nerve |
| **Vas Deferens**<br>**Vas Deferens, Bilateral**<br>**Vas Deferens, Left**<br>**Vas Deferens, Right** | **Includes:**<br>Ductus deferens<br>Ejaculatory duct |
| **Ventricle, Right** | **Includes:**<br>Conus arteriosus |
| **Ventricular Septum** | **Includes:**<br>Interventricular septum |
| **Vertebral Artery, Left**<br>**Vertebral Artery, Right** | **Includes:**<br>Anterior spinal artery<br>Posterior spinal artery |
| **Vertebral Vein, Left**<br>**Vertebral Vein, Right** | **Includes:**<br>Deep cervical vein<br>Suboccipital venous plexus |
| **Vestibular Gland** | **Includes:**<br>Bartholin's (greater vestibular) gland<br>Greater vestibular (Bartholin's) gland<br>Paraurethral (Skene's) gland<br>Skene's (paraurethral) gland |
| **Vitreous, Left**<br>**Vitreous, Right** | **Includes:**<br>Vitreous body |
| **Vocal Cord, Left**<br>**Vocal Cord, Right** | **Includes:**<br>Vocal fold |
| **Vulva** | **Includes:**<br>Labia majora<br>Labia minora |
| **Wrist Bursa and Ligament, Left**<br>**Wrist Bursa and Ligament, Right** | **Includes:**<br>Palmar ulnocarpal ligament<br>Radial collateral carpal ligament<br>Radiocarpal ligament<br>Radioulnar ligament<br>Ulnar collateral carpal ligament |
| **Wrist Joint, Left**<br>**Wrist Joint, Right** | **Includes:**<br>Distal radioulnar joint<br>Radiocarpal joint |

# Appendix F: Device Key and Aggregation Table

## Device Key

| Term | ICD-10-PCS Value |
|---|---|
| 3f (Aortic) Bioprosthesis valve | Zooplastic Tissue in Heart and Great Vessels |
| AbioCor® Total Replacement Heart | Synthetic Substitute |
| Absolute Pro Vascular (OTW) Self-Expanding Stent System | Intraluminal Device |
| Acculink (RX) Carotid Stent System | Intraluminal Device |
| Acellular Hydrated Dermis | Nonautologous Tissue Substitute |
| Acetabular cup | Liner in Lower Joints |
| Activa PC neurostimulator | Stimulator Generator, Multiple Array for Insertion in Subcutaneous Tissue and Fascia |
| Activa RC neurostimulator | Stimulator Generator, Multiple Array Rechargeable for Insertion in Subcutaneous Tissue and Fascia |
| Activa SC neurostimulator | Stimulator Generator, Single Array for Insertion in Subcutaneous Tissue and Fascia |
| ACUITY™ Steerable Lead | Cardiac Lead, Pacemaker for Insertion in Heart and Great Vessels<br>Cardiac Lead, Defibrillator for Insertion in Heart and Great Vessels |
| Advisa (MRI) | Pacemaker, Dual Chamber for Insertion in Subcutaneous Tissue and Fascia |
| AFX® Endovascular AAA System | Intraluminal Device |
| AMPLATZER® Muscular VSD Occluder | Synthetic Substitute |
| AMS 800® Urinary Control System | Artificial Sphincter in Urinary System |
| AneuRx® AAA Advantage® | Intraluminal Device |
| Annuloplasty ring | Synthetic Substitute |
| Artificial anal sphincter (AAS) | Artificial Sphincter in Gastrointestinal System |
| Artificial bowel sphincter (neosphincter) | Artificial Sphincter in Gastrointestinal System |
| Artificial urinary sphincter (AUS) | Artificial Sphincter in Urinary System |
| Ascenda Intrathecal Catheter | Infusion Device |
| Assurant (Cobalt) stent | Intraluminal Device |
| AtriClip LAA Exclusion System | Extraluminal Device |
| Attain Ability® Lead | Cardiac Lead, Pacemaker for Insertion in Heart and Great Vessels<br>Cardiac Lead, Defibrillator for Insertion in Heart and Great Vessels |
| Attain StarFix® (OTW) Lead | Cardiac Lead, Pacemaker for Insertion in Heart and Great Vessels<br>Cardiac Lead, Defibrillator for Insertion in Heart and Great Vessels |
| Autograft | Autologous Tissue Substitute |
| Autologous artery graft | Autologous Arterial Tissue in Heart and Great Vessels<br>Autologous Arterial Tissue in Upper Arteries<br>Autologous Arterial Tissue in Lower Arteries<br>Autologous Arterial Tissue in Upper Veins<br>Autologous Arterial Tissue in Lower Veins |

| Term | ICD-10-PCS Value |
|---|---|
| Autologous vein graft | Autologous Venous Tissue in Heart and Great Vessels<br>Autologous Venous Tissue in Upper Arteries<br>Autologous Venous Tissue in Lower Arteries<br>Autologous Venous Tissue in Upper Veins<br>Autologous Venous Tissue in Lower Veins |
| Axial Lumbar Interbody Fusion System | Interbody Fusion Device in Lower Joints |
| AxiaLIF® System | Interbody Fusion Device in Lower Joints |
| BAK/C® Interbody Cervical Fusion System | Interbody Fusion Device in Upper Joints |
| Bard® Composix® (E/X)(LP) mesh | Synthetic Substitute |
| Bard® Composix® Kugel® patch | Synthetic Substitute |
| Bard® Dulex™ mesh | Synthetic Substitute |
| Bard® Ventralex™ hernia patch | Synthetic Substitute |
| Baroreflex Activation Therapy® (BAT®) | Stimulator Lead in Upper Arteries<br>Stimulator Generator in Subcutaneous Tissue and Fascia |
| Berlin Heart Ventricular Assist Device | Implantable Heart Assist System in Heart and Great Vessels |
| Bioactive embolization coil(s) | Intraluminal Device, Bioactive in Upper Arteries |
| Biventricular external heart assist system | Short-term External Heart Assist System in Heart and Great Vessels |
| Blood glucose monitoring system | Monitoring Device |
| Bone anchored hearing device | Hearing Device, Bone Conduction for Insertion in Ear, Nose, Sinus<br>Hearing Device, in Head and Facial Bones |
| Bone bank bone graft | Nonautologous Tissue Substitute |
| Bone screw (interlocking)(lag)(pedicle)(recessed) | Internal Fixation Device in Head and Facial Bones<br>Internal Fixation Device in Upper Bones<br>Internal Fixation Device in Lower Bones |
| Bovine pericardial valve | Zooplastic Tissue in Heart and Great Vessels |
| Bovine pericardium graft | Zooplastic Tissue in Heart and Great Vessels |
| Brachytherapy seeds | Radioactive Element |
| BRYAN® Cervical Disc System | Synthetic Substitute |
| BVS 5000 Ventricular Assist Device | Short-term External Heart Assist System in Heart and Great Vessels |
| Cardiac contractility modulation lead | Cardiac Lead in Heart and Great Vessels |
| Cardiac event recorder | Monitoring Device |
| Cardiac resynchronization therapy (CRT) lead | Cardiac Lead, Pacemaker for Insertion in Heart and Great Vessels<br>Cardiac Lead, Defibrillator for Insertion in Heart and Great Vessels |
| CardioMEMS® pressure sensor | Monitoring Device, Pressure Sensor for Insertion in Heart and Great Vessels |
| Carotid (artery) sinus (baroreceptor) lead | Stimulator Lead in Upper Arteries |

| Term | ICD-10-PCS Value |
|---|---|
| Carotid WALLSTENT® Monorail® Endoprosthesis | Intraluminal Device |
| Centrimag® Blood Pump | Short-term External Heart Assist System in Heart and Great Vessels |
| Ceramic on ceramic bearing surface | Synthetic Substitute, Ceramic for Replacement in Lower Joints |
| Cesium-131 Collagen Implant | Radioactive Element, Cesium-131 Collagen Implant for Insertion in Central Nervous System and Cranial Nerves |
| Clamp and rod internal fixation system (CRIF) | Internal Fixation Device in Upper Bones<br>Internal Fixation Device in Lower Bones |
| COALESCE® radiolucent interbody fusion device | Interbody Fusion Device, Radiolucent Porous in New Technology |
| CoAxia NeuroFlo catheter | Intraluminal Device |
| Cobalt/chromium head and polyethylene socket | Synthetic Substitute, Metal on Polyethylene for Replacement in Lower Joints |
| Cobalt/chromium head and socket | Synthetic Substitute, Metal for Replacement in Lower Joints |
| Cochlear implant (CI), multiple channel (electrode) | Hearing Device, Multiple Channel Cochlear Prosthesis for Insertion in Ear, Nose, Sinus |
| Cochlear implant (CI), single channel (electrode) | Hearing Device, Single Channel Cochlear Prosthesis for Insertion in Ear, Nose, Sinus |
| COGNIS® CRT-D | Cardiac Resynchronization Defibrillator Pulse Generator for Insertion in Subcutaneous Tissue and Fascia |
| COHERE® radiolucent interbody fusion device | Interbody Fusion Device, Radiolucent Porous in New Technology |
| Colonic Z-Stent® | Intraluminal Device |
| Complete (SE) stent | Intraluminal Device |
| Concerto II CRT-D | Cardiac Resynchronization Defibrillator Pulse Generator for Insertion in Subcutaneous Tissue and Fascia |
| CONSERVE® PLUS Total Resurfacing Hip System | Resurfacing Device in Lower Joints |
| Consulta CRT-D | Cardiac Resynchronization Defibrillator Pulse Generator for Insertion in Subcutaneous Tissue and Fascia |
| Consulta CRT-P | Cardiac Resynchronization Pacemaker Pulse Generator for Insertion in Subcutaneous Tissue and Fascia |
| CONTAK RENEWAL® 3 RF (HE) CRT-D | Cardiac Resynchronization Defibrillator Pulse Generator for Insertion in Subcutaneous Tissue and Fascia |
| Contegra Pulmonary Valved Conduit | Zooplastic Tissue in Heart and Great Vessels |
| Continuous Glucose Monitoring (CGM) device | Monitoring Device |
| Cook Biodesign® Fistula Plug(s) | Nonautologous Tissue Substitute |
| Cook Biodesign® Hernia Graft(s) | Nonautologous Tissue Substitute |
| Cook Biodesign® Layered Graft(s) | Nonautologous Tissue Substitute |
| Cook Zenapro™ Layered Graft(s) | Nonautologous Tissue Substitute |

| Term | ICD-10-PCS Value |
|---|---|
| Cook Zenith AAA Endovascular Graft | Intraluminal Device<br>Intraluminal Device, Branched or Fenestrated, One or Two Arteries for Restriction in Lower Arteries<br>Intraluminal Device, Branched or Fenestrated, Three or More Arteries for Restriction in Lower Arteries |
| CoreValve transcatheter aortic valve | Zooplastic Tissue in Heart and Great Vessels |
| Cormet Hip Resurfacing System | Resurfacing Device in Lower Joints |
| CoRoent® XL | Interbody Fusion Device in Lower Joints |
| Corox (OTW) Bipolar Lead | Cardiac Lead, Pacemaker for Insertion in Heart and Great Vessels<br>Cardiac Lead, Defibrillator for Insertion in Heart and Great Vessels |
| Cortical strip neurostimulator lead | Neurostimulator Lead in Central Nervous System and Cranial Nerves |
| Cultured epidermal cell autograft | Autologous Tissue Substitute |
| CYPHER® Stent | Intraluminal Device, Drug-eluting in Heart and Great Vessels |
| Cystostomy tube | Drainage Device |
| DBS lead | Neurostimulator Lead in Central Nervous System and Cranial Nerves |
| DeBakey Left Ventricular Assist Device | Implantable Heart Assist System in Heart and Great Vessels |
| Deep brain neurostimulator lead | Neurostimulator Lead in Central Nervous System and Cranial Nerves |
| Delta frame external fixator | External Fixation Device, Hybrid for Insertion in Upper Bones<br>External Fixation Device, Hybrid for Reposition in Upper Bones<br>External Fixation Device, Hybrid for Insertion in Lower Bones<br>External Fixation Device, Hybrid for Reposition in Lower Bones |
| Delta III Reverse shoulder prosthesis | Synthetic Substitute, Reverse Ball and Socket for Replacement in Upper Joints |
| Diaphragmatic pacemaker generator | Stimulator Generator in Subcutaneous Tissue and Fascia |
| Direct Lateral Interbody Fusion (DLIF) device | Interbody Fusion Device in Lower Joints |
| Driver stent (RX) (OTW) | Intraluminal Device |
| DuraHeart Left Ventricular Assist System | Implantable Heart Assist System in Heart and Great Vessels |
| Durata® Defibrillation Lead | Cardiac Lead, Defibrillator for Insertion in Heart and Great Vessels |
| Dynesys® Dynamic Stabilization System | Spinal Stabilization Device, Pedicle-Based for Insertion in Upper Joints<br>Spinal Stabilization Device, Pedicle-Based for Insertion in Lower Joints |
| E-Luminexx™ (Biliary)(Vascular) Stent | Intraluminal Device |
| EDWARDS INTUITY Elite valve system | Zooplastic Tissue, Rapid Deployment Technique in New Technology |
| Electrical bone growth stimulator (EBGS) | Bone Growth Stimulator in Head and Facial Bones<br>Bone Growth Stimulator in Upper Bones<br>Bone Growth Stimulator in Lower Bones |

| Term | ICD-10-PCS Value |
|---|---|
| Electrical muscle stimulation (EMS) lead | Stimulator Lead in Muscles |
| Electronic muscle stimulator lead | Stimulator Lead in Muscles |
| Embolization coil(s) | Intraluminal Device |
| Endeavor® (III)(IV) (Sprint) Zotarolimus-eluting Coronary Stent System | Intraluminal Device, Drug-eluting in Heart and Great Vessels |
| Endologix AFX® Endovascular AAA System | Intraluminal Device |
| EndoSure® sensor | Monitoring Device, Pressure Sensor for Insertion in Heart and Great Vessels |
| ENDOTAK RELIANCE® (G) Defibrillation Lead | Cardiac Lead, Defibrillator for Insertion in Heart and Great Vessels |
| Endotracheal tube (cuffed)(double-lumen) | Intraluminal Device, Endotracheal Airway in Respiratory System |
| Endurant® Endovascular Stent Graft | Intraluminal Device |
| Endurant® II AAA stent graft system | Intraluminal Device |
| EnRhythm | Pacemaker, Dual Chamber for Insertion in Subcutaneous Tissue and Fascia |
| Enterra gastric neurostimulator | Stimulator Generator, Multiple Array for Insertion in Subcutaneous Tissue and Fascia |
| Epic™ Stented Tissue Valve (aortic) | Zooplastic Tissue in Heart and Great Vessels |
| Epicel® cultured epidermal autograft | Autologous Tissue Substitute |
| Esophageal obturator airway (EOA) | Intraluminal Device, Airway in Gastrointestinal System |
| Esteem® implantable hearing system | Hearing Device in Ear, Nose, Sinus |
| Evera (XT)(S)(DR/VR) | Defibrillator Generator for Insertion in Subcutaneous Tissue and Fascia |
| Everolimus-eluting coronary stent | Intraluminal Device, Drug-eluting in Heart and Great Vessels |
| Ex-PRESS™ mini glaucoma shunt | Synthetic Substitute |
| EXCLUDER® AAA Endoprosthesis | Intraluminal Device<br>Intraluminal Device, Branched or Fenestrated, One or Two Arteries for Restriction in Lower Arteries<br>Intraluminal Device, Branched or Fenestrated, Three or More Arteries for Restriction in Lower Arteries |
| EXCLUDER® IBE Endoprosthesis | Intraluminal Device, Branched or Fenestrated, One or Two Arteries for Restriction in Lower Arteries |
| Express® (LD) Premounted Stent System | Intraluminal Device |
| Express® Biliary SD Monorail® Premounted Stent System | Intraluminal Device |
| Express® SD Renal Monorail® Premounted Stent System | Intraluminal Device |

| Term | ICD-10-PCS Value |
|---|---|
| External fixator | External Fixation Device in Head and Facial Bones<br>External Fixation Device in Upper Bones<br>External Fixation Device in Lower Bones<br>External Fixation Device in Upper Joints<br>External Fixation Device in Lower Joints |
| EXtreme Lateral Interbody Fusion (XLIF) device | Interbody Fusion Device in Lower Joints |
| Facet replacement spinal stabilization device | Spinal Stabilization Device, Facet Replacement for Insertion in Upper Joints<br>Spinal Stabilization Device, Facet Replacement for Insertion in Lower Joints |
| FLAIR® Endovascular Stent Graft | Intraluminal Device |
| Flexible Composite Mesh | Synthetic Substitute |
| Foley catheter | Drainage Device |
| Formula™ Balloon-Expandable Renal Stent System | Intraluminal Device |
| Freestyle (Stentless) Aortic Root Bioprosthesis | Zooplastic Tissue in Heart and Great Vessels |
| Fusion screw (compression)(lag)(locking) | Internal Fixation Device in Upper Joints<br>Internal Fixation Device in Lower Joints |
| GammaTile™ | Radioactive Element, Cesium-131 Collagen Implant for Insertion in Central Nervous System and Cranial Nerves |
| Gastric electrical stimulation (GES) lead | Stimulator Lead in Gastrointestinal System |
| Gastric pacemaker lead | Stimulator Lead in Gastrointestinal System |
| GORE EXCLUDER® AAA Endoprosthesis | Intraluminal Device<br>Intraluminal Device, Branched or Fenestrated, One or Two Arteries for Restriction in Lower Arteries<br>Intraluminal Device, Branched or Fenestrated, Three or More Arteries for Restriction in Lower Arteries |
| GORE EXCLUDER® IBE Endoprosthesis | Intraluminal Device, Branched or Fenestrated, One or Two Arteries for Restriction in Lower Arteries |
| GORE TAG® Thoracic Endoprosthesis | Intraluminal Device |
| GORE® DUALMESH® | Synthetic Substitute |
| Guedel airway | Intraluminal Device, Airway in Mouth and Throat |
| Hancock Bioprosthesis (aortic)(mitral) valve | Zooplastic Tissue in Heart and Great Vessels |
| Hancock Bioprosthetic Valved Conduit | Zooplastic Tissue in Heart and Great Vessels |
| HeartMate 3™ LVAS | Implantable Heart Assist System in Heart and Great Vessels |
| HeartMate II® Left Ventricular Assist Device (LVAD) | Implantable Heart Assist System in Heart and Great Vessels |
| HeartMate XVE® Left Ventricular Assist Device (LVAD) | Implantable Heart Assist System in Heart and Great Vessels |
| Herculink (RX) Elite Renal Stent System | Intraluminal Device |

| Term | ICD-10-PCS Value |
|---|---|
| Hip (joint) liner | Liner in Lower Joints |
| Holter valve ventricular shunt | Synthetic Substitute |
| Ilizarov external fixator | External Fixation Device, Ring for Insertion in Upper Bones<br>External Fixation Device, Ring for Reposition in Upper Bones<br>External Fixation Device, Ring for Insertion in Lower Bones<br>External Fixation Device, Ring for Reposition in Lower Bones |
| Ilizarov-Vecklich device | External Fixation Device, Limb Lengthening for Insertion in Upper Bones<br>External Fixation Device, Limb Lengthening for Insertion in Lower Bones |
| Impella® heart pump | Short-term External Heart Assist System in Heart and Great Vessels |
| Implantable cardioverter-defibrillator (ICD) | Defibrillator Generator for Insertion in Subcutaneous Tissue and Fascia |
| Implantable drug infusion pump (anti-spasmodic) (chemotherapy)(pain) | Infusion Device, Pump in Subcutaneous Tissue and Fascia |
| Implantable glucose monitoring device | Monitoring Device |
| Implantable hemodynamic monitor (IHM) | Monitoring Device, Hemodynamic for Insertion in Subcutaneous Tissue and Fascia |
| Implantable hemodynamic monitoring system (IHMS) | Monitoring Device, Hemodynamic for Insertion in Subcutaneous Tissue and Fascia |
| Implantable Miniature Telescope™ (IMT) | Synthetic Substitute, Intraocular Telescope for Replacement in Eye |
| Implanted (venous)(access) port | Vascular Access Device, Totally Implantable in Subcutaneous Tissue and Fascia |
| InDura, intrathecal catheter (1P) (spinal) | Infusion Device |
| Injection reservoir, port | Vascular Access Device, Totally Implantable in Subcutaneous Tissue and Fascia |
| Injection reservoir, pump | Infusion Device, Pump in Subcutaneous Tissue and Fascia |
| Interbody fusion (spine) cage | Interbody Fusion Device in Upper Joints<br>Interbody Fusion Device in Lower Joints |
| Interspinous process spinal stabilization device | Spinal Stabilization Device, Interspinous Process for Insertion in Upper Joints<br>Spinal Stabilization Device, Interspinous Process for Insertion in Lower Joints |
| InterStim® Therapy lead | Neurostimulator Lead in Peripheral Nervous System |
| InterStim® Therapy neurostimulator | Stimulator Generator, Single Array for Insertion in Subcutaneous Tissue and Fascia |
| Intramedullary (IM) rod (nail) | Internal Fixation Device, Intramedullary in Upper Bones<br>Internal Fixation Device, Intramedullary in Lower Bones |

| Term | ICD-10-PCS Value |
|---|---|
| Intramedullary skeletal kinetic distractor (ISKD) | Internal Fixation Device, Intramedullary in Upper Bones<br>Internal Fixation Device, Intramedullary in Lower Bones |
| Intrauterine Device (IUD) | Contraceptive Device in Female Reproductive System |
| INTUITY Elite valve system, EDWARDS | Zooplastic Tissue, Rapid Deployment Technique in New Technology |
| Itrel (3)(4) neurostimulator | Stimulator Generator, Single Array for Insertion in Subcutaneous Tissue and Fascia |
| Joint fixation plate | Internal Fixation Device in Upper Joints<br>Internal Fixation Device in Lower Joints |
| Joint liner (insert) | Liner in Lower Joints |
| Joint spacer (antibiotic) | Spacer in Upper Joints<br>Spacer in Lower Joints |
| Kappa | Pacemaker, Dual Chamber for Insertion in Subcutaneous Tissue and Fascia |
| Kirschner wire (K-wire) | Internal Fixation Device in Head and Facial Bones<br>Internal Fixation Device in Upper Bones<br>Internal Fixation Device in Lower Bones<br>Internal Fixation Device in Upper Joints<br>Internal Fixation Device in Lower Joints |
| Knee (implant) insert | Liner in Lower Joints |
| Kuntscher nail | Internal Fixation Device, Intramedullary in Upper Bones<br>Internal Fixation Device, Intramedullary in Lower Bones |
| LAP-BAND® adjustable gastric banding system | Extraluminal Device |
| LifeStent® (Flexstar)(XL) Vascular Stent System | Intraluminal Device |
| LIVIAN™ CRT-D | Cardiac Resynchronization Defibrillator Pulse Generator for Insertion in Subcutaneous Tissue and Fascia |
| Loop recorder, implantable | Monitoring Device |
| MAGEC® Spinal Bracing and Distraction System | Magnetically Controlled Growth Rod(s) in New Technology |
| Mark IV Breathing Pacemaker System | Stimulator Generator in Subcutaneous Tissue and Fascia |
| Maximo II DR (VR) | Defibrillator Generator for Insertion in Subcutaneous Tissue and Fascia |
| Maximo II DR CRT-D | Cardiac Resynchronization Defibrillator Pulse Generator for Insertion in Subcutaneous Tissue and Fascia |
| Medtronic Endurant® II AAA stent graft system | Intraluminal Device |
| Melody® transcatheter pulmonary valve | Zooplastic Tissue in Heart and Great Vessels |
| Metal on metal bearing surface | Synthetic Substitute, Metal for Replacement in Lower Joints |
| Micro-Driver stent (RX) (OTW) | Intraluminal Device |
| MicroMed HeartAssist | Implantable Heart Assist System in Heart and Great Vessels |
| Micrus CERECYTE microcoil | Intraluminal Device, Bioactive in Upper Arteries |
| MIRODERM™ Biologic Wound Matrix | Skin Substitute, Porcine Liver Derived in New Technology |
| MitraClip valve repair system | Synthetic Substitute |

| Term | ICD-10-PCS Value |
|---|---|
| Mitroflow® Aortic Pericardial Heart Valve | Zooplastic Tissue in Heart and Great Vessels |
| Mosaic Bioprosthesis (aortic) (mitral) valve | Zooplastic Tissue in Heart and Great Vessels |
| MULTI-LINK (VISION)(MINI-VISION)(ULTRA) Coronary Stent System | Intraluminal Device |
| nanoLOCK™ interbody fusion device | Interbody Fusion Device, Nanotextured Surface in New Technology |
| Nasopharyngeal airway (NPA) | Intraluminal Device, Airway in Ear, Nose, Sinus |
| Neuromuscular electrical stimulation (NEMS) lead | Stimulator Lead in Muscles |
| Neurostimulator generator, multiple channel | Stimulator Generator, Multiple Array for Insertion in Subcutaneous Tissue and Fascia |
| Neurostimulator generator, multiple channel rechargeable | Stimulator Generator, Multiple Array Rechargeable for Insertion in Subcutaneous Tissue and Fascia |
| Neurostimulator generator, single channel | Stimulator Generator, Single Array for Insertion in Subcutaneous Tissue and Fascia |
| Neurostimulator generator, single channel rechargeable | Stimulator Generator, Single Array Rechargeable for Insertion in Subcutaneous Tissue and Fascia |
| Neutralization plate | Internal Fixation Device in Head and Facial Bones<br>Internal Fixation Device in Upper Bones<br>Internal Fixation Device in Lower Bones |
| Nitinol framed polymer mesh | Synthetic Substitute |
| Non-tunneled central venous catheter | Infusion Device |
| Novacor Left Ventricular Assist Device | Implantable Heart Assist System in Heart and Great Vessels |
| Novation® Ceramic AHS® (Articulation Hip System) | Synthetic Substitute, Ceramic for Replacement in Lower Joints |
| Omnilink Elite Vascular Balloon Expandable Stent System | Intraluminal Device |
| Open Pivot Aortic Valve Graft (AVG) | Synthetic Substitute |
| Open Pivot (mechanical) Valve | Synthetic Substitute |
| Optimizer™ III implantable pulse generator | Contractility Modulation Device for Insertion in Subcutaneous Tissue and Fascia |
| Oropharyngeal airway (OPA) | Intraluminal Device, Airway in Mouth and Throat |
| Ovatio™ CRT-D | Cardiac Resynchronization Defibrillator Pulse Generator for Insertion in Subcutaneous Tissue and Fascia |
| OXINIUM | Synthetic Substitute, Oxidized Zirconium on Polyethylene for Replacement in Lower Joints |
| Paclitaxel-eluting coronary stent | Intraluminal Device, Drug-eluting in Heart and Great Vessels |
| Paclitaxel-eluting peripheral stent | Intraluminal Device, Drug-eluting in Upper Arteries<br>Intraluminal Device, Drug-eluting in Lower Arteries |
| Partially absorbable mesh | Synthetic Substitute |

| Term | ICD-10-PCS Value |
|---|---|
| Pedicle-based dynamic stabilization device | Spinal Stabilization Device, Pedicle-Based for Insertion in Upper Joints<br>Spinal Stabilization Device, Pedicle-Based for Insertion in Lower Joints |
| Perceval sutureless valve | Zooplastic Tissue, Rapid Deployment Technique in New Technology |
| Percutaneous endoscopic gastrojejunostomy (PEG/J) tube | Feeding Device in Gastrointestinal System |
| Percutaneous endoscopic gastrostomy (PEG) tube | Feeding Device in Gastrointestinal System |
| Percutaneous nephrostomy catheter | Drainage Device |
| Peripherally inserted central catheter (PICC) | Infusion Device |
| Pessary ring | Intraluminal Device, Pessary in Female Reproductive System |
| Phrenic nerve stimulator generator | Stimulator Generator in Subcutaneous Tissue and Fascia |
| Phrenic nerve stimulator lead | Diaphragmatic Pacemaker Lead in Respiratory System |
| PHYSIOMESH™ Flexible Composite Mesh | Synthetic Substitute |
| Pipeline™ Embolization device (PED) | Intraluminal Device |
| Polyethylene socket | Synthetic Substitute, Polyethylene for Replacement in Lower Joints |
| Polymethylmethacrylate (PMMA) | Synthetic Substitute |
| Polypropylene mesh | Synthetic Substitute |
| Porcine (bioprosthetic) valve | Zooplastic Tissue in Heart and Great Vessels |
| PRESTIGE® Cervical Disc | Synthetic Substitute |
| PrimeAdvanced neurostimulator (SureScan)(MRI Safe) | Stimulator Generator, Multiple Array for Insertion in Subcutaneous Tissue and Fascia |
| PROCEED™ Ventral Patch | Synthetic Substitute |
| Prodisc-C | Synthetic Substitute |
| Prodisc-L | Synthetic Substitute |
| PROLENE Polypropylene Hernia System (PHS) | Synthetic Substitute |
| Protecta XT CRT-D | Cardiac Resynchronization Defibrillator Pulse Generator for Insertion in Subcutaneous Tissue and Fascia |
| Protecta XT DR (XT VR) | Defibrillator Generator for Insertion in Subcutaneous Tissue and Fascia |
| Protégé® RX Carotid Stent System | Intraluminal Device |
| Pump reservoir | Infusion Device, Pump in Subcutaneous Tissue and Fascia |
| REALIZE® Adjustable Gastric Band | Extraluminal Device |
| Rebound HRD® (Hernia Repair Device) | Synthetic Substitute |
| RestoreAdvanced neurostimulator (SureScan)(MRI Safe) | Stimulator Generator, Multiple Array Rechargeable for Insertion in Subcutaneous Tissue and Fascia |
| RestoreSensor neurostimulator (SureScan)(MRI Safe) | Stimulator Generator, Multiple Array Rechargeable for Insertion in Subcutaneous Tissue and Fascia |
| RestoreUltra neurostimulator (SureScan)(MRI Safe) | Stimulator Generator, Multiple Array Rechargeable for Insertion in Subcutaneous Tissue and Fascia |

| Term | ICD-10-PCS Value |
|---|---|
| Reveal (DX)(XT) | Monitoring Device |
| Reverse® Shoulder Prosthesis | Synthetic Substitute, Reverse Ball and Socket for Replacement in Upper Joints |
| Revo MRI™ SureScan® pacemaker | Pacemaker, Dual Chamber for Insertion in Subcutaneous Tissue and Fascia |
| Rheos® System device | Stimulator Generator in Subcutaneous Tissue and Fascia |
| Rheos® System lead | Stimulator Lead in Upper Arteries |
| RNS System lead | Neurostimulator Lead in Central Nervous System and Cranial Nerves |
| RNS system neurostimulator generator | Neurostimulator Generator in Head and Facial Bones |
| Sacral nerve modulation (SNM) lead | Stimulator Lead in Urinary System |
| Sacral neuromodulation lead | Stimulator Lead in Urinary System |
| SAPIEN transcatheter aortic valve | Zooplastic Tissue in Heart and Great Vessels |
| Secura (DR) (VR) | Defibrillator Generator for Insertion in Subcutaneous Tissue and Fascia |
| Sheffield hybrid external fixator | External Fixation Device, Hybrid for Insertion in Upper Bones<br>External Fixation Device, Hybrid for Reposition in Upper Bones<br>External Fixation Device, Hybrid for Insertion in Lower Bones<br>External Fixation Device, Hybrid for Reposition in Lower Bones |
| Sheffield ring external fixator | External Fixation Device, Ring for Insertion in Upper Bones<br>External Fixation Device, Ring for Reposition in Upper Bones<br>External Fixation Device, Ring for Insertion in Lower Bones<br>External Fixation Device, Ring for Reposition in Lower Bones |
| Single lead pacemaker (atrium)(ventricle) | Pacemaker, Single Chamber for Insertion in Subcutaneous Tissue and Fascia |
| Single lead rate responsive pacemaker (atrium)(ventricle) | Pacemaker, Single Chamber Rate Responsive for Insertion in Subcutaneous Tissue and Fascia |
| Sirolimus-eluting coronary stent | Intraluminal Device, Drug-eluting in Heart and Great Vessels |
| SJM Biocor® Stented Valve System | Zooplastic Tissue in Heart and Great Vessels |
| Spinal cord neurostimulator lead | Neurostimulator Lead in Central Nervous System and Cranial Nerves |
| Spinal growth rods, magnetically controlled | Magnetically Controlled Growth Rod(s) in New Technology |
| Spiration IBV™ Valve System | Intraluminal Device, Endobronchial Valve in Respiratory System |
| Stent, Intraluminal (cardiovascular)(gastrointestinal)(hepatobiliary)(urinary) | Intraluminal Device |
| Stented tissue valve | Zooplastic Tissue in Heart and Great Vessels |
| Stratos LV | Cardiac Resynchronization Pacemaker Pulse Generator for Insertion in Subcutaneous Tissue and Fascia |
| Subcutaneous injection reservoir, port | Vascular Access Device, Totally Implantable in Subcutaneous Tissue and Fascia |
| Subcutaneous injection reservoir, pump | Infusion Device, Pump in Subcutaneous Tissue and Fascia |
| Subdermal progesterone implant | Contraceptive Device in Subcutaneous Tissue and Fascia |
| Sutureless valve, Perceval | Zooplastic Tissue, Rapid Deployment Technique in New Technology |
| SynCardia Total Artificial Heart | Synthetic Substitute |
| Synchra CRT-P | Cardiac Resynchronization Pacemaker Pulse Generator for Insertion in Subcutaneous Tissue and Fascia |
| SyncroMed Pump | Infusion Device, Pump in Subcutaneous Tissue and Fascia |
| Talent® Converter | Intraluminal Device |
| Talent® Occluder | Intraluminal Device |
| Talent® Stent Graft (abdominal)(thoracic) | Intraluminal Device |
| TandemHeart® System | Short-term External Heart Assist System in Heart and Great Vessels |
| TAXUS® Liberté® Paclitaxel-eluting Coronary Stent System | Intraluminal Device, Drug-eluting in Heart and Great Vessels |
| Therapeutic occlusion coil(s) | Intraluminal Device |
| Thoracostomy tube | Drainage Device |
| Thoratec IVAD (Implantable Ventricular Assist Device) | Implantable Heart Assist System in Heart and Great Vessels |
| Thoratec Paracorporeal Ventricular Assist Device | Short-term External Heart Assist System in Heart and Great Vessels |
| Tibial insert | Liner in Lower Joints |
| Tissue bank graft | Nonautologous Tissue Substitute |
| Tissue expander (inflatable)(injectable) | Tissue Expander in Skin and Breast<br>Tissue Expander in Subcutaneous Tissue and Fascia |
| Titanium Sternal Fixation System (TSFS) | Internal Fixation Device, Rigid Plate for Insertion in Upper Bones<br>Internal Fixation Device, Rigid Plate for Reposition in Upper Bones |
| Total artificial (replacement) heart | Synthetic Substitute |
| Tracheostomy tube | Tracheostomy Device in Respiratory System |
| Trifecta™ Valve (aortic) | Zooplastic Tissue in Heart and Great Vessels |
| Tunneled central venous catheter | Vascular Access Device, Tunneled in Subcutaneous Tissue and Fascia |
| Tunneled spinal (intrathecal) catheter | Infusion Device |
| Two lead pacemaker | Pacemaker, Dual Chamber for Insertion in Subcutaneous Tissue and Fascia |
| Ultraflex™ Precision Colonic Stent System | Intraluminal Device |
| ULTRAPRO Hernia System (UHS) | Synthetic Substitute |
| ULTRAPRO Partially Absorbable Lightweight Mesh | Synthetic Substitute |
| ULTRAPRO Plug | Synthetic Substitute |
| Ultrasonic osteogenic stimulator | Bone Growth Stimulator in Head and Facial Bones<br>Bone Growth Stimulator in Upper Bones<br>Bone Growth Stimulator in Lower Bones |

| Term | ICD-10-PCS Value |
|---|---|
| Ultrasound bone healing system | Bone Growth Stimulator in Head and Facial Bones<br>Bone Growth Stimulator in Upper Bones<br>Bone Growth Stimulator in Lower Bones |
| Uniplanar external fixator | External Fixation Device, Monoplanar for Insertion in Upper Bones<br>External Fixation Device, Monoplanar for Reposition in Upper Bones<br>External Fixation Device, Monoplanar for Insertion in Lower Bones<br>External Fixation Device, Monoplanar for Reposition in Lower Bones |
| Urinary incontinence stimulator lead | Stimulator Lead in Urinary System |
| Vaginal pessary | Intraluminal Device, Pessary in Female Reproductive System |
| Valiant Thoracic Stent Graft | Intraluminal Device |
| Vectra® Vascular Access Graft | Vascular Access Device, Tunneled in Subcutaneous Tissue and Fascia |
| Ventrio™ Hernia Patch | Synthetic Substitute |
| Versa | Pacemaker, Dual Chamber for Insertion in Subcutaneous Tissue and Fascia |
| Virtuoso (II) (DR) (VR) | Defibrillator Generator for Insertion in Subcutaneous Tissue and Fascia |
| Viva(XT)(S) | Cardiac Resynchronization Defibrillator Pulse Generator for Insertion in Subcutaneous Tissue and Fascia |
| WALLSTENT® Endoprosthesis | Intraluminal Device |
| X-STOP® Spacer | Spinal Stabilization Device, Interspinous Process for Insertion in Upper Joints<br>Spinal Stabilization Device, Interspinous Process for Insertion in Lower Joints |
| Xact Carotid Stent System | Intraluminal Device |
| Xenograft | Zooplastic Tissue in Heart and Great Vessels |
| XIENCE Everolimus Eluting Coronary Stent System | Intraluminal Device, Drug-eluting in Heart and Great Vessels |
| XLIF® System | Interbody Fusion Device in Lower Joints |
| Zenith AAA Endovascular Graft | Intraluminal Device, Branched or Fenestrated, One or Two Arteries for Restriction in Lower Arteries<br>Intraluminal Device, Branched or Fenestrated, Three or More Arteries for Restriction in Lower Arteries<br>Intraluminal Device |
| Zenith Flex® AAA Endovascular Graft | Intraluminal Device |
| Zenith TX2® TAA Endovascular Graft | Intraluminal Device |
| Zenith® Renu™ AAA Ancillary Graft | Intraluminal Device |
| Zilver® PTX® (paclitaxel) Drug-Eluting Peripheral Stent | Intraluminal Device, Drug-eluting in Upper Arteries<br>Intraluminal Device, Drug-eluting in Lower Arteries |
| Zimmer® NexGen® LPS Mobile Bearing Knee | Synthetic Substitute |
| Zimmer® NexGen® LPS-Flex Mobile Knee | Synthetic Substitute |
| Zotarolimus-eluting coronary stent | Intraluminal Device, Drug-eluting in Heart and Great Vessels |

## Device Aggregation Table

This table crosswalks specific device character value definitions for specific root operations in a specific body system to the more general device character value to be used when the root operation covers a wide range of body parts and the device character represents an entire family of devices.

| Specific Device | for Operation | in Body System | General Device |
|---|---|---|---|
| Autologous Arterial Tissue (A) | All applicable | Heart and Great Vessels<br>Lower Arteries<br>Lower Veins<br>Upper Arteries<br>Upper Veins | **7** Autologous Tissue Substitute |
| Autologous Venous Tissue (9) | All applicable | Heart and Great Vessels<br>Lower Arteries<br>Lower Veins<br>Upper Arteries<br>Upper Veins | **7** Autologous Tissue Substitute |
| Cardiac Lead, Defibrillator (K) | Insertion | Heart and Great Vessels | **M** Cardiac Lead |
| Cardiac Lead, Pacemaker (J) | Insertion | Heart and Great Vessels | **M** Cardiac Lead |
| Cardiac Resynchronization Defibrillator Pulse Generator (9) | Insertion | Subcutaneous Tissue and Fascia | **P** Cardiac Rhythm Related Device |
| Cardiac Resynchronization Pacemaker Pulse Generator (7) | Insertion | Subcutaneous Tissue and Fascia | **P** Cardiac Rhythm Related Device |
| Contractility Modulation Device (A) | Insertion | Subcutaneous Tissue and Fascia | **P** Cardiac Rhythm Related Device |
| Defibrillator Generator (8) | Insertion | Subcutaneous Tissue and Fascia | **P** Cardiac Rhythm Related Device |
| Epiretinal Visual Prosthesis (5) | All applicable | Eye | **J** Synthetic Substitute |
| External Fixation Device, Hybrid (D) | Insertion | Lower Bones<br>Upper Bones | **5** External Fixation Device |
| External Fixation Device, Hybrid (D) | Reposition | Lower Bones<br>Upper Bones | **5** External Fixation Device |
| External Fixation Device, Limb Lengthening (8) | Insertion | Lower Bones<br>Upper Bones | **5** External Fixation Device |
| External Fixation Device, Monoplanar (B) | Insertion | Lower Bones<br>Upper Bones | **5** External Fixation Device |
| External Fixation Device, Monoplanar (B) | Reposition | Lower Bones<br>Upper Bones | **5** External Fixation Device |
| External Fixation Device, Ring (C) | Insertion | Lower Bones<br>Upper Bones | **5** External Fixation Device |
| External Fixation Device, Ring (C) | Reposition | Lower Bones<br>Upper Bones | **5** External Fixation Device |
| Hearing Device, Bone Conduction (4) | Insertion | Ear, Nose, Sinus | **S** Hearing Device |
| Hearing Device, Multiple Channel Cochlear Prosthesis (6) | Insertion | Ear, Nose, Sinus | **S** Hearing Device |
| Hearing Device, Single Channel Cochlear Prosthesis (5) | Insertion | Ear, Nose, Sinus | **S** Hearing Device |
| Internal Fixation Device, Intramedullary (6) | All applicable | Lower Bones<br>Upper Bones | **4** Internal Fixation Device |
| Internal Fixation Device, Rigid Plate (Ø) | Insertion | Upper Bones | **4** Internal Fixation Device |
| Internal Fixation Device, Rigid Plate (Ø) | Reposition | Upper Bones | **4** Internal Fixation Device |
| Intraluminal Device, Airway (B) | All applicable | Ear, Nose, Sinus<br>Gastrointestinal System<br>Mouth and Throat | **D** Intraluminal Device |
| Intraluminal Device, Bioactive (B) | All applicable | Upper Arteries | **D** Intraluminal Device |
| Intraluminal Device, Branched or Fenestrated, One or Two Arteries (E) | Restriction | Heart and Great Vessels<br>Lower Arteries | **D** Intraluminal Device |
| Intraluminal Device, Branched or Fenestrated, Three or More Arteries (F) | Restriction | Heart and Great Vessels<br>Lower Arteries | **D** Intraluminal Device |
| Intraluminal Device, Drug-eluting (4) | All applicable | Heart and Great Vessels<br>Lower Arteries<br>Upper Arteries | **D** Intraluminal Device |
| Intraluminal Device, Drug-eluting, Four or More (7) | All applicable | Heart and Great Vessels<br>Lower Arteries<br>Upper Arteries | **D** Intraluminal Device |
| Intraluminal Device, Drug-eluting, Three (6) | All applicable | Heart and Great Vessels<br>Lower Arteries<br>Upper Arteries | **D** Intraluminal Device |

| Specific Device | for Operation | in Body System | General Device |
|---|---|---|---|
| Intraluminal Device, Drug-eluting, Two (5) | All applicable | Heart and Great Vessels<br>Lower Arteries<br>Upper Arteries | **D** Intraluminal Device |
| Intraluminal Device, Endobronchial Valve (G) | All applicable | Respiratory System | **D** Intraluminal Device |
| Intraluminal Device, Endotracheal Airway (E) | All applicable | Respiratory System | **D** Intraluminal Device |
| Intraluminal Device, Four or More (G) | All applicable | Heart and Great Vessels<br>Lower Arteries<br>Upper Arteries | **D** Intraluminal Device |
| Intraluminal Device, Pessary (G) | All applicable | Female Reproductive System | **D** Intraluminal Device |
| Intraluminal Device, Radioactive (T) | All applicable | Heart and Great Vessels | **D** Intraluminal Device |
| Intraluminal Device, Three (F) | All applicable | Heart and Great Vessels<br>Lower Arteries<br>Upper Arteries | **D** Intraluminal Device |
| Intraluminal Device, Two (E) | All applicable | Heart and Great Vessels<br>Lower Arteries<br>Upper Arteries | **D** Intraluminal Device |
| Monitoring Device, Hemodynamic (Ø) | Insertion | Subcutaneous Tissue and Fascia | **2** Monitoring Device |
| Monitoring Device, Pressure Sensor (Ø) | Insertion | Heart and Great Vessels | **2** Monitoring Device |
| Pacemaker, Dual Chamber (6) | Insertion | Subcutaneous Tissue and Fascia | **P** Cardiac Rhythm Related Device |
| Pacemaker, Single Chamber (4) | Insertion | Subcutaneous Tissue and Fascia | **P** Cardiac Rhythm Related Device |
| Pacemaker, Single Chamber Rate Responsive (5) | Insertion | Subcutaneous Tissue and Fascia | **P** Cardiac Rhythm Related Device |
| Spinal Stabilization Device, Facet Replacement (D) | Insertion | Lower Joints<br>Upper Joints | **4** Internal Fixation Device |
| Spinal Stabilization Device, Interspinous Process (B) | Insertion | Lower Joints<br>Upper Joints | **4** Internal Fixation Device |
| Spinal Stabilization Device, Pedicle-Based (C) | Insertion | Lower Joints<br>Upper Joints | **4** Internal Fixation Device |
| Stimulator Generator, Multiple Array (D) | Insertion | Subcutaneous Tissue and Fascia | **M** Stimulator Generator |
| Stimulator Generator, Multiple Array Rechargeable (E) | Insertion | Subcutaneous Tissue and Fascia | **M** Stimulator Generator |
| Stimulator Generator, Single Array (B) | Insertion | Subcutaneous Tissue and Fascia | **M** Stimulator Generator |
| Stimulator Generator, Single Array Rechargeable (C) | Insertion | Subcutaneous Tissue and Fascia | **M** Stimulator Generator |
| Synthetic Substitute, Ceramic (3) | Replacement | Lower Joints | **J** Synthetic Substitute |
| Synthetic Substitute, Ceramic on Polyethylene (4) | Replacement | Lower Joints | **J** Synthetic Substitute |
| Synthetic Substitute, Intraocular Telescope (Ø) | Replacement | Eye | **J** Synthetic Substitute |
| Synthetic Substitute, Metal (1) | Replacement | Lower Joints | **J** Synthetic Substitute |
| Synthetic Substitute, Metal on Polyethylene (2) | Replacement | Lower Joints | **J** Synthetic Substitute |
| Synthetic Substitute, Oxidized Zirconium on Polyethylene (6) | Replacement | Lower Joints | **J** Synthetic Substitute |
| Synthetic Substitute, Polyethylene (Ø) | Replacement | Lower Joints | **J** Synthetic Substitute |
| Synthetic Substitute, Reverse Ball and Socket (Ø) | Replacement | Upper Joints | **J** Synthetic Substitute |
| Synthetic Substitute, Unicondylar (L) | Replacement | Lower Joints | **J** Synthetic Substitute |

# Appendix G: Device Definitions

| ICD-10-PCS Value | Definition |
|---|---|
| **Artificial Sphincter in Gastrointestinal System** | **Includes:**<br>Artificial anal sphincter (AAS)<br>Artificial bowel sphincter (neosphincter) |
| **Artificial Sphincter in Urinary System** | **Includes:**<br>AMS 800® Urinary Control System<br>Artificial urinary sphincter (AUS) |
| **Autologous Arterial Tissue in Heart and Great Vessels** | **Includes:**<br>Autologous artery graft |
| **Autologous Arterial Tissue in Lower Arteries** | **Includes:**<br>Autologous artery graft |
| **Autologous Arterial Tissue in Lower Veins** | **Includes:**<br>Autologous artery graft |
| **Autologous Arterial Tissue in Upper Arteries** | **Includes:**<br>Autologous artery graft |
| **Autologous Arterial Tissue in Upper Veins** | **Includes:**<br>Autologous artery graft |
| **Autologous Tissue Substitute** | **Includes:**<br>Autograft<br>Cultured epidermal cell autograft<br>Epicel® cultured epidermal autograft |
| **Autologous Venous Tissue in Heart and Great Vessels** | **Includes:**<br>Autologous vein graft |
| **Autologous Venous Tissue in Lower Arteries** | **Includes:**<br>Autologous vein graft |
| **Autologous Venous Tissue in Lower Veins** | **Includes:**<br>Autologous vein graft |
| **Autologous Venous Tissue in Upper Arteries** | **Includes:**<br>Autologous vein graft |
| **Autologous Venous Tissue in Upper Veins** | **Includes:**<br>Autologous vein graft |
| **Bone Growth Stimulator in Head and Facial Bones** | **Includes:**<br>Electrical bone growth stimulator (EBGS)<br>Ultrasonic osteogenic stimulator<br>Ultrasound bone healing system |
| **Bone Growth Stimulator in Lower Bones** | **Includes:**<br>Electrical bone growth stimulator (EBGS)<br>Ultrasonic osteogenic stimulator<br>Ultrasound bone healing system |
| **Bone Growth Stimulator in Upper Bones** | **Includes:**<br>Electrical bone growth stimulator (EBGS)<br>Ultrasonic osteogenic stimulator<br>Ultrasound bone healing system |
| **Cardiac Lead in Heart and Great Vessels** | **Includes:**<br>Cardiac contractility modulation lead |
| **Cardiac Lead, Defibrillator for Insertion in Heart and Great Vessels** | **Includes:**<br>ACUITY™ Steerable Lead<br>Attain Ability® lead<br>Attain StarFix® (OTW) lead<br>Cardiac resynchronization therapy (CRT) lead<br>Corox (OTW) Bipolar Lead<br>Durata® Defibrillation Lead<br>ENDOTAK RELIANCE® (G) Defibrillation Lead |
| **Cardiac Lead, Pacemaker for Insertion in Heart and Great Vessels** | **Includes:**<br>ACUITY™ Steerable Lead<br>Attain Ability® lead<br>Attain StarFix® (OTW) lead<br>Cardiac resynchronization therapy (CRT) lead<br>Corox (OTW) Bipolar Lead |
| **Cardiac Resynchronization Defibrillator Pulse Generator for Insertion in Subcutaneous Tissue and Fascia** | **Includes:**<br>COGNIS® CRT-D<br>Concerto II CRT-D<br>Consulta CRT-D<br>CONTAK RENEWA® 3 RF (HE) CRT-D<br>LIVIAN™ CRT-D<br>Maximo II DR CRT-D<br>Ovatio™ CRT-D<br>Protecta XT CRT-D<br>Viva (XT)(S) |
| **Cardiac Resynchronization Pacemaker Pulse Generator for Insertion in Subcutaneous Tissue and Fascia** | **Includes:**<br>Consulta CRT-P<br>Stratos LV<br>Synchra CRT-P |
| **Contraceptive Device in Female Reproductive System** | **Includes:**<br>Intrauterine device (IUD) |
| **Contraceptive Device in Subcutaneous Tissue and Fascia** | **Includes:**<br>Subdermal progesterone implant |
| **Contractility Modulation Device for Insertion in Subcutaneous Tissue and Fascia** | **Includes:**<br>Optimizer™ III implantable pulse generator |
| **Defibrillator Generator for Insertion in Subcutaneous Tissue and Fascia** | **Includes:**<br>Evera (XT)(S)(DR/VR)<br>Implantable cardioverter-defibrillator (ICD)<br>Maximo II DR (VR)<br>Protecta XT DR (XT VR)<br>Secura (DR) (VR)<br>Virtuoso (II) (DR) (VR) |
| **Diaphragmatic Pacemaker Lead in Respiratory System** | **Includes:**<br>Phrenic nerve stimulator lead |
| **Drainage Device** | **Includes:**<br>Cystostomy tube<br>Foley catheter<br>Percutaneous nephrostomy catheter<br>Thoracostomy tube |
| **External Fixation Device in Head and Facial Bones** | **Includes:**<br>External fixator |
| **External Fixation Device in Lower Bones** | **Includes:**<br>External fixator |
| **External Fixation Device in Lower Joints** | **Includes:**<br>External fixator |
| **External Fixation Device in Upper Bones** | **Includes:**<br>External fixator |
| **External Fixation Device in Upper Joints** | **Includes:**<br>External fixator |
| **External Fixation Device, Hybrid for Insertion in Lower Bones** | **Includes:**<br>Delta frame external fixator<br>Sheffield hybrid external fixator |
| **External Fixation Device, Hybrid for Insertion in Upper Bones** | **Includes:**<br>Delta frame external fixator<br>Sheffield hybrid external fixator |

| ICD-10-PCS Value | Definition |
|---|---|
| **External Fixation Device, Hybrid for Reposition in Lower Bones** | **Includes:**<br>Delta frame external fixator<br>Sheffield hybrid external fixator |
| **External Fixation Device, Hybrid for Reposition in Upper Bones** | **Includes:**<br>Delta frame external fixator<br>Sheffield hybrid external fixator |
| **External Fixation Device, Limb Lengthening for Insertion in Lower Bones** | **Includes:**<br>Ilizarov-Vecklich device |
| **External Fixation Device, Limb Lengthening for Insertion in Upper Bones** | **Includes:**<br>Ilizarov-Vecklich device |
| **External Fixation Device, Monoplanar for Insertion in Lower Bones** | **Includes:**<br>Uniplanar external fixator |
| **External Fixation Device, Monoplanar for Insertion in Upper Bones** | **Includes:**<br>Uniplanar external fixator |
| **External Fixation Device, Monoplanar for Reposition in Lower Bones** | **Includes:**<br>Uniplanar external fixator |
| **External Fixation Device, Monoplanar for Reposition in Upper Bones** | **Includes:**<br>Uniplanar external fixator |
| **External Fixation Device, Ring for Insertion in Lower Bones** | **Includes:**<br>Ilizarov external fixator<br>Sheffield ring external fixator |
| **External Fixation Device, Ring for Insertion in Upper Bones** | **Includes:**<br>Ilizarov external fixator<br>Sheffield ring external fixator |
| **External Fixation Device, Ring for Reposition in Lower Bones** | **Includes:**<br>Ilizarov external fixator<br>Sheffield ring external fixator |
| **External Fixation Device, Ring for Reposition in Upper Bones** | **Includes:**<br>Ilizarov external fixator<br>Sheffield ring external fixator |
| **Extraluminal Device** | **Includes:**<br>AtriClip LAA Exclusion System<br>LAP-BAND® adjustable gastric banding system<br>REALIZE® Adjustable Gastric Band |
| **Feeding Device in Gastrointestinal System** | **Includes:**<br>Percutaneous endoscopic gastrojejunostomy (PEG/J) tube<br>Percutaneous endoscopic gastrostomy (PEG) tube |
| **Hearing Device in Ear, Nose, Sinus** | **Includes:**<br>Esteem® implantable hearing system |
| **Hearing Device in Head and Facial Bones** | **Includes:**<br>Bone anchored hearing device |
| **Hearing Device, Bone Conduction for Insertion in Ear, Nose, Sinus** | **Includes:**<br>Bone anchored hearing device |
| **Hearing Device, Multiple Channel Cochlear Prosthesis for Insertion in Ear, Nose, Sinus** | **Includes:**<br>Cochlear implant (CI), multiple channel (electrode) |
| **Hearing Device, Single Channel Cochlear Prosthesis for Insertion in Ear, Nose, Sinus** | **Includes:**<br>Cochlear implant (CI), single channel (electrode) |

| ICD-10-PCS Value | Definition |
|---|---|
| **Implantable Heart Assist System in Heart and Great Vessels** | **Includes:**<br>Berlin Heart Ventricular Assist Device<br>DeBakey Left Ventricular Assist Device<br>DuraHeart Left Ventricular Assist System<br>HeartMate 3™ LVAS<br>HeartMate II® Left Ventricular Assist Device (LVAD)<br>HeartMate XVE® Left Ventricular Assist Device (LVAD)<br>MicroMed HeartAssist<br>Novacor Left Ventricular Assist Device<br>Thoratec IVAD (Implantable Ventricular Assist Device) |
| **Infusion Device** | **Includes:**<br>Ascenda Intrathecal Catheter<br>InDura, intrathecal catheter (1P) (spinal)<br>Non-tunneled central venous catheter<br>Peripherally inserted central catheter (PICC)<br>Tunneled spinal (intrathecal) catheter |
| **Infusion Device, Pump in Subcutaneous Tissue and Fascia** | **Includes:**<br>Implantable drug infusion pump (anti-spasmodic)(chemotherapy) (pain)<br>Injection reservoir, pump<br>Pump reservoir<br>Subcutaneous injection reservoir, pump<br>SynchroMed pump |
| **Interbody Fusion Device in Lower Joints** | **Includes:**<br>Axial Lumbar Interbody Fusion System<br>AxiaLIF® System<br>CoRoent® XL<br>Direct Lateral Interbody Fusion (DLIF) device<br>EXtreme Lateral Interbody Fusion (XLIF) device<br>Interbody fusion (spine) cage<br>XLIF® System |
| **Interbody Fusion Device in Upper Joints** | **Includes:**<br>BAK/C® Interbody Cervical Fusion System<br>Interbody fusion (spine) cage |
| **Internal Fixation Device in Head and Facial Bones** | **Includes:**<br>Bone screw (interlocking)(lag)(pedicle) (recessed)<br>Kirschner wire (K-wire)<br>Neutralization plate |
| **Internal Fixation Device in Lower Bones** | **Includes:**<br>Bone screw (interlocking)(lag)(pedicle) (recessed)<br>Clamp and rod internal fixation system (CRIF)<br>Kirschner wire (K-wire)<br>Neutralization plate |

| ICD-10-PCS Value | Definition |
|---|---|
| **Internal Fixation Device in Lower Joints** | **Includes:**<br>Fusion screw (compression)(lag)(locking)<br>Joint fixation plate<br>Kirschner wire (K-wire) |
| **Internal Fixation Device in Upper Bones** | **Includes:**<br>Bone screw (interlocking)(lag)(pedicle)(recessed)<br>Clamp and rod internal fixation system (CRIF)<br>Kirschner wire (K-wire)<br>Neutralization plate |
| **Internal Fixation Device in Upper Joints** | **Includes:**<br>Fusion screw (compression)(lag)(locking)<br>Joint fixation plate<br>Kirschner wire (K-wire) |
| **Internal Fixation Device, Intramedullary in Lower Bones** | **Includes:**<br>Intramedullary (IM) rod (nail)<br>Intramedullary skeletal kinetic distractor (ISKD)<br>Kuntscher nail |
| **Internal Fixation Device, Intramedullary in Upper Bones** | **Includes:**<br>Intramedullary (IM) rod (nail)<br>Intramedullary skeletal kinetic distractor (ISKD)<br>Kuntscher nail |
| **Internal Fixation Device, Rigid Plate for Insertion in Upper Bones** | **Includes:**<br>Titanium Sternal Fixation System (TSFS) |
| **Internal Fixation Device, Rigid Plate for Reposition in Upper Bones** | **Includes:**<br>Titanium Sternal Fixation System (TSFS) |
| **Intraluminal Device** | **Includes:**<br>Absolute Pro Vascular (OTW) Self-Expanding Stent System<br>Acculink (RX) Carotid Stent System<br>AFX® Endovascular AAA System<br>AneuRx® AAA Advantage®<br>Assurant (Cobalt) stent<br>Carotid WALLSTENT® Monorail® Endoprosthesis<br>CoAxia NeuroFlo catheter<br>Colonic Z-Stent®<br>Complete (SE) stent<br>Cook Zenith AAA Endovascular Graft<br>Driver stent (RX) (OTW)<br>E-Luminexx™ (Biliary)(Vascular) Stent<br>Embolization coil(s)<br>Endologix AFX® Endovascular AAA System<br>Endurant® Endovascular Stent Graft<br>Endurant® II AAA stent graft system<br>EXCLUDER® AAA Endoprosthesis |

Continued on next column

| ICD-10-PCS Value | Definition |
|---|---|
| **Intraluminal Device (continued)** | Express® (LD) Premounted Stent System<br>Express® Biliary SD Monorail® Premounted Stent System<br>Express® SD Renal Monorail® Premounted Stent System<br>FLAIR® Endovascular Stent Graft<br>Formula™ Balloon-Expandable Renal Stent System<br>GORE EXCLUDER® AAA Endoprosthesis<br>GORE TAG® Thoracic Endoprosthesis<br>Herculink (RX) Elite Renal Stent System<br>LifeStent® (Flexstar)(XL) Vascular Stent System<br>Medtronic Endurant® II AAA stent graft system<br>Micro-Driver stent (RX) (OTW)<br>MULTI-LINK (VISION)(MINI-VISION)(ULTRA) Coronary Stent System<br>Omnilink Elite Vascular Balloon Expandable Stent System<br>Pipeline™ Embolization device (PED)<br>Protege® RX Carotid Stent System<br>Stent, intraluminal (cardiovascular)(gastrointestinal)(hepatobiliary)(urinary)<br>Talent® Converter<br>Talent® Occluder<br>Talent® Stent Graft (abdominal)(thoracic)<br>Therapeutic occlusion coil(s)<br>Ultraflex™ Precision Colonic Stent System<br>Valiant Thoracic Stent Graft<br>WALLSTENT® Endoprosthesis<br>Xact Carotid Stent System<br>Zenith AAA Endovascular Graft<br>Zenith Flex® AAA Endovascular Graft<br>Zenith TX2® TAA Endovascular Graft<br>Zenith® Renu™ AAA Ancillary Graft |
| **Intraluminal Device, Airway in Ear, Nose, Sinus** | **Includes:**<br>Nasopharyngeal airway (NPA) |
| **Intraluminal Device, Airway in Gastrointestinal System** | **Includes:**<br>Esophageal obturator airway (EOA) |
| **Intraluminal Device, Airway in Mouth and Throat** | **Includes:**<br>Guedel airway<br>Oropharyngeal airway (OPA) |
| **Intraluminal Device, Bioactive in Upper Arteries** | **Includes:**<br>Bioactive embolization coil(s)<br>Micrus CERECYTE microcoil |
| **Intraluminal Device, Branched or Fenestrated, One or Two Arteries for Restriction in Lower Arteries** | **Includes:**<br>Cook Zenith AAA Endovascular Graft<br>EXCLUDER® AAA Endoprosthesis<br>EXCLUDER® IBE Endoprosthesis<br>GORE EXCLUDER® AAA Endoprosthesis<br>GORE EXCLUDER®IBE Endoprosthesis<br>Zenith AAA Endovascular Graft |
| **Intraluminal Device, Branched or Fenestrated, Three or More Arteries for Restriction in Lower Arteries** | **Includes:**<br>Cook Zenith AAA Endovascular Graft<br>EXCLUDER® AAA Endoprosthesis<br>GORE EXCLUDER® AAA Endoprosthesis<br>Zenith AAA Endovascular Graft |

| ICD-10-PCS Value | Definition |
|---|---|
| **Intraluminal Device, Drug-eluting in Heart and Great Vessels** | **Includes:**<br>CYPHER® Stent<br>Endeavor® (III)(IV) (Sprint) Zotarolimus-eluting Coronary Stent System<br>Everolimus-eluting coronary stent<br>Paclitaxel-eluting coronary stent<br>Sirolimus-eluting coronary stent<br>TAXUS® Liberte® Paclitaxel-eluting Coronary Stent System<br>XIENCE Everolimus Eluting Coronary Stent System<br>Zotarolimus-eluting coronary stent |
| **Intraluminal Device, Drug-eluting in Lower Arteries** | **Includes:**<br>Paclitaxel-eluting peripheral stent<br>Zilver® PTX® (paclitaxel) Drug-Eluting Peripheral Stent |
| **Intraluminal Device, Drug-eluting in Upper Arteries** | **Includes:**<br>Paclitaxel-eluting peripheral stent<br>Zilver® PTX® (paclitaxel) Drug-Eluting Peripheral Stent |
| **Intraluminal Device, Endobronchial Valve in Respiratory System** | **Includes:**<br>Spiration IBV™ Valve System |
| **Intraluminal Device, Endotracheal Airway in Respiratory System** | **Includes:**<br>Endotracheal tube (cuffed)(double-lumen) |
| **Intraluminal Device, Pessary in Female Reproductive System** | **Includes:**<br>Pessary ring<br>Vaginal pessary |
| **Liner in Lower Joints** | **Includes:**<br>Acetabular cup<br>Hip (joint) liner<br>Joint liner (insert)<br>Knee (implant) insert<br>Tibial insert |
| **Monitoring Device** | **Includes:**<br>Blood glucose monitoring system<br>Cardiac event recorder<br>Continuous Glucose Monitoring (CGM) device<br>Implantable glucose monitoring device<br>Loop recorder, implantable<br>Reveal (DX)(XT) |
| **Monitoring Device, Hemodynamic for Insertion in Subcutaneous Tissue and Fascia** | **Includes:**<br>Implantable hemodynamic monitor (IHM)<br>Implantable hemodynamic monitoring system (IHMS) |
| **Monitoring Device, Pressure Sensor for Insertion in Heart and Great Vessels** | **Includes:**<br>CardioMEMS® pressure sensor<br>EndoSure® sensor |
| **Neurostimulator Generator in Head and Facial Bones** | **Includes:**<br>RNS system neurostimulator generator |
| **Neurostimulator Lead in Central Nervous System and Cranial Nerves** | **Includes:**<br>Cortical strip neurostimulator lead<br>DBS lead<br>Deep brain neurostimulator lead<br>RNS System lead<br>Spinal cord neurostimulator lead |
| **Neurostimulator Lead in Peripheral Nervous System** | **Includes:**<br>InterStim® Therapy lead |

| ICD-10-PCS Value | Definition |
|---|---|
| **Nonautologous Tissue Substitute** | **Includes:**<br>Acellular Hydrated Dermis<br>Bone bank bone graft<br>Cook Biodesign® Fistula Plug(s)<br>Cook Biodesign® Hernia Graft(s)<br>Cook Biodesign® Layered Graft(s)<br>Cook Zenapro™ Layered Graft(s)<br>Tissue bank graft |
| **Pacemaker, Dual Chamber for Insertion in Subcutaneous Tissue and Fascia** | **Includes:**<br>Advisa (MRI)<br>EnRhythm<br>Kappa<br>Revo MRI™ SureScan® pacemaker<br>Two lead pacemaker<br>Versa |
| **Pacemaker, Single Chamber for Insertion in Subcutaneous Tissue and Fascia** | **Includes:**<br>Single lead pacemaker (atrium)(ventricle) |
| **Pacemaker, Single Chamber Rate Responsive for Insertion in Subcutaneous Tissue and Fascia** | **Includes:**<br>Single lead rate responsive pacemaker (atrium)(ventricle) |
| **Radioactive Element** | **Includes:**<br>Brachytherapy seeds |
| **Radioactive Element, Cesium-131 Collagen Implant for Insertion in Central Nervous System and Cranial Nerves** | **Includes:**<br>Cesium-131 Collagen Implant<br>GammaTile™ |
| **Resurfacing Device in Lower Joints** | **Includes:**<br>CONSERVE® PLUS Total Resurfacing Hip System<br>Cormet Hip Resurfacing System |
| **Short-term External Heart Assist System in Heart and Great Vessels** | **Includes:**<br>Biventricular external heart assist system<br>BVS 5000 Ventricular Assist Device<br>Centrimag® Blood Pump<br>Impella® heart pump<br>TandemHeart® System<br>Thoratec Paracorporeal Ventricular Assist Device |
| **Spacer in Lower Joints** | **Includes:**<br>Joint spacer (antibiotic) |
| **Spacer in Upper Joints** | **Includes:**<br>Joint spacer (antibiotic) |
| **Spinal Stabilization Device, Facet Replacement for Insertion in Lower Joints** | **Includes:**<br>Facet replacement spinal stabilization device |
| **Spinal Stabilization Device, Facet Replacement for Insertion in Upper Joints** | **Includes:**<br>Facet replacement spinal stabilization device |
| **Spinal Stabilization Device, Interspinous Process for Insertion in Lower Joints** | **Includes:**<br>Interspinous process spinal stabilization device<br>X-STOP® Spacer |
| **Spinal Stabilization Device, Interspinous Process for Insertion in Upper Joints** | **Includes:**<br>Interspinous process spinal stabilization device<br>X-STOP® Spacer |

| ICD-10-PCS Value | Definition |
|---|---|
| **Spinal Stabilization Device, Pedicle- Based for Insertion in Lower Joints** | **Includes:**<br>Dynesys® Dynamic Stabilization System<br>Pedicle-based dynamic stabilization device |
| **Spinal Stabilization Device, Pedicle-Based for Insertion in Upper Joints** | **Includes:**<br>Dynesys® Dynamic Stabilization System<br>Pedicle-based dynamic stabilization device |
| **Stimulator Generator in Subcutaneous Tissue and Fascia** | **Includes:**<br>Baroreflex Activation Therapy® (BAT®)<br>Diaphragmatic pacemaker generator<br>Mark IV Breathing Pacemaker System<br>Phrenic nerve stimulator generator<br>Rheos® System device |
| **Stimulator Generator, Multiple Array for Insertion in Subcutaneous Tissue and Fascia** | **Includes:**<br>Activa PC neurostimulator<br>Enterra gastric neurostimulator<br>Neurostimulator generator, multiple channel<br>PrimeAdvanced neurostimulator (SureScan)(MRI Safe) |
| **Stimulator Generator, Multiple Array Rechargeable for Insertion in Subcutaneous Tissue and Fascia** | **Includes:**<br>Activa RC neurostimulator<br>Neurostimulator generator, multiple channel rechargeable<br>RestoreAdvanced neurostimulator (SureScan)(MRI Safe)<br>RestoreSensor neurostimulator (SureScan)(MRI Safe)<br>RestoreUltra neurostimulator (SureScan)(MRI Safe) |
| **Stimulator Generator, Single Array for Insertion in Subcutaneous Tissue and Fascia** | **Includes:**<br>Activa SC neurostimulator<br>InterStim® Therapy neurostimulator<br>Itrel (3)(4) neurostimulator<br>Neurostimulator generator, single channel |
| **Stimulator Generator, Single Array Rechargeable for Insertion in Subcutaneous Tissue and Fascia** | **Includes:**<br>Neurostimulator generator, single channel rechargeable |
| **Stimulator Lead in Gastrointestinal System** | **Includes:**<br>Gastric electrical stimulation (GES) lead<br>Gastric pacemaker lead |
| **Stimulator Lead in Muscles** | **Includes:**<br>Electrical muscle stimulation (EMS) lead<br>Electronic muscle stimulator lead<br>Neuromuscular electrical stimulation (NEMS) lead |
| **Stimulator Lead in Upper Arteries** | **Includes:**<br>Baroreflex Activation Therapy® (BAT®)<br>Carotid (artery) sinus (baroreceptor) lead<br>Rheos® System lead |
| **Stimulator Lead in Urinary System** | **Includes:**<br>Sacral nerve modulation (SNM) lead<br>Sacral neuromodulation lead<br>Urinary incontinence stimulator lead |

| ICD-10-PCS Value | Definition |
|---|---|
| **Synthetic Substitute** | **Includes:**<br>AbioCor® Total Replacement Heart<br>AMPLATZER® Muscular VSD Occluder<br>Annuloplasty ring<br>Bard® Composix® (E/X) (LP) mesh<br>Bard® Composix® Kugel® patch<br>Bard® Dulex™ mesh<br>Bard® Ventralex™ hernia patch<br>BRYAN® Cervical Disc System<br>Ex-PRESS™ mini glaucoma shunt<br>Flexible Composite Mesh<br>GORE® DUALMESH®<br>Holter valve ventricular shunt<br>MitraClip valve repair system<br>Nitinol framed polymer mesh<br>Open Pivot (mechanical) valve<br>Open Pivot Aortic Valve Graft (AVG)<br>Partially absorbable mesh<br>PHYSIOMESH™ Flexible Composite Mesh<br>Polymethylmethacrylate (PMMA)<br>Polypropylene mesh<br>PRESTIGE® Cervical Disc<br>PROCEED™ Ventral Patch<br>Prodisc-C<br>Prodisc-L<br>PROLENE Polypropylene Hernia System (PHS)<br>Rebound HRD® (Hernia Repair Device)<br>SynCardia Total Artificial Heart<br>Total artificial (replacement) heart<br>ULTRAPRO Hernia System (UHS)<br>ULTRAPRO Partially Absorbable Lightweight Mesh<br>ULTRAPRO Plug<br>Ventrio™ Hernia Patch<br>Zimmer® NexGen® LPS Mobile Bearing Knee<br>Zimmer® NexGen® LPS-Flex Mobile Knee |
| **Synthetic Substitute, Ceramic for Replacement in Lower Joints** | **Includes:**<br>Ceramic on ceramic bearing surface<br>Novation® Ceramic AHS® (Articulation Hip System) |
| **Synthetic Substitute, Intraocular Telescope for Replacement in Eye** | **Includes:**<br>Implantable Miniature Telescope™ (IMT) |
| **Synthetic Substitute, Metal for Replacement in Lower Joints** | **Includes:**<br>Cobalt/chromium head and socket<br>Metal on metal bearing surface |
| **Synthetic Substitute, Metal on Polyethylene for Replacement in Lower Joints** | **Includes:**<br>Cobalt/chromium head and polyethylene socket |
| **Synthetic Substitute, Oxidized Zirconium on Polyethylene for Replacement in Lower Joints** | **Includes:**<br>OXINIUM |
| **Synthetic Substitute, Polyethylene for Replacement in Lower Joints** | **Includes:**<br>Polyethylene socket |
| **Synthetic Substitute, Reverse Ball and Socket for Replacement in Upper Joints** | **Includes:**<br>Delta III Reverse shoulder prosthesis<br>Reverse® Shoulder Prosthesis |
| **Tissue Expander in Skin and Breast** | **Includes:**<br>Tissue expander (inflatable) (injectable) |

| ICD-10-PCS Value | Definition |
|---|---|
| **Tissue Expander in Subcutaneous Tissue and Fascia** | **Includes:**<br>Tissue expander (inflatable) (injectable) |
| **Tracheostomy Device in Respiratory System** | **Includes:**<br>Tracheostomy tube |
| **Vascular Access Device, Totally Implantable in Subcutaneous Tissue and Fascia** | **Includes:**<br>Implanted (venous)(access) port<br>Injection reservoir, port<br>Subcutaneous injection reservoir, port |
| **Vascular Access Device, Tunneled in Subcutaneous Tissue and Fascia** | **Includes:**<br>Tunneled central venous catheter<br>Vectra® Vascular Access Graft |

| ICD-10-PCS Value | Definition |
|---|---|
| **Zooplastic Tissue in Heart and Great Vessels** | **Includes:**<br>3f (Aortic) Bioprosthesis valve<br>Bovine pericardial valve<br>Bovine pericardium graft<br>Contegra Pulmonary Valved Conduit<br>CoreValve transcatheter aortic valve<br>Epic™ Stented Tissue Valve (aortic)<br>Freestyle (Stentless) Aortic Root Bioprosthesis<br>Hancock Bioprosthesis (aortic) (mitral) valve<br>Hancock Bioprosthetic Valved Conduit<br>Melody® transcatheter pulmonary valve<br>Mitroflow® Aortic Pericardial Heart Valve<br>Mosaic Bioprosthesis (aortic) (mitral) valve<br>Porcine (bioprosthetic) valve<br>SAPIEN transcatheter aortic valve<br>SJM Biocor® Stented Valve System<br>Stented tissue valve<br>Trifecta™ Valve (aortic)<br>Xenograft |

# Appendix H: Substance Key/Substance Definitions



## Substance Key

This key classifies substances listed by trade name or synonym to a PCS character in the Administration or New Technology section indicated in the sixth-character Substance or seventh-character Qualifier column.

| Term | ICD-10-PCS Value |
|---|---|
| **AIGISRx Antibacterial Envelope** | Anti-Infective Envelope |
| **Antimicrobial envelope** | Anti-Infective Envelope |
| **Axicabtagene Ciloeucel** | Engineered Autologous Chimeric Antigen Receptor T-cell Immunotherapy |
| **Bone morphogenetic protein 2 (BMP 2)** | Recombinant Bone Morphogenetic Protein |
| **CBMA (Concentrated Bone Marrow Aspirate)** | Concentrated Bone Marrow Aspirate |
| **Clolar** | Clofarabine |
| **Defitelio** | Defibrotide Sodium Anticoagulant |
| **DuraGraft® Endothelial Damage Inhibitor** | Endothelial Damage Inhibitor |
| **Factor Xa Inhibitor Reversal Agent, Andexanet Alfa** | Andexanet Alfa, Factor Xa Inhibitor Reversal Agent |
| **Kcentra** | 4-Factor Prothrombin Complex Concentrate |
| **Nesiritide** | Human B-type Natriutretic Peptide |
| **rhBMP-2** | Recombinant Bone Morphogenetic Protein |
| **Seprafilm** | Adhesion Barrier |
| **STELARA®** | Other New Technology Therapeutic Substance |
| **Tissue Plasminogen Activator (tPA)(r-tPA)** | Other Thrombolytic |
| **Ustekinumab** | Other New Technology Therapeutic Substance |
| **Vistogard®** | Uridine Triacetate |
| **Voraxaze** | Glucarpidase |
| **VYXEOS™** | Cytarabine and Daunorubicin Liposome Antineoplastic |
| **ZINPLAVA™** | Bezlotoxumab Monoclonal Antibody |
| **Zyvox** | Oxazolidinones |

## Substance Definitions

| ICD-10-PCS Value | Definition |
|---|---|
| **4-Factor Prothrombin Complex Concentrate** | **Includes:**<br>Kcentra |
| **Adhesion Barrier** | **Includes:**<br>Seprafilm |
| **Andexanet Alfa, Factor Xa Inhibitor Reversal Agent** | **Includes:**<br>Factor Xa Inhibitor Reversal Agent, Andexanet Alfa |
| **Anti-Infective Envelope** | **Includes:**<br>AIGISRx Antibacterial Envelope<br>Antimicrobial envelope |
| **Bezlotoxumab Monoclonal Antibody** | **Includes:**<br>ZINPLAVA™ |
| **Clofarabine** | **Includes:**<br>Clolar |
| **Concentrated Bone Marrow Aspirate** | **Includes:**<br>CBMA (Concentrated Bone Marrow Aspirate) |
| **Cytarabine and Daunorubicin Liposome Antineoplastic** | **Includes:**<br>VYXEOS™ |
| **Defibrotide Sodium Anticoagulant** | **Includes:**<br>Defitelio |
| **Endothelial Damage Inhibitor** | **Includes:**<br>DuraGraft® Endothelial Damage Inhibitor |
| **Engineered Autologous Chimeric Antigen Receptor T-cell Immunotherapy** | **Includes:**<br>Axicabtagene Ciloeucel |
| **Glucarpidase** | **Includes:**<br>Voraxaze |

| ICD-10-PCS Value | Definition |
|---|---|
| **Human B-type Natriuretic Peptide** | **Includes:**<br>Nesiritide |
| **Other New Technology Therapeutic Substance** | **Includes:**<br>STELARA®<br>Ustekinumab |
| **Other Thrombolytic** | **Includes:**<br>Tissue Plasminogen Activator (tPA) (r-tPA) |
| **Oxazolidinones** | **Includes:**<br>Zyvox |
| **Recombinant Bone Morphogenetic Protein** | **Includes:**<br>Bone morphogenetic protein 2 (BMP 2)<br>rhBMP-2 |
| **Uridine Triacetate** | **Includes:**<br>Vistogard® |

# Appendix I: Sections B–H Character Definitions



## Section B–Imaging

| ICD-10-PCS Value (Character 3) | Definition |
|---|---|
| Computerized Tomography (CT Scan) (2) | Computer reformatted digital display of multiplanar images developed from the capture of multiple exposures of external ionizing radiation |
| Fluoroscopy (1) | Single plane or bi-plane real time display of an image developed from the capture of external ionizing radiation on a fluorescent screen. The image may also be stored by either digital or analog means. |
| Magnetic Resonance Imaging (MRI) (3) | Computer reformatted digital display of multiplanar images developed from the capture of radiofrequency signals emitted by nuclei in a body site excited within a magnetic field |
| Plain Radiography (Ø) | Planar display of an image developed from the capture of external ionizing radiation on photographic or photoconductive plate |
| Ultrasonography (4) | Real time display of images of anatomy or flow information developed from the capture of reflected and attenuated high frequency sound waves |

## Section C–Nuclear Medicine

| ICD-10-PCS Value (Character 3) | Definition |
|---|---|
| Nonimaging Nuclear Medicine Assay (6) | Introduction of radioactive materials into the body for the study of body fluids and blood elements, by the detection of radioactive emissions |
| Nonimaging Nuclear Medicine Probe (5) | Introduction of radioactive materials into the body for the study of distribution and fate of certain substances by the detection of radioactive emissions; or, alternatively, measurement of absorption of radioactive emissions from an external source |
| Nonimaging Nuclear Medicine Uptake (4) | Introduction of radioactive materials into the body for measurements of organ function, from the detection of radioactive emissions |
| Planar Nuclear Medicine Imaging (1) | Introduction of radioactive materials into the body for single plane display of images developed from the capture of radioactive emissions |
| Positron Emission Tomographic (PET) Imaging (3) | Introduction of radioactive materials into the body for three dimensional display of images developed from the simultaneous capture, 18Ø degrees apart, of radioactive emissions |
| Systemic Nuclear Medicine Therapy (7) | Introduction of unsealed radioactive materials into the body for treatment |
| Tomographic (Tomo) Nuclear Medicine Imaging (2) | Introduction of radioactive materials into the body for three dimensional display of images developed from the capture of radioactive emissions |

## Section F–Physical Rehabilitation and Diagnostic Audiology

| ICD-10-PCS Value (Character 3) | Definition |
|---|---|
| Activities of Daily Living Assessment (2) | Measurement of functional level for activities of daily living |
| Activities of Daily Living Treatment (8) | Exercise or activities to facilitate functional competence for activities of daily living |
| Caregiver Training (F) | Training in activities to support patient's optimal level of function |
| Cochlear Implant Treatment (B) | Application of techniques to improve the communication abilities of individuals with cochlear implant |
| Device Fitting (D) | Fitting of a device designed to facilitate or support achievement of a higher level of function |
| Hearing Aid Assessment (4) | Measurement of the appropriateness and/or effectiveness of a hearing device |
| Hearing Assessment (3) | Measurement of hearing and related functions |
| Hearing Treatment (9) | Application of techniques to improve, augment, or compensate for hearing and related functional impairment |
| Motor and/or Nerve Function Assessment (1) | Measurement of motor, nerve, and related functions |
| Motor Treatment (7) | Exercise or activities to increase or facilitate motor function |

*Continued on next page*

## Section F–Physical Rehabilitation and Diagnostic Audiology

*Continued from previous page*

| ICD-10-PCS Value (Character 3) | Definition |
|---|---|
| Speech Assessment (Ø) | Measurement of speech and related functions |
| Speech Treatment (6) | Application of techniques to improve, augment, or compensate for speech and related functional impairment |
| Vestibular Assessment (5) | Measurement of the vestibular system and related functions |
| Vestibular Treatment (C) | Application of techniques to improve, augment, or compensate for vestibular and related functional impairment |

## Section F–Physical Rehabilitation and Diagnostic Audiology

| ICD-10-PCS Value Qualifier (Character 5) | Definition |
|---|---|
| Acoustic Reflex Decay (J) | Measures reduction in size/strength of acoustic reflex over time<br>Includes/Examples: Includes site of lesion test |
| Acoustic Reflex Patterns (G) | Defines site of lesion based upon presence/absence of acoustic reflexes with ipsilateral vs. contralateral stimulation |
| Acoustic Reflex Threshold (H) | Determines minimal intensity that acoustic reflex occurs with ipsilateral and/or contralateral stimulation |
| Aerobic Capacity and Endurance (7) | Measures autonomic responses to positional changes; perceived exertion, dyspnea or angina during activity; performance during exercise protocols; standard vital signs; and blood gas analysis or oxygen consumption |
| Alternate Binaural or Monaural Loudness Balance (7) | Determines auditory stimulus parameter that yields the same objective sensation<br>Includes/Examples: Sound intensities that yield same loudness perception |
| Anthropometric Characteristics (B) | Measures edema, body fat composition, height, weight, length and girth |
| Aphasia (Assessment) (C) | Measures expressive and receptive speech and language function including reading and writing |
| Aphasia (Treatment) (3) | Applying techniques to improve, augment, or compensate for receptive/ expressive language impairments |
| Articulation/Phonology (Assessment) (9) | Measures speech production |
| Articulation/Phonology (Treatment) (4) | Applying techniques to correct, improve, or compensate for speech productive impairment |
| Assistive Listening Device (5) | Assists in use of effective and appropriate assistive listening device/system |
| Assistive Listening System/Device Selection (4) | Measures the effectiveness and appropriateness of assistive listening systems/devices |
| Assistive, Adaptive, Supportive or Protective Devices (9) | Explanation: Devices to facilitate or support achievement of a higher level of function in wheelchair mobility; bed mobility; transfer or ambulation ability; bath and showering ability; dressing; grooming; personal hygiene; play or leisure |
| Auditory Evoked Potentials (L) | Measures electric responses produced by the VIIIth cranial nerve and brainstem following auditory stimulation |
| Auditory Processing (Assessment) (Q) | Evaluates ability to receive and process auditory information and comprehension of spoken language |
| Auditory Processing (Treatment) (2) | Applying techniques to improve the receiving and processing of auditory information and comprehension of spoken language |
| Augmentative/Alternative Communication System (Assessment) (L) | Determines the appropriateness of aids, techniques, symbols, and/or strategies to augment or replace speech and enhance communication<br>Includes/Examples: Includes the use of telephones, writing equipment, emergency equipment, and TDD |
| Augmentative/Alternative Communication System (Treatment) (3) | Includes/Examples: Includes augmentative communication devices and aids |
| Aural Rehabilitation (5) | Applying techniques to improve the communication abilities associated with hearing loss |
| Aural Rehabilitation Status (P) | Measures impact of a hearing loss including evaluation of receptive and expressive communication skills |
| Bathing/Showering (Ø) | Includes/Examples: Includes obtaining and using supplies; soaping, rinsing, and drying body parts; maintaining bathing position; and transferring to and from bathing positions |

*Continued on next page*

## Section F–Physical Rehabilitation and Diagnostic Audiology

*Continued from previous page*

| ICD-10-PCS Value Qualifier (Character 5) | Definition |
|---|---|
| Bathing/Showering Techniques (Ø) | Activities to facilitate obtaining and using supplies, soaping, rinsing and drying body parts, maintaining bathing position, and transferring to and from bathing positions |
| Bed Mobility (Assessment) (B) | Transitional movement within bed |
| Bed Mobility (Treatment) (5) | Exercise or activities to facilitate transitional movements within bed |
| Bedside Swallowing and Oral Function (H) | Includes/Examples: Bedside swallowing includes assessment of sucking, masticating, coughing, and swallowing. Oral function includes assessment of musculature for controlled movements, structures, and functions to determine coordination and phonation. |
| Bekesy Audiometry (3) | Uses an instrument that provides a choice of discrete or continuously varying pure tones; choice of pulsed or continuous signal |
| Binaural Electroacoustic Hearing Aid Check (6) | Determines mechanical and electroacoustic function of bilateral hearing aids using hearing aid test box |
| Binaural Hearing Aid (Assessment) (3) | Measures the candidacy, effectiveness, and appropriateness of a hearing aid<br>Explanation: Measures bilateral fit |
| Binaural Hearing Aid (Treatment) (2) | Explanation: Assists in achieving maximum understanding and performance |
| Bithermal, Binaural Caloric Irrigation (Ø) | Measures the rhythmic eye movements stimulated by changing the temperature of the vestibular system |
| Bithermal, Monaural Caloric Irrigation (1) | Measures the rhythmic eye movements stimulated by changing the temperature of the vestibular system in one ear |
| Brief Tone Stimuli (R) | Measures specific central auditory process |
| Cerumen Management (3) | Includes examination of external auditory canal and tympanic membrane and removal of cerumen from external ear canal |
| Cochlear Implant (Ø) | Measures candidacy for cochlear implant |
| Cochlear Implant Rehabilitation (Ø) | Applying techniques to improve the communication abilities of individuals with cochlear implant; includes programming the device, providing patients/families with information |
| Communicative/Cognitive Integration Skills (Assessment) (G) | Measures ability to use higher cortical functions<br>Includes/Examples: Includes orientation, recognition, attention span, initiation and termination of activity, memory, sequencing, categorizing, concept formation, spatial operations, judgment, problem solving, generalization and pragmatic communication |
| Communicative/Cognitive Integration Skills (Treatment) (6) | Activities to facilitate the use of higher cortical functions<br>Includes/Examples: Includes level of arousal, orientation, recognition, attention span, initiation and termination of activity, memory sequencing, judgment and problem solving, learning and generalization, and pragmatic communication |
| Computerized Dynamic Posturography (6) | Measures the status of the peripheral and central vestibular system and the sensory/motor component of balance; evaluates the efficacy of vestibular rehabilitation |
| Conditioned Play Audiometry (4) | Behavioral measures using nonspeech and speech stimuli to obtain frequency-specific and ear-specific information on auditory status from the patient<br>Explanation: Obtains speech reception threshold by having patient point to pictures of spondaic words |
| Coordination/Dexterity (Assessment) (3) | Measures large and small muscle groups for controlled goal-directed movements<br>Explanation: Dexterity includes object manipulation |
| Coordination/Dexterity (Treatment) (2) | Exercise or activities to facilitate gross coordination and fine coordination |
| Cranial Nerve Integrity (9) | Measures cranial nerve sensory and motor functions, including tastes, smell and facial expression |
| Dichotic Stimuli (T) | Measures specific central auditory process |
| Distorted Speech (S) | Measures specific central auditory process |
| Dix-Hallpike Dynamic (5) | Measures nystagmus following Dix-Hallpike maneuver |
| Dressing (1) | Includes/Examples: Includes selecting clothing and accessories, obtaining clothing from storage, dressing, fastening and adjusting clothing and shoes, and applying and removing personal devices, prosthesis or orthosis |

*Continued on next page*

## Section F–Physical Rehabilitation and Diagnostic Audiology

*Continued from previous page*

| ICD-10-PCS Value Qualifier (Character 5) | Definition |
|---|---|
| Dressing Techniques (1) | Activities to facilitate selecting clothing and accessories, dressing and undressing, adjusting clothing and shoes, applying and removing devices, prostheses or orthoses |
| Dynamic Orthosis (6) | Includes/Examples: Includes customized and prefabricated splints, inhibitory casts, spinal and other braces, and protective devices; allows motion through transfer of movement from other body parts or by use of outside forces |
| Ear Canal Probe Microphone (1) | Real ear measures |
| Ear Protector Attentuation (7) | Measures ear protector fit and effectiveness |
| Electrocochleography (K) | Measures the VIII$^{th}$ cranial nerve action potential |
| Environmental, Home, Work Barriers (B) | Measures current and potential barriers to optimal function, including safety hazards, access problems and home or office design |
| Ergonomics and Body Mechanics (C) | Ergonomic measurement of job tasks, work hardening or work conditioning needs; functional capacity; and body mechanics |
| Eustachian Tube Function (F) | Measures eustachian tube function and patency of eustachian tube |
| Evoked Otoacoustic Emissions, Diagnostic (N) | Measures auditory evoked potentials in a diagnostic format |
| Evoked Otoacoustic Emissions, Screening (M) | Measures auditory evoked potentials in a screening format |
| Facial Nerve Function (7) | Measures electrical activity of the VII$^{th}$ cranial nerve (facial nerve) |
| Feeding/Eating (Assessment) (2) | Includes/Examples: Includes setting up food, selecting and using utensils and tableware, bringing food or drink to mouth, cleaning face, hands, and clothing, and management of alternative methods of nourishment |
| Feeding/Eating (Treatment) (3) | Exercise or activities to facilitate setting up food, selecting and using utensils and tableware, bringing food or drink to mouth, cleaning face, hands, and clothing, and management of alternative methods of nourishment |
| Filtered Speech (Ø) | Uses high or low pass filtered speech stimuli to assess central auditory processing disorders, site of lesion testing |
| Fluency (Assessment) (D) | Measures speech fluency or stuttering |
| Fluency (Treatment) (7) | Applying techniques to improve and augment fluent speech |
| Gait and/or Balance (D) | Measures biomechanical, arthrokinematic and other spatial and temporal characteristics of gait and balance |
| Gait Training/Functional Ambulation (9) | Exercise or activities to facilitate ambulation on a variety of surfaces and in a variety of environments |
| Grooming/Personal Hygiene (Assessment) (3) | Includes/Examples: Includes ability to obtain and use supplies in a sequential fashion, general grooming, oral hygiene, toilet hygiene, personal care devices, including care for artificial airways |
| Grooming/Personal Hygiene (Treatment) (2) | Activities to facilitate obtaining and using supplies in a sequential fashion: general grooming, oral hygiene, toilet hygiene, cleaning body, and personal care devices, including artificial airways |
| Hearing and Related Disorders Counseling (Ø) | Provides patients/families/caregivers with information, support, referrals to facilitate recovery from a communication disorder<br>Includes/Examples: Includes strategies for psychosocial adjustment to hearing loss for clients and families/caregivers |
| Hearing and Related Disorders Prevention (1) | Provides patients/families/caregivers with information and support to prevent communication disorders |
| Hearing Screening (Ø) | Pass/refer measures designed to identify need for further audiologic assessment |
| Home Management (Assessment) (4) | Obtaining and maintaining personal and household possessions and environment<br>Includes/Examples: Includes clothing care, cleaning, meal preparation and cleanup, shopping, money management, household maintenance, safety procedures, and childcare/parenting |
| Home Management (Treatment) (4) | Activities to facilitate obtaining and maintaining personal household possessions and environment<br>Includes/Examples: Includes clothing care, cleaning, meal preparation and clean-up, shopping, money management, household maintenance, safety procedures, childcare/parenting |

*Continued on next page*

## Section F–Physical Rehabilitation and Diagnostic Audiology

Continued from previous page

| ICD-10-PCS Value Qualifier (Character 5) | Definition |
|---|---|
| Instrumental Swallowing and Oral Function (J) | Measures swallowing function using instrumental diagnostic procedures<br>Explanation: Methods include videofluoroscopy, ultrasound, manometry, endoscopy |
| Integumentary Integrity (1) | Includes/Examples: Includes burns, skin conditions, ecchymosis, bleeding, blisters, scar tissue, wounds and other traumas, tissue mobility, turgor and texture |
| Manual Therapy Techniques (7) | Techniques in which the therapist uses his/her hands to administer skilled movements<br>Includes/Examples: Includes connective tissue massage, joint mobilization and manipulation, manual lymph drainage, manual traction, soft tissue mobilization and manipulation |
| Masking Patterns (W) | Measures central auditory processing status |
| Monaural Electroacoustic Hearing Aid Check (8) | Determines mechanical and electroacoustic function of one hearing aid using hearing aid test box |
| Monaural Hearing Aid (Assessment) (2) | Measures the candidacy, effectiveness, and appropriateness of a hearing aid<br>Explanation: Measures unilateral fit |
| Monaural Hearing Aid (Treatment) (1) | Explanation: Assists in achieving maximum understanding and performance |
| Motor Function (Assessment) (4) | Measures the body's functional and versatile movement patterns<br>Includes/Examples: Includes motor assessment scales, analysis of head, trunk and limb movement, and assessment of motor learning |
| Motor Function (Treatment) (3) | Exercise or activities to facilitate crossing midline, laterality, bilateral integration, praxis, neuromuscular relaxation, inhibition, facilitation, motor function and motor learning |
| Motor Speech (Assessment) (B) | Measures neurological motor aspects of speech production |
| Motor Speech (Treatment) (8) | Applying techniques to improve and augment the impaired neurological motor aspects of speech production |
| Muscle Performance (Assessment) (Ø) | Measures muscle strength, power and endurance using manual testing, dynamometry or computer-assisted electromechanical muscle test; functional muscle strength, power and endurance; muscle pain, tone, or soreness; or pelvic-floor musculature<br>Explanation: Muscle endurance refers to the ability to contract a muscle repeatedly over time |
| Muscle Performance (Treatment) (1) | Exercise or activities to increase the capacity of a muscle to do work in terms of strength, power, and/or endurance<br>Explanation: Muscle strength is the force exerted to overcome resistance in one maximal effort. Muscle power is work produced per unit of time, or the product of strength and speed. Muscle endurance is the ability to contract a muscle repeatedly over time. |
| Neuromotor Development (D) | Measures motor development, righting and equilibrium reactions, and reflex and equilibrium reactions |
| Non-invasive Instrumental Status (N) | Instrumental measures of oral, nasal, vocal, and velopharyngeal functions as they pertain to speech production |
| Nonspoken Language (Assessment) (7) | Measures nonspoken language (print, sign, symbols) for communication |
| Nonspoken Language (Treatment) (Ø) | Applying techniques that improve, augment, or compensate spoken communication |
| Oral Peripheral Mechanism (P) | Structural measures of face, jaw, lips, tongue, teeth, hard and soft palate, pharynx as related to speech production |
| Orofacial Myofunctional (Assessment) (K) | Measures orofacial myofunctional patterns for speech and related functions |
| Orofacial Myofunctional (Treatment) (9) | Applying techniques to improve, alter, or augment impaired orofacial myofunctional patterns and related speech production errors |
| Oscillating Tracking (3) | Measures ability to visually track |
| Pain (F) | Measures muscle soreness, pain and soreness with joint movement, and pain perception<br>Includes/Examples: Includes questionnaires, graphs, symptom magnification scales or visual analog scales |
| Perceptual Processing (Assessment) (5) | Measures stereognosis, kinesthesia, body schema, right-left discrimination, form constancy, position in space, visual closure, figure-ground, depth perception, spatial relations and topographical orientation |

Continued on next page

## Section F–Physical Rehabilitation and Diagnostic Audiology

*Continued from previous page*

| ICD-10-PCS Value Qualifier (Character 5) | Definition |
|---|---|
| Perceptual Processing (Treatment)<br>(1) | Exercise and activities to facilitate perceptual processing<br>Explanation: Includes stereognosis, kinesthesia, body schema, right-left discrimination, form constancy, position in space, visual closure, figure-ground, depth perception, spatial relations, and topographical orientation<br>Includes/Examples: Includes stereognosis, kinesthesia, body schema, right-left discrimination, form constancy, position in space, visual closure, figure-ground, depth perception, spatial relations, and topographical orientation |
| Performance Intensity Phonetically Balanced Speech Discrimination<br>(Q) | Measures word recognition over varying intensity levels |
| Postural Control<br>(3) | Exercise or activities to increase postural alignment and control |
| Prosthesis<br>(8) | Explanation: Artificial substitutes for missing body parts that augment performance or function<br>Includes/Examples: Limb prosthesis, ocular prosthesis |
| Psychosocial Skills (Assessment)<br>(6) | The ability to interact in society and to process emotions<br>Includes/Examples: Includes psychological (values, interests, self-concept); social (role performance, social conduct, interpersonal skills, self expression); self-management (coping skills, time management, self-control) |
| Psychosocial Skills (Treatment)<br>(6) | The ability to interact in society and to process emotions<br>Includes/Examples: Includes psychological (values, interests, self-concept); social (role performance, social conduct, interpersonal skills, self expression); self-management (coping skills, time management, self-control) |
| Pure Tone Audiometry, Air<br>(1) | Air-conduction pure tone threshold measures with appropriate masking |
| Pure Tone Audiometry, Air and Bone<br>(2) | Air-conduction and bone-conduction pure tone threshold measures with appropriate masking |
| Pure Tone Stenger<br>(C) | Measures unilateral nonorganic hearing loss based on simultaneous presentation of pure tones of differing volume |
| Range of Motion and Joint Integrity<br>(5) | Measures quantity, quality, grade, and classification of joint movement and/or mobility<br>Explanation: Range of Motion is the space, distance or angle through which movement occurs at a joint or series of joints. Joint integrity is the conformance of joints to expected anatomic, biomechanical and kinematic norms. |
| Range of Motion and Joint Mobility<br>(Ø) | Exercise or activities to increase muscle length and joint mobility |
| Receptive/Expressive Language (Assessment)<br>(8) | Measures receptive and expressive language |
| Receptive/Expressive Language (Treatment)<br>(B) | Applying techniques to improve and augment receptive/expressive language |
| Reflex Integrity<br>(G) | Measures the presence, absence, or exaggeration of developmentally appropriate, pathologic or normal reflexes |
| Select Picture Audiometry<br>(5) | Establishes hearing threshold levels for speech using pictures |
| Sensorineural Acuity Level<br>(4) | Measures sensorineural acuity masking presented via bone conduction |
| Sensory Aids<br>(5) | Determines the appropriateness of a sensory prosthetic device, other than a hearing aid or assistive listening system/device |
| Sensory Awareness/ Processing/ Integrity<br>(6) | Includes/Examples: Includes light touch, pressure, temperature, pain, sharp/dull, proprioception, vestibular, visual, auditory, gustatory, and olfactory |
| Short Increment Sensitivity Index<br>(9) | Measures the ear's ability to detect small intensity changes; site of lesion test requiring a behavioral response |
| Sinusoidal Vertical Axis Rotational<br>(4) | Measures nystagmus following rotation |
| Somatosensory Evoked Potentials<br>(9) | Measures neural activity from sites throughout the body |
| Speech/Language Screening<br>(6) | Identifies need for further speech and/or language evaluation |
| Speech Threshold<br>(1) | Measures minimal intensity needed to repeat spondaic words |

*Continued on next page*

## Section F–Physical Rehabilitation and Diagnostic Audiology

*Continued from previous page*

| ICD-10-PCS Value Qualifier (Character 5) | Definition |
|---|---|
| Speech-Language Pathology and Related Disorders Counseling (1) | Provides patients/families with information, support, referrals to facilitate recovery from a communication disorder |
| Speech-Language Pathology and Related Disorders Prevention (2) | Applying techniques to avoid or minimize onset and/or development of a communication disorder |
| Speech/Word Recognition (2) | Measures ability to repeat/identify single syllable words; scores given as a percentage; includes word recognition/speech discrimination |
| Staggered Spondaic Word (3) | Measures central auditory processing site of lesion based upon dichotic presentation of spondaic words |
| Static Orthosis (7) | Includes/Examples: Includes customized and prefabricated splints, inhibitory casts, spinal and other braces, and protective devices; has no moving parts, maintains joint(s) in desired position |
| Stenger (B) | Measures unilateral nonorganic hearing loss based on simultaneous presentation of signals of differing volume |
| Swallowing Dysfunction (D) | Activities to improve swallowing function in coordination with respiratory function<br>Includes/Examples: Includes function and coordination of sucking, mastication, coughing, swallowing |
| Synthetic Sentence Identification (5) | Measures central auditory dysfunction using identification of third order approximations of sentences and competing messages |
| Temporal Ordering of Stimuli (V) | Measures specific central auditory process |
| Therapeutic Exercise (6) | Exercise or activities to facilitate sensory awareness, sensory processing, sensory integration, balance training, conditioning, reconditioning<br>Includes/Examples: Includes developmental activities, breathing exercises, aerobic endurance activities, aquatic exercises, stretching and ventilatory muscle training |
| Tinnitus Masker (Assessment) (7) | Determines candidacy for tinnitus masker |
| Tinnitus Masker (Treatment) (Ø) | Explanation: Used to verify physical fit, acoustic appropriateness, and benefit; assists in achieving maximum benefit |
| Tone Decay (8) | Measures decrease in hearing sensitivity to a tone; site of lesion test requiring a behavioral response |
| Transfer (C) | Transitional movement from one surface to another |
| Transfer Training (8) | Exercise or activities to facilitate movement from one surface to another |
| Tympanometry (D) | Measures the integrity of the middle ear; measures ease at which sound flows through the tympanic membrane while air pressure against the membrane is varied |
| Unithermal Binaural Screen (2) | Measures the rhythmic eye movements stimulated by changing the temperature of the vestibular system in both ears using warm water, screening format |
| Ventilation/Respiration/Circulation (G) | Measures ventilatory muscle strength, power and endurance, pulmonary function and ventilatory mechanics<br>Includes/Examples: Includes ability to clear airway, activities that aggravate or relieve edema, pain, dyspnea or other symptoms, chest wall mobility, cardiopulmonary response to performance of ADL and IAD, cough and sputum, standard vital signs |
| Vestibular (Ø) | Applying techniques to compensate for balance disorders; includes habituation, exercise therapy, and balance retraining |
| Visual Motor Integration (Assessment) (2) | Coordinating the interaction of information from the eyes with body movement during activity |
| Visual Motor Integration (Treatment) (2) | Exercise or activities to facilitate coordinating the interaction of information from eyes with body movement during activity |
| Visual Reinforcement Audiometry (6) | Behavioral measures using nonspeech and speech stimuli to obtain frequency/ear-specific information on auditory status<br>Includes/Examples: Includes a conditioned response of looking toward a visual reinforcer (e.g., lights, animated toy) every time auditory stimuli are heard |
| Vocational Activities and Functional Community or Work Reintegration Skills (Assessment) (H) | Measures environmental, home, work (job/school/play) barriers that keep patients from functioning optimally in their environment<br>Includes/Examples: Includes assessment of vocational skills and interests, environment of work (job/school/play), injury potential and injury prevention or reduction, ergonomic stressors, transportation skills, and ability to access and use community resources |

*Continued on next page*

## Section F–Physical Rehabilitation and Diagnostic Audiology

*Continued from previous page*

| ICD-10-PCS Value Qualifier (Character 5) | Definition |
|---|---|
| Vocational Activities and Functional Community or Work Reintegration Skills (Treatment)<br>(7) | Activities to facilitate vocational exploration, body mechanics training, job acquisition, and environmental or work (job/school/play) task adaptation<br>Includes/Examples: Includes injury prevention and reduction, ergonomic stressor reduction, job coaching and simulation, work hardening and conditioning, driving training, transportation skills, and use of community resources |
| Voice (Assessment)<br>(F) | Measures vocal structure, function and production |
| Voice (Treatment)<br>(C) | Applying techniques to improve voice and vocal function |
| Voice Prosthetic (Assessment)<br>(M) | Determines the appropriateness of voice prosthetic/adaptive device to enhance or facilitate communication |
| Voice Prosthetic (Treatment)<br>(4) | Includes/Examples: Includes electrolarynx, and other assistive, adaptive, supportive devices |
| Wheelchair Mobility (Assessment)<br>(F) | Measures fit and functional abilities within wheelchair in a variety of environments |
| Wheelchair Mobility (Treatment)<br>(4) | Management, maintenance and controlled operation of a wheelchair, scooter or other device, in and on a variety of surfaces and environments |
| Wound Management<br>(5) | Includes/Examples: Includes non-selective and selective debridement (enzymes, autolysis, sharp debridement), dressings (wound coverings, hydrogel, vacuum-assisted closure), topical agents, etc. |

## Section G–Mental Health

| ICD-10-PCS Value (Character 3) | Definition |
|---|---|
| Biofeedback<br>(C) | Provision of information from the monitoring and regulating of physiological processes in conjunction with cognitive-behavioral techniques to improve patient functioning or well-being<br>Includes/Examples: Includes EEG, blood pressure, skin temperature or peripheral blood flow, ECG, electrooculogram, EMG, respirometry or capnometry, GSR/EDR, perineometry to monitor/regulate bowel/bladder activity, electrogastrogram to monitor/regulate gastric motility |
| Counseling<br>(6) | The application of psychological methods to treat an individual with normal developmental issues and psychological problems in order to increase function, improve well-being, alleviate distress, maladjustment or resolve crises |
| Crisis Intervention<br>(2) | Treatment of a traumatized, acutely disturbed or distressed individual for the purpose of short-term stabilization<br>Includes/Examples: Includes defusing, debriefing, counseling, psychotherapy and/or coordination of care with other providers or agencies |
| Electroconvulsive Therapy<br>(B) | The application of controlled electrical voltages to treat a mental health disorder<br>Includes/Examples: Includes appropriate sedation and other preparation of the individual |
| Family Psychotherapy<br>(7) | Treatment that includes one or more family members of an individual with a mental health disorder by behavioral, cognitive, psychoanalytic, psychodynamic or psychophysiological means to improve functioning or well-being<br>Explanation: Remediation of emotional or behavioral problems presented by one or more family members in cases where psychotherapy with more than one family member is indicated |
| Group Psychotherapy<br>(H) | Treatment of two or more individuals with a mental health disorder by behavioral, cognitive, psychoanalytic, psychodynamic or psychophysiological means to improve functioning or well-being |
| Hypnosis<br>(F) | Induction of a state of heightened suggestibility by auditory, visual and tactile techniques to elicit an emotional or behavioral response |
| Individual Psychotherapy<br>(5) | Treatment of an individual with a mental health disorder by behavioral, cognitive, psychoanalytic, psychodynamic or psychophysiological means to improve functioning or well-being |
| Light Therapy<br>(J) | Application of specialized light treatments to improve functioning or well-being |
| Medication Management<br>(3) | Monitoring and adjusting the use of medications for the treatment of a mental health disorder |
| Narcosynthesis<br>(G) | Administration of intravenous barbiturates in order to release suppressed or repressed thoughts |
| Psychological Tests<br>(1) | The administration and interpretation of standardized psychological tests and measurement instruments for the assessment of psychological function |

*Continued on next page*

## Section G–Mental Health

| ICD-10-PCS Value Qualifier (Character 4) | Definition |
|---|---|
| Behavioral<br>(1) | Primarily to modify behavior<br>Includes/Examples: Includes modeling and role playing, positive reinforcement of target behaviors, response cost, and training of self-management skills |
| Cognitive<br>(2) | Primarily to correct cognitive distortions and errors |
| Cognitive-Behavioral<br>(8) | Combining cognitive and behavioral treatment strategies to improve functioning<br>Explanation: Maladaptive responses are examined to determine how cognitions relate to behavior patterns in response to an event. Uses learning principles and information-processing models. |
| Developmental<br>(Ø) | Age-normed developmental status of cognitive, social and adaptive behavior skills |
| Intellectual and Psychoeducational<br>(2) | Intellectual abilities, academic achievement and learning capabilities (including behaviors and emotional factors affecting learning) |
| Interactive<br>(Ø) | Uses primarily physical aids and other forms of non-oral interaction with a patient who is physically, psychologically or developmentally unable to use ordinary language for communication<br>Includes/Examples: Includes the use of toys in symbolic play |
| Interpersonal<br>(3) | Helps an individual make changes in interpersonal behaviors to reduce psychological dysfunction<br>Includes/Examples: Includes exploratory techniques, encouragement of affective expression, clarification of patient statements, analysis of communication patterns, use of therapy relationship and behavior change techniques |
| Neurobehavioral and Cognitive Status<br>(4) | Includes neurobehavioral status exam, interview(s), and observation for the clinical assessment of thinking, reasoning and judgment, acquired knowledge, attention, memory, visual spatial abilities, language functions, and planning |
| Neuropsychological<br>(3) | Thinking, reasoning and judgment, acquired knowledge, attention, memory, visual spatial abilities, language functions, planning |
| Personality and Behavioral<br>(1) | Mood, emotion, behavior, social functioning, psychopathological conditions, personality traits and characteristics |
| Psychoanalysis<br>(4) | Methods of obtaining a detailed account of past and present mental and emotional experiences to determine the source and eliminate or diminish the undesirable effects of unconscious conflicts<br>Explanation: Accomplished by making the individual aware of their existence, origin, and inappropriate expression in emotions and behavior |
| Psychodynamic<br>(5) | Exploration of past and present emotional experiences to understand motives and drives using insight-oriented techniques to reduce the undesirable effects of internal conflicts on emotions and behavior<br>Explanation: Techniques include empathetic listening, clarifying self-defeating behavior patterns, and exploring adaptive alternatives |
| Psychophysiological<br>(9) | Monitoring and alteration of physiological processes to help the individual associate physiological reactions combined with cognitive and behavioral strategies to gain improved control of these processes to help the individual cope more effectively |
| Supportive<br>(6) | Formation of therapeutic relationship primarily for providing emotional support to prevent further deterioration in functioning during periods of particular stress<br>Explanation: Often used in conjunction with other therapeutic approaches |
| Vocational<br>(1) | Exploration of vocational interests, aptitudes and required adaptive behavior skills to develop and carry out a plan for achieving a successful vocational placement<br>Includes/Examples: Includes enhancing work related adjustment and/or pursuing viable options in training education or preparation |

## Section H - Substance Abuse Treatment

| ICD-10-PCS Value (Character 3) | Definition |
|---|---|
| Detoxification Services<br>(2) | Detoxification from alcohol and/or drugs<br>Explanation: Not a treatment modality, but helps the patient stabilize physically and psychologically until the body becomes free of drugs and the effects of alcohol |
| Family Counseling<br>(6) | The application of psychological methods that includes one or more family members to treat an individual with addictive behavior<br>Explanation: Provides support and education for family members of addicted individuals. Family member participation is seen as a critical area of substance abuse treatment. |
| Group Counseling<br>(4) | The application of psychological methods to treat two or more individuals with addictive behavior<br>Explanation: Provides structured group counseling sessions and healing power through the connection with others |
| Individual Counseling<br>(3) | The application of psychological methods to treat an individual with addictive behavior<br>Explanation: Comprised of several different techniques, which apply various strategies to address drug addiction |
| Individual Psychotherapy<br>(5) | Treatment of an individual with addictive behavior by behavioral, cognitive, psychoanalytic, psychodynamic or psychophysiological means |
| Medication Management<br>(8) | Monitoring and adjusting the use of replacement medications for the treatment of addiction |
| Pharmacotherapy<br>(9) | The use of replacement medications for the treatment of addiction |

# Appendix J: Hospital Acquired Conditions

Hospital-acquired conditions (HACs) are conditions considered reasonably preventable through the application of evidence-based guidelines. Although it is the ICD-10-CM code that drives a HAC designation, in some cases a specific ICD-10-PCS code must also be present before that ICD-10-CM code can be considered a HAC. For example, the yellow color bar identifies ØJH63XZ as a HAC in the tabular section of this manual. In the annotation box below table ØJH it is noted that when the ICD-1Ø-CM code J95.811 is reported as a secondary diagnosis, not present on admission, AND ØJH63XZ is also reported during that same admission, J95.811 would be considered a hospital-acquired condition. This resource provides all 14 HAC categories, as well as the specific ICD-10-CM codes and, when applicable, the specific ICD-10-PCS codes applicable to each category.

**Note:** The resource used to compile this list is the fiscal 2017 ICD-10 MS-DRG Definitions Manual Files v34. The most current version, v35, of ICD-10 MS-DRG Definitions Manual was not available at the time this book was printed. For the most current files related to IPPS please refer to the following: https://www.cms.gov/Medicare/Medicare-Fee-for-Service-Payment/AcuteInpatientPPS/IPPS-Regulations-and-Notices.html.

**HAC 01: Foreign Object Retained After Surgery**

Secondary diagnosis not POA:

T81.5ØØA
T81.5Ø1A
T81.5Ø2A
T81.5Ø3A
T81.5Ø4A
T81.5Ø5A
T81.5Ø6A
T81.5Ø7A
T81.5Ø8A
T81.5Ø9A
T81.51ØA
T81.511A
T81.512A
T81.513A
T81.514A
T81.515A
T81.516A
T81.517A
T81.518A
T81.519A
T81.52ØA
T81.521A
T81.522A
T81.523A
T81.524A
T81.525A
T81.526A
T81.527A
T81.528A
T81.529A
T81.53ØA
T81.531A
T81.532A
T81.533A
T81.534A
T81.535A
T81.536A
T81.537A
T81.538A
T81.539A
T81.59ØA
T81.591A
T81.592A
T81.593A
T81.594A
T81.595A
T81.596A
T81.597A
T81.598A
T81.599A
T81.6ØXA
T81.61XA
T81.69XA

**HAC 02: Air Embolism**

Secondary diagnosis not POA:

T8Ø.ØXXA

**HAC 03: Blood Incompatibility**

Secondary diagnosis not POA:

T8Ø.3ØXA
T8Ø.31ØA
T8Ø.311A
T8Ø.319A
T8Ø.39XA

**HAC 04: Stage III and IV Pressure Ulcers**

Secondary diagnosis not POA:

L89.ØØ3
L89.ØØ4
L89.Ø13
L89.Ø14
L89.Ø23
L89.Ø24
L89.1Ø3
L89.1Ø4
L89.113
L89.114
L89.123
L89.124
L89.133
L89.134
L89.143
L89.144
L89.153
L89.154
L89.2Ø3
L89.2Ø4
L89.213
L89.214
L89.223
L89.224
L89.3Ø3
L89.3Ø4
L89.313
L89.314
L89.323
L89.324
L89.43
L89.44
L89.5Ø3
L89.5Ø4
L89.513
L89.514
L89.523
L89.524
L89.6Ø3
L89.6Ø4
L89.613
L89.614
L89.623
L89.624
L89.813
L89.814
L89.893
L89.894
L89.93
L89.94

**HAC 05: Falls and Trauma**

Secondary diagnosis not POA:

M99.1Ø
M99.11
M99.18
SØ2.ØXXA
SØ2.ØXXB
SØ2.1Ø1A
SØ2.1Ø1B
SØ2.1Ø2A
SØ2.1Ø2B
SØ2.1Ø9A
SØ2.1Ø9B
SØ2.11ØA
SØ2.11ØB
SØ2.111A
SØ2.111B
SØ2.112A
SØ2.112B
SØ2.113A
SØ2.113B
SØ2.118A
SØ2.118B
SØ2.119A
SØ2.119B
SØ2.11AA
SØ2.11AB
SØ2.11BA
SØ2.11BB
SØ2.11CA
SØ2.11CB
SØ2.11DA
SØ2.11DB
SØ2.11EA
SØ2.11EB
SØ2.11FA
SØ2.11FB
SØ2.11GA
SØ2.11GB
SØ2.11HA
SØ2.11HB
SØ2.19XA
SØ2.19XB
SØ2.2XXB
SØ2.3ØXA
SØ2.3ØXB
SØ2.31XA
SØ2.31XB
SØ2.32XA
SØ2.32XB
SØ2.4ØØA
SØ2.4ØØB
SØ2.4Ø1A
SØ2.4Ø1B
SØ2.4Ø2A
SØ2.4Ø2B
SØ2.4ØAA
SØ2.4ØAB
SØ2.4ØBA
SØ2.4ØBB
SØ2.4ØCA
SØ2.4ØCB
SØ2.4ØDA
SØ2.4ØDB
SØ2.4ØEA
SØ2.4ØEB
SØ2.4ØFA
SØ2.4ØFB
SØ2.411A
SØ2.411B
SØ2.412A
SØ2.412B
SØ2.413A
SØ2.413B
SØ2.42XA
SØ2.42XB
SØ2.6ØØA
SØ2.6ØØB
SØ2.6Ø1A
SØ2.6Ø1B
SØ2.6Ø2A
SØ2.6Ø2B
SØ2.6Ø9A
SØ2.6Ø9B
SØ2.61ØA
SØ2.61ØB
SØ2.611A
SØ2.611B
SØ2.612A
SØ2.612B
SØ2.62ØA
SØ2.62ØB
SØ2.621A
SØ2.621B
SØ2.622A
SØ2.622B
SØ2.63ØA
SØ2.63ØB
SØ2.631A
SØ2.631B
SØ2.632A
SØ2.632B
SØ2.64ØA
SØ2.64ØB
SØ2.641A
SØ2.641B
SØ2.642A
SØ2.642B
SØ2.65ØA
SØ2.65ØB
SØ2.651A
SØ2.651B
SØ2.652A
SØ2.652B
SØ2.66XA
SØ2.66XB
SØ2.67ØA
SØ2.67ØB
SØ2.671A
SØ2.671B
SØ2.672A
SØ2.672B
SØ2.69XA
SØ2.69XB
SØ2.8ØXA
SØ2.8ØXB
SØ2.81XA
SØ2.81XB
SØ2.82XA
SØ2.82XB
SØ2.91XA
SØ2.91XB
SØ2.92XA
SØ2.92XB
SØ6.ØX1A
SØ6.ØX9A
SØ6.1X1A
SØ6.1X2A
SØ6.1X3A
SØ6.1X4A
SØ6.1X5A
SØ6.1X6A
SØ6.1X7A
SØ6.1X8A
SØ6.1X9A
SØ6.2X1A
SØ6.2X2A
SØ6.2X3A
SØ6.2X4A
SØ6.2X5A
SØ6.2X6A
SØ6.2X7A
SØ6.2X8A
SØ6.2X9A
SØ6.3Ø1A
SØ6.3Ø2A
SØ6.3Ø3A
SØ6.3Ø4A
SØ6.3Ø5A
SØ6.3Ø6A
SØ6.3Ø7A
SØ6.3Ø8A
SØ6.3Ø9A
SØ6.31ØA
SØ6.311A
SØ6.312A
SØ6.313A
SØ6.314A
SØ6.315A
SØ6.316A
SØ6.317A
SØ6.318A
SØ6.319A
SØ6.32ØA
SØ6.321A
SØ6.322A
SØ6.323A
SØ6.324A
SØ6.325A
SØ6.326A
SØ6.327A
SØ6.328A
SØ6.329A
SØ6.33ØA
SØ6.331A
SØ6.332A
SØ6.333A
SØ6.334A
SØ6.335A
SØ6.336A
SØ6.337A
SØ6.338A
SØ6.339A
SØ6.34ØA
SØ6.341A
SØ6.342A
SØ6.343A
SØ6.344A
SØ6.345A
SØ6.346A
SØ6.347A
SØ6.348A
SØ6.349A
SØ6.35ØA
SØ6.351A
SØ6.352A
SØ6.353A
SØ6.354A
SØ6.355A
SØ6.356A
SØ6.357A
SØ6.358A
SØ6.359A
SØ6.36ØA
SØ6.361A
SØ6.362A
SØ6.363A
SØ6.364A
SØ6.365A
SØ6.366A
SØ6.367A
SØ6.368A
SØ6.369A
SØ6.37ØA

**HAC 05: Falls and Trauma (continued)**

S06.371A
S06.372A
S06.373A
S06.374A
S06.375A
S06.376A
S06.377A
S06.378A
S06.379A
S06.380A
S06.381A
S06.382A
S06.383A
S06.384A
S06.385A
S06.386A
S06.387A
S06.388A
S06.389A
S06.4X0A
S06.4X1A
S06.4X2A
S06.4X3A
S06.4X4A
S06.4X5A
S06.4X6A
S06.4X7A
S06.4X8A
S06.4X9A
S06.5X0A
S06.5X1A
S06.5X2A
S06.5X3A
S06.5X4A
S06.5X5A
S06.5X6A
S06.5X7A
S06.5X8A
S06.5X9A
S06.6X0A
S06.6X1A
S06.6X2A
S06.6X3A
S06.6X4A
S06.6X5A
S06.6X6A
S06.6X7A
S06.6X8A
S06.6X9A
S06.811A
S06.812A
S06.813A
S06.814A
S06.815A
S06.816A
S06.817A
S06.818A
S06.819A
S06.821A
S06.822A
S06.823A
S06.824A
S06.825A
S06.826A
S06.827A
S06.828A
S06.829A
S06.891A
S06.892A
S06.893A
S06.894A
S06.895A
S06.896A
S06.897A
S06.898A
S06.899A
S06.9X1A
S06.9X2A
S06.9X3A
S06.9X4A
S06.9X5A
S06.9X6A
S06.9X7A
S06.9X8A
S06.9X9A
S07.0XXA
S07.1XXA
S07.8XXA
S07.9XXA
S12.000A
S12.000B
S12.001A
S12.001B
S12.01XA
S12.01XB
S12.02XA
S12.02XB
S12.030A
S12.030B
S12.031A
S12.031B
S12.040A
S12.040B
S12.041A
S12.041B
S12.090A
S12.090B
S12.091A
S12.091B
S12.100A
S12.100B
S12.101A
S12.101B
S12.110A
S12.110B
S12.111A
S12.111B
S12.112A
S12.112B
S12.120A
S12.120B
S12.121A
S12.121B
S12.130A
S12.130B
S12.131A
S12.131B
S12.14XA
S12.14XB
S12.150A
S12.150B
S12.151A
S12.151B
S12.190A
S12.190B
S12.191A
S12.191B
S12.200A
S12.200B
S12.201A
S12.201B
S12.230A
S12.230B
S12.231A
S12.231B
S12.24XA
S12.24XB
S12.250A
S12.250B
S12.251A
S12.251B
S12.290A
S12.290B
S12.291A
S12.291B
S12.300A
S12.300B
S12.301A
S12.301B
S12.330A
S12.330B
S12.331A
S12.331B
S12.34XA
S12.34XB
S12.350A
S12.350B
S12.351A
S12.351B
S12.390A
S12.390B
S12.391A
S12.391B
S12.400A
S12.400B
S12.401A
S12.401B
S12.430A
S12.430B
S12.431A
S12.431B
S12.44XA
S12.44XB
S12.450A
S12.450B
S12.451A
S12.451B
S12.490A
S12.490B
S12.491A
S12.491B
S12.500A
S12.500B
S12.501A
S12.501B
S12.530A
S12.530B
S12.531A
S12.531B
S12.54XA
S12.54XB
S12.550A
S12.550B
S12.551A
S12.551B
S12.590A
S12.590B
S12.591A
S12.591B
S12.600A
S12.600B
S12.601A
S12.601B
S12.630A
S12.630B
S12.631A
S12.631B
S12.64XA
S12.64XB
S12.650A
S12.650B
S12.651A
S12.651B
S12.690A
S12.690B
S12.691A
S12.691B
S12.8XXA
S12.9XXA
S13.0XXA
S13.100A
S13.101A
S13.110A
S13.111A
S13.120A
S13.121A
S13.130A
S13.131A
S13.140A
S13.141A
S13.150A
S13.151A
S13.160A
S13.161A
S13.170A
S13.171A
S13.180A
S13.181A
S13.20XA
S13.29XA
S14.101A
S14.102A
S14.103A
S14.104A
S14.105A
S14.106A
S14.107A
S14.109A
S14.111A
S14.112A
S14.113A
S14.114A
S14.115A
S14.116A
S14.117A
S14.121A
S14.122A
S14.123A
S14.124A
S14.125A
S14.126A
S14.127A
S14.131A
S14.132A
S14.133A
S14.134A
S14.135A
S14.136A
S14.137A
S14.151A
S14.152A
S14.153A
S14.154A
S14.155A
S14.156A
S14.157A
S17.0XXA
S17.8XXA
S17.9XXA
S22.000A
S22.000B
S22.001A
S22.001B
S22.002A
S22.002B
S22.008A
S22.008B
S22.009A
S22.009B
S22.010A
S22.010B
S22.011A
S22.011B
S22.012A
S22.012B
S22.018A
S22.018B
S22.019A
S22.019B
S22.020A
S22.020B
S22.021A
S22.021B
S22.022A
S22.022B
S22.028A
S22.028B
S22.029A
S22.029B
S22.030A
S22.030B
S22.031A
S22.031B
S22.032A
S22.032B
S22.038A
S22.038B
S22.039A
S22.039B
S22.040A
S22.040B
S22.041A
S22.041B
S22.042A
S22.042B
S22.048A
S22.048B
S22.049A
S22.049B
S22.050A
S22.050B
S22.051A
S22.051B
S22.052A
S22.052B
S22.058A
S22.058B
S22.059A
S22.059B
S22.060A
S22.060B
S22.061A
S22.061B
S22.062A
S22.062B
S22.068A
S22.068B
S22.069A
S22.069B
S22.070A
S22.070B
S22.071A
S22.071B
S22.072A
S22.072B
S22.078A
S22.078B
S22.079A
S22.079B
S22.080A
S22.080B
S22.081A
S22.081B
S22.082A
S22.082B
S22.088A
S22.088B
S22.089A
S22.089B
S22.20XA
S22.20XB
S22.21XA
S22.21XB
S22.22XA
S22.22XB
S22.23XA
S22.23XB
S22.24XA
S22.24XB
S22.31XA
S22.31XB
S22.32XA
S22.32XB
S22.39XA
S22.39XB
S22.41XA
S22.41XB
S22.42XA
S22.42XB
S22.43XA
S22.43XB
S22.49XA
S22.49XB
S22.5XXA
S22.5XXB
S22.9XXA
S22.9XXB
S24.101A
S24.102A
S24.103A
S24.104A
S24.109A
S24.111A
S24.112A
S24.113A
S24.114A
S24.131A
S24.132A
S24.133A
S24.134A
S24.151A
S24.152A
S24.153A
S24.154A
S32.000A
S32.000B
S32.001A
S32.001B
S32.002A
S32.002B
S32.008A
S32.008B
S32.009A
S32.009B
S32.010A
S32.010B
S32.011A
S32.011B
S32.012A
S32.012B
S32.018A
S32.018B
S32.019A
S32.019B
S32.020A
S32.020B
S32.021A
S32.021B
S32.022A
S32.022B
S32.028A
S32.028B
S32.029A
S32.029B

**HAC 05: Falls and Trauma (continued)**

S32.030A
S32.030B
S32.031A
S32.031B
S32.032A
S32.032B
S32.038A
S32.038B
S32.039A
S32.039B
S32.040A
S32.040B
S32.041A
S32.041B
S32.042A
S32.042B
S32.048A
S32.048B
S32.049A
S32.049B
S32.050A
S32.050B
S32.051A
S32.051B
S32.052A
S32.052B
S32.058A
S32.058B
S32.059A
S32.059B
S32.10XA
S32.10XB
S32.110A
S32.110B
S32.111A
S32.111B
S32.112A
S32.112B
S32.119A
S32.119B
S32.120A
S32.120B
S32.121A
S32.121B
S32.122A
S32.122B
S32.129A
S32.129B
S32.130A
S32.130B
S32.131A
S32.131B
S32.132A
S32.132B
S32.139A
S32.139B
S32.14XA
S32.14XB
S32.15XA
S32.15XB
S32.16XA
S32.16XB
S32.17XA
S32.17XB
S32.19XA
S32.19XB
S32.2XXA
S32.2XXB
S32.301A
S32.301B
S32.302A
S32.302B
S32.309A
S32.309B
S32.311A
S32.311B
S32.312A
S32.312B
S32.313A
S32.313B
S32.314A
S32.314B
S32.315A
S32.315B
S32.316A
S32.316B
S32.391A
S32.391B
S32.392A
S32.392B
S32.399A
S32.399B
S32.401A
S32.401B
S32.402A
S32.402B
S32.409A
S32.409B
S32.411A
S32.411B
S32.412A
S32.412B
S32.413A
S32.413B
S32.414A
S32.414B
S32.415A
S32.415B
S32.416A
S32.416B
S32.421A
S32.421B
S32.422A
S32.422B
S32.423A
S32.423B
S32.424A
S32.424B
S32.425A
S32.425B
S32.426A
S32.426B
S32.431A
S32.431B
S32.432A
S32.432B
S32.433A
S32.433B
S32.434A
S32.434B
S32.435A
S32.435B
S32.436A
S32.436B
S32.441A
S32.441B
S32.442A
S32.442B
S32.443A
S32.443B
S32.444A
S32.444B
S32.445A
S32.445B
S32.446A
S32.446B
S32.451A
S32.451B
S32.452A
S32.452B
S32.453A
S32.453B
S32.454A
S32.454B
S32.455A
S32.455B
S32.456A
S32.456B
S32.461A
S32.461B
S32.462A
S32.462B
S32.463A
S32.463B
S32.464A
S32.464B
S32.465A
S32.465B
S32.466A
S32.466B
S32.471A
S32.471B
S32.472A
S32.472B
S32.473A
S32.473B
S32.474A
S32.474B
S32.475A
S32.475B
S32.476A
S32.476B
S32.481A
S32.481B
S32.482A
S32.482B
S32.483A
S32.483B
S32.484A
S32.484B
S32.485A
S32.485B
S32.486A
S32.486B
S32.491A
S32.491B
S32.492A
S32.492B
S32.499A
S32.499B
S32.501A
S32.501B
S32.502A
S32.502B
S32.509A
S32.509B
S32.511A
S32.511B
S32.512A
S32.512B
S32.519A
S32.519B
S32.591A
S32.591B
S32.592A
S32.592B
S32.599A
S32.599B
S32.601A
S32.601B
S32.602A
S32.602B
S32.609A
S32.609B
S32.611A
S32.611B
S32.612A
S32.612B
S32.613A
S32.613B
S32.614A
S32.614B
S32.615A
S32.615B
S32.616A
S32.616B
S32.691A
S32.691B
S32.692A
S32.692B
S32.699A
S32.699B
S32.810A
S32.810B
S32.811A
S32.811B
S32.82XA
S32.82XB
S32.89XA
S32.89XB
S32.9XXA
S32.9XXB
S34.101A
S34.102A
S34.103A
S34.104A
S34.105A
S34.109A
S34.111A
S34.112A
S34.113A
S34.114A
S34.115A
S34.119A
S34.121A
S34.122A
S34.123A
S34.124A
S34.125A
S34.129A
S34.131A
S34.132A
S34.139A
S34.3XXA
S42.001B
S42.002B
S42.009B
S42.011B
S42.012B
S42.013B
S42.014B
S42.015B
S42.016B
S42.017B
S42.018B
S42.019B
S42.021B
S42.022B
S42.023B
S42.024B
S42.025B
S42.026B
S42.031B
S42.032B
S42.033B
S42.034B
S42.035B
S42.036B
S42.101B
S42.102B
S42.109B
S42.111B
S42.112B
S42.113B
S42.114B
S42.115B
S42.116B
S42.121B
S42.122B
S42.123B
S42.124B
S42.125B
S42.126B
S42.131B
S42.132B
S42.133B
S42.134B
S42.135B
S42.136B
S42.141B
S42.142B
S42.143B
S42.144B
S42.145B
S42.146B
S42.151B
S42.152B
S42.153B
S42.154B
S42.155B
S42.156B
S42.191B
S42.192B
S42.199B
S42.201A
S42.201B
S42.202A
S42.202B
S42.209A
S42.209B
S42.211A
S42.211B
S42.212A
S42.212B
S42.213A
S42.213B
S42.214A
S42.214B
S42.215A
S42.215B
S42.216A
S42.216B
S42.221A
S42.221B
S42.222A
S42.222B
S42.223A
S42.223B
S42.224A
S42.224B
S42.225A
S42.225B
S42.226A
S42.226B
S42.231A
S42.231B
S42.232A
S42.232B
S42.239A
S42.239B
S42.241A
S42.241B
S42.242A
S42.242B
S42.249A
S42.249B
S42.251A
S42.251B
S42.252A
S42.252B
S42.253A
S42.253B
S42.254A
S42.254B
S42.255A
S42.255B
S42.256A
S42.256B
S42.261A
S42.261B
S42.262A
S42.262B
S42.263A
S42.263B
S42.264A
S42.264B
S42.265A
S42.265B
S42.266A
S42.266B
S42.271A
S42.272A
S42.279A
S42.291A
S42.291B
S42.292A
S42.292B
S42.293A
S42.293B
S42.294A
S42.294B
S42.295A
S42.295B
S42.296A
S42.296B
S42.301A
S42.301B
S42.302A
S42.302B
S42.309A
S42.309B
S42.311A
S42.312A
S42.319A
S42.321A
S42.321B
S42.322A
S42.322B
S42.323A
S42.323B
S42.324A
S42.324B
S42.325A
S42.325B
S42.326A
S42.326B
S42.331A
S42.331B
S42.332A
S42.332B
S42.333A
S42.333B
S42.334A
S42.334B
S42.335A
S42.335B
S42.336A
S42.336B
S42.341A
S42.341B
S42.342A
S42.342B
S42.343A
S42.343B

**HAC 05: Falls and Trauma (continued)**

S42.344A
S42.344B
S42.345A
S42.345B
S42.346A
S42.346B
S42.351A
S42.351B
S42.352A
S42.352B
S42.353A
S42.353B
S42.354A
S42.354B
S42.355A
S42.355B
S42.356A
S42.356B
S42.361A
S42.361B
S42.362A
S42.362B
S42.363A
S42.363B
S42.364A
S42.364B
S42.365A
S42.365B
S42.366A
S42.366B
S42.391A
S42.391B
S42.392A
S42.392B
S42.399A
S42.399B
S42.401A
S42.401B
S42.402A
S42.402B
S42.409A
S42.409B
S42.411A
S42.411B
S42.412A
S42.412B
S42.413A
S42.413B
S42.414A
S42.414B
S42.415A
S42.415B
S42.416A
S42.416B
S42.421A
S42.421B
S42.422A
S42.422B
S42.423A
S42.423B
S42.424A
S42.424B
S42.425A
S42.425B
S42.426A
S42.426B
S42.431A
S42.431B
S42.432A
S42.432B
S42.433A
S42.433B
S42.434A
S42.434B
S42.435A
S42.435B
S42.436A
S42.436B
S42.441A
S42.441B
S42.442A
S42.442B
S42.443A
S42.443B
S42.444A
S42.444B
S42.445A
S42.445B
S42.446A
S42.446B
S42.447A
S42.447B
S42.448A
S42.448B
S42.449A
S42.449B
S42.451A
S42.451B
S42.452A
S42.452B
S42.453A
S42.453B
S42.454A
S42.454B
S42.455A
S42.455B
S42.456A
S42.456B
S42.461A
S42.461B
S42.462A
S42.462B
S42.463A
S42.463B
S42.464A
S42.464B
S42.465A
S42.465B
S42.466A
S42.466B
S42.471A
S42.471B
S42.472A
S42.472B
S42.473A
S42.473B
S42.474A
S42.474B
S42.475A
S42.475B
S42.476A
S42.476B
S42.481A
S42.482A
S42.489A
S42.491A
S42.491B
S42.492A
S42.492B
S42.493A
S42.493B
S42.494A
S42.494B
S42.495A
S42.495B
S42.496A
S42.496B
S42.90XA
S42.90XB
S42.91XA
S42.91XB
S42.92XA
S42.92XB
S43.201A
S43.202A
S43.203A
S43.204A
S43.205A
S43.206A
S43.211A
S43.212A
S43.213A
S43.214A
S43.215A
S43.216A
S43.221A
S43.222A
S43.223A
S43.224A
S43.225A
S43.226A
S49.001A
S49.002A
S49.009A
S49.011A
S49.012A
S49.019A
S49.021A
S49.022A
S49.029A
S49.031A
S49.032A
S49.039A
S49.041A
S49.042A
S49.049A
S49.091A
S49.092A
S49.099A
S49.101A
S49.102A
S49.109A
S49.111A
S49.112A
S49.119A
S49.121A
S49.122A
S49.129A
S49.131A
S49.132A
S49.139A
S49.141A
S49.142A
S49.149A
S49.191A
S49.192A
S49.199A
S52.001B
S52.001C
S52.002B
S52.002C
S52.009B
S52.009C
S52.011A
S52.012A
S52.019A
S52.021B
S52.021C
S52.022B
S52.022C
S52.023B
S52.023C
S52.024B
S52.024C
S52.025B
S52.025C
S52.026B
S52.026C
S52.031B
S52.031C
S52.032B
S52.032C
S52.033B
S52.033C
S52.034B
S52.034C
S52.035B
S52.035C
S52.036B
S52.036C
S52.041B
S52.041C
S52.042B
S52.042C
S52.043B
S52.043C
S52.044B
S52.044C
S52.045B
S52.045C
S52.046B
S52.046C
S52.091B
S52.091C
S52.092B
S52.092C
S52.099B
S52.099C
S52.101B
S52.101C
S52.102B
S52.102C
S52.109B
S52.109C
S52.111A
S52.112A
S52.119A
S52.121B
S52.121C
S52.122B
S52.122C
S52.123B
S52.123C
S52.124B
S52.124C
S52.125B
S52.125C
S52.126B
S52.126C
S52.131B
S52.131C
S52.132B
S52.132C
S52.133B
S52.133C
S52.134B
S52.134C
S52.135B
S52.135C
S52.136B
S52.136C
S52.181B
S52.181C
S52.182B
S52.182C
S52.189B
S52.189C
S52.201A
S52.201B
S52.201C
S52.202A
S52.202B
S52.202C
S52.209A
S52.209B
S52.209C
S52.211A
S52.212A
S52.219A
S52.221A
S52.221B
S52.221C
S52.222A
S52.222B
S52.222C
S52.223A
S52.223B
S52.223C
S52.224A
S52.224B
S52.224C
S52.225A
S52.225B
S52.225C
S52.226A
S52.226B
S52.226C
S52.231A
S52.231B
S52.231C
S52.232A
S52.232B
S52.232C
S52.233A
S52.233B
S52.233C
S52.234A
S52.234B
S52.234C
S52.235A
S52.235B
S52.235C
S52.236A
S52.236B
S52.236C
S52.241A
S52.241B
S52.241C
S52.242A
S52.242B
S52.242C
S52.243A
S52.243B
S52.243C
S52.244A
S52.244B
S52.244C
S52.245A
S52.245B
S52.245C
S52.246A
S52.246B
S52.246C
S52.251A
S52.251B
S52.251C
S52.252A
S52.252B
S52.252C
S52.253A
S52.253B
S52.253C
S52.254A
S52.254B
S52.254C
S52.255A
S52.255B
S52.255C
S52.256A
S52.256B
S52.256C
S52.261A
S52.261B
S52.261C
S52.262A
S52.262B
S52.262C
S52.263A
S52.263B
S52.263C
S52.264A
S52.264B
S52.264C
S52.265A
S52.265B
S52.265C
S52.266A
S52.266B
S52.266C
S52.271B
S52.271C
S52.272B
S52.272C
S52.279B
S52.279C
S52.281A
S52.281B
S52.281C
S52.282A
S52.282B
S52.282C
S52.283A
S52.283B
S52.283C
S52.291A
S52.291B
S52.291C
S52.292A
S52.292B
S52.292C
S52.299A
S52.299B
S52.299C
S52.301A
S52.301B
S52.301C
S52.302A
S52.302B
S52.302C
S52.309A
S52.309B
S52.309C
S52.311A
S52.312A
S52.319A
S52.321A
S52.321B
S52.321C
S52.322A
S52.322B
S52.322C
S52.323A
S52.323B
S52.323C
S52.324A
S52.324B
S52.324C
S52.325A
S52.325B
S52.325C
S52.326A
S52.326B
S52.326C
S52.331A

**HAC 05: Falls and Trauma (continued)**

S52.331B
S52.331C
S52.332A
S52.332B
S52.332C
S52.333A
S52.333B
S52.333C
S52.334A
S52.334B
S52.334C
S52.335A
S52.335B
S52.335C
S52.336A
S52.336B
S52.336C
S52.341A
S52.341B
S52.341C
S52.342A
S52.342B
S52.342C
S52.343A
S52.343B
S52.343C
S52.344A
S52.344B
S52.344C
S52.345A
S52.345B
S52.345C
S52.346A
S52.346B
S52.346C
S52.351A
S52.351B
S52.351C
S52.352A
S52.352B
S52.352C
S52.353A
S52.353B
S52.353C
S52.354A
S52.354B
S52.354C
S52.355A
S52.355B
S52.355C
S52.356A
S52.356B
S52.356C
S52.361A
S52.361B
S52.361C
S52.362A
S52.362B
S52.362C
S52.363A
S52.363B
S52.363C
S52.364A
S52.364B
S52.364C
S52.365A
S52.365B
S52.365C
S52.366A
S52.366B
S52.366C
S52.371A
S52.371B
S52.371C
S52.372A
S52.372B
S52.372C
S52.379A
S52.379B
S52.379C
S52.381A
S52.381B
S52.381C
S52.382A
S52.382B
S52.382C
S52.389A
S52.389B
S52.389C
S52.391A
S52.391B
S52.391C
S52.392A
S52.392B
S52.392C
S52.399A
S52.399B
S52.399C
S52.501A
S52.501B
S52.501C
S52.502A
S52.502B
S52.502C
S52.509A
S52.509B
S52.509C
S52.511A
S52.511B
S52.511C
S52.512A
S52.512B
S52.512C
S52.513A
S52.513B
S52.513C
S52.514A
S52.514B
S52.514C
S52.515A
S52.515B
S52.515C
S52.516A
S52.516B
S52.516C
S52.521A
S52.522A
S52.529A
S52.531A
S52.531B
S52.531C
S52.532A
S52.532B
S52.532C
S52.539A
S52.539B
S52.539C
S52.541A
S52.541B
S52.541C
S52.542A
S52.542B
S52.542C
S52.549A
S52.549B
S52.549C
S52.551A
S52.551B
S52.551C
S52.552A
S52.552B
S52.552C
S52.559A
S52.559B
S52.559C
S52.561A
S52.561B
S52.561C
S52.562A
S52.562B
S52.562C
S52.569A
S52.569B
S52.569C
S52.571A
S52.571B
S52.571C
S52.572A
S52.572B
S52.572C
S52.579A
S52.579B
S52.579C
S52.591A
S52.591B
S52.591C
S52.592A
S52.592B
S52.592C
S52.599A
S52.599B
S52.599C
S52.601A
S52.601B
S52.601C
S52.602A
S52.602B
S52.602C
S52.609A
S52.609B
S52.609C
S52.611A
S52.611B
S52.611C
S52.612A
S52.612B
S52.612C
S52.613A
S52.613B
S52.613C
S52.614A
S52.614B
S52.614C
S52.615A
S52.615B
S52.615C
S52.616A
S52.616B
S52.616C
S52.621A
S52.622A
S52.629A
S52.691A
S52.691B
S52.691C
S52.692A
S52.692B
S52.692C
S52.699A
S52.699B
S52.699C
S52.90XA
S52.90XB
S52.90XC
S52.91XA
S52.91XB
S52.91XC
S52.92XA
S52.92XB
S52.92XC
S59.001A
S59.002A
S59.009A
S59.011A
S59.012A
S59.019A
S59.021A
S59.022A
S59.029A
S59.031A
S59.032A
S59.039A
S59.041A
S59.042A
S59.049A
S59.091A
S59.092A
S59.099A
S59.201A
S59.202A
S59.209A
S59.211A
S59.212A
S59.219A
S59.221A
S59.222A
S59.229A
S59.231A
S59.232A
S59.239A
S59.241A
S59.242A
S59.249A
S59.291A
S59.292A
S59.299A
S62.001B
S62.002B
S62.009B
S62.011B
S62.012B
S62.013B
S62.014B
S62.015B
S62.016B
S62.021B
S62.022B
S62.023B
S62.024B
S62.025B
S62.026B
S62.031B
S62.032B
S62.033B
S62.034B
S62.035B
S62.036B
S62.101B
S62.102B
S62.109B
S62.111B
S62.112B
S62.113B
S62.114B
S62.115B
S62.116B
S62.121B
S62.122B
S62.123B
S62.124B
S62.125B
S62.126B
S62.131B
S62.132B
S62.133B
S62.134B
S62.135B
S62.136B
S62.141B
S62.142B
S62.143B
S62.144B
S62.145B
S62.146B
S62.151B
S62.152B
S62.153B
S62.154B
S62.155B
S62.156B
S62.161B
S62.162B
S62.163B
S62.164B
S62.165B
S62.166B
S62.171B
S62.172B
S62.173B
S62.174B
S62.175B
S62.176B
S62.181B
S62.182B
S62.183B
S62.184B
S62.185B
S62.186B
S62.201B
S62.202B
S62.209B
S62.211B
S62.212B
S62.213B
S62.221B
S62.222B
S62.223B
S62.224B
S62.225B
S62.226B
S62.231B
S62.232B
S62.233B
S62.234B
S62.235B
S62.236B
S62.241B
S62.242B
S62.243B
S62.244B
S62.245B
S62.246B
S62.251B
S62.252B
S62.253B
S62.254B
S62.255B
S62.256B
S62.291B
S62.292B
S62.299B
S62.300B
S62.301B
S62.302B
S62.303B
S62.304B
S62.305B
S62.306B
S62.307B
S62.308B
S62.309B
S62.310B
S62.311B
S62.312B
S62.313B
S62.314B
S62.315B
S62.316B
S62.317B
S62.318B
S62.319B
S62.320B
S62.321B
S62.322B
S62.323B
S62.324B
S62.325B
S62.326B
S62.327B
S62.328B
S62.329B
S62.330B
S62.331B
S62.332B
S62.333B
S62.334B
S62.335B
S62.336B
S62.337B
S62.338B
S62.339B
S62.340B
S62.341B
S62.342B
S62.343B
S62.344B
S62.345B
S62.346B
S62.347B
S62.348B
S62.349B
S62.350B
S62.351B
S62.352B
S62.353B
S62.354B
S62.355B
S62.356B
S62.357B
S62.358B
S62.359B
S62.360B
S62.361B
S62.362B
S62.363B
S62.364B
S62.365B
S62.366B
S62.367B
S62.368B
S62.369B
S62.390B
S62.391B
S62.392B
S62.393B
S62.394B
S62.395B
S62.396B
S62.397B
S62.398B
S62.399B
S62.501B
S62.502B
S62.509B

**HAC 05: Falls and Trauma (continued)**

S62.511B
S62.512B
S62.513B
S62.514B
S62.515B
S62.516B
S62.521B
S62.522B
S62.523B
S62.524B
S62.525B
S62.526B
S62.6ØØB
S62.6Ø1B
S62.6Ø2B
S62.6Ø3B
S62.6Ø4B
S62.6Ø5B
S62.6Ø6B
S62.6Ø7B
S62.6Ø8B
S62.6Ø9B
S62.61ØB
S62.611B
S62.612B
S62.613B
S62.614B
S62.615B
S62.616B
S62.617B
S62.618B
S62.619B
S62.62ØB
S62.621B
S62.622B
S62.623B
S62.624B
S62.625B
S62.626B
S62.627B
S62.628B
S62.629B
S62.63ØB
S62.631B
S62.632B
S62.633B
S62.634B
S62.635B
S62.636B
S62.637B
S62.638B
S62.639B
S62.64ØB
S62.641B
S62.642B
S62.643B
S62.644B
S62.645B
S62.646B
S62.647B
S62.648B
S62.649B
S62.65ØB
S62.651B
S62.652B
S62.653B
S62.654B
S62.655B
S62.656B
S62.657B
S62.658B
S62.659B
S62.66ØB
S62.661B
S62.662B
S62.663B
S62.664B
S62.665B
S62.666B
S62.667B
S62.668B
S62.669B
S62.9ØXB
S62.91XB
S62.92XB
S72.ØØ1A
S72.ØØ1B
S72.ØØ1C
S72.ØØ2A
S72.ØØ2B
S72.ØØ2C
S72.ØØ9A
S72.ØØ9B
S72.ØØ9C
S72.Ø11A
S72.Ø11B
S72.Ø11C
S72.Ø12A
S72.Ø12B
S72.Ø12C
S72.Ø19A
S72.Ø19B
S72.Ø19C
S72.Ø21A
S72.Ø21B
S72.Ø21C
S72.Ø22A
S72.Ø22B
S72.Ø22C
S72.Ø23A
S72.Ø23B
S72.Ø23C
S72.Ø24A
S72.Ø24B
S72.Ø24C
S72.Ø25A
S72.Ø25B
S72.Ø25C
S72.Ø26A
S72.Ø26B
S72.Ø26C
S72.Ø31A
S72.Ø31B
S72.Ø31C
S72.Ø32A
S72.Ø32B
S72.Ø32C
S72.Ø33A
S72.Ø33B
S72.Ø33C
S72.Ø34A
S72.Ø34B
S72.Ø34C
S72.Ø35A
S72.Ø35B
S72.Ø35C
S72.Ø36A
S72.Ø36B
S72.Ø36C
S72.Ø41A
S72.Ø41B
S72.Ø41C
S72.Ø42A
S72.Ø42B
S72.Ø42C
S72.Ø43A
S72.Ø43B
S72.Ø43C
S72.Ø44A
S72.Ø44B
S72.Ø44C
S72.Ø45A
S72.Ø45B
S72.Ø45C
S72.Ø46A
S72.Ø46B
S72.Ø46C
S72.Ø51A
S72.Ø51B
S72.Ø51C
S72.Ø52A
S72.Ø52B
S72.Ø52C
S72.Ø59A
S72.Ø59B
S72.Ø59C
S72.Ø61A
S72.Ø61B
S72.Ø61C
S72.Ø62A
S72.Ø62B
S72.Ø62C
S72.Ø63A
S72.Ø63B
S72.Ø63C
S72.Ø64A
S72.Ø64B
S72.Ø64C
S72.Ø65A
S72.Ø65B
S72.Ø65C
S72.Ø66A
S72.Ø66B
S72.Ø66C
S72.Ø91A
S72.Ø91B
S72.Ø91C
S72.Ø92A
S72.Ø92B
S72.Ø92C
S72.Ø99A
S72.Ø99B
S72.Ø99C
S72.1Ø1A
S72.1Ø1B
S72.1Ø1C
S72.1Ø2A
S72.1Ø2B
S72.1Ø2C
S72.1Ø9A
S72.1Ø9B
S72.1Ø9C
S72.111A
S72.111B
S72.111C
S72.112A
S72.112B
S72.112C
S72.113A
S72.113B
S72.113C
S72.114A
S72.114B
S72.114C
S72.115A
S72.115B
S72.115C
S72.116A
S72.116B
S72.116C
S72.121A
S72.121B
S72.121C
S72.122A
S72.122B
S72.122C
S72.123A
S72.123B
S72.123C
S72.124A
S72.124B
S72.124C
S72.125A
S72.125B
S72.125C
S72.126A
S72.126B
S72.126C
S72.131A
S72.131B
S72.131C
S72.132A
S72.132B
S72.132C
S72.133A
S72.133B
S72.133C
S72.134A
S72.134B
S72.134C
S72.135A
S72.135B
S72.135C
S72.136A
S72.136B
S72.136C
S72.141A
S72.141B
S72.141C
S72.142A
S72.142B
S72.142C
S72.143A
S72.143B
S72.143C
S72.144A
S72.144B
S72.144C
S72.145A
S72.145B
S72.145C
S72.146A
S72.146B
S72.146C
S72.21XA
S72.21XB
S72.21XC
S72.22XA
S72.22XB
S72.22XC
S72.23XA
S72.23XB
S72.23XC
S72.24XA
S72.24XB
S72.24XC
S72.25XA
S72.25XB
S72.25XC
S72.26XA
S72.26XB
S72.26XC
S72.3Ø1A
S72.3Ø1B
S72.3Ø1C
S72.3Ø2A
S72.3Ø2B
S72.3Ø2C
S72.3Ø9A
S72.3Ø9B
S72.3Ø9C
S72.321A
S72.321B
S72.321C
S72.322A
S72.322B
S72.322C
S72.323A
S72.323B
S72.323C
S72.324A
S72.324B
S72.324C
S72.325A
S72.325B
S72.325C
S72.326A
S72.326B
S72.326C
S72.331A
S72.331B
S72.331C
S72.332A
S72.332B
S72.332C
S72.333A
S72.333B
S72.333C
S72.334A
S72.334B
S72.334C
S72.335A
S72.335B
S72.335C
S72.336A
S72.336B
S72.336C
S72.341A
S72.341B
S72.341C
S72.342A
S72.342B
S72.342C
S72.343A
S72.343B
S72.343C
S72.344A
S72.344B
S72.344C
S72.345A
S72.345B
S72.345C
S72.346A
S72.346B
S72.346C
S72.351A
S72.351B
S72.351C
S72.352A
S72.352B
S72.352C
S72.353A
S72.353B
S72.353C
S72.354A
S72.354B
S72.354C
S72.355A
S72.355B
S72.355C
S72.356A
S72.356B
S72.356C
S72.361A
S72.361B
S72.361C
S72.362A
S72.362B
S72.362C
S72.363A
S72.363B
S72.363C
S72.364A
S72.364B
S72.364C
S72.365A
S72.365B
S72.365C
S72.366A
S72.366B
S72.366C
S72.391A
S72.391B
S72.391C
S72.392A
S72.392B
S72.392C
S72.399A
S72.399B
S72.399C
S72.4Ø1A
S72.4Ø1B
S72.4Ø1C
S72.4Ø2A
S72.4Ø2B
S72.4Ø2C
S72.4Ø9A
S72.4Ø9B
S72.4Ø9C
S72.411A
S72.411B
S72.411C
S72.412A
S72.412B
S72.412C
S72.413A
S72.413B
S72.413C
S72.414A
S72.414B
S72.414C
S72.415A
S72.415B
S72.415C
S72.416A
S72.416B
S72.416C
S72.421A
S72.421B
S72.421C
S72.422A
S72.422B
S72.422C
S72.423A
S72.423B
S72.423C
S72.424A
S72.424B
S72.424C
S72.425A
S72.425B
S72.425C
S72.426A
S72.426B
S72.426C
S72.431A
S72.431B
S72.431C
S72.432A
S72.432B
S72.432C
S72.433A
S72.433B
S72.433C

**HAC 05: Falls and Trauma (continued)**

S72.434A
S72.434B
S72.434C
S72.435A
S72.435B
S72.435C
S72.436A
S72.436B
S72.436C
S72.441A
S72.441B
S72.441C
S72.442A
S72.442B
S72.442C
S72.443A
S72.443B
S72.443C
S72.444A
S72.444B
S72.444C
S72.445A
S72.445B
S72.445C
S72.446A
S72.446B
S72.446C
S72.451A
S72.451B
S72.451C
S72.452A
S72.452B
S72.452C
S72.453A
S72.453B
S72.453C
S72.454A
S72.454B
S72.454C
S72.455A
S72.455B
S72.455C
S72.456A
S72.456B
S72.456C
S72.461A
S72.461B
S72.461C
S72.462A
S72.462B
S72.462C
S72.463A
S72.463B
S72.463C
S72.464A
S72.464B
S72.464C
S72.465A
S72.465B
S72.465C
S72.466A
S72.466B
S72.466C
S72.471A
S72.472A
S72.479A
S72.491A
S72.491B
S72.491C
S72.492A
S72.492B
S72.492C
S72.499A
S72.499B
S72.499C
S72.8X1A
S72.8X1B
S72.8X1C
S72.8X2A
S72.8X2B
S72.8X2C
S72.8X9A
S72.8X9B
S72.8X9C
S72.9ØXA
S72.9ØXB
S72.9ØXC
S72.91XA
S72.91XB
S72.91XC
S72.92XA
S72.92XB
S72.92XC
S73.ØØ1A
S73.ØØ2A
S73.ØØ3A
S73.ØØ4A
S73.ØØ5A
S73.ØØ6A
S73.Ø11A
S73.Ø12A
S73.Ø13A
S73.Ø14A
S73.Ø15A
S73.Ø16A
S73.Ø21A
S73.Ø22A
S73.Ø23A
S73.Ø24A
S73.Ø25A
S73.Ø26A
S73.Ø31A
S73.Ø32A
S73.Ø33A
S73.Ø34A
S73.Ø35A
S73.Ø36A
S73.Ø41A
S73.Ø42A
S73.Ø43A
S73.Ø44A
S73.Ø45A
S73.Ø46A
S77.ØØXA
S77.Ø1XA
S77.Ø2XA
S77.1ØXA
S77.11XA
S77.12XA
S79.ØØ1A
S79.ØØ2A
S79.ØØ9A
S79.Ø11A
S79.Ø12A
S79.Ø19A
S79.Ø91A
S79.Ø92A
S79.Ø99A
S79.1Ø1A
S79.1Ø2A
S79.1Ø9A
S79.111A
S79.112A
S79.119A
S79.121A
S79.122A
S79.129A
S79.131A
S79.132A
S79.139A
S79.141A
S79.142A
S79.149A
S79.191A
S79.192A
S79.199A
S82.ØØ1A
S82.ØØ1B
S82.ØØ1C
S82.ØØ2A
S82.ØØ2B
S82.ØØ2C
S82.ØØ9A
S82.ØØ9B
S82.ØØ9C
S82.Ø11A
S82.Ø11B
S82.Ø11C
S82.Ø12A
S82.Ø12B
S82.Ø12C
S82.Ø13A
S82.Ø13B
S82.Ø13C
S82.Ø14A
S82.Ø14B
S82.Ø14C
S82.Ø15A
S82.Ø15B
S82.Ø15C
S82.Ø16A
S82.Ø16B
S82.Ø16C
S82.Ø21A
S82.Ø21B
S82.Ø21C
S82.Ø22A
S82.Ø22B
S82.Ø22C
S82.Ø23A
S82.Ø23B
S82.Ø23C
S82.Ø24A
S82.Ø24B
S82.Ø24C
S82.Ø25A
S82.Ø25B
S82.Ø25C
S82.Ø26A
S82.Ø26B
S82.Ø26C
S82.Ø31A
S82.Ø31B
S82.Ø31C
S82.Ø32A
S82.Ø32B
S82.Ø32C
S82.Ø33A
S82.Ø33B
S82.Ø33C
S82.Ø34A
S82.Ø34B
S82.Ø34C
S82.Ø35A
S82.Ø35B
S82.Ø35C
S82.Ø36A
S82.Ø36B
S82.Ø36C
S82.Ø41A
S82.Ø41B
S82.Ø41C
S82.Ø42A
S82.Ø42B
S82.Ø42C
S82.Ø43A
S82.Ø43B
S82.Ø43C
S82.Ø44A
S82.Ø44B
S82.Ø44C
S82.Ø45A
S82.Ø45B
S82.Ø45C
S82.Ø46A
S82.Ø46B
S82.Ø46C
S82.Ø91A
S82.Ø91B
S82.Ø91C
S82.Ø92A
S82.Ø92B
S82.Ø92C
S82.Ø99A
S82.Ø99B
S82.Ø99C
S82.1Ø1A
S82.1Ø1B
S82.1Ø1C
S82.1Ø2A
S82.1Ø2B
S82.1Ø2C
S82.1Ø9A
S82.1Ø9B
S82.1Ø9C
S82.111A
S82.111B
S82.111C
S82.112A
S82.112B
S82.112C
S82.113A
S82.113B
S82.113C
S82.114A
S82.114B
S82.114C
S82.115A
S82.115B
S82.115C
S82.116A
S82.116B
S82.116C
S82.121A
S82.121B
S82.121C
S82.122A
S82.122B
S82.122C
S82.123A
S82.123B
S82.123C
S82.124A
S82.124B
S82.124C
S82.125A
S82.125B
S82.125C
S82.126A
S82.126B
S82.126C
S82.131A
S82.131B
S82.131C
S82.132A
S82.132B
S82.132C
S82.133A
S82.133B
S82.133C
S82.134A
S82.134B
S82.134C
S82.135A
S82.135B
S82.135C
S82.136A
S82.136B
S82.136C
S82.141A
S82.141B
S82.141C
S82.142A
S82.142B
S82.142C
S82.143A
S82.143B
S82.143C
S82.144A
S82.144B
S82.144C
S82.145A
S82.145B
S82.145C
S82.146A
S82.146B
S82.146C
S82.151A
S82.151B
S82.151C
S82.152A
S82.152B
S82.152C
S82.153A
S82.153B
S82.153C
S82.154A
S82.154B
S82.154C
S82.155A
S82.155B
S82.155C
S82.156A
S82.156B
S82.156C
S82.161A
S82.162A
S82.169A
S82.191A
S82.191B
S82.191C
S82.192A
S82.192B
S82.192C
S82.199A
S82.199B
S82.199C
S82.2Ø1A
S82.2Ø1B
S82.2Ø1C
S82.2Ø2A
S82.2Ø2B
S82.2Ø2C
S82.2Ø9A
S82.2Ø9B
S82.2Ø9C
S82.221A
S82.221B
S82.221C
S82.222A
S82.222B
S82.222C
S82.223A
S82.223B
S82.223C
S82.224A
S82.224B
S82.224C
S82.225A
S82.225B
S82.225C
S82.226A
S82.226B
S82.226C
S82.231A
S82.231B
S82.231C
S82.232A
S82.232B
S82.232C
S82.233A
S82.233B
S82.233C
S82.234A
S82.234B
S82.234C
S82.235A
S82.235B
S82.235C
S82.236A
S82.236B
S82.236C
S82.241A
S82.241B
S82.241C
S82.242A
S82.242B
S82.242C
S82.243A
S82.243B
S82.243C
S82.244A
S82.244B
S82.244C
S82.245A
S82.245B
S82.245C
S82.246A
S82.246B
S82.246C
S82.251A
S82.251B
S82.251C
S82.252A
S82.252B
S82.252C
S82.253A
S82.253B
S82.253C
S82.254A
S82.254B
S82.254C
S82.255A
S82.255B
S82.255C
S82.256A
S82.256B
S82.256C
S82.261A
S82.261B
S82.261C
S82.262A
S82.262B
S82.262C
S82.263A
S82.263B
S82.263C
S82.264A
S82.264B
S82.264C
S82.265A
S82.265B
S82.265C
S82.266A

**HAC 05: Falls and Trauma (continued)**

S82.266B
S82.266C
S82.291A
S82.291B
S82.291C
S82.292A
S82.292B
S82.292C
S82.299A
S82.299B
S82.299C
S82.3Ø1B
S82.3Ø1C
S82.3Ø2B
S82.3Ø2C
S82.3Ø9B
S82.3Ø9C
S82.311A
S82.312A
S82.319A
S82.391B
S82.391C
S82.392B
S82.392C
S82.399B
S82.399C
S82.4Ø1B
S82.4Ø1C
S82.4Ø2B
S82.4Ø2C
S82.4Ø9B
S82.4Ø9C
S82.421B
S82.421C
S82.422B
S82.422C
S82.423B
S82.423C
S82.424B
S82.424C
S82.425B
S82.425C
S82.426B
S82.426C
S82.431B
S82.431C
S82.432B
S82.432C
S82.433B
S82.433C
S82.434B
S82.434C
S82.435B
S82.435C
S82.436B
S82.436C
S82.441B
S82.441C
S82.442B
S82.442C
S82.443B
S82.443C
S82.444B
S82.444C
S82.445B
S82.445C
S82.446B
S82.446C
S82.451B
S82.451C
S82.452B
S82.452C
S82.453B
S82.453C
S82.454B
S82.454C
S82.455B
S82.455C
S82.456B
S82.456C
S82.461B
S82.461C
S82.462B
S82.462C
S82.463B
S82.463C
S82.464B
S82.464C
S82.465B
S82.465C
S82.466B
S82.466C
S82.491B
S82.491C
S82.492B
S82.492C
S82.499B
S82.499C
S82.51XB
S82.51XC
S82.52XB
S82.52XC
S82.53XB
S82.53XC
S82.54XB
S82.54XC
S82.55XB
S82.55XC
S82.56XB
S82.56XC
S82.61XB
S82.61XC
S82.62XB
S82.62XC
S82.63XB
S82.63XC
S82.64XB
S82.64XC
S82.65XB
S82.65XC
S82.66XB
S82.66XC
S82.831B
S82.831C
S82.832B
S82.832C
S82.839B
S82.839C
S82.841B
S82.841C
S82.842B
S82.842C
S82.843B
S82.843C
S82.844B
S82.844C
S82.845B
S82.845C
S82.846B
S82.846C
S82.851B
S82.851C
S82.852B
S82.852C
S82.853B
S82.853C
S82.854B
S82.854C
S82.855B
S82.855C
S82.856B
S82.856C
S82.861B
S82.861C
S82.862B
S82.862C
S82.863B
S82.863C
S82.864B
S82.864C
S82.865B
S82.865C
S82.866B
S82.866C
S82.871B
S82.871C
S82.872B
S82.872C
S82.873B
S82.873C
S82.874B
S82.874C
S82.875B
S82.875C
S82.876B
S82.876C
S82.891B
S82.891C
S82.892B
S82.892C
S82.899B
S82.899C
S82.9ØXB
S82.9ØXC
S82.91XB
S82.91XC
S82.92XB
S82.92XC
S89.ØØ1A
S89.ØØ2A
S89.ØØ9A
S89.Ø11A
S89.Ø12A
S89.Ø19A
S89.Ø21A
S89.Ø22A
S89.Ø29A
S89.Ø31A
S89.Ø32A
S89.Ø39A
S89.Ø41A
S89.Ø42A
S89.Ø49A
S89.Ø91A
S89.Ø92A
S89.Ø99A
S92.ØØ1B
S92.ØØ2B
S92.ØØ9B
S92.Ø11B
S92.Ø12B
S92.Ø13B
S92.Ø14B
S92.Ø15B
S92.Ø16B
S92.Ø21B
S92.Ø22B
S92.Ø23B
S92.Ø24B
S92.Ø25B
S92.Ø26B
S92.Ø31B
S92.Ø32B
S92.Ø33B
S92.Ø34B
S92.Ø35B
S92.Ø36B
S92.Ø41B
S92.Ø42B
S92.Ø43B
S92.Ø44B
S92.Ø45B
S92.Ø46B
S92.Ø51B
S92.Ø52B
S92.Ø53B
S92.Ø54B
S92.Ø55B
S92.Ø56B
S92.Ø61B
S92.Ø62B
S92.Ø63B
S92.Ø64B
S92.Ø65B
S92.Ø66B
S92.1Ø1B
S92.1Ø2B
S92.1Ø9B
S92.111B
S92.112B
S92.113B
S92.114B
S92.115B
S92.116B
S92.121B
S92.122B
S92.123B
S92.124B
S92.125B
S92.126B
S92.131B
S92.132B
S92.133B
S92.134B
S92.135B
S92.136B
S92.141B
S92.142B
S92.143B
S92.144B
S92.145B
S92.146B
S92.151B
S92.152B
S92.153B
S92.154B
S92.155B
S92.156B
S92.191B
S92.192B
S92.199B
S92.2Ø1B
S92.2Ø2B
S92.2Ø9B
S92.211B
S92.212B
S92.213B
S92.214B
S92.215B
S92.216B
S92.221B
S92.222B
S92.223B
S92.224B
S92.225B
S92.226B
S92.231B
S92.232B
S92.233B
S92.234B
S92.235B
S92.236B
S92.241B
S92.242B
S92.243B
S92.244B
S92.245B
S92.246B
S92.251B
S92.252B
S92.253B
S92.254B
S92.255B
S92.256B
S92.3Ø1B
S92.3Ø2B
S92.3Ø9B
S92.311B
S92.312B
S92.313B
S92.314B
S92.315B
S92.316B
S92.321B
S92.322B
S92.323B
S92.324B
S92.325B
S92.326B
S92.331B
S92.332B
S92.333B
S92.334B
S92.335B
S92.336B
S92.341B
S92.342B
S92.343B
S92.344B
S92.345B
S92.346B
S92.351B
S92.352B
S92.353B
S92.354B
S92.355B
S92.356B
S92.811B
S92.812B
S92.819B
S92.9Ø1B
S92.9Ø2B
S92.9Ø9B
T2Ø.3ØXA
T2Ø.311A
T2Ø.312A
T2Ø.319A
T2Ø.32XA
T2Ø.33XA
T2Ø.34XA
T2Ø.35XA
T2Ø.36XA
T2Ø.37XA
T2Ø.39XA
T2Ø.7ØXA
T2Ø.711A
T2Ø.712A
T2Ø.719A
T2Ø.72XA
T2Ø.73XA
T2Ø.74XA
T2Ø.75XA
T2Ø.76XA
T2Ø.77XA
T2Ø.79XA
T21.3ØXA
T21.31XA
T21.32XA
T21.33XA
T21.34XA
T21.35XA
T21.36XA
T21.37XA
T21.39XA
T21.7ØXA
T21.71XA
T21.72XA
T21.73XA
T21.74XA
T21.75XA
T21.76XA
T21.77XA
T21.79XA
T22.3ØXA
T22.311A
T22.312A
T22.319A
T22.321A
T22.322A
T22.329A
T22.331A
T22.332A
T22.339A
T22.341A
T22.342A
T22.349A
T22.351A
T22.352A
T22.359A
T22.361A
T22.362A
T22.369A
T22.391A
T22.392A
T22.399A
T22.7ØXA
T22.711A
T22.712A
T22.719A
T22.721A
T22.722A
T22.729A
T22.731A
T22.732A
T22.739A
T22.741A
T22.742A
T22.749A
T22.751A
T22.752A
T22.759A
T22.761A
T22.762A
T22.769A
T22.791A
T22.792A
T22.799A
T23.3Ø1A
T23.3Ø2A
T23.3Ø9A
T23.311A
T23.312A
T23.319A
T23.321A
T23.322A
T23.329A
T23.331A
T23.332A
T23.339A
T23.341A
T23.342A
T23.349A
T23.351A
T23.352A

**HAC 05: Falls and Trauma (continued)**

T23.359A
T23.361A
T23.362A
T23.369A
T23.371A
T23.372A
T23.379A
T23.391A
T23.392A
T23.399A
T23.701A
T23.702A
T23.709A
T23.711A
T23.712A
T23.719A
T23.721A
T23.722A
T23.729A
T23.731A
T23.732A
T23.739A
T23.741A
T23.742A
T23.749A
T23.751A
T23.752A
T23.759A
T23.761A
T23.762A
T23.769A
T23.771A
T23.772A
T23.779A
T23.791A
T23.792A
T23.799A
T24.301A
T24.302A
T24.309A
T24.311A
T24.312A
T24.319A
T24.321A
T24.322A
T24.329A
T24.331A
T24.332A
T24.339A
T24.391A
T24.392A
T24.399A
T24.701A
T24.702A
T24.709A
T24.711A
T24.712A
T24.719A
T24.721A
T24.722A
T24.729A
T24.731A
T24.732A
T24.739A
T24.791A
T24.792A
T24.799A
T25.311A
T25.312A
T25.319A
T25.321A
T25.322A
T25.329A
T25.331A
T25.332A
T25.339A
T25.391A
T25.392A
T25.399A
T25.711A
T25.712A
T25.719A
T25.721A
T25.722A
T25.729A
T25.731A
T25.732A
T25.739A
T25.791A
T25.792A
T25.799A
T26.20XA
T26.21XA
T26.22XA
T26.70XA
T26.71XA
T26.72XA
T27.0XXA
T27.1XXA
T27.2XXA
T27.3XXA
T27.4XXA
T27.5XXA
T27.6XXA
T27.7XXA
T28.1XXA
T28.2XXA
T28.6XXA
T28.7XXA
T31.10
T31.11
T31.20
T31.21
T31.22
T31.30
T31.31
T31.32
T31.33
T31.40
T31.41
T31.42
T31.43
T31.44
T31.50
T31.51
T31.52
T31.53
T31.54
T31.55
T31.60
T31.61
T31.62
T31.63
T31.64
T31.65
T31.66
T31.70
T31.71
T31.72
T31.73
T31.74
T31.75
T31.76
T31.77
T31.80
T31.81
T31.82
T31.83
T31.84
T31.85
T31.86
T31.87
T31.88
T31.90
T31.91
T31.92
T31.93
T31.94
T31.95
T31.96
T31.97
T31.98
T31.99
T32.10
T32.11
T32.20
T32.21
T32.22
T32.30
T32.31
T32.32
T32.33
T32.40
T32.41
T32.42
T32.43
T32.44
T32.50
T32.51
T32.52
T32.53
T32.54
T32.55
T32.60
T32.61
T32.62
T32.63
T32.64
T32.65
T32.66
T32.70
T32.71
T32.72
T32.73
T32.74
T32.75
T32.76
T32.77
T32.80
T32.81
T32.82
T32.83
T32.84
T32.85
T32.86
T32.87
T32.88
T32.90
T32.91
T32.92
T32.93
T32.94
T32.95
T32.96
T32.97
T32.98
T32.99
T33.011A
T33.012A
T33.019A
T33.02XA
T33.09XA
T33.1XXA
T33.2XXA
T33.3XXA
T33.40XA
T33.41XA
T33.42XA
T33.511A
T33.512A
T33.519A
T33.521A
T33.522A
T33.529A
T33.531A
T33.532A
T33.539A
T33.60XA
T33.61XA
T33.62XA
T33.70XA
T33.71XA
T33.72XA
T33.811A
T33.812A
T33.819A
T33.821A
T33.822A
T33.829A
T33.831A
T33.832A
T33.839A
T33.90XA
T33.99XA
T34.011A
T34.012A
T34.019A
T34.02XA
T34.09XA
T34.1XXA
T34.2XXA
T34.3XXA
T34.40XA
T34.41XA
T34.42XA
T34.511A
T34.512A
T34.519A
T34.521A
T34.522A
T34.529A
T34.531A
T34.532A
T34.539A
T34.60XA
T34.61XA
T34.62XA
T34.70XA
T34.71XA
T34.72XA
T34.811A
T34.812A
T34.819A
T34.821A
T34.822A
T34.829A
T34.831A
T34.832A
T34.839A
T34.90XA
T34.99XA
T67.0XXA
T69.021A
T69.022A
T69.029A
T70.3XXA
T71.111A
T71.112A
T71.113A
T71.114A
T71.121A
T71.122A
T71.123A
T71.124A
T71.131A
T71.132A
T71.133A
T71.134A
T71.141A
T71.143A
T71.144A
T71.151A
T71.152A
T71.153A
T71.154A
T71.161A
T71.162A
T71.163A
T71.164A
T71.191A
T71.192A
T71.193A
T71.194A
T71.20XA
T71.21XA
T71.29XA
T71.9XXA
T75.1XXA

**HAC 06: Catheter Associated Urinary Tract Infection (UTI)**

Secondary diagnosis not POA:

T83.511A
T83.518A

**With or Without**

Secondary diagnosis (also not POA) of:

B37.41
B37.49
N10
N11.9
N12
N13.6
N15.1
N28.84
N28.85
N28.86
N30.00
N30.01
N34.0
N39.0

**HAC 07: Vascular Catheter Associated Infection**

Secondary diagnosis not POA:

T80.211A
T80.212A
T80.218A
T80.219A

**HAC 08: Surgical Site Infection of Mediastinitis Following Coronary Bypass Graft (CABG) Procedures**

Secondary diagnosis not POA:

J98.51
J98.59

**AND**

Any of the following procedures:

Ø21ØØ83 Bypass Coronary Artery, One Artery from Coronary Artery with Zooplastic Tissue, Open Approach
Ø21ØØ88 Bypass Coronary Artery, One Artery from Right Internal Mammary with Zooplastic Tissue, Open Approach
Ø21ØØ89 Bypass Coronary Artery, One Artery from Left Internal Mammary with Zooplastic Tissue, Open Approach
Ø21ØØ8C Bypass Coronary Artery, One Artery from Thoracic Artery with Zooplastic Tissue, Open Approach
Ø21ØØ8F Bypass Coronary Artery, One Artery from Abdominal Artery with Zooplastic Tissue, Open Approach
Ø21ØØ8W Bypass Coronary Artery, One Artery from Aorta with Zooplastic Tissue, Open Approach
Ø21ØØ93 Bypass Coronary Artery, One Artery from Coronary Artery with Autologous Venous Tissue, Open Approach
Ø21ØØ98 Bypass Coronary Artery, One Artery from Right Internal Mammary with Autologous Venous Tissue, Open Approach
Ø21ØØ99 Bypass Coronary Artery, One Artery from Left Internal Mammary with Autologous Venous Tissue, Open Approach
Ø21ØØ9C Bypass Coronary Artery, One Artery from Thoracic Artery with Autologous Venous Tissue, Open Approach
Ø21ØØ9F Bypass Coronary Artery, One Artery from Abdominal Artery with Autologous Venous Tissue, Open Approach
Ø21ØØ9W Bypass Coronary Artery, One Artery from Aorta with Autologous Venous Tissue, Open Approach
Ø21ØØA3 Bypass Coronary Artery, One Artery from Coronary Artery with Autologous Arterial Tissue, Open Approach
Ø21ØØA8 Bypass Coronary Artery, One Artery from Right Internal Mammary with Autologous Arterial Tissue, Open Approach
Ø21ØØA9 Bypass Coronary Artery, One Artery from Left Internal Mammary with Autologous Arterial Tissue, Open Approach
Ø21ØØAC Bypass Coronary Artery, One Artery from Thoracic Artery with Autologous Arterial Tissue, Open Approach
Ø21ØØAF Bypass Coronary Artery, One Artery from Abdominal Artery with Autologous Arterial Tissue, Open Approach
Ø21ØØAW Bypass Coronary Artery, One Artery from Aorta with Autologous Arterial Tissue, Open Approach
Ø21ØØJ3 Bypass Coronary Artery, One Artery from Coronary Artery with Synthetic Substitute, Open Approach
Ø21ØØJ8 Bypass Coronary Artery, One Artery from Right Internal Mammary with Synthetic Substitute, Open Approach
Ø21ØØJ9 Bypass Coronary Artery, One Artery from Left Internal Mammary with Synthetic Substitute, Open Approach
Ø21ØØJC Bypass Coronary Artery, One Artery from Thoracic Artery with Synthetic Substitute, Open Approach
Ø21ØØJF Bypass Coronary Artery, One Artery from Abdominal Artery with Synthetic Substitute, Open Approach
Ø21ØØJW Bypass Coronary Artery, One Artery from Aorta with Synthetic Substitute, Open Approach
Ø21ØØK3 Bypass Coronary Artery, One Artery from Coronary Artery with Nonautologous Tissue Substitute, Open Approach
Ø21ØØK8 Bypass Coronary Artery, One Artery from Right Internal Mammary with Nonautologous Tissue Substitute, Open Approach
Ø21ØØK9 Bypass Coronary Artery, One Artery from Left Internal Mammary with Nonautologous Tissue Substitute, Open Approach
Ø21ØØKC Bypass Coronary Artery, One Artery from Thoracic Artery with Nonautologous Tissue Substitute, Open Approach
Ø21ØØKF Bypass Coronary Artery, One Artery from Abdominal Artery with Nonautologous Tissue Substitute, Open Approach
Ø21ØØKW Bypass Coronary Artery, One Artery from Aorta with Nonautologous Tissue Substitute, Open Approach
Ø21ØØZ3 Bypass Coronary Artery, One Artery from Coronary Artery, Open Approach
Ø21ØØZ8 Bypass Coronary Artery, One Artery from Right Internal Mammary, Open Approach
Ø21ØØZ9 Bypass Coronary Artery, One Artery from Left Internal Mammary, Open Approach
Ø21ØØZC Bypass Coronary Artery, One Artery from Thoracic Artery, Open Approach
Ø21ØØZF Bypass Coronary Artery, One Artery from Abdominal Artery, Open Approach
Ø21Ø483 Bypass Coronary Artery, One Artery from Coronary Artery with Zooplastic Tissue, Percutaneous Endoscopic Approach
Ø21Ø488 Bypass Coronary Artery, One Artery from Right Internal Mammary with Zooplastic Tissue, Percutaneous Endoscopic Approach
Ø21Ø489 Bypass Coronary Artery, One Artery from Left Internal Mammary with Zooplastic Tissue, Percutaneous Endoscopic Approach
Ø21Ø48C Bypass Coronary Artery, One Artery from Thoracic Artery with Zooplastic Tissue, Percutaneous Endoscopic Approach
Ø21Ø48F Bypass Coronary Artery, One Artery from Abdominal Artery with Zooplastic Tissue, Percutaneous Endoscopic Approach
Ø21Ø48W Bypass Coronary Artery, One Artery from Aorta with Zooplastic Tissue, Percutaneous Endoscopic Approach
Ø21Ø493 Bypass Coronary Artery, One Artery from Coronary Artery with Autologous Venous Tissue, Percutaneous Endoscopic Approach
Ø21Ø498 Bypass Coronary Artery, One Artery from Right Internal Mammary with Autologous Venous Tissue, Percutaneous Endoscopic Approach
Ø21Ø499 Bypass Coronary Artery, One Artery from Left Internal Mammary with Autologous Venous Tissue, Percutaneous Endoscopic Approach
Ø21Ø49C Bypass Coronary Artery, One Artery from Thoracic Artery with Autologous Venous Tissue, Percutaneous Endoscopic Approach
Ø21Ø49F Bypass Coronary Artery, One Artery from Abdominal Artery with Autologous Venous Tissue, Percutaneous Endoscopic Approach
Ø21Ø49W Bypass Coronary Artery, One Artery from Aorta with Autologous Venous Tissue, Percutaneous Endoscopic Approach
Ø21Ø4A3 Bypass Coronary Artery, One Artery from Coronary Artery with Autologous Arterial Tissue, Percutaneous Endoscopic Approach
Ø21Ø4A8 Bypass Coronary Artery, One Artery from Right Internal Mammary with Autologous Arterial Tissue, Percutaneous Endoscopic Approach
Ø21Ø4A9 Bypass Coronary Artery, One Artery from Left Internal Mammary with Autologous Arterial Tissue, Percutaneous Endoscopic Approach
Ø21Ø4AC Bypass Coronary Artery, One Artery from Thoracic Artery with Autologous Arterial Tissue, Percutaneous Endoscopic Approach
Ø21Ø4AF Bypass Coronary Artery, One Artery from Abdominal Artery with Autologous Arterial Tissue, Percutaneous Endoscopic Approach
Ø21Ø4AW Bypass Coronary Artery, One Artery from Aorta with Autologous Arterial Tissue, Percutaneous Endoscopic Approach
Ø21Ø4J3 Bypass Coronary Artery, One Artery from Coronary Artery with Synthetic Substitute, Percutaneous Endoscopic Approach
Ø21Ø4J8 Bypass Coronary Artery, One Artery from Right Internal Mammary with Synthetic Substitute, Percutaneous Endoscopic Approach
Ø21Ø4J9 Bypass Coronary Artery, One Artery from Left Internal Mammary with Synthetic Substitute, Percutaneous Endoscopic Approach
Ø21Ø4JC Bypass Coronary Artery, One Artery from Thoracic Artery with Synthetic Substitute, Percutaneous Endoscopic Approach
Ø21Ø4JF Bypass Coronary Artery, One Artery from Abdominal Artery with Synthetic Substitute, Percutaneous Endoscopic Approach
Ø21Ø4JW Bypass Coronary Artery, One Artery from Aorta with Synthetic Substitute, Percutaneous Endoscopic Approach
Ø21Ø4K3 Bypass Coronary Artery, One Artery from Coronary Artery with Nonautologous Tissue Substitute, Percutaneous Endoscopic Approach
Ø21Ø4K8 Bypass Coronary Artery, One Artery from Right Internal Mammary with Nonautologous Tissue Substitute, Percutaneous Endoscopic Approach
Ø21Ø4K9 Bypass Coronary Artery, One Artery from Left Internal Mammary with Nonautologous Tissue Substitute, Percutaneous Endoscopic Approach
Ø21Ø4KC Bypass Coronary Artery, One Artery from Thoracic Artery with Nonautologous Tissue Substitute, Percutaneous Endoscopic Approach

**HAC 08: Surgical Artery Infection of Mediastinitis Following Coronary Bypass Graft (CABG) Procedures (continued)**

- Ø2104KF Bypass Coronary Artery, One Artery from Abdominal Artery with Nonautologous Tissue Substitute, Percutaneous Endoscopic Approach
- Ø2104KW Bypass Coronary Artery, One Artery from Aorta with Nonautologous Tissue Substitute, Percutaneous Endoscopic Approach
- Ø2104Z3 Bypass Coronary Artery, One Artery from Coronary Artery, Percutaneous Endoscopic Approach
- Ø2104Z8 Bypass Coronary Artery, One Artery from Right Internal Mammary, Percutaneous Endoscopic Approach
- Ø2104Z9 Bypass Coronary Artery, One Artery from Left Internal Mammary, Percutaneous Endoscopic Approach
- Ø2104ZC Bypass Coronary Artery, One Artery from Thoracic Artery, Percutaneous Endoscopic Approach
- Ø2104ZF Bypass Coronary Artery, One Artery from Abdominal Artery, Percutaneous Endoscopic Approach
- Ø211Ø83 Bypass Coronary Artery, Two Arteries from Coronary Artery with Zooplastic Tissue, Open Approach
- Ø211Ø88 Bypass Coronary Artery, Two Arteries from Right Internal Mammary with Zooplastic Tissue, Open Approach
- Ø211Ø89 Bypass Coronary Artery, Two Arteries from Left Internal Mammary with Zooplastic Tissue, Open Approach
- Ø211Ø8C Bypass Coronary Artery, Two Arteries from Thoracic Artery with Zooplastic Tissue, Open Approach
- Ø211Ø8F Bypass Coronary Artery, Two Arteries from Abdominal Artery with Zooplastic Tissue, Open Approach
- Ø211Ø8W Bypass Coronary Artery, Two Arteries from Aorta with Zooplastic Tissue, Open Approach
- Ø211Ø93 Bypass Coronary Artery, Two Arteries from Coronary Artery with Autologous Venous Tissue, Open Approach
- Ø211Ø98 Bypass Coronary Artery, Two Arteries from Right Internal Mammary with Autologous Venous Tissue, Open Approach
- Ø211Ø99 Bypass Coronary Artery, Two Arteries from Left Internal Mammary with Autologous Venous Tissue, Open Approach
- Ø211Ø9C Bypass Coronary Artery, Two Arteries from Thoracic Artery with Autologous Venous Tissue, Open Approach
- Ø211Ø9F Bypass Coronary Artery, Two Arteries from Abdominal Artery with Autologous Venous Tissue, Open Approach
- Ø211Ø9W Bypass Coronary Artery, Two Arteries from Aorta with Autologous Venous Tissue, Open Approach
- Ø211ØA3 Bypass Coronary Artery, Two Arteries from Coronary Artery with Autologous Arterial Tissue, Open Approach
- Ø211ØA8 Bypass Coronary Artery, Two Arteries from Right Internal Mammary with Autologous Arterial Tissue, Open Approach
- Ø211ØA9 Bypass Coronary Artery, Two Arteries from Left Internal Mammary with Autologous Arterial Tissue, Open Approach
- Ø211ØAC Bypass Coronary Artery, Two Arteries from Thoracic Artery with Autologous Arterial Tissue, Open Approach
- Ø211ØAF Bypass Coronary Artery, Two Arteries from Abdominal Artery with Autologous Arterial Tissue, Open Approach
- Ø211ØAW Bypass Coronary Artery, Two Arteries from Aorta with Autologous Arterial Tissue, Open Approach
- Ø211ØJ3 Bypass Coronary Artery, Two Arteries from Coronary Artery with Synthetic Substitute, Open Approach
- Ø211ØJ8 Bypass Coronary Artery, Two Arteries from Right Internal Mammary with Synthetic Substitute, Open Approach
- Ø211ØJ9 Bypass Coronary Artery, Two Arteries from Left Internal Mammary with Synthetic Substitute, Open Approach
- Ø211ØJC Bypass Coronary Artery, Two Arteries from Thoracic Artery with Synthetic Substitute, Open Approach
- Ø211ØJF Bypass Coronary Artery, Two Arteries from Abdominal Artery with Synthetic Substitute, Open Approach
- Ø211ØJW Bypass Coronary Artery, Two Arteries from Aorta with Synthetic Substitute, Open Approach
- Ø211ØK3 Bypass Coronary Artery, Two Arteries from Coronary Artery with Nonautologous Tissue Substitute, Open Approach
- Ø211ØK8 Bypass Coronary Artery, Two Arteries from Right Internal Mammary with Nonautologous Tissue Substitute, Open Approach
- Ø211ØK9 Bypass Coronary Artery, Two Arteries from Left Internal Mammary with Nonautologous Tissue Substitute, Open Approach
- Ø211ØKC Bypass Coronary Artery, Two Arteries from Thoracic Artery with Nonautologous Tissue Substitute, Open Approach
- Ø211ØKF Bypass Coronary Artery, Two Arteries from Abdominal Artery with Nonautologous Tissue Substitute, Open Approach
- Ø211ØKW Bypass Coronary Artery, Two Arteries from Aorta with Nonautologous Tissue Substitute, Open Approach
- Ø211ØZ3 Bypass Coronary Artery, Two Arteries from Coronary Artery, Open Approach
- Ø211ØZ8 Bypass Coronary Artery, Two Arteries from Right Internal Mammary, Open Approach
- Ø211ØZ9 Bypass Coronary Artery, Two Arteries from Left Internal Mammary, Open Approach
- Ø211ØZC Bypass Coronary Artery, Two Arteries from Thoracic Artery, Open Approach
- Ø211ØZF Bypass Coronary Artery, Two Arteries from Abdominal Artery, Open Approach
- Ø211483 Bypass Coronary Artery, Two Arteries from Coronary Artery with Zooplastic Tissue, Percutaneous Endoscopic Approach
- Ø211488 Bypass Coronary Artery, Two Arteries from Right Internal Mammary with Zooplastic Tissue, Percutaneous Endoscopic Approach
- Ø211489 Bypass Coronary Artery, Two Arteries from Left Internal Mammary with Zooplastic Tissue, Percutaneous Endoscopic Approach
- Ø21148C Bypass Coronary Artery, Two Arteries from Thoracic Artery with Zooplastic Tissue, Percutaneous Endoscopic Approach
- Ø21148F Bypass Coronary Artery, Two Arteries from Abdominal Artery with Zooplastic Tissue, Percutaneous Endoscopic Approach
- Ø21148W Bypass Coronary Artery, Two Arteries from Aorta with Zooplastic Tissue, Percutaneous Endoscopic Approach
- Ø211493 Bypass Coronary Artery, Two Arteries from Coronary Artery with Autologous Venous Tissue, Percutaneous Endoscopic Approach
- Ø211498 Bypass Coronary Artery, Two Arteries from Right Internal Mammary with Autologous Venous Tissue, Percutaneous Endoscopic Approach
- Ø211499 Bypass Coronary Artery, Two Arteries from Left Internal Mammary with Autologous Venous Tissue, Percutaneous Endoscopic Approach
- Ø21149C Bypass Coronary Artery, Two Arteries from Thoracic Artery with Autologous Venous Tissue, Percutaneous Endoscopic Approach
- Ø21149F Bypass Coronary Artery, Two Arteries from Abdominal Artery with Autologous Venous Tissue, Percutaneous Endoscopic Approach
- Ø21149W Bypass Coronary Artery, Two Arteries from Aorta with Autologous Venous Tissue, Percutaneous Endoscopic Approach
- Ø2114A3 Bypass Coronary Artery, Two Arteries from Coronary Artery with Autologous Arterial Tissue, Percutaneous Endoscopic Approach
- Ø2114A8 Bypass Coronary Artery, Two Arteries from Right Internal Mammary with Autologous Arterial Tissue, Percutaneous Endoscopic Approach
- Ø2114A9 Bypass Coronary Artery, Two Arteries from Left Internal Mammary with Autologous Arterial Tissue, Percutaneous Endoscopic Approach
- Ø2114AC Bypass Coronary Artery, Two Arteries from Thoracic Artery with Autologous Arterial Tissue, Percutaneous Endoscopic Approach
- Ø2114AF Bypass Coronary Artery, Two Arteries from Abdominal Artery with Autologous Arterial Tissue, Percutaneous Endoscopic Approach
- Ø2114AW Bypass Coronary Artery, Two Arteries from Aorta with Autologous Arterial Tissue, Percutaneous Endoscopic Approach
- Ø2114J3 Bypass Coronary Artery, Two Arteries from Coronary Artery with Synthetic Substitute, Percutaneous Endoscopic Approach
- Ø2114J8 Bypass Coronary Artery, Two Arteries from Right Internal Mammary with Synthetic Substitute, Percutaneous Endoscopic Approach
- Ø2114J9 Bypass Coronary Artery, Two Arteries from Left Internal Mammary with Synthetic Substitute, Percutaneous Endoscopic Approach
- Ø2114JC Bypass Coronary Artery, Two Arteries from Thoracic Artery with Synthetic Substitute, Percutaneous Endoscopic Approach

**HAC 08: Surgical Site Infection of Mediastinitis Following Coronary Bypass Graft (CABG) Procedures (continued)**

| | |
|---|---|
| Ø2114JF | Bypass Coronary Artery, Two Arteries from Abdominal Artery with Synthetic Substitute, Percutaneous Endoscopic Approach |
| Ø2114JW | Bypass Coronary Artery, Two Arteries from Aorta with Synthetic Substitute, Percutaneous Endoscopic Approach |
| Ø2114K3 | Bypass Coronary Artery, Two Arteries from Coronary Artery with Nonautologous Tissue Substitute, Percutaneous Endoscopic Approach |
| Ø2114K8 | Bypass Coronary Artery, Two Arteries from Right Internal Mammary with Nonautologous Tissue Substitute, Percutaneous Endoscopic Approach |
| Ø2114K9 | Bypass Coronary Artery, Two Arteries from Left Internal Mammary with Nonautologous Tissue Substitute, Percutaneous Endoscopic Approach |
| Ø2114KC | Bypass Coronary Artery, Two Arteries from Thoracic Artery with Nonautologous Tissue Substitute, Percutaneous Endoscopic Approach |
| Ø2114KF | Bypass Coronary Artery, Two Arteries from Abdominal Artery with Nonautologous Tissue Substitute, Percutaneous Endoscopic Approach |
| Ø2114KW | Bypass Coronary Artery, Two Arteries from Aorta with Nonautologous Tissue Substitute, Percutaneous Endoscopic Approach |
| Ø2114Z3 | Bypass Coronary Artery, Two Arteries from Coronary Artery, Percutaneous Endoscopic Approach |
| Ø2114Z8 | Bypass Coronary Artery, Two Arteries from Right Internal Mammary, Percutaneous Endoscopic Approach |
| Ø2114Z9 | Bypass Coronary Artery, Two Arteries from Left Internal Mammary, Percutaneous Endoscopic Approach |
| Ø2114ZC | Bypass Coronary Artery, Two Arteries from Thoracic Artery, Percutaneous Endoscopic Approach |
| Ø2114ZF | Bypass Coronary Artery, Two Arteries from Abdominal Artery, Percutaneous Endoscopic Approach |
| Ø212Ø83 | Bypass Coronary Artery, Three Arteries from Coronary Artery with Zooplastic Tissue, Open Approach |
| Ø212Ø88 | Bypass Coronary Artery, Three Arteries from Right Internal Mammary with Zooplastic Tissue, Open Approach |
| Ø212Ø89 | Bypass Coronary Artery, Three Arteries from Left Internal Mammary with Zooplastic Tissue, Open Approach |
| Ø212Ø8C | Bypass Coronary Artery, Three Arteries from Thoracic Artery with Zooplastic Tissue, Open Approach |
| Ø212Ø8F | Bypass Coronary Artery, Three Arteries from Abdominal Artery with Zooplastic Tissue, Open Approach |
| Ø212Ø8W | Bypass Coronary Artery, Three Arteries from Aorta with Zooplastic Tissue, Open Approach |
| Ø212Ø93 | Bypass Coronary Artery, Three Arteries from Coronary Artery with Autologous Venous Tissue, Open Approach |
| Ø212Ø98 | Bypass Coronary Artery, Three Arteries from Right Internal Mammary with Autologous Venous Tissue, Open Approach |
| Ø212Ø99 | Bypass Coronary Artery, Three Arteries from Left Internal Mammary with Autologous Venous Tissue, Open Approach |
| Ø212Ø9C | Bypass Coronary Artery, Three Arteries from Thoracic Artery with Autologous Venous Tissue, Open Approach |
| Ø212Ø9F | Bypass Coronary Artery, Three Arteries from Abdominal Artery with Autologous Venous Tissue, Open Approach |
| Ø212Ø9W | Bypass Coronary Artery, Three Arteries from Aorta with Autologous Venous Tissue, Open Approach |
| Ø212ØA3 | Bypass Coronary Artery, Three Arteries from Coronary Artery with Autologous Arterial Tissue, Open Approach |
| Ø212ØA8 | Bypass Coronary Artery, Three Arteries from Right Internal Mammary with Autologous Arterial Tissue, Open Approach |
| Ø212ØA9 | Bypass Coronary Artery, Three Arteries from Left Internal Mammary with Autologous Arterial Tissue, Open Approach |
| Ø212ØAC | Bypass Coronary Artery, Three Arteries from Thoracic Artery with Autologous Arterial Tissue, Open Approach |
| Ø212ØAF | Bypass Coronary Artery, Three Arteries from Abdominal Artery with Autologous Arterial Tissue, Open Approach |
| Ø212ØAW | Bypass Coronary Artery, Three Arteries from Aorta with Autologous Arterial Tissue, Open Approach |
| Ø212ØJ3 | Bypass Coronary Artery, Three Arteries from Coronary Artery with Synthetic Substitute, Open Approach |
| Ø212ØJ8 | Bypass Coronary Artery, Three Arteries from Right Internal Mammary with Synthetic Substitute, Open Approach |
| Ø212ØJ9 | Bypass Coronary Artery, Three Arteries from Left Internal Mammary with Synthetic Substitute, Open Approach |
| Ø212ØJC | Bypass Coronary Artery, Three Arteries from Thoracic Artery with Synthetic Substitute, Open Approach |
| Ø212ØJF | Bypass Coronary Artery, Three Arteries from Abdominal Artery with Synthetic Substitute, Open Approach |
| Ø212ØJW | Bypass Coronary Artery, Three Arteries from Aorta with Synthetic Substitute, Open Approach |
| Ø212ØK3 | Bypass Coronary Artery, Three Arteries from Coronary Artery with Nonautologous Tissue Substitute, Open Approach |
| Ø212ØK8 | Bypass Coronary Artery, Three Arteries from Right Internal Mammary with Nonautologous Tissue Substitute, Open Approach |
| Ø212ØK9 | Bypass Coronary Artery, Three Arteries from Left Internal Mammary with Nonautologous Tissue Substitute, Open Approach |
| Ø212ØKC | Bypass Coronary Artery, Three Arteries from Thoracic Artery with Nonautologous Tissue Substitute, Open Approach |
| Ø212ØKF | Bypass Coronary Artery, Three Arteries from Abdominal Artery with Nonautologous Tissue Substitute, Open Approach |
| Ø212ØKW | Bypass Coronary Artery, Three Arteries from Aorta with Nonautologous Tissue Substitute, Open Approach |
| Ø212ØZ3 | Bypass Coronary Artery, Three Arteries from Coronary Artery, Open Approach |
| Ø212ØZ8 | Bypass Coronary Artery, Three Arteries from Right Internal Mammary, Open Approach |
| Ø212ØZ9 | Bypass Coronary Artery, Three Arteries from Left Internal Mammary, Open Approach |
| Ø212ØZC | Bypass Coronary Artery, Three Arteries from Thoracic Artery, Open Approach |
| Ø212ØZF | Bypass Coronary Artery, Three Arteries from Abdominal Artery, Open Approach |
| Ø212483 | Bypass Coronary Artery, Three Arteries from Coronary Artery with Zooplastic Tissue, Percutaneous Endoscopic Approach |
| Ø212488 | Bypass Coronary Artery, Three Arteries from Right Internal Mammary with Zooplastic Tissue, Percutaneous Endoscopic Approach |
| Ø212489 | Bypass Coronary Artery, Three Arteries from Left Internal Mammary with Zooplastic Tissue, Percutaneous Endoscopic Approach |
| Ø21248C | Bypass Coronary Artery, Three Arteries from Thoracic Artery with Zooplastic Tissue, Percutaneous Endoscopic Approach |
| Ø21248F | Bypass Coronary Artery, Three Arteries from Abdominal Artery with Zooplastic Tissue, Percutaneous Endoscopic Approach |
| Ø21248W | Bypass Coronary Artery, Three Arteries from Aorta with Zooplastic Tissue, Percutaneous Endoscopic Approach |
| Ø212493 | Bypass Coronary Artery, Three Arteries from Coronary Artery with Autologous Venous Tissue, Percutaneous Endoscopic Approach |
| Ø212498 | Bypass Coronary Artery, Three Arteries from Right Internal Mammary with Autologous Venous Tissue, Percutaneous Endoscopic Approach |
| Ø212499 | Bypass Coronary Artery, Three Arteries from Left Internal Mammary with Autologous Venous Tissue, Percutaneous Endoscopic Approach |
| Ø21249C | Bypass Coronary Artery, Three Arteries from Thoracic Artery with Autologous Venous Tissue, Percutaneous Endoscopic Approach |
| Ø21249F | Bypass Coronary Artery, Three Arteries from Abdominal Artery with Autologous Venous Tissue, Percutaneous Endoscopic Approach |
| Ø21249W | Bypass Coronary Artery, Three Arteries from Aorta with Autologous Venous Tissue, Percutaneous Endoscopic Approach |
| Ø2124A3 | Bypass Coronary Artery, Three Arteries from Coronary Artery with Autologous Arterial Tissue, Percutaneous Endoscopic Approach |
| Ø2124A8 | Bypass Coronary Artery, Three Arteries from Right Internal Mammary with Autologous Arterial Tissue, Percutaneous Endoscopic Approach |
| Ø2124A9 | Bypass Coronary Artery, Three Arteries from Left Internal Mammary with Autologous Arterial Tissue, Percutaneous Endoscopic Approach |
| Ø2124AC | Bypass Coronary Artery, Three Arteries from Thoracic Artery with Autologous Arterial Tissue, Percutaneous Endoscopic Approach |

**HAC 08: Surgical Site Infection of Mediastinitis Following Coronary Bypass Graft (CABG) Procedures (continued)**

Ø2124AF Bypass Coronary Artery, Three Arteries from Abdominal Artery with Autologous Arterial Tissue, Percutaneous Endoscopic Approach
Ø2124AW Bypass Coronary Artery, Three Arteries from Aorta with Autologous Arterial Tissue, Percutaneous Endoscopic Approach
Ø2124J3 Bypass Coronary Artery, Three Arteries from Coronary Artery with Synthetic Substitute, Percutaneous Endoscopic Approach
Ø2124J8 Bypass Coronary Artery, Three Arteries from Right Internal Mammary with Synthetic Substitute, Percutaneous Endoscopic Approach
Ø2124J9 Bypass Coronary Artery, Three Arteries from Left Internal Mammary with Synthetic Substitute, Percutaneous Endoscopic Approach
Ø2124JC Bypass Coronary Artery, Three Arteries from Thoracic Artery with Synthetic Substitute, Percutaneous Endoscopic Approach
Ø2124JF Bypass Coronary Artery, Three Arteries from Abdominal Artery with Synthetic Substitute, Percutaneous Endoscopic Approach
Ø2124JW Bypass Coronary Artery, Three Arteries from Aorta with Synthetic Substitute, Percutaneous Endoscopic Approach
Ø2124K3 Bypass Coronary Artery, Three Arteries from Coronary Artery with Nonautologous Tissue Substitute, Percutaneous Endoscopic Approach
Ø2124K8 Bypass Coronary Artery, Three Arteries from Right Internal Mammary with Nonautologous Tissue Substitute, Percutaneous Endoscopic Approach
Ø2124K9 Bypass Coronary Artery, Three Arteries from Left Internal Mammary with Nonautologous Tissue Substitute, Percutaneous Endoscopic Approach
Ø2124KC Bypass Coronary Artery, Three Arteries from Thoracic Artery with Nonautologous Tissue Substitute, Percutaneous Endoscopic Approach
Ø2124KF Bypass Coronary Artery, Three Arteries from Abdominal Artery with Nonautologous Tissue Substitute, Percutaneous Endoscopic Approach
Ø2124KW Bypass Coronary Artery, Three Arteries from Aorta with Nonautologous Tissue Substitute, Percutaneous Endoscopic Approach
Ø2124Z3 Bypass Coronary Artery, Three Arteries from Coronary Artery, Percutaneous Endoscopic Approach
Ø2124Z8 Bypass Coronary Artery, Three Arteries from Right Internal Mammary, Percutaneous Endoscopic Approach
Ø2124Z9 Bypass Coronary Artery, Three Arteries from Left Internal Mammary, Percutaneous Endoscopic Approach
Ø2124ZC Bypass Coronary Artery, Three Arteries from Thoracic Artery, Percutaneous Endoscopic Approach
Ø2124ZF Bypass Coronary Artery, Three Arteries from Abdominal Artery, Percutaneous Endoscopic Approach
Ø213Ø83 Bypass Coronary Artery, Four or More Arteries from Coronary Artery with Zooplastic Tissue, Open Approach
Ø213Ø88 Bypass Coronary Artery, Four or More Arteries from Right Internal Mammary with Zooplastic Tissue, Open Approach
Ø213Ø89 Bypass Coronary Artery, Four or More Arteries from Left Internal Mammary with Zooplastic Tissue, Open Approach
Ø213Ø8C Bypass Coronary Artery, Four or More Arteries from Thoracic Artery with Zooplastic Tissue, Open Approach
Ø213Ø8F Bypass Coronary Artery, Four or More Arteries from Abdominal Artery with Zooplastic Tissue, Open Approach
Ø213Ø8W Bypass Coronary Artery, Four or More Arteries from Aorta with Zooplastic Tissue, Open Approach
Ø213Ø93 Bypass Coronary Artery, Four or More Arteries from Coronary Artery with Autologous Venous Tissue, Open Approach
Ø213Ø98 Bypass Coronary Artery, Four or More Arteries from Right Internal Mammary with Autologous Venous Tissue, Open Approach
Ø213Ø99 Bypass Coronary Artery, Four or More Arteries from Left Internal Mammary with Autologous Venous Tissue, Open Approach
Ø213Ø9C Bypass Coronary Artery, Four or More Arteries from Thoracic Artery with Autologous Venous Tissue, Open Approach
Ø213Ø9F Bypass Coronary Artery, Four or More Arteries from Abdominal Artery with Autologous Venous Tissue, Open Approach
Ø213Ø9W Bypass Coronary Artery, Four or More Arteries from Aorta with Autologous Venous Tissue, Open Approach
Ø213ØA3 Bypass Coronary Artery, Four or More Arteries from Coronary Artery with Autologous Arterial Tissue, Open Approach
Ø213ØA8 Bypass Coronary Artery, Four or More Arteries from Right Internal Mammary with Autologous Arterial Tissue, Open Approach
Ø213ØA9 Bypass Coronary Artery, Four or More Arteries from Left Internal Mammary with Autologous Arterial Tissue, Open Approach
Ø213ØAC Bypass Coronary Artery, Four or More Arteries from Thoracic Artery with Autologous Arterial Tissue, Open Approach
Ø213ØAF Bypass Coronary Artery, Four or More Arteries from Abdominal Artery with Autologous Arterial Tissue, Open Approach
Ø213ØAW Bypass Coronary Artery, Four or More Arteries from Aorta with Autologous Arterial Tissue, Open Approach
Ø213ØJ3 Bypass Coronary Artery, Four or More Arteries from Coronary Artery with Synthetic Substitute, Open Approach
Ø213ØJ8 Bypass Coronary Artery, Four or More Arteries from Right Internal Mammary with Synthetic Substitute, Open Approach
Ø213ØJ9 Bypass Coronary Artery, Four or More Arteries from Left Internal Mammary with Synthetic Substitute, Open Approach
Ø213ØJC Bypass Coronary Artery, Four or More Arteries from Thoracic Artery with Synthetic Substitute, Open Approach
Ø213ØJF Bypass Coronary Artery, Four or More Arteries from Abdominal Artery with Synthetic Substitute, Open Approach
Ø213ØJW Bypass Coronary Artery, Four or More Arteries from Aorta with Synthetic Substitute, Open Approach
Ø213ØK3 Bypass Coronary Artery, Four or More Arteries from Coronary Artery with Nonautologous Tissue Substitute, Open Approach
Ø213ØK8 Bypass Coronary Artery, Four or More Arteries from Right Internal Mammary with Nonautologous Tissue Substitute, Open Approach
Ø213ØK9 Bypass Coronary Artery, Four or More Arteries from Left Internal Mammary with Nonautologous Tissue Substitute, Open Approach
Ø213ØKC Bypass Coronary Artery, Four or More Arteries from Thoracic Artery with Nonautologous Tissue Substitute, Open Approach
Ø213ØKF Bypass Coronary Artery, Four or More Arteries from Abdominal Artery with Nonautologous Tissue Substitute, Open Approach
Ø213ØKW Bypass Coronary Artery, Four or More Arteries from Aorta with Nonautologous Tissue Substitute, Open Approach
Ø213ØZ3 Bypass Coronary Artery, Four or More Arteries from Coronary Artery, Open Approach
Ø213ØZ8 Bypass Coronary Artery, Four or More Arteries from Right Internal Mammary, Open Approach
Ø213ØZ9 Bypass Coronary Artery, Four or More Arteries from Left Internal Mammary, Open Approach
Ø213ØZC Bypass Coronary Artery, Four or More Arteries from Thoracic Artery, Open Approach
Ø213ØZF Bypass Coronary Artery, Four or More Arteries from Abdominal Artery, Open Approach
Ø213483 Bypass Coronary Artery, Four or More Arteries from Coronary Artery with Zooplastic Tissue, Percutaneous Endoscopic Approach
Ø213488 Bypass Coronary Artery, Four or More Arteries from Right Internal Mammary with Zooplastic Tissue, Percutaneous Endoscopic Approach
Ø213489 Bypass Coronary Artery, Four or More Arteries from Left Internal Mammary with Zooplastic Tissue, Percutaneous Endoscopic Approach
Ø21348C Bypass Coronary Artery, Four or More Arteries from Thoracic Artery with Zooplastic Tissue, Percutaneous Endoscopic Approach
Ø21348F Bypass Coronary Artery, Four or More Arteries from Abdominal Artery with Zooplastic Tissue, Percutaneous Endoscopic Approach
Ø21348W Bypass Coronary Artery, Four or More Arteries from Aorta with Zooplastic Tissue, Percutaneous Endoscopic Approach
Ø213493 Bypass Coronary Artery, Four or More Arteries from Coronary Artery with Autologous Venous Tissue, Percutaneous Endoscopic Approach
Ø213498 Bypass Coronary Artery, Four or More Arteries from Right Internal Mammary with Autologous Venous Tissue, Percutaneous Endoscopic Approach

**HAC 08: Surgical Site Infection of Mediastinitis Following Coronary Bypass Graft (CABG) Procedures (continued)**

- Ø213499 Bypass Coronary Artery, Four or More Arteries from Left Internal Mammary with Autologous Venous Tissue, Percutaneous Endoscopic Approach
- Ø21349C Bypass Coronary Artery, Four or More Arteries from Thoracic Artery with Autologous Venous Tissue, Percutaneous Endoscopic Approach
- Ø21349F Bypass Coronary Artery, Four or More Arteries from Abdominal Artery with Autologous Venous Tissue, Percutaneous Endoscopic Approach
- Ø21349W Bypass Coronary Artery, Four or More Arteries from Aorta with Autologous Venous Tissue, Percutaneous Endoscopic Approach
- Ø2134A3 Bypass Coronary Artery, Four or More Arteries from Coronary Artery with Autologous Arterial Tissue, Percutaneous Endoscopic Approach
- Ø2134A8 Bypass Coronary Artery, Four or More Arteries from Right Internal Mammary with Autologous Arterial Tissue, Percutaneous Endoscopic Approach
- Ø2134A9 Bypass Coronary Artery, Four or More Arteries from Left Internal Mammary with Autologous Arterial Tissue, Percutaneous Endoscopic Approach
- Ø2134AC Bypass Coronary Artery, Four or More Arteries from Thoracic Artery with Autologous Arterial Tissue, Percutaneous Endoscopic Approach
- Ø2134AF Bypass Coronary Artery, Four or More Arteries from Abdominal Artery with Autologous Arterial Tissue, Percutaneous Endoscopic Approach
- Ø2134AW Bypass Coronary Artery, Four or More Arteries from Aorta with Autologous Arterial Tissue, Percutaneous Endoscopic Approach
- Ø2134J3 Bypass Coronary Artery, Four or More Arteries from Coronary Artery with Synthetic Substitute, Percutaneous Endoscopic Approach
- Ø2134J8 Bypass Coronary Artery, Four or More Arteries from Right Internal Mammary with Synthetic Substitute, Percutaneous Endoscopic Approach
- Ø2134J9 Bypass Coronary Artery, Four or More Arteries from Left Internal Mammary with Synthetic Substitute, Percutaneous Endoscopic Approach
- Ø2134JC Bypass Coronary Artery, Four or More Arteries from Thoracic Artery with Synthetic Substitute, Percutaneous Endoscopic Approach
- Ø2134JF Bypass Coronary Artery, Four or More Arteries from Abdominal Artery with Synthetic Substitute, Percutaneous Endoscopic Approach
- Ø2134JW Bypass Coronary Artery, Four or More Arteries from Aorta with Synthetic Substitute, Percutaneous Endoscopic Approach
- Ø2134K3 Bypass Coronary Artery, Four or More Arteries from Coronary Artery with Nonautologous Tissue Substitute, Percutaneous Endoscopic Approach
- Ø2134K8 Bypass Coronary Artery, Four or More Arteries from Right Internal Mammary with Nonautologous Tissue Substitute, Percutaneous Endoscopic Approach
- Ø2134K9 Bypass Coronary Artery, Four or More Arteries from Left Internal Mammary with Nonautologous Tissue Substitute, Percutaneous Endoscopic Approach
- Ø2134KC Bypass Coronary Artery, Four or More Arteries from Thoracic Artery with Nonautologous Tissue Substitute, Percutaneous Endoscopic Approach
- Ø2134KF Bypass Coronary Artery, Four or More Arteries from Abdominal Artery with Nonautologous Tissue Substitute, Percutaneous Endoscopic Approach
- Ø2134KW Bypass Coronary Artery, Four or More Arteries from Aorta with Nonautologous Tissue Substitute, Percutaneous Endoscopic Approach
- Ø2134Z3 Bypass Coronary Artery, Four or More Arteries from Coronary Artery, Percutaneous Endoscopic Approach
- Ø2134Z8 Bypass Coronary Artery, Four or More Arteries from Right Internal Mammary, Percutaneous Endoscopic Approach
- Ø2134Z9 Bypass Coronary Artery, Four or More Arteries from Left Internal Mammary, Percutaneous Endoscopic Approach
- Ø2134ZC Bypass Coronary Artery, Four or More Arteries from Thoracic Artery, Percutaneous Endoscopic Approach
- Ø2134ZF Bypass Coronary Artery, Four or More Arteries from Abdominal Artery, Percutaneous Endoscopic Approach

**HAC 09: Manifestations of Poor Glycemic Control**

Secondary diagnosis not POA:

E08.ØØ
E08.Ø1
E08.1Ø
E09.ØØ
E09.Ø1
E09.1Ø
E1Ø.1Ø
E11.ØØ
E11.Ø1
E13.ØØ
E13.Ø1
E13.1Ø
E15

**HAC 10: Deep Vein Thrombosis (DVT) or Pulmonary Embolism (PE) with Total Knee or Hip Replacement**

Secondary diagnosis not POA:

I26.Ø2
I26.Ø9
I26.92
I26.99
I82.4Ø1
I82.4Ø2
I82.4Ø3
I82.4Ø9
I82.411
I82.412
I82.413
I82.419
I82.421
I82.422
I82.423
I82.429
I82.431
I82.432
I82.433
I82.439
I82.441
I82.442
I82.443
I82.449
I82.491
I82.492
I82.493
I82.499
I82.4Y1
I82.4Y2
I82.4Y3
I82.4Y9
I82.4Z1
I82.4Z2
I82.4Z3
I82.4Z9

**AND**

Any of the following procedures:

- ØSR9Ø19 Replacement of Right Hip Joint with Metal Synthetic Substitute, Cemented, Open Approach
- ØSR9Ø1A Replacement of Right Hip Joint with Metal Synthetic Substitute, Uncemented, Open Approach
- ØSR9Ø1Z Replacement of Right Hip Joint with Metal Synthetic Substitute, Open Approach
- ØSR9Ø29 Replacement of Right Hip Joint with Metal on Polyethylene Synthetic Substitute, Cemented, Open Approach
- ØSR9Ø2A Replacement of Right Hip Joint with Metal on Polyethylene Synthetic Substitute, Uncemented, Open Approach
- ØSR9Ø2Z Replacement of Right Hip Joint with Metal on Polyethylene Synthetic Substitute, Open Approach
- ØSR9Ø39 Replacement of Right Hip Joint with Ceramic Synthetic Substitute, Cemented, Open Approach
- ØSR9Ø3A Replacement of Right Hip Joint with Ceramic Synthetic Substitute, Uncemented, Open Approach
- ØSR9Ø3Z Replacement of Right Hip Joint with Ceramic Synthetic Substitute, Open Approach
- ØSR9Ø49 Replacement of Right Hip Joint with Ceramic on Polyethylene Synthetic Substitute, Cemented, Open Approach
- ØSR9Ø4A Replacement of Right Hip Joint with Ceramic on Polyethylene Synthetic Substitute, Uncemented, Open Approach
- ØSR9Ø4Z Replacement of Right Hip Joint with Ceramic on Polyethylene Synthetic Substitute, Open Approach
- ØSR9Ø7Z Replacement of Right Hip Joint with Autologous Tissue Substitute, Open Approach
- ØSR9ØJ9 Replacement of Right Hip Joint with Synthetic Substitute, Cemented, Open Approach
- ØSR9ØJA Replacement of Right Hip Joint with Synthetic Substitute, Uncemented, Open Approach
- ØSR9ØJZ Replacement of Right Hip Joint with Synthetic Substitute, Open Approach
- ØSR9ØKZ Replacement of Right Hip Joint with Nonautologous Tissue Substitute, Open Approach
- ØSRAØØ9 Replacement of Right Hip Joint, Acetabular Surface with Polyethylene Synthetic Substitute, Cemented, Open Approach
- ØSRAØØA Replacement of Right Hip Joint, Acetabular Surface with Polyethylene Synthetic Substitute, Uncemented, Open Approach

**HAC 10: Deep Vein Thrombosis (DVT) or Pulmonary Embolism (PE) with Total Knee or Hip Replacement (continued)**

ØSRAØØZ Replacement of Right Hip Joint, Acetabular Surface with Polyethylene Synthetic Substitute, Open Approach
ØSRAØ19 Replacement of Right Hip Joint, Acetabular Surface with Metal Synthetic Substitute, Cemented, Open Approach
ØSRAØ1A Replacement of Right Hip Joint, Acetabular Surface with Metal Synthetic Substitute, Uncemented, Open Approach
ØSRAØ1Z Replacement of Right Hip Joint, Acetabular Surface with Metal Synthetic Substitute, Open Approach
ØSRAØ39 Replacement of Right Hip Joint, Acetabular Surface with Ceramic Synthetic Substitute, Cemented, Open Approach
ØSRAØ3A Replacement of Right Hip Joint, Acetabular Surface with Ceramic Synthetic Substitute, Uncemented, Open Approach
ØSRAØ3Z Replacement of Right Hip Joint, Acetabular Surface with Ceramic Synthetic Substitute, Open Approach
ØSRAØ7Z Replacement of Right Hip Joint, Acetabular Surface with Autologous Tissue Substitute, Open Approach
ØSRAØJ9 Replacement of Right Hip Joint, Acetabular Surface with Synthetic Substitute, Cemented, Open Approach
ØSRAØJA Replacement of Right Hip Joint, Acetabular Surface with Synthetic Substitute, Uncemented, Open Approach
ØSRAØJZ Replacement of Right Hip Joint, Acetabular Surface with Synthetic Substitute, Open Approach
ØSRAØKZ Replacement of Right Hip Joint, Acetabular Surface with Nonautologous Tissue Substitute, Open Approach
ØSRBØ19 Replacement of Left Hip Joint with Metal Synthetic Substitute, Cemented, Open Approach
ØSRBØ1A Replacement of Left Hip Joint with Metal Synthetic Substitute, Uncemented, Open Approach
ØSRBØ1Z Replacement of Left Hip Joint with Metal Synthetic Substitute, Open Approach
ØSRBØ29 Replacement of Left Hip Joint with Metal on Polyethylene Synthetic Substitute, Cemented, Open Approach
ØSRBØ2A Replacement of Left Hip Joint with Metal on Polyethylene Synthetic Substitute, Uncemented, Open Approach
ØSRBØ2Z Replacement of Left Hip Joint with Metal on Polyethylene Synthetic Substitute, Open Approach
ØSRBØ39 Replacement of Left Hip Joint with Ceramic Synthetic Substitute, Cemented, Open Approach
ØSRBØ3A Replacement of Left Hip Joint with Ceramic Synthetic Substitute, Uncemented, Open Approach
ØSRBØ3Z Replacement of Left Hip Joint with Ceramic Synthetic Substitute, Open Approach
ØSRBØ49 Replacement of Left Hip Joint with Ceramic on Polyethylene Synthetic Substitute, Cemented, Open Approach
ØSRBØ4A Replacement of Left Hip Joint with Ceramic on Polyethylene Synthetic Substitute, Uncemented, Open Approach
ØSRBØ4Z Replacement of Left Hip Joint with Ceramic on Polyethylene Synthetic Substitute, Open Approach
ØSRBØ7Z Replacement of Left Hip Joint with Autologous Tissue Substitute, Open Approach
ØSRBØJ9 Replacement of Left Hip Joint with Synthetic Substitute, Cemented, Open Approach
ØSRBØJA Replacement of Left Hip Joint with Synthetic Substitute, Uncemented, Open Approach
ØSRBØJZ Replacement of Left Hip Joint with Synthetic Substitute, Open Approach
ØSRBØKZ Replacement of Left Hip Joint with Nonautologous Tissue Substitute, Open Approach
ØSRCØ7Z Replacement of Right Knee Joint with Autologous Tissue Substitute, Open Approach
ØSRCØJ9 Replacement of Right Knee Joint with Synthetic Substitute, Cemented, Open Approach
ØSRCØJA Replacement of Right Knee Joint with Synthetic Substitute, Uncemented, Open Approach
ØSRCØJZ Replacement of Right Knee Joint with Synthetic Substitute, Open Approach
ØSRCØKZ Replacement of Right Knee Joint with Nonautologous Tissue Substitute, Open Approach
ØSRCØL9 Replacement of Right Knee Joint with Unicondylar Synthetic Substitute, Cemented, Open Approach
ØSRCØLA Replacement of Right Knee Joint with Unicondylar Synthetic Substitute, Uncemented, Open Approach
ØSRCØLZ Replacement of Right Knee Joint with Unicondylar Synthetic Substitute, Open Approach
ØSRDØ7Z Replacement of Left Knee Joint with Autologous Tissue Substitute, Open Approach
ØSRDØJ9 Replacement of Left Knee Joint with Synthetic Substitute, Cemented, Open Approach
ØSRDØJA Replacement of Left Knee Joint with Synthetic Substitute, Uncemented, Open Approach
ØSRDØJZ Replacement of Left Knee Joint with Synthetic Substitute, Open Approach
ØSRDØKZ Replacement of Left Knee Joint with Nonautologous Tissue Substitute, Open Approach
ØSRDØL9 Replacement of Left Knee Joint with Unicondylar Synthetic Substitute, Cemented, Open Approach
ØSRDØLA Replacement of Left Knee Joint with Unicondylar Synthetic Substitute, Uncemented, Open Approach
ØSRDØLZ Replacement of Left Knee Joint with Unicondylar Synthetic Substitute, Open Approach
ØSREØØ9 Replacement of Left Hip Joint, Acetabular Surface with Polyethylene Synthetic Substitute, Cemented, Open Approach
ØSREØØA Replacement of Left Hip Joint, Acetabular Surface with Polyethylene Synthetic Substitute, Uncemented, Open Approach
ØSREØØZ Replacement of Left Hip Joint, Acetabular Surface with Polyethylene Synthetic Substitute, Open Approach
ØSREØ19 Replacement of Left Hip Joint, Acetabular Surface with Metal Synthetic Substitute, Cemented, Open Approach
ØSREØ1A Replacement of Left Hip Joint, Acetabular Surface with Metal Synthetic Substitute, Uncemented, Open Approach
ØSREØ1Z Replacement of Left Hip Joint, Acetabular Surface with Metal Synthetic Substitute, Open Approach
ØSREØ39 Replacement of Left Hip Joint, Acetabular Surface with Ceramic Synthetic Substitute, Cemented, Open Approach
ØSREØ3A Replacement of Left Hip Joint, Acetabular Surface with Ceramic Synthetic Substitute, Uncemented, Open Approach
ØSREØ3Z Replacement of Left Hip Joint, Acetabular Surface with Ceramic Synthetic Substitute, Open Approach
ØSREØ7Z Replacement of Left Hip Joint, Acetabular Surface with Autologous Tissue Substitute, Open Approach
ØSREØJ9 Replacement of Left Hip Joint, Acetabular Surface with Synthetic Substitute, Cemented, Open Approach
ØSREØJA Replacement of Left Hip Joint, Acetabular Surface with Synthetic Substitute, Uncemented, Open Approach
ØSREØJZ Replacement of Left Hip Joint, Acetabular Surface with Synthetic Substitute, Open Approach
ØSREØKZ Replacement of Left Hip Joint, Acetabular Surface with Nonautologous Tissue Substitute, Open Approach
ØSRRØ19 Replacement of Right Hip Joint, Femoral Surface with Metal Synthetic Substitute, Cemented, Open Approach
ØSRRØ1A Replacement of Right Hip Joint, Femoral Surface with Metal Synthetic Substitute, Uncemented, Open Approach
ØSRRØ1Z Replacement of Right Hip Joint, Femoral Surface with Metal Synthetic Substitute, Open Approach
ØSRRØ39 Replacement of Right Hip Joint, Femoral Surface with Ceramic Synthetic Substitute, Cemented, Open Approach
ØSRRØ3A Replacement of Right Hip Joint, Femoral Surface with Ceramic Synthetic Substitute, Uncemented, Open Approach
ØSRRØ3Z Replacement of Right Hip Joint, Femoral Surface with Ceramic Synthetic Substitute, Open Approach
ØSRRØ7Z Replacement of Right Hip Joint, Femoral Surface with Autologous Tissue Substitute, Open Approach
ØSRRØJ9 Replacement of Right Hip Joint, Femoral Surface with Synthetic Substitute, Cemented, Open Approach
ØSRRØJA Replacement of Right Hip Joint, Femoral Surface with Synthetic Substitute, Uncemented, Open Approach
ØSRRØJZ Replacement of Right Hip Joint, Femoral Surface with Synthetic Substitute, Open Approach
ØSRRØKZ Replacement of Right Hip Joint, Femoral Surface with Nonautologous Tissue Substitute, Open Approach

**HAC 10: Deep Vein Thrombosis (DVT) or Pulmonary Embolism (PE) with Total Knee or Hip Replacement (continued)**

ØSRSØ19 Replacement of Left Hip Joint, Femoral Surface with Metal Synthetic Substitute, Cemented, Open Approach
ØSRSØ1A Replacement of Left Hip Joint, Femoral Surface with Metal Synthetic Substitute, Uncemented, Open Approach
ØSRSØ1Z Replacement of Left Hip Joint, Femoral Surface with Metal Synthetic Substitute, Open Approach
ØSRSØ39 Replacement of Left Hip Joint, Femoral Surface with Ceramic Synthetic Substitute, Cemented, Open Approach
ØSRSØ3A Replacement of Left Hip Joint, Femoral Surface with Ceramic Synthetic Substitute, Uncemented, Open Approach
ØSRSØ3Z Replacement of Left Hip Joint, Femoral Surface with Ceramic Synthetic Substitute, Open Approach
ØSRSØ7Z Replacement of Left Hip Joint, Femoral Surface with Autologous Tissue Substitute, Open Approach
ØSRSØJ9 Replacement of Left Hip Joint, Femoral Surface with Synthetic Substitute, Cemented, Open Approach
ØSRSØJA Replacement of Left Hip Joint, Femoral Surface with Synthetic Substitute, Uncemented, Open Approach
ØSRSØJZ Replacement of Left Hip Joint, Femoral Surface with Synthetic Substitute, Open Approach
ØSRSØKZ Replacement of Left Hip Joint, Femoral Surface with Nonautologous Tissue Substitute, Open Approach
ØSRTØ7Z Replacement of Right Knee Joint, Femoral Surface with Autologous Tissue Substitute, Open Approach
ØSRTØJ9 Replacement of Right Knee Joint, Femoral Surface with Synthetic Substitute, Cemented, Open Approach
ØSRTØJA Replacement of Right Knee Joint, Femoral Surface with Synthetic Substitute, Uncemented, Open Approach
ØSRTØJZ Replacement of Right Knee Joint, Femoral Surface with Synthetic Substitute, Open Approach
ØSRTØKZ Replacement of Right Knee Joint, Femoral Surface with Nonautologous Tissue Substitute, Open Approach
ØSRUØ7Z Replacement of Left Knee Joint, Femoral Surface with Autologous Tissue Substitute, Open Approach
ØSRUØJ9 Replacement of Left Knee Joint, Femoral Surface with Synthetic Substitute, Cemented, Open Approach
ØSRUØJA Replacement of Left Knee Joint, Femoral Surface with Synthetic Substitute, Uncemented, Open Approach
ØSRUØJZ Replacement of Left Knee Joint, Femoral Surface with Synthetic Substitute, Open Approach
ØSRUØKZ Replacement of Left Knee Joint, Femoral Surface with Nonautologous Tissue Substitute, Open Approach
ØSRVØ7Z Replacement of Right Knee Joint, Tibial Surface with Autologous Tissue Substitute, Open Approach
ØSRVØJ9 Replacement of Right Knee Joint, Tibial Surface with Synthetic Substitute, Cemented, Open Approach
ØSRVØJA Replacement of Right Knee Joint, Tibial Surface with Synthetic Substitute, Uncemented, Open Approach
ØSRVØJZ Replacement of Right Knee Joint, Tibial Surface with Synthetic Substitute, Open Approach
ØSRVØKZ Replacement of Right Knee Joint, Tibial Surface with Nonautologous Tissue Substitute, Open Approach
ØSRWØ7Z Replacement of Left Knee Joint, Tibial Surface with Autologous Tissue Substitute, Open Approach
ØSRWØJ9 Replacement of Left Knee Joint, Tibial Surface with Synthetic Substitute, Cemented, Open Approach
ØSRWØJA Replacement of Left Knee Joint, Tibial Surface with Synthetic Substitute, Uncemented, Open Approach
ØSRWØJZ Replacement of Left Knee Joint, Tibial Surface with Synthetic Substitute, Open Approach
ØSRWØKZ Replacement of Left Knee Joint, Tibial Surface with Nonautologous Tissue Substitute, Open Approach
ØSU9ØBZ Supplement Right Hip Joint with Resurfacing Device, Open Approach
ØSUAØBZ Supplement Right Hip Joint, Acetabular Surface with Resurfacing Device, Open Approach
ØSUBØBZ Supplement Left Hip Joint with Resurfacing Device, Open Approach
ØSUEØBZ Supplement Left Hip Joint, Acetabular Surface with Resurfacing Device, Open Approach
ØSURØBZ Supplement Right Hip Joint, Femoral Surface with Resurfacing Device, Open Approach
ØSUSØBZ Supplement Left Hip Joint, Femoral Surface with Resurfacing Device, Open Approach

**HAC 11: Surgical Site Infection Following Bariatric Surgery**

Principal diagnosis of:
E66.Ø1

**AND**

Secondary diagnosis not POA:
K68.11
K95.Ø1
K95.81
T81.4XXA

**AND**

Any of the following procedures:
ØD16Ø79 Bypass Stomach to Duodenum with Autologous Tissue Substitute, Open Approach
ØD16Ø7A Bypass Stomach to Jejunum with Autologous Tissue Substitute, Open Approach
ØD16Ø7B Bypass Stomach to Ileum with Autologous Tissue Substitute, Open Approach
ØD16Ø7L Bypass Stomach to Transverse Colon with Autologous Tissue Substitute, Open Approach
ØD16ØJ9 Bypass Stomach to Duodenum with Synthetic Substitute, Open Approach
ØD16ØJA Bypass Stomach to Jejunum with Synthetic Substitute, Open Approach
ØD16ØJB Bypass Stomach to Ileum with Synthetic Substitute, Open Approach
ØD16ØJL Bypass Stomach to Transverse Colon with Synthetic Substitute, Open Approach
ØD16ØK9 Bypass Stomach to Duodenum with Nonautologous Tissue Substitute, Open Approach
ØD16ØKA Bypass Stomach to Jejunum with Nonautologous Tissue Substitute, Open Approach
ØD16ØKB Bypass Stomach to Ileum with Nonautologous Tissue Substitute, Open Approach
ØD16ØKL Bypass Stomach to Transverse Colon with Nonautologous Tissue Substitute, Open Approach
ØD16ØZ9 Bypass Stomach to Duodenum, Open Approach
ØD16ØZA Bypass Stomach to Jejunum, Open Approach
ØD16ØZB Bypass Stomach to Ileum, Open Approach
ØD16ØZL Bypass Stomach to Transverse Colon, Open Approach
ØD16479 Bypass Stomach to Duodenum with Autologous Tissue Substitute, Percutaneous Endoscopic Approach
ØD1647A Bypass Stomach to Jejunum with Autologous Tissue Substitute, Percutaneous Endoscopic Approach
ØD1647B Bypass Stomach to Ileum with Autologous Tissue Substitute, Percutaneous Endoscopic Approach
ØD1647L Bypass Stomach to Transverse Colon with Autologous Tissue Substitute, Percutaneous Endoscopic Approach
ØD164J9 Bypass Stomach to Duodenum with Synthetic Substitute, Percutaneous Endoscopic Approach
ØD164JA Bypass Stomach to Jejunum with Synthetic Substitute, Percutaneous Endoscopic Approach
ØD164JB Bypass Stomach to Ileum with Synthetic Substitute, Percutaneous Endoscopic Approach
ØD164JL Bypass Stomach to Transverse Colon with Synthetic Substitute, Percutaneous Endoscopic Approach
ØD164K9 Bypass Stomach to Duodenum with Nonautologous Tissue Substitute, Percutaneous Endoscopic Approach
ØD164KA Bypass Stomach to Jejunum with Nonautologous Tissue Substitute, Percutaneous Endoscopic Approach
ØD164KB Bypass Stomach to Ileum with Nonautologous Tissue Substitute, Percutaneous Endoscopic Approach
ØD164KL Bypass Stomach to Transverse Colon with Nonautologous Tissue Substitute, Percutaneous Endoscopic Approach
ØD164Z9 Bypass Stomach to Duodenum, Percutaneous Endoscopic Approach
ØD164ZA Bypass Stomach to Jejunum, Percutaneous Endoscopic Approach
ØD164ZB Bypass Stomach to Ileum, Percutaneous Endoscopic Approach
ØD164ZL Bypass Stomach to Transverse Colon, Percutaneous Endoscopic Approach
ØD16879 Bypass Stomach to Duodenum with Autologous Tissue Substitute, Via Natural or Artificial Opening Endoscopic
ØD1687A Bypass Stomach to Jejunum with Autologous Tissue Substitute, Via Natural or Artificial Opening Endoscopic
ØD1687B Bypass Stomach to Ileum with Autologous Tissue Substitute, Via Natural or Artificial Opening Endoscopic
ØD1687L Bypass Stomach to Transverse Colon with Autologous Tissue Substitute, Via Natural or Artificial Opening Endoscopic

**HAC 11: Surgical Site Infection Following Bariatric Surgery (continued)**

ØD168J9 Bypass Stomach to Duodenum with Synthetic Substitute, Via Natural or Artificial Opening Endoscopic
ØD168JA Bypass Stomach to Jejunum with Synthetic Substitute, Via Natural or Artificial Opening Endoscopic
ØD168JB Bypass Stomach to Ileum with Synthetic Substitute, Via Natural or Artificial Opening Endoscopic
ØD168JL Bypass Stomach to Transverse Colon with Synthetic Substitute, Via Natural or Artificial Opening Endoscopic
ØD168K9 Bypass Stomach to Duodenum with Nonautologous Tissue Substitute, Via Natural or Artificial Opening Endoscopic
ØD168KA Bypass Stomach to Jejunum with Nonautologous Tissue Substitute, Via Natural or Artificial Opening Endoscopic
ØD168KB Bypass Stomach to Ileum with Nonautologous Tissue Substitute, Via Natural or Artificial Opening Endoscopic
ØD168KL Bypass Stomach to Transverse Colon with Nonautologous Tissue Substitute, Via Natural or Artificial Opening Endoscopic
ØD168Z9 Bypass Stomach to Duodenum, Via Natural or Artificial Opening Endoscopic
ØD168ZA Bypass Stomach to Jejunum, Via Natural or Artificial Opening Endoscopic
ØD168ZB Bypass Stomach to Ileum, Via Natural or Artificial Opening Endoscopic
ØD168ZL Bypass Stomach to Transverse Colon, Via Natural or Artificial Opening Endoscopic
ØDV64CZ Restriction of Stomach with Extraluminal Device, Percutaneous Endoscopic Approach

**HAC 12: Surgical Site Infection Following Certain Orthopedic Procedures of the Spine, Shoulder, and Elbow**

Secondary diagnosis not POA:

K68.11
T81.4XXA
T84.6ØXA
T84.61ØA
T84.611A
T84.612A
T84.613A
T84.614A
T84.615A
T84.619A
T84.63XA
T84.69XA
T84.7XXA

**AND**

Any of the following procedures:

ØRGØØ7Ø Fusion of Occipital-cervical Joint with Autologous Tissue Substitute, Anterior Approach, Anterior Column, Open Approach
ØRGØØ71 Fusion of Occipital-cervical Joint with Autologous Tissue Substitute, Posterior Approach, Posterior Column, Open Approach
ØRGØØ7J Fusion of Occipital-cervical Joint with Autologous Tissue Substitute, Posterior Approach, Anterior Column, Open Approach
ØRGØØAØ Fusion of Occipital-cervical Joint with Interbody Fusion Device, Anterior Approach, Anterior Column, Open Approach
ØRGØØA1 Fusion of Occipital-cervical Joint with Interbody Fusion Device, Posterior Approach, Posterior Column, Open Approach
ØRGØØAJ Fusion of Occipital-cervical Joint with Interbody Fusion Device, Posterior Approach, Anterior Column, Open Approach
ØRGØØJØ Fusion of Occipital-cervical Joint with Synthetic Substitute, Anterior Approach, Anterior Column, Open Approach
ØRGØØJ1 Fusion of Occipital-cervical Joint with Synthetic Substitute, Posterior Approach, Posterior Column, Open Approach
ØRGØØJJ Fusion of Occipital-cervical Joint with Synthetic Substitute, Posterior Approach, Anterior Column, Open Approach
ØRGØØKØ Fusion of Occipital-cervical Joint with Nonautologous Tissue Substitute, Anterior Approach, Anterior Column, Open Approach
ØRGØØK1 Fusion of Occipital-cervical Joint with Nonautologous Tissue Substitute, Posterior Approach, Posterior Column, Open Approach
ØRGØØKJ Fusion of Occipital-cervical Joint with Nonautologous Tissue Substitute, Posterior Approach, Anterior Column, Open Approach
ØRGØØZØ Fusion of Occipital-cervical Joint, Anterior Approach, Anterior Column, Open Approach
ØRGØØZ1 Fusion of Occipital-cervical Joint, Posterior Approach, Posterior Column, Open Approach
ØRGØØZJ Fusion of Occipital-cervical Joint, Posterior Approach, Anterior Column, Open Approach
ØRGØ37Ø Fusion of Occipital-cervical Joint with Autologous Tissue Substitute, Anterior Approach, Anterior Column, Percutaneous Approach
ØRGØ371 Fusion of Occipital-cervical Joint with Autologous Tissue Substitute, Posterior Approach, Posterior Column, Percutaneous Approach
ØRGØ37J Fusion of Occipital-cervical Joint with Autologous Tissue Substitute, Posterior Approach, Anterior Column, Percutaneous Approach
ØRGØ3AØ Fusion of Occipital-cervical Joint with Interbody Fusion Device, Anterior Approach, Anterior Column, Percutaneous Approach
ØRGØ3A1 Fusion of Occipital-cervical Joint with Interbody Fusion Device, Posterior Approach, Posterior Column, Percutaneous Approach
ØRGØ3AJ Fusion of Occipital-cervical Joint with Interbody Fusion Device, Posterior Approach, Anterior Column, Percutaneous Approach
ØRGØ3JØ Fusion of Occipital-cervical Joint with Synthetic Substitute, Anterior Approach, Anterior Column, Percutaneous Approach
ØRGØ3J1 Fusion of Occipital-cervical Joint with Synthetic Substitute, Posterior Approach, Posterior Column, Percutaneous Approach
ØRGØ3JJ Fusion of Occipital-cervical Joint with Synthetic Substitute, Posterior Approach, Anterior Column, Percutaneous Approach
ØRGØ3KØ Fusion of Occipital-cervical Joint with Nonautologous Tissue Substitute, Anterior Approach, Anterior Column, Percutaneous Approach
ØRGØ3K1 Fusion of Occipital-cervical Joint with Nonautologous Tissue Substitute, Posterior Approach, Posterior Column, Percutaneous Approach
ØRGØ3KJ Fusion of Occipital-cervical Joint with Nonautologous Tissue Substitute, Posterior Approach, Anterior Column, Percutaneous Approach
ØRGØ3ZØ Fusion of Occipital-cervical Joint, Anterior Approach, Anterior Column, Percutaneous Approach
ØRGØ3Z1 Fusion of Occipital-cervical Joint, Posterior Approach, Posterior Column, Percutaneous Approach
ØRGØ3ZJ Fusion of Occipital-cervical Joint, Posterior Approach, Anterior Column, Percutaneous Approach
ØRGØ47Ø Fusion of Occipital-cervical Joint with Autologous Tissue Substitute, Anterior Approach, Anterior Column, Percutaneous Endoscopic Approach
ØRGØ471 Fusion of Occipital-cervical Joint with Autologous Tissue Substitute, Posterior Approach, Posterior Column, Percutaneous Endoscopic Approach
ØRGØ47J Fusion of Occipital-cervical Joint with Autologous Tissue Substitute, Posterior Approach, Anterior Column, Percutaneous Endoscopic Approach
ØRGØ4AØ Fusion of Occipital-cervical Joint with Interbody Fusion Device, Anterior Approach, Anterior Column, Percutaneous Endoscopic Approach
ØRGØ4A1 Fusion of Occipital-cervical Joint with Interbody Fusion Device, Posterior Approach, Posterior Column, Percutaneous Endoscopic Approach
ØRGØ4AJ Fusion of Occipital-cervical Joint with Interbody Fusion Device, Posterior Approach, Anterior Column, Percutaneous Endoscopic Approach
ØRGØ4JØ Fusion of Occipital-cervical Joint with Synthetic Substitute, Anterior Approach, Anterior Column, Percutaneous Endoscopic Approach
ØRGØ4J1 Fusion of Occipital-cervical Joint with Synthetic Substitute, Posterior Approach, Posterior Column, Percutaneous Endoscopic Approach
ØRGØ4JJ Fusion of Occipital-cervical Joint with Synthetic Substitute, Posterior Approach, Anterior Column, Percutaneous Endoscopic Approach
ØRGØ4KØ Fusion of Occipital-cervical Joint with Nonautologous Tissue Substitute, Anterior Approach, Anterior Column, Percutaneous Endoscopic Approach
ØRGØ4K1 Fusion of Occipital-cervical Joint with Nonautologous Tissue Substitute, Posterior Approach, Posterior Column, Percutaneous Endoscopic Approach
ØRGØ4KJ Fusion of Occipital-cervical Joint with Nonautologous Tissue Substitute, Posterior Approach, Anterior Column, Percutaneous Endoscopic Approach
ØRGØ4ZØ Fusion of Occipital-cervical Joint, Anterior Approach, Anterior Column, Percutaneous Endoscopic Approach
ØRGØ4Z1 Fusion of Occipital-cervical Joint, Posterior Approach, Posterior Column, Percutaneous Endoscopic Approach

**HAC 12: Surgical Site Infection Following Certain Orthopedic Procedures of the Spine, Shoulder, and Elbow (continued)**

ØRGØ4ZJ Fusion of Occipital-cervical Joint, Posterior Approach, Anterior Column, Percutaneous Endoscopic Approach
ØRG1Ø7Ø Fusion of Cervical Vertebral Joint with Autologous Tissue Substitute, Anterior Approach, Anterior Column, Open Approach
ØRG1Ø71 Fusion of Cervical Vertebral Joint with Autologous Tissue Substitute, Posterior Approach, Posterior Column, Open Approach
ØRG1Ø7J Fusion of Cervical Vertebral Joint with Autologous Tissue Substitute, Posterior Approach, Anterior Column, Open Approach
ØRG1ØAØ Fusion of Cervical Vertebral Joint with Interbody Fusion Device, Anterior Approach, Anterior Column, Open Approach
ØRG1ØA1 Fusion of Cervical Vertebral Joint with Interbody Fusion Device, Posterior Approach, Posterior Column, Open Approach
ØRG1ØAJ Fusion of Cervical Vertebral Joint with Interbody Fusion Device, Posterior Approach, Anterior Column, Open Approach
ØRG1ØJØ Fusion of Cervical Vertebral Joint with Synthetic Substitute, Anterior Approach, Anterior Column, Open Approach
ØRG1ØJ1 Fusion of Cervical Vertebral Joint with Synthetic Substitute, Posterior Approach, Posterior Column, Open Approach
ØRG1ØJJ Fusion of Cervical Vertebral Joint with Synthetic Substitute, Posterior Approach, Anterior Column, Open Approach
ØRG1ØKØ Fusion of Cervical Vertebral Joint with Nonautologous Tissue Substitute, Anterior Approach, Anterior Column, Open Approach
ØRG1ØK1 Fusion of Cervical Vertebral Joint with Nonautologous Tissue Substitute, Posterior Approach, Posterior Column, Open Approach
ØRG1ØKJ Fusion of Cervical Vertebral Joint with Nonautologous Tissue Substitute, Posterior Approach, Anterior Column, Open Approach
ØRG1ØZØ Fusion of Cervical Vertebral Joint, Anterior Approach, Anterior Column, Open Approach
ØRG1ØZ1 Fusion of Cervical Vertebral Joint, Posterior Approach, Posterior Column, Open Approach
ØRG1ØZJ Fusion of Cervical Vertebral Joint, Posterior Approach, Anterior Column, Open Approach
ØRG137Ø Fusion of Cervical Vertebral Joint with Autologous Tissue Substitute, Anterior Approach, Anterior Column, Percutaneous Approach
ØRG1371 Fusion of Cervical Vertebral Joint with Autologous Tissue Substitute, Posterior Approach, Posterior Column, Percutaneous Approach
ØRG137J Fusion of Cervical Vertebral Joint with Autologous Tissue Substitute, Posterior Approach, Anterior Column, Percutaneous Approach
ØRG13AØ Fusion of Cervical Vertebral Joint with Interbody Fusion Device, Anterior Approach, Anterior Column, Percutaneous Approach
ØRG13A1 Fusion of Cervical Vertebral Joint with Interbody Fusion Device, Posterior Approach, Posterior Column, Percutaneous Approach
ØRG13AJ Fusion of Cervical Vertebral Joint with Interbody Fusion Device, Posterior Approach, Anterior Column, Percutaneous Approach
ØRG13JØ Fusion of Cervical Vertebral Joint with Synthetic Substitute, Anterior Approach, Anterior Column, Percutaneous Approach
ØRG13J1 Fusion of Cervical Vertebral Joint with Synthetic Substitute, Posterior Approach, Posterior Column, Percutaneous Approach
ØRG13JJ Fusion of Cervical Vertebral Joint with Synthetic Substitute, Posterior Approach, Anterior Column, Percutaneous Approach
ØRG13KØ Fusion of Cervical Vertebral Joint with Nonautologous Tissue Substitute, Anterior Approach, Anterior Column, Percutaneous Approach
ØRG13K1 Fusion of Cervical Vertebral Joint with Nonautologous Tissue Substitute, Posterior Approach, Posterior Column, Percutaneous Approach
ØRG13KJ Fusion of Cervical Vertebral Joint with Nonautologous Tissue Substitute, Posterior Approach, Anterior Column, Percutaneous Approach
ØRG13ZØ Fusion of Cervical Vertebral Joint, Anterior Approach, Anterior Column, Percutaneous Approach
ØRG13Z1 Fusion of Cervical Vertebral Joint, Posterior Approach, Posterior Column, Percutaneous Approach
ØRG13ZJ Fusion of Cervical Vertebral Joint, Posterior Approach, Anterior Column, Percutaneous Approach
ØRG147Ø Fusion of Cervical Vertebral Joint with Autologous Tissue Substitute, Anterior Approach, Anterior Column, Percutaneous Endoscopic Approach
ØRG1471 Fusion of Cervical Vertebral Joint with Autologous Tissue Substitute, Posterior Approach, Posterior Column, Percutaneous Endoscopic Approach
ØRG147J Fusion of Cervical Vertebral Joint with Autologous Tissue Substitute, Posterior Approach, Anterior Column, Percutaneous Endoscopic Approach
ØRG14AØ Fusion of Cervical Vertebral Joint with Interbody Fusion Device, Anterior Approach, Anterior Column, Percutaneous Endoscopic Approach
ØRG14A1 Fusion of Cervical Vertebral Joint with Interbody Fusion Device, Posterior Approach, Posterior Column, Percutaneous Endoscopic Approach
ØRG14AJ Fusion of Cervical Vertebral Joint with Interbody Fusion Device, Posterior Approach, Anterior Column, Percutaneous Endoscopic Approach
ØRG14JØ Fusion of Cervical Vertebral Joint with Synthetic Substitute, Anterior Approach, Anterior Column, Percutaneous Endoscopic Approach
ØRG14J1 Fusion of Cervical Vertebral Joint with Synthetic Substitute, Posterior Approach, Posterior Column, Percutaneous Endoscopic Approach
ØRG14JJ Fusion of Cervical Vertebral Joint with Synthetic Substitute, Posterior Approach, Anterior Column, Percutaneous Endoscopic Approach
ØRG14KØ Fusion of Cervical Vertebral Joint with Nonautologous Tissue Substitute, Anterior Approach, Anterior Column, Percutaneous Endoscopic Approach
ØRG14K1 Fusion of Cervical Vertebral Joint with Nonautologous Tissue Substitute, Posterior Approach, Posterior Column, Percutaneous Endoscopic Approach
ØRG14KJ Fusion of Cervical Vertebral Joint with Nonautologous Tissue Substitute, Posterior Approach, Anterior Column, Percutaneous Endoscopic Approach
ØRG14ZØ Fusion of Cervical Vertebral Joint, Anterior Approach, Anterior Column, Percutaneous Endoscopic Approach
ØRG14Z1 Fusion of Cervical Vertebral Joint, Posterior Approach, Posterior Column, Percutaneous Endoscopic Approach
ØRG14ZJ Fusion of Cervical Vertebral Joint, Posterior Approach, Anterior Column, Percutaneous Endoscopic Approach
ØRG2Ø7Ø Fusion of 2 or more Cervical Vertebral Joints with Autologous Tissue Substitute, Anterior Approach, Anterior Column, Open Approach
ØRG2Ø71 Fusion of 2 or more Cervical Vertebral Joints with Autologous Tissue Substitute, Posterior Approach, Posterior Column, Open Approach
ØRG2Ø7J Fusion of 2 or more Cervical Vertebral Joints with Autologous Tissue Substitute, Posterior Approach, Anterior Column, Open Approach
ØRG2ØAØ Fusion of 2 or more Cervical Vertebral Joints with Interbody Fusion Device, Anterior Approach, Anterior Column, Open Approach
ØRG2ØA1 Fusion of 2 or more Cervical Vertebral Joints with Interbody Fusion Device, Posterior Approach, Posterior Column, Open Approach
ØRG2ØAJ Fusion of 2 or more Cervical Vertebral Joints with Interbody Fusion Device, Posterior Approach, Anterior Column, Open Approach
ØRG2ØJØ Fusion of 2 or more Cervical Vertebral Joints with Synthetic Substitute, Anterior Approach, Anterior Column, Open Approach
ØRG2ØJ1 Fusion of 2 or more Cervical Vertebral Joints with Synthetic Substitute, Posterior Approach, Posterior Column, Open Approach
ØRG2ØJJ Fusion of 2 or more Cervical Vertebral Joints with Synthetic Substitute, Posterior Approach, Anterior Column, Open Approach
ØRG2ØKØ Fusion of 2 or more Cervical Vertebral Joints with Nonautologous Tissue Substitute, Anterior Approach, Anterior Column, Open Approach
ØRG2ØK1 Fusion of 2 or more Cervical Vertebral Joints with Nonautologous Tissue Substitute, Posterior Approach, Posterior Column, Open Approach

**HAC 12: Surgical Site Infection Following Certain Orthopedic Procedures of the Spine, Shoulder, and Elbow (continued)**

ØRG2ØKJ Fusion of 2 or more Cervical Vertebral Joints with Nonautologous Tissue Substitute, Posterior Approach, Anterior Column, Open Approach
ØRG2ØZØ Fusion of 2 or more Cervical Vertebral Joints, Anterior Approach, Anterior Column, Open Approach
ØRG2ØZ1 Fusion of 2 or more Cervical Vertebral Joints, Posterior Approach, Posterior Column, Open Approach
ØRG2ØZJ Fusion of 2 or more Cervical Vertebral Joints, Posterior Approach, Anterior Column, Open Approach
ØRG237Ø Fusion of 2 or more Cervical Vertebral Joints with Autologous Tissue Substitute, Anterior Approach, Anterior Column, Percutaneous Approach
ØRG2371 Fusion of 2 or more Cervical Vertebral Joints with Autologous Tissue Substitute, Posterior Approach, Posterior Column, Percutaneous Approach
ØRG237J Fusion of 2 or more Cervical Vertebral Joints with Autologous Tissue Substitute, Posterior Approach, Anterior Column, Percutaneous Approach
ØRG23AØ Fusion of 2 or more Cervical Vertebral Joints with Interbody Fusion Device, Anterior Approach, Anterior Column, Percutaneous Approach
ØRG23A1 Fusion of 2 or more Cervical Vertebral Joints with Interbody Fusion Device, Posterior Approach, Posterior Column, Percutaneous Approach
ØRG23AJ Fusion of 2 or more Cervical Vertebral Joints with Interbody Fusion Device, Posterior Approach, Anterior Column, Percutaneous Approach
ØRG23JØ Fusion of 2 or more Cervical Vertebral Joints with Synthetic Substitute, Anterior Approach, Anterior Column, Percutaneous Approach
ØRG23J1 Fusion of 2 or more Cervical Vertebral Joints with Synthetic Substitute, Posterior Approach, Posterior Column, Percutaneous Approach
ØRG23JJ Fusion of 2 or more Cervical Vertebral Joints with Synthetic Substitute, Posterior Approach, Anterior Column, Percutaneous Approach
ØRG23KØ Fusion of 2 or more Cervical Vertebral Joints with Nonautologous Tissue Substitute, Anterior Approach, Anterior Column, Percutaneous Approach
ØRG23K1 Fusion of 2 or more Cervical Vertebral Joints with Nonautologous Tissue Substitute, Posterior Approach, Posterior Column, Percutaneous Approach
ØRG23KJ Fusion of 2 or more Cervical Vertebral Joints with Nonautologous Tissue Substitute, Posterior Approach, Anterior Column, Percutaneous Approach
ØRG23ZØ Fusion of 2 or more Cervical Vertebral Joints, Anterior Approach, Anterior Column, Percutaneous Approach
ØRG23Z1 Fusion of 2 or more Cervical Vertebral Joints, Posterior Approach, Posterior Column, Percutaneous Approach
ØRG23ZJ Fusion of 2 or more Cervical Vertebral Joints, Posterior Approach, Anterior Column, Percutaneous Approach
ØRG247Ø Fusion of 2 or more Cervical Vertebral Joints with Autologous Tissue Substitute, Anterior Approach, Anterior Column, Percutaneous Endoscopic Approach
ØRG2471 Fusion of 2 or more Cervical Vertebral Joints with Autologous Tissue Substitute, Posterior Approach, Posterior Column, Percutaneous Endoscopic Approach
ØRG247J Fusion of 2 or more Cervical Vertebral Joints with Autologous Tissue Substitute, Posterior Approach, Anterior Column, Percutaneous Endoscopic Approach
ØRG24AØ Fusion of 2 or more Cervical Vertebral Joints with Interbody Fusion Device, Anterior Approach, Anterior Column, Percutaneous Endoscopic Approach
ØRG24A1 Fusion of 2 or more Cervical Vertebral Joints with Interbody Fusion Device, Posterior Approach, Posterior Column, Percutaneous Endoscopic Approach
ØRG24AJ Fusion of 2 or more Cervical Vertebral Joints with Interbody Fusion Device, Posterior Approach, Anterior Column, Percutaneous Endoscopic Approach
ØRG24JØ Fusion of 2 or more Cervical Vertebral Joints with Synthetic Substitute, Anterior Approach, Anterior Column, Percutaneous Endoscopic Approach
ØRG24J1 Fusion of 2 or more Cervical Vertebral Joints with Synthetic Substitute, Posterior Approach, Posterior Column, Percutaneous Endoscopic Approach
ØRG24JJ Fusion of 2 or more Cervical Vertebral Joints with Synthetic Substitute, Posterior Approach, Anterior Column, Percutaneous Endoscopic Approach
ØRG24KØ Fusion of 2 or more Cervical Vertebral Joints with Nonautologous Tissue Substitute, Anterior Approach, Anterior Column, Percutaneous Endoscopic Approach
ØRG24K1 Fusion of 2 or more Cervical Vertebral Joints with Nonautologous Tissue Substitute, Posterior Approach, Posterior Column, Percutaneous Endoscopic Approach
ØRG24KJ Fusion of 2 or more Cervical Vertebral Joints with Nonautologous Tissue Substitute, Posterior Approach, Anterior Column, Percutaneous Endoscopic Approach
ØRG24ZØ Fusion of 2 or more Cervical Vertebral Joints, Anterior Approach, Anterior Column, Percutaneous Endoscopic Approach
ØRG24Z1 Fusion of 2 or more Cervical Vertebral Joints, Posterior Approach, Posterior Column, Percutaneous Endoscopic Approach
ØRG24ZJ Fusion of 2 or more Cervical Vertebral Joints, Posterior Approach, Anterior Column, Percutaneous Endoscopic Approach
ØRG4Ø7Ø Fusion of Cervicothoracic Vertebral Joint with Autologous Tissue Substitute, Anterior Approach, Anterior Column, Open Approach
ØRG4Ø71 Fusion of Cervicothoracic Vertebral Joint with Autologous Tissue Substitute, Posterior Approach, Posterior Column, Open Approach
ØRG4Ø7J Fusion of Cervicothoracic Vertebral Joint with Autologous Tissue Substitute, Posterior Approach, Anterior Column, Open Approach
ØRG4ØAØ Fusion of Cervicothoracic Vertebral Joint with Interbody Fusion Device, Anterior Approach, Anterior Column, Open Approach
ØRG4ØA1 Fusion of Cervicothoracic Vertebral Joint with Interbody Fusion Device, Posterior Approach, Posterior Column, Open Approach
ØRG4ØAJ Fusion of Cervicothoracic Vertebral Joint with Interbody Fusion Device, Posterior Approach, Anterior Column, Open Approach
ØRG4ØJØ Fusion of Cervicothoracic Vertebral Joint with Synthetic Substitute, Anterior Approach, Anterior Column, Open Approach
ØRG4ØJ1 Fusion of Cervicothoracic Vertebral Joint with Synthetic Substitute, Posterior Approach, Posterior Column, Open Approach
ØRG4ØJJ Fusion of Cervicothoracic Vertebral Joint with Synthetic Substitute, Posterior Approach, Anterior Column, Open Approach
ØRG4ØKØ Fusion of Cervicothoracic Vertebral Joint with Nonautologous Tissue Substitute, Anterior Approach, Anterior Column, Open Approach
ØRG4ØK1 Fusion of Cervicothoracic Vertebral Joint with Nonautologous Tissue Substitute, Posterior Approach, Posterior Column, Open Approach
ØRG4ØKJ Fusion of Cervicothoracic Vertebral Joint with Nonautologous Tissue Substitute, Posterior Approach, Anterior Column, Open Approach
ØRG4ØZØ Fusion of Cervicothoracic Vertebral Joint, Anterior Approach, Anterior Column, Open Approach
ØRG4ØZ1 Fusion of Cervicothoracic Vertebral Joint, Posterior Approach, Posterior Column, Open Approach
ØRG4ØZJ Fusion of Cervicothoracic Vertebral Joint, Posterior Approach, Anterior Column, Open Approach
ØRG437Ø Fusion of Cervicothoracic Vertebral Joint with Autologous Tissue Substitute, Anterior Approach, Anterior Column, Percutaneous Approach
ØRG4371 Fusion of Cervicothoracic Vertebral Joint with Autologous Tissue Substitute, Posterior Approach, Posterior Column, Percutaneous Approach
ØRG437J Fusion of Cervicothoracic Vertebral Joint with Autologous Tissue Substitute, Posterior Approach, Anterior Column, Percutaneous Approach
ØRG43AØ Fusion of Cervicothoracic Vertebral Joint with Interbody Fusion Device, Anterior Approach, Anterior Column, Percutaneous Approach
ØRG43A1 Fusion of Cervicothoracic Vertebral Joint with Interbody Fusion Device, Posterior Approach, Posterior Column, Percutaneous Approach
ØRG43AJ Fusion of Cervicothoracic Vertebral Joint with Interbody Fusion Device, Posterior Approach, Anterior Column, Percutaneous Approach

**HAC 12: Surgical Site Infection Following Certain Orthopedic Procedures of the Spine, Shoulder, and Elbow (continued)**

ØRG43JØ Fusion of Cervicothoracic Vertebral Joint with Synthetic Substitute, Anterior Approach, Anterior Column, Percutaneous Approach
ØRG43J1 Fusion of Cervicothoracic Vertebral Joint with Synthetic Substitute, Posterior Approach, Posterior Column, Percutaneous Approach
ØRG43JJ Fusion of Cervicothoracic Vertebral Joint with Synthetic Substitute, Posterior Approach, Anterior Column, Percutaneous Approach
ØRG43KØ Fusion of Cervicothoracic Vertebral Joint with Nonautologous Tissue Substitute, Anterior Approach, Anterior Column, Percutaneous Approach
ØRG43K1 Fusion of Cervicothoracic Vertebral Joint with Nonautologous Tissue Substitute, Posterior Approach, Posterior Column, Percutaneous Approach
ØRG43KJ Fusion of Cervicothoracic Vertebral Joint with Nonautologous Tissue Substitute, Posterior Approach, Anterior Column, Percutaneous Approach
ØRG43ZØ Fusion of Cervicothoracic Vertebral Joint, Anterior Approach, Anterior Column, Percutaneous Approach
ØRG43Z1 Fusion of Cervicothoracic Vertebral Joint, Posterior Approach, Posterior Column, Percutaneous Approach
ØRG43ZJ Fusion of Cervicothoracic Vertebral Joint, Posterior Approach, Anterior Column, Percutaneous Approach
ØRG447Ø Fusion of Cervicothoracic Vertebral Joint with Autologous Tissue Substitute, Anterior Approach, Anterior Column, Percutaneous Endoscopic Approach
ØRG4471 Fusion of Cervicothoracic Vertebral Joint with Autologous Tissue Substitute, Posterior Approach, Posterior Column, Percutaneous Endoscopic Approach
ØRG447J Fusion of Cervicothoracic Vertebral Joint with Autologous Tissue Substitute, Posterior Approach, Anterior Column, Percutaneous Endoscopic Approach
ØRG44AØ Fusion of Cervicothoracic Vertebral Joint with Interbody Fusion Device, Anterior Approach, Anterior Column, Percutaneous Endoscopic Approach
ØRG44A1 Fusion of Cervicothoracic Vertebral Joint with Interbody Fusion Device, Posterior Approach, Posterior Column, Percutaneous Endoscopic Approach
ØRG44AJ Fusion of Cervicothoracic Vertebral Joint with Interbody Fusion Device, Posterior Approach, Anterior Column, Percutaneous Endoscopic Approach
ØRG44JØ Fusion of Cervicothoracic Vertebral Joint with Synthetic Substitute, Anterior Approach, Anterior Column, Percutaneous Endoscopic Approach
ØRG44J1 Fusion of Cervicothoracic Vertebral Joint with Synthetic Substitute, Posterior Approach, Posterior Column, Percutaneous Endoscopic Approach
ØRG44JJ Fusion of Cervicothoracic Vertebral Joint with Synthetic Substitute, Posterior Approach, Anterior Column, Percutaneous Endoscopic Approach
ØRG44KØ Fusion of Cervicothoracic Vertebral Joint with Nonautologous Tissue Substitute, Anterior Approach, Anterior Column, Percutaneous Endoscopic Approach
ØRG44K1 Fusion of Cervicothoracic Vertebral Joint with Nonautologous Tissue Substitute, Posterior Approach, Posterior Column, Percutaneous Endoscopic Approach
ØRG44KJ Fusion of Cervicothoracic Vertebral Joint with Nonautologous Tissue Substitute, Posterior Approach, Anterior Column, Percutaneous Endoscopic Approach
ØRG44ZØ Fusion of Cervicothoracic Vertebral Joint, Anterior Approach, Anterior Column, Percutaneous Endoscopic Approach
ØRG44Z1 Fusion of Cervicothoracic Vertebral Joint, Posterior Approach, Posterior Column, Percutaneous Endoscopic Approach
ØRG44ZJ Fusion of Cervicothoracic Vertebral Joint, Posterior Approach, Anterior Column, Percutaneous Endoscopic Approach
ØRG6Ø7Ø Fusion of Thoracic Vertebral Joint with Autologous Tissue Substitute, Anterior Approach, Anterior Column, Open Approach
ØRG6Ø71 Fusion of Thoracic Vertebral Joint with Autologous Tissue Substitute, Posterior Approach, Posterior Column, Open Approach
ØRG6Ø7J Fusion of Thoracic Vertebral Joint with Autologous Tissue Substitute, Posterior Approach, Anterior Column, Open Approach
ØRG6ØAØ Fusion of Thoracic Vertebral Joint with Interbody Fusion Device, Anterior Approach, Anterior Column, Open Approach
ØRG6ØA1 Fusion of Thoracic Vertebral Joint with Interbody Fusion Device, Posterior Approach, Posterior Column, Open Approach
ØRG6ØAJ Fusion of Thoracic Vertebral Joint with Interbody Fusion Device, Posterior Approach, Anterior Column, Open Approach
ØRG6ØJØ Fusion of Thoracic Vertebral Joint with Synthetic Substitute, Anterior Approach, Anterior Column, Open Approach
ØRG6ØJ1 Fusion of Thoracic Vertebral Joint with Synthetic Substitute, Posterior Approach, Posterior Column, Open Approach
ØRG6ØJJ Fusion of Thoracic Vertebral Joint with Synthetic Substitute, Posterior Approach, Anterior Column, Open Approach
ØRG6ØKØ Fusion of Thoracic Vertebral Joint with Nonautologous Tissue Substitute, Anterior Approach, Anterior Column, Open Approach
ØRG6ØK1 Fusion of Thoracic Vertebral Joint with Nonautologous Tissue Substitute, Posterior Approach, Posterior Column, Open Approach
ØRG6ØKJ Fusion of Thoracic Vertebral Joint with Nonautologous Tissue Substitute, Posterior Approach, Anterior Column, Open Approach
ØRG6ØZØ Fusion of Thoracic Vertebral Joint, Anterior Approach, Anterior Column, Open Approach
ØRG6ØZ1 Fusion of Thoracic Vertebral Joint, Posterior Approach, Posterior Column, Open Approach
ØRG6ØZJ Fusion of Thoracic Vertebral Joint, Posterior Approach, Anterior Column, Open Approach
ØRG637Ø Fusion of Thoracic Vertebral Joint with Autologous Tissue Substitute, Anterior Approach, Anterior Column, Percutaneous Approach
ØRG6371 Fusion of Thoracic Vertebral Joint with Autologous Tissue Substitute, Posterior Approach, Posterior Column, Percutaneous Approach
ØRG637J Fusion of Thoracic Vertebral Joint with Autologous Tissue Substitute, Posterior Approach, Anterior Column, Percutaneous Approach
ØRG63AØ Fusion of Thoracic Vertebral Joint with Interbody Fusion Device, Anterior Approach, Anterior Column, Percutaneous Approach
ØRG63A1 Fusion of Thoracic Vertebral Joint with Interbody Fusion Device, Posterior Approach, Posterior Column, Percutaneous Approach
ØRG63AJ Fusion of Thoracic Vertebral Joint with Interbody Fusion Device, Posterior Approach, Anterior Column, Percutaneous Approach
ØRG63JØ Fusion of Thoracic Vertebral Joint with Synthetic Substitute, Anterior Approach, Anterior Column, Percutaneous Approach
ØRG63J1 Fusion of Thoracic Vertebral Joint with Synthetic Substitute, Posterior Approach, Posterior Column, Percutaneous Approach
ØRG63JJ Fusion of Thoracic Vertebral Joint with Synthetic Substitute, Posterior Approach, Anterior Column, Percutaneous Approach
ØRG63KØ Fusion of Thoracic Vertebral Joint with Nonautologous Tissue Substitute, Anterior Approach, Anterior Column, Percutaneous Approach
ØRG63K1 Fusion of Thoracic Vertebral Joint with Nonautologous Tissue Substitute, Posterior Approach, Posterior Column, Percutaneous Approach
ØRG63KJ Fusion of Thoracic Vertebral Joint with Nonautologous Tissue Substitute, Posterior Approach, Anterior Column, Percutaneous Approach
ØRG63ZØ Fusion of Thoracic Vertebral Joint, Anterior Approach, Anterior Column, Percutaneous Approach
ØRG63Z1 Fusion of Thoracic Vertebral Joint, Posterior Approach, Posterior Column, Percutaneous Approach
ØRG63ZJ Fusion of Thoracic Vertebral Joint, Posterior Approach, Anterior Column, Percutaneous Approach
ØRG647Ø Fusion of Thoracic Vertebral Joint with Autologous Tissue Substitute, Anterior Approach, Anterior Column, Percutaneous Endoscopic Approach
ØRG6471 Fusion of Thoracic Vertebral Joint with Autologous Tissue Substitute, Posterior Approach, Posterior Column, Percutaneous Endoscopic Approach
ØRG647J Fusion of Thoracic Vertebral Joint with Autologous Tissue Substitute, Posterior Approach, Anterior Column, Percutaneous Endoscopic Approach
ØRG64AØ Fusion of Thoracic Vertebral Joint with Interbody Fusion Device, Anterior Approach, Anterior Column, Percutaneous Endoscopic Approach

**HAC 12: Surgical Site Infection Following Certain Orthopedic Procedures of the Spine, Shoulder, and Elbow (continued)**

ØRG64A1 Fusion of Thoracic Vertebral Joint with Interbody Fusion Device, Posterior Approach, Posterior Column, Percutaneous Endoscopic Approach
ØRG64AJ Fusion of Thoracic Vertebral Joint with Interbody Fusion Device, Posterior Approach, Anterior Column, Percutaneous Endoscopic Approach
ØRG64JØ Fusion of Thoracic Vertebral Joint with Synthetic Substitute, Anterior Approach, Anterior Column, Percutaneous Endoscopic Approach
ØRG64J1 Fusion of Thoracic Vertebral Joint with Synthetic Substitute, Posterior Approach, Posterior Column, Percutaneous Endoscopic Approach
ØRG64JJ Fusion of Thoracic Vertebral Joint with Synthetic Substitute, Posterior Approach, Anterior Column, Percutaneous Endoscopic Approach
ØRG64KØ Fusion of Thoracic Vertebral Joint with Nonautologous Tissue Substitute, Anterior Approach, Anterior Column, Percutaneous Endoscopic Approach
ØRG64K1 Fusion of Thoracic Vertebral Joint with Nonautologous Tissue Substitute, Posterior Approach, Posterior Column, Percutaneous Endoscopic Approach
ØRG64KJ Fusion of Thoracic Vertebral Joint with Nonautologous Tissue Substitute, Posterior Approach, Anterior Column, Percutaneous Endoscopic Approach
ØRG64ZØ Fusion of Thoracic Vertebral Joint, Anterior Approach, Anterior Column, Percutaneous Endoscopic Approach
ØRG64Z1 Fusion of Thoracic Vertebral Joint, Posterior Approach, Posterior Column, Percutaneous Endoscopic Approach
ØRG64ZJ Fusion of Thoracic Vertebral Joint, Posterior Approach, Anterior Column, Percutaneous Endoscopic Approach
ØRG7Ø7Ø Fusion of 2 to 7 Thoracic Vertebral Joints with Autologous Tissue Substitute, Anterior Approach, Anterior Column, Open Approach
ØRG7Ø71 Fusion of 2 to 7 Thoracic Vertebral Joints with Autologous Tissue Substitute, Posterior Approach, Posterior Column, Open Approach
ØRG7Ø7J Fusion of 2 to 7 Thoracic Vertebral Joints with Autologous Tissue Substitute, Posterior Approach, Anterior Column, Open Approach
ØRG7ØAØ Fusion of 2 to 7 Thoracic Vertebral Joints with Interbody Fusion Device, Anterior Approach, Anterior Column, Open Approach
ØRG7ØA1 Fusion of 2 to 7 Thoracic Vertebral Joints with Interbody Fusion Device, Posterior Approach, Posterior Column, Open Approach
ØRG7ØAJ Fusion of 2 to 7 Thoracic Vertebral Joints with Interbody Fusion Device, Posterior Approach, Anterior Column, Open Approach
ØRG7ØJØ Fusion of 2 to 7 Thoracic Vertebral Joints with Synthetic Substitute, Anterior Approach, Anterior Column, Open Approach
ØRG7ØJ1 Fusion of 2 to 7 Thoracic Vertebral Joints with Synthetic Substitute, Posterior Approach, Posterior Column, Open Approach
ØRG7ØJJ Fusion of 2 to 7 Thoracic Vertebral Joints with Synthetic Substitute, Posterior Approach, Anterior Column, Open Approach
ØRG7ØKØ Fusion of 2 to 7 Thoracic Vertebral Joints with Nonautologous Tissue Substitute, Anterior Approach, Anterior Column, Open Approach
ØRG7ØK1 Fusion of 2 to 7 Thoracic Vertebral Joints with Nonautologous Tissue Substitute, Posterior Approach, Posterior Column, Open Approach
ØRG7ØKJ Fusion of 2 to 7 Thoracic Vertebral Joints with Nonautologous Tissue Substitute, Posterior Approach, Anterior Column, Open Approach
ØRG7ØZØ Fusion of 2 to 7 Thoracic Vertebral Joints, Anterior Approach, Anterior Column, Open Approach
ØRG7ØZ1 Fusion of 2 to 7 Thoracic Vertebral Joints, Posterior Approach, Posterior Column, Open Approach
ØRG7ØZJ Fusion of 2 to 7 Thoracic Vertebral Joints, Posterior Approach, Anterior Column, Open Approach
ØRG737Ø Fusion of 2 to 7 Thoracic Vertebral Joints with Autologous Tissue Substitute, Anterior Approach, Anterior Column, Percutaneous Approach
ØRG7371 Fusion of 2 to 7 Thoracic Vertebral Joints with Autologous Tissue Substitute, Posterior Approach, Posterior Column, Percutaneous Approach
ØRG737J Fusion of 2 to 7 Thoracic Vertebral Joints with Autologous Tissue Substitute, Posterior Approach, Anterior Column, Percutaneous Approach
ØRG73AØ Fusion of 2 to 7 Thoracic Vertebral Joints with Interbody Fusion Device, Anterior Approach, Anterior Column, Percutaneous Approach
ØRG73A1 Fusion of 2 to 7 Thoracic Vertebral Joints with Interbody Fusion Device, Posterior Approach, Posterior Column, Percutaneous Approach
ØRG73AJ Fusion of 2 to 7 Thoracic Vertebral Joints with Interbody Fusion Device, Posterior Approach, Anterior Column, Percutaneous Approach
ØRG73JØ Fusion of 2 to 7 Thoracic Vertebral Joints with Synthetic Substitute, Anterior Approach, Anterior Column, Percutaneous Approach
ØRG73J1 Fusion of 2 to 7 Thoracic Vertebral Joints with Synthetic Substitute, Posterior Approach, Posterior Column, Percutaneous Approach
ØRG73JJ Fusion of 2 to 7 Thoracic Vertebral Joints with Synthetic Substitute, Posterior Approach, Anterior Column, Percutaneous Approach
ØRG73KØ Fusion of 2 to 7 Thoracic Vertebral Joints with Nonautologous Tissue Substitute, Anterior Approach, Anterior Column, Percutaneous Approach
ØRG73K1 Fusion of 2 to 7 Thoracic Vertebral Joints with Nonautologous Tissue Substitute, Posterior Approach, Posterior Column, Percutaneous Approach
ØRG73KJ Fusion of 2 to 7 Thoracic Vertebral Joints with Nonautologous Tissue Substitute, Posterior Approach, Anterior Column, Percutaneous Approach
ØRG73ZØ Fusion of 2 to 7 Thoracic Vertebral Joints, Anterior Approach, Anterior Column, Percutaneous Approach
ØRG73Z1 Fusion of 2 to 7 Thoracic Vertebral Joints, Posterior Approach, Posterior Column, Percutaneous Approach
ØRG73ZJ Fusion of 2 to 7 Thoracic Vertebral Joints, Posterior Approach, Anterior Column, Percutaneous Approach
ØRG747Ø Fusion of 2 to 7 Thoracic Vertebral Joints with Autologous Tissue Substitute, Anterior Approach, Anterior Column, Percutaneous Endoscopic Approach
ØRG7471 Fusion of 2 to 7 Thoracic Vertebral Joints with Autologous Tissue Substitute, Posterior Approach, Posterior Column, Percutaneous Endoscopic Approach
ØRG747J Fusion of 2 to 7 Thoracic Vertebral Joints with Autologous Tissue Substitute, Posterior Approach, Anterior Column, Percutaneous Endoscopic Approach
ØRG74AØ Fusion of 2 to 7 Thoracic Vertebral Joints with Interbody Fusion Device, Anterior Approach, Anterior Column, Percutaneous Endoscopic Approach
ØRG74A1 Fusion of 2 to 7 Thoracic Vertebral Joints with Interbody Fusion Device, Posterior Approach, Posterior Column, Percutaneous Endoscopic Approach
ØRG74AJ Fusion of 2 to 7 Thoracic Vertebral Joints with Interbody Fusion Device, Posterior Approach, Anterior Column, Percutaneous Endoscopic Approach
ØRG74JØ Fusion of 2 to 7 Thoracic Vertebral Joints with Synthetic Substitute, Anterior Approach, Anterior Column, Percutaneous Endoscopic Approach
ØRG74J1 Fusion of 2 to 7 Thoracic Vertebral Joints with Synthetic Substitute, Posterior Approach, Posterior Column, Percutaneous Endoscopic Approach
ØRG74JJ Fusion of 2 to 7 Thoracic Vertebral Joints with Synthetic Substitute, Posterior Approach, Anterior Column, Percutaneous Endoscopic Approach
ØRG74KØ Fusion of 2 to 7 Thoracic Vertebral Joints with Nonautologous Tissue Substitute, Anterior Approach, Anterior Column, Percutaneous Endoscopic Approach
ØRG74K1 Fusion of 2 to 7 Thoracic Vertebral Joints with Nonautologous Tissue Substitute, Posterior Approach, Posterior Column, Percutaneous Endoscopic Approach
ØRG74KJ Fusion of 2 to 7 Thoracic Vertebral Joints with Nonautologous Tissue Substitute, Posterior Approach, Anterior Column, Percutaneous Endoscopic Approach
ØRG74ZØ Fusion of 2 to 7 Thoracic Vertebral Joints, Anterior Approach, Anterior Column, Percutaneous Endoscopic Approach
ØRG74Z1 Fusion of 2 to 7 Thoracic Vertebral Joints, Posterior Approach, Posterior Column, Percutaneous Endoscopic Approach
ØRG74ZJ Fusion of 2 to 7 Thoracic Vertebral Joints, Posterior Approach, Anterior Column, Percutaneous Endoscopic Approach
ØRG8Ø7Ø Fusion of 8 or More Thoracic Vertebral Joints with Autologous Tissue Substitute, Anterior Approach, Anterior Column, Open Approach
ØRG8Ø71 Fusion of 8 or More Thoracic Vertebral Joints with Autologous Tissue Substitute, Posterior Approach, Posterior Column, Open Approach

**HAC 12: Surgical Site Infection Following Certain Orthopedic Procedures of the Spine, Shoulder, and Elbow (continued)**

ØRG807J Fusion of 8 or More Thoracic Vertebral Joints with Autologous Tissue Substitute, Posterior Approach, Anterior Column, Open Approach
ØRG80AØ Fusion of 8 or More Thoracic Vertebral Joints with Interbody Fusion Device, Anterior Approach, Anterior Column, Open Approach
ØRG80A1 Fusion of 8 or More Thoracic Vertebral Joints with Interbody Fusion Device, Posterior Approach, Posterior Column, Open Approach
ØRG80AJ Fusion of 8 or More Thoracic Vertebral Joints with Interbody Fusion Device, Posterior Approach, Anterior Column, Open Approach
ØRG80JØ Fusion of 8 or More Thoracic Vertebral Joints with Synthetic Substitute, Anterior Approach, Anterior Column, Open Approach
ØRG80J1 Fusion of 8 or More Thoracic Vertebral Joints with Synthetic Substitute, Posterior Approach, Posterior Column, Open Approach
ØRG80JJ Fusion of 8 or More Thoracic Vertebral Joints with Synthetic Substitute, Posterior Approach, Anterior Column, Open Approach
ØRG80KØ Fusion of 8 or More Thoracic Vertebral Joints with Nonautologous Tissue Substitute, Anterior Approach, Anterior Column, Open Approach
ØRG80K1 Fusion of 8 or More Thoracic Vertebral Joints with Nonautologous Tissue Substitute, Posterior Approach, Posterior Column, Open Approach
ØRG80KJ Fusion of 8 or More Thoracic Vertebral Joints with Nonautologous Tissue Substitute, Posterior Approach, Anterior Column, Open Approach
ØRG80ZØ Fusion of 8 or More Thoracic Vertebral Joints, Anterior Approach, Anterior Column, Open Approach
ØRG80Z1 Fusion of 8 or More Thoracic Vertebral Joints, Posterior Approach, Posterior Column, Open Approach
ØRG80ZJ Fusion of 8 or More Thoracic Vertebral Joints, Posterior Approach, Anterior Column, Open Approach
ØRG837Ø Fusion of 8 or More Thoracic Vertebral Joints with Autologous Tissue Substitute, Anterior Approach, Anterior Column, Percutaneous Approach
ØRG8371 Fusion of 8 or More Thoracic Vertebral Joints with Autologous Tissue Substitute, Posterior Approach, Posterior Column, Percutaneous Approach
ØRG837J Fusion of 8 or More Thoracic Vertebral Joints with Autologous Tissue Substitute, Posterior Approach, Anterior Column, Percutaneous Approach
ØRG83AØ Fusion of 8 or More Thoracic Vertebral Joints with Interbody Fusion Device, Anterior Approach, Anterior Column, Percutaneous Approach
ØRG83A1 Fusion of 8 or More Thoracic Vertebral Joints with Interbody Fusion Device, Posterior Approach, Posterior Column, Percutaneous Approach
ØRG83AJ Fusion of 8 or More Thoracic Vertebral Joints with Interbody Fusion Device, Posterior Approach, Anterior Column, Percutaneous Approach
ØRG83JØ Fusion of 8 or More Thoracic Vertebral Joints with Synthetic Substitute, Anterior Approach, Anterior Column, Percutaneous Approach
ØRG83J1 Fusion of 8 or More Thoracic Vertebral Joints with Synthetic Substitute, Posterior Approach, Posterior Column, Percutaneous Approach
ØRG83JJ Fusion of 8 or More Thoracic Vertebral Joints with Synthetic Substitute, Posterior Approach, Anterior Column, Percutaneous Approach
ØRG83KØ Fusion of 8 or More Thoracic Vertebral Joints with Nonautologous Tissue Substitute, Anterior Approach, Anterior Column, Percutaneous Approach
ØRG83K1 Fusion of 8 or More Thoracic Vertebral Joints with Nonautologous Tissue Substitute, Posterior Approach, Posterior Column, Percutaneous Approach
ØRG83KJ Fusion of 8 or More Thoracic Vertebral Joints with Nonautologous Tissue Substitute, Posterior Approach, Anterior Column, Percutaneous Approach
ØRG83ZØ Fusion of 8 or More Thoracic Vertebral Joints, Anterior Approach, Anterior Column, Percutaneous Approach
ØRG83Z1 Fusion of 8 or More Thoracic Vertebral Joints, Posterior Approach, Posterior Column, Percutaneous Approach
ØRG83ZJ Fusion of 8 or More Thoracic Vertebral Joints, Posterior Approach, Anterior Column, Percutaneous Approach
ØRG847Ø Fusion of 8 or More Thoracic Vertebral Joints with Autologous Tissue Substitute, Anterior Approach, Anterior Column, Percutaneous Endoscopic Approach
ØRG8471 Fusion of 8 or More Thoracic Vertebral Joints with Autologous Tissue Substitute, Posterior Approach, Posterior Column, Percutaneous Endoscopic Approach
ØRG847J Fusion of 8 or More Thoracic Vertebral Joints with Autologous Tissue Substitute, Posterior Approach, Anterior Column, Percutaneous Endoscopic Approach
ØRG84AØ Fusion of 8 or More Thoracic Vertebral Joints with Interbody Fusion Device, Anterior Approach, Anterior Column, Percutaneous Endoscopic Approach
ØRG84A1 Fusion of 8 or More Thoracic Vertebral Joints with Interbody Fusion Device, Posterior Approach, Posterior Column, Percutaneous Endoscopic Approach
ØRG84AJ Fusion of 8 or More Thoracic Vertebral Joints with Interbody Fusion Device, Posterior Approach, Anterior Column, Percutaneous Endoscopic Approach
ØRG84JØ Fusion of 8 or More Thoracic Vertebral Joints with Synthetic Substitute, Anterior Approach, Anterior Column, Percutaneous Endoscopic Approach
ØRG84J1 Fusion of 8 or More Thoracic Vertebral Joints with Synthetic Substitute, Posterior Approach, Posterior Column, Percutaneous Endoscopic Approach
ØRG84JJ Fusion of 8 or More Thoracic Vertebral Joints with Synthetic Substitute, Posterior Approach, Anterior Column, Percutaneous Endoscopic Approach
ØRG84KØ Fusion of 8 or More Thoracic Vertebral Joints with Nonautologous Tissue Substitute, Anterior Approach, Anterior Column, Percutaneous Endoscopic Approach
ØRG84K1 Fusion of 8 or More Thoracic Vertebral Joints with Nonautologous Tissue Substitute, Posterior Approach, Posterior Column, Percutaneous Endoscopic Approach
ØRG84KJ Fusion of 8 or More Thoracic Vertebral Joints with Nonautologous Tissue Substitute, Posterior Approach, Anterior Column, Percutaneous Endoscopic Approach
ØRG84ZØ Fusion of 8 or More Thoracic Vertebral Joints, Anterior Approach, Anterior Column, Percutaneous Endoscopic Approach
ØRG84Z1 Fusion of 8 or More Thoracic Vertebral Joints, Posterior Approach, Posterior Column, Percutaneous Endoscopic Approach
ØRG84ZJ Fusion of 8 or More Thoracic Vertebral Joints, Posterior Approach, Anterior Column, Percutaneous Endoscopic Approach
ØRGA07Ø Fusion of Thoracolumbar Vertebral Joint with Autologous Tissue Substitute, Anterior Approach, Anterior Column, Open Approach
ØRGA071 Fusion of Thoracolumbar Vertebral Joint with Autologous Tissue Substitute, Posterior Approach, Posterior Column, Open Approach
ØRGA07J Fusion of Thoracolumbar Vertebral Joint with Autologous Tissue Substitute, Posterior Approach, Anterior Column, Open Approach
ØRGAØAØ Fusion of Thoracolumbar Vertebral Joint with Interbody Fusion Device, Anterior Approach, Anterior Column, Open Approach
ØRGAØA1 Fusion of Thoracolumbar Vertebral Joint with Interbody Fusion Device, Posterior Approach, Posterior Column, Open Approach
ØRGAØAJ Fusion of Thoracolumbar Vertebral Joint with Interbody Fusion Device, Posterior Approach, Anterior Column, Open Approach
ØRGAØJØ Fusion of Thoracolumbar Vertebral Joint with Synthetic Substitute, Anterior Approach, Anterior Column, Open Approach
ØRGAØJ1 Fusion of Thoracolumbar Vertebral Joint with Synthetic Substitute, Posterior Approach, Posterior Column, Open Approach
ØRGAØJJ Fusion of Thoracolumbar Vertebral Joint with Synthetic Substitute, Posterior Approach, Anterior Column, Open Approach
ØRGAØKØ Fusion of Thoracolumbar Vertebral Joint with Nonautologous Tissue Substitute, Anterior Approach, Anterior Column, Open Approach
ØRGAØK1 Fusion of Thoracolumbar Vertebral Joint with Nonautologous Tissue Substitute, Posterior Approach, Posterior Column, Open Approach

**HAC 12: Surgical Site Infection Following Certain Orthopedic Procedures of the Spine, Shoulder, and Elbow (continued)**

ØRGAØKJ Fusion of Thoracolumbar Vertebral Joint with Nonautologous Tissue Substitute, Posterior Approach, Anterior Column, Open Approach
ØRGAØZØ Fusion of Thoracolumbar Vertebral Joint, Anterior Approach, Anterior Column, Open Approach
ØRGAØZ1 Fusion of Thoracolumbar Vertebral Joint, Posterior Approach, Posterior Column, Open Approach
ØRGAØZJ Fusion of Thoracolumbar Vertebral Joint, Posterior Approach, Anterior Column, Open Approach
ØRGA37Ø Fusion of Thoracolumbar Vertebral Joint with Autologous Tissue Substitute, Anterior Approach, Anterior Column, Percutaneous Approach
ØRGA371 Fusion of Thoracolumbar Vertebral Joint with Autologous Tissue Substitute, Posterior Approach, Posterior Column, Percutaneous Approach
ØRGA37J Fusion of Thoracolumbar Vertebral Joint with Autologous Tissue Substitute, Posterior Approach, Anterior Column, Percutaneous Approach
ØRGA3AØ Fusion of Thoracolumbar Vertebral Joint with Interbody Fusion Device, Anterior Approach, Anterior Column, Percutaneous Approach
ØRGA3A1 Fusion of Thoracolumbar Vertebral Joint with Interbody Fusion Device, Posterior Approach, Posterior Column, Percutaneous Approach
ØRGA3AJ Fusion of Thoracolumbar Vertebral Joint with Interbody Fusion Device, Posterior Approach, Anterior Column, Percutaneous Approach
ØRGA3JØ Fusion of Thoracolumbar Vertebral Joint with Synthetic Substitute, Anterior Approach, Anterior Column, Percutaneous Approach
ØRGA3J1 Fusion of Thoracolumbar Vertebral Joint with Synthetic Substitute, Posterior Approach, Posterior Column, Percutaneous Approach
ØRGA3JJ Fusion of Thoracolumbar Vertebral Joint with Synthetic Substitute, Posterior Approach, Anterior Column, Percutaneous Approach
ØRGA3KØ Fusion of Thoracolumbar Vertebral Joint with Nonautologous Tissue Substitute, Anterior Approach, Anterior Column, Percutaneous Approach
ØRGA3K1 Fusion of Thoracolumbar Vertebral Joint with Nonautologous Tissue Substitute, Posterior Approach, Posterior Column, Percutaneous Approach
ØRGA3KJ Fusion of Thoracolumbar Vertebral Joint with Nonautologous Tissue Substitute, Posterior Approach, Anterior Column, Percutaneous Approach
ØRGA3ZØ Fusion of Thoracolumbar Vertebral Joint, Anterior Approach, Anterior Column, Percutaneous Approach
ØRGA3Z1 Fusion of Thoracolumbar Vertebral Joint, Posterior Approach, Posterior Column, Percutaneous Approach
ØRGA3ZJ Fusion of Thoracolumbar Vertebral Joint, Posterior Approach, Anterior Column, Percutaneous Approach
ØRGA47Ø Fusion of Thoracolumbar Vertebral Joint with Autologous Tissue Substitute, Anterior Approach, Anterior Column, Percutaneous Endoscopic Approach
ØRGA471 Fusion of Thoracolumbar Vertebral Joint with Autologous Tissue Substitute, Posterior Approach, Posterior Column, Percutaneous Endoscopic Approach
ØRGA47J Fusion of Thoracolumbar Vertebral Joint with Autologous Tissue Substitute, Posterior Approach, Anterior Column, Percutaneous Endoscopic Approach
ØRGA4AØ Fusion of Thoracolumbar Vertebral Joint with Interbody Fusion Device, Anterior Approach, Anterior Column, Percutaneous Endoscopic Approach
ØRGA4A1 Fusion of Thoracolumbar Vertebral Joint with Interbody Fusion Device, Posterior Approach, Posterior Column, Percutaneous Endoscopic Approach
ØRGA4AJ Fusion of Thoracolumbar Vertebral Joint with Interbody Fusion Device, Posterior Approach, Anterior Column, Percutaneous Endoscopic Approach
ØRGA4JØ Fusion of Thoracolumbar Vertebral Joint with Synthetic Substitute, Anterior Approach, Anterior Column, Percutaneous Endoscopic Approach
ØRGA4J1 Fusion of Thoracolumbar Vertebral Joint with Synthetic Substitute, Posterior Approach, Posterior Column, Percutaneous Endoscopic Approach
ØRGA4JJ Fusion of Thoracolumbar Vertebral Joint with Synthetic Substitute, Posterior Approach, Anterior Column, Percutaneous Endoscopic Approach
ØRGA4KØ Fusion of Thoracolumbar Vertebral Joint with Nonautologous Tissue Substitute, Anterior Approach, Anterior Column, Percutaneous Endoscopic Approach
ØRGA4K1 Fusion of Thoracolumbar Vertebral Joint with Nonautologous Tissue Substitute, Posterior Approach, Posterior Column, Percutaneous Endoscopic Approach
ØRGA4KJ Fusion of Thoracolumbar Vertebral Joint with Nonautologous Tissue Substitute, Posterior Approach, Anterior Column, Percutaneous Endoscopic Approach
ØRGA4ZØ Fusion of Thoracolumbar Vertebral Joint, Anterior Approach, Anterior Column, Percutaneous Endoscopic Approach
ØRGA4Z1 Fusion of Thoracolumbar Vertebral Joint, Posterior Approach, Posterior Column, Percutaneous Endoscopic Approach
ØRGA4ZJ Fusion of Thoracolumbar Vertebral Joint, Posterior Approach, Anterior Column, Percutaneous Endoscopic Approach
ØRGEØ4Z Fusion of Right Sternoclavicular Joint with Internal Fixation Device, Open Approach
ØRGEØ7Z Fusion of Right Sternoclavicular Joint with Autologous Tissue Substitute, Open Approach
ØRGEØJZ Fusion of Right Sternoclavicular Joint with Synthetic Substitute, Open Approach
ØRGEØKZ Fusion of Right Sternoclavicular Joint with Nonautologous Tissue Substitute, Open Approach
ØRGEØZZ Fusion of Right Sternoclavicular Joint, Open Approach
ØRGE34Z Fusion of Right Sternoclavicular Joint with Internal Fixation Device, Percutaneous Approach
ØRGE37Z Fusion of Right Sternoclavicular Joint with Autologous Tissue Substitute, Percutaneous Approach
ØRGE3JZ Fusion of Right Sternoclavicular Joint with Synthetic Substitute, Percutaneous Approach
ØRGE3KZ Fusion of Right Sternoclavicular Joint with Nonautologous Tissue Substitute, Percutaneous Approach
ØRGE3ZZ Fusion of Right Sternoclavicular Joint, Percutaneous Approach
ØRGE44Z Fusion of Right Sternoclavicular Joint with Internal Fixation Device, Percutaneous Endoscopic Approach
ØRGE47Z Fusion of Right Sternoclavicular Joint with Autologous Tissue Substitute, Percutaneous Endoscopic Approach
ØRGE4JZ Fusion of Right Sternoclavicular Joint with Synthetic Substitute, Percutaneous Endoscopic Approach
ØRGE4KZ Fusion of Right Sternoclavicular Joint with Nonautologous Tissue Substitute, Percutaneous Endoscopic Approach
ØRGE4ZZ Fusion of Right Sternoclavicular Joint, Percutaneous Endoscopic Approach
ØRGFØ4Z Fusion of Left Sternoclavicular Joint with Internal Fixation Device, Open Approach
ØRGFØ7Z Fusion of Left Sternoclavicular Joint with Autologous Tissue Substitute, Open Approach
ØRGFØJZ Fusion of Left Sternoclavicular Joint with Synthetic Substitute, Open Approach
ØRGFØKZ Fusion of Left Sternoclavicular Joint with Nonautologous Tissue Substitute, Open Approach
ØRGFØZZ Fusion of Left Sternoclavicular Joint, Open Approach
ØRGF34Z Fusion of Left Sternoclavicular Joint with Internal Fixation Device, Percutaneous Approach
ØRGF37Z Fusion of Left Sternoclavicular Joint with Autologous Tissue Substitute, Percutaneous Approach
ØRGF3JZ Fusion of Left Sternoclavicular Joint with Synthetic Substitute, Percutaneous Approach
ØRGF3KZ Fusion of Left Sternoclavicular Joint with Nonautologous Tissue Substitute, Percutaneous Approach
ØRGF3ZZ Fusion of Left Sternoclavicular Joint, Percutaneous Approach
ØRGF44Z Fusion of Left Sternoclavicular Joint with Internal Fixation Device, Percutaneous Endoscopic Approach
ØRGF47Z Fusion of Left Sternoclavicular Joint with Autologous Tissue Substitute, Percutaneous Endoscopic Approach
ØRGF4JZ Fusion of Left Sternoclavicular Joint with Synthetic Substitute, Percutaneous Endoscopic Approach
ØRGF4KZ Fusion of Left Sternoclavicular Joint with Nonautologous Tissue Substitute, Percutaneous Endoscopic Approach
ØRGF4ZZ Fusion of Left Sternoclavicular Joint, Percutaneous Endoscopic Approach
ØRGGØ4Z Fusion of Right Acromioclavicular Joint with Internal Fixation Device, Open Approach
ØRGGØ7Z Fusion of Right Acromioclavicular Joint with Autologous Tissue Substitute, Open Approach

Appendix J: Hospital Acquired Conditions

**HAC 12: Surgical Site Infection Following Certain Orthopedic Procedures of the Spine, Shoulder, and Elbow (continued)**

ØRGGØJZ Fusion of Right Acromioclavicular Joint with Synthetic Substitute, Open Approach
ØRGGØKZ Fusion of Right Acromioclavicular Joint with Nonautologous Tissue Substitute, Open Approach
ØRGGØZZ Fusion of Right Acromioclavicular Joint, Open Approach
ØRGG34Z Fusion of Right Acromioclavicular Joint with Internal Fixation Device, Percutaneous Approach
ØRGG37Z Fusion of Right Acromioclavicular Joint with Autologous Tissue Substitute, Percutaneous Approach
ØRGG3JZ Fusion of Right Acromioclavicular Joint with Synthetic Substitute, Percutaneous Approach
ØRGG3KZ Fusion of Right Acromioclavicular Joint with Nonautologous Tissue Substitute, Percutaneous Approach
ØRGG3ZZ Fusion of Right Acromioclavicular Joint, Percutaneous Approach
ØRGG44Z Fusion of Right Acromioclavicular Joint with Internal Fixation Device, Percutaneous Endoscopic Approach
ØRGG47Z Fusion of Right Acromioclavicular Joint with Autologous Tissue Substitute, Percutaneous Endoscopic Approach
ØRGG4JZ Fusion of Right Acromioclavicular Joint with Synthetic Substitute, Percutaneous Endoscopic Approach
ØRGG4KZ Fusion of Right Acromioclavicular Joint with Nonautologous Tissue Substitute, Percutaneous Endoscopic Approach
ØRGG4ZZ Fusion of Right Acromioclavicular Joint, Percutaneous Endoscopic Approach
ØRGHØ4Z Fusion of Left Acromioclavicular Joint with Internal Fixation Device, Open Approach
ØRGHØ7Z Fusion of Left Acromioclavicular Joint with Autologous Tissue Substitute, Open Approach
ØRGHØJZ Fusion of Left Acromioclavicular Joint with Synthetic Substitute, Open Approach
ØRGHØKZ Fusion of Left Acromioclavicular Joint with Nonautologous Tissue Substitute, Open Approach
ØRGHØZZ Fusion of Left Acromioclavicular Joint, Open Approach
ØRGH34Z Fusion of Left Acromioclavicular Joint with Internal Fixation Device, Percutaneous Approach
ØRGH37Z Fusion of Left Acromioclavicular Joint with Autologous Tissue Substitute, Percutaneous Approach
ØRGH3JZ Fusion of Left Acromioclavicular Joint with Synthetic Substitute, Percutaneous Approach
ØRGH3KZ Fusion of Left Acromioclavicular Joint with Nonautologous Tissue Substitute, Percutaneous Approach
ØRGH3ZZ Fusion of Left Acromioclavicular Joint, Percutaneous Approach
ØRGH44Z Fusion of Left Acromioclavicular Joint with Internal Fixation Device, Percutaneous Endoscopic Approach
ØRGH47Z Fusion of Left Acromioclavicular Joint with Autologous Tissue Substitute, Percutaneous Endoscopic Approach
ØRGH4JZ Fusion of Left Acromioclavicular Joint with Synthetic Substitute, Percutaneous Endoscopic Approach
ØRGH4KZ Fusion of Left Acromioclavicular Joint with Nonautologous Tissue Substitute, Percutaneous Endoscopic Approach
ØRGH4ZZ Fusion of Left Acromioclavicular Joint, Percutaneous Endoscopic Approach
ØRGJØ4Z Fusion of Right Shoulder Joint with Internal Fixation Device, Open Approach
ØRGJØ7Z Fusion of Right Shoulder Joint with Autologous Tissue Substitute, Open Approach
ØRGJØJZ Fusion of Right Shoulder Joint with Synthetic Substitute, Open Approach
ØRGJØKZ Fusion of Right Shoulder Joint with Nonautologous Tissue Substitute, Open Approach
ØRGJØZZ Fusion of Right Shoulder Joint, Open Approach
ØRGJ34Z Fusion of Right Shoulder Joint with Internal Fixation Device, Percutaneous Approach
ØRGJ37Z Fusion of Right Shoulder Joint with Autologous Tissue Substitute, Percutaneous Approach
ØRGJ3JZ Fusion of Right Shoulder Joint with Synthetic Substitute, Percutaneous Approach
ØRGJ3KZ Fusion of Right Shoulder Joint with Nonautologous Tissue Substitute, Percutaneous Approach
ØRGJ3ZZ Fusion of Right Shoulder Joint, Percutaneous Approach
ØRGJ44Z Fusion of Right Shoulder Joint with Internal Fixation Device, Percutaneous Endoscopic Approach
ØRGJ47Z Fusion of Right Shoulder Joint with Autologous Tissue Substitute, Percutaneous Endoscopic Approach
ØRGJ4JZ Fusion of Right Shoulder Joint with Synthetic Substitute, Percutaneous Endoscopic Approach
ØRGJ4KZ Fusion of Right Shoulder Joint with Nonautologous Tissue Substitute, Percutaneous Endoscopic Approach
ØRGJ4ZZ Fusion of Right Shoulder Joint, Percutaneous Endoscopic Approach
ØRGKØ4Z Fusion of Left Shoulder Joint with Internal Fixation Device, Open Approach
ØRGKØ7Z Fusion of Left Shoulder Joint with Autologous Tissue Substitute, Open Approach
ØRGKØJZ Fusion of Left Shoulder Joint with Synthetic Substitute, Open Approach
ØRGKØKZ Fusion of Left Shoulder Joint with Nonautologous Tissue Substitute, Open Approach
ØRGKØZZ Fusion of Left Shoulder Joint, Open Approach
ØRGK34Z Fusion of Left Shoulder Joint with Internal Fixation Device, Percutaneous Approach
ØRGK37Z Fusion of Left Shoulder Joint with Autologous Tissue Substitute, Percutaneous Approach
ØRGK3JZ Fusion of Left Shoulder Joint with Synthetic Substitute, Percutaneous Approach
ØRGK3KZ Fusion of Left Shoulder Joint with Nonautologous Tissue Substitute, Percutaneous Approach
ØRGK3ZZ Fusion of Left Shoulder Joint, Percutaneous Approach
ØRGK44Z Fusion of Left Shoulder Joint with Internal Fixation Device, Percutaneous Endoscopic Approach
ØRGK47Z Fusion of Left Shoulder Joint with Autologous Tissue Substitute, Percutaneous Endoscopic Approach
ØRGK4JZ Fusion of Left Shoulder Joint with Synthetic Substitute, Percutaneous Endoscopic Approach
ØRGK4KZ Fusion of Left Shoulder Joint with Nonautologous Tissue Substitute, Percutaneous Endoscopic Approach
ØRGK4ZZ Fusion of Left Shoulder Joint, Percutaneous Endoscopic Approach
ØRGLØ4Z Fusion of Right Elbow Joint with Internal Fixation Device, Open Approach
ØRGLØ5Z Fusion of Right Elbow Joint with External Fixation Device, Open Approach
ØRGLØ7Z Fusion of Right Elbow Joint with Autologous Tissue Substitute, Open Approach
ØRGLØJZ Fusion of Right Elbow Joint with Synthetic Substitute, Open Approach
ØRGLØKZ Fusion of Right Elbow Joint with Nonautologous Tissue Substitute, Open Approach
ØRGLØZZ Fusion of Right Elbow Joint, Open Approach
ØRGL34Z Fusion of Right Elbow Joint with Internal Fixation Device, Percutaneous Approach
ØRGL35Z Fusion of Right Elbow Joint with External Fixation Device, Percutaneous Approach
ØRGL37Z Fusion of Right Elbow Joint with Autologous Tissue Substitute, Percutaneous Approach
ØRGL3JZ Fusion of Right Elbow Joint with Synthetic Substitute, Percutaneous Approach
ØRGL3KZ Fusion of Right Elbow Joint with Nonautologous Tissue Substitute, Percutaneous Approach
ØRGL3ZZ Fusion of Right Elbow Joint, Percutaneous Approach
ØRGL44Z Fusion of Right Elbow Joint with Internal Fixation Device, Percutaneous Endoscopic Approach
ØRGL45Z Fusion of Right Elbow Joint with External Fixation Device, Percutaneous Endoscopic Approach
ØRGL47Z Fusion of Right Elbow Joint with Autologous Tissue Substitute, Percutaneous Endoscopic Approach
ØRGL4JZ Fusion of Right Elbow Joint with Synthetic Substitute, Percutaneous Endoscopic Approach
ØRGL4KZ Fusion of Right Elbow Joint with Nonautologous Tissue Substitute, Percutaneous Endoscopic Approach
ØRGL4ZZ Fusion of Right Elbow Joint, Percutaneous Endoscopic Approach
ØRGMØ4Z Fusion of Left Elbow Joint with Internal Fixation Device, Open Approach
ØRGMØ5Z Fusion of Left Elbow Joint with External Fixation Device, Open Approach
ØRGMØ7Z Fusion of Left Elbow Joint with Autologous Tissue Substitute, Open Approach
ØRGMØJZ Fusion of Left Elbow Joint with Synthetic Substitute, Open Approach
ØRGMØKZ Fusion of Left Elbow Joint with Nonautologous Tissue Substitute, Open Approach
ØRGMØZZ Fusion of Left Elbow Joint, Open Approach
ØRGM34Z Fusion of Left Elbow Joint with Internal Fixation Device, Percutaneous Approach

**HAC 12: Surgical Site Infection Following Certain Orthopedic Procedures of the Spine, Shoulder, and Elbow (continued)**

ØRGM35Z Fusion of Left Elbow Joint with External Fixation Device, Percutaneous Approach
ØRGM37Z Fusion of Left Elbow Joint with Autologous Tissue Substitute, Percutaneous Approach
ØRGM3JZ Fusion of Left Elbow Joint with Synthetic Substitute, Percutaneous Approach
ØRGM3KZ Fusion of Left Elbow Joint with Nonautologous Tissue Substitute, Percutaneous Approach
ØRGM3ZZ Fusion of Left Elbow Joint, Percutaneous Approach
ØRGM44Z Fusion of Left Elbow Joint with Internal Fixation Device, Percutaneous Endoscopic Approach
ØRGM45Z Fusion of Left Elbow Joint with External Fixation Device, Percutaneous Endoscopic Approach
ØRGM47Z Fusion of Left Elbow Joint with Autologous Tissue Substitute, Percutaneous Endoscopic Approach
ØRGM4JZ Fusion of Left Elbow Joint with Synthetic Substitute, Percutaneous Endoscopic Approach
ØRGM4KZ Fusion of Left Elbow Joint with Nonautologous Tissue Substitute, Percutaneous Endoscopic Approach
ØRGM4ZZ Fusion of Left Elbow Joint, Percutaneous Endoscopic Approach
ØRQEØZZ Repair Right Sternoclavicular Joint, Open Approach
ØRQE3ZZ Repair Right Sternoclavicular Joint, Percutaneous Approach
ØRQE4ZZ Repair Right Sternoclavicular Joint, Percutaneous Endoscopic Approach
ØRQEXZZ Repair Right Sternoclavicular Joint, External Approach
ØRQFØZZ Repair Left Sternoclavicular Joint, Open Approach
ØRQF3ZZ Repair Left Sternoclavicular Joint, Percutaneous Approach
ØRQF4ZZ Repair Left Sternoclavicular Joint, Percutaneous Endoscopic Approach
ØRQFXZZ Repair Left Sternoclavicular Joint, External Approach
ØRQGØZZ Repair Right Acromioclavicular Joint, Open Approach
ØRQG3ZZ Repair Right Acromioclavicular Joint, Percutaneous Approach
ØRQG4ZZ Repair Right Acromioclavicular Joint, Percutaneous Endoscopic Approach
ØRQGXZZ Repair Right Acromioclavicular Joint, External Approach
ØRQHØZZ Repair Left Acromioclavicular Joint, Open Approach
ØRQH3ZZ Repair Left Acromioclavicular Joint, Percutaneous Approach
ØRQH4ZZ Repair Left Acromioclavicular Joint, Percutaneous Endoscopic Approach
ØRQHXZZ Repair Left Acromioclavicular Joint, External Approach
ØRQJØZZ Repair Right Shoulder Joint, Open Approach
ØRQJ3ZZ Repair Right Shoulder Joint, Percutaneous Approach
ØRQJ4ZZ Repair Right Shoulder Joint, Percutaneous Endoscopic Approach
ØRQJXZZ Repair Right Shoulder Joint, External Approach
ØRQKØZZ Repair Left Shoulder Joint, Open Approach
ØRQK3ZZ Repair Left Shoulder Joint, Percutaneous Approach
ØRQK4ZZ Repair Left Shoulder Joint, Percutaneous Endoscopic Approach
ØRQKXZZ Repair Left Shoulder Joint, External Approach
ØRQLØZZ Repair Right Elbow Joint, Open Approach
ØRQL3ZZ Repair Right Elbow Joint, Percutaneous Approach
ØRQL4ZZ Repair Right Elbow Joint, Percutaneous Endoscopic Approach
ØRQLXZZ Repair Right Elbow Joint, External Approach
ØRQMØZZ Repair Left Elbow Joint, Open Approach
ØRQM3ZZ Repair Left Elbow Joint, Percutaneous Approach
ØRQM4ZZ Repair Left Elbow Joint, Percutaneous Endoscopic Approach
ØRQMXZZ Repair Left Elbow Joint, External Approach
ØRUEØ7Z Supplement Right Sternoclavicular Joint with Autologous Tissue Substitute, Open Approach
ØRUEØJZ Supplement Right Sternoclavicular Joint with Synthetic Substitute, Open Approach
ØRUEØKZ Supplement Right Sternoclavicular Joint with Nonautologous Tissue Substitute, Open Approach
ØRUE37Z Supplement Right Sternoclavicular Joint with Autologous Tissue Substitute, Percutaneous Approach
ØRUE3JZ Supplement Right Sternoclavicular Joint with Synthetic Substitute, Percutaneous Approach
ØRUE3KZ Supplement Right Sternoclavicular Joint with Nonautologous Tissue Substitute, Percutaneous Approach
ØRUE47Z Supplement Right Sternoclavicular Joint with Autologous Tissue Substitute, Percutaneous Endoscopic Approach
ØRUE4JZ Supplement Right Sternoclavicular Joint with Synthetic Substitute, Percutaneous Endoscopic Approach
ØRUE4KZ Supplement Right Sternoclavicular Joint with Nonautologous Tissue Substitute, Percutaneous Endoscopic Approach
ØRUFØ7Z Supplement Left Sternoclavicular Joint with Autologous Tissue Substitute, Open Approach
ØRUFØJZ Supplement Left Sternoclavicular Joint with Synthetic Substitute, Open Approach
ØRUFØKZ Supplement Left Sternoclavicular Joint with Nonautologous Tissue Substitute, Open Approach
ØRUF37Z Supplement Left Sternoclavicular Joint with Autologous Tissue Substitute, Percutaneous Approach
ØRUF3JZ Supplement Left Sternoclavicular Joint with Synthetic Substitute, Percutaneous Approach
ØRUF3KZ Supplement Left Sternoclavicular Joint with Nonautologous Tissue Substitute, Percutaneous Approach
ØRUF47Z Supplement Left Sternoclavicular Joint with Autologous Tissue Substitute, Percutaneous Endoscopic Approach
ØRUF4JZ Supplement Left Sternoclavicular Joint with Synthetic Substitute, Percutaneous Endoscopic Approach
ØRUF4KZ Supplement Left Sternoclavicular Joint with Nonautologous Tissue Substitute, Percutaneous Endoscopic Approach
ØRUGØ7Z Supplement Right Acromioclavicular Joint with Autologous Tissue Substitute, Open Approach
ØRUGØJZ Supplement Right Acromioclavicular Joint with Synthetic Substitute, Open Approach
ØRUGØKZ Supplement Right Acromioclavicular Joint with Nonautologous Tissue Substitute, Open Approach
ØRUG37Z Supplement Right Acromioclavicular Joint with Autologous Tissue Substitute, Percutaneous Approach
ØRUG3JZ Supplement Right Acromioclavicular Joint with Synthetic Substitute, Percutaneous Approach
ØRUG3KZ Supplement Right Acromioclavicular Joint with Nonautologous Tissue Substitute, Percutaneous Approach
ØRUG47Z Supplement Right Acromioclavicular Joint with Autologous Tissue Substitute, Percutaneous Endoscopic Approach
ØRUG4JZ Supplement Right Acromioclavicular Joint with Synthetic Substitute, Percutaneous Endoscopic Approach
ØRUG4KZ Supplement Right Acromioclavicular Joint with Nonautologous Tissue Substitute, Percutaneous Endoscopic Approach
ØRUHØ7Z Supplement Left Acromioclavicular Joint with Autologous Tissue Substitute, Open Approach
ØRUHØJZ Supplement Left Acromioclavicular Joint with Synthetic Substitute, Open Approach
ØRUHØKZ Supplement Left Acromioclavicular Joint with Nonautologous Tissue Substitute, Open Approach
ØRUH37Z Supplement Left Acromioclavicular Joint with Autologous Tissue Substitute, Percutaneous Approach
ØRUH3JZ Supplement Left Acromioclavicular Joint with Synthetic Substitute, Percutaneous Approach
ØRUH3KZ Supplement Left Acromioclavicular Joint with Nonautologous Tissue Substitute, Percutaneous Approach
ØRUH47Z Supplement Left Acromioclavicular Joint with Autologous Tissue Substitute, Percutaneous Endoscopic Approach
ØRUH4JZ Supplement Left Acromioclavicular Joint with Synthetic Substitute, Percutaneous Endoscopic Approach
ØRUH4KZ Supplement Left Acromioclavicular Joint with Nonautologous Tissue Substitute, Percutaneous Endoscopic Approach
ØRUJØ7Z Supplement Right Shoulder Joint with Autologous Tissue Substitute, Open Approach
ØRUJØJZ Supplement Right Shoulder Joint with Synthetic Substitute, Open Approach
ØRUJØKZ Supplement Right Shoulder Joint with Nonautologous Tissue Substitute, Open Approach
ØRUJ37Z Supplement Right Shoulder Joint with Autologous Tissue Substitute, Percutaneous Approach
ØRUJ3JZ Supplement Right Shoulder Joint with Synthetic Substitute, Percutaneous Approach
ØRUJ3KZ Supplement Right Shoulder Joint with Nonautologous Tissue Substitute, Percutaneous Approach
ØRUJ47Z Supplement Right Shoulder Joint with Autologous Tissue Substitute, Percutaneous Endoscopic Approach
ØRUJ4JZ Supplement Right Shoulder Joint with Synthetic Substitute, Percutaneous Endoscopic Approach

**HAC 12: Surgical Site Infection Following Certain Orthopedic Procedures of the Spine, Shoulder, and Elbow (continued)**

ØRUJ4KZ Supplement Right Shoulder Joint with Nonautologous Tissue Substitute, Percutaneous Endoscopic Approach
ØRUKØ7Z Supplement Left Shoulder Joint with Autologous Tissue Substitute, Open Approach
ØRUKØJZ Supplement Left Shoulder Joint with Synthetic Substitute, Open Approach
ØRUKØKZ Supplement Left Shoulder Joint with Nonautologous Tissue Substitute, Open Approach
ØRUK37Z Supplement Left Shoulder Joint with Autologous Tissue Substitute, Percutaneous Approach
ØRUK3JZ Supplement Left Shoulder Joint with Synthetic Substitute, Percutaneous Approach
ØRUK3KZ Supplement Left Shoulder Joint with Nonautologous Tissue Substitute, Percutaneous Approach
ØRUK47Z Supplement Left Shoulder Joint with Autologous Tissue Substitute, Percutaneous Endoscopic Approach
ØRUK4JZ Supplement Left Shoulder Joint with Synthetic Substitute, Percutaneous Endoscopic Approach
ØRUK4KZ Supplement Left Shoulder Joint with Nonautologous Tissue Substitute, Percutaneous Endoscopic Approach
ØRULØ7Z Supplement Right Elbow Joint with Autologous Tissue Substitute, Open Approach
ØRULØJZ Supplement Right Elbow Joint with Synthetic Substitute, Open Approach
ØRULØKZ Supplement Right Elbow Joint with Nonautologous Tissue Substitute, Open Approach
ØRUL37Z Supplement Right Elbow Joint with Autologous Tissue Substitute, Percutaneous Approach
ØRUL3JZ Supplement Right Elbow Joint with Synthetic Substitute, Percutaneous Approach
ØRUL3KZ Supplement Right Elbow Joint with Nonautologous Tissue Substitute, Percutaneous Approach
ØRUL47Z Supplement Right Elbow Joint with Autologous Tissue Substitute, Percutaneous Endoscopic Approach
ØRUL4JZ Supplement Right Elbow Joint with Synthetic Substitute, Percutaneous Endoscopic Approach
ØRUL4KZ Supplement Right Elbow Joint with Nonautologous Tissue Substitute, Percutaneous Endoscopic Approach
ØRUMØ7Z Supplement Left Elbow Joint with Autologous Tissue Substitute, Open Approach
ØRUMØJZ Supplement Left Elbow Joint with Synthetic Substitute, Open Approach
ØRUMØKZ Supplement Left Elbow Joint with Nonautologous Tissue Substitute, Open Approach
ØRUM37Z Supplement Left Elbow Joint with Autologous Tissue Substitute, Percutaneous Approach
ØRUM3JZ Supplement Left Elbow Joint with Synthetic Substitute, Percutaneous Approach
ØRUM3KZ Supplement Left Elbow Joint with Nonautologous Tissue Substitute, Percutaneous Approach
ØRUM47Z Supplement Left Elbow Joint with Autologous Tissue Substitute, Percutaneous Endoscopic Approach
ØRUM4JZ Supplement Left Elbow Joint with Synthetic Substitute, Percutaneous Endoscopic Approach
ØRUM4KZ Supplement Left Elbow Joint with Nonautologous Tissue Substitute, Percutaneous Endoscopic Approach
ØSGØØ7Ø Fusion of Lumbar Vertebral Joint with Autologous Tissue Substitute, Anterior Approach, Anterior Column, Open Approach
ØSGØØ71 Fusion of Lumbar Vertebral Joint with Autologous Tissue Substitute, Posterior Approach, Posterior Column, Open Approach
ØSGØØ7J Fusion of Lumbar Vertebral Joint with Autologous Tissue Substitute, Posterior Approach, Anterior Column, Open Approach
ØSGØØAØ Fusion of Lumbar Vertebral Joint with Interbody Fusion Device, Anterior Approach, Anterior Column, Open Approach
ØSGØØA1 Fusion of Lumbar Vertebral Joint with Interbody Fusion Device, Posterior Approach, Posterior Column, Open Approach
ØSGØØAJ Fusion of Lumbar Vertebral Joint with Interbody Fusion Device, Posterior Approach, Anterior Column, Open Approach
ØSGØØJØ Fusion of Lumbar Vertebral Joint with Synthetic Substitute, Anterior Approach, Anterior Column, Open Approach
ØSGØØJ1 Fusion of Lumbar Vertebral Joint with Synthetic Substitute, Posterior Approach, Posterior Column, Open Approach
ØSGØØJJ Fusion of Lumbar Vertebral Joint with Synthetic Substitute, Posterior Approach, Anterior Column, Open Approach
ØSGØØKØ Fusion of Lumbar Vertebral Joint with Nonautologous Tissue Substitute, Anterior Approach, Anterior Column, Open Approach
ØSGØØK1 Fusion of Lumbar Vertebral Joint with Nonautologous Tissue Substitute, Posterior Approach, Posterior Column, Open Approach
ØSGØØKJ Fusion of Lumbar Vertebral Joint with Nonautologous Tissue Substitute, Posterior Approach, Anterior Column, Open Approach
ØSGØØZØ Fusion of Lumbar Vertebral Joint, Anterior Approach, Anterior Column, Open Approach
ØSGØØZ1 Fusion of Lumbar Vertebral Joint, Posterior Approach, Posterior Column, Open Approach
ØSGØØZJ Fusion of Lumbar Vertebral Joint, Posterior Approach, Anterior Column, Open Approach
ØSGØ37Ø Fusion of Lumbar Vertebral Joint with Autologous Tissue Substitute, Anterior Approach, Anterior Column, Percutaneous Approach
ØSGØ371 Fusion of Lumbar Vertebral Joint with Autologous Tissue Substitute, Posterior Approach, Posterior Column, Percutaneous Approach
ØSGØ37J Fusion of Lumbar Vertebral Joint with Autologous Tissue Substitute, Posterior Approach, Anterior Column, Percutaneous Approach
ØSGØ3AØ Fusion of Lumbar Vertebral Joint with Interbody Fusion Device, Anterior Approach, Anterior Column, Percutaneous Approach
ØSGØ3A1 Fusion of Lumbar Vertebral Joint with Interbody Fusion Device, Posterior Approach, Posterior Column, Percutaneous Approach
ØSGØ3AJ Fusion of Lumbar Vertebral Joint with Interbody Fusion Device, Posterior Approach, Anterior Column, Percutaneous Approach
ØSGØ3JØ Fusion of Lumbar Vertebral Joint with Synthetic Substitute, Anterior Approach, Anterior Column, Percutaneous Approach
ØSGØ3J1 Fusion of Lumbar Vertebral Joint with Synthetic Substitute, Posterior Approach, Posterior Column, Percutaneous Approach
ØSGØ3JJ Fusion of Lumbar Vertebral Joint with Synthetic Substitute, Posterior Approach, Anterior Column, Percutaneous Approach
ØSGØ3KØ Fusion of Lumbar Vertebral Joint with Nonautologous Tissue Substitute, Anterior Approach, Anterior Column, Percutaneous Approach
ØSGØ3K1 Fusion of Lumbar Vertebral Joint with Nonautologous Tissue Substitute, Posterior Approach, Posterior Column, Percutaneous Approach
ØSGØ3KJ Fusion of Lumbar Vertebral Joint with Nonautologous Tissue Substitute, Posterior Approach, Anterior Column, Percutaneous Approach
ØSGØ3ZØ Fusion of Lumbar Vertebral Joint, Anterior Approach, Anterior Column, Percutaneous Approach
ØSGØ3Z1 Fusion of Lumbar Vertebral Joint, Posterior Approach, Posterior Column, Percutaneous Approach
ØSGØ3ZJ Fusion of Lumbar Vertebral Joint, Posterior Approach, Anterior Column, Percutaneous Approach
ØSGØ47Ø Fusion of Lumbar Vertebral Joint with Autologous Tissue Substitute, Anterior Approach, Anterior Column, Percutaneous Endoscopic Approach
ØSGØ471 Fusion of Lumbar Vertebral Joint with Autologous Tissue Substitute, Posterior Approach, Posterior Column, Percutaneous Endoscopic Approach
ØSGØ47J Fusion of Lumbar Vertebral Joint with Autologous Tissue Substitute, Posterior Approach, Anterior Column, Percutaneous Endoscopic Approach
ØSGØ4AØ Fusion of Lumbar Vertebral Joint with Interbody Fusion Device, Anterior Approach, Anterior Column, Percutaneous Endoscopic Approach
ØSGØ4A1 Fusion of Lumbar Vertebral Joint with Interbody Fusion Device, Posterior Approach, Posterior Column, Percutaneous Endoscopic Approach
ØSGØ4AJ Fusion of Lumbar Vertebral Joint with Interbody Fusion Device, Posterior Approach, Anterior Column, Percutaneous Endoscopic Approach

**HAC 12: Surgical Site Infection Following Certain Orthopedic Procedures of the Spine, Shoulder, and Elbow (continued)**

ØSGØ4JØ Fusion of Lumbar Vertebral Joint with Synthetic Substitute, Anterior Approach, Anterior Column, Percutaneous Endoscopic Approach
ØSGØ4J1 Fusion of Lumbar Vertebral Joint with Synthetic Substitute, Posterior Approach, Posterior Column, Percutaneous Endoscopic Approach
ØSGØ4JJ Fusion of Lumbar Vertebral Joint with Synthetic Substitute, Posterior Approach, Anterior Column, Percutaneous Endoscopic Approach
ØSGØ4KØ Fusion of Lumbar Vertebral Joint with Nonautologous Tissue Substitute, Anterior Approach, Anterior Column, Percutaneous Endoscopic Approach
ØSGØ4K1 Fusion of Lumbar Vertebral Joint with Nonautologous Tissue Substitute, Posterior Approach, Posterior Column, Percutaneous Endoscopic Approach
ØSGØ4KJ Fusion of Lumbar Vertebral Joint with Nonautologous Tissue Substitute, Posterior Approach, Anterior Column, Percutaneous Endoscopic Approach
ØSGØ4ZØ Fusion of Lumbar Vertebral Joint, Anterior Approach, Anterior Column, Percutaneous Endoscopic Approach
ØSGØ4Z1 Fusion of Lumbar Vertebral Joint, Posterior Approach, Posterior Column, Percutaneous Endoscopic Approach
ØSGØ4ZJ Fusion of Lumbar Vertebral Joint, Posterior Approach, Anterior Column, Percutaneous Endoscopic Approach
ØSG1Ø7Ø Fusion of 2 or More Lumbar Vertebral Joints with Autologous Tissue Substitute, Anterior Approach, Anterior Column, Open Approach
ØSG1Ø71 Fusion of 2 or More Lumbar Vertebral Joints with Autologous Tissue Substitute, Posterior Approach, Posterior Column, Open Approach
ØSG1Ø7J Fusion of 2 or More Lumbar Vertebral Joints with Autologous Tissue Substitute, Posterior Approach, Anterior Column, Open Approach
ØSG1ØAØ Fusion of 2 or More Lumbar Vertebral Joints with Interbody Fusion Device, Anterior Approach, Anterior Column, Open Approach
ØSG1ØA1 Fusion of 2 or More Lumbar Vertebral Joints with Interbody Fusion Device, Posterior Approach, Posterior Column, Open Approach
ØSG1ØAJ Fusion of 2 or More Lumbar Vertebral Joints with Interbody Fusion Device, Posterior Approach, Anterior Column, Open Approach
ØSG1ØJØ Fusion of 2 or More Lumbar Vertebral Joints with Synthetic Substitute, Anterior Approach, Anterior Column, Open Approach
ØSG1ØJ1 Fusion of 2 or More Lumbar Vertebral Joints with Synthetic Substitute, Posterior Approach, Posterior Column, Open Approach
ØSG1ØJJ Fusion of 2 or More Lumbar Vertebral Joints with Synthetic Substitute, Posterior Approach, Anterior Column, Open Approach
ØSG1ØKØ Fusion of 2 or More Lumbar Vertebral Joints with Nonautologous Tissue Substitute, Anterior Approach, Anterior Column, Open Approach
ØSG1ØK1 Fusion of 2 or More Lumbar Vertebral Joints with Nonautologous Tissue Substitute, Posterior Approach, Posterior Column, Open Approach
ØSG1ØKJ Fusion of 2 or More Lumbar Vertebral Joints with Nonautologous Tissue Substitute, Posterior Approach, Anterior Column, Open Approach
ØSG1ØZØ Fusion of 2 or More Lumbar Vertebral Joints, Anterior Approach, Anterior Column, Open Approach
ØSG1ØZ1 Fusion of 2 or More Lumbar Vertebral Joints, Posterior Approach, Posterior Column, Open Approach
ØSG1ØZJ Fusion of 2 or More Lumbar Vertebral Joints, Posterior Approach, Anterior Column, Open Approach
ØSG137Ø Fusion of 2 or More Lumbar Vertebral Joints with Autologous Tissue Substitute, Anterior Approach, Anterior Column, Percutaneous Approach
ØSG1371 Fusion of 2 or More Lumbar Vertebral Joints with Autologous Tissue Substitute, Posterior Approach, Posterior Column, Percutaneous Approach
ØSG137J Fusion of 2 or More Lumbar Vertebral Joints with Autologous Tissue Substitute, Posterior Approach, Anterior Column, Percutaneous Approach
ØSG13AØ Fusion of 2 or More Lumbar Vertebral Joints with Interbody Fusion Device, Anterior Approach, Anterior Column, Percutaneous Approach
ØSG13A1 Fusion of 2 or More Lumbar Vertebral Joints with Interbody Fusion Device, Posterior Approach, Posterior Column, Percutaneous Approach
ØSG13AJ Fusion of 2 or More Lumbar Vertebral Joints with Interbody Fusion Device, Posterior Approach, Anterior Column, Percutaneous Approach
ØSG13JØ Fusion of 2 or More Lumbar Vertebral Joints with Synthetic Substitute, Anterior Approach, Anterior Column, Percutaneous Approach
ØSG13J1 Fusion of 2 or More Lumbar Vertebral Joints with Synthetic Substitute, Posterior Approach, Posterior Column, Percutaneous Approach
ØSG13JJ Fusion of 2 or More Lumbar Vertebral Joints with Synthetic Substitute, Posterior Approach, Anterior Column, Percutaneous Approach
ØSG13KØ Fusion of 2 or More Lumbar Vertebral Joints with Nonautologous Tissue Substitute, Anterior Approach, Anterior Column, Percutaneous Approach
ØSG13K1 Fusion of 2 or More Lumbar Vertebral Joints with Nonautologous Tissue Substitute, Posterior Approach, Posterior Column, Percutaneous Approach
ØSG13KJ Fusion of 2 or More Lumbar Vertebral Joints with Nonautologous Tissue Substitute, Posterior Approach, Anterior Column, Percutaneous Approach
ØSG13ZØ Fusion of 2 or More Lumbar Vertebral Joints, Anterior Approach, Anterior Column, Percutaneous Approach
ØSG13Z1 Fusion of 2 or More Lumbar Vertebral Joints, Posterior Approach, Posterior Column, Percutaneous Approach
ØSG13ZJ Fusion of 2 or More Lumbar Vertebral Joints, Posterior Approach, Anterior Column, Percutaneous Approach
ØSG147Ø Fusion of 2 or More Lumbar Vertebral Joints with Autologous Tissue Substitute, Anterior Approach, Anterior Column, Percutaneous Endoscopic Approach
ØSG1471 Fusion of 2 or More Lumbar Vertebral Joints with Autologous Tissue Substitute, Posterior Approach, Posterior Column, Percutaneous Endoscopic Approach
ØSG147J Fusion of 2 or More Lumbar Vertebral Joints with Autologous Tissue Substitute, Posterior Approach, Anterior Column, Percutaneous Endoscopic Approach
ØSG14AØ Fusion of 2 or More Lumbar Vertebral Joints with Interbody Fusion Device, Anterior Approach, Anterior Column, Percutaneous Endoscopic Approach
ØSG14A1 Fusion of 2 or More Lumbar Vertebral Joints with Interbody Fusion Device, Posterior Approach, Posterior Column, Percutaneous Endoscopic Approach
ØSG14AJ Fusion of 2 or More Lumbar Vertebral Joints with Interbody Fusion Device, Posterior Approach, Anterior Column, Percutaneous Endoscopic Approach
ØSG14JØ Fusion of 2 or More Lumbar Vertebral Joints with Synthetic Substitute, Anterior Approach, Anterior Column, Percutaneous Endoscopic Approach
ØSG14J1 Fusion of 2 or More Lumbar Vertebral Joints with Synthetic Substitute, Posterior Approach, Posterior Column, Percutaneous Endoscopic Approach
ØSG14JJ Fusion of 2 or More Lumbar Vertebral Joints with Synthetic Substitute, Posterior Approach, Anterior Column, Percutaneous Endoscopic Approach
ØSG14KØ Fusion of 2 or More Lumbar Vertebral Joints with Nonautologous Tissue Substitute, Anterior Approach, Anterior Column, Percutaneous Endoscopic Approach
ØSG14K1 Fusion of 2 or More Lumbar Vertebral Joints with Nonautologous Tissue Substitute, Posterior Approach, Posterior Column, Percutaneous Endoscopic Approach
ØSG14KJ Fusion of 2 or More Lumbar Vertebral Joints with Nonautologous Tissue Substitute, Posterior Approach, Anterior Column, Percutaneous Endoscopic Approach
ØSG14ZØ Fusion of 2 or More Lumbar Vertebral Joints, Anterior Approach, Anterior Column, Percutaneous Endoscopic Approach
ØSG14Z1 Fusion of 2 or More Lumbar Vertebral Joints, Posterior Approach, Posterior Column, Percutaneous Endoscopic Approach
ØSG14ZJ Fusion of 2 or More Lumbar Vertebral Joints, Posterior Approach, Anterior Column, Percutaneous Endoscopic Approach
ØSG3Ø7Ø Fusion of Lumbosacral Joint with Autologous Tissue Substitute, Anterior Approach, Anterior Column, Open Approach
ØSG3Ø71 Fusion of Lumbosacral Joint with Autologous Tissue Substitute, Posterior Approach, Posterior Column, Open Approach

**HAC 12: Surgical Site Infection Following Certain Orthopedic Procedures of the Spine, Shoulder, and Elbow (continued)**

ØSG3Ø7J Fusion of Lumbosacral Joint with Autologous Tissue Substitute, Posterior Approach, Anterior Column, Open Approach
ØSG3ØAØ Fusion of Lumbosacral Joint with Interbody Fusion Device, Anterior Approach, Anterior Column, Open Approach
ØSG3ØA1 Fusion of Lumbosacral Joint with Interbody Fusion Device, Posterior Approach, Posterior Column, Open Approach
ØSG3ØAJ Fusion of Lumbosacral Joint with Interbody Fusion Device, Posterior Approach, Anterior Column, Open Approach
ØSG3ØJØ Fusion of Lumbosacral Joint with Synthetic Substitute, Anterior Approach, Anterior Column, Open Approach
ØSG3ØJ1 Fusion of Lumbosacral Joint with Synthetic Substitute, Posterior Approach, Posterior Column, Open Approach
ØSG3ØJJ Fusion of Lumbosacral Joint with Synthetic Substitute, Posterior Approach, Anterior Column, Open Approach
ØSG3ØKØ Fusion of Lumbosacral Joint with Nonautologous Tissue Substitute, Anterior Approach, Anterior Column, Open Approach
ØSG3ØK1 Fusion of Lumbosacral Joint with Nonautologous Tissue Substitute, Posterior Approach, Posterior Column, Open Approach
ØSG3ØKJ Fusion of Lumbosacral Joint with Nonautologous Tissue Substitute, Posterior Approach, Anterior Column, Open Approach
ØSG3ØZØ Fusion of Lumbosacral Joint, Anterior Approach, Anterior Column, Open Approach
ØSG3ØZ1 Fusion of Lumbosacral Joint, Posterior Approach, Posterior Column, Open Approach
ØSG3ØZJ Fusion of Lumbosacral Joint, Posterior Approach, Anterior Column, Open Approach
ØSG337Ø Fusion of Lumbosacral Joint with Autologous Tissue Substitute, Anterior Approach, Anterior Column, Percutaneous Approach
ØSG3371 Fusion of Lumbosacral Joint with Autologous Tissue Substitute, Posterior Approach, Posterior Column, Percutaneous Approach
ØSG337J Fusion of Lumbosacral Joint with Autologous Tissue Substitute, Posterior Approach, Anterior Column, Percutaneous Approach
ØSG33AØ Fusion of Lumbosacral Joint with Interbody Fusion Device, Anterior Approach, Anterior Column, Percutaneous Approach
ØSG33A1 Fusion of Lumbosacral Joint with Interbody Fusion Device, Posterior Approach, Posterior Column, Percutaneous Approach
ØSG33AJ Fusion of Lumbosacral Joint with Interbody Fusion Device, Posterior Approach, Anterior Column, Percutaneous Approach
ØSG33JØ Fusion of Lumbosacral Joint with Synthetic Substitute, Anterior Approach, Anterior Column, Percutaneous Approach
ØSG33J1 Fusion of Lumbosacral Joint with Synthetic Substitute, Posterior Approach, Posterior Column, Percutaneous Approach
ØSG33JJ Fusion of Lumbosacral Joint with Synthetic Substitute, Posterior Approach, Anterior Column, Percutaneous Approach
ØSG33KØ Fusion of Lumbosacral Joint with Nonautologous Tissue Substitute, Anterior Approach, Anterior Column, Percutaneous Approach
ØSG33K1 Fusion of Lumbosacral Joint with Nonautologous Tissue Substitute, Posterior Approach, Posterior Column, Percutaneous Approach
ØSG33KJ Fusion of Lumbosacral Joint with Nonautologous Tissue Substitute, Posterior Approach, Anterior Column, Percutaneous Approach
ØSG33ZØ Fusion of Lumbosacral Joint, Anterior Approach, Anterior Column, Percutaneous Approach
ØSG33Z1 Fusion of Lumbosacral Joint, Posterior Approach, Posterior Column, Percutaneous Approach
ØSG33ZJ Fusion of Lumbosacral Joint, Posterior Approach, Anterior Column, Percutaneous Approach
ØSG347Ø Fusion of Lumbosacral Joint with Autologous Tissue Substitute, Anterior Approach, Anterior Column, Percutaneous Endoscopic Approach
ØSG3471 Fusion of Lumbosacral Joint with Autologous Tissue Substitute, Posterior Approach, Posterior Column, Percutaneous Endoscopic Approach
ØSG347J Fusion of Lumbosacral Joint with Autologous Tissue Substitute, Posterior Approach, Anterior Column, Percutaneous Endoscopic Approach
ØSG34AØ Fusion of Lumbosacral Joint with Interbody Fusion Device, Anterior Approach, Anterior Column, Percutaneous Endoscopic Approach
ØSG34A1 Fusion of Lumbosacral Joint with Interbody Fusion Device, Posterior Approach, Posterior Column, Percutaneous Endoscopic Approach
ØSG34AJ Fusion of Lumbosacral Joint with Interbody Fusion Device, Posterior Approach, Anterior Column, Percutaneous Endoscopic Approach
ØSG34JØ Fusion of Lumbosacral Joint with Synthetic Substitute, Anterior Approach, Anterior Column, Percutaneous Endoscopic Approach
ØSG34J1 Fusion of Lumbosacral Joint with Synthetic Substitute, Posterior Approach, Posterior Column, Percutaneous Endoscopic Approach
ØSG34JJ Fusion of Lumbosacral Joint with Synthetic Substitute, Posterior Approach, Anterior Column, Percutaneous Endoscopic Approach
ØSG34KØ Fusion of Lumbosacral Joint with Nonautologous Tissue Substitute, Anterior Approach, Anterior Column, Percutaneous Endoscopic Approach
ØSG34K1 Fusion of Lumbosacral Joint with Nonautologous Tissue Substitute, Posterior Approach, Posterior Column, Percutaneous Endoscopic Approach
ØSG34KJ Fusion of Lumbosacral Joint with Nonautologous Tissue Substitute, Posterior Approach, Anterior Column, Percutaneous Endoscopic Approach
ØSG34ZØ Fusion of Lumbosacral Joint, Anterior Approach, Anterior Column, Percutaneous Endoscopic Approach
ØSG34Z1 Fusion of Lumbosacral Joint, Posterior Approach, Posterior Column, Percutaneous Endoscopic Approach
ØSG34ZJ Fusion of Lumbosacral Joint, Posterior Approach, Anterior Column, Percutaneous Endoscopic Approach
ØSG7Ø4Z Fusion of Right Sacroiliac Joint with Internal Fixation Device, Open Approach
ØSG7Ø7Z Fusion of Right Sacroiliac Joint with Autologous Tissue Substitute, Open Approach
ØSG7ØJZ Fusion of Right Sacroiliac Joint with Synthetic Substitute, Open Approach
ØSG7ØKZ Fusion of Right Sacroiliac Joint with Nonautologous Tissue Substitute, Open Approach
ØSG7ØZZ Fusion of Right Sacroiliac Joint, Open Approach
ØSG734Z Fusion of Right Sacroiliac Joint with Internal Fixation Device, Percutaneous Approach
ØSG737Z Fusion of Right Sacroiliac Joint with Autologous Tissue Substitute, Percutaneous Approach
ØSG73JZ Fusion of Right Sacroiliac Joint with Synthetic Substitute, Percutaneous Approach
ØSG73KZ Fusion of Right Sacroiliac Joint with Nonautologous Tissue Substitute, Percutaneous Approach
ØSG73ZZ Fusion of Right Sacroiliac Joint, Percutaneous Approach
ØSG744Z Fusion of Right Sacroiliac Joint with Internal Fixation Device, Percutaneous Endoscopic Approach
ØSG747Z Fusion of Right Sacroiliac Joint with Autologous Tissue Substitute, Percutaneous Endoscopic Approach
ØSG74JZ Fusion of Right Sacroiliac Joint with Synthetic Substitute, Percutaneous Endoscopic Approach
ØSG74KZ Fusion of Right Sacroiliac Joint with Nonautologous Tissue Substitute, Percutaneous Endoscopic Approach
ØSG74ZZ Fusion of Right Sacroiliac Joint, Percutaneous Endoscopic Approach
ØSG8Ø4Z Fusion of Left Sacroiliac Joint with Internal Fixation Device, Open Approach
ØSG8Ø7Z Fusion of Left Sacroiliac Joint with Autologous Tissue Substitute, Open Approach
ØSG8ØJZ Fusion of Left Sacroiliac Joint with Synthetic Substitute, Open Approach
ØSG8ØKZ Fusion of Left Sacroiliac Joint with Nonautologous Tissue Substitute, Open Approach
ØSG8ØZZ Fusion of Left Sacroiliac Joint, Open Approach
ØSG834Z Fusion of Left Sacroiliac Joint with Internal Fixation Device, Percutaneous Approach
ØSG837Z Fusion of Left Sacroiliac Joint with Autologous Tissue Substitute, Percutaneous Approach

**HAC 12: Surgical Site Infection Following Certain Orthopedic Procedures of the Spine, Shoulder, and Elbow (continued)**

ØSG83JZ Fusion of Left Sacroiliac Joint with Synthetic Substitute, Percutaneous Approach
ØSG83KZ Fusion of Left Sacroiliac Joint with Nonautologous Tissue Substitute, Percutaneous Approach
ØSG83ZZ Fusion of Left Sacroiliac Joint, Percutaneous Approach
ØSG844Z Fusion of Left Sacroiliac Joint with Internal Fixation Device, Percutaneous Endoscopic Approach
ØSG847Z Fusion of Left Sacroiliac Joint with Autologous Tissue Substitute, Percutaneous Endoscopic Approach
ØSG84JZ Fusion of Left Sacroiliac Joint with Synthetic Substitute, Percutaneous Endoscopic Approach
ØSG84KZ Fusion of Left Sacroiliac Joint with Nonautologous Tissue Substitute, Percutaneous Endoscopic Approach
ØSG84ZZ Fusion of Left Sacroiliac Joint, Percutaneous Endoscopic Approach
XRGØØ92 Fusion of Occipital-cervical Joint using Nanotextured Surface Interbody Fusion Device, Open Approach, New Technology Group 2
XRG1Ø92 Fusion of Cervical Vertebral Joint using Nanotextured Surface Interbody Fusion Device, Open Approach, New Technology Group 2
XRG2Ø92 Fusion of 2 or more Cervical Vertebral Joints using Nanotextured Surface Interbody Fusion Device, Open Approach, New Technology Group 2
XRG4Ø92 Fusion of Cervicothoracic Vertebral Joint using Nanotextured Surface Interbody Fusion Device, Open Approach, New Technology Group 2
XRG6Ø92 Fusion of Thoracic Vertebral Joint using Nanotextured Surface Interbody Fusion Device, Open Approach, New Technology Group 2
XRG7Ø92 Fusion of 2 to 7 Thoracic Vertebral Joints using Nanotextured Surface Interbody Fusion Device, Open Approach, New Technology Group 2
XRG8Ø92 Fusion of 8 or more Thoracic Vertebral Joints using Nanotextured Surface Interbody Fusion Device, Open Approach, New Technology Group 2
XRGAØ92 Fusion of Thoracolumbar Vertebral Joint using Nanotextured Surface Interbody Fusion Device, Open Approach, New Technology Group 2
XRGBØ92 Fusion of Lumbar Vertebral Joint using Nanotextured Surface Interbody Fusion Device, Open Approach, New Technology Group 2
XRGCØ92 Fusion of 2 or more Lumbar Vertebral Joints using Nanotextured Surface Interbody Fusion Device, Open Approach, New Technology Group 2
XRGDØ92 Fusion of Lumbosacral Joint using Nanotextured Surface Interbody Fusion Device, Open Approach, New Technology Group 2

**HAC 13: Surgical Site Infection (SSI) Following Cardiac Implantable Electronic Device (CIED) Procedures**

Secondary diagnosis not POA:
K68.11
T81.4XXA
T82.6XXA
T82.7XXA

**AND**

Any of the following procedures:
Ø2H43JZ Insertion of Pacemaker Lead into Coronary Vein, Percutaneous Approach
Ø2H43KZ Insertion of Defibrillator Lead into Coronary Vein, Percutaneous Approach
Ø2H43MZ Insertion of Cardiac Lead into Coronary Vein, Percutaneous Approach
Ø2H63JZ Insertion of Pacemaker Lead into Right Atrium, Percutaneous Approach
Ø2H63MZ Insertion of Cardiac Lead into Right Atrium, Percutaneous Approach
Ø2H73JZ Insertion of Pacemaker Lead into Left Atrium, Percutaneous Approach
Ø2H73MZ Insertion of Cardiac Lead into Left Atrium, Percutaneous Approach
Ø2HK3JZ Insertion of Pacemaker Lead into Right Ventricle, Percutaneous Approach
Ø2HL3JZ Insertion of Pacemaker Lead into Left Ventricle, Percutaneous Approach
Ø2HNØJZ Insertion of Pacemaker Lead into Pericardium, Open Approach
Ø2HNØMZ Insertion of Cardiac Lead into Pericardium, Open Approach
Ø2HN3JZ Insertion of Pacemaker Lead into Pericardium, Percutaneous Approach
Ø2HN3MZ Insertion of Cardiac Lead into Pericardium, Percutaneous Approach
Ø2HN4JZ Insertion of Pacemaker Lead into Pericardium, Percutaneous Endoscopic Approach
Ø2HN4MZ Insertion of Cardiac Lead into Pericardium, Percutaneous Endoscopic Approach
Ø2PAØMZ Removal of Cardiac Lead from Heart, Open Approach
Ø2PA3MZ Removal of Cardiac Lead from Heart, Percutaneous Approach
Ø2PA4MZ Removal of Cardiac Lead from Heart, Percutaneous Endoscopic Approach
Ø2PAXMZ Removal of Cardiac Lead from Heart, External Approach
Ø2WAØMZ Revision of Cardiac Lead in Heart, Open Approach
Ø2WA3MZ Revision of Cardiac Lead in Heart, Percutaneous Approach
Ø2WA4MZ Revision of Cardiac Lead in Heart, Percutaneous Endoscopic Approach
ØJH6Ø4Z Insertion of Pacemaker, Single Chamber into Chest Subcutaneous Tissue and Fascia, Open Approach
ØJH6Ø5Z Insertion of Pacemaker, Single Chamber Rate Responsive into Chest Subcutaneous Tissue and Fascia, Open Approach
ØJH6Ø6Z Insertion of Pacemaker, Dual Chamber into Chest Subcutaneous Tissue and Fascia, Open Approach
ØJH6Ø7Z Insertion of Cardiac Resynchronization Pacemaker Pulse Generator into Chest Subcutaneous Tissue and Fascia, Open Approach
ØJH6Ø8Z Insertion of Defibrillator Generator into Chest Subcutaneous Tissue and Fascia, Open Approach
ØJH6Ø9Z Insertion of Cardiac Resynchronization Defibrillator Pulse Generator into Chest Subcutaneous Tissue and Fascia, Open Approach
ØJH6ØPZ Insertion of Cardiac Rhythm Related Device into Chest Subcutaneous Tissue and Fascia, Open Approach
ØJH634Z Insertion of Pacemaker, Single Chamber into Chest Subcutaneous Tissue and Fascia, Percutaneous Approach
ØJH635Z Insertion of Pacemaker, Single Chamber Rate Responsive into Chest Subcutaneous Tissue and Fascia, Percutaneous Approach
ØJH636Z Insertion of Pacemaker, Dual Chamber into Chest Subcutaneous Tissue and Fascia, Percutaneous Approach
ØJH637Z Insertion of Cardiac Resynchronization Pacemaker Pulse Generator into Chest Subcutaneous Tissue and Fascia, Percutaneous Approach
ØJH638Z Insertion of Defibrillator Generator into Chest Subcutaneous Tissue and Fascia, Percutaneous Approach
ØJH639Z Insertion of Cardiac Resynchronization Defibrillator Pulse Generator into Chest Subcutaneous Tissue and Fascia, Percutaneous Approach
ØJH63PZ Insertion of Cardiac Rhythm Related Device into Chest Subcutaneous Tissue and Fascia, Percutaneous Approach
ØJH8Ø4Z Insertion of Pacemaker, Single Chamber into Abdomen Subcutaneous Tissue and Fascia, Open Approach
ØJH8Ø5Z Insertion of Pacemaker, Single Chamber Rate Responsive into Abdomen Subcutaneous Tissue and Fascia, Open Approach
ØJH8Ø6Z Insertion of Pacemaker, Dual Chamber into Abdomen Subcutaneous Tissue and Fascia, Open Approach
ØJH8Ø7Z Insertion of Cardiac Resynchronization Pacemaker Pulse Generator into Abdomen Subcutaneous Tissue and Fascia, Open Approach
ØJH8Ø8Z Insertion of Defibrillator Generator into Abdomen Subcutaneous Tissue and Fascia, Open Approach
ØJH8Ø9Z Insertion of Cardiac Resynchronization Defibrillator Pulse Generator into Abdomen Subcutaneous Tissue and Fascia, Open Approach
ØJH8ØPZ Insertion of Cardiac Rhythm Related Device into Abdomen Subcutaneous Tissue and Fascia, Open Approach
ØJH834Z Insertion of Pacemaker, Single Chamber into Abdomen Subcutaneous Tissue and Fascia, Percutaneous Approach
ØJH835Z Insertion of Pacemaker, Single Chamber Rate Responsive into Abdomen Subcutaneous Tissue and Fascia, Percutaneous Approach
ØJH836Z Insertion of Pacemaker, Dual Chamber into Abdomen Subcutaneous Tissue and Fascia, Percutaneous Approach
ØJH837Z Insertion of Cardiac Resynchronization Pacemaker Pulse Generator into Abdomen Subcutaneous Tissue and Fascia, Percutaneous Approach
ØJH838Z Insertion of Defibrillator Generator into Abdomen Subcutaneous Tissue and Fascia, Percutaneous Approach
ØJH839Z Insertion of Cardiac Resynchronization Defibrillator Pulse Generator into Abdomen Subcutaneous Tissue and Fascia, Percutaneous Approach
ØJH83PZ Insertion of Cardiac Rhythm Related Device into Abdomen Subcutaneous Tissue and Fascia, Percutaneous Approach
ØJPTØPZ Removal of Cardiac Rhythm Related Device from Trunk Subcutaneous Tissue and Fascia, Open Approach

**HAC 13: Surgical Site Infection (SSI) Following Cardiac Implantable Electronic Device (CIED) Procedures (continued)**

ØJPT3PZ Removal of Cardiac Rhythm Related Device from Trunk Subcutaneous Tissue and Fascia, Percutaneous Approach
ØJWTØPZ Revision of Cardiac Rhythm Related Device in Trunk Subcutaneous Tissue and Fascia, Open Approach
ØJWT3PZ Revision of Cardiac Rhythm Related Device in Trunk Subcutaneous Tissue and Fascia, Percutaneous Approach

**HAC 14: Iatrogenic Pneumothorax with Venous Catheterization**

Secondary diagnosis not POA:
J95.811

**AND**

Any of the following procedures:

Ø2H633Z Insertion of Infusion Device into Right Atrium, Percutaneous Approach
Ø2HK33Z Insertion of Infusion Device into Right Ventricle, Percutaneous Approach
Ø2HS33Z Insertion of Infusion Device into Right Pulmonary Vein, Percutaneous Approach
Ø2HS43Z Insertion of Infusion Device into Right Pulmonary Vein, Percutaneous Endoscopic Approach
Ø2HT33Z Insertion of Infusion Device into Left Pulmonary Vein, Percutaneous Approach
Ø2HT43Z Insertion of Infusion Device into Left Pulmonary Vein, Percutaneous Endoscopic Approach
Ø2HV33Z Insertion of Infusion Device into Superior Vena Cava, Percutaneous Approach
Ø2HV43Z Insertion of Infusion Device into Superior Vena Cava, Percutaneous Endoscopic Approach
Ø5HØ33Z Insertion of Infusion Device into Azygos Vein, Percutaneous Approach
Ø5HØ43Z Insertion of Infusion Device into Azygos Vein, Percutaneous Endoscopic Approach
Ø5H133Z Insertion of Infusion Device into Hemiazygos Vein, Percutaneous Approach
Ø5H143Z Insertion of Infusion Device into Hemiazygos Vein, Percutaneous Endoscopic Approach
Ø5H333Z Insertion of Infusion Device into Right Innominate Vein, Percutaneous Approach
Ø5H343Z Insertion of Infusion Device into Right Innominate Vein, Percutaneous Endoscopic Approach
Ø5H433Z Insertion of Infusion Device into Left Innominate Vein, Percutaneous Approach
Ø5H443Z Insertion of Infusion Device into Left Innominate Vein, Percutaneous Endoscopic Approach
Ø5H533Z Insertion of Infusion Device into Right Subclavian Vein, Percutaneous Approach
Ø5H543Z Insertion of Infusion Device into Right Subclavian Vein, Percutaneous Endoscopic Approach
Ø5H633Z Insertion of Infusion Device into Left Subclavian Vein, Percutaneous Approach
Ø5H643Z Insertion of Infusion Device into Left Subclavian Vein, Percutaneous Endoscopic Approach
Ø5HM33Z Insertion of Infusion Device into Right Internal Jugular Vein, Percutaneous Approach
Ø5HN33Z Insertion of Infusion Device into Left Internal Jugular Vein, Percutaneous Approach
Ø5HP33Z Insertion of Infusion Device into Right External Jugular Vein, Percutaneous Approach
Ø5HQ33Z Insertion of Infusion Device into Left External Jugular Vein, Percutaneous Approach
ØJH63XZ Insertion of Vascular Access Device into Chest Subcutaneous Tissue and Fascia, Percutaneous Approach

# Appendix K: Coding Exercises and Answers



Using the ICD-10-PCS tables construct the code that accurately represents the procedure performed.

## Medical Surgical Section

| Procedure | Code |
|---|---|
| 1. Excision of malignant melanoma from skin of right ear | |
| 2. Laparoscopy with excision of endometrial implant from left ovary | |
| 3. Percutaneous needle core biopsy of right kidney | |
| 4. EGD with gastric biopsy | |
| 5. Open endarterectomy of left common carotid artery | |
| 6. Excision of basal cell carcinoma of lower lip | |
| 7. Open excision of tail of pancreas | |
| 8. Percutaneous biopsy of right gastrocnemius muscle | |
| 9. Sigmoidoscopy with sigmoid polypectomy | |
| 10. Open excision of lesion from right Achilles tendon | |
| 11. Open resection of cecum | |
| 12. Total excision of pituitary gland, open | |
| 13. Explantation of left failed kidney, open | |
| 14. Open left axillary total lymphadenectomy | |
| 15. Laparoscopic-assisted vaginal hysterectomy | |
| 16. Right total mastectomy, open | |
| 17. Open resection of papillary muscle | |
| 18. Total retropubic prostatectomy, open | |
| 19. Laparoscopic cholecystectomy | |
| 20. Endoscopic bilateral total maxillary sinusectomy | |
| 21. Amputation at right elbow level | |
| 22. Right below-knee amputation, proximal tibia/fibula | |
| 23. Fifth ray carpometacarpal joint amputation, left hand | |
| 24. Right leg and hip amputation through ischium | |
| 25. DIP joint amputation of right thumb | |
| 26. Right wrist joint amputation | |
| 27. Trans-metatarsal amputation of foot at left big toe | |
| 28. Mid-shaft amputation, right humerus | |
| 29. Left fourth toe amputation, mid-proximal phalanx | |
| 30. Right above-knee amputation, distal femur | |
| 31. Cryotherapy of wart on left hand | |
| 32. Percutaneous radiofrequency ablation of right vocal cord lesion | |
| 33. Left heart catheterization with laser destruction of arrhythmogenic focus, A-V node | |
| 34. Cautery of nosebleed | |
| 35. Transurethral endoscopic laser ablation of prostate | |
| 36. Percutaneous cautery of oozing varicose vein, left calf | |

| Procedure | Code |
|---|---|
| 37. Laparoscopy with destruction of endometriosis, bilateral ovaries | |
| 38. Laser coagulation of right retinal vessel hemorrhage, percutaneous | |
| 39. Thoracoscopic pleurodesis, left side | |
| 40. Percutaneous insertion of Greenfield IVC filter | |
| 41. Forceps total mouth extraction, upper and lower teeth | |
| 42. Removal of left thumbnail | |
| 43. Extraction of right intraocular lens without replacement, percutaneous | |
| 44. Laparoscopy with needle aspiration of ova for in vitro fertilization | |
| 45. Nonexcisional debridement of skin ulcer, right foot | |
| 46. Open stripping of abdominal fascia, right side | |
| 47. Hysteroscopy with D&C, diagnostic | |
| 48. Liposuction for medical purposes, left upper arm | |
| 49. Removal of tattered right ear drum fragments with tweezers | |
| 50. Microincisional phlebectomy of spider veins, right lower leg | |
| 51. Routine Foley catheter placement | |
| 52. Incision and drainage of external anal abscess | |
| 53. Percutaneous drainage of ascites | |
| 54. Laparoscopy with left ovarian cystotomy and drainage | |
| 55. Laparotomy and drain placement for liver abscess, right lobe | |
| 56. Right knee arthrotomy with drain placement | |
| 57. Thoracentesis of left pleural effusion | |
| 58. Phlebotomy of left median cubital vein for polycythemia vera | |
| 59. Percutaneous chest tube placement for right pneumothorax | |
| 60. Endoscopic drainage of left ethmoid sinus | |
| 61. External ventricular CSF drainage catheter placement via burr hole | |
| 62. Removal of foreign body, right cornea | |
| 63. Percutaneous mechanical thrombectomy, left brachial artery | |
| 64. Esophagogastroscopy with removal of bezoar from stomach | |
| 65. Foreign body removal, skin of left thumb | |
| 66. Transurethral cystoscopy with removal of bladder stone | |
| 67. Forceps removal of foreign body in right nostril | |
| 68. Laparoscopy with excision of old suture from mesentery | |
| 69. Incision and removal of right lacrimal duct stone | |
| 70. Nonincisional removal of intraluminal foreign body from vagina | |
| 71. Right common carotid endarterectomy, open | |
| 72. Open excision of retained sliver, subcutaneous tissue of left foot | |
| 73. Extracorporeal shockwave lithotripsy (ESWL), bilateral ureters | |

| Procedure | Code |
|---|---|
| 74. Endoscopic retrograde cholangiopancreatography (ERCP) with lithotripsy of common bile duct stone | |
| 75. Thoracotomy with crushing of pericardial calcifications | |
| 76. Transurethral cystoscopy with fragmentation of bladder calculus | |
| 77. Hysteroscopy with intraluminal lithotripsy of left fallopian tube calcification | |
| 78. Division of right foot tendon, percutaneous | |
| 79. Left heart catheterization with division of bundle of HIS | |
| 80. Open osteotomy of capitate, left hand | |
| 81. EGD with esophagotomy of esophagogastric junction | |
| 82. Sacral rhizotomy for pain control, percutaneous | |
| 83. Laparotomy with exploration and adhesiolysis of right ureter | |
| 84. Incision of scar contracture, right elbow | |
| 85. Frenulotomy for treatment of tongue-tie syndrome | |
| 86. Right shoulder arthroscopy with coracoacromial ligament release | |
| 87. Mitral valvulotomy for release of fused leaflets, open approach | |
| 88. Percutaneous left Achilles tendon release | |
| 89. Laparoscopy with lysis of peritoneal adhesions | |
| 90. Manual rupture of right shoulder joint adhesions under general anesthesia | |
| 91. Open posterior tarsal tunnel release | |
| 92. Laparoscopy with freeing of left ovary and fallopian tube | |
| 93. Liver transplant with donor matched liver | |
| 94. Orthotopic heart transplant using porcine heart | |
| 95. Right lung transplant, open, using organ donor match | |
| 96. Transplant of large intestine, organ donor match | |
| 97. Left kidney/pancreas organ bank transplant | |
| 98. Replantation of avulsed scalp | |
| 99. Reattachment of severed right ear | |
| 100. Reattachment of traumatic left gastrocnemius avulsion, open | |
| 101. Closed replantation of three avulsed teeth, lower jaw | |
| 102. Reattachment of severed left hand | |
| 103. Right open palmaris longus tendon transfer | |
| 104. Endoscopic radial to median nerve transfer | |
| 105. Fasciocutaneous flap closure of left thigh, open | |
| 106. Transfer left index finger to left thumb position, open | |
| 107. Percutaneous fascia transfer to fill defect, anterior neck | |
| 108. Trigeminal to facial nerve transfer, percutaneous endoscopic | |
| 109. Endoscopic left leg flexor hallucis longus tendon transfer | |
| 110. Right scalp advancement flap to right temple | |

| Procedure | Code |
|---|---|
| 111. Bilateral TRAM pedicle flap reconstruction status post mastectomy, muscle only, open | |
| 112. Skin transfer flap closure of complex open wound, left lower back | |
| 113. Open fracture reduction, right tibia | |
| 114. Laparoscopy with gastropexy for malrotation | |
| 115. Left knee arthroscopy with reposition of anterior cruciate ligament | |
| 116. Open transposition of ulnar nerve | |
| 117. Closed reduction with percutaneous internal fixation of right femoral neck fracture | |
| 118. Trans-vaginal intraluminal cervical cerclage | |
| 119. Cervical cerclage using Shirodkar technique | |
| 120. Thoracotomy with banding of left pulmonary artery using extraluminal device | |
| 121. Restriction of thoracic duct with intraluminal stent, percutaneous | |
| 122. Craniotomy with clipping of cerebral aneurysm | |
| 123. Nonincisional, transnasal placement of restrictive stent in right lacrimal duct | |
| 124. Catheter-based temporary restriction of blood flow in abdominal aorta for treatment of cerebral ischemia | |
| 125. Percutaneous ligation of esophageal vein | |
| 126. Percutaneous embolization of left internal carotid-cavernous fistula | |
| 127. Laparoscopy with bilateral occlusion of fallopian tubes using Hulka extraluminal clips | |
| 128. Open suture ligation of failed AV graft, left brachial artery | |
| 129. Percutaneous embolization of vascular supply, intracranial meningioma | |
| 130. Percutaneous embolization of right uterine artery, using coils | |
| 131. Open occlusion of left atrial appendage, using extraluminal pressure clips | |
| 132. Percutaneous suture exclusion of left atrial appendage, via femoral artery access | |
| 133. ERCP with balloon dilation of common bile duct | |
| 134. PTCA of two coronary arteries, LAD with stent placement, RCA with no stent | |
| 135. Cystoscopy with intraluminal dilation of bladder neck stricture | |
| 136. Open dilation of old anastomosis, left femoral artery | |
| 137. Dilation of upper esophageal stricture, direct visualization, with Bougie sound | |
| 138. PTA of right brachial artery stenosis | |
| 139. Transnasal dilation and stent placement in right lacrimal duct | |
| 140. Hysteroscopy with balloon dilation of bilateral fallopian tubes | |
| 141. Tracheoscopy with intraluminal dilation of tracheal stenosis | |
| 142. Cystoscopy with dilation of left ureteral stricture, with stent placement | |
| 143. Open gastric bypass with Roux-en-Y limb to jejunum | |
| 144. Right temporal artery to intracranial artery bypass using Gore-Tex graft, open | |

| Procedure | Code |
|---|---|
| 145. Tracheostomy formation with tracheostomy tube placement, percutaneous | |
| 146. PICVA (percutaneous in situ coronary venous arterialization) of single coronary artery | |
| 147. Open left femoral-popliteal artery bypass using cadaver vein graft | |
| 148. Shunting of intrathecal cerebrospinal fluid to peritoneal cavity using synthetic shunt | |
| 149. Colostomy formation, open, transverse colon to abdominal wall | |
| 150. Open urinary diversion, left ureter, using ileal conduit to skin | |
| 151. CABG of LAD using left internal mammary artery, open off-bypass | |
| 152. Open pleuroperitoneal shunt, right pleural cavity, using synthetic device | |
| 153. Percutaneous placement of ventriculoperitoneal shunt for treatment of hydrocephalus | |
| 154. End-of-life replacement of spinal neurostimulator generator, multiple array, in lower abdomen | |
| 155. Percutaneous insertion of spinal neurostimulator lead, lumbar spinal cord | |
| 156. Percutaneous replacement of broken pacemaker lead in left atrium | |
| 157. Open placement of dual chamber pacemaker generator in chest wall | |
| 158. Percutaneous placement of venous central line in right internal jugular, with tip in superior vena cava | |
| 159. Open insertion of multiple channel cochlear implant, left ear | |
| 160. Percutaneous placement of Swan-Ganz catheter in pulmonary trunk | |
| 161. Bronchoscopy with insertion of Low Dose, Pd-103 brachytherapy seeds, right main bronchus | |
| 162. Open insertion of interspinous process device into lumbar vertebral joint | |
| 163. Open placement of bone growth stimulator, left femoral shaft | |
| 164. Cystoscopy with placement of brachytherapy seeds in prostate gland | |
| 165. Percutaneous insertion of Greenfield IVC filter | |
| 166. Full-thickness skin graft to right lower arm, autograft (do not code graft harvest for this exercise) | |
| 167. Excision of necrosed left femoral head with bone bank bone graft to fill the defect, open | |
| 168. Penetrating keratoplasty of right cornea with donor matched cornea, percutaneous approach | |
| 169. Bilateral mastectomy with concomitant saline breast implants, open | |
| 170. Excision of abdominal aorta with Gore-Tex graft replacement, open | |
| 171. Total right knee arthroplasty with insertion of total knee prosthesis | |
| 172. Bilateral mastectomy with free TRAM flap reconstruction | |
| 173. Tenonectomy with graft to right ankle using cadaver graft, open | |

| Procedure | Code |
|---|---|
| 174. Mitral valve replacement using porcine valve, open | |
| 175. Percutaneous phacoemulsification of right eye cataract with prosthetic lens insertion | |
| 176. Transcatheter replacement of pulmonary valve using of bovine jugular vein valve | |
| 177. Total left hip replacement using ceramic on ceramic prosthesis, without bone cement | |
| 178. Aortic valve annuloplasty using ring, open | |
| 179. Laparoscopic repair of left inguinal hernia with marlex plug | |
| 180. Autograft nerve graft to right median nerve, percutaneous endoscopic (do not code graft harvest for this exercise) | |
| 181. Exchange of liner in femoral component of previous left hip replacement, open approach | |
| 182. Anterior colporrhaphy with polypropylene mesh reinforcement, open approach | |
| 183. Implantation of CorCap cardiac support device, open approach | |
| 184. Abdominal wall herniorrhaphy, open, using synthetic mesh | |
| 185. Tendon graft to strengthen injured left shoulder using autograft, open (do not code graft harvest for this exercise) | |
| 186. Onlay lamellar keratoplasty of left cornea using autograft, external approach | |
| 187. Resurfacing procedure on right femoral head, open approach | |
| 188. Exchange of drainage tube from right hip joint | |
| 189. Tracheostomy tube exchange | |
| 190. Change chest tube for left pneumothorax | |
| 191. Exchange of cerebral ventriculostomy drainage tube | |
| 192. Foley urinary catheter exchange | |
| 193. Open removal of lumbar sympathetic neurostimulator lead | |
| 194. Nonincisional removal of Swan-Ganz catheter from right pulmonary artery | |
| 195. Laparotomy with removal of pancreatic drain | |
| 196. Extubation, endotracheal tube | |
| 197. Nonincisional PEG tube removal | |
| 198. Transvaginal removal of brachytherapy seeds | |
| 199. Transvaginal removal of extraluminal cervical cerclage | |
| 200. Incision with removal of K-wire fixation, right first metatarsal | |
| 201. Cystoscopy with retrieval of left ureteral stent | |
| 202. Removal of nasogastric drainage tube for decompression | |
| 203. Removal of external fixator, left radial fracture | |
| 204. Trimming and reanastomosis of stenosed femorofemoral synthetic bypass graft, open | |
| 205. Open revision of right hip replacement, with readjustment of prosthesis | |
| 206. Adjustment of position, pacemaker lead in left ventricle, percutaneous | |
| 207. External repositioning of Foley catheter to bladder | |
| 208. Taking out loose screw and putting larger screw in fracture repair plate, left tibia | |

| Procedure | Code |
|---|---|
| 209. Revision of totally implantable VAD port placement in chest wall, causing patient discomfort, open | |
| 210. Thoracotomy with exploration of right pleural cavity | |
| 211. Diagnostic laryngoscopy | |
| 212. Exploratory arthrotomy of left knee | |
| 213. Colposcopy with diagnostic hysteroscopy | |
| 214. Digital rectal exam | |
| 215. Diagnostic arthroscopy of right shoulder | |
| 216. Endoscopy of maxillary sinus | |
| 217. Laparotomy with palpation of liver | |
| 218. Transurethral diagnostic cystoscopy | |
| 219. Colonoscopy, discontinued at sigmoid colon | |
| 220. Percutaneous mapping of basal ganglia | |
| 221. Heart catheterization with cardiac mapping | |
| 222. Intraoperative whole brain mapping via craniotomy | |
| 223. Mapping of left cerebral hemisphere, percutaneous endoscopic | |
| 224. Intraoperative cardiac mapping during open heart surgery | |
| 225. Hysteroscopy with cautery of post-hysterectomy oozing and evacuation of clot | |
| 226. Open exploration and ligation of post-op arterial bleeder, left forearm | |
| 227. Control of post-operative retroperitoneal bleeding via laparotomy | |
| 228. Reopening of thoracotomy site with drainage and control of post-op hemopericardium | |
| 229. Arthroscopy with drainage of hemarthrosis at previous operative site, right knee | |
| 230. Radiocarpal fusion of left hand with internal fixation, open | |
| 231. Posterior spinal fusion at L1-L3 level with BAK cage interbody fusion device, open | |
| 232. Intercarpal fusion of right hand with bone bank bone graft, open | |
| 233. Sacrococcygeal fusion with bone graft from same operative site, open | |
| 234. Interphalangeal fusion of left great toe, percutaneous pin fixation | |
| 235. Suture repair of left radial nerve laceration | |
| 236. Laparotomy with suture repair of blunt force duodenal laceration | |
| 237. Perineoplasty with repair of old obstetric laceration, open | |
| 238. Suture repair of right biceps tendon (upper arm) laceration, open | |
| 239. Closure of abdominal wall stab wound | |
| 240. Cosmetic face lift, open, no other information available | |
| 241. Bilateral breast augmentation with silicone implants, open | |
| 242. Cosmetic rhinoplasty with septal reduction and tip elevation using local tissue graft, open | |
| 243. Abdominoplasty (tummy tuck), open | |
| 244. Liposuction of bilateral thighs | |
| 245. Creation of penis in female patient using tissue bank donor graft | |
| 246. Creation of vagina in male patient using synthetic material | |
| 247. Laparoscopic vertical (sleeve) gastrectomy | |
| 248. Left uterine artery embolization with intraluminal biosphere injection | |

## Obstetrics

| Procedure | Code |
|---|---|
| 1. Abortion by dilation and evacuation following laminaria insertion | |
| 2. Manually assisted spontaneous abortion | |
| 3. Abortion by abortifacient insertion | |
| 4. Bimanual pregnancy examination | |
| 5. Extraperitoneal C-section, low transverse incision | |
| 6. Fetal spinal tap, percutaneous | |
| 7. Fetal kidney transplant, laparoscopic | |
| 8. Open in utero repair of congenital diaphragmatic hernia | |
| 9. Laparoscopy with total excision of tubal pregnancy | |
| 10. Transvaginal removal of fetal monitoring electrode | |

## Placement

| Procedure | Code |
|---|---|
| 1. Placement of packing material, right ear | |
| 2. Mechanical traction of entire left leg | |
| 3. Removal of splint, right shoulder | |
| 4. Placement of neck brace | |
| 5. Change of vaginal packing | |
| 6. Packing of wound, chest wall | |
| 7. Sterile dressing placement to left groin region | |
| 8. Removal of packing material from pharynx | |
| 9. Placement of intermittent pneumatic compression device, covering entire right arm | |
| 10. Exchange of pressure dressing to left thigh | |

## Administration

| Procedure | Code |
|---|---|
| 1. Peritoneal dialysis via indwelling catheter | |
| 2. Transvaginal artificial insemination | |
| 3. Infusion of total parenteral nutrition via central venous catheter | |
| 4. Esophagogastroscopy with Botox injection into esophageal sphincter | |
| 5. Percutaneous irrigation of knee joint | |
| 6. Systemic infusion of recombinant tissue plasminogen activator (r-tPA) via peripheral venous catheter | |
| 7. Transfusion of antihemophilic factor, (nonautologous) via arterial central line | |
| 8. Transabdominal in vitro fertilization, implantation of donor ovum | |
| 9. Autologous bone marrow transplant via central venous line | |
| 10. Implantation of anti-microbial envelope with cardiac defibrillator placement, open | |

| Procedure | Code |
|---|---|
| 11. Sclerotherapy of brachial plexus lesion, alcohol injection | |
| 12. Percutaneous peripheral vein injection, glucarpidase | |
| 13. Introduction of anti-infective envelope into subcutaneous tissue, open | |

## Measurement and Monitoring

| Procedure | Code |
|---|---|
| 1. Cardiac stress test, single measurement | |
| 2. EGD with biliary flow measurement | |
| 3. Right and left heart cardiac catheterization with bilateral sampling and pressure measurements | |
| 4. Temperature monitoring, rectal | |
| 5. Peripheral venous pulse, external, single measurement | |
| 6. Holter monitoring | |
| 7. Respiratory rate, external, single measurement | |
| 8. Fetal heart rate monitoring, transvaginal | |
| 9. Visual mobility test, single measurement | |
| 10. Left ventricular cardiac output monitoring from pulmonary artery wedge (Swan-Ganz) catheter | |
| 11. Olfactory acuity test, single measurement | |

## Extracorporeal or Systemic Assistance and Performance

| Procedure | Code |
|---|---|
| 1. Intermittent mechanical ventilation, 16 hours | |
| 2. Liver dialysis, single encounter | |
| 3. Cardiac countershock with successful conversion to sinus rhythm | |
| 4. IPPB (intermittent positive pressure breathing) for mobilization of secretions, 22 hours | |
| 5. Renal dialysis, 12 hours | |
| 6. IABP (intra-aortic balloon pump) continuous | |
| 7. Intra-operative cardiac pacing, continuous | |
| 8. ECMO (extracorporeal membrane oxygenation), continuous | |
| 9. Controlled mechanical ventilation (CMV), 45 hours | |
| 10. Pulsatile compression boot with intermittent inflation | |

## Extracorporeal or Systemic Therapies

| Procedure | Code |
|---|---|
| 1. Donor thrombocytapheresis, single encounter | |
| 2. Bili-lite phototherapy, series treatment | |
| 3. Whole body hypothermia, single treatment | |
| 4. Circulatory phototherapy, single encounter | |
| 5. Shock wave therapy of plantar fascia, single treatment | |
| 6. Antigen-free air conditioning, series treatment | |
| 7. TMS (transcranial magnetic stimulation), series treatment | |
| 8. Therapeutic ultrasound of peripheral vessels, single treatment | |
| 9. Plasmapheresis, series treatment | |
| 10. Extracorporeal electromagnetic stimulation (EMS) for urinary incontinence, single treatment | |

## Osteopathic

| Procedure | Code |
|---|---|
| 1. Isotonic muscle energy treatment of right leg | |
| 2. Low velocity-high amplitude osteopathic treatment of head | |
| 3. Lymphatic pump osteopathic treatment of left axilla | |
| 4. Indirect osteopathic treatment of sacrum | |
| 5. Articulatory osteopathic treatment of cervical region | |

## Other Procedures

| Procedure | Code |
|---|---|
| 1. Near infrared spectroscopy of leg vessels | |
| 2. CT computer assisted sinus surgery | |
| 3. Suture removal, abdominal wall | |
| 4. Isolation after infectious disease exposure | |
| 5. Robotic assisted open prostatectomy | |
| 6. In vitro fertilization | |

## Chiropractic

| Procedure | Code |
|---|---|
| 1. Chiropractic treatment of lumbar region using long lever specific contact | |
| 2. Chiropractic manipulation of abdominal region, indirect visceral | |
| 3. Chiropractic extra-articular treatment of hip region | |
| 4. Chiropractic treatment of sacrum using long and short lever specific contact | |
| 5. Mechanically-assisted chiropractic manipulation of head | |

## Imaging

| Procedure | Code |
|---|---|
| 1. Noncontrast CT of abdomen and pelvis | |
| 2. Intravascular ultrasound, left subclavian artery | |
| 3. Fluoroscopic guidance for insertion of central venous catheter in SVC, low osmolar contrast | |
| 4. Chest x-ray, AP/PA and lateral views | |

| Procedure | Code |
|---|---|
| 5. Endoluminal ultrasound of gallbladder and bile ducts | |
| 6. MRI of thyroid gland, contrast unspecified | |
| 7. Esophageal videofluoroscopy study with oral barium contrast | |
| 8. Portable x-ray study of right radius/ulna shaft, standard series | |
| 9. Routine fetal ultrasound, second trimester twin gestation | |
| 10. CT scan of bilateral lungs, high osmolar contrast with densitometry | |
| 11. Fluoroscopic guidance for percutaneous transluminal angioplasty (PTA) of left common femoral artery, low osmolar contrast | |

## Nuclear Medicine

| Procedure | Code |
|---|---|
| 1. Tomo scan of right and left heart, unspecified radiopharmaceutical, qualitative gated rest | |
| 2. Technetium pentetate assay of kidneys, ureters, and bladder | |
| 3. Uniplanar scan of spine using technetium oxidronate, with first-pass study | |
| 4. Thallous chloride tomographic scan of bilateral breasts | |
| 5. PET scan of myocardium using rubidium | |
| 6. Gallium citrate scan of head and neck, single plane imaging | |
| 7. Xenon gas nonimaging probe of brain | |
| 8. Upper GI scan, radiopharmaceutical unspecified, for gastric emptying | |
| 9. Carbon 11 PET scan of brain with quantification | |
| 10. Iodinated albumin nuclear medicine assay, blood plasma volume study | |

## Radiation Therapy

| Procedure | Code |
|---|---|
| 1. Plaque radiation of left eye, single port | |
| 2. 8 MeV photon beam radiation to brain | |
| 3. IORT of colon, 3 ports | |
| 4. HDR brachytherapy of prostate using palladium-103 | |
| 5. Electron radiation treatment of right breast, with custom device | |
| 6. Hyperthermia oncology treatment of pelvic region | |
| 7. Contact radiation of tongue | |
| 8. Heavy particle radiation treatment of pancreas, four risk sites | |
| 9. LDR brachytherapy to spinal cord using iodine | |
| 10. Whole body Phosphorus 32 administration with risk to hematopoetic system | |

## Physical Rehabilitation and Diagnostic Audiology

| Procedure | Code |
|---|---|
| 1. Bekesy assessment using audiometer | |
| 2. Individual fitting of left eye prosthesis | |
| 3. Physical therapy for range of motion and mobility, patient right hip, no special equipment | |
| 4. Bedside swallow assessment using assessment kit | |
| 5. Caregiver training in airway clearance techniques | |
| 6. Application of short arm cast in rehabilitation setting | |
| 7. Verbal assessment of patient's pain level | |
| 8. Caregiver training in communication skills using manual communication board | |
| 9. Group musculoskeletal balance training exercises, whole body, no special equipment | |
| 10. Individual therapy for auditory processing using tape recorder | |

## Mental Health

| Procedure | Code |
|---|---|
| 1. Cognitive-behavioral psychotherapy, individual | |
| 2. Narcosynthesis | |
| 3. Light therapy | |
| 4. ECT (electroconvulsive therapy), unilateral, multiple seizure | |
| 5. Crisis intervention | |
| 6. Neuropsychological testing | |
| 7. Hypnosis | |
| 8. Developmental testing | |
| 9. Vocational counseling | |
| 10. Family psychotherapy | |

## Substance Abuse Treatment

| Procedure | Code |
|---|---|
| 1. Naltrexone treatment for drug dependency | |
| 2. Substance abuse treatment family counseling | |
| 3. Medication monitoring of patient on methadone maintenance | |
| 4. Individual interpersonal psychotherapy for drug abuse | |
| 5. Patient in for alcohol detoxification treatment | |
| 6. Group motivational counseling | |
| 7. Individual 12-step psychotherapy for substance abuse | |
| 8. Post-test infectious disease counseling for IV drug abuser | |
| 9. Psychodynamic psychotherapy for drug dependent patient | |
| 10. Group cognitive-behavioral counseling for substance abuse | |

## New Technology

| Procedure | Code |
|---|---|
| 1. Infusion of ceftazidime via peripheral venous catheter | |

# Answers to Coding Exercises

## Medical Surgical Section

| Procedure | Code |
|---|---|
| 1. Excision of malignant melanoma from skin of right ear | ØHB2XZZ |
| 2. Laparoscopy with excision of endometrial implant from left ovary | ØUB14ZZ |
| 3. Percutaneous needle core biopsy of right kidney | ØTBØ3ZX |
| 4. EGD with gastric biopsy | ØDB68ZX |
| 5. Open endarterectomy of left common carotid artery | Ø3CJØZZ |
| 6. Excision of basal cell carcinoma of lower lip | ØCB1XZZ |
| 7. Open excision of tail of pancreas | ØFBGØZZ |
| 8. Percutaneous biopsy of right gastrocnemius muscle | ØKBS3ZX |
| 9. Sigmoidoscopy with sigmoid polypectomy | ØDBN8ZZ |
| 10. Open excision of lesion from right Achilles tendon | ØLBNØZZ |
| 11. Open resection of cecum | ØDTHØZZ |
| 12. Total excision of pituitary gland, open | ØGTØØZZ |
| 13. Explantation of left failed kidney, open | ØTT1ØZZ |
| 14. Open left axillary total lymphadenectomy | Ø7T6ØZZ (RESECTION is coded for cutting out a chain of lymph nodes.) |
| 15. Laparoscopic-assisted vaginal hysterectomy | ØUT9FZZ |
| 16. Right total mastectomy, open | ØHTTØZZ |
| 17. Open resection of papillary muscle | Ø2TDØZZ (The papillary muscle refers to the heart and is found in the *Heart and Great Vessels* body system.) |
| 18. Total retropubic prostatectomy, open | ØVTØØZZ |
| 19. Laparoscopic cholecystectomy | ØFT44ZZ |
| 20. Endoscopic bilateral total maxillary sinusectomy | Ø9TQ4ZZ, Ø9TR4ZZ |
| 21. Amputation at right elbow level | ØX6BØZZ |
| 22. Right below-knee amputation, proximal tibia/fibula | ØY6HØZ1 (The qualifier *High* here means the portion of the tib/fib closest to the knee.) |
| 23. Fifth ray carpometacarpal joint amputation, left hand | ØX6KØZ8 (A *complete* ray amputation is through the carpometacarpal joint.) |
| 24. Right leg and hip amputation through ischium | ØY62ØZZ (The *Hindquarter* body part includes amputation along any part of the hip bone.) |
| 25. DIP joint amputation of right thumb | ØX6LØZ3 (The qualifier *low* here means through the distal interphalangeal joint.) |
| 26. Right wrist joint amputation | ØX6JØZØ (Amputation at the wrist joint is actually complete amputation of the hand.) |
| 27. Trans-metatarsal amputation of foot at left big toe | ØY6NØZ9 (A *partial* amputation is through the shaft of the metatarsal bone.) |
| 28. Mid-shaft amputation, right humerus | ØX68ØZ2 |

| Procedure | Code |
|---|---|
| 29. Left fourth toe amputation, mid-proximal phalanx | ØY6WØZ1 (The qualifier *High* here means anywhere along the proximal phalanx.) |
| 30. Right above-knee amputation, distal femur | ØY6CØZ3 |
| 31. Cryotherapy of wart on left hand | ØH5GXZZ |
| 32. Percutaneous radiofrequency ablation of right vocal cord lesion | ØC5T3ZZ |
| 33. Left heart catheterization with laser destruction of arrhythmogenic focus, A-V node | Ø2583ZZ |
| 34. Cautery of nosebleed | Ø95KXZZ |
| 35. Transurethral endoscopic laser ablation of prostate | ØV5Ø8ZZ |
| 36. Percutaneous cautery of oozing varicose vein, left calf | Ø65Y3ZZ |
| 37. Laparoscopy with destruction of endometriosis, bilateral ovaries | ØU524ZZ |
| 38. Laser coagulation of right retinal vessel hemorrhage, percutaneous | Ø85G3ZZ (The *Retinal Vessel* body-part values are in the *Eye* body system.) |
| 39. Thoracoscopic pleurodesis, left side | ØB5P4ZZ |
| 40. Percutaneous insertion of Greenfield IVC filter | Ø6HØ3DZ |
| 41. Forceps total mouth extraction, upper and lower teeth | ØCDWXZ2, ØCDXXZ2 |
| 42. Removal of left thumbnail | ØHDQXZZ (No separate body-part value is given for thumbnail, so this is coded to *Fingernail*.) |
| 43. Extraction of right intraocular lens without replacement, percutaneous | Ø8DJ3ZZ |
| 44. Laparoscopy with needle aspiration of ova for in vitro fertilization | ØUDN4ZZ |
| 45. Nonexcisional debridement of skin ulcer, right foot | ØHDMXZZ |
| 46. Open stripping of abdominal fascia, right side | ØJD8ØZZ |
| 47. Hysteroscopy with D&C, diagnostic | ØUDB8ZX |
| 48. Liposuction for medical purposes, left upper arm | ØJDF3ZZ (The *Percutaneous* approach is inherent in the liposuction technique.) |
| 49. Removal of tattered right ear drum fragments with tweezers | Ø9D77ZZ |
| 50. Microincisional phlebectomy of spider veins, right lower leg | Ø6DY3ZZ |
| 51. Routine Foley catheter placement | ØT9B7ØZ |
| 52. Incision and drainage of external anal abscess | ØD9QXZZ |
| 53. Percutaneous drainage of ascites | ØW9G3ZZ (This is drainage of the cavity and not the peritoneal membrane itself.) |
| 54. Laparoscopy with left ovarian cystotomy and drainage | ØU914ZZ |
| 55. Laparotomy and drain placement for liver abscess, right lobe | ØF91ØØZ |
| 56. Right knee arthrotomy with drain placement | ØS9CØØZ |
| 57. Thoracentesis of left pleural effusion | ØW9B3ZZ (This is drainage of the pleural cavity) |
| 58. Phlebotomy of left median cubital vein for polycythemia vera | Ø59C3ZZ (The median cubital vein is a branch of the basilic vein) |

| Procedure | Code |
|---|---|
| 59. Percutaneous chest tube placement for right pneumothorax | ØW993ØZ |
| 60. Endoscopic drainage of left ethmoid sinus | Ø99V4ZZ |
| 61. External ventricular CSF drainage catheter placement via burr hole | ØØ963ØZ |
| 62. Removal of foreign body, right cornea | Ø8C8XZZ |
| 63. Percutaneous mechanical thrombectomy, left brachial artery | Ø3C83ZZ |
| 64. Esophagogastroscopy with removal of bezoar from stomach | ØDC68ZZ |
| 65. Foreign body removal, skin of left thumb | ØHCGXZZ (There is no specific value for thumb skin, so the procedure is coded to *Hand*.) |
| 66. Transurethral cystoscopy with removal of bladder stone | ØTCB8ZZ |
| 67. Forceps removal of foreign body in right nostril | Ø9CKXZZ (Nostril is coded to the *Nose* body-part value.) |
| 68. Laparoscopy with excision of old suture from mesentery | ØDCV4ZZ |
| 69. Incision and removal of right lacrimal duct stone | Ø8CXØZZ |
| 70. Nonincisional removal of intraluminal foreign body from vagina | ØUCG7ZZ (The approach *External* is also a possibility. It is assumed here that since the patient went to the doctor to have the object removed, that it was not in the vaginal orifice.) |
| 71. Right common carotid endarterectomy, open | Ø3CHØZZ |
| 72. Open excision of retained sliver, subcutaneous tissue of left foot | ØJCRØZZ |
| 73. Extracorporeal shockwave lithotripsy (ESWL), bilateral ureters | ØTF6XZZ, ØTF7XZZ (The *Bilateral Ureter* body-part value is not available for the root operation FRAGMENTATION, so the procedures are coded separately.) |
| 74. Endoscopic retrograde cholangiopancreatography (ERCP) with lithotripsy of common bile duct stone | ØFF98ZZ (ERCP is performed through the mouth to the biliary system via the duodenum, so the approach value is *Via Natural or Artificial Opening Endoscopic*.) |
| 75. Thoracotomy with crushing of pericardial calcifications | Ø2FNØZZ |
| 76. Transurethral cystoscopy with fragmentation of bladder calculus | ØTFB8ZZ |
| 77. Hysteroscopy with intraluminal lithotripsy of left fallopian tube calcification | ØUF68ZZ |
| 78. Division of right foot tendon, percutaneous | ØL8V3ZZ |
| 79. Left heart catheterization with division of bundle of HIS | Ø2883ZZ |
| 80. Open osteotomy of capitate, left hand | ØP8NØZZ (The capitate is one of the carpal bones of the hand.) |
| 81. EGD with esophagotomy of esophagogastric junction | ØD948ZZ |
| 82. Sacral rhizotomy for pain control, percutaneous | Ø18R3ZZ |
| 83. Laparotomy with exploration and adhesiolysis of right ureter | ØTN6ØZZ |
| 84. Incision of scar contracture, right elbow | ØHNDXZZ (The skin of the elbow region is coded to *Lower Arm*.) |
| 85. Frenulotomy for treatment of tongue-tie syndrome | ØCN7XZZ (The frenulum is coded to the body-part value *Tongue*.) |
| 86. Right shoulder arthroscopy with coracoacromial ligament release | ØMN14ZZ |
| 87. Mitral valvulotomy for release of fused leaflets, open approach | Ø2NGØZZ |
| 88. Percutaneous left Achilles tendon release | ØLNP3ZZ |
| 89. Laparoscopy with lysis of peritoneal adhesions | ØDNW4ZZ |
| 90. Manual rupture of right shoulder joint adhesions under general anesthesia | ØRNJXZZ |
| 91. Open posterior tarsal tunnel release | Ø1NGØZZ (The nerve released in the posterior tarsal tunnel is the tibial nerve.) |
| 92. Laparoscopy with freeing of left ovary and fallopian tube | ØUN14ZZ, ØUN64ZZ |
| 93. Liver transplant with donor matched liver | ØFYØØZØ |
| 94. Orthotopic heart transplant using porcine heart | Ø2YAØZ2 (The donor heart comes from an animal [pig], so the qualifier value is *Zooplastic.*) |
| 95. Right lung transplant, open, using organ donor match | ØBYKØZØ |
| 96. Transplant of large intestine, organ donor match | ØDYEØZØ |
| 97. Left kidney/pancreas organ bank transplant | ØFYGØZØ, ØTY1ØZØ |
| 98. Replantation of avulsed scalp | ØHMØXZZ |
| 99. Reattachment of severed right ear | Ø9MØXZZ |
| 100. Reattachment of traumatic left gastrocnemius avulsion, open | ØKMTØZZ |
| 101. Closed replantation of three avulsed teeth, lower jaw | ØCMXXZ1 |
| 102. Reattachment of severed left hand | ØXMKØZZ |
| 103. Right open palmaris longus tendon transfer | ØLX5ØZZ |
| 104. Endoscopic radial to median nerve transfer | Ø1X64Z5 |
| 105. Fasciocutaneous flap closure of left thigh, open | ØJXMØZC (The qualifier identifies the body layers in addition to fascia included in the procedure.) |
| 106. Transfer left index finger to left thumb position, open | ØXXPØZM |
| 107. Percutaneous fascia transfer to fill defect, anterior neck | ØJX43ZZ |
| 108. Trigeminal to facial nerve transfer, percutaneous endoscopic | ØØXK4ZM |
| 109. Endoscopic left leg flexor hallucis longus tendon transfer | ØLXP4ZZ |
| 110. Right scalp advancement flap to right temple | ØHXØXZZ |
| 111. Bilateral TRAM pedicle flap reconstruction status post mastectomy, muscle only, open | ØKXKØZ6, ØKXLØZ6 (The transverse rectus abdominus muscle (TRAM) flap is coded for each flap developed.) |
| 112. Skin transfer flap closure of complex open wound, left lower back | ØHX6XZZ |
| 113. Open fracture reduction, right tibia | ØQSGØZZ |
| 114. Laparoscopy with gastropexy for malrotation | ØDS64ZZ |
| 115. Left knee arthroscopy with reposition of anterior cruciate ligament | ØMSP4ZZ |

| Procedure | Code |
|---|---|
| 116. Open transposition of ulnar nerve | Ø1S4ØZZ |
| 117. Closed reduction with percutaneous internal fixation of right femoral neck fracture | ØQS634Z |
| 118. Trans-vaginal intraluminal cervical cerclage | ØUVC7DZ |
| 119. Cervical cerclage using Shirodkar technique | ØUVC7ZZ |
| 120. Thoracotomy with banding of left pulmonary artery using extraluminal device | Ø2VRØCZ |
| 121. Restriction of thoracic duct with intraluminal stent, percutaneous | Ø7VK3DZ |
| 122. Craniotomy with clipping of cerebral aneurysm | Ø3VGØCZ (The clip is placed lengthwise on the outside wall of the widened portion of the vessel.) |
| 123. Nonincisional, transnasal placement of restrictive stent in right lacrimal duct | Ø8VX7DZ |
| 124. Catheter-based temporary restriction of blood flow in abdominal aorta for treatment of cerebral ischemia | Ø4VØ3DJ |
| 125. Percutaneous ligation of esophageal vein | Ø6L33ZZ |
| 126. Percutaneous embolization of left internal carotid-cavernous fistula | Ø3LL3DZ |
| 127. Laparoscopy with bilateral occlusion of fallopian tubes using Hulka extraluminal clips | ØUL74CZ |
| 128. Open suture ligation of failed AV graft, left brachial artery | Ø3L8ØZZ |
| 129. Percutaneous embolization of vascular supply, intracranial meningioma | Ø3LG3DZ |
| 130. Percutaneous embolization of right uterine artery, using coils | Ø4LE3DT |
| 131. Open occlusion of left atrial appendage, using extraluminal pressure clips | Ø2L7ØCK |
| 132. Percutaneous suture exclusion of left atrial appendage, via femoral artery access | Ø2L73ZK |
| 133. ERCP with balloon dilation of common bile duct | ØF798ZZ |
| 134. PTCA of two coronary arteries, LAD with stent placement, RCA with no stent | Ø27Ø3DZ, Ø27Ø3ZZ (A separate procedure is coded for each artery dilated, since the device value differs for each artery.) |
| 135. Cystoscopy with intraluminal dilation of bladder neck stricture | ØT7C8ZZ |
| 136. Open dilation of old anastomosis, left femoral artery | Ø47LØZZ |
| 137. Dilation of upper esophageal stricture, direct visualization, with Bougie sound | ØD717ZZ |
| 138. PTA of right brachial artery stenosis | Ø3773ZZ |
| 139. Transnasal dilation and stent placement in right lacrimal duct | Ø87X7DZ |
| 140. Hysteroscopy with balloon dilation of bilateral fallopian tubes | ØU778ZZ |
| 141. Tracheoscopy with intraluminal dilation of tracheal stenosis | ØB718ZZ |
| 142. Cystoscopy with dilation of left ureteral stricture, with stent placement | ØT778DZ |
| 143. Open gastric bypass with Roux-en-Y limb to jejunum | ØD16ØZA |
| 144. Right temporal artery to intracranial artery bypass using Gore-Tex graft, open | Ø31SØJG |
| 145. Tracheostomy formation with tracheostomy tube placement, percutaneous | ØB113F4 |
| 146. PICVA (percutaneous in situ coronary venous arterialization) of single coronary artery | Ø21Ø3D4 |
| 147. Open left femoral-popliteal artery bypass using cadaver vein graft | Ø41LØKL |
| 148. Shunting of intrathecal cerebrospinal fluid to peritoneal cavity using synthetic shunt | ØØ16ØJ6 |
| 149. Colostomy formation, open, transverse colon to abdominal wall | ØD1LØZ4 |
| 150. Open urinary diversion, left ureter, using ileal conduit to skin | ØT17ØZC |
| 151. CABG of LAD using left internal mammary artery, open off-bypass | Ø21ØØZ9 |
| 152. Open pleuroperitoneal shunt, right pleural cavity, using synthetic device | ØW19ØJG |
| 153. Percutaneous placement of ventriculoperitoneal shunt for treatment of hydrocephalus | ØØ163J6 |
| 154. End-of-life replacement of spinal neurostimulator generator, multiple array, in lower abdomen | ØJH8ØDZ (Taking out of the old generator is coded separately to the root operation *Removal*) |
| 155. Percutaneous insertion of spinal neurostimulator lead, lumbar spinal cord | ØØHV3MZ |
| 156. Percutaneous replacement of broken pacemaker lead in left atrium | Ø2H73JZ (Taking out the broken pacemaker lead is coded separately to the root operation *Removal*.) |
| 157. Open placement of dual chamber pacemaker generator in chest wall | ØJH6Ø6Z |
| 158. Percutaneous placement of venous central line in right internal jugular, with tip in superior vena cava | Ø2HV33Z |
| 159. Open insertion of multiple channel cochlear implant, left ear | Ø9HEØ6Z |
| 160. Percutaneous placement of Swan-Ganz catheter in pulmonary trunk | Ø2HP32Z (The Swan-Ganz catheter is coded to the device value *Monitoring Device* because it monitors pulmonary artery output.) |
| 161. Bronchoscopy with insertion of Low Dose Pd-103 brachytherapy seeds, right main bronchus | ØBHØ81Z, DB11BB2 |
| 162. Open insertion of interspinous process device into lumbar vertebral joint | ØSHØØBZ |
| 163. Open placement of bone growth stimulator, left femoral shaft | ØQHYØMZ |
| 164. Cystoscopy with placement of brachytherapy seeds in prostate gland | ØVHØ81Z |
| 165. Percutaneous insertion of Greenfield IVC filter | Ø6HØ3DZ |
| 166. Full-thickness skin graft to right lower arm, autograft (do not code graft harvest for this exercise) | ØHRDX73 |
| 167. Excision of necrosed left femoral head with bone bank bone graft to fill the defect, open | ØQR7ØKZ |
| 168. Penetrating keratoplasty of right cornea with donor matched cornea, percutaneous approach | Ø8R83KZ |
| 169. Bilateral mastectomy with concomitant saline breast implants, open | ØHRVØJZ |
| 170. Excision of abdominal aorta with Gore-Tex graft replacement, open | Ø4RØØJZ |
| 171. Total right knee arthroplasty with insertion of total knee prosthesis | ØSRCØJZ |
| 172. Bilateral mastectomy with free TRAM flap reconstruction | ØHRVØ76 |
| 173. Tenonectomy with graft to right ankle using cadaver graft, open | ØLRSØKZ |

| Procedure | Code |
|---|---|
| 174. Mitral valve replacement using porcine valve, open | Ø2RGØ8Z |
| 175. Percutaneous phacoemulsification of right eye cataract with prosthetic lens insertion | Ø8RJ3JZ |
| 176. Transcatheter replacement of pulmonary valve using of bovine jugular vein valve | Ø2RH38Z |
| 177. Total left hip replacement using ceramic on ceramic prosthesis, without bone cement | ØSRBØ3A |
| 178. Aortic valve annuloplasty using ring, open | Ø2UFØJZ |
| 179. Laparoscopic repair of left inguinal hernia with marlex plug | ØYU64JZ |
| 180. Autograft nerve graft to right median nerve, percutaneous endoscopic (do not code graft harvest for this exercise) | Ø1U547Z |
| 181. Exchange of liner in femoral component of previous left hip replacement, open approach | ØSUSØ9Z (Taking out of the old liner is coded separately to the root operation *Removal*) |
| 182. Anterior colporrhaphy with polypropylene mesh reinforcement, open approach | ØJUCØJZ |
| 183. Implantation of CorCap cardiac support device, open approach | Ø2UAØJZ |
| 184. Abdominal wall herniorrhaphy, open, using synthetic mesh | ØWUFØJZ |
| 185. Tendon graft to strengthen injured left shoulder using autograft, open (do not code graft harvest for this exercise) | ØLU2Ø7Z |
| 186. Onlay lamellar keratoplasty of left cornea using autograft, external approach | Ø8U9X7Z |
| 187. Resurfacing procedure on right femoral head, open approach | ØSURØBZ |
| 188. Exchange of drainage tube from right hip joint | ØS2YXØZ |
| 189. Tracheostomy tube exchange | ØB21XFZ |
| 190. Change chest tube for left pneumothorax | ØW2BXØZ |
| 191. Exchange of cerebral ventriculostomy drainage tube | ØØ2ØXØZ |
| 192. Foley urinary catheter exchange | ØT2BXØZ (This is coded to *Drainage Device* because urine is being drained.) |
| 193. Open removal of lumbar sympathetic neurostimulator lead | Ø1PYØMZ |
| 194. Nonincisional removal of Swan-Ganz catheter from right pulmonary artery | Ø2PYX2Z |
| 195. Laparotomy with removal of pancreatic drain | ØFPGØØZ |
| 196. Extubation, endotracheal tube | ØBP1XDZ |
| 197. Nonincisional PEG tube removal | ØDP6XUZ |
| 198. Transvaginal removal of brachytherapy seeds | ØUPH71Z |
| 199. Transvaginal removal of extraluminal cervical cerclage | ØUPD7CZ |
| 200. Incision with removal of K-wire fixation, right first metatarsal | ØQPNØ4Z |
| 201. Cystoscopy with retrieval of left ureteral stent | ØTP98DZ |
| 202. Removal of nasogastric drainage tube for decompression | ØDP6XØZ |
| 203. Removal of external fixator, left radial fracture | ØPPJX5Z |
| 204. Trimming and reanastomosis of stenosed femorofemoral synthetic bypass graft, open | Ø4WYØJZ |
| 205. Open revision of right hip replacement, with readjustment of prosthesis | ØSW9ØJZ |
| 206. Adjustment of position, pacemaker lead in left ventricle, percutaneous | Ø2WA3MZ |
| 207. External repositioning of Foley catheter to bladder | ØTWBXØZ |
| 208. Taking out loose screw and putting larger screw in fracture repair plate, left tibia | ØQWHØ4Z |
| 209. Revision of totally implantable VAD port placement in chest wall, causing patient discomfort, open | ØJWTØXZ |
| 210. Thoracotomy with exploration of right pleural cavity | ØWJ9ØZZ |
| 211. Diagnostic laryngoscopy | ØCJS8ZZ |
| 212. Exploratory arthrotomy of left knee | ØSJDØZZ |
| 213. Colposcopy with diagnostic hysteroscopy | ØUJD8ZZ |
| 214. Digital rectal exam | ØDJD7ZZ |
| 215. Diagnostic arthroscopy of right shoulder | ØRJJ4ZZ |
| 216. Endoscopy of maxillary sinus | Ø9JY4ZZ |
| 217. Laparotomy with palpation of liver | ØFJØØZZ |
| 218. Transurethral diagnostic cystoscopy | ØTJB8ZZ |
| 219. Colonoscopy, discontinued at sigmoid colon | ØDJD8ZZ |
| 220. Percutaneous mapping of basal ganglia | ØØK83ZZ |
| 221. Heart catheterization with cardiac mapping | Ø2K83ZZ |
| 222. Intraoperative whole brain mapping via craniotomy | ØØKØØZZ |
| 223. Mapping of left cerebral hemisphere, percutaneous endoscopic | ØØK74ZZ |
| 224. Intraoperative cardiac mapping during open heart surgery | Ø2K8ØZZ |
| 225. Hysteroscopy with cautery of post-hysterectomy oozing and evacuation of clot | ØW3R8ZZ |
| 226. Open exploration and ligation of post-op arterial bleeder, left forearm | ØX3FØZZ |
| 227. Control of post-operative retroperitoneal bleeding via laparotomy | ØW3HØZZ |
| 228. Reopening of thoracotomy site with drainage and control of post-op hemopericardium | ØW3DØZZ |
| 229. Arthroscopy with drainage of hemarthrosis at previous operative site, right knee | ØY3F4ZZ |
| 230. Radiocarpal fusion of left hand with internal fixation, open | ØRGPØ4Z |
| 231. Posterior spinal fusion at L1-L3 level with BAK cage interbody fusion device, open | ØSG1ØAJ |
| 232. Intercarpal fusion of right hand with bone bank bone graft, open | ØRGQØKZ |
| 233. Sacrococcygeal fusion with bone graft from same operative site, open | ØSG5Ø7Z |
| 234. Interphalangeal fusion of left great toe, percutaneous pin fixation | ØSGQ34Z |
| 235. Suture repair of left radial nerve laceration | Ø1Q6ØZZ (The approach value is *Open*, though the surgical exposure may have been created by the wound itself.) |
| 236. Laparotomy with suture repair of blunt force duodenal laceration | ØDQ9ØZZ |
| 237. Perineoplasty with repair of old obstetric laceration, open | ØWQNØZZ |
| 238. Suture repair of right biceps tendon (upper arm) laceration, open | ØLQ3ØZZ |
| 239. Closure of abdominal wall stab wound | ØWQFØZZ |
| 240. Cosmetic face lift, open, no other information available | ØWØ2ØZZ |
| 241. Bilateral breast augmentation with silicone implants, open | ØHØVØJZ |
| 242. Cosmetic rhinoplasty with septal reduction and tip elevation using local tissue graft, open | Ø9ØKØ7Z |
| 243. Abdominoplasty (tummy tuck), open | ØWØFØZZ |

| Procedure | Code |
|---|---|
| 244. Liposuction of bilateral thighs | ØJØL3ZZ, ØJØM3ZZ |
| 245. Creation of penis in female patient using tissue bank donor graft | ØW4NØK1 |
| 246. Creation of vagina in male patient using synthetic material | ØW4MØJØ |
| 247. Laparoscopic vertical (sleeve) gastrectomy | ØDB64Z3 |
| 248. Left uterine artery embolization with intraluminal biosphere injection | Ø4LF3DU |

## Obstetrics

| Procedure | Code |
|---|---|
| 1. Abortion by dilation and evacuation following laminaria insertion | 1ØAØ7ZW |
| 2. Manually assisted spontaneous abortion | 1ØEØXZZ (Since the pregnancy was not artificially terminated, this is coded to *Delivery* because it captures the procedure objective. The fact that it was an abortion will be identified in the diagnosis code.) |
| 3. Abortion by abortifacient insertion | 1ØAØ7ZX |
| 4. Bimanual pregnancy examination | 1ØJØ7ZZ |
| 5. Extraperitoneal C-section, low transverse incision | 1ØDØØZ2 |
| 6. Fetal spinal tap, percutaneous | 1Ø9Ø3ZA |
| 7. Fetal kidney transplant, laparoscopic | 1ØYØ4ZS |
| 8. Open in utero repair of congenital diaphragmatic hernia | 1ØQØØZK (Diaphragm is classified to the *Respiratory* body system in the *Medical and Surgical* section.) |
| 9. Laparoscopy with total excision of tubal pregnancy | 1ØT24ZZ |
| 10. Transvaginal removal of fetal monitoring electrode | 1ØPØ73Z |

## Placement

| Procedure | Code |
|---|---|
| 1. Placement of packing material, right ear | 2Y42X5Z |
| 2. Mechanical traction of entire left leg | 2W6MXØZ |
| 3. Removal of splint, right shoulder | 2W5AX1Z |
| 4. Placement of neck brace | 2W32X3Z |
| 5. Change of vaginal packing | 2YØ4X5Z |
| 6. Packing of wound, chest wall | 2W44X5Z |
| 7. Sterile dressing placement to left groin region | 2W27X4Z |
| 8. Removal of packing material from pharynx | 2Y5ØX5Z |
| 9. Placement of intermittent pneumatic compression device, covering entire right arm | 2W18X7Z |
| 10. Exchange of pressure dressing to left thigh | 2WØPX6Z |

## Administration

| Procedure | Code |
|---|---|
| 1. Peritoneal dialysis via indwelling catheter | 3E1M39Z |
| 2. Transvaginal artificial insemination | 3EØP7LZ |
| 3. Infusion of total parenteral nutrition via central venous catheter | 3EØ436Z |
| 4. Esophagogastroscopy with Botox injection into esophageal sphincter | 3EØG8GC (Botulinum toxin is a paralyzing agent with temporary effects; it does not sclerose or destroy the nerve.) |
| 5. Percutaneous irrigation of knee joint | 3E1U38Z |
| 6. Systemic infusion of recombinant tissue plasminogen activator (r-tPA) via peripheral venous catheter | 3EØ3317 |
| 7. Transfusion of antihemophilic factor, (nonautologous) via arterial central line | 3Ø263V1 |
| 8. Transabdominal in vitro fertilization, implantation of donor ovum | 3EØP3Q1 |
| 9. Autologous bone marrow transplant via central venous line | 3Ø243GØ |
| 10. Implantation of anti-microbial envelope with cardiac defibrillator placement, open | 3EØ1Ø2A |
| 11. Sclerotherapy of brachial plexus lesion, alcohol injection | 3EØT3TZ |
| 12. Percutaneous peripheral vein injection, glucarpidase | 3EØ33GQ |
| 13. Introduction of anti-infective envelope into subcutaneous tissue, open | 3EØ1Ø2A |

## Measurement and Monitoring

| Procedure | Code |
|---|---|
| 1. Cardiac stress test, single measurement | 4AØ2XM4 |
| 2. EGD with biliary flow measurement | 4AØC85Z |
| 3. Right and left heart cardiac catheterization with bilateral sampling and pressure measurements | 4AØ23N8 |
| 4. Temperature monitoring, rectal | 4A1Z7KZ |
| 5. Peripheral venous pulse, external, single measurement | 4AØ4XJ1 |
| 6. Holter monitoring | 4A12X45 |
| 7. Respiratory rate, external, single measurement | 4AØ9XCZ |
| 8. Fetal heart rate monitoring, transvaginal | 4A1H7CZ |
| 9. Visual mobility test, single measurement | 4AØ7X7Z |
| 10. Left ventricular cardiac output monitoring from pulmonary artery wedge (Swan-Ganz) catheter | 4A1239Z |
| 11. Olfactory acuity test, single measurement | 4AØ8XØZ |

## Extracorporeal or Systemic Assistance and Performance

| Procedure | Code |
|---|---|
| 1. Intermittent mechanical ventilation, 16 hours | 5A1935Z |
| 2. Liver dialysis, single encounter | 5A1CØØZ |
| 3. Cardiac countershock with successful conversion to sinus rhythm | 5A22Ø4Z |
| 4. IPPB (intermittent positive pressure breathing) for mobilization of secretions, 22 hours | 5AØ9358 |
| 5. Renal dialysis, 12 hours | 5A1D8ØZ |
| 6. IABP (intra-aortic balloon pump) continuous | 5AØ221Ø |
| 7. Intra-operative cardiac pacing, continuous | 5A1223Z |
| 8. ECMO (extracorporeal membrane oxygenation), continuous | 5A15223 |
| 9. Controlled mechanical ventilation (CMV), 45 hours | 5A1945Z |
| 10. Pulsatile compression boot with intermittent inflation | 5AØ2115 (This is coded to the function value *Cardiac Output*, because the purpose of such compression devices is to return blood to the heart faster.) |

## Extracorporeal or Systemic Therapies

| Procedure | Code |
|---|---|
| 1. Donor thrombocytapheresis, single encounter | 6A55ØZ2 |
| 2. Bili-lite phototherapy, series treatment | 6A6Ø1ZZ |
| 3. Whole body hypothermia, single treatment | 6A4ZØZZ |
| 4. Circulatory phototherapy, single encounter | 6A65ØZZ |
| 5. Shock wave therapy of plantar fascia, single treatment | 6A93ØZZ |
| 6. Antigen-free air conditioning, series treatment | 6AØZ1ZZ |
| 7. TMS (transcranial magnetic stimulation), series treatment | 6A221ZZ |
| 8. Therapeutic ultrasound of peripheral vessels, single treatment | 6A75ØZ6 |
| 9. Plasmapheresis, series treatment | 6A551Z3 |
| 10. Extracorporeal electromagnetic stimulation (EMS) for urinary incontinence, single treatment | 6A21ØZZ |

## Osteopathic

| Procedure | Code |
|---|---|
| 1. Isotonic muscle energy treatment of right leg | 7WØ6X8Z |
| 2. Low velocity-high amplitude osteopathic treatment of head | 7WØØX5Z |
| 3. Lymphatic pump osteopathic treatment of left axilla | 7WØ7X6Z |
| 4. Indirect osteopathic treatment of sacrum | 7WØ4X4Z |
| 5. Articulatory osteopathic treatment of cervical region | 7WØ1XØZ |

## Other Procedures

| Procedure | Code |
|---|---|
| 1. Near infrared spectroscopy of leg vessels | 8EØ23DZ |
| 2. CT computer assisted sinus surgery | 8EØ9XBG (The primary procedure is coded separately.) |
| 3. Suture removal, abdominal wall | 8EØWXY8 |
| 4. Isolation after infectious disease exposure | 8EØZXY6 |
| 5. Robotic assisted open prostatectomy | 8EØWØCZ (The primary procedure is coded separately.) |
| 6. In vitro fertilization | 8EØZXY1 |

## Chiropractic

| Procedure | Code |
|---|---|
| 1. Chiropractic treatment of lumbar region using long lever specific contact | 9WB3XGZ |
| 2. Chiropractic manipulation of abdominal region, indirect visceral | 9WB9XCZ |
| 3. Chiropractic extra-articular treatment of hip region | 9WB6XDZ |
| 4. Chiropractic treatment of sacrum using long and short lever specific contact | 9WB4XJZ |
| 5. Mechanically-assisted chiropractic manipulation of head | 9WBØXKZ |

## Imaging

| Procedure | Code |
|---|---|
| 1. Noncontrast CT of abdomen and pelvis | BW21ZZZ |
| 2. Intravascular ultrasound, left subclavian artery | B342ZZ3 |
| 3. Fluoroscopic guidance for insertion of central venous catheter in SVC, low osmolar contrast | B5181ZA |
| 4. Chest x-ray, AP/PA and lateral views | BWØ3ZZZ |
| 5. Endoluminal ultrasound of gallbladder and bile ducts | BF43ZZZ |
| 6. MRI of thyroid gland, contrast unspecified | BG34YZZ |
| 7. Esophageal videofluoroscopy study with oral barium contrast | BD11YZZ |
| 8. Portable x-ray study of right radius/ulna shaft, standard series | BPØJZZZ |
| 9. Routine fetal ultrasound, second trimester twin gestation | BY4DZZZ |
| 10. CT scan of bilateral lungs, high osmolar contrast with densitometry | BB24ØZZ |
| 11. Fluoroscopic guidance for percutaneous transluminal angioplasty (PTA) of left common femoral artery, low osmolar contrast | B41G1ZZ |

## Nuclear Medicine

| Procedure | Code |
|---|---|
| 1. Tomo scan of right and left heart, unspecified radiopharmaceutical, qualitative gated rest | C226YZZ |
| 2. Technetium pentetate assay of kidneys, ureters, and bladder | CT631ZZ |
| 3. Uniplanar scan of spine using technetium oxidronate, with first-pass study | CP151ZZ |
| 4. Thallous chloride tomographic scan of bilateral breasts | CH22SZZ |
| 5. PET scan of myocardium using rubidium | C23GQZZ |
| 6. Gallium citrate scan of head and neck, single plane imaging | CW1BLZZ |
| 7. Xenon gas nonimaging probe of brain | CØ5ØVZZ |
| 8. Upper GI scan, radiopharmaceutical unspecified, for gastric emptying | CD15YZZ |
| 9. Carbon 11 PET scan of brain with quantification | CØ3ØBZZ |
| 10. Iodinated albumin nuclear medicine assay, blood plasma volume study | C763HZZ |

## Radiation Therapy

| Procedure | Code |
|---|---|
| 1. Plaque radiation of left eye, single port | D8YØFZZ |
| 2. 8 MeV photon beam radiation to brain | DØØ11ZZ |
| 3. IORT of colon, 3 ports | DDY5CZZ |
| 4. HDR brachytherapy of prostate using palladium-103 | DV1Ø9BZ |
| 5. Electron radiation treatment of right breast, with custom device | DMØ13ZZ |
| 6. Hyperthermia oncology treatment of pelvic region | DWY68ZZ |
| 7. Contact radiation of tongue | D9Y57ZZ |
| 8. Heavy particle radiation treatment of pancreas, four risk sites | DFØ34ZZ |
| 9. LDR brachytherapy to spinal cord using iodine | DØ16B9Z |
| 10. Whole body Phosphorus 32 administration with risk to hematopoetic system | DWY5GFZ |

## Physical Rehabilitation and Diagnostic Audiology

| Procedure | Code |
|---|---|
| 1. Bekesy assessment using audiometer | F13Z31Z |
| 2. Individual fitting of left eye prosthesis | FØDZ8UZ |
| 3. Physical therapy for range of motion and mobility, patient right hip, no special equipment | FØ7LØZZ |
| 4. Bedside swallow assessment using assessment kit | FØØZHYZ |
| 5. Caregiver training in airway clearance techniques | FØFZ8ZZ |
| 6. Application of short arm cast in rehabilitation setting | FØDZ7EZ (Inhibitory cast is listed in the equipment reference table under E, *Orthosis*.) |
| 7. Verbal assessment of patient's pain level | FØ2ZFZZ |
| 8. Caregiver training in communication skills using manual communication board | FØFZJMZ (Manual communication board is listed in the equipment reference table under M, *Augmentative/ Alternative Communication*.) |
| 9. Group musculoskeletal balance training exercises, whole body, no special equipment | FØ7M6ZZ (Balance training is included in the motor treatment reference table under *Therapeutic Exercise*.) |
| 10. Individual therapy for auditory processing using tape recorder | FØ9Z2KZ (Tape recorder is listed in the equipment reference table under *Audiovisual Equipment*.) |

## Mental Health

| Procedure | Code |
|---|---|
| 1. Cognitive-behavioral psychotherapy, individual | GZ58ZZZ |
| 2. Narcosynthesis | GZGZZZZ |
| 3. Light therapy | GZJZZZZ |
| 4. ECT (electroconvulsive therapy), unilateral, multiple seizure | GZB1ZZZ |
| 5. Crisis intervention | GZ2ZZZZ |
| 6. Neuropsychological testing | GZ13ZZZ |
| 7. Hypnosis | GZFZZZZ |
| 8. Developmental testing | GZ1ØZZZ |
| 9. Vocational counseling | GZ61ZZZ |
| 10. Family psychotherapy | GZ72ZZZ |

## Substance Abuse Treatment

| Procedure | Code |
|---|---|
| 1. Naltrexone treatment for drug dependency | HZ94ZZZ |
| 2. Substance abuse treatment family counseling | HZ63ZZZ |
| 3. Medication monitoring of patient on methadone maintenance | HZ81ZZZ |
| 4. Individual interpersonal psychotherapy for drug abuse | HZ54ZZZ |
| 5. Patient in for alcohol detoxification treatment | HZ2ZZZZ |
| 6. Group motivational counseling | HZ47ZZZ |
| 7. Individual 12-step psychotherapy for substance abuse | HZ53ZZZ |
| 8. Post-test infectious disease counseling for IV drug abuser | HZ3CZZZ |
| 9. Psychodynamic psychotherapy for drug dependent patient | HZ5CZZZ |
| 10. Group cognitive-behavioral counseling for substance abuse | HZ42ZZZ |

## New Technology

| Procedure | Code |
|---|---|
| 1. Infusion of ceftazidime via peripheral venous catheter | XWØ3321 |

# Appendix L: Procedure Combination Tables

The tables below were developed to help simplify the relationship between ICD-10-PCS coding and MS-DRG assignment. The Centers for Medicare & Medicaid Services (CMS) has identified in the MS-DRG v34 Definitions Manual certain procedure combinations that must occur in order to assign a specific MS-DRG. There are many factors influencing MS-DRG assignment, including principal and secondary diagnoses, MCC or CC use, sex of the patient, and discharge status. These tables should be used only as a guide.

## DRG ØØ1-ØØ2 Heart Transplant or Implant of Heart Assist System

### Heart Transplant

**Replacement of Right and Left Ventricle Ø2RKØJZ and Ø2RLØJZ**

**Insertion With Removal of Heart Assist System**

| Type of Heart Assist System | Code as appropriate Insertion by approach | Code also as appropriate Removal of Heart Assist System by approach |
|---|---|---|
| Biventricular External | Ø2HA[Ø,3,4]RS | Ø2PA[Ø,3,4]RZ |
| External | Ø2HA[Ø,4]RZ | Ø2PA[Ø,3,4]RZ |

**Revision With Removal of Heart Assist System**

| Type of Heart Assist System | Code as appropriate Revision by approach | Code also as appropriate Removal of Heart Assist System by approach |
|---|---|---|
| Implantable | Ø2WA[Ø,3,4]QZ | Ø2PA[Ø,3,4]RZ |
| External | Ø2WA[Ø,3,4]RZ | Ø2PA[Ø,3,4]RZ |

## DRG ØØ8 Simultaneous Pancreas/Kidney Transplant

| Transplanted Body Part Laterality | Code Transplant as appropriate by tissue type | | | Code also Pancreas Transplant as appropriate by tissue type | | |
|---|---|---|---|---|---|---|
| | Allogeneic | Syngeneic | Zooplastic | Allogeneic | Syngeneic | Zooplastic |
| Kidney, Right | ØTYØØZØ | ØTYØØZ1 | ØTYØØZ2 | ØFYGØZØ | ØFYGØZ1 | ØFYGØZ2 |
| Kidney, Left | ØTY1ØZØ | ØTY1ØZ1 | ØTY1ØZ2 | ØFYGØZØ | ØFYGØZ1 | ØFYGØZ2 |

## DRG Ø23-Ø27 Craniotomy

| Site of Neurostimulator Lead | Code as appropriate Insertion of Lead by approach | Code also as appropriate Insertion of Device by type and subcutaneous site | | | | | | |
|---|---|---|---|---|---|---|---|---|
| | | Neuro-stimulator Generator | Stimulator Multiple Array Code as appropriate by approach | | | Stimulator Multiple Array, Rechargeable Code as appropriate by approach | | |
| | | Skull | Chest | Back | Abdomen | Chest | Back | Abdomen |
| Brain | ØØHØ[Ø,3,4]MZ | ØNHØØNZ | ØJH6[Ø,3]DZ | ØJH7[Ø,3]DZ | ØJH8[Ø,3]DZ | ØJH6[Ø,3]EZ | ØJH7[Ø,3]EZ | ØJH8[Ø,3]EZ |
| Cerebral Ventricle | ØØH6[Ø,3,4]MZ | ØNHØØNZ | ØJH6[Ø,3]DZ | ØJH7[Ø,3]DZ | ØJH8[Ø,3]DZ | ØJH6[Ø,3]EZ | ØJH7[Ø,3]EZ | ØJH8[Ø,3]EZ |

## DRG Ø28-Ø3Ø Spinal Procedures

| Generator Type | Insertion of Generator by Site | | | Code also as appropriate Insertion of Neurostimulator Lead by approach | |
|---|---|---|---|---|---|
| | Chest | Abdomen | Back | Spinal Canal | Spinal Cord |
| Single Array | ØJH6[Ø,3]BZ | ØJH8[Ø,3]BZ | ØJH7[Ø,3]BZ | ØØHU[Ø,3,4]MZ | ØØHV[Ø,3,4]MZ |
| Single Array, Rechargeable | ØJH6[Ø,3]CZ | ØJH8[Ø,3]CZ | ØJH7[Ø,3]CZ | ØØHU[Ø,3,4]MZ | ØØHV[Ø,3,4]MZ |
| Multiple Array | ØJH6[Ø,3]DZ | ØJH8[Ø,3]DZ | ØJH7[Ø,3]DZ | ØØHU[Ø,3,4]MZ | ØØHV[Ø,3,4]MZ |
| Multiple Array, Rechargable | ØJH6[Ø,3]EZ | — | ØJH7[Ø,3]EZ | ØØHU[Ø,3,4]MZ | ØØHV[Ø,3,4]MZ |
| Multiple Array, Rechargable | — | ØJH8[Ø,3]EZ | — | ØØHU[Ø,3,4]MZ | ØØHVØMZ |
| Multiple Array, Rechargable | — | ØJH8ØEZ | — | — | ØØHV[3,4]MZ |

# DRG Ø4Ø-Ø42 Peripheral and Cranial Nerve and Other Nervous System Procedures

**Insertion of Neurostimulator Lead With Device**

| Site of Neurostimulator Lead | Code as appropriate Insertion by approach | Code also as appropriate Insertion of Device by type and subcutaneous site | | | | | |
|---|---|---|---|---|---|---|---|
| | | Stimulator Single Array Code as appropriate by approach | | | Stimulator Single Array, Rechargeable Code as appropriate by approach | | |
| | | Chest | Back | Abdomen | Chest | Back | Abdomen |
| **Cranial Nerve** | ØØHE[Ø,3,4]MZ | ØJH6[Ø,3]BZ | ØJH7[Ø,3]BZ | ØJH8[Ø,3]BZ | ØJH6[Ø,3]CZ | ØJH7[Ø,3]CZ | ØJH8[Ø,3]CZ |
| **Peripheral Nerve** | Ø1HY[Ø,3,4]MZ | ØJH6[Ø,3]BZ | ØJH7[Ø,3]BZ | ØJH8[Ø,3]BZ | ØJH6[Ø,3]CZ | ØJH7[Ø,3]CZ | ØJH8[Ø,3]CZ |
| **Stomach** | ØDH6[Ø,3,4]MZ | ØJH6[Ø,3]BZ | ØJH7[Ø,3]BZ | ØJH8[Ø,3]BZ | ØJH6[Ø,3]CZ | ØJH7[Ø,3]CZ | ØJH8[Ø,3]CZ |
| **Azygos vein** | Ø5HØ[Ø,3,4]MZ | ØJH6[Ø,3]BZ | ØJH7[Ø,S]BZ | ØJH8[Ø,3]BZ | ØJH6[Ø,3]CZ | ØJH7[Ø,S]CZ | ØJH8[Ø,3]CZ |
| **Innominate Vein, Right** | Ø5H3[Ø,3,4]MZ | ØJH6[Ø,3]BZ | ØJH7[Ø,S]BZ | ØJH8[Ø,3]BZ | ØJH6[Ø,3]CZ | ØJH7[Ø,S]CZ | ØJH8[Ø,3]CZ |
| **Innominate Vein, Left** | Ø5H4[Ø,3,4]MZ | ØJH6[Ø,3]BZ | ØJH7[Ø,S]BZ | ØJH8[Ø,3]BZ | ØJH6[Ø,3]CZ | ØJH7[Ø,S]CZ | ØJH8[Ø,3]CZ |
| | | Stimulator Multiple Array Code as appropriate by approach | | | Stimulator Multiple Array, Rechargeable Code as appropriate by approach | | |
| | | Chest | Back | Abdomen | Chest | Back | Abdomen |
| **Cranial Nerve** | ØØHE[Ø,3,4]MZ | ØJH6[Ø,3]DZ | ØJH7[Ø,3]DZ | ØJH8[Ø,3]DZ | ØJH6[Ø,3]EZ | ØJH7[Ø,3]EZ | ØJH8[Ø,3]EZ |
| **Peripheral Nerve** | Ø1HY[Ø,3,4]MZ | ØJH6[Ø,3]DZ | ØJH7[Ø,3]DZ | ØJH8[Ø,3]DZ | ØJH6[Ø,3]EZ | ØJH7[Ø,3]EZ | ØJH8[Ø,3]EZ |
| **Stomach** | ØDH6[Ø,3,4]MZ | ØJH6[Ø,3]DZ | ØJH7[Ø,3]DZ | ØJH8[Ø,3]DZ | ØJH6[Ø,3]EZ | ØJH7[Ø,3]EZ | ØJH8[Ø,3]EZ |
| **Azygos vein** | Ø5HØ[Ø,3,4]MZ | ØJH6[Ø,3]DZ | ØJH7[Ø,S]DZ | ØJH8[Ø,3]DZ | ØJH6[Ø,3]EZ | ØJH7[Ø,S]EZ | ØJH8[Ø,3]EZ |
| **Innominate Vein, Right** | Ø5H3[Ø,3,4]MZ | ØJH6[Ø,3]DZ | ØJH7[Ø,S]DZ | ØJH8[Ø,3]DZ | ØJH6[Ø,3]EZ | ØJH7[Ø,S]EZ | ØJH8[Ø,3]EZ |
| **Innominate Vein, Left** | Ø5H4[Ø,3,4]MZ | ØJH6[Ø,3]DZ | ØJH7[Ø,S]DZ | ØJH8[Ø,3]DZ | ØJH6[Ø,3]EZ | ØJH7[Ø,S]EZ | ØJH8[Ø,3]EZ |

# DRG 222-227 Cardiac Defibrillator Implant

**Insertion of Generator With Insertion of Lead(s) into Coronary Vein, Atrium or Ventricle**

| Generator Type | Insertion of Generator by Site | | Code also as appropriate Insertion of Leads by site | | | | |
|---|---|---|---|---|---|---|---|
| | Chest | Abdomen | Coronary Vein | Atrium | | Ventricle | |
| | | | | Right | Left | Right | Left |
| **Defibrillator** | ØJH6[Ø,3]8Z | ØJH8[Ø,3]8Z | Ø2H4[Ø,4]KZ | Ø2H6[Ø,3,4]KZ | Ø2H7[Ø,3,4]KZ | Ø2HK[Ø,3,4]KZ | Ø2HL[Ø,3,4]KZ |
| **Cardiac Resynch Defibrillator Pulse Generator** | ØJH6[Ø,3]9Z | ØJH8[Ø,3]9Z | Ø2H4[Ø,3,4]KZ or Ø2H43[J,M]Z | Ø2H6[Ø,3,4]KZ | Ø2H7[Ø,3,4]KZ | Ø2HK[Ø,3,4]KZ | Ø2HL[Ø,3,4]KZ |
| **Contractility Modulation Device** | ØJH6[Ø,3]AZ | ØJH8[Ø,3]AZ | — | — | — | — | Ø2HL[Ø,3,4]MZ |

**Insertion of Generator with Insertion of Lead(s) into Pericardium**

| Generator Type | Insertion of Generator by Site | | Code also as appropriate Insertion of Leads by Type | | |
|---|---|---|---|---|---|
| | Chest | Abdomen | Pericardium | | |
| | | | Pacemaker | Defibrillator | Cardiac |
| **Defibrillator** | ØJH6[Ø,3]8Z | ØJH8[Ø,3]8Z | Ø2HN[Ø,3,4]JZ | Ø2HN[Ø,3,4]KZ | Ø2HN[Ø,3,4]MZ |
| **Cardiac Resynch Defibrillator Pulse Generator** | ØJH6[Ø,3]9Z | ØJH8[Ø,3]9Z | Ø2HN[Ø,3,4]JZ | Ø2HN[Ø,3,4]KZ | Ø2HN[Ø,3,4]MZ |

# DRG 326-328 Stomach, Esophageal and Duodenal Procedures

| Site | Resection by Open Approach | Code also as appropriate Resection of Pancreas by Open Approach |
|---|---|---|
| **Duodenum** | ØDT9ØZZ | ØFTGØZZ |

# DRG 344-346 Minor Small and Large Bowel Procedures

| Site | Repair by Open Approach | Code also as appropriate Repair by external approach of Abdominal Wall Stoma |
|---|---|---|
| **Small Intestine** | ØDQ8ØZZ | ØWQFXZ2 |
| **Duodenum** | ØDQ9ØZZ | ØWQFXZ2 |
| **Jejunum** | ØDQAØZZ | ØWQFXZ2 |
| **Ileum** | ØDQBØZZ | ØWQFXZ2 |
| **Large Intestine** | ØDQEØZZ | ØWQFXZ2 |
| **Large Intestine, Right** | ØDQFØZZ | ØWQFXZ2 |
| **Large Intestine, Left** | ØDQGØZZ | ØWQFXZ2 |
| **Cecum** | ØDQHØZZ | ØWQFXZ2 |
| **Ascending Colon** | ØDQKØZZ | ØWQFXZ2 |
| **Transverse Colon** | ØDQLØZZ | ØWQFXZ2 |
| **Descending Colon** | ØDQMØZZ | ØWQFXZ2 |
| **Sigmoid Colon** | ØDQNØZZ | ØWQFXZ2 |

# DRG 456-458 Spinal Fusion Except Cervical with Spinal Curvature/Malignancy/ Infection or Extensive Fusions

**Fusion of Thoracic and Lumbar Vertebra, Anterior Column**

| 2 to 7 Thoracic Vertebra | Code also 2 or more Lumbar Vertebra |
|---|---|
| ØRG7[Ø,3,4][7,A,J,K,Z]Ø | ØSG1[Ø,3,4][7,A,J,K,Z]Ø |

**Fusion of Thoracic and Lumbar Vertebra, Posterior Column**

| 2 to 7 Thoracic Vertebra | | Code also 2 or more Lumbar Vertebra | |
|---|---|---|---|
| **Posterior Approach** | **Anterior Approach** | **Posterior Approach** | **Anterior Approach** |
| ØRG7[Ø,3,4][7,A,J,K,Z]1 | ØRG7[Ø,3,4][7,A,J,K,Z]J | ØSG1[Ø,3,4][7,A,J,K,Z]1 | ØSG1[Ø,3,4][7,A,J,K,Z]J |

# DRG 466-468 Revision of Hip or Knee Replacement

**Open Removal of Hip Joint Spacer, Liner, or Resurfacing Device With Supplement of Liner**

| Body Part | Removal Spacer/Liner/Resurfacing Device | Code also as appropriate Supplement of Body Part by Site | | |
|---|---|---|---|---|
| | | **Joint** | **Acetabular Surface** | **Femoral Surface** |
| **Hip, RT** | ØSP9Ø[8,9,B]Z | ØSU9Ø9Z | ØSUAØ9Z | ØSURØ9Z |
| **Hip, LT** | ØSPBØ[8,9,B]Z | ØSUBØ9Z | ØSUEØ9Z | ØSUSØ9Z |

**Open Removal of Hip Joint Spacer, Liner, Resurfacing Device, or Synthetic Substitute With Replacement**

| Body Part | Removal Spacer/Liner/ Resurfacing Device/Synthetic Substitute | Code also as appropriate Replacement of Body Part by Device Type | | | | | |
|---|---|---|---|---|---|---|---|
| | | **Polyethylene** | **Metal** | **Metal on Poly** | **Ceramic** | **Ceramic on Poly** | **Synth Subst** |
| **Hip, RT** | ØSP9Ø[8,9,B,J]Z | — | ØSR9Ø1[9,A,Z] | ØSR9Ø2[9,A,Z] | ØSR9Ø3[9,A,Z] | ØSR9Ø4[9,A,Z] | ØSR9ØJ[9,A,Z] |
| **Hip, LT** | ØSPBØ[8,9,B,J]Z | — | ØSRBØ1[9,A,Z] | ØSRBØ2[9,A,Z] | ØSRBØ3[9,A,Z] | ØSRBØ4[9,A,Z] | ØSRBØJ[9,A,Z] |
| **Acetabular Surface, RT** | ØSP9Ø[8,9,B,J]Z | ØSRAØØ[9,A,Z] | ØSRAØ1[9,A,Z] | — | ØSRAØ3[9,A,Z] | — | ØSRAØJ[9,A,Z] |
| **Acetabular Surface, LT** | ØSPBØ[8,9,B,J]Z | ØSREØØ[9,A,Z] | ØSREØ1[9,A,Z] | — | ØSREØ3[9,A,Z] | — | ØSREØJ[9,A,Z] |
| **Femoral Surface, RT** | ØSP9Ø[8,9,B,J]Z | — | ØSRRØ1[9,A,Z] | — | ØSRRØ3[9,A,Z] | — | ØSRRØJ[9,A,Z] |
| **Femoral Surface, LT** | ØSPBØ[8,9,B,J]Z | — | ØSRSØ1[9,A,Z] | — | ØSRSØ3[9,A,Z] | — | ØSRSØJ[9,A,Z] |

## DRG 466-468 Revision of Hip or Knee Replacement *(Continued)*

### Percutaneous Endoscopic Removal of Hip Joint Spacer or Synthetic Substitute With Supplement of Liner

| Body Part | Removal Spacer/Synthetic Substitute | Code also as appropriate Supplement of Body Part by Site | | |
|---|---|---|---|---|
| | | Joint | Acetabular Surface | Femoral Surface |
| Hip, RT | ØSP94[8,J]Z | ØSU9Ø9Z | ØSUAØ9Z | ØSURØ9Z |
| Hip, LT | ØSPB4[8,J]Z | ØSUBØ9Z | ØSUEØ9Z | ØSUSØ9Z |

### Percutaneous Endoscopic Removal of Hip Joint Spacer or Synthetic Substitute With Replacement

| Body Part | Removal Spacer/Synthetic Substitute | Code also as appropriate Replacement of Body Part by Device Type | | | | | |
|---|---|---|---|---|---|---|---|
| | | Polyethylene | Metal | Metal on Poly | Ceramic | Ceramic on Poly | Synth Subst |
| Hip, RT | ØSP94[8,J]Z | — | ØSR9Ø1[9,A,Z] | ØSR9Ø2[9,A,Z] | ØSR9Ø3[9,A,Z] | ØSR9Ø4[9,A,Z] | ØSR9ØJ[9,A,Z] |
| Hip, LT | ØSPB4[8,J]Z | — | ØSRBØ1[9,A,Z] | ØSRBØ2[9,A,Z] | ØSRBØ3[9,A,Z] | ØSRBØ4[9,A,Z] | ØSRBØJ[9,A,Z] |
| Acetabular Surface, RT | ØSP94[8,J]Z | ØSRAØØ[9,A,Z] | ØSRAØ1[9,A,Z] | — | ØSRAØ3[9,A,Z] | — | ØSRAØJ[9,A,Z] |
| Acetabular Surface, LT | ØSPB4[8,J]Z | ØSREØØ[9,A,Z] | ØSREØ1[9,A,Z] | — | ØSREØ3[9,A,Z] | — | ØSREØJ[9,A,Z] |
| Femoral Surface, RT | ØSP94[8,J]Z | — | ØSRRØ1[9,A,Z] | — | ØSRRØ3[9,A,Z] | — | ØSRRØJ[9,A,Z] |
| Femoral Surface, LT | ØSPB4[8,J]Z | — | ØSRSØ1[9,A,Z] | — | ØSRSØ3[9,A,Z] | — | ØSRSØJ[9,A,Z] |

### Removal of Hip Joint Surface With Hip Joint Replacement

| Body Part | Removal of Spacer/Liner/Resurfacing Device/Synthetic Substitute | Code also as appropriate Replacement of Hip Joint | | | | |
|---|---|---|---|---|---|---|
| | | Metal | Metal on Poly | Ceramic | Ceramic on Poly | Synth Subst |
| Acetabular Surface, RT | ØSPA[Ø,4]JZ | ØSR9Ø1[9,A,Z] | ØSR9Ø2[9,A,Z] | ØSR9Ø3[9,A,Z] | ØSR9Ø4[9,A,Z] | ØSR9ØJ[9,A,Z] |
| Acetabular Surface, LT | ØSPE[Ø,4]JZ | ØSRBØ1[9,A,Z] | ØSRBØ2[9,A,Z] | ØSRBØ3[9,A,Z] | ØSRBØ4[9,A,Z] | ØSRBØJ[9,A,Z] |
| Femoral Surface, RT | ØSPR[Ø,4]JZ | ØSR9Ø1[9,A,Z] | ØSR9Ø2[9,A,Z] | ØSR9Ø3[9,A,Z] | ØSR9Ø4[9,A,Z] | ØSR9ØJ[9,A,Z] |
| Femoral Surface, LT | ØSPS[Ø,4]JZ | ØSRBØ1[9,A,Z] | ØSRBØ2[9,A,Z] | ØSRBØ3[9,A,Z] | ØSRBØ4[9,A,Z] | ØSRBØJ[9,A,Z] |

### Removal of Hip Joint Surface with Replacement with New Joint Acetabular Surface

| Body Part | Removal of Spacer/Liner/Resurfacing Device/Synthetic Substitute | Code also as appropriate Replacement of Acetabular Surface | | | |
|---|---|---|---|---|---|
| | | Polyethylene | Metal | Ceramic | Synth Subst |
| Acetabular Surface, RT | ØSPA[Ø,4]JZ | ØSRAØØ[9,A,Z] | ØSRAØ1[9,A,Z] | ØSRAØ3[9,A,Z] | ØSRAØJ[9,A,Z] |
| Acetabular Surface, LT | ØSPE[Ø,4]JZ | ØSREØØ[9,A,Z] | ØSREØ1[9,A,Z] | ØSREØ3[9,A,Z] | ØSREØJ[9,A,Z] |
| Femoral Surface, RT | ØSPR[Ø,4]JZ | ØSRAØØ[9,A,Z] | ØSRAØ1[9,A,Z] | ØSRAØ3[9,A,Z] | ØSRAØJ[9,A,Z] |
| Femoral Surface, LT | ØSPS[Ø,4]JZ | ØSREØØ[9,A,Z] | ØSREØ1[9,A,Z] | ØSREØ3[9,A,Z] | ØSREØJ[9,A,Z] |

### Removal of Hip Joint Surface With Replacement with New Joint Femoral Surface

| Body Part | Removal of Spacer/Liner/Resurfacing Device/Synthetic Substitute | Code also as appropriate Replacement of Femoral Surface | | |
|---|---|---|---|---|
| | | Metal | Ceramic | Synth Subst |
| Acetabular Surface, RT | ØSPA[Ø,4]JZ | ØSRRØ1[9,A,Z] | ØSRRØ3[9,A,Z] | ØSRRØJ[9,A,Z] |
| Acetabular Surface, LT | ØSPE[Ø,4]JZ | ØSRSØ1[9,A,Z] | ØSRSØ3[9,A,Z] | ØSRSØJ[9,A,Z] |
| Femoral Surface, RT | ØSPR[Ø,4]JZ | ØSRRØ1[9,A,Z] | ØSRRØ3[9,A,Z] | ØSRRØJ[9,A,Z] |
| Femoral Surface, LT | ØSPS[Ø,4]JZ | ØSRSØ1[9,A,Z] | ØSRSØ3[9,A,Z] | ØSRSØJ[9,A,Z] |

### Percutaneous Endoscopic Removal of Hip Joint Surface With Supplement of Liner

| Body Part | Removal of Spacer/Liner/Resurfacing Device/Synthetic Substitute | Code also as appropriate Body Part by Site | | |
|---|---|---|---|---|
| | | Joint | Acetabular Surface | Femoral Surface |
| Acetabular Surface, RT | ØSPA4JZ | ØSU9Ø9Z | ØSUAØ9Z | ØSURØ9Z |
| Acetabular Surface, LT | ØSPE4JZ | ØSUBØ9Z | ØSUEØ9Z | ØSUSØ9Z |
| Femoral Surface, RT | ØSPR4JZ | ØSU9Ø9Z | ØSUAØ9Z | ØSURØ9Z |
| Femoral Surface, LT | ØSPS4JZ | ØSUBØ9Z | ØSUEØ9Z | ØSUSØ9Z |

## DRG 466-468 Revision of Hip or Knee Replacement *(Continued)*

**Removal of Knee Joint, Liner, With Replacment**

| Body Part | Removal of Liner | Code also as appropriate Replacement of Body Part | | | |
|---|---|---|---|---|---|
| | | Joint | Unicondylar | Femoral Surface | Tibial Surface |
| Knee, RT | ØSPCØ9Z | ØSRCØJ[9,A,Z] | ØSRCØL[9,A,Z] | ØSRTØJ[9,A,Z] | ØSRVØJ[9,A,Z] |
| Knee, LT | ØSPDØ9Z | ØSRDØJ[9,A,Z] | ØSRDØL[9,A,Z] | ØSRUØJ[9,A,Z] | ØSRWØJ[9,A,Z] |

**Removal of Knee Joint, Spacer, With Replacment**

| Body Part | Removal of Spacer | Code also as appropriate Replacement of Body Part | | |
|---|---|---|---|---|
| | | Joint | Femoral Surface | Tibial Surface |
| Knee, RT | ØSPC[Ø,3,4]8Z | ØSRCØJ[9,A,Z] | ØSRTØJ[9,A,Z] | ØSRVØJ[9,A,Z] |
| Knee, LT | ØSPD[Ø,3,4]8Z | ØSRDØJ[9,A,Z] | ØSRUØJ[9,A,Z] | ØSRWØJ[9,A,Z] |

**Removal of Knee Joint, Synthetic Substitute, With Replacment**

| Body Part | Removal of Synthetic Substitute | Code also as appropriate Replacement of Body Part | | | |
|---|---|---|---|---|---|
| | | Joint | Unicondylar | Femoral Surface | Tibial Surface |
| Knee, RT | ØSPC[Ø,4]JZ | ØSRCØJ[9,A,Z] | ØSRCØL[9,A,Z] | ØSRTØJ[9,A,Z] | ØSRVØJ[9,A,Z] |
| Knee, LT | ØSPD[Ø,4]JZ | ØSRDØJ[9,A,Z] | ØSRDØL[9,A,Z] | ØSRUØJ[9,A,Z] | ØSRWØJ[9,A,Z] |

**Open Removal of Knee Joint, Patellar Surface, With Replacment**

| Body Part | Removal of Patellar Surface | Code also as appropriate Replacement of Body Part | | |
|---|---|---|---|---|
| | | Joint | Femoral Surface | Tibial Surface |
| Knee, RT | ØSPCØJC | ØSRCØJ[9,A,Z] | ØSRTØJ[9,A,Z] | ØSRVØJ[9,A,Z] |
| Knee, LT | ØSPDØJC | ØSRDØJ[9,A,Z] | ØSRUØJ[9,A,Z] | ØSRWØJ[9,A,Z] |

**Percutaneous Removal of Knee Joint, Patellar Surface, With Replacment**

| Body Part | Removal of Patellar Surface | Code also as appropriate Replacement of Body Part | | |
|---|---|---|---|---|
| | | Joint | Femoral Surface | Tibial Surface |
| Knee, RT | ØSPC4JC | ØSRCØJ[9,A,Z] | — | — |
| Knee, LT | ØSPD4JC | ØSRDØJ[9,A,Z] | — | — |

**Removal of Knee Joint, Synthetic Substitute, With Replacment**

| Body Part | Removal of Synthetic Sustitute | Code also as appropriate Replacement of Body Part | | |
|---|---|---|---|---|
| | | Joint | Femoral Surface | Tibial Surface |
| Femoral Surface, RT | ØSPT[Ø,4]JZ | ØSRCØJ[9,A,Z] | ØSRTØJ[9,A,Z] | ØSRVØJ[9,A,Z] |
| Femoral Surface, LT | ØSPU[Ø,4]JZ | ØSRDØJ[9,A,Z] | ØSRUØJ[9,A,Z] | ØSRWØJ[9,A,Z] |
| Tibial Surface, RT | ØSPV[Ø,4]JZ | ØSRCØJ[9,A,Z] | ØSRTØJ[9,A,Z] | ØSRVØJ[9,A,Z] |
| Tibial Surface, LT | ØSPW[Ø,4]JZ | ØSRDØJ[9,A,Z] | ØSRUØJ[9,A,Z] | ØSRWØJ[9,A,Z] |

## DRG 485-489 Knee Procedures

| Joint | Removal of Liner by open approach | Code also as appropriate Supplement of Tibial Surface by Site |
|---|---|---|
| Knee, RT | ØSPCØ9Z | ØSUVØ9Z |
| Knee, LT | ØSPDØ9Z | ØSUWØ9Z |

# DRG 515-517 Other Musculoskeletal System and Connective Tissue Procedures

| Site | Reposition of Vertebra by percutaneous approach | Code also as appropriate Supplement With Synthetic Substitute by Percutaneous Approach at site of Repositioned Vertebra |
|---|---|---|
| Cervical | ØPS33ZZ | ØPU33JZ |
| Coccyx | ØQSS3ZZ | ØQUS3JZ |
| Lumbar | ØQSØ3ZZ | ØQUØ3JZ |
| Sacrum | ØQS13ZZ | ØQU13JZ |
| Thoracic | ØPS43ZZ | ØPU43JZ |

# DRG 518-52Ø Back and Neck Procedures, Except Spinal Fusion, or Disc Devices/Neurostimulators

| Generator Type | Insertion of Generator by Site | | | Code also as appropriate Insertion Neurostimulator Lead by approach and Site | |
|---|---|---|---|---|---|
| | Chest | Abdomen | Back | Spinal Canal | Spinal Cord |
| Single Array | ØJH6[Ø,3]BZ | ØJH8[Ø,3]BZ | ØJH7[Ø,3]BZ | ØØHU[Ø,3,4]MZ | ØØHV[Ø,3,4]MZ |
| Single Array, Rechargeable | ØJH6[Ø,3]CZ | ØJH8[Ø,3]CZ | ØJH7[Ø,3]CZ | ØØHU[Ø,3,4]MZ | ØØHV[Ø,3,4]MZ |
| Multiple Array | ØJH6[Ø,3]DZ | ØJH8[Ø,3]DZ | ØJH7[Ø,3]DZ | ØØHU[Ø,3,4]MZ | ØØHV[Ø,3,4]MZ |
| Multiple Array, Rechargable | ØJH6[Ø,3]EZ | — | ØJH7[Ø,3]EZ | ØØHU[Ø,3,4]MZ | ØØHV[Ø,3,4]MZ |
| Multiple Array, Rechargable | — | ØJH8[Ø,3]EZ | — | ØØHU[Ø,3,4]MZ | ØØHVØMZ |
| Multiple Array, Rechargable | — | ØJH8ØEZ | — | — | ØØHV[3,4]MZ |

# DRG 582-583 Mastectomy for Malignancy

| Site | Resection by Open approach | Code also as appropriate Resection of Lymph Nodes by Open approach by site | | | Code also as appropriate Resection of Thorax Muscle by Open approach | |
|---|---|---|---|---|---|---|
| | | Axillary | Internal Mammary | Thorax | Right | Left |
| Breast, Right | ØHTTØZZ | Ø7T5ØZZ | Ø7T8ØZZ | Ø7T7ØZZ | ØKTHØZZ | — |
| Breast, Left | ØHTUØZZ | Ø7T6ØZZ | Ø7T9ØZZ | Ø7T7ØZZ | — | ØKTJØZZ |
| Breast, Bilateral | ØHTVØZZ | Ø7T5ØZZ and Ø7T6ØZZ | Ø7T8ØZZ and Ø7T9ØZZ | Ø7T7ØZZ | ØKTHØZZ | ØKTJØZZ |

# DRG 584-585 Breast Biopsy, Local Excision and Other Breast procedures

**Resection of Breast With Resection of Lymph Nodes and Thorax Muscle**

| Site | Resection by Open approach | Code also as appropriate Resection of Lymph Nodes by Open approach by site | | | Code also as appropriate Resection of Thorax Muscle by Open approach | |
|---|---|---|---|---|---|---|
| | | Axillary | Internal Mammary | Thorax | Right | Left |
| Breast, Right | ØHTTØZZ | Ø7T5ØZZ | Ø7T8ØZZ | Ø7T7ØZZ | ØKTHØZZ | — |
| Breast, Left | ØHTUØZZ | Ø7T6ØZZ | Ø7T9ØZZ | Ø7T7ØZZ | — | ØKTJØZZ |
| Breast, Bilateral | ØHTVØZZ | Ø7T5ØZZ and Ø7T6ØZZ | Ø7T8ØZZ and Ø7T9ØZZ | Ø7T7ØZZ | ØKTHØZZ | ØKTJØZZ |

**Replacement of Breast Tissue**

| Site | Replacement by Percutaneous approach with Autologous Tissue | Code also as appropriate Extraction of Subcutaneous Tissue by Percutaneous approach | | | | | |
|---|---|---|---|---|---|---|---|
| | | Abdomen | Back | Buttock | Chest | Leg, Upper, Right | Leg, Upper, Left |
| Breast, Right | ØHRT37Z | ØJD83ZZ | ØJD73ZZ | ØJD93ZZ | ØJD63ZZ | ØJDL3ZZ | ØJDM3ZZ |
| Breast, Left | ØHRU37Z | ØJD83ZZ | ØJD73ZZ | ØJD93ZZ | ØJD63ZZ | ØJDL3ZZ | ØJDM3ZZ |
| Breast, Bilateral | ØHRV37Z | ØJD83ZZ | ØJD73ZZ | ØJD93ZZ | ØJD63ZZ | ØJDL3ZZ | ØJDM3ZZ |

# DRG 628-63Ø Other Endocrine, Nutritional and Metabolic Procedures

## Open Removal of Hip Joint Spacer, Liner, Resurfacing Device, or Synthetic Substitute With Replacement

| Body Part | Removal Spacer/ Liner/Resurfacing Device/Synthetic Substitute | Code also as appropriate Replacement of Body Part by Device Type | | | | | |
|---|---|---|---|---|---|---|---|
| | | Polyethylene | Metal | Metal on Poly | Ceramic | Ceramic on Poly | Synth Subst |
| Hip, RT | ØSP9Ø[8,9,B,J]Z | — | ØSR9Ø1[9,A,Z] | ØSR9Ø2[9,A,Z] | ØSR9Ø3[9,A,Z] | ØSR9Ø4[9,A,Z] | ØSR9ØJ[9,A,Z] |
| Hip, LT | ØSPBØ[8,9,B,J]Z | — | ØSRBØ1[9,A,Z] | ØSRBØ2[9,A,Z] | ØSRBØ3[9,A,Z] | ØSRBØ4[9,A,Z] | ØSRBØJ[9,A,Z] |
| Acetabular Surface, RT | ØSP9Ø[8,9,B,J]Z | ØSRAØØ[9,A,Z] | ØSRAØ1[9,A,Z] | — | ØSRAØ3[9,A,Z] | — | ØSRAØJ[9,A,Z] |
| Acetabular Surface, LT | ØSPBØ[8,9,B,J]Z | ØSREØØ[9,A,Z] | ØSREØ1[9,A,Z] | — | ØSREØ3[9,A,Z] | — | ØSREØJ[9,A,Z] |
| Femoral Surface, RT | ØSP9Ø[8,9,B,J]Z | — | ØSRRØ1[9,A,Z] | — | ØSRRØ3[9,A,Z] | — | ØSRRØJ[9,A,Z] |
| Femoral Surface, LT | ØSPBØ[8,9,B,J]Z | — | ØSRSØ1[9,A,Z] | — | ØSRSØ3[9,A,Z] | — | ØSRSØJ[9,A,Z] |

## Open Removal of Hip Joint Spacer, Liner, or Resurfacing Device With Supplement of Liner

| Body Part | Removal Spacer/Liner/ Resurfacing Device | Code also as appropriate Supplement of Body Part | | |
|---|---|---|---|---|
| | | Joint | Acetabular Surface | Femoral Surface |
| Hip, RT | ØSP9Ø[8,9,B]Z | ØSU9Ø9Z | ØSUAØ9Z | ØSURØ9Z |
| Hip, LT | ØSPBØ[8,9,B]Z | ØSUBØ9Z | ØSUEØ9Z | ØSUSØ9Z |

## Percutaneous Endoscopic Removal of Hip Joint Spacer or Synthetic Substitute With Replacement

| Body Part | Removal Spacer/Synthetic Substitute | Code also as appropriate Replacement of Body Part by Device Type | | | | | |
|---|---|---|---|---|---|---|---|
| | | Polyethylene | Metal | Metal on Poly | Ceramic | Ceramic on Poly | Synth Subst |
| Hip, RT | ØSP94[8,J]Z | — | ØSR9Ø1[9,A,Z] | ØSR9Ø2[9,A,Z] | ØSR9Ø3[9,A,Z] | ØSR9Ø4[9,A,Z] | ØSR9ØJ[9,A,Z] |
| Hip, LT | ØSPB4[8,J]Z | — | ØSRBØ1[9,A,Z] | ØSRBØ2[9,A,Z] | ØSRBØ3[9,A,Z] | ØSRBØ4[9,A,Z] | ØSRBØJ[9,A,Z] |
| Acetabular Surface, RT | ØSP94[8,J]Z | ØSRAØØ[9,A,Z] | ØSRAØ1[9,A,Z] | — | ØSRAØ3[9,A,Z] | — | ØSRAØJ[9,A,Z] |
| Acetabular Surface, LT | ØSPB4[8,J]Z | ØSREØØ[9,A,Z] | ØSREØ1[9,A,Z] | — | ØSREØ3[9,A,Z] | — | ØSREØJ[9,A,Z] |
| Femoral Surface, RT | ØSP94[8,J]Z | — | ØSRRØ1[9,A,Z] | — | ØSRRØ3[9,A,Z] | — | ØSRRØJ[9,A,Z] |
| Femoral Surface, LT | ØSPB4[8,J]Z | — | ØSRSØ1[9,A,Z] | — | ØSRSØ3[9,A,Z] | — | ØSRSØJ[9,A,Z] |

## Percutaneous Endoscopic Removal of Hip Joint Spacer or Synthetic Substitute With Supplement of Liner

| Body Part | Removal Spacer/Synthetic Substitute | Code also as appropriate Supplement of Body Part by Site | | |
|---|---|---|---|---|
| | | Joint | Acetabular Surface | Femoral Surface |
| Hip, RT | ØSP94[8,J]Z | ØSU9Ø9Z | ØSUAØ9Z | ØSURØ9Z |
| Hip, LT | ØSPB4[8,J]Z | ØSUBØ9Z | ØSUEØ9Z | ØSUSØ9Z |

## Removal of Hip Joint Surface with Replacement with New Joint Acetabular Surface

| Body Part | Removal of Spacer/ Liner/Resurfacing Device/Synthetic Substitute | Code also as appropriate Replacement of Acetabular Surface | | | |
|---|---|---|---|---|---|
| | | Polyethylene | Metal | Ceramic | Synth Subst |
| Acetabular Surface, RT | ØSPA[Ø,4]JZ | ØSRAØØ[9,A,Z] | ØSRAØ1[9,A,Z] | ØSRAØ3[9,A,Z] | ØSRAØJ[9,A,Z] |
| Acetabular Surface, LT | ØSPE[Ø,4]JZ | ØSREØØ[9,A,Z] | ØSREØ1[9,A,Z] | ØSREØ3[9,A,Z] | ØSREØJ[9,A,Z] |
| Femoral Surface, RT | ØSPR[Ø,4]JZ | ØSRAØØ[9,A,Z] | ØSRAØ1[9,A,Z] | ØSRAØ3[9,A,Z] | ØSRAØJ[9,A,Z] |
| Femoral Surface, LT | ØSPS[Ø,4]JZ | ØSREØØ[9,A,Z] | ØSREØ1[9,A,Z] | ØSREØ3[9,A,Z] | ØSREØJ[9,A,Z] |

## DRG 628-630 Other Endocrine, Nutritional and Metabolic Procedures *(Continued)*

**Removal of Hip Joint Surface With Replacement with New Joint Femoral Surface**

| Body Part | Removal of Spacer/ Liner/Resurfacing Device/Synthetic Substitute | Code also as appropriate Replacement of Femoral Surface | | |
|---|---|---|---|---|
| | | Metal | Ceramic | Synth Subst |
| Acetabular Surface, RT | ØSPA[Ø,4]JZ | ØSRRØ1[9,A,Z] | ØSRRØ3[9,A,Z] | ØSRRØJ[9,A,Z] |
| Acetabular Surface, LT | ØSPE[Ø,4]JZ | ØSRSØ1[9,A,Z] | ØSRSØ3[9,A,Z] | ØSRSØJ[9,A,Z] |
| Femoral Surface, RT | ØSPR[Ø,4]JZ | ØSRRØ1[9,A,Z] | ØSRRØ3[9,A,Z] | ØSRRØJ[9,A,Z] |
| Femoral Surface, LT | ØSPS[Ø,4]JZ | ØSRSØ1[9,A,Z] | ØSRSØ3[9,A,Z] | ØSRSØJ[9,A,Z] |

**Percutaneous Endoscopic Removal of Hip Joint Surface With Supplement of Liner**

| Body Part | Removal of Spacer/ Liner/Resurfacing Device/Synthetic Substitute | Code also as appropriate Body Part by Site | | |
|---|---|---|---|---|
| | | Joint | Acetabular Surface | Femoral Surface |
| Acetabular Surface, RT | ØSPA4JZ | ØSU9Ø9Z | ØSUAØ9Z | ØSURØ9Z |
| Acetabular Surface, LT | ØSPE4JZ | ØSUBØ9Z | ØSUEØ9Z | ØSUSØ9Z |
| Femoral Surface, RT | ØSPR4JZ | ØSU9Ø9Z | ØSUAØ9Z | ØSURØ9Z |
| Femoral Surface, LT | ØSPS4JZ | ØSUBØ9Z | ØSUEØ9Z | ØSUSØ9Z |

**Removal of Knee Joint, Liner, With Replacment**

| Body Part | Removal of Liner | Code also as appropriate Replacement of Body Part | | | |
|---|---|---|---|---|---|
| | | Joint | Unicondylar | Femoral Surface | Tibial Surface |
| Knee, RT | ØSPCØ9Z | ØSRCØJ[9,A,Z] | ØSRCØL[9,A,Z] | ØSRTØJ[9,A,Z] | ØSRVØJ[9,A,Z] |
| Knee, LT | ØSPDØ9Z | ØSRDØJ[9,A,Z] | ØSRDØL[9,A,Z] | ØSRUØJ[9,A,Z] | ØSRWØJ[9,A,Z] |

**Removal of Knee Joint, Patellar Surface, With Replacment**

| Body Part | Removal of Patellar Surface | Code also as appropriate Replacement of Body Part | |
|---|---|---|---|
| | | Femoral Surface | Tibial Surface |
| Knee, RT | ØSPC[Ø,4]JC | ØSRTØJ[9,A] | ØSRVØJ[9,A] |
| Knee, LT | ØSPD[Ø,4]JC | ØSRUØJ[9,A] | ØSRWØJ[9,A,Z] |

**Removal of Knee Joint, Synthetic Substitute, With Replacment**

| Body Part | Removal of Synthetic Sustitute | Code also as appropriate Replacement of Body Part | |
|---|---|---|---|
| | | Femoral Surface | Tibial Surface |
| Knee, RT | ØSPC[Ø,4]JZ | ØSRTØJ[9,A] | ØSRVØJ[9,A] |
| Knee, LT | ØSPD[Ø,4]JZ | ØSRUØJ[9,A] | ØSRWØJ[9,A,Z] |
| Femoral Surface, RT | ØSPT[Ø,4]JZ | ØSRTØJ[9,A] | ØSRVØJ[9,A] |
| Femoral Surface, LT | ØSPU[Ø,4]JZ | ØSRUØJ[9,A] | ØSRWØJ[9,A,Z] |
| Tibial Surface, RT | ØSPV[Ø,4]JZ | ØSRTØJ[9,A] | ØSRVØJ[9,A] |
| Tibial Surface, LT | ØSPW[Ø,4]JZ | ØSRUØJ[9,A] | ØSRWØJ[9,A,Z] |

## DRG 662-664 Minor Bladder Procedure

| Repair of Bladder | Code also as appropriate Repair of Abdominal Wall | |
|---|---|---|
| | with Stoma | without Stoma |
| ØTQB[Ø,3,4]ZZ | ØWQFXZ2 | ØWQFXZZ |

## DRG 665-667 Prostatectomy

| Site | Resection by approach | | | | Code also as appropriate Resection of Seminal Vesicles, Bilateral by approach | |
|---|---|---|---|---|---|---|
| | Open | Percutaneous Endoscopic | Via Natural or Artificial Opening | Via Natural or Artificial Opening Endoscopic | Open | Percutaneous Endoscopic |
| Prostate | ØVTØØZZ | ØVTØ4ZZ | ØVTØ7ZZ | ØVTØ8ZZ | ØVT3ØZZ | ØVT34ZZ |

## DRG 7Ø7-7Ø8 Major Male Pelvic Procedures

| Site | Resection by approach | | | | Code also as appropriate Resection of Seminal Vesicles, Bilateral by approach | |
|---|---|---|---|---|---|---|
| | Open | Percutaneous Endoscopic | Via Natural or Artificial Opening | Via Natural or Artificial Opening Endoscopic | Open | Percutaneous Endoscopic |
| Prostate | ØVTØØZZ | ØVTØ4ZZ | ØVTØ7ZZ | ØVTØ8ZZ | ØVT3ØZZ | ØVT34ZZ |

## DRG 734-735 Pelvic Evisceration, Radical Hysterectomy and Radical Vulvectomy

**Pelvic Evisceration**

| Resection by Site | | | | | | |
|---|---|---|---|---|---|---|
| Bladder | Cervix | Fallopian Tubes, Bilateral | Ovaries, Bilateral | Urethra | Uterus | Vagina |
| ØTTBØZZ | ØUTCØZZ | ØUT7ØZZ | ØUT2ØZZ | ØTTDØZZ | ØUT9ØZZ | ØUTGØZZ |

**Radical Hysterectomy**

| Approach | Resection by Site | | |
|---|---|---|---|
| | Cervix | Uterus | Uterine Support Structure |
| Vaginal | ØUTC[7,8]ZZ | ØUT9[7,8]ZZ | ØUT4[7,8]ZZ |
| Abdominal, Endoscopic | ØUTC4ZZ | ØUT9[4,F]ZZ | ØUT44ZZ |
| Abdominal, Open | ØUTCØZZ | ØUT9ØZZ | ØUT4ØZZ |

**Radical Vulvectomy**

| Resection by Site | Code also as appropriate Excision of Inguinal Lymph Nodes by Approach | |
|---|---|---|
| Vulva | Right | Left |
| ØUTM[Ø,X]ZZ | Ø7BH[Ø,4]ZZ | Ø7BJ[Ø,4]ZZ |

# Non-OR procedure combinations

**Note:** The following table identifies procedure combinations that are considered Non-OR even though one or more procedures of the combination are considered valid DRG OR procedures

### Dilation With Removal of Intraluminal Device - Via Natural or Artificial Opening

| Code as appropriate Dilation by Site | | | | | Code also as appropriate Removal of Intraluminal Device by Site | |
|---|---|---|---|---|---|---|
| Hepatic Duct, Right | Hepatic Duct, Left | Cystic Duct | Common Bile Duct | Pancreatic Duct | Hepatobiliary Duct | Pancreatic Duct |
| ØF75[7,8]DZ | ØF76[7,8]DZ | ØF78[7,8]DZ | ØF79[7,8]DZ | ØF7D[7,8]DZ | ØFPB[7,8]DZ | ØFPD[7,8]DZ |

### Insertion With Removal of Intraluminal Device

| Code as appropriate Insertion of Intraluminal Device into Hepatobiliary Duct | Code also as appropriate Removal of Intraluminal Device by Approach and Site | | | |
|---|---|---|---|---|
| | Via Natural or Artificial Opening | | External | |
| | Hepatobiliary Duct | Pancreatic Duct | Hepatobiliary Duct | Pancreatic Duct |
| ØFHB[7,8]DZ | ØFPB[7,8]DZ | ØFPD[7,8]DZ | — | — |
| ØFHB7DZ | — | — | ØFPBXDZ | ØFPDXDZ |

# NOTES

## NOTES